TEXTBOOK *of* CHRONIC WOUND CARE

An Evidence-Based Approach to Diagnosis and Treatment

TEXTBOOK *of* CHRONIC WOUND CARE

An Evidence-Based Approach to Diagnosis and Treatment

Jayesh B. Shah, MD
Paul J. Sheffield, PhD
Caroline E. Fife, MD
Editors

BEST PUBLISHING COMPANY

Cover photos courtesy of Jayesh B. Shah, MD and Caroline E. Fife, MD

Photos included in this edition without specific recognition were provided by the specific chapter authors.

International Standard Book Number: 978-1-947239-07-4
Library of Congress Control Number: 2018930683

Best Publishing Company
631 US Highway 1, Suite 307
North Palm Beach, FL 33408

Printed in the United States of America

CONTENTS

SECTION 2: Essentials of Wound Healing

Editor - Robert J. Snyder

SECTION 3: Pathophysiology, Diagnosis, and Management of Special Wound Patients
Editor - Kelly Johnson-Arbor

SECTION 4: Atypical Wounds and Burns
Editor - Jayesh B. Shah

SECTION 5: Wound Care in Special Populations

Editor - Dianne Rudolph

SECTION 6: Wound Care in Different Settings

Editor - Helen B. Gelly

SECTION 7: Challenges and Opportunities in Wound Care Practice in the New Era

Editor - Caroline E. Fife

SECTION 8: Wound Care in Other Countries
Editor - Julio E. Garcia

FOREWORD

Chronic wounds may have cost the U.S. Medicare system as much as $95 billion dollars in 2014, which rivals the gross domestic product (GDP) of a small European country. Nearly 15% of all Medicare patients are affected, far more than have heart failure, although unlike heart disease, there are no recognized specialty training programs producing wound care experts to manage the growing epidemic of problem wounds. This is in part because a nonhealing wound is not actually a *disease* so much as it is a *symptom*. The typical patient with a nonhealing wound has an average of six serious comorbid conditions and takes an average of ten medications. If a wound fails to achieve healing, there is always a reason, and often more than one reason, with several different organ systems involved.

The most common reason wounds fail to heal is tissue hypoxia. There was a time when we did not know that basic fact. The critical role of hypoxia in chronic wounds was identified in the 1970s through the pioneering work of Paul Sheffield and his colleagues at Brooks Air Force Base in San Antonio, Texas, some of whom implanted gas permeable electrodes in the subcutaneous tissue of their own thighs to better understand oxygen diffusion. It has been four decades since Paul first helped to elucidate the role of oxygen in healing, during which new methods of improving vascular supply have become available. Yet, we continue to struggle with implementing simple, noninvasive vascular screening to identify patients with ischemia. In some ways we have advanced very far, and in other ways, we have made little progress. In the absence of a recognized medical specialty, the training programs and textbooks developed by pioneers like Paul Sheffield continue to fill a vital role in moving the field forward. Jay Shah and I are immeasurably grateful for Paul's guidance and leadership in this latest contribution to the field of wound care. We will borrow a quote from him to express our gratitude to say that in working with him on this project, we have been, "strutting in high cotton."

With Paul's guidance, Jay and I have tried, although perhaps not always succeeded, to do justice to those predecessor texts. With the advent of the Quality Payment Program on January 1, 2017, practitioners have a new focus—how to heal wounds in the shortest period of time at the lowest cost. We hope this textbook will help prepare clinicians for their new role as stewards of resources, providing the right care to the right patient at the right time.

Caroline E. Fife, MD
Editor

PREFACE

The co-editors of this book, Paul J. Sheffield, PhD and Caroline E. Fife, MD, have also edited the *Wound Care Practice*'s first edition in 2004 and its second edition in 2007. Instead of a third edition of *Wound Care Practice*, we decided to write a new textbook focused on evidence-based pathways and that is how the *Textbook of Chronic Wound Care* was created. We realized the traditional experienced-based criteria for selecting wound care interventions is being replaced with evidence-based practice. This textbook has made an attempt to focus on the evidence-based practice approach with case studies, pathways, and key concepts outlined in a majority of the chapters.

The value of evidence-based approach for providing optimal care is established, but the process used to generate this evidence continues to evolve. Many guidelines for wound care are published on *clinicalguidelines.gov* but a textbook that can put all those guidelines in a simple manner to help wound care practitioners in their daily practice was lacking. This book makes a sincere attempt to help the reader apply those guidelines into their clinical practice.

Another reason for this new textbook was to create a companion to our study guide, *Wound Care Certification Study Guide, 2nd edition* (Best Publishing Company, 2016), which will give in-depth knowledge and evidence-based pathway to handle different kinds of chronic wounds. I want to thank all my colleagues and the chapter contributors for their outstanding support for *Wound Care Certification Study Guide, 2nd edition*. Their response to our study guide gave strength to the present editors to venture into this new textbook. All editors and more than 50 contributors are committed in the field of wound care and they believe in making a difference in the lives of our patients through education.

This textbook is organized into eight sections. The first section explores the anatomy, physiology, and biochemistry of wound healing. The second section explores all essentials of wound healing including discussion on etiology of wound, nutritional assessment and management, wound assessment, wound bed preparation, evidence-based selection of wound dressings, advanced wound modalities, and advanced plastic surgical techniques in wound care. The third section discusses pathophysiology, diagnosis, and management of special wound patients including discussion of diabetic foot ulcer, pressure ulcers, venous insufficiency ulcers, lymphedema, and arterial insufficiency ulcers. The fourth section explores atypical wounds, arthropod bites, stings and infestation, radiation wounds, and burns.

The fifth section discusses wound care in special populations like pediatrics, geriatrics and patients with fistulae. The sixth section discusses wound care in different settings like outpatient hospital wound clinic, physician's outpatient office, acute long-term care facility, and nursing home setting. It also discusses ways to incorporate research in wound care practice. The seventh section explores challenges and opportunities in wound care practice in the new era, discusses use of telemedicine in wound care, and presents challenges and opportunities with electronic health records. There is also a discussion on the future of wound care moving from volume to value in the wound care arena and a discussion on patient-centered decision making in wound care and hyperbaric medicine. Finally, section eight looks at disparities in health care in different countries and how wound care is being done in other countries.

A disclaimer by Dr. Fife concerning the NPUAP 2016 Terminology controversy is provided to give you some clarification on certain terminology regarding pressure ulcer throughout the textbook.

Thank you for the opportunity to present this textbook that will assist wound care professionals, caregivers, patients, and their families. By working as a team, we can drastically improve the care of our wound care patients globally.

With regards,

Jayesh B. Shah, MD
Editor

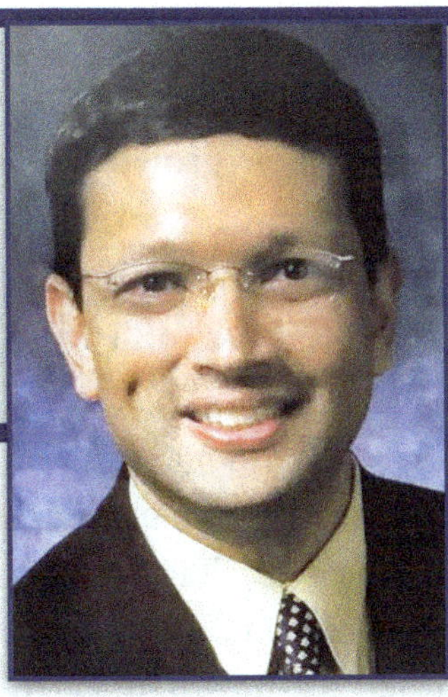

JAYESH B. SHAH MD, UHM(ABPM), CWSP, FAPWCA, FCCWS, FUHM, FACP, FACHM

Dr. Jayesh B. Shah is President of South Texas Wound Associates, PA, San Antonio, Texas, where he has provided clinical wound care services in San Antonio and the surrounding communities for the past 17 years. He is also President of TIMEO2 Healing Concepts, LLC, in San Antonio, Texas, through which he provides consulting and education services in wound care and hyperbaric medicine both nationally and internationally. His degrees include MBBS from M. S. University, India, and MD in Internal Medicine from St. Luke's Roosevelt Hospital, Columbia University, New York. He is board certified in internal medicine, board certified in undersea and hyperbaric medicine, certified in wound management, and certified in hyperbaric medicine. He is the past chair of American College of Clinical Wound Specialists, past president of American Association of Physicians of Indian Origin, past chair of American Medical Association, International Medical Graduates Section, 2016 President of the Bexar County Medical Society, and 2017 President of American College of Hyperbaric Medicine. He is an adjunct professor in the Department of Family and Community Medicine at the University of Texas Health Science Center and an associate professor at the Osteopathic School of Medicine for the University of Incarnate Word in San Antonio, Texas.

He has been the recipient of the Entrepreneur of the Year Award by the Alamo Asia Chamber of Commerce (2016); the Paul James Sheffield Education Award for Lifetime Dedication to Education in the Field of Undersea and Hyperbaric Medicine (2014); Jefferson C. Davis Memorial Award for Excellence in Clinical Hyperbaric Medicine (2007 and 2011); Carolyn Sue Award (2009); Young Scientist/Medical Doctor Award (2008); and Community Service and Leadership Award by Alamo Asian American Chamber of Commerce (2008).

Dr. Jayesh Shah has 20 years of experience in wound care and hyperbaric medicine practice and 14 years of experience as program director for continuing medical education courses. As Medical Director of the Wound Care Centers, Dr. Shah has helped these centers from startup through their growth up to their maximum potential. Since 2010, he has served as the Medical Director for the Northeast Baptist Wound Healing Center, which recently became accredited by the UHMS within its first four years of inception. He is also the co-medical director for the Mission Trail Baptist Wound Healing Center since 2014.

He is the co-editor of the first and second editions of *Wound Care Certification Study Guide* and created *WoundDoctor App*, a comprehensive wound care resource tool for physicians, nurses, and physical therapists for iPhone, Android, and iPad. He has authored over 40 chapters on various wound topics in 4 books in addition to 30+ scientific articles in wound care and hyperbaric medicine. As an assistant editor of the *Journal of ACCWS*, he regularly writes a column on certification exam in wound care.

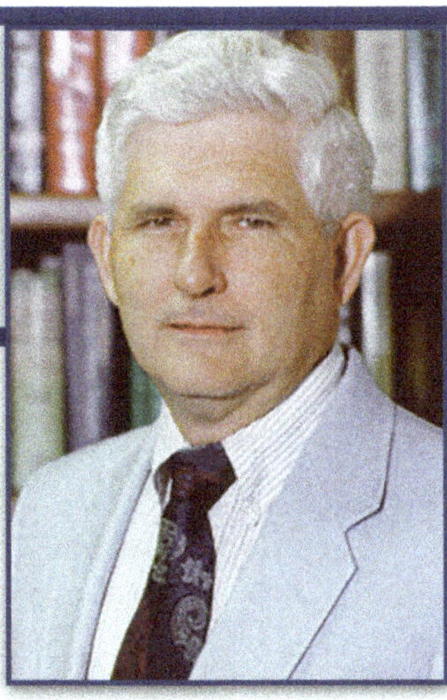

PAUL J. SHEFFIELD PhD, CAsP, CHT-ADMIN, FAsMA, FUHM

Dr. Paul Sheffield is President, International ATMO, Inc. of San Antonio, Texas, which provides wound care and hyperbaric medicine management, consulting, and education services. His degrees include BS (Chemistry) from University of Florida, and MS & PhD (Physiology) from University of Southern California. He is a certified aerospace physiologist and certified hyperbaric technologist.

Dr. Sheffield began his career as a US Air Force aerospace physiologist, with primary responsibilities in aircrew training, research, and hyperbaric medicine. He was on the original team that established the USAF Hyperbaric Center at Brooks Air Force Base, Texas in 1974 where he was one of the originators of the use of tissue oximetry for wound assessment and patient selection for hyperbaric oxygen therapy. He completed his Air Force career as Chief of Aerospace Physiology at the Office of the Air Force Surgeon General in Washington, DC and retired in the grade of colonel after 30 years of military service. He joined International ATMO as Director of Research and Education and eventually became president in 2000.

For over 50 years, Dr. Sheffield has been educating physicians, nurses, and technologists in aerospace physiology, undersea and hyperbaric medicine, and wound care. He authored over 145 publications, including 12 book chapters and edited several books, including *Proceedings of the XIV International Congress on Hyperbaric Medicine* (Best Publishing Company), first and second editions of *Wound Care Practice* (Best Publishing Company), and first and second editions of *Wound Care Certification Study Guide* (Best Publishing Company).

The Gulf Coast Chapter of the Undersea and Hyperbaric Medical Society (UHMS) honored him in 2009 by creating the Paul James Sheffield Education Award, which is presented annually to an individual who made significant contributions to science and education in undersea and hyperbaric medicine.

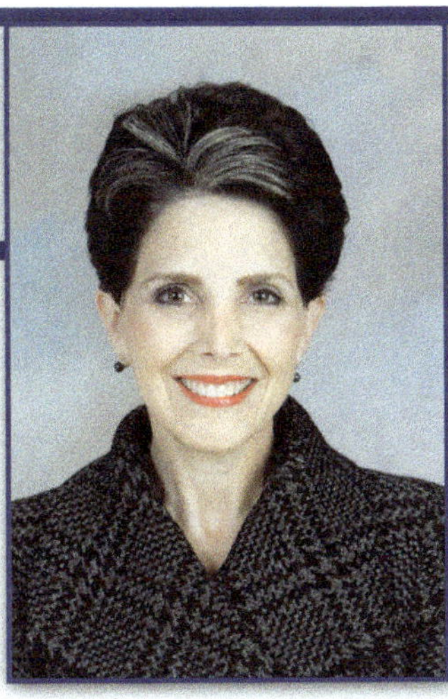

CAROLINE E. FIFE MD, FAAFP, CWS, FUHM

Dr. Fife completed a family medicine residency at the University of Texas, Southwestern in Dallas followed by a two-year fellowship in undersea and hyperbaric medicine at Duke University. Until 2013 she was a professor of medicine at the University of Texas Health Science Center, Houston, where she initiated the Memorial Hermann Center for Wound Healing and Hyperbaric Medicine and the Lymphedema Center. She is now a professor of geriatrics at Baylor College of Medicine in Houston and the medical director of the CHI St. Luke's Wound Care Clinic in The Woodlands, Texas.

She is also the chief medical officer of Intellicure, Inc., a health information technology company, and the executive director of the U.S. Wound Registry, a nonprofit organization recognized by CMS as a qualified clinical data registry. The USWR develops quality measures and helps wound care and hyperbaric practitioners meet the requirements of Medicare's Quality Payment Program.

She has been a certified wound specialist since 1998. Past and present board activities include the Alliance of Wound Care Stakeholders (current co-chair), the American Academy of Wound Management, the Association for the Advancement of Wound Care and the American Professional Wound Care Association. She is a past president of the Undersea and Hyperbaric Medical Society.

Dr. Fife is co-editor of the books *Wound Care Practice*, *Women and Pressure: Diving and Flying*, and both editions of *Wound Care Certification Study Guide*, all published by Best Publishing Company. She is the author of more than 100 peer-reviewed articles and book chapters and is a popular speaker. Her research contributions include altitude decompression studies enabling the construction of the International Space Station by decreasing the time needed for oxygen prebreathe as part of a NASA lead research consortium; the development of real time lymphatic imaging with Dr. Eva Sevick using near infrared technology; and more recently, the use of real-world data for comparative effectiveness studies to understand what works best for patients with chronic wounds and ulcers.

CONTRIBUTORS LIST

A

J. Javier Soldevilla Agreda, RN, MsG, BAsc, PhD

B

Dimitri Beeckman, RN, PhD
Samih Bittar, MD
Robyn Bjork, MPT, CWS, CLT-LANA, CLWT

C

Apirag Chuangsuwanich, MD
Kevin K. Chung, MD
Cherison Cuffy, DPM, CWS

E

Joey K. Ead, MS
Dirk Elston, MD

F

Regina M. Fearmonti, MD
John J. Feldmeier, DO, FACRO, FUHM
Caroline E. Fife, MD, FAAFP, CWS, FUHM
John Fish, MD
Elizabeth Friedrich, MPH, RDN, CSG, LDN, FAND

G

Aimee D. Garcia, MD, CWS, FACCWS
Julio Garcia, RN, MD, AAPWCA
Helen B. Gelly, MD, FUHM, FCCWS
Daniel J. Gibson, PhD
Timothy M. Graham, DPM
Stephen D. Guthrie, MD, PhD
Barbara R. Guthrie, MD

H

Heather Hettrick, PT, PhD, CWS, CLT-LANA, CLWT
JoonPio (JP) Hong, MD, PhD, MMM

J

David A. Johnson, MD, FAAFP, CWSP
Kelly Johnson-Arbor, MD, FACEP, FUHM, FACMT

L

Javier La Fontaine, DPM, MS
Lawrence Lavery, DPM, MPH
Iestyn Marc Lewis, BS, MB, FACEM, DHM
Fedor Lurie, MD, PhD

N

Harikrishna K. R. Nair, MD, FMSWCP

O

Supaporn Opasanon, MD, FRCST, FICS, FACS

P

Arun Prasad, MD

R

Christina Ramsey, RN, MSN, GNP-BC, LNCC, CWS
Julie A. Rizzo, MD
Margie Rodriguez, RN, MSN, WCC
Matthew P. Rowan, PhD
Dianne Rudolph, DNP, GNP-BC, CWOCN

S

Tarun Sahni, MD
Pamela Scarborough, PT, DPT, MS, CDE, CWS, CEEAA
Gregory S. Schultz, PhD
Thomas E. Serena, MD, FACS, FACHM, MAPWCA
Jayesh B. Shah, MD, UHM(ABPM), CWSP, FAPWCA, FCCWS, FUHM, FACP, FACHM
Herbert B. Slade, MD, FAAAAI
Jamie M. Slade, MD
Robert J. Snyder, DPM, MSc, CWS
Hyunsuk (Peter) Suh, MD, PhD
Mellick T. Sykes MD, FACS

T

Abhishek Tiwari, MD
Boulos Toursarkissian, MD, RPVI, FACS
Terry Treadwell, MD, FACS

V

Suzanne Van Asten, MD

W

Dot Weir, RN, CWON, CWS
Michael White, MD, MMM
Jaime Wise, MD, CWSP
Kevin Y. Woo, RN, PhD, FAPWCA

Z

Pedram Zendehrouh, MD, PhD, FACS

ACKNOWLEDGMENTS

I am sincerely thankful to the co-editors of this book, Dr. Paul Sheffield and Dr. Caroline Fife, for supporting and encouraging my idea of creating the companion textbook to accompany *Wound Care Certification Study Guide*. I greatly admire their friendship, mentorship and guidance in making this project successful.

I am greatly thankful to all authors who have shared their knowledge, experience, expertise, and valuable time by contributing the chapters in this book.

Finally, a special thanks to Lorraine Fico White, publishing editor, and the entire staff of Best Publishing Company, for patiently and diligently editing, formatting, and presenting the material in an organized manner for the readers.

Jayesh B. Shah, MD
Editor

DEDICATION

To my loving and supportive wife, Neha, for her understanding and patience with my hectic schedule.

To my two beautiful children, Prachi and Aj, for giving me the space to write and edit this book, and for giving me the emotional support to persevere through a challenging year.

To my mother, Jaivanti, for keeping me spiritually uplifted.

To my late father, Bipinchandra, for inspiring me to be a physician. His spirit is with me every day.

To my wonderful team of wound care staff and colleagues at Northeast Baptist Wound Healing Center and Mission Trail Baptist Wound Healing Center in San Antonio, for helping me care for chronic wounds.

And finally, to my patients and their caregivers, for their trust in me.

Jayesh B. Shah, MD
Editor

CONTROVERSY OVER NATIONAL PRESSURE ULCER ADVISORY PANEL (NPUAP) 2016 TERMINOLOGY

Disclaimer and Editorial Viewpoint from Caroline E. Fife, MD

In May of 2016 at its consensus conference, the National Pressure Ulcer Advisory Panel (NPUAP) released new definitions for pressure ulcer staging, replacing the term pressure "ulcer" with pressure "injury." The debate regarding this change has been heated. For decades, CMS has segregated all cutaneous lesions into two broad categories: "wounds" which are caused by surgical procedures or accidents, and "ulcers" which are skin lesions related to underlying medical problems (e.g. diabetic foot ulcers, arterial ulcers, etc.). From a diagnosis coding standpoint, an open lesion caused by an "injury" would actually be a "wound." Thus, one possible outcome of the terminology change by the NPUAP is that pressure ulcers are now pressure wounds. Wounds must be subsequently identified by the surgical procedure or accident to which they are related. The "injury codes" of ICD-10 are the source of much levity since they encompass all the misadventures sustained by cartoon characters including injuries caused by an animal-drawn vehicle and being sucked into a jet engine. It will be necessary to add new ICD-10 codes in order to identify the cause of these "wounds due to injuries", opening the door to a set of causation codes that might include "inadequate clinical care," "failure to turn," and injuries due to specific (named) medical devices, all with serious legal implications.

Pressure ulcers are already the main reason for malpractice lawsuits against long-term care institutions. Because tort reform caps on punitive damages enacted by many states do not apply in cases of elder abuse, plaintiff's attorneys successfully equate pressure ulcers with elder abuse in order to increase potential monetary awards. Making pressure ulcers synonymous with elder abuse has resulted in *criminal* litigation related to their formation, and the successful conviction of some family members and at least one nursing home owner with manslaughter and prison sentences. The use of the term "injury" in relation to all pressure-related events could make defending these cases more difficult and perhaps increase the risk of criminal charges related to them because of the implication of intentional harm.

An alternative possibility of the NPUAP's terminology change is to create a previously unknown, third category of skin lesion called the "skin injuries." While it may be true that tissue "injury" (describing a causal factor) is involved in the causation of these lesions, we have not adopted a naming convention for other types of skin ulcers based on their etiologies. If so, we should create a new category for arterial ulcers called "ischemics," and diabetic foot ulcers called "neuropathics."

It is true that a glaringly obvious semantic problem has existed for years with the NPUAP staging system because it used the term "ulcer" to refer to skin discoloration in the absence of epithelial breakdown (e.g. a Stage 1 pressure ulcer). The NPUAP may have hoped to address this issue by changing the term "ulcer" to "injury." Unfortunately, the term "injury" makes it impossible to determine whether the lesion now being described is actually an open sore, effectively creating the opposite of the problem it was designed to fix, in which some closed lesions were called ulcers. Instead, now some open sores are called "pressure injuries."

For example, if tasked with describing the tissue injury sustained from a motor vehicle accident, we would diagnose the precise manifestation of the injury (e.g. abrasion, laceration, purpura, etc.), rather than the cause. The term "pressure injury" will confound current classification systems (e.g. ICD-11 and the Systematized Nomenclature of Medicine), which are designed to improve diagnostic specificity and which do not conflate the cause of a lesion with its manifestation. Although the NPUAP staging system requires improvement, many respected clinical associations in the United States and abroad do not support this particular change until there has been further discussion regarding the unintended consequences. In this textbook, a skin lesion related to an underlying medical problem that presents as an open draining defect on the body is defined as an ulcer.

Caroline E. Fife, MD

Section 1

ANATOMY, PHYSIOLOGY AND BIOCHEMISTRY OF WOUND HEALING

Editor - Herbert B. Slade, MD, FAAAAI

Chapter 1

ANATOMY OF THE SKIN

Herbert B. Slade, MD, FAAAAI
Jamie M. Slade, MD

KEY CONCEPTS

1. Skin is arranged over subcutaneous fatty tissue in six distinct layers:
   a) Reticular (deep) dermis
   b) Papillary dermis
   c) Epidermal basal layer (stratum basale)
   d) Epidermal mitotic layer (stratum spinosum)
   e) Epidermal differentiation layer (stratum granulosum)*
   f) Epidermal terminal differentiation layer (stratum corneum)
2. Approximately 20 different cell types are found in skin, each with unique roles.
3. The functions of skin include waterproofing, insulation, temperature regulation, barrier against toxins and pathogens, protection against solar radiation, and sensation of the environment.
4. Skin is a dynamic organ, with respect to structural changes throughout life and the movement and interactions of cells within the skin at any point in time.

**An additional layer is seen above the stratum granulosum (stratum lucidum) beneath friction ridges.*

CONTENTS

Introduction

Skin is an integumentary system at the interface between the human organism and its environment (Table 1). The boundary limits of skin are found at its transition to mucosal surfaces of the respiratory, alimentary, and urogenital systems; at the conjunctival epithelium of the eye; at the ductal epithelium of the lacrimal and mammary ducts; and at the tympanic membrane of the ear.

Anatomically, skin is organized into an outer layer of epidermis covering a deeper layer of dermis, which is further subdivided into papillary dermis and reticular dermis. The epidermal epithelium gives rise during fetal development to the skin appendages, namely the hair follicles and associated sebaceous glands (pilosebaceous units), eccrine and apocrine sweat glands, and nails. Beneath the dermis is the hypodermis or subcutaneous fat layer (the panniculus adiposus). Connections between skin and its underlying hypodermis include ligaments, nerves, blood vessels, and lymphatic vessels.

The gross appearance of skin varies between individuals, within an individual by anatomic location at any point in time and within an individual over a lifetime. Variation is found with respect to texture, tone, distribution and amount of pigmentation, and expression of hair. For example, scrotal skin is very thin, with readily visible hair roots, specialized sebaceous glands, and few or no elastic fibers, but considerably greater laxity compared with skin covering the trunk. By contrast, the glabrous skin of the palms and soles is tightly fixed to the underlying fascia, lacks hair follicles and sebaceous glands, and contains sweat pores opening into ostia located along prominent friction ridges. The epidermis is considerably thicker.

The overall thickness of skin across the body is determined by the thickness of the several layers of epidermis and the thickness of the underlying dermis. Typical thickness in a young adult ranges from the eyelids (epidermis ~50 μm, dermis ~1,000 μm) to the back (epidermis ~40 μm, dermis ~5,000 μm), to the palms of the hands (epidermis ~600 μm).[1-2] The thickness of the outermost cornified layer (the stratum corneum) is greatest in areas of callous but also varies among flexor forearm, thigh, back and abdomen across a range of ~13μm (flexor forearm) to ~8μm (abdomen).[3] Published values for these measurements differ considerably, likely as a result of differences in location of sampling, methods of visualization, and methods of preservation in the case of biopsy material.[4-5]

The structure of the skin (Figure 1) is established through the orchestrated arrival, arrangement, and differentiation of a broad array of cell lineages during embryogenesis and fetal development.[6] When it is fully developed, approximately 20 different types of cells are found in association with a complex extracellular matrix that provides both strength and flexibility[7] (Table 2).

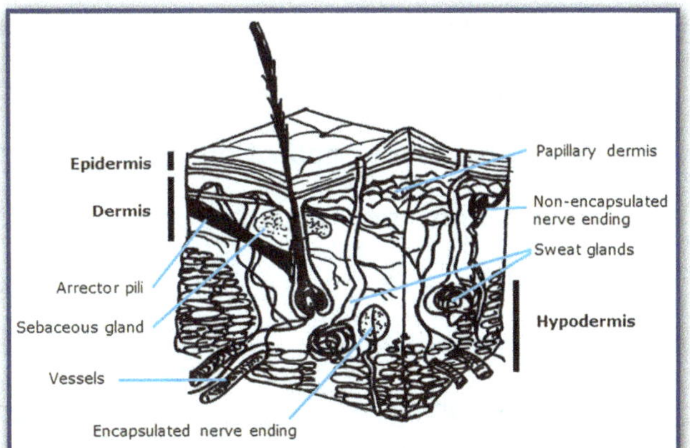

FIGURE 1. Organization of the skin
Courtesy of Jessica A. Slade, ME

I. Epidermis

Full keratinization of the outermost keratinocytes is achieved prior to birth, by gestational weeks 26-28. The epidermis at birth is still relatively thin with only two to three cell layers in the stratum spinosum and five to six layers in the stratum corneum.[8] The thick whitish "vernix caseosa" covering the epidermis at birth is a product of the sebaceous glands combined with shed periderm and squames. A mixture of water, proteins, antimicrobial enzymes and lipids, the vernix is thought to provide a degree of protection against maceration while the skin is exposed to amniotic fluid, while allowing the skin to hydrate itself more rapidly following birth.[9] Removal of the vernix at birth leaves the stratum corneum drier than adult skin for some time.

Four distinct epidermal layers persist into adult life, with a basal germinative layer resting upon a basement membrane elaborated through cooperative effort between the basal keratinocytes and the underlying mesodermal fibroblasts. A fifth layer of cells can be found beneath friction ridges on the palms of the hand and soles of the feet, between the granular and horny layers. Fully developed epidermis is thus a stratified squamous arrangement consisting of a basal layer of stem and transit-amplifying cells,[10-11] above which are the spinous, granular, clear, and horny layers. The corresponding Latin descriptive terms – stratum basale, stratum spinosum, stratum granulosum, stratum lucidum, and stratum corneum – remain in use. The integrity of epidermis is maintained by various connections between cells and at the basal layer, with the basement membrane. Basal cells use hemidesmosomes, integrins, and anchoring fibrils to maintain contact with the basement membrane, while desmosomes, gap junctions, and adherens junctions keep them connected

TABLE 1. Functions of the integumentary system

Function	Major structure(s) or cells
Waterproofing	Stratum corneum
Protection against minor trauma	Stratum corneum
Prevent entry of toxins	Stratum corneum
Moisture balance	Epidermis
Vitamin D, hormone production	Keratinocytes
Prevention of invasion by pathogens	Epidermis, dermis, lymphatics
Regeneration	Basal epithelium, hair follicles, blood vessels
UV radiation protection	Melanocytes
Physical cushioning	Dermis, subcutaneous fat
Insulation	Hair, subcutaneous fat, arrector pili muscles
Temperature regulation	Vasculature, sweat glands, motor nerves
Sensation	Sensory nerves
Immunity	Dendritic cells, lymphocytes, lymphatic channels

with each other and with cells of the spinous layer. Desmosome, gap junctions, and adherens junctions persist in the spinous layer, while in the granular layer the gap junctions give way to tight junctions. Adherens junctions and desmosomes persist in the granular layer, while in the stratum corneum the predominant connections are corneodesmosomes and tight junctions. Although epidermis is commonly thought of in terms of a "bricks and mortar" organization, cells other than keratinocytes make their way into the epidermis, some of them sending dendritic extensions between the keratinocytes (melanocytes, Langerhans cells) or crawling into and through the epidermis to perform immunologic surveillance.

Melanocytes have a remarkably different shape compared with resting keratinocytes, with long extensions termed "dendrites" passing between and around their keratinocyte neighbors. These cells take up residence in the stratum basale and in the hair bulb. Within the stratum basale, the ratio of melanocytes to basal keratinocytes is approximately 1:10, with each melanocyte associating with 30-40 keratinocytes above the basal layer through dendritic extensions.[12] An essential role of melanocytes is to protect the basal cells from ultraviolet radiation, accomplished through the production and transfer of melanin via melanosomes. The darkness of skin pigmentation does not depend on the number of melanocytes, which is constant across all skin tones, but rather on the extent to which melanin is produced and the size of the melanosomes, which serve as transport vehicles from the melanocytes to the keratinocytes.

Epidermal Langerhans cells are found in the epidermis, replicating there to replace dying cells and cells which have migrated to the draining lymph nodes. There does not appear to be any need for replenishment from the circulation, although circulating monocytes can enter the skin and differentiate into scavenging and antigen presenting dendritic cells.

II. Dermis

Development of the dermis is largely controlled by fibroblasts. Each of the embryonic fibroblast precursor lines is thought to split into distinct lineages, giving rise to "upper lineage" fibroblasts, which include fibroblasts of the papillary dermis, the hair follicle dermal papilla, dermal sheath cells surrounding hair shafts, and the arrector pili muscle. It also includes "lower lineage" reticular fibroblasts, pre-adipocytes, and adipocytes. Cells of the lower lineage are primarily involved in replacement of extracellular matrix following wounding, while cells of the upper lineage support re-epithelialization.[13] The depth of injury determines the types of cells, which become engaged in repair, with lacerations extending into the middle depth of reticular dermis leading to a scarring response. Lacerations of the superficial dermis can repair themselves without visible scarring.[14] In addition to depth of injury, the amount of tension experienced by fibroblasts and the duration of inflammation also affect scarring. Primary closure of lacerations reduces tension, while control of infection limits inflammation, resulting in reduced scarring.

Hair follicles are widely distributed in skin. Epidermal cells form the primitive hair germ, penetrating as a column into the underlying dermis. An invagination or papilla is formed at the column tip into which mesodermal blood vessels and nerve endings develop. Fibroblasts within this dermal papilla seem to induce the follicular epithelial cells in the center of the follicle to undergo differentiation into central cortex cells, which generate the keratinized hair shafts. The dermal papilla and surrounding epithelial matrix cells constitute the bulb of the hair follicle. The hair shaft itself eventually

TABLE 2. Cells found in healthy adult skin

Name	Location	Function	Subsets
Keratinocyte	Epidermis	Regeneration of the stratum corneum, re-epithelialization of denuded skin, acidification of the skin surface, antimicrobial peptide production, inflammatory signaling. Terminally differentiated keratinocyte providing a physical and chemical barrier	Basal, transit amplifying, granular, corneocyte
Fibroblast	Dermis	Generation of extracellular matrix, repair	Papillary, reticular, myofibroblast
Melanocyte	Basal layer of epidermis, hair follicle bulb	Protection against ultraviolet radiation, hair coloration	---
Merkel cell	Epidermis at dermal-epidermal boundary, upper portion of hair follicle	Touch sensation through connection with nerve endings in touch domes	---
Endothelial cell	Blood vessel lining, lymphatic vessel lining	Vascular channels	Blood vascular, lymphatic vascular
Pericyte	Abluminal basement membrane of endothelial cells	Support endothelial cells, participate in angiogenesis	---
Neuronal axons	Nerves	Sensory and motor nervous functions	Based on neurotransmitters, end structures, efferent or afferent function
Schwann cell	Surrounding neuronal axons	Create myelin sheaths to insulate nerves	---
Endoneural cell	Surrounding Schwann cells	Protect and support Schwann cells	---
Perineurial cell	Surrounding endoneural cells	Create nerve fascicles	---
Myocytes	Smooth muscles	Express the contents of glands, cause "goosebumps" and hair erection, modulate blood flow	Arrector pili, vascular smooth muscle, glandular smooth muscle
Mast cell	Near blood vessels	Innate immune defense, immune modulation, wound healing, angiogenesis	---
Macrophage	Near blood vessels	Immune surveillance, cell killing, phagocytosis of cell debris	M1, M2
Dendritic cell	Epidermis and dermis	Immune surveillance	Langerhans cells, conventional dendritic cells, plasmacytoid dendritic cells
Lymphocyte	Epidermis and dermis	Immune surveillance, cell killing, regulation of adaptive immune responses	Memory CD4+, memory CD8+, $\gamma\delta$-T cell, invariant $\alpha\beta$-NKT, variant $\alpha\beta$-NKT, anergic CD4+, Tr1 T-regulatory, Th3 T-regulatory
Adipocyte	Hypodermis	Energy storage (triglycerides), thermal insulation, modulation of inflammation (adipokines)	Pre-adipocytes, adipocytes
Stem cell	Hypodermis, basal epithelium, hair follicle "bulge region"	Regeneration of various cell lines	Keratinocyte stem cells, mesenchymal stem cells, skin-derived precursor cells

consists of a medullary core, surrounded by the cortex and hair shaft cuticle.[15]

Along the upper portion of the hair follicle, superficial to what will become the upper cutaneous plexus of blood and lymphatic vessels, one or more small out buddings of the epithelial follicular sheath develop into the dermal sebaceous glands. These glands generate a lipid-rich material (sebum) that rises to the skin surface alongside the hair shaft, lubricating the skin and occluding the shaft. Deeper along the hair follicle below the forming vascular plexus, mesodermal cells give rise to smooth muscle fibers which develop into the arrector pili muscles.[16] These muscle fibers are anchored to the follicle at the "bulge region" of the outer root sheath and superficially to connective tissue beneath the basement membrane, such that a sebaceous gland is often located between the muscle and the hair follicle. Activation of these muscles results in the hairs becoming more vertical and a small amount of sebum being expressed from the glands between the shaft and muscle.

A single hair follicle with its associated sebaceous gland(s), arrector pili muscle, and papilla is termed a pilosebaceous unit. Arrector pili muscles may attach to several adjacent follicles within a follicular unit consisting of 2-6 follicles. Pilosebaceous units serve as reservoirs of Langerhans cells. They are normally absent from the glabrous skin of the palms and soles. Pilosebaceous units differ between the scalp and beard region (terminal units), the axilla and groin (apopilosebaceous units), the face, back, and chest (sebaceous units), and the remainder of the skin (vellus units). Vellus hair follicles extend to the upper or middle reticular dermis, while terminal hair follicles and surrounding dermis protrude down through the interface with the hypodermis.

Eccrine sweat glands ("true" sweat glands) develop over most parts of the skin, beginning in a similar manner to hair follicles with an extension of germinative epidermal cells down into the developing dermis. The coiled secretory gland is located at or below the level of the hair follicle bulb, with a relatively straight dermal portion of duct becoming a spiraled duct as it passes through the epidermis (the acrocyringium).

Apocrine sweat glands develop normally as a third bud from hair follicles, superficial to the sebaceous glands. These are notably present in the axilla and pubic regions, areola and nipple of the breast, eyelids, and circumanal region. With the exception of the modified apocrine glands forming the ciliary glands in the eyelids and the ceruminous glands in the auditory canal, these specialized structures do not begin development until puberty. Other distinguishing features are that the secreted product of apocrine glands normally exit the skin from the hair follicle and includes remnants of the secretory vesicles which are released from the glandular cells. The milk-producing mammary glands are modified apocrine glands. Myoepithelial cells arising from the basal layer of the glands provide a smooth muscle shroud that can squeeze the contents of the gland out through the duct.[17]

Multipotential hematopoietic stem cells arising from the fetal liver and bone marrow give rise to mast cell committed progenitors, which interact with fibroblasts in their environment to determine their differentiation into connective tissue mast cells which are found associated with blood vessels, nerves, and skin appendages of the subpapillary dermis.[18]

III. Dermal-epidermal junction

The boundary separating the epidermis from the dermis is marked by a basement membrane, occupied along its superior border by basal keratinocytes, which bind to basement membrane anchoring filaments. On the inferior aspect of the basement membrane are anchoring fibrils attaching into the extracellular matrix of the papillary dermis. Including the anchoring elements, the "basement membrane zone" is typically described as having four layers:

- A basal keratinocyte hemidesmosome layer
- The lamina lucida
- The lamina densa
- A lamina reticularis (or fibroreticularis)

The epidermis extends into the papillary dermis at regular intervals to form rete pegs, thus increasing the amount of contact between epidermis and dermis. The rete pegs deepen following term birth. On the palms and soles, the dermal-epidermal boundary forms extended ridges and troughs termed friction ridges, most prominently visible at the fingertips (fingerprints).[(19)]

IV. Hypodermis and dermal attachment

The loose connective tissue beneath the dermis is termed the hypodermis or subcutaneous layer. A prominent feature of this layer is adipocytes (fat cells) organized into prominent lobules separated by fibrous septa containing the blood and lymphatic vessels. Fibroblasts, macrophages, mast cells, and mesenchymal stem cells are also found in the hypodermis. A thin layer of smooth muscle termed the tunica dartos scroti (male) and tunica dartos labia majora (female) is found within the subcutaneous fascia of the genital region, where it will contract in response to cold temperatures to tighten and wrinkle the skin. Muscle fibers are also found in reticular dermis adjacent to the nipple, in the penis, and perineum. Immediately beneath the hypodermis is a more densely fibrous deep fascia. Human skin attaches to underlying skeletal muscle groups indirectly via small fibrous bands termed skin ligaments (retinacular ligaments), extending through the hypodermis to connect the deep reticular dermis with the underlying fascia.[(20)] Although widely distributed, the skin ligaments are not uniform across the body. In the upper trunk, limbs, head, and neck, the ligaments provide a close association with underlying muscles. Elsewhere, such as the abdominal region and buttocks, attachments are less dense. In particular regions these ligamentous structures are prominent, as with Cooper's suspensory ligaments in the breast. Various degrees of tethering create greater or lesser limits to the movement of skin over the underlying fascial planes.

The depth of sharp debridement can be gauged by key differences in the appearance of these distinctive layers. Bleeding occurs at the papillary dermis and deeper, white collagen bundles are prominent in the reticular dermis, yellow bundles of adipocytes mark the hypodermis, while fascial planes, ligaments, and muscle fibers indicate the lower boundary of the skin.

V. Vascularization

The epidermis contains no blood vessels (Figure 2). Nutrients arrive by diffusion from capillaries in the papillary dermis, while oxygen arrives both by diffusion through tissue and by direct uptake from the atmosphere. It is currently estimated that atmospheric oxygen penetrates to a depth of 250 – 400 μm, which includes the full epidermis and much of the papillary dermis.[(21)] Atmospheric oxygen flux through skin decreases when more skin capillaries open up, but shutting off capillary flow results in only a small increase in oxygen flux directly from the atmosphere.[(22)] Thus a lack of vascular perfusion cannot be overcome by direct diffusion except under hyperbaric conditions.

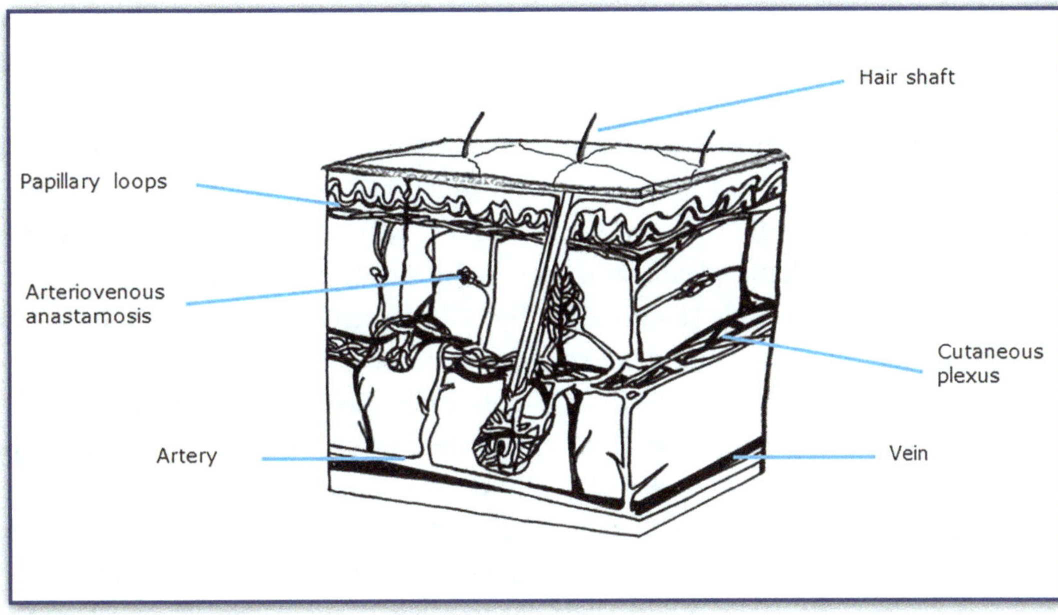

FIGURE 2. Blood vessels
Courtesy of Jessica A. Slade, ME

The blood vasculature of skin develops in two horizontally oriented networks or plexa, the superficial plexus being 1-1,500 μm beneath the surface within the papillary dermis, with the deeper plexus located near the dermal-hypodermal border, connected to perforating vessels emerging from beneath subcutaneous fat.[23] Arterioles ascend from the upper plexus to form a single capillary loop within each of the papillae, with corresponding venules descending to the superficial plexus. Each of these plexa is in communication with the deeper plexus, with capillary networks intermediate in depth between the plexa associated with hair bulbs and sweat glands. Anatomic regions of skin supplied by a single source artery are termed angiosomes.

The density of blood vessels is dictated in part by the metabolic demands of the tissue at any point in time. For example, the density of vessels associated with the hair follicle bulb fluctuates with the phase of the follicle. However, the number of blood vessels found in skin is considerably greater than what would be needed to provide oxygen and nutrients, revealing a secondary function of skin vasculature in heat loss and temperature control. It is estimated that ~60% of normal cutaneous blood flow occurs through capillary shunts rather than through the full capillary network. Circumferential vascular smooth muscle cells adjust the lumen diameter of arterioles and, to a lesser extent, venules, providing control over the distribution of blood flow.

Special arteriovenous shunts are contained within encapsulated, innervated formations termed glomus bodies. These temperature-regulating structures are located in the reticular dermis of the pads and nail beds of the fingers and toes, volar aspects of the hands and feet, the skin of the ears, and the skin of the central face.

The development of blood vessels through angiogenesis is intimately associated with pericytes, a specialized cell found at the budding ends of new vessels and wrapped around mature vessels adjacent to the basement membrane.[24] Similar to smooth muscle cells, pericytes are able to modulate the diameter of blood vessels through α-smooth muscle actin (αSMA) fibers, except for pericytes associated with capillaries, which lack αSMA. They continue throughout life to serve as, or give rise to, mesenchymal stem cells, which participate in tissue formation and regeneration.[25-26]

Lymphatic vessels are organized into a superficial and a deep lymphatic plexus adjacent to the cutaneous blood vessels (Figure 2). The superficial lymphatic plexus is found below the subpapillary venous plexus, while the deep lymphatic plexus is located in the deep dermis/hypodermis. Terminal lymphatics consist of a typically discontinuous endothelium, which lacks a basement membrane and pericytes, allowing junctions to open between endothelial cells for the ingress of fluid and cells. The vessels are typically collapsed but are surrounded and supported by a network of elastic fibers, which serve to open the lymphatics when tissue fluid levels increase. Lymphatic vasculature provides a route for egress from the skin of water, macromolecules, and antigen-presenting cells to the draining lymph nodes.[27] Leukocyte trafficking through the lymphatics is controlled by a combination of cell surface receptor expression by lymphatic endothelial cells and leukocytes, in combination with chemokine gradients, which are altered by inflammatory cytokines produced in the skin.[28] New lymphatic vessels can form through lymphangiogenesis in a process similar to angiogenesis.[29]

VI. Innervation

Innervation of the skin comes from both the sensory nervous system and the autonomic portion of the peripheral nervous system. Both myelinated and non-myelinated axonal extensions of afferent sensory neurons provide for detection and monitoring of a range of external signals, while non-myelinated efferent nerve fibers connecting with blood vessel, glandular, and follicular smooth muscle fibers serve to modulate skin function independent of conscious thought (Table 3).

Grossly visible nerves are made up of neural functional units consisting of a neural axon (nerve fiber) and its enveloping Schwann cell (myelin sheath). Each nerve fiber is surrounded by a basement membrane and endoneurium made up of connective tissue and endoneurial cells. Individual nerve fibers gather together into fascicles, wrapped by a multilayered perineurium of connective tissue and perineurial cells (epithelioid myofibroblasts) plus their basement membrane. Larger nerves contain collections of fascicles, connective tissue, and blood vessels further encased by a layer of epineurium.

A superficial nerve plexus and deep nerve plexus form in association with cutaneous blood vessels. In the papillary dermis, only a small endoneurium and a single layer of perineurial cells surround myelinated nerve fibers.

A. Afferent (sensory) nerves

Sensory nerves arise from the developing spinal cord in a segmental manner, resulting in sensory dermatomes as they send their axonal extensions out into the skin. Adjacent spinal sensory nerves produce adjacent sensory dermatomes, with some degree of overlap across the boundaries as well as physical peripheral nerve communications. There is no overlap or physical intercommunication across axial lines in the extremities.[30]

The nerve cells themselves (neurons) remain within dorsal root ganglia adjacent to the spinal cord, where transmission of signals to the central nervous system occurs via communications within the spinal cord. Through signals arriving from their axonal extensions in the skin (afferent fibers), dorsal root neurons transmit a range of sensations including pain (nociceptors),

TABLE 3. Sensory nerve endings in the skin

Receptor type	Location	Function
Free nerve endings	Epidermis	Pain, temperature, itch, crude touch
Free nerve endings	Dermis	Light touch
Touch domes, Merkel discs (free nerve endings)	Dermal-epidermal boundary of all skin; upper portions (infundibulum, isthmus) of hair follicles	Touch, static indentation/pressure
Meissner's corpuscles (Nonencapsulated†)	Papillary dermis at the dermal-epidermal boundary of glabrous skin	Light touch, pressure, low frequency vibration
Ruffini's corpuscles (encapsulated)	Dermis, oriented along stretch lines	Stretching of skin
Pacinian corpuscles (encapsulated)	Dermis, hypodermis	Deep pressure, high frequency vibration/ flutter
End bulbs of Krause (encapsulated)	Dermis of the vermillion border, eyelids, clitoris, labia minora, prepuce, glans penis, and perianal region.	Light touch, pressure, temperature

† May be partially encapsulated

temperature (thermoceptors) and itch (pruriceptors). The ability to distinguish different sensations in the skin is based on structural and functional differences of the nerve endings, of which 11 distinct structural types have been described in primates.[31]

Nerve endings and structures are found in all layers of skin. Free nerve endings are found in both the epidermis and the dermis, providing the sensations of pain, heat, cold, itch, and crude touch. Corpuscular nerve endings, some of which are encapsulated, are found in the epidermis, at the dermal-epidermal boundary, within the dermis, and within the hypodermis. In the epidermis, specialized epithelial cells termed Merkel cells form desmosomal connections with columnar "touch dome" keratinocytes. Touch domes appear to attract innervation through the release of neuroactive substances, with Merkel cells eventually developing synapse-like contact with their associated nerve endings.[32] The corpuscular, nonencapsulated touch domes respond to static pressure on the skin.[33]

Meissner corpuscles are found primarily in the dermal papillae beneath papillary ridges, with multiple innervations, providing sensations of touch, pressure, and movement of the skin. The neural axon terminating as a Meissner corpuscle is always coated by Schwann-related cells and sometimes also by an external capsule continuous with the perineurium of the nerve trunk.[34] Ruffini's corpuscles are located within glabrous skin at the dermal-epidermal boundary, where they detect stretching of the skin. Fully encapsulated Pacinian corpuscles form in the deeper layers of the skin, providing vibratory and pressure perception through a single innervation. Known as Golgi-Mazzoni corpuscles in the fingertips, these are organized in a lamellar structure similar to Ruffini corpuscles.

Receptors that respond to movement of the skin typically adapt rapidly, allowing for detection of dynamic changes. The encapsulated end-bulbs of Krause (including mucocutaneous end organs, termed genital corpuscles in the genital skin) provide touch, pressure, and/or cold temperature sensation. The presence and density of the various receptors varies by location.

The combination of receptor stimulus responsiveness, threshold, adaptation, and axonal transmission provides a discriminating perceptual representation of the world at the interface with the integument. In the case of pain receptors, the threshold for depolarization is lowered by cutaneous injury, causing normally painless stimuli to be perceived as painful and exaggerating the sense of pain with normally painful stimuli.

B. Efferent (motor) nerves

Nerves of the autonomic system reach the skin from postganglionic fibers in the sympathetic chain. These codistribute with afferent sensory nerves until the point where they branch out to make terminal contact with glands, blood vessels, and arrector pili muscles. The sympathetic division of the autonomic system only innervates these structures, without dual innervation from the parasympathetic division. Classifying the neurons according to their use of neurotransmitters, adrenergic (epinephrine, norepinephrine), cholinergic (acetylcholine), and purinergic (adenosine, adenosine triphosphate) fibers are all found in the skin.

Adrenergic fibers of vasomotor neurons mediate vasoconstriction, while cholinergic fibers mediate vasodilation. Neuropeptides may also be involved in vascular permeability. Similar to vascular smooth muscle, arrector pili muscles are in very intimate contact with adrenergic nerve endings. Sebaceous gland secretion does not appear to be under the control of neuronal signals but rather is controlled by circulating hormones.

VII. Cells of the immune system

A large number of different cell types are involved in immune responses within the skin. Normally the epidermis is able to block, repel, or neutralize chemical and microbial threats. Keratinocytes, for example, can kill bacteria through release of antimicrobial peptides. Langerhans cells provide active surveillance in the epidermis through probing with dendrites and lateral migration. These dendritic cells (DC) can capture antigens through phagocytosis and are seen to continuously leave the skin via lymphatic channels to deliver information to the draining lymph nodes.[35-36] The dermis contains various subtypes of conventional DC which appear to require higher antigen loads to stimulate an adaptive response and which seem to move more quickly to draining lymph nodes.[36] A small number of tissue resident macrophages are normally found in the dermis associated with blood vessels, lymphatic vessels, or within the intervascular spaces.[37] These cell types work in intact skin to respond to and minimize a range of threats.

Dermal lymphocytes expressing the gamma and delta chains of the T-cell receptor ($\gamma\delta$-Tcells) may be found in the skin at low levels, increased by inflammation. They behave somewhat like antigen presenting cells of the monocyte lineage but can also engage in destruction of various targets.[38] Two subsets of natural killer T-cells (NKT) are found in normal skin, where they recognize lipid antigens including lysophospholipids from human cell membranes, using specific $\alpha\beta$-Tcell receptors. These cells engage in both the destruction of target cells and the regulation of immune responses within the skin.[39]

Damage to the skin causes keratinocytes and mast cells to release cytokines that attract an inflammatory response, in part by causing venules to grab cells out of the circulation and allow them to pass through the vessel wall into the skin. Microbial invasion leads to a greater release of inflammatory mediators from resident immune cells. Polymorphonuclear neutrophils enter skin very rapidly in response to inflammatory chemokine signaling. Their normally very short lifespan, measured in hours, is extended to a day or more following entry into inflamed skin where they eventually die through apoptosis.[40]

Plasmacytoid DC, which arises along a separate lineage from the conventional DC, is rarely found in uninflamed skin. When attracted by inflammatory signals, the cells are particularly responsive to viral nucleic acid, to which they respond by releasing large amounts of interferon.[41] Monocytes derived from committed dendritic cell precursors enter the skin as monocyte derived DC.[42] Macrophages, arising from uncommitted monocytes that enter from the circulation, can either participate in the inflammatory response (M1 macrophages) or help to resolve inflammation (M2 macrophages).[43-44] Monocyte recruitment and differential polarization to M1or M2 subsets is mediated by different combinations of chemokine signals,[45-46] with exit via lymphatic channels being similarly controlled by receptor-ligand interactions.[47]

Lymphocytes bearing αβT-cell receptors can home specifically to skin through the expression of cutaneous lymphocyte antigen (CLA), where they engage in target killing.[48] As with M2 macrophages, various subsets of regulatory T-cells also respond to skin injury, providing antigen-specific downregulation of adaptive responses both locally and in the draining lymph nodes.[49]

VIII. Skin proteins

Proteomic studies of microdissected skin have identified more than 150 different proteins[2]. Actin, catenins, cadherins (desmogleins), and desmoplakin are important components of the connections between basal cells, with keratins also interacting with desmosomal cadherins to create a cross-cellular mechanical framework. Involucrin, filaggrin (filament aggregating protein), and loricrin are found in the epidermal granular layer, being produced as keratinocytes undergoing terminal differentiation to the keratinized squames with cornified envelopes.[7,50]

The extracellular matrix of the dermis consists predominantly of gel-forming proteoglycans and structural fibrous proteins (collagens, elastin, fibronectin, vitronectin, tenascins, osteopontin, and laminins), intermingled in a structurally relaxed network.[51] By weight, collagens are the most prominent protein making up 75% of the dry weight of dermis (80-90% Type I, 10-20% Type III).[1]

Large diameter fibers of Types I and III collagen are found arranged in parallel bundles within the reticular dermis. The interrelationship between elastic fibers and the collagen fibers, and the anchorage of collagen bundles to each other, gives rise to the cleavage or tension lines also known as Langer's lines.[52] Injury to the skin, which moves these bundles apart without breaking them, or is parallel to the bundles, results in the least amount of scarring. Injuries, which break or disrupt these bundles, cause a greater amount of fibrosis and visible scar.

IX. Aging

From the earliest migration of ectodermal cells during embryogenesis until the end of life, the skin never stops changing.[53] The most remarkable and rapid changes occur prior to birth, but emergence from the womb does not mark any sharp boundary in skin development. Infants born prematurely have few cornified layers of epidermis and a relative deficiency of dermal structural proteins.[9] The stratum corneum continues to mature through the first 12 months following full-term birth based on studies of skin electrical conductance and transepidermal water loss.[54] Dermal thickness and collagen concentration take considerably longer to reach adult levels, increasing from birth to adolescence.[55] At its peak, it is estimated that the suprabasal layers of the epidermis turn over every 40–56 days.[56]

Until the end of the third decade, adult skin retains a stable anatomical structure with vigorous capacity for responsiveness and self-renewal. Keratinocyte proliferation then begins to slow, with mitotic rates eventually dropping to half their maximum rate earlier in life. Epidermal turnover continues but at a slower pace, resulting in longer persistence of the stratum corneum associated with changes in the shape and size of the squames. Epidermal thickness consequently declines with advancing age.[57-58] The levels of epidermal junctional proteins also decrease, leading to compromised junctional integrity.[51] The number of nerve fiber endings in epidermis and dermis also declines with age, except perhaps in photoaged skin.[53]

The number and functioning of sweat glands diminishes with age, with a reduced sweating rate eventually leading to heat intolerance. As sebaceous gland output also diminishes, the moisture content of the thinning stratum corneum decreases, leading to xerosis. Rete pegs become less deep, and dermal collagen gradually decreases in content with a corresponding increase in stability. A progressively more haphazard organization of thickening collagen fibers results in a reduced capacity for swelling. Elastin fibers are also altered, leaving the skin simultaneously stiffer but with a more lax appearance.[59] Different dermal fibroblast lineages may shift in relative proportion to one another, with expansion of the adipocyte layer over time, indicating a relatively greater abundance of reticular fibroblasts and pre-adipocytes. The number of blood vessels diminishes, while decreased cushioning of vessels results in easier vessel rupture with bruising following minor trauma.

In both sun-exposed and nonexposed areas of skin, the number of melanocytes decreases by ~8% to 20% of the surviving population per decade after the age of 30 years. The number of mast cells and density of native Langerhans cells are substantially reduced from the 3rd to 7th decade. Expression of delayed type hypersensitivity also diminishes with advancing age, as does the ability to induce new cell mediated adaptive immune responses. The changes in skin vasculature and decreasing number of native Langerhans cells may each contribute,[60] although Langerhans cells which arise from circulating monocytes appear to remain responsive to inflammatory signals through the 8th decade.[61]

X. Cellular therapies

The management of chronic wounds involves removing barriers to healing, supporting the natural healing process, and driving healing through the provision of stimulants. Drug development experience to date indicates that singular pharmacologic or biologic factors having highly targeted effects are seldom beneficial. More complex products composed of decellularized extracellular dermal matrix, relevant composed matrices containing living cells, and skin cells suspended in a delivery vehicle have yielded more promising results. Products containing both fibroblasts and keratinocytes may address each of the key goals – reducing inflammation, which is a barrier to healing; supporting the natural process through delivery of repair-associated proteins, cytokine, and chemokines; and driving healing through the provision or stimulation of growth factors. Allogeneic cell-based products composed of only a single cell type or of peripheral blood mononuclear cells or platelets have shown less promise,[62] but any allogeneic cell-based product, as with matrix products, can be used in any depth of wound as the cells will not engraft or persist.[63] A clean, well-granulated, and adequately perfused wound can be covered with an autologous graft with a high expectation of success, bearing in mind that failure to control underlying pathologies invites recurrence of the wound.

Summary

Our skin is a remarkable organ, with a richly complex structure. The ability of skin to react to its environment, and to repair itself through regeneration or fibrosis, is critical to survival. Chronic cutaneous wounds seem to represent a disordered state in which the repair program has failed, leaving the patient at grave risk. Such a view offers little opportunity for the discovery of new therapeutics. Greater progress will be made by appreciating the dynamic interplay among the many cell types found in skin, seeking ways to remove impediments and resolve inflammatory states such that the repair process can again dominate.

Review questions

1. ***True/False.*** Persons with darker skin pigmentation have a greater number of melanocytes compared with persons of fair complexion.

2. ***True/False.*** Capillaries extend through the basement membrane into the epidermis, to provide nutrients and oxygen to keratinocytes.

3. ***True/False.*** Epidermal turnover slows with advancing age, resulting in thinning of the skin.

4. ***True/False.*** Keratinocytes are held together by extracellular matrix and do not normally make contact with other keratinocytes.

5. ***True/False.*** Neutrophils that enter the skin during an inflammatory response only live for about one day.

ANSWERS: 1) False
2) False
3) True
4) False
5) True

References

1. McGrath JA, Eady RAJ, Pope FM. Anatomy and organization of human skin. In: Rook AH, editor. 2016.
2. Wong R, Geyer S, Weninger W, Guimberteau JC, Wong JK. The dynamic anatomy and patterning of skin. Exp Dermatol. 2016 Feb;25(2):92-8.
3. Holbrook KA, Odland GF. Regional differences in the thickness (cell layers) of the human stratum corneum: an ultrastructural analysis. J Invest Dermatol. 1974 Apr;62(4):415-22.
4. Whitton JT, Everall JD. The thickness of the epidermis. Br J Dermatol. 1973 Nov;89(5):467-76.
5. Josse G, George J, Black D. Automatic measurement of epidermal thickness from optical coherence tomography images using a new algorithm. Skin Res Technol. 2011 Aug;17(3):314-9.
6. Loomis CA. Development and morphogenesis of the skin. Adv Dermatol. 2001;17:183-210.
7. Blanpain C, Fuchs E. Epidermal stem cells of the skin. Annu Rev Cell Dev Biol. 2006;22:339-73.
8. Visscher M, Narendran V. The ontogeny of skin. Adv Wound Care (New Rochelle). 2014 Apr 1;3(4):291-303.
9. Visscher MO, Adam R, Brink S, Odio M. Newborn infant skin: physiology, development, and care. Clin Dermatol. 2015 May;33(3):271-80.
10. Fuchs E, Raghavan S. Getting under the skin of epidermal morphogenesis. Nat Rev Genet. 2002 Mar;3(3):199-209.
11. Barrandon Y, Green H. Three clonal types of keratinocyte with different capacities for multiplication. Proc Natl Acad Sci USA. 1987 Apr;84(8):2302-6.
12. Cichorek M, Wachulska M, Stasiewicz A, Tyminska A. Skin melanocytes: biology and development. Postepy Derm Alergol. 2013;30(1):30-41.
13. Driskell RR, Lichtenberger BM, Hoste E, Kretzschmar K, Simons BD, Charalambous M, et al. Distinct fibroblast lineages determine dermal architecture in skin development and repair. Nature. 2013 Dec 12;504(7479):277-81.
14. Dunkin CS, Pleat JM, Gillespie PH, Tyler MP, Roberts AH, McGrouther DA. Scarring occurs at a critical depth of skin injury: precise measurement in a graduated dermal scratch in human volunteers. Plast Reconstr Surg. 2007 May;119(6):1722-32.
15. Stenn KS, Paus R. Controls of hair follicle cycling. Physiol Rev. 2001;81:450-81.
16. Torkamani N, Rufaut NW, Jones L, Sinclair RD. Beyond goosebumps: does the arrector pili muscle have a role in hair loss? Int J Trichology. 2014 Jul;6(3):88-94.
17. Shelley WB, Hurley HJ Jr. The physiology of the human axillary apocrine sweat gland. J Invest Dermatol. 1953 Apr;20(4):285-97.
18. Kitamura Y, Oboki K, Ito A. Development of mast cells. Proc Jpn Acad Ser B Phys Biol Sci. 2007 Sep;83(6):164-74.
19. Wertheim K. Embryology and morphology of friction ridge skin. In: McRoberts A, editor. Fingerprint sourcebook. Rockville MD: U.S. Department of Justice, Office of Justice Programs; 2011. p. 1-26.
20. Nash LG, Phillips MN, Nicholson H, Barnett R, Zhang M. Skin ligaments: regional distribution and variation in morphology. Clin Anat. 2004 May;17(4):287-93.
21. Stucker M, Struk A, Altmeyer P, Herde M, Baumgartl H, Lubbers DW. The cutaneous uptake of atmospheric oxygen contributes significantly to the oxygen supply of human dermis and epidermis. J Physiol. 2002 Feb 1;538(Pt 3):985-94.

22. Stucker M, Struk PA, Hoffmann K, Schulze L, Rochling A, Lubbers DW. The transepidermal oxygen flux from the environment is in balance with the capillary oxygen supply. J Invest Dermatol. 2000 Mar;114(3):533-40.

23. Braverman IM. The cutaneous microcirculation. J Investig Dermatol Symp Proc. 2000 Dec;5(1):3-9.

24. Armulik A, Genove G, Betsholtz C. Pericytes: developmental, physiological, and pathological perspectives, problems, and promises. Dev Cell. 2011 Aug 16;21(2):193-215.

25. Birbrair A, Zhang T, Wang ZM, Messi ML, Mintz A, Delbono O. Pericytes at the intersection between tissue regeneration and pathology. Clin Sci (Lond). 2015 Jan;128(2):81-93.

26. Paquet-Fifield S, Schluter H, Li A, Aitken T, Gangatirkar P, Blashki D, et al. A role for pericytes as microenvironmental regulators of human skin tissue regeneration. J Clin Invest. 2009 Sep;119(9):2795-806.

27. Ryan TJ. Structure and function of lymphatics. J Invest Dermatol. 1989 Aug;93(2 Suppl):18S-24S.

28. Teijeira A, Rouzaut A, Melero I. Initial afferent lymphatic vessels controlling outbound leukocyte traffic from skin to lymph nodes. Front Immunol. 2013 Dec 9;4:433.

29. Varricchi G, Granata F, Loffredo S, Genovese A, Marone G. Angiogenesis and lymphangiogenesis in inflammatory skin disorders. J Am Acad Dermatol. 2015 Jul;73(1):144-53.

30. Ladak A, Tubbs RS, Spinner RJ. Mapping sensory nerve communications between peripheral nerve territories. Clin Anat. 2014 Jul;27(5):681-90.

31. Malinovsky L. Sensory nerve formations in the skin and their classification. Microsc Res Tech. 1996 Jul 1;34(4):283-301.

32. Xiao Y, Williams JS, Brownell I. Merkel cells and touch domes: more than mechanosensory functions? Exp Dermatol. 2014 Oct;23(10):692-5.

33. Doucet YS, Woo SH, Ruiz ME, Owens DM. The touch dome defines an epidermal niche specialized for mechanosensory signaling. Cell Rep. 2013 Jun 27;3(6):1759-65.

34. Vega JA, Garcia-Suarez O, Montano JA, Pardo B, Cobo JM. The Meissner and Pacinian sensory corpuscles revisited new data from the last decade. Microsc Res Tech. 2009 Apr;72(4):299-309.

35. Nishibu A, Ward BR, Jester JV, Ploegh HL, Boes M, Takashima A. Behavioral responses of epidermal Langerhans cells in situ to local pathological stimuli. J Invest Dermatol. 2006 Apr;126(4):787-96.

36. Scott CL, Henri S, Guilliams M. Mononuclear phagocytes of the intestine, the skin, and the lung. Immunol Rev. 2014 Nov;262(1):9-24.

37. Tay SS, Roediger B, Tong PL, Tikoo S, Weninger W. The skin-resident immune network. Curr Dermatol Rep. 2013 Nov 28;3:13-22.

38. Wu Y, Wu W, Wong WM, Ward E, Thrasher AJ, Goldblatt D, et al. Human gamma delta T cells: a lymphoid lineage cell capable of professional phagocytosis. J Immunol. 2009 Nov 1;183(9):5622-9.

39. Macho-Fernandez E, Brigl M. The extended family of CD1d-restricted NKT cells: sifting through a mixed bag of TCRs, antigens, and functions. Front Immunol. 2015 Jul 28;6:362.

40. Ortega-Gomez A, Perretti M, Soehnlein O. Resolution of inflammation: an integrated view. EMBO Mol Med. 2013 May;5(5):661-74.

41. Conrad C, Meller S, Gilliet M. Plasmacytoid dendritic cells in the skin: to sense or not to sense nucleic acids. Semin Immunol. 2009 Jun;21(3):101-9.

42. Malissen B, Tamoutounour S, Henri S. The origins and functions of dendritic cells and macrophages in the skin. Nat Rev Immunol. 2014 Jun;14(6):417-28.

43. Hristodorov D, Mladenov R, Huhn M, Barth S, Thepen T. Macrophage-targeted therapy: CD64-based immunotoxins for treatment of chronic inflammatory diseases. Toxins (Basel). 2012 Sep 14;4(9):676-94.

44. Mosser DM, Edwards JP. Exploring the full spectrum of macrophage activation. Nat Rev Immunol. 2008 Dec;8(12):958-69.

45. Xuan W, Qu Q, Zheng B, Xiong S, Fan GH. The chemotaxis of M1 and M2 macrophages is regulated by different chemokines. J Leukoc Biol. 2015 Jan;97(1):61-9.

46. Italiani P, Boraschi D. From monocytes to M1/M2 macrophages: phenotypical vs. functional differentiation. Front Immunol. 2014 Oct 17;5:514.

47. Schif-Zuck S, Gross N, Assi S, Rostoker R, Serhan CN, Ariel A. Saturated-efferocytosis generates pro-resolving CD11b low macrophages: modulation by resolvins and glucocorticoids. Eur J Immunol. 2011 Feb;41(2):366-79.

48. Nomura T, Kabashima K, Miyachi Y. The panoply of alphabetaT cells in the skin. J Dermatol Sci. 2014 Oct;76(1):3-9.

49. MacConmara MP, Tajima G, O'Leary F, Delisle AJ, McKenna AM, Stallwood CG, et al. Regulatory T cells suppress antigen-driven CD4 T cell reactivity following injury. J Leukoc Biol. 2011 Jan;89(1):137-47.

50. Kalinin A, Marekov LN, Steinert PM. Assembly of the epidermal cornified cell envelope. J Cell Sci. 2001 Sep;114(Pt 17):3069-70.

51. Frantz C, Stewart KM, Weaver VM. The extracellular matrix at a glance. J Cell Sci. 2010 Dec 15;123(Pt 24):4195-200.

52. Carmichael SW. The tangled web of Langer's lines. Clin Anat. 2014 Mar;27(2):162-8.

53. Rittie L, Fisher GJ. Natural and sun-induced aging of human skin. Cold Spring Harb Perspect Med. 2015 Jan 5;5(1):1-14.

54. Nikolovski J, Stamatas GN, Kollias N, Wiegand BC. Barrier function and water-holding and transport properties of infant stratum corneum are different from adult and continue to develop through the first year of life. J Invest Dermatol. 2008 Jul;128(7):1728-36.

55. Saitoh A, Aizawa Y, Sato I, Hirano H, Sakai T, Mori M. Skin thickness in young infants and adolescents: Applications for intradermal vaccination. Vaccine. 2015 Jun 26;33(29):3384-91.

56. Koster MI. Making an epidermis. Ann N Y Acad Sci. 2009 Jul;1170:7-10.

57. Gambichler T, Matip R, Moussa G, Altmeyer P, Hoffmann K. In vivo data of epidermal thickness evaluated by optical coherence tomography: effects of age, gender, skin type, and anatomic site. J Dermatol Sci. 2006 Dec;44(3):145-52.

58. Hwang K, Kim DJ, Kim SK. Does the upper eyelid skin become thinner with age? J Craniofac Surg. 2006 May;17(3):474-6.

59. Richey ML, Richey HK, Fenske NA. Aging-related skin changes: development and clinical meaning. Geriatrics. 1988 Apr;43(4):49-52, 57-9, 63-4.

60. Gilchrest BA, Murphy GF, Soter NA. Effect of chronologic aging and ultraviolet irradiation on Langerhans cells in human epidermis. J Invest Dermatol. 1982 Aug;79(2):85-8.

61. Ogden S, Dearman RJ, Kimber I, Griffiths CE. The effect of ageing on phenotype and function of monocyte-derived Langerhans cells. Br J Dermatol. 2011 Jul;165(1):184-8.

62. Slade HB, Jacobson N, Lu E. Human cell therapy for venous leg ulcers. Phlebological Rev. 2015;23(2):1-10.

63. Dickerson JE, Planz JV, Reece BT, Weedon KA, Kirkpatrick SD, Slade HB. Cell persistence of allogeneic keratinocytes and fibroblasts applied in a fibrin matrix to acute, full thickness wounds. Cell Medicine. 2013;4(3):149-52.

Chapter 2

PHYSIOLOGY AND BIOCHEMISTRY OF WOUND HEALING

Gregory S. Schultz, PhD
Daniel J. Gibson, PhD

KEY CONCEPTS

1. Normal wound healing in the skin proceeds through four major phases that have some temporal overlap.

   a) **Hemostasis Phase** - Fibrin clotting cascade is activated, preventing hemorrhage, and platelets trapped in the fibrin clot release multiple cytokines and growth factors that stimulate the initial chemotactic migration of inflammatory cells into the wound bed.

   b) **In ammation Phase** – Neutrophils migrate into the wound, followed by macrophages, which engulf contaminating bacteria and generate reactive oxygen species (ROS) that kill bacteria in phagosomes. Inflammatory cells also secrete proteases (matrix metalloproteases [MMPs] and neutrophil elastase) that break down damaged extracellular matrix molecules (ECM). Inflammation spontaneously resolves in the absence of continued bioburden.

   c) **Repair Phase** – Quiescent fibroblasts adjacent to the injury proliferate and migrate into the provisional fibrin matrix, where they synthesize new collagen and other ECM components that constitute the initial scar. Some fibroblasts differentiate into myofibroblasts that contract the developing new scar tissue. Vascular endothelial cells also proliferate and migrate into the provisional fibrin matrix generating new capillaries (granulation tissue). Epithelial stem cells in hair follicles proliferate and migrate over the initial scar matrix, completing the initial healing of the wound.

   d) **Remodeling Phase** – During the next 6 to 12 months, the initial scar matrix is slowly remodeled by the controlled action of secreted proteases (MMPs) that remove the irregular ECM, which is replaced by more normally organized collagen fibers and other ECM molecules. The density of cells in the scar tissue decreases through controlled apoptosis.

2. Acute wounds can convert into chronic wounds when the inflammatory phase becomes excessively prolonged, usually due to persistently elevated levels of bacterial bioburden, including biofilms, that lead to chronically elevated levels of proteases and ROS that destroy proteins essential for healing.

3. Wound bed preparation is a process that removes the major barriers to healing and restores the correct balance of bioburden, proteases, growth factors, cytokines, and ECM components that allows healing to proceed.

CONTENTS

Introduction

Acute wounds normally heal in an orderly and efficient manner and progress smoothly through the four distinct but overlapping phases of wound healing: hemostasis, inflammation, repair, and remodeling[1-6] (Figure 1). The process of wound healing is complex and involves a variety of specialized cells, such as macrophages, fibroblasts, and epithelial and endothelial cells. These cells interact with each other and with the extracellular matrix. In addition to the various cellular interactions, healing is also influenced by the action of proteins and glycoproteins, such as cytokines, chemokines, growth factors, inhibitors, and their receptors. Each stage of wound healing has certain milestones that must occur in order for normal healing to progress.

In the following sections, we first review the key molecular and cellular regulators of the four distinct phases of normal acute wound healing. We then present data that show that most acute wounds fail to progress through the four phases of healing and become "stuck" in a chronic inflammatory phase that is due to the presence of a persistent bioburden of both planktonic bacteria and especially biofilm bacteria. We explain that bacteria present in the biofilm phenotype are highly tolerant to the antibodies and phagocytic inflammatory cells (neutrophils and macrophages) of the patient's immune system, as well as antibiotics and many antiseptics. We emphasize the "down-stream" consequence of the chronic inflammatory status is the presence of elevated levels of proteases (especially matrix metalloproteases, MMPs) and reactive oxygen species (ROS) that degrade proteins that are essential for healing and leads to impaired healing. Finally, we discuss the concepts of wound bed preparation and emphasize techniques and new therapies that

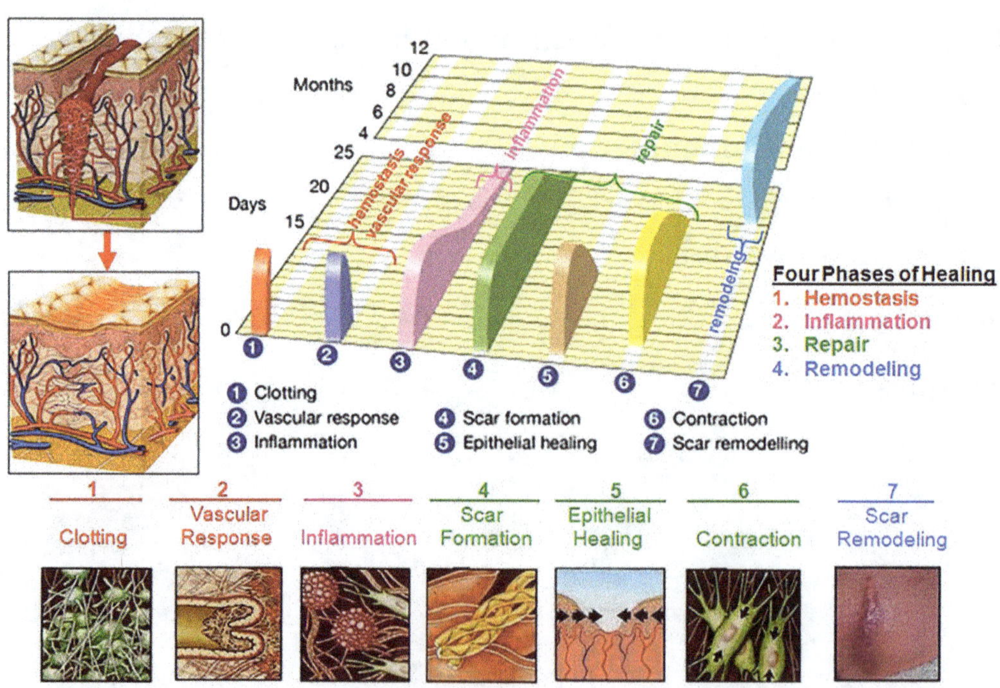

FIGURE 1. Sequence of wound healing. Normal skin wound healing proceeds through the four phases of hemostasis, inflammation, repair, and remodeling. Most chronic wounds get "stuck" in a prolonged inflammatory phase that prevents the wound from moving into an effective repair phase.

Reprinted with permission from HMP Communications. *Chronic Wound Care: The Essentials*. 2005.

TABLE 1. Major growth factor families

GROWTH FACTOR FAMILY	SOURCE	ACTIONS
Transforming Growth Factor B TGF-β1, TGF-β2 TGF-β3	Platelets Fibroblasts Macrophages	Fibroblast Chemotaxis and Activation ECM Deposition ☐ Collagen Synthesis ☐ TIMP Synthesis ☐ MMP Synthesis Reduces Scarring ☐ Collagen ☐ Fibronectin
Platelet Derived Growth Factor PDGF-AA, PDGF-BB, VEGF	Platelets Macrophages Keratinocytes Fibroblasts	Activation of Immune Cells and Fibroblasts ECM Deposition ☐ Collagen Synthesis ☐ TIMP Synthesis ☐ MMP Synthesis Angiogenesis
Fibroblast Growth Factor Acidic FGF, Basic FGF, KGF	Macrophages Endothelial Cells Fibroblasts	Angiogenesis Endothelial Cell Activation Keratinocyte Proliferation and Migration ECM Deposition
Insulin-like Growth Factor IGF-I, IGF-II, Insulin	Liver Skeletal Muscle Fibroblasts Macrophages Neutrophils	Keratinocyte Proliferation Fibroblast Proliferation Endothelial Cell Activation Angiogenesis ☐ Collagen Synthesis ECM Deposition Cell Metabolism
Epidermal Growth Factor EGF, HB-EGF, TGF-α, Amphiregulin, Betacellulin	Keratinocytes Macrophages	Keratinocyte Proliferation and Migration ECM Deposition
Connective Tissue Growth Factor CTGF	Fibroblasts Endothelial Cells Epithelial Cells	Mediates Action of TGF-βs on Collagen Synthesis

correct the molecular abnormalities in chronic wounds that are barriers to healing.

I. Overview of the four stages of normal skin wound healing

In order to identify the differences inherent in chronic wounds that prevent healing, it is important to review the process of healing in normal wounds.

A. Hemostasis phase

Hemostasis occurs immediately following an injury.[7] To prevent exsanguination, vasoconstriction occurs and platelets undergo activation, adhesion, and aggregation at the site of injury. Platelets become activated when exposed to extravascular collagen (such as Type I collagen), which they detect via specific integrin receptors, cell surface receptors that mediate a cell's interactions with the extracellular matrix.

Once in contact with collagen, platelets release the soluble mediators (growth factors and cyclic AMP) and adhesive glycoproteins, which signal them to become sticky and aggregate. The key glycoproteins released from the platelet alpha granules include fibrinogen, fibronectin, thrombospondin, and von Willebrand factor. As platelet aggregation proceeds, clotting factors are released, resulting in the deposition of a fibrin clot at the site of injury. The fibrin clot serves as a provisional matrix.[8] The aggregated platelets become trapped in the fibrin web and provide the bulk of the clot. Their membranes provide a surface on which inactive clotting enzyme proteases are bound, become activated, and accelerate the clotting cascade.

Growth factors are also released from the platelet alpha granules and include platelet-derived growth factor (PDGF), transforming growth factor beta (TGF-β), transforming growth factor alpha (TGF-α), basic fibroblast growth factor (bFGF), insulin-like growth factor-1 (IGF-1), and vascular endothelial growth factor (VEGF). Major growth factor families are presented in Table 1. Neutrophils and monocytes are then recruited by PDGF and TGF-β from the vasculature to initiate the inflammatory response. A breakdown fragment generated from complement, C5a, and a bacterial waste product, f-Met-Leu-Phe, also provide additional chemotactic signals for the recruitment of neutrophils to the site of injury. Meanwhile, endothelial cells are activated by VEGF, TGF-α, and bFGF to initiate angiogenesis. Fibroblasts are then activated and recruited by PDGF to migrate to the wound site and begin production of collagen and glycosaminoglycans, proteins in the extracellular matrix, which facilitate cellular migration and interactions with the matrix supporting framework. Thus, the healing process begins with hemostasis, platelet deposition at the site of injury, and interactions of soluble mediators and growth factors with the extracellular matrix to set the stage for subsequent healing events.[9]

B. Inflammation phase

Inflammation, the next stage of wound healing, develops over the first 24 hours after injury and can last for up to 2 weeks in normal wounds and significantly longer in chronic nonhealing wounds. Mast cells release contents filled with enzymes, histamine, and other active amines, which are responsible for the characteristic signs of inflammation, the *rubor* (redness), *calor* (heat), *tumor* (swelling), and *dolor* (pain) around the wound site. Neutrophils, monocytes, and macrophages are the key cells during the inflammatory phase. They cleanse the wound of infection and debris and release soluble mediators such as proinflammatory cytokines (including IL-1, IL-6, IL-8, and TNF-α), and growth factors (such as PDGF, TGF-β, TGF-α, IGF-1, and FGF) that are involved in the recruitment and activation of fibroblasts and epithelial cells in preparation for the next phase in healing. Cytokines that play important roles in regulating inflammation in wound healing are described in Table 2.

In addition to the growth factors and cytokines, a third important group of small regulatory proteins, listed in Table 3, has been identified, and are collectively named chemokines, from a contraction of chemoattractive cytokine(s).[10-12] The structural and functional similarities among chemokines were not initially appreciated. This has led to an idiosyncratic nomenclature consisting of many acronyms that were based on their biological functions. Some examples are monocyte chemoattractant protein 1 (MCP-1), macrophage inflammatory protein 1 (MIP-1) their source for isolation (platelet factor 4 [PF-4]) or their biochemical properties (interferon-inducible protein of 10 kDa [IP-10]), or regulated upon

TABLE 2. Cytokines involved in wound healing

CYTOKINE	CELL SOURCE	BIOLOGICAL ACTIVITY
PRO-INFLAMMATORY CYTOKINES		
TNF-α	Macrophages	PMN margination and cytotoxicity, ± collagen synthesis; provides metabolic substrate
IL-1	Macrophages Keratinocytes	Fibroblast and keratinocyte chemotaxis, collagen synthesis
IL-2	T lymphocytes	Increases fibroblast infiltration and metabolism
IL-6	Macrophages PMNs Fibroblasts	Fibroblast proliferation, hepatic acute-phase protein synthesis
IL-8	Macrophages Fibroblasts	Macrophage and PMN chemotaxis, keratinocyte maturation
IFN-γ	T lymphocytes Macrophages	Macrophage and PMN activation; retards collagen synthesis and cross-linking; stimulates collagenase activity
ANTI-INFLAMMATORY CYTOKINES		
IL-4	T lymphocytes Basophils Mast cells	Inhibition of TNF, IL-1, IL-6 production; fibroblast proliferation, collagen synthesis
IL-10	T lymphocytes Macrophages Keratinocytes	Inhibition of TNF, IL-1, IL-6 production; inhibits macrophage and PMN activation

activation normal T-cell expressed and secreted, RANTES.

As their biochemical properties were established, it was recognized that the approximately 40 chemokines could be grouped into four major classes based on the pattern of cysteine residues located near the N-terminus. In fact, there has been a recent trend to re-establish a more organized nomenclature system based on these four major classes. In general, chemokines have two primary functions: 1) they regulate the trafficking of leukocyte populations during normal health and development, and 2) they direct the recruitment and activation of neutrophils, lymphocytes, macrophages, eosinophils, and basophils during inflammation.

1. *Neutrophils*

Neutrophils are the first inflammatory cells to respond to the soluble mediators released by platelets and the coagulation cascade. They serve as the first line of defense against infection by phagocytosing and killing bacteria and by removing foreign materials and devitalized tissue. During the process of extravasation of inflammatory cells into a wound, important interactions occur between adhesion molecules (selectins, cell adhesion molecules [CAMs],

TABLE 3. Chemokine families involved in wound healing

CHEMOKINES	CELLS AFFECTED
α-CHEMOKINES (CXC) With glutamic acid-leucine-arginine near the N-terminal Interleukin-8 (IL-8)	Neutrophils
α-CHEMOKINES (CXC) *Without* glutamic acid-leucine-arginine near the N-terminal Interferon -inducible protein of 10 kd (IP-10) Monokine induced by interferon-γ (MIG) Stromal-cell-derived factor 1 (SDF-1)	Activated T lymphocytes
β-CHEMOKINES (CC) Monocyte chemoattractant proteins (MCPs): MCP-1, -2, -3, -4, -5 Regulated upon activation normal T-cell expressed and secreted (RANTES) Macrophage inflammatory protein (MIP-1α) Exotoxin	Eosinophils Basophils Monocytes Activated T lymphocytes
γ-CHEMOKINES (C) Lymphotactin	Resting T lymphocytes
δ-CHEMOKINES (CXXXC) Fractalkine	Natural killer cells

and cadherins) and receptors (integrins) that are associated with the plasma membranes of circulating leukocytes and vascular endothelial cells[13]. Initially, leukocytes weakly adhere to the endothelial cell walls via their selectin molecules, which causes them to decelerate and begin to roll on the surface of endothelial cells. While rolling, leukocytes can become activated by chemoattractants (cytokines, growth factors, or bacterial products). After activation, leukocytes firmly adhere to endothelial cells as a result of the binding between their integrin receptors and ligands such as VCAM and ICAM that are expressed on activated endothelial cells. Chemotactic signals present outside the venule then induce leukocytes to squeeze between endothelial cells of the venule and migrate into the wounded tissue using their integrin receptors to recognize and bind to extracellular matrix components. The inflammatory cells release elastase and collagenase to help them migrate through the endothelial cell basement membrane and to migrate into the ECM at the site of the wound. Neutrophils also produce and release inflammatory mediators such as TNF-α and IL-1 that further recruit and activate fibroblasts and epithelial cells. After the neutrophils migrate into the wound site, they generate oxygen free radicals, which kill phagocytized bacteria, and they release high levels of proteases (neutrophil elastase and neutrophil collagenase) which remove components of the extracellular matrix that were damaged by the injury. The persistent presence of bacteria in a wound may contribute to chronicity through continued recruitment of neutrophils and their release of proteases, cytokines, and reactive oxygen species. Usually neutrophils are depleted in the wound after two to three days by the process of apoptosis, and they are replaced by tissue monocytes.

2. *Macrophages*

Activated macrophages play pivotal roles in the regulation of healing, and the healing process does not proceed normally without macrophages. Macrophages begin as circulating monocytes that are attracted to the wound site beginning about 24 hours after injury. They extravasate by the mechanism described for neutrophils and are stimulated to differentiate into activated tissue macrophages in response to chemokines, cytokines, growth factors, and soluble fragments of extracellular matrix components produced by proteolytic degradation of collagen and fibronectin.[14] Similar to neutrophils, tissue macrophages have a dual role in the healing process. They patrol the wound area, ingesting and killing bacteria and removing devitalized tissue through the actions of secreted MMPs and elastase. Macrophages differ from neutrophils in their ability to more closely regulate the proteolytic destruction of wound tissue by secreting inhibitors for the proteases. As important as their phagocytic role, macrophages also mediate the transition from the inflammatory phase to the proliferative phase of healing. They release a wide variety of growth factors and cytokines including PDGF, TGF-β, TGF-α, FGF, IGF-1, TNFα, IL-1, and IL-6. Some of these soluble mediators recruit and activate fibroblasts, which will then synthesize, deposit, and organize the new tissue matrix, while others promote angiogenesis. The absence of neutrophils and a decrease in the number of macrophages in the wound is an indication that the inflammatory phase is nearing an end and that the proliferative phase is beginning.

C. Repair phase

The milestones during the proliferative phase include replacement of the provisional fibrin matrix with a new matrix of collagen fibers, proteoglycans, and fibronectin to restore the structure and function to the tissue. Another important event in healing is angiogenesis, the in-growth of new capillaries to replace the previously damaged vessels and restore circulation. Other significant events in this phase of healing are the formation of granulation tissue and epithelialization. Fibroblasts are the key cells in the proliferative phase of healing.

1. *Fibroblast migration*

Fibroblasts migrate into the wound in response to multiple soluble mediators released initially by platelets and later by macrophages.[5] Fibroblast migration in the extracellular matrix depends on precise recognition and interaction with specific components of the matrix. Fibroblasts in normal dermis are typically quiescent and sparsely distributed, whereas in the provisional matrix of the wound site and in the granulation tissue, they are quite active and numerous. Their migration and accumulation in the wound site requires them to change their morphology and to produce and secrete proteases to clear a path for their movement from the ECM into the wound site.

Fibroblasts begin moving by first binding to matrix components such as fibronectin, vitronectin, and fibrin via their integrin receptors. Integrin receptors attach to specific amino acid sequences (such as R-G-D or arginine-glycine-aspartic acid) or binding sites in these matrix components. While one end of the fibroblast remains bound to the matrix component, the cell extends a cytoplasmic projection to find another binding site. When the next site is found, the original site is released (apparently by local protease activity), and the cell uses its cytoskeleton network of actin fibers to pull itself forward.

The direction of fibroblast movement is determined by the concentration gradient of chemotactic growth factors, cytokines and chemokines, and by the alignment of the fibrils in the ECM and provisional matrix. Fibroblasts tend to migrate along these fibrils as opposed to across them. Fibroblasts secrete proteolytic enzymes locally to facilitate their forward motion through the matrix. The enzymes secreted by the fibroblasts include three types of MMPs: collagenase (MMP-1); gelatinases (MMP-2 and MMP-9), which degrade gelatin substrates; and stromelysin (MMP-3), which has multiple protein substrates in the ECM.

2. *Collagen and extracellular matrix production*

The collagen, proteoglycans, and other components that comprise granulation tissue are synthesized and deposited primarily by fibroblasts. PDGF and TGF-β are two of the most important growth factors that regulate fibroblast activity. PDGF, which predominantly originates from platelets and macrophages, stimulates a number of fibroblast functions including proliferation, chemotaxis, and collagenase expression. TGF-β, also secreted by platelets and macrophages, is considered to be the master control signal that regulates extracellular matrix deposition. Through the stimulation of gene transcription for collagen, proteoglycans, and fibronectin, TGF-β increases the overall production of matrix proteins. At the same time, TGF-β downregulates the secretion of proteases responsible for matrix degradation and also stimulates synthesis of tissue inhibitor of metalloproteinases (TIMP) to further inhibit breakdown of the matrix. Recent data indicate that a new growth factor named connective tissue growth factor (CTGF) mediates many of the effects of TGF-β on the synthesis of extracellular matrix.[15]

Once the fibroblasts have migrated into the matrix, they again change their morphology, settle down, and begin to proliferate and to synthesize granulation tissue components including collagen, elastin and proteoglycans. Fibroblasts attach to the cables of the provisional fibrin matrix and begin to produce collagen. At least 20 individual types of collagen have been identified to date. Type III collagen is initially synthesized at high levels, along with other extracellular matrix proteins and proteoglycans. After transcription and processing of the collagen mRNA, it is attached to polyribosomes on the endoplasmic reticulum where the new collagen chains are produced. During this process, there is an important step involving hydroxylation of proline and lysine residues. Three protein chains associate and begin to form the characteristic triple helical structure of the fibrillar collagen molecule, and the nascent chains undergo further modification by the process of glycosylation. Hydroxyproline in collagen is important because it plays a major role in stabilizing the triple helical conformation of collagen molecules. Fully hydroxylated collagen has a higher melting temperature. When levels of hydroxyproline are low, for example in vitamin C-deficient conditions (scurvy), the collagen triple helix has an altered structure and denatures (unwinds) much more rapidly and at lower temperatures. To ensure optimal wound healing, wound care specialists should be sure patients are receiving good nutritional support with a diet with ample protein and vitamin C.

Finally, procollagen molecules are secreted into the extracellular space where they undergo further processing by proteolytic cleavage of the short, non-helical segments at the N- and C-termini. The collagen molecules then spontaneously associate in a head-to-tail and side-by-side arrangement forming collagen fibrils, which associate into larger bundles that form collagen fibers. In the extra-cellular spaces an important enzyme, lysyl oxidase, acts on the collagen molecules to form stable, covalent, cross-links. As the collagen matures and becomes older, more and more of these intramolecular and intermolecular cross-links are placed in the molecules. This important cross-linking step gives collagen its strength and stability, and the older the collagen the more cross-link formation has occurred.

Dermal collagen on a per-weight basis approaches the tensile strength of steel. In normal tissue, it is a strong molecule and highly organized. In contrast, collagen fibers formed in scar tissue are much smaller and have a random appearance. Scar tissue is always weaker and will break apart before the surrounding normal tissue.

3. *Angiogenesis*

Damaged vasculature must be replaced to maintain tissue viability. The process of angiogenesis is stimulated by local factors of the microenvironment, including low oxygen tension, low pH, and high lactate levels. [16] Also, certain soluble mediators are potent angiogenic signals for endothelial cells. Many of these are produced by epidermal cells, fibroblasts, vascular endothelial cells, and macrophages, and include bFGF, TGF-β, and VEGF. It is now recognized that oxygen levels in tissues directly regulate angiogenesis by interacting with oxygen-sensing proteins that regulate transcription of angiogenic and anti-angiogenic genes. For example, synthesis of VEGF by capillary endothelial cells is directly increased by hypoxia through the activation of the transcription factor, hypoxia-inducible factor (HIF), which binds oxygen.[17] When oxygen levels surrounding capillary endothelial cells drop, levels of HIF increase inside the cells. HIF-1 binds to specific DNA sequences and stimulates transcription of specific genes such as VEGF that promote angiogenesis. When oxygen levels in wound tissue increase, oxygen binds to HIF, leading to the destruction of HIF molecules in cells and decreased synthesis of angiogenic factors. Regulation of angiogenesis involves both stimulatory factors like VEGF and anti-angiogenic factors like angiostatin, endostatin, thrombospondin, and pigment epithelium-derived factor (PEDF).

Binding of angiogenic factors causes endothelial cells of the capillaries adjacent to the devascularized site to begin to migrate into the matrix and then proliferate to form buds or sprouts. Once again, the migration of these cells into the matrix requires the local secretion of proteolytic enzymes, especially MMPs. As the tips of the sprouts extends from endothelial cells and encounter other sprouts, they develop a cleft that subsequently becomes the lumen of the evolving vessel and completes a new vascular loop. This process continues until the capillary system is sufficiently repaired, and the tissue oxygenation and metabolic needs are met. It is these new capillary tuffs that give granulation tissue its characteristic bumpy or granular appearance.

Granulation tissue is a transitional replacement for normal dermis, which eventually matures into a scar during the remodeling phase of healing. It is characterized from unwounded dermis by an extremely dense network of blood vessels and capillaries, elevated cellular density of fibroblasts and macrophages, and randomly organized collagen fibers. It also has an elevated metabolic rate compared to normal dermis, which reflects the activity required for cellular migration and division and protein synthesis.

4. *Epithelialization*

All dermal wounds heal by three basic mechanisms: contraction, connective tissue matrix deposition, and epithelialization. Wounds that remain open heal by contraction; the interaction between cells and matrix results in movement of tissue toward the center of the wound. As previously described, matrix deposition is the process by which collagen, proteoglycans, and attachment proteins are deposited to form a new extracellular matrix. Epithelialization is the process where epithelial cells around the margin of the wound or in residual skin appendages such as hair follicles and sebaceous glands lose contact inhibition and begin to migrate into the wound area by the process of epiboly. As migration proceeds, cells in the basal layers begin to proliferate to provide additional epithelial cells.

Epithelialization is a multi-step process that involves epithelial cell detachment and change in their internal structure, migration, proliferation, and differentiation.[18] The intact mature epidermis consists of 5 layers of differentiated epithelial cells ranging from the cuboidal basal keratinocytes nearest the dermis up to the flattened, hexagonal, tough squames in the uppermost layer. Only the basal epithelial cells and the transit amplifying cells are capable of proliferation. These basal cells are normally attached to their neighboring cells by intercellular connectors called desmosomes and to the basement membrane by hemi-desmosomes. When growth factors such as EGF, keratinocyte growth factor (KGF), and TGF-α are released during the healing process, they bind to receptors on these epithelial cells and stimulate migration and proliferation. The binding of the growth factors triggers the desmosomes and hemi-desmosomes to dissolve so the cells can detach in preparation for migration. Integrin receptors are then expressed, and the normally cuboidal basal epithelial cells flatten in shape and begin to migrate as a monolayer over the newly deposited granulation tissue, following along collagen fibers. Proliferation of the basal epithelial cells near the wound margin supplies new cells to the advancing monolayer apron of cells (cells that are actively migrating are incapable of proliferation). Epithelial cells in the leading edge of the monolayer produce and secrete proteolytic enzymes (MMPs), which enable the cells to penetrate scab, surface necrosis, or eschar. Migration continues until the epithelial cells contact other advancing cells to form a confluent sheet. Once this contact has been made, the entire epithelial monolayer enters a proliferative mode and the stratified layers of the epidermis are re-established and begin to mature to restore barrier function. TGF-β is one growth factor that can speed up the maturation (differentiation and keratinization) of the epidermal layers. The intercellular desmosomes and the hemi-desmosome attachments to the newly formed basement membrane are also re-established. Epithelialization is the clinical hallmark of healing, but it is not the final event—remodeling of the granulation tissue is yet to occur.

Recent studies by Sen, et al. have demonstrated that under conditions of hypoxia, HIF-1alpha is stabilized, which in turn induces the expression of specific micro RNAs that then downregulate epithelial cell proliferation.[19-20] Therefore, it appears that there are very complex mechanisms involved in the role of oxygen and hypoxia during the process of wound healing.

D. Remodeling phase

Remodeling is the final phase of the healing process, in which the granulation tissue matures into scar, and tissue tensile strength is increased. The maturation of granulation tissue also involves a reduction in the number of capillaries via aggregation into larger vessels and a decrease in the amount of glycosaminoglycans and the water associated with the GAGs and proteoglycans. Cell density and metabolic activity in the granulation tissue decrease during maturation. Changes also occur in the type, amount, and organization of collagen, which enhance tensile strength. Initially, Type III collagen was synthesized at high levels, but it becomes replaced by Type I collagen, the dominant fibrillar collagen in skin. The tensile strength of a newly epithelialized wound is only about 25% of normal tissue. Healed or repaired tissue is never as strong as normal tissues that have never been wounded. Primarily the reorganization of collagen fibers that were deposited randomly during granulation and increased covalent cross-linking of collagen molecules by the enzyme, lysyl oxidase, which is secreted into the ECM by fibroblasts, enhances tissue tensile strength. Over several months or more, changes in collagen organization in the repaired tissue will slowly increase the tensile strength to a maximum of about 80% of normal tissue.

Remodeling of the extracellular matrix proteins occurs through the actions of several different classes of proteolytic enzymes produced by cells in the wound bed at different times during the healing process. Two of the most important families are the matrix metalloproteinases (MMPs) (Table 4) and serine proteases. Specific MMP proteases that are necessary for wound healing are the collagenases (which degrade

TABLE 4. Matrix metalloproteinases and tissue inhibitors of metalloproteinases

PROTEIN	PSEUDONYM	SUBSTRATES
MMP-1	INTERSTITIAL COLLAGENASEFIBRO-BLAST COLLAGENASE	TYPE I, II, III, VII, AND X COLLAGENS
MMP-2	72 kDa GELATINASEGELATINASE ATYPE IV COLLAGENASE	TYPE IV, V, VII, AND X COLLAGENS
MMP-3	STROMELYSIN-1	TYPE III, IV, IX, AND X COLLA-GENSTYPE I, III, IV, AND V GELA-TINSFIBRONECTIN, LAMININ AND PRO-COLLAGENASE
MMP-7	MATRILYSINUTERINE METALLOPROTEINASE	TYPE I, III, IV AND V GELATIN-SCASEIN, FIBRONECTIN AND PRO-COLLAGENASE
MMP-8	NEUTROPHIL COLLAGENASE	TYPE I, II, AND III COLLAGENS
MMP-9	92 kDa GELATINASEGELATINASE BTYPE IV COLLAGENASE	TYPE IV AND V COLLAGENSTYPE I AND V GELATINS
MMP-10	STROMELYSIN-2	TYPE III, IV, V, IX, AND X COL-LAGENSTYPE I, III, AND IV GELA-TINSFIBRONECTIN, LAMININ AND PRO-COLLAGENASE
MMP-11	STROMELYSIN -3	NOT DETERMINED
MMP-12	MACROPHAGE METALLOELASTASE	SOLUBLE AND INSOLUBLE ELASTIN
MT-MMP-1	MEMBRANE TYPE MMP-1	PRO-MMP-2
MT-MMP-2	MEMBRANE TYPE MMP-2	NOT DETERMINED
TIMP-1	TISSUE INHIBITOR OF METALLOPROTEINASES-1	COLLAGENASES
TIMP-2	TISSUE INHIBITOR OF METALLOPROTEINASES-2	COLLAGENASES
TIMP-3	TISSUE INHIBITOR OF METALLOPROTEINASES-3	COLLAGENASES

intact fibrillar collagen molecules), the gelatinases (which degrade damaged fibrillar collagen molecules), and the stromelysins (which very effectively degrade proteoglycans). An important serine protease is neutrophil elastase, which can degrade almost all types of protein molecules. Under normal conditions, the destructive actions of the proteolytic enzymes are tightly regulated by specific enzyme inhibitors, which are also produced by cells in the wound bed. The specific inhibitors of the MMPs are the tissue inhibitors of metalloproteinases (TIMPs), and specific inhibitors of serine protease are α1-protease inhibitor (α1-PI) and α2 macroglobulin.

E. Summary of acute wound healing

Four phases of wound healing:

1. **Hemostasis** – This phase establishes the fibrin provisional wound matrix, and platelets provide initial release of cytokines and growth factors in the wound.

2. **Inflammation** – This phase is mediated by neutrophils, and macrophages remove bacteria and denatured matrix components that retard healing and are the second source of growth factors and cytokines. Prolonged, elevated inflammation retards healing due to excessive levels of proteases and reactive oxygen that destroy essential factors.

3. **Repair** – Fibroblasts, supported by new capillaries, proliferate and synthesize disorganized ECM. Basal epithelial cells proliferate and migrate over the granulation tissue to close the wound surface.

4. **Remodeling** – Fibroblast and capillary density decreases, and initial scar tissue is removed and replaced by ECM that is more similar to normal skin. ECM remodeling is the result of the balanced, regulated activity of proteases.

Cellular functions during the different phases of wound healing are regulated by key cytokines, chemokines, and growth factors. Cell actions are also influenced by interaction with components of the ECM through their integrin receptors and adhesion molecules. MMPs produced by epidermal cells, fibroblasts, and vascular endothelial cells assist in migration of the cells, while proteolytic enzymes produced by neutrophils and macrophages remove denatured ECM components and assist in remodeling.

II. Overview of molecular and cellular abnormalities in chronic wounds

All chronic wounds begin as acute wounds, but an acute wound becomes a chronic wound when it fails to progress through the sequential phases of healing as expected.[4,21] A key question to ask is, are there common molecular and cellular patterns in chronic wounds that indicate the stage of the wound healing sequence where most chronic wounds get stalled? The simple answer is yes. As shown in Figure 2, cellular and molecular data from numerous clinical studies suggest that most chronic wounds get "stuck" in a prolonged inflammatory phase that is due to the presence of both planktonic and biofilm bacteria in the wound[22] (Figure 4). The bacteria stimulate production of pro-inflammatory cytokines like tumor necrosis factor alpha (TNFa) and interleukin 1 (IL-1) that act as chemotactic factors (chemical messengers) to recruit neutrophils, macrophages, and mast cells into the wound. The inflammatory cells, which are drawn into the wound, secrete proteases (matrix metalloproteinases MMPs, neutrophil elastase, plasmin) and reactive oxygen species (ROS) in an attempt to kill bacteria and detach biofilm colonies that are tightly attached to the wound bed. However, because biofilm bacteria colonies are very tolerant to ROS, as well as antibodies, antibiotics, and even antiseptics, the biofilm colonies persist and continue to stimulate inflammation. This results in chronically elevated levels of proteases and ROS that eventually begin to destroy essential proteins that are necessary for healing, including growth factors, their receptors, and extracellular matrix proteins (ECM). These "off-target" effects of proteases and ROS combine to reduce cell proliferation, migration, and generation of functional scar matrix.[23-25] The "biological sum" of this prolonged inflammatory state is a very distorted molecular and cellular wound environment that prevents wound healing. In the simplest terms, the molecular and cellular environment between acute healing wounds and chronic wounds is totally different. As shown in Figure 3, these "imbalances" must be corrected by clinical therapies or the wound will not progress to healing. Strategies designed to reverse these imbalances would be expected to promote healing, and indeed, innovative new treatments are being developed and tested, and some have already been shown to clinically improve healing of chronic wounds. Of utmost importance is attention to evidence-based wound care, adequate wound bed preparation, appropriate management of underlying disease, and correction of other contributing factors (such as inadequate nutrition) which may impair wound healing. [21]

A. Repeated tissue injury

Clinical observations indicate that acute wounds which develop into chronic wounds are frequently subjected to repeated episodes of tissue injury that leads to ischemia such as prolonged pressure in spinal cord injury patients (pressure ulcers) or vasculopathies (venous leg ulcer) or

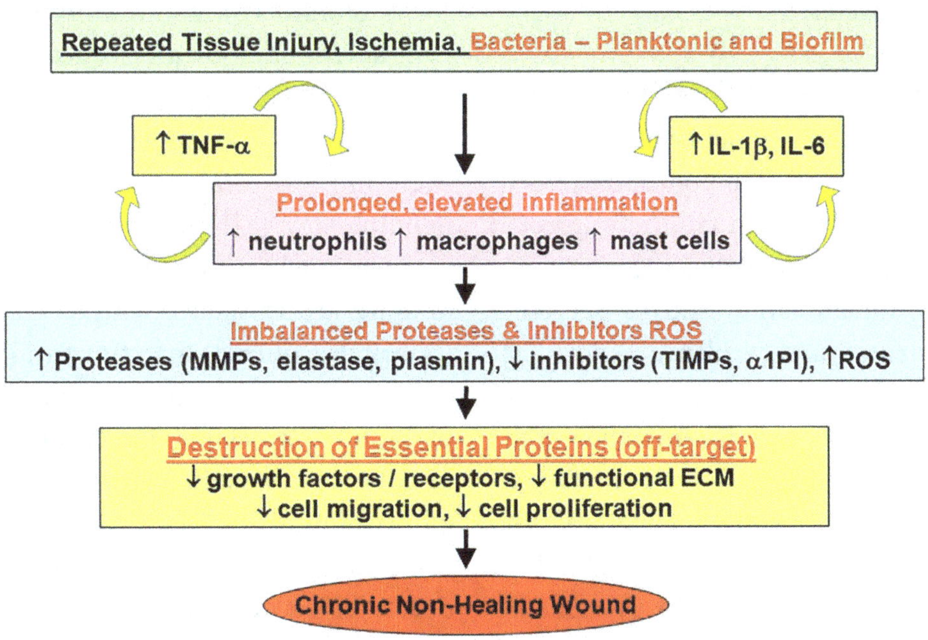

FIGURE 2. Molecular and cellular pathology of chronic wounds. Acute wounds that become critically colonized by planktonic and biofilm bacteria develop chronic inflammation that is characterized by high levels of proteases and ROS that destroy "off-target" proteins that are essential for healing, resulting in a chronic wound.

Courtesy of Gregory Schultz, MD

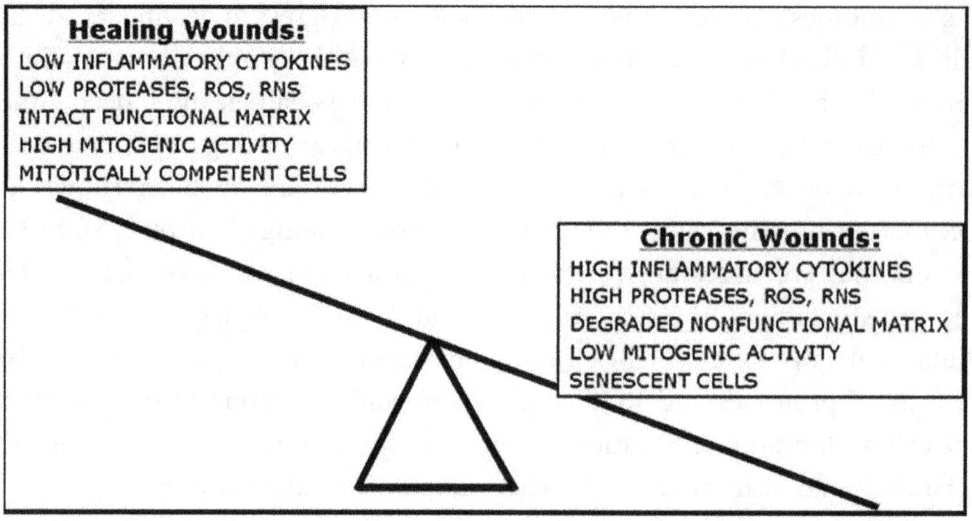

FIGURE 3. Imbalanced molecular and cellular environments of healing and chronic wounds. The molecular and cellular environment of acute healing wounds is dramatically different than that of chronic wounds and must be "rebalanced" to approximate the environment of healing wounds before healing can progress.
Courtesy of Mast and Schultz, Wound Repair Regen. 1996;4(4):411.

blunt trauma that occurs on plantar foot surfaces of neuropathic diabetic patients.[26, 22] This causes the epidermis to break down, generating an open wound that quickly becomes colonized with planktonic bacteria.

B. Bacterial bioburden and biofilms

Decades of clinical and laboratory research have conclusively shown that high concentrations of planktonic bacteria found in clinically infected wounds can impair wound healing, primarily by stimulating inflammation and by secreting exotoxins, proteases, and virulence factors that impair inflammatory cell functions and break down host tissue to promote dissemination of the bacteria and provide nutrients for the rapidly proliferating bacteria. Historically, many nonhealing wounds were not reported to have high levels of planktonic bacteria when assessed by standard clinical microbiology assays. However, aggressive debridement and systemic and topical treatments designed to reduce bacterial bioburden were frequently found to improve healing. This led to the concept of "critical colonization," which was an attempt to recognize that something about the bioburden was impairing healing (Figure 5). New data suggests the critical factor determining wound bioburden is usually the presence of bacteria in polymicrobial biofilm communities.[27]

A biofilm is a community of microorganisms surrounded by an extracellular polymeric matrix (EPM), which attaches to a surface.[28-30] Recent studies demonstrate that biofilms are becoming a significant component of infections in humans.[31-33] The Centers for Disease Control and National Institutes of Health project that biofilms are associated with 65% of nosocomial (hospital-acquired) infections and up to 80% of all US human infections. In addition, treatment of biofilm-associated infections costs billions of dollars and results in hundreds of thousands of deaths annually in the United States.[31] Both acute and chronic wounds are susceptible to the development of biofilms within the wound bed.

Open wounds provide a perfect environment for opportunistic organisms such as bacteria to reside and reproduce. Analyses of the microflora of chronic wounds (such as pressure and diabetic foot ulcers) demonstrate a phenomenon known as "chronic wound pathogenic

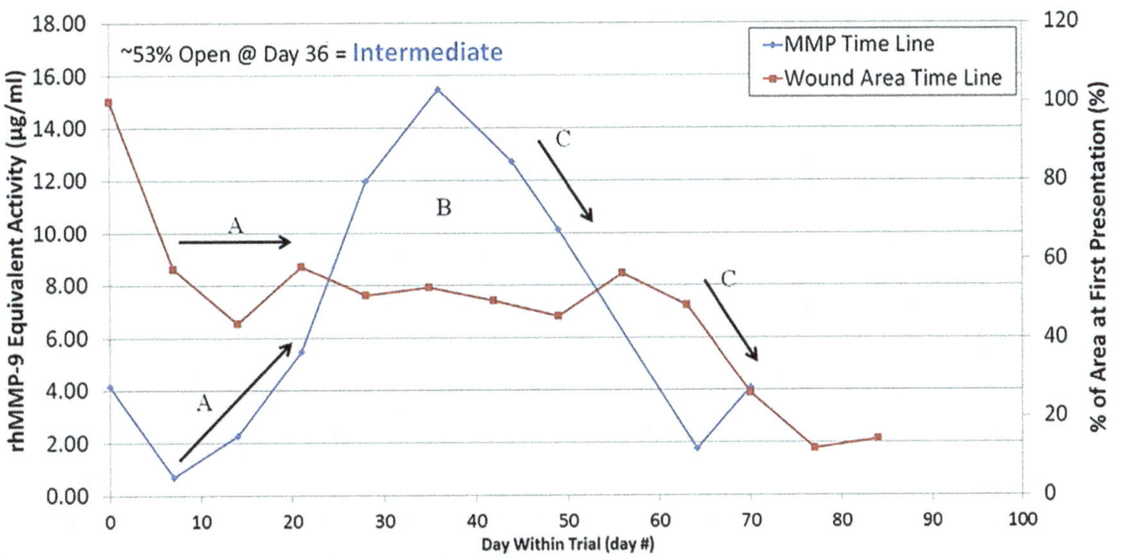

FIGURE 4. Changes in MMPs predict wound closure changes. A co-plotted time course of MMP activity versus wound area. A) A rise in MMPs anticipates wound stalling. B) Elevated MMPs coincident with wound closure stalling. C) A reduction of MMP activities precedes continuance of wound closure.
Adapted with permission from G.Bohn, B.Liden, G. Schultz, Q. Yang, D.J. Gibson. *Advances In Wound Care, Vol 5* (1) 1-10, 2016.

biofilms" (CWPB).[31-33] Typical mechanisms by which biofilms impede wound healing progress involve heightening the level of inflammation (increasing the amount of ROS and proteases in the wound bed), stimulating overly aggressive immune responses, producing detrimental exogenous toxins within the wound environment, and impairing normal chemokine signalling pathways.[34] Aerobic organisms within biofilms use oxygen and help to create anaerobic niches within the biofilm matrix that support the development of anaerobes within the biofilm.[31] Importantly, the presence of biofilm in a wound may affect the wound healing process without visible clinical signs of infection. However, there may be indications of bacterial imbalance (e.g., change in wound color or odor together with the presence of devitalized tissue and ischemia).[34]

Studies suggest certain bacterial groups, which by themselves are considered essentially harmless (such as Corynebacterium spp.), tend to form symbiotic communities with other bacteria and fungi in chronic wounds. These polymicrobial groups in biofilm are termed "functional equivalent pathogroups" (FEPs) because they have been shown to have functionally detrimental effects on wound healing similar to other well-known pathogens, such as Staphylococcus aureus.[31] In addition, biofilm colonies may extend 2mm beneath the wound bed and into surrounding healthy tissue, making them difficult to eradicate by many traditional bedside debridement methods.[32] Treatment options to consider include debridement and the use of a broad-spectrum topical antimicrobial agent directly after debridement to control the planktonic bacterial load and reduce the progression into biofilms. Importantly, recent data indicate that mature biofilm communities can re-establish in wounds within three days following debridement.[27] If control of microbial progression from planktonic to mature biofilms is not achieved, a change from an early stage biofilm to a polymicrobial "complex" mature wound biofilm may develop and ultimately lead to a compromised state.[34]

Biofilm experts suggest traditional culturing methods as a diagnostic tool (which involve inoculating a culture medium with a swab sample obtained from the patient) are insufficient to identify true components of the polymicrobial mature biofilm colonies.[31] The exact microbial composition of biofilm is largely undetectable by traditional cotton swab culture techniques due to the protective polymeric coating that biofilms produce. This self-protective coating encapsulates the colony and is also impervious to most systemic and topical antimicrobials/antibiotics. Other limitations of the traditional clinical swab sampling approach include the facts that cotton swab cultures typically query only the most common aerobic organisms, culture results are often unavailable for two to three days, and the culture is naturally biased toward identifying only those hardy bacterial species which are easily cultured under standard laboratory conditions.[31] Recent literature suggests the PCR assay is a cost-effective and more sensitive and rapid method to detect microbial pathogens (particularly biofilm microbes) in clinical specimens.[35]

C. Elevated pro-inflammatory cytokines

Closely linked to the bacterial bioburden in a wound is the profile of pro-inflammatory cytokines. In general, fluids from acute healing wounds tend to have an early peak of major pro-inflammatory cytokines, TNF-α and IL-1β, and their natural inhibitors, P55 and IL-1 receptor antagonist, within the first few days after injury, which corresponds to the rapid increase in inflammatory cells in the acute wound.[36] However, the levels of pro-inflammatory cytokines begin to decrease after six to seven days as the inflammatory stimuli in acute wounds decrease. However, in chronic leg ulcers, levels of inflammatory cytokines, IL-1β, IL-6, and TNF-α were significantly higher than acute healing wounds, and as the chronic ulcers began to heal, the levels decreased.[22] These findings indicate that chronic wounds have persistently elevated levels of pro-inflammatory cytokines, but as chronic wounds heal, the molecular environment changes to a less pro-inflammatory wound environment.

D. Elevated proteases

Another major concept to emerge from wound fluid analyses is that levels of proteases, especially MMPs and neutrophil elastase, are much higher in chronic wounds than in acute wound fluids.[4, 36-37] During the early phase of acute wound healing, the average level of protease activity in mastectomy fluids was found to be low, suggesting that protease activity is tightly controlled during the early phase of wound healing.[38] However, in chronic wounds the average level of protease activity was found to be approximately 116-fold higher than in acute mastectomy wound fluids. Furthermore, as chronic venous ulcers begin to heal, the levels of protease activity decreased. Similar results were reported for fluids or biopsies of chronic pressure ulcers, where levels of MMP-2, MMP-9, and MMP-1 were 10 to 25 times higher than levels in acute, surgical wound fluids.[39-40] Levels of the tissue inhibitors of metalloproteinases (TIMPs), which are the natural inhibitors of MMPs, were found to be decreased in wound fluids from chronic venous ulcers compared to acute mastectomy wound fluids.[41]

In nonhealing chronic pressure ulcers, MMP-8, the neutrophil-derived collagenase, was elevated indicating there may be a persistent influx of neutrophils releasing MMP-8 and elastase, which could contribute to destruction of ECM proteins and growth factors that are essential for healing.[42] Chronic venous ulcers were found to have 10-fold to 40-fold higher levels of neutrophil elastase activity and to have degraded a1-antitrypsin. Elevated MMP-2 and MMP-9 levels in chronic venous ulcers were also observed to coincide with degradation of fibronectin in the wound bed.[43-44] Fibronectin is an important multidomain adhesion protein that is present in the ECM and granulation tissue and is very important in promoting epithelial cell migration. Proteases in chronic wound fluids were shown to rapidly degrade exogenously added growth factors such as TGF-a, EGF, or PDGF using *in vitro* laboratory tests. In contrast, exogenously added growth factors were stable when added to acute surgical wound fluids.[23, 45-46]

Recent clinical data further supports the important correlation between wound healing and the levels of proteases in wound fluid.[47] Levels of MMP activities were measured in samples of wound fluid that were collected weekly for up to 12 weeks of treatment in a series of 11 patients with chronic wounds. Levels of MMP activities correlated closely with the healing status of the wound bed. When MMP activites were high or were increasing, wounds did not heal, but when MMP activities were low or decreasing, the wound beds showed healing (decrease in wound area). More importantly, as shown in Figure 4, when a chronic wound that had decreasing levels of MMPs and was healing began to "stall" and did not progress in healing, the levels of MMP activities in the wound fluid samples began rapidly increasing the week before the wound stalled. Only when the levels of MMP activites began to drop to levels that were more compatible with healing did the stalled wound begin to heal again with decreased wound area.

E. Reduced mitogenic activity of chronic wound fluids

Another key concept that emerged from laboratory analysis of acute and chronic wound fluids demonstrates that the mitogenic activity of chronic wound fluids is dramatically less than levels in acute wound fluids. For example, fluids from chronic leg ulcers did not stimulate DNA synthesis of cells in culture, while acute wound fluids strongly stimulate proliferation of cells in culture. Furthermore, when acute and chronic wound fluids were combined, the mitotic activity of acute wound fluids were inhibited.[48] These results show that the proteases in chronic wound fluid degrade growth factors normally present in acute wound fluids, and without the essential actions of these growth factors, wound healing will not progress.

F. Factors affecting cell senescence

In chronic wounds, the capacity of the wound cells to respond to cytokines and growth factors is altered. Research suggests fibroblasts (white cells which manufacture collagen and perform other essential functions in wound healing) in chronic wounds have a diminished response to growth factors. For example, fibroblast cultures established from chronic venous leg ulcers proliferated very slowly and formed less dense confluent cultures when compared to normal fibroblast cultures established from uninjured dermis[46]. In another study of chronic venous leg ulcers that were present for more than three years' duration, fibroblasts proliferated poorly in response to platelet-derived growth factors (PDGF) added to the culture medium and rapidly approached senescence compared to fibroblasts cultured from venous ulcers that had been present for less than three years.[48]

In summary, the molecular environments of acute and chronic wounds are dramatically different (Figure 3). Healing wounds have low bacterial bioburden and no biofilms, low levels of inflammatory cytokines, low levels of proteases, high levels of growth factors, and cells that divide rapidly in response to growth factors. The molecular and cellular environment of chronic wounds is exactly the opposite. Chronic wounds have high levels of bacterial biofilm, elevated levels of inflammatory cytokines, high levels of proteases, low levels of growth factors, and cells that are approaching senescence.

III. Wound bed preparation: removing the barriers to healing

The concept of wound bed preparation and the TIME acronym (tissue, infection/inflammation, moisture imbalance, and edge of wound) was first developed and published in 2003 by an international group of experts in wound healing. It provided a framework for a structured approach to identifying and removing the barriers to wound healing[49] (Figure 5). Since then, the TIME acronym has been widely used as a practical guide for the assessment and management of chronic wounds. The clinical observations and interventions relating to wound bed preparation are grouped into the four areas, all of which need to be addressed at each wound assessment:

Tissue - assessment and debridement of nonviable or foreign material (including host necrotic tissue, adherent dressing material, multiple organism-related biofilm or slough, exudate, and debris) on the surface of the wound

Infection/Inflammation - assessment of the etiology of each wound, need for topical antiseptic and/or systemic antibiotic use to control infection, and management of inappropriate inflammation unrelated to infection

Moisture imbalance – assessment of the etiology and management of wound exudate

Edge of wound - assessment of nonadvancing or undermined wound edges (and state of the surrounding skin)

Since the initial publication on wound bed preparation, substantial additional laboratory and clinical research has helped to expand the

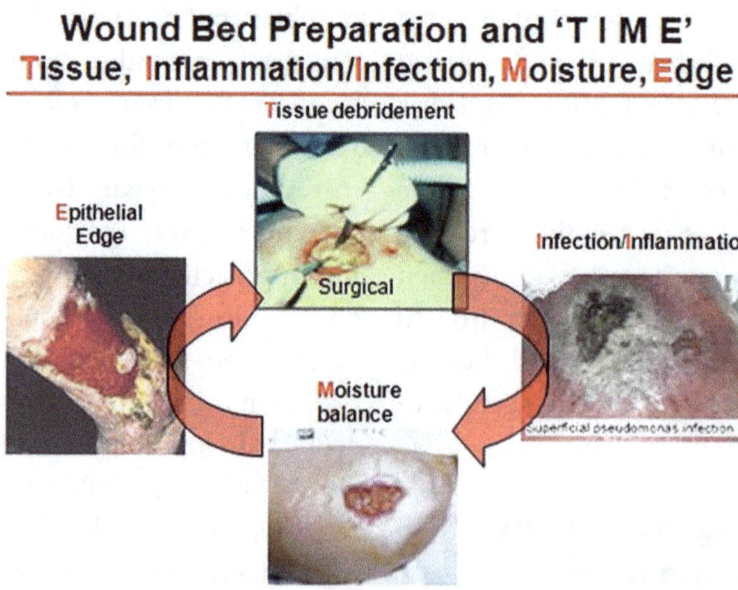

FIGURE 5. Imbalanced molecular and cellular environments of healing and chronic wounds. The molecular and cellular environment of acute healing wounds is dramatically different than that of chronic wounds and must be "rebalanced" to approximate the environment of healing wounds before healing can progress.

Modified with permission from Mast and Schultz, Wound Repair Regen. 1996;4(4):411.

concepts of TIME and how it is translated into current best practice.[50] Four developments stand out: recognition of the importance of biofilms (and the need for a simple diagnostic), use of negative pressure wound therapy (NPWT), evolution of topical antiseptic therapy as dressings and for wound lavage (notably, silver and polyhexamethylene biguanide), and expanded insight of the role of molecular biological processes in chronic wounds (with emerging diagnostics and theranostics).

A. Tissue

A major advance has been the recognition of the value of repetitive and maintenance debridement and wound cleansing, both in time-honored and novel methods (notably using NPWT and hydrosurgery). This was demonstrated in a clinical study performed by Steed et al.[51] That showed healing of chronic diabetic foot ulcers (treated at 10 different centers) was closely correlated with the frequency of debridement. The benefit of wound debridement was seen both in patients that received standard care and in patients who were treated with topical platelet derived growth factor (PDGF). It is possible that frequent sharp debridement of diabetic ulcers may reduce the level of inflammation in the wound by mechanically removing biofilm as well as converting the chronic wound into a pseudo-acute wound molecular environment. Therefore, appropriate wound debridement should be considered a vital component in the care of patients with chronic diabetic foot ulcers.

B. Infection/inflammation

Clinical recognition of infection (and noninfective causes of persisting inflammation) is critical. The concept of a bacterial continuum though contamination, colonization, and infection is now widely accepted, together with the understanding of biofilm presence. There has been a return to topical antiseptics to control bioburden in wounds, emphasized by the awareness of increasing antibiotic resistance.

C. Moisture

The relevance of excessive or insufficient wound exudate and its molecular components has led to the development and use of a wide range of dressings to regulate moisture balance and to protect periwound skin and optimize healing.

D. Edge of wound

Several treatment modalities are being investigated and introduced to improve epithelial advancement, which can be regarded as the clearest sign of wound healing.

The TIME principles remain highly relevant with continuing important developments, which incorporate new evidence for wound care, which is discussed at length in Chapter 6: Wound Bed Preparation.

Summary

Wound healing occurs through four phases. These phases are sequentially regulated by the actions of cytokines, growth factors, ECM proteins, and proteases. If an acute wound fails to move through a phase of healing, molecular imbalances will occur, leading to a chronic wound. Bacterial biofilms, elevated inflammatory cytokines and proteases, low levels of mitogenic activity, and senescent cells that are unable to respond to growth factors characterize chronic wounds. Healing of chronic wounds occurs as the molecular environment of the wound shifts to the environment of an acute wound. New therapies are designed to correct the molecular abnormalities of chronic wounds and correspond to the principles of wound bed preparation.

Review questions

1. **What are the four sequential phases of normal wound healing in skin wounds?**

    a. repair, inflammation, hemostasis, remodeling

    b. hemostasis, repair, inflammation, remodeling

    c. remodeling, hemostasis, repair, inflammation

    d. hemostasis, inflammation, repair, remodeling

    e. inflammation, hemostasis, repair, remodeling

2. ***True/False.*** Acute wounds that fail to progress through normal healing typically get stuck in the inflammatory phase of healing.

3. ***True/False.*** Bacteria in biofilm structures are highly tolerant to the patient's immune system and to antibiotics and most antiseptics.

4. **The molecular environment of healing wounds typically have:**

    a. low levels of pro-inflammatory cytokines

    b. low levels of proteases

    c. high levels of active growth factors

    d. mitotically competent wound cells

    e. all the above

5. **Wound bed preparation of chronic wounds is based on the principle(s) of:**

    a. debridement to remove necrotic tissue and biofilm

    b. reducing chronic inflammation/infection which reduces high levels of protease and ROS

    c. maintaining proper moisture balance in the wound

    d. enhancing epithelial cell migration at the edge of the chronic wound bed

    e. all the above

ANSWERS: 1) d
2) True
3) True
4) e
5) e

References

1. Bennett NT, Schultz GS. Growth factors and wound healing: biochemical properties of growth factors and their receptors. Am J Surg. 1993;165(6):728-37.
2. Bennett NT, Schultz GS. Growth factors and wound healing: part II. Role in normal and chronic wound healing. Am J Surg. 1993;166(1):74-81.
3. Lawrence WT. Physiology of the acute wound. Clin Plast Surg. 1998;25(3):321-40.
4. Mast BA, Schultz GS. Interactions of cytokines, growth factors, and proteases in acute and chronic wounds. Wound Repair Regen. 1996;4(4):411-20.
5. Schultz G, Chin GA, Moldawer LL, Diegelmann RF. Principles of wound healing. In: Fitridge R, Thompson A, editors. Mechanisms of vascular disease. Adelaide, Australia: University of Adelaide Press; 2011. p. 423-49.
6. Cowan L, Stechmiller J, Phillips P, Schultz G. Science of wound healing: translation of bench science into advances for chronic wound care. In: Krasner DL, Rodeheaver GT, Sibbald RG, Woo KY, editors. Chronic wound care. Malvern, PA: HMP Communications; 2012. p. 25-35.
7. Schultz GS. Molecular regulation of wound healing. In: Bryant, RA, editor. Acute and chronic wounds: nursing management. Philadelphia: Mosby; 2000. p. 413-29.
8. Gailit J, Clark RAF. Wound repair in context of extracellular matrix. Curr Opin Cell Biol. 1994;6(5):717-25.
9. Rumalla VK, Borah GL. Cytokines, growth factors, and plastic surgery. Plast Reconstr Surg. 2001;108(3):719-33.
10. Luster AD. Chemokines--chemotactic cytokines that mediate inflammation. N Engl J Med. 1998;338(7):436-45.
11. Gillitzer R, Goebeler M. Chemokines in cutaneous wound healing. J Leukoc Biol. 2001;69(4):513-21.
12. Dinarello CA, Moldawer LL. Proinflammatory and anti-inflammatory cytokines in rheumatoid arthritis. Thousand Oaks, CA: Amgen Inc.; 2000. Cytokines and the Inflammatory Response; p. 3-22.
13. Frenette PS, Wagner DD. Adhesion molecules—part 1. N Engl J Med. 1996;334(23):1526-9.
14. Diegelmann RF, Cohen IK, Kaplan AM. The role of macrophages in wound repair: a review. Plast Reconstr Surg. 1981;68(1):107-13.
15. Duncan MR, Frazier KS, Abramson S, Williams S, Klapper H, Huang X, Grotendorst GR. Connective tissue growth factor mediates transforming growth factor beta-induced collagen synthesis: down-regulation by cAMP. FASEB J. 1999;13(13):1774-86.
16. Bhushan M, Young HS, Brenchley PE, Griffiths CE. Recent advances in cutaneous angiogenesis. Br J Dermatol. 2002;147(3):418-25.
17. Semenza GL. HIF-1 and tumor progression: pathophysiology and therapeutics. Trends Mol Med. 2002;8(4 Suppl):S62-S67.
18. O'Toole EA. Extracellular matrix and keratinocyte migration. Clin Exp Dermatol. 2001;26(6):525-30.
19. Sen CK. MicroRNAs as new maestro conducting the expanding symphony orchestra of regenerative and reparative medicine. Physiol Genomics. 2011;43(10):517-20.
20. Sen CK, Gordillo GM, Khanna S, Roy S. Micromanaging vascular biology: tiny microRNAs play big band. J Vasc Res. 2009;46(6):527-40.
21. Doughty DB, Sparkes-DeFriese B. Wound healing physiology. In: Bryant RA, Nix DP, editors. Acute & chronic wounds. St. Louis, Missouri: Elsevier Mosby, 2009:63-82.
22. Trengove NJ, Bielefeldt-Ohmann H, Stacey MC. Mitogenic activity and cytokine levels in nonhealing and healing chronic leg ulcers. Wound Repair Regen. 2000;8(1):13-25.

23. Trengove NJ, Stacey MC, Macauley S, Bennett N, Gibson J, Burslem F, Murphy G, Schultz G. Analysis of the acute and chronic wound environments: the role of proteases and their inhibitors. Wound Repair Regen. 1999;7(6):442-52.

24. Tarnuzzer RW, Schultz GS. Biochemical analysis of acute and chronic wound environments. Wound Repair Regen. 1996;4(3):321-5.

25. Yager DR, Chen SM, Ward SI, Olutoye OO, Diegelmann RF, Cohen IK. Ability of chronic wound fluids to degrade peptide growth factors is associated with increased levels of elastase activity and diminished levels of proteinase inhibitors. Wound Repair Regen. 1997;5(1):23-32.

26. Harris IR, Yee KC, Walters CE, Cunliffe WJ, Kearney JN, Wood EJ, Ingham E. Cytokine and protease levels in healing and nonhealing chronic venous leg ulcers. Exp Dermatol. 1995;4(6):342-9.

27. Wolcott RD, Rumbaugh KP, James G, Schultz G, Phillips P, Yang Q, Watters C, Stewart PS, Dowd SE. Biofilm maturity studies indicate sharp debridement opens a time-dependent therapeutic window. J Wound Care. 2010;19(8):320-8.

28. Costerton JW. Introduction to biofilm. Int J Antimicrob Agents. 1999;11(3-4):217-21.

29. Costerton JW, Lewandowski Z, Caldwell DE, Korber DR, Lappin-Scott HM. Microbial biofilms. Annu Rev Microbiol. 1995;49:711-45.

30. Costerton JW, Stewart PS, Greenberg EP. Bacterial biofilms: a common cause of persistent infections. Science. 1999;284(5418):1318-22.

31. Dowd SE, Wolcott RD, Sun Y, McKeehan T, Smith E, Rhoads D. Polymicrobial nature of chronic diabetic foot ulcer biofilm infections determined using bacterial tag encoded FLX amplicon pyrosequencing (bTEFAP). PLoS ONE. 2008;3(10):e3326.

32. James GA, Swogger E, Wolcott R, Pulcini ED, Secor P, Sestrich J, Costerton JW, Stewart PS. Biofilms in chronic wounds. Wound Repair Regen. 2008;16(1):37-44.

33. Smith DM, Snow DE, Rees E, Zischkau AM, Hanson JD, Wolcott RD, Sun Y, White J, Kumar S, Dowd SE. Evaluation of the bacterial diversity of pressure ulcers using bTEFAP pyrosequencing. BMC Med Genomics. 2010;3(1):41.

34. Phillips P, Sampson E, Yang Q, Antonelli A, Progulske-Fox A, Schultz G. Bacterial biofilms in wounds. Wound Healing Southern Africa. 2008;1(2):10-2.

35. Wolcott RD, Hanson JD, Rees EJ, Koenig LD, Phillips CD, Wolcott RA, Cox SB, White JS. Analysis of the chronic wound microbiota of 2,963 patients by 16S rDNA pyrosequencing. Wound Repair Regen. 2016;24(1):163-74.

36. Schreml S, Szeimies RM, Prantl L, Landthaler M, Babilas P. Wound healing in the 21st century. J Am Acad Dermatol. 2010;63(5):866-81.

37. Yager DR, Nwomeh BC. The proteolytic environment of chronic wounds. Wound Repair Regen. 1999;7(6):433-41.

38. Yager DR, Zhang LY, Liang HX, Diegelmann RF, Cohen IK. Wound fluids from human pressure ulcers contain elevated matrix metalloproteinase levels and activity compared to surgical wound fluids. J Invest Dermatol. 1996;107(5):743-8.

39. Rogers AA, Burnett S, Moore JC, Shakespeare PG, Chen WY. Involvement of proteolytic enzymes—plasminogen activators and matrix metalloproteinases—in the pathophysiology of pressure ulcers. Wound Repair Regen. 1995;3(3):273-83.

40. Bullen, E. C., Longaker, M. T., Updike, D. L., Benton, R., Ladin, D., and Hou, Z. Tissue inhibitor of metalloproteinases-1 is decreased and activated gelatinases are increased in chronic wounds. J Invest Dermatol. 1995;104(2):236-240.

41. Ladwig GP, Robson MC, Liu R, Kuhn MA, Muir DF, Schultz GS. Ratios of activated matrix metalloproteinase-9 to tissue inhibitor of matrix metalloproteinase-1 in wound fluids are inversely correlated with healing of pressure ulcers. Wound Repair Regen. 2002;10(1):26-37.

42. Wysocki AB, Staiano-Coico L, Grinnell F. Wound fluid from chronic leg ulcers contains elevated levels of metalloproteinases MMP-2 and MMP-9. J Invest Dermatol. 1993;101(1):64-8.

43. Grinnell F, Zhu M. Fibronectin degradation in chronic wounds depends on the relative levels of elastase, alpha1-proteinase inhibitor, and alpha2-macroglobulin. J Invest Dermatol. 1996;106(2):335-41.

44. Bucalo B, Eaglstein WH, Falanga V. Inhibition of cell proliferation by chronic wound fluid. Wound Repair Regen. 1993;1:181-6.

45. Katz MH, Alvarez AF, Kirsner RS, Eaglstein WH, Falanga V. Human wound fluid from acute wounds stimulates fibroblast and endothelial cell growth. J Am Acad Dermatol. 1991;25(6 Pt 1):1054-8.

46. Agren MS, Eaglstein WH, Ferguson MW, Harding KG, Moore K, Saarialho-Kere UK, Schultz GS. Causes and effects of the chronic inflammation in venous leg ulcers. Acta Derm Venereol Suppl (Stockh). 2000;210:3-17.

47. Bohn G, Liden B, Schultz G, Yang Q, Gibson DJ. Ovine-based collagen matrix dressing: next-generation collagen dressing for wound care. Adv Wound Care (New Rochelle). 2016;5(1):1-10.

48. Trengove NJ, Langton SR, Stacey MC. Biochemical analysis of wound fluid from non-healing and healing chronic leg ulcers. Wound Repair Regen. 1996;4(2):234-9.

49. Schultz GS, Sibbald RG, Falanga V, Ayello EA, Dowsett C, Harding K, Romanelli M, Stacey MC, Teot L, Vanscheidt W. Wound bed preparation: a systematic approach to wound management. Wound Repair Regen. 2003;11(Suppl s1):S1-S28.

50. Leaper DJ, Schultz G, Carville K, Fletcher J, Swanson T, Drake R. Extending the TIME concept: what have we learned in the past 10 years?. Int Wound J. 2012;9(Suppl 2):1-19.

51. Steed DL, Donohoe D, Webster MW, Lindsley L. Effect of extensive debridement and treatment on the healing of diabetic foot ulcers. Diabetic Ulcer Study Group. J Am Coll Surg. 1996;183(1):61-4.

Section 2

ESSENTIALS OF WOUND HEALING

Editor - Robert J. Snyder, DPM, MSc, CWS

Chapter 3

ETIOLOGY OF WOUNDS

Robert J. Snyder, DPM, MSc, CWS
Timothy M. Graham, DPM

KEY CONCEPTS

1. Identifying the underlying cause(s) of wound development should be the foundation for treatment planning.
2. All wound care patients should receive a customized treatment plan based on wound etiology.
3. Obtaining an accurate History and Physical (H&P) plays an integral role within quality patient care.
4. The mnemonic PROBLEM WOUND could be used to determine etiology of the wounds.
5. Different case scenarios are incorporated as part of this chapter for further understanding on different etiology of wounds.

CONTENTS

Introduction

Chronic, nonhealing wounds have a prevalence of 2% among the U.S. population. Spending on chronic wound care for this patient subset costs an estimated $50 billion annually.[1] Chronic wounds of the lower extremity currently affect 6 million persons in the United States. Approximately 15% of the elderly community suffer from lower-extremity ulcerations and are predicted to rise to 25% by the year 2050.[2]

Cost to care for patients is at an all-time high. This trend continues to grow with morbidity rates on the rise, such as diabetes. From 1980–2014, the number of Americans diagnosed with diabetes increased from 5.5 million to 22.0 million.[3] During 2000–2002, an estimated 11.8% of the diabetic population had a history of foot ulceration. In the United States, roughly 60% of all lower-extremity amputations are among the diabetic population; of these amputations, approximately 85% are preceded by foot ulcerations.[4]

Excellent patient care with a multispecialty approach is paramount to the success of medicine's future. Lowering the cost of health care is on the shoulders of all practitioners. Proper screening and examinations will mitigate the negative effects of disease, by recognizing signs and symptoms before secondary pathology develops. In this chapter, we will discuss strategies of quality patient care, which begins with a good history and physical.

I. History taking

Obtaining an accurate history and physical (H&P) plays an integral role within quality patient care. Oftentimes a patient presents with a primary purpose of seeking medical attention. This is commonly referred to as the patient's chief complaint (CC). After learning the patient's CC, the next logical step is to find out more about this particular ailment's history. Historical inquiries of any particular ailment may include questions such as, "How long have you been dealing with this problem?", "Since this issue began, has it been constant or has it gone through periods of getting better versus worse?", "Does this ailment cause you pain? If so, does anything exacerbate or relieve the pain?", and "How much pain does this ailment cause you, on a scale of 1 to 10?"[5]

One guideline for the questioning of a patient's CC can be summarized with a helpful acronym: NLDOCAT.[6]

<u>N</u>*ature* – In what ways does the CC affect the patient's life?

<u>L</u>*ocation* – Is the patient's CC localized or widespread?

<u>D</u>*uration* – How long has the patient been dealing with this particular CC?

<u>O</u>*nset* – When did the CC begin? Has the CC been constant?

<u>C</u>haracter – How does the patient characterize the CC? (Painful, irritating, burning, etc.)

<u>A</u>lleviate/Aggravate – Does anything make the CC better or worse?

<u>T</u>reatment – Has the patient been doing anything at home to self-treat this CC?

It is important to keep in mind what is already known about the patient's current medical condition, as this may guide the clinician down a path of fruitful historical findings. A standard of broadly approaching patients' past medical history is referred to as the review of systems (ROS).[7] When performing a ROS, it is best to ask opening questions such as, "Have you had any recent changes or significant medical history involving your health?" A thorough ROS should include all, but not limited to the following systems:

Constitutional – fever / chills / sweats / weakness / fatigue / decreased activity

Eyes – recent visual problems / discharge / blurring / double vision

Ears/Nose/Mouth/Throat (ENMT) – ear pain / nasal congestion / sore throat

Respiratory – shortness of breath / cough / hemoptysis / wheezing / apnea / sputum

Cardiovascular – chest pain / palpitations / bradycardia / tachycardia / edema

Gastrointestinal – nausea / vomiting / diarrhea / constipation / heartburn

Genitourinary – dysuria / urethral discharge / hematuria / lesions

Hematologic/Lymphatic – bleeding tendency / bruising tendency / swollen lymph nodes

Endocrine – excessive thirst / cold intolerance / heat intolerance / excessive hunger

Allergic/Immunologic – recurrent fevers / recurrent infections / immunocompromised

Musculoskeletal – back pain / decreased ROM / joint pain / muscle pain / claudication

Integumentary/Breast – rash / pruritus / abrasion / burns / lesions / dryness

Neurological – balance / confusion / numbness / tingling / headache

Psychiatric – anxiety / depression / mania / delusions / hallucinations

ROS is an efficient way of approaching a patient with questions regarding his or her overall health. Subconsciously for the patient, the review of systems also allows our patients to understand that we are concerned with their overall health and not just their CC.[8] A timely ROS can also make for an excellent segue from the original, problem-focused history taking to a broader scope of history taking.

Additional review of a patient's past medical history (PMH) includes personal medical issues that may or may not be linked to the CC in question. It is best to approach this issue broadly by asking if the patient has ever been hospitalized or undergone surgery or if he or she is currently taking medication. If the answer to any of these questions is yes, appropriate follow-up questions would be, "When did that happen?", "Do you remember the name of the doctor who treated you?", "Do you remember your diagnosis?", and "What medications are/were you taking, and for what period of time?"

An accurate family medical history (FMH) is an important part of patient history taking. A relative of the patient who may have suffered from the same or similar ailments can be of great benefit to the clinical investigator. With the luxury of FMH in hand, days and even weeks of valuable time can be spared. Knowledge of a previously diagnosed family member can guide health-care providers down a shortened path of ordering tests, finding a diagnosis, and providing treatments. It is important to remember that this does not pertain only to blood relatives, especially if a condition has arisen due to environmental factors.[9]

Social history taking is a very important and often overlooked portion of the health history taking process. Many social factors in the patient's life will inevitably affect his or her overall health. Having a grasp on our patient's overall socioeconomic status can give health-care providers an understanding about the patient's accessibility to health care and the ability of the patient to effectively use the resources available. As health-care providers, it is necessary to understand the patient's life at work, home, and leisure. Crafting questions to inform oneself without violating the patient's privacy is a desired skill. Regarding work, questions such as, "What do you do for a living?", "How many hours per week do you work?", "Is that a physically demanding line of work?", and "How long have you been retired?" can be very informative. Regarding life at home, questions such as, "Are you married?", "Do you have children?", and "How long have you lived in the area?" can all be of much use when building trust and gaining information which may be helpful in treatment planning. Regarding leisure time, questions such as, "Do you have any hobbies?", or "What do you like to do for fun?" are great icebreakers and allow the patient to understand that he or she is being well cared for. While performing a social history, other topics to ask about are alcohol/tobacco/drug usage, travel, diet, and exercise. Ultimately, it should be every health-care provider's goal to gain perspective about a patient in order to understand how to better treat that individual in the future.[9-10]

A. Problem-focused history taking in a patient with a wound

Consider a patient who presents with a lower-extremity ulceration of unknown etiology. When performing a problem-focused history on a patient with a wound, some key inquiries should be made:

- Has the patient had an arterial/venous workup? Examples include arterial ultrasounds, venous reflux ultrasounds, angiogram, ankle brachial index, or toe brachial index.
- Has the patient had the periwound transcutaneous oxygen pressure measured?
- Has the microbiological burden of the wound been identified or addressed? Examples include tissue culture, wound culture, antibiotic therapy.
- Has the patient undergone debridement for this wound in the past? Examples include sharp excisional versus mechanical versus enzymatic.

The answers to these questions should follow the guidelines of the DIME wound care model that is later discussed in this chapter.[11]

II. Physical examination

While performing a physical evaluation of a patient, it is important to maintain a systematic routine. What will be discussed in this chapter is a guideline to performing a physical examination. It is important to develop a personal approach to performing a physical exam, one that is tailored to the individual examiner.[9]

As a general principle, patients should receive one annual comprehensive exam. However, return visits by a patient seeking medical attention for a specific ailment may require only a problem-focused physical exam, which would be comprised of select portions of the comprehensive exam. The physical examination process is composed of observation and testing of the major bodily systems which can be examined with non-invasive approaches. Some bodily systems are further examined by specialists, such as the genitourinary system. And other systems of the body aren't physically examinable, such as the psychiatric system. The systems involved in the comprehensive physical exam should include: [9,11-12]

Constitutional – Obtain the patient's vital signs (heart rate, respiratory rate, blood pressure, and body temperature).

Eyes – General physical inspection of the patient's conjunctiva, sclera, and eyelids.

Use a Snellen chart to test for visual acuity. Test ocular motility by having the patient follow the finger of the clinician with his or her eyes in a "figure eight" pattern. Use a pen light to test pupillary reaction to light. Use an ophthalmoscope to examine the fundus.

Ears/Nose/Mouth/Throat (ENMT) – Use an otoscope to inspect that the ears are free of cerumen build up, free of infection, and the eardrum is intact. Conduct Webber and Rinne hearing test with the use of a tuning fork. Use an otoscope to visualize the nasal cavity, looking for obstruction or congestion. Use an otoscope to visualize the oral cavity, observing the mucous membranes, dentition, and the presence or absence of lesions. Percuss the frontal and paranasal sinuses, while asking if the patient feels pressure or pain. Palpate the lymph nodes, while trying to detect enlargement or irregularity. Palpate the temporomandibular joint, while asking the patient if there is pain when opening and closing his or her jaw. Palpate the thyroid, while trying to detect enlargement or irregularity. Auscultate carotid artery for bruits.

Respiratory – Observe the patient's breathing pattern, depth, and rate. Observe the patient's trachea for deviation. Observe the patient's extremities for any clinical signs of cyanosis or clubbing. Observe and palpate the patient's lung expansion, examining for bilateral equality. Palpate lung fields for vibratory consolidation. Percuss for hyper/hypo-resonance over the lung fields. Auscultate over the lung fields, listening for wheezes, rhonchi, crackles, etc.

Cardiovascular – Observe cardiac rate and rhythm. Palpate peripheral pulses. Palpate the cardiac apex's point of maximum impulse. Auscultate over all four heart valves, listening for murmurs, rubs, or gallops.

Gastrointestinal – Observe the patient's abdomen in general appearance, looking for distension, masses, lesions, etc. Auscultate and listen for sounds of obstruction or bruits. Apply light palpation, all nine regions. Apply deep palpation, all nine regions. From the palpation portion of the exam note guarding, rebound pain, and possible herniation. Percuss all nine regions, noting possible enlarged organs or fluid accumulation.

Musculoskeletal – Observe the patient walk and perform actions on command, such as "balance on one leg." Test the patient's passive and active range of motions to all four limbs. Test the patient's ability to perform motion in flexion, extension, abduction, adduction, internal rotation, and external rotation. Testing should include active free-range motions and motions against resistance, in which the clinician tests the patient's ability to create force against resistance. A similar test should be run for multiplane axis of the patient's head and neck.

Neurological – Assess consciousness, often on the level of the Glasgow Coma Scale. Mini-mental state examination, which includes testing the patient's ability to reason with time, place, registration, attenuation/calculation, recall, language, repetition, and complex commands. Cranial nerve examination: sense of smell (I), visual fields and acuity (II), eye movements (III, IV, VI), sensory function of the face (V), strength of facial muscles (VII), hearing (VII, VIII), taste (VII, XI, X), pharyngeal movement/reflex (IX, X), strength of shoulder girdle muscles (XI), tongue movements (XII). Motor system testing: muscle strength, muscle tone, overall posture, resting tremors, abnormal movements, etc. Deep tendon reflexes: biceps (C5/C6), triceps (C7/C8), patellar (L2-L4), Achilles (S1/S2). Eliciting appropriate versus inappropriate pain, temperature, and fine touch sensation over various dermatomes.

A. Problem-focused physical exam in a patient with a wound

When performing a problem-focused physical exam on a patient with a wound, it is important to determine the location, depth, and extent. Wound location is a vital determinant on the future treatment. As an example, a traumatic wound located on the face of a 15-year-old girl will be treated much differently than a pressure wound on the heel of an 80-year-old man.

Wound measurements should be taken upon every evaluation, to track the wound's progression. The first measurement taken is length (proximal to distal). The next measurement is width (medial to lateral). And the final measurement is depth. Sheehan et al.[13] shows that a 50% area reduction in diabetic foot ulcerations at Week 4 of treatment provides for a positive predictor of healing with a 12-week period.

The depth of a wound and the underlying structures can dictate future treatment as well. Superficial wounds will be treated much differently than wounds that extend to the level of tendon and bone. Also, the extent of a wound upon initial presentation can lead to a false impression, leading clinicians to believe the patient's wounds are less extensive than they are in reality. It is important to examine a wound for undermining, tunneling, and probing. An in-depth discussion of these topics will take place in Chapter 5: Wound Assessment of this textbook.[11-12]

Consider a patient with a lower-extremity wound of unknown etiology. When performing a problem-focused lower-extremity examination, the following functions need to be addressed:

Dermatological assessment:

- Skin
  - Texture/turgor/temperature
  - With or without defect?
  - Visual signs of infection?
- Nails
  - Elongated/incurved/mycotic
- Callus
  - Present versus absent
  - What anatomical location?

Vascular assessment:

- Pedal pulses
  - Palpability rated on a scale 0 (non-palpable) to +2 (normal)
- Digital capillary refill time (normal < 3 seconds)
- Hair growth
  - Present versus absent
  - To what level?
- Varicosities
  - Present versus absent
  - At what anatomical location?
- Temperature
  - Does the gradient change drastically from proximal to distal?

- Edema (pitting versus non-pitting)
  - 0 not present
  - 1+ minimal
  - 2+ moderate
  - 3+ severe
- How is the coloration?
  - Ischemia can appear pale and mottled.
  - Venous insufficiency can appear blue/purple (which may dissipate when the extremity is elevated). Hemosiderin deposits can also be visualized in chronic venous insufficiency.
  - Gangrenous tissue appears darkened and nonviable.
- Consider handheld Doppler to access major foot vessels.
- Consider performing an ankle-brachial index(ABI), toe-brachial index(TBI), and Skin Perfusion Pressure (SSP) when instrumentation is available.

Neurological assessment:

- Vibration sensation testing, absent versus present
- Proprioceptive position sensing
  - With the eyes closed, can the patient report position changes "up versus down" at the 1st metatarsophalangeal joint?
- Protective threshold testing
  - Semmes Weinstein monofilament
- Deep tendon reflexive testing
  - Patellar (L2-L4)
  - Achilles (S1/S2)
- Superficial reflexes
  - Babinski, Chaddock, Clonus

Orthopedic assessment:

- Gait analysis
- Range of motion testing
- Muscle strength testing
  - 0/5 No contraction present
  - 1/5 Palpable or observable contraction, without movement
  - 2/5 Movement without gravity as a factor
  - 3/5 Movement against gravity, without resistance
  - 4/5 Movement against gravity, with some resistance
  - 5/5 Movement against gravity, with full resistance

III. Components of the Wound Bed Preparation Model including the DIME in wound care

The Wound Bed Preparation Model represents a simplistic yet powerful and holistic algorithm to evaluate and treat chronic wounds. Patients with wounds should have an initial workup that covers the evaluation that establishes etiology and patient-centered concerns (i.e. vascularity, nutrition, and underlying comorbidities) prior to wound evaluation and treatment. Once these parameters have been recognized, the wound may be addressed through removal of devitalized tissue, control of infection and inflammation, moisture balance, and the need for wound edge preparation and depth management. As a patient progresses through a practitioner's wound care protocols, the same parameters should continually be used to reevaluate a patient on subsequent visits. It is of the utmost importance to keep in mind the patient's individual quality of life, medication use, and financial restraints.(14)

Devitalized tissue
- nonviable tissue that is no longer receiving adequate nutrient supply

Infection/Inflammation
- immunological response to pathogens or a foreign body

Moisture balance
- providing a moisture barrier for a proper wound-healing environment

Edge preparation and wound depth
- debridement protocols that promote wound healing

IV. Case studies

Mnemonic PROBLEM WOUNDS
(Courtesy Jayesh B. Shah, MD)

Pressure
Radiation
Oxygenation/Perfusion/Arterial/ Compromised STSG/Flaps
Burns
Lymphedema/Venous
Edema
Medications

Weird (Psychosocial)
Obesity
Unusual Wounds
Nutrition and Hydration
Diabetes
Socioeconomic Issues/Surgical Wounds

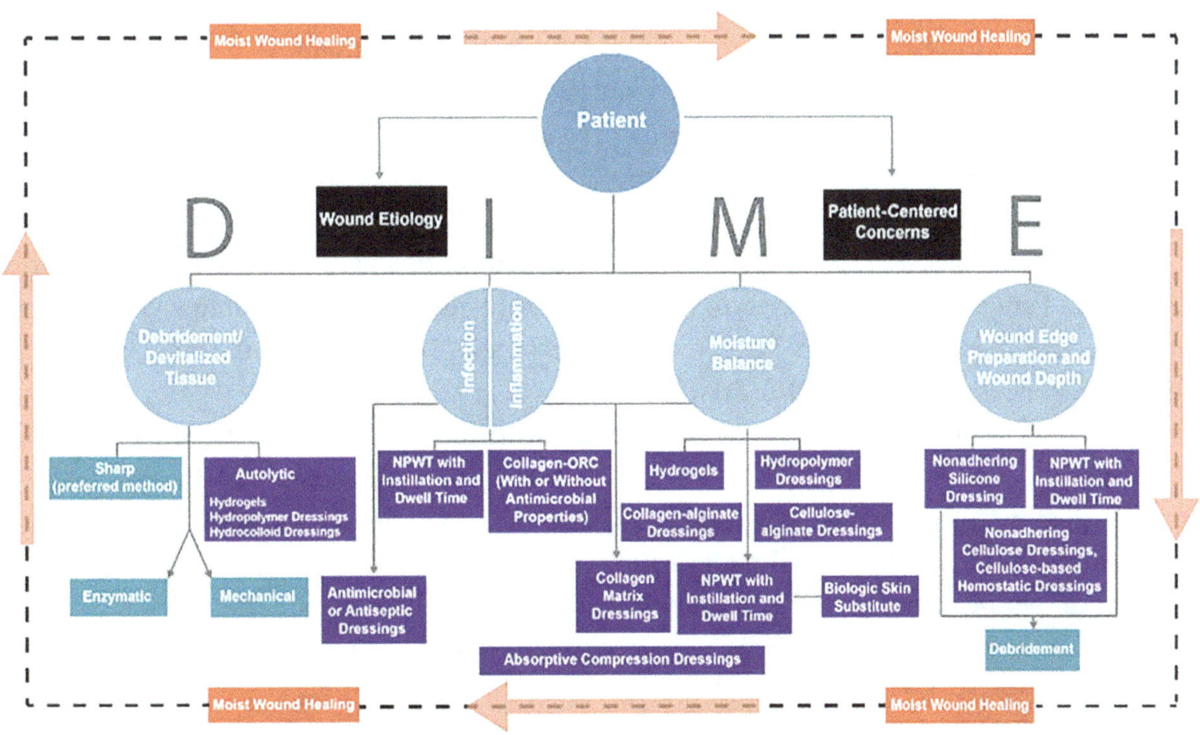

FIGURE 1. Abbreviations: NPWT, negative-pressure wound therapy; ORC, oxidized regenerated cellulose.
Reprinted with permission: Snyder RJ, Fife C, Moore Z. Adv Skin Wound Care 2016; 29:205-215. (14)

A. Problem wounds—"P" Pressure

1. *Case study–Pressure*

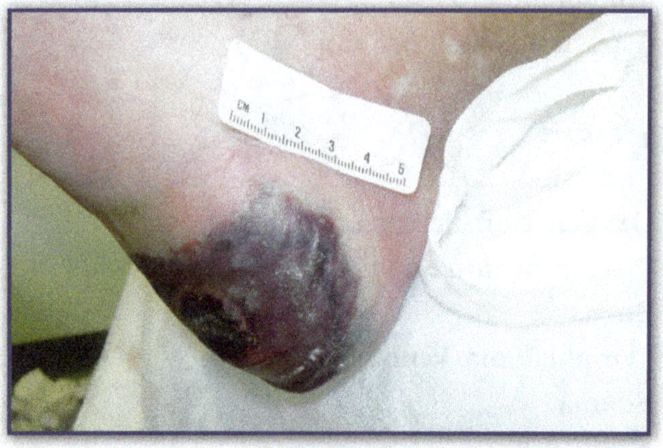

FIGURE 2.
Courtesy of Robert J. Snyder, DPM

History: This patient is a resident of a long-term-care facility. Upon initial consult the nursing staff states that this 6' 6" patient regularly slides to the foot of his bed, applying pressure to the heel.

General: This is a 56-year-old male, in no acute distress (NAD), and vital signs stable (VSS). Patient is mentally aberrant.

Physical:
Dermatological: Early dermal degradation with underlying lividity, right heel. Without clinical signs of infection (CSI)

Neurological: Patient is unable to perform interactive protective threshold testing. Patient with positive within normal limits (WNL) deep tendon reflex (DTR) testing.

Vascular: Positive pedal pulses to bilateral Lower Extremities (LE) +2. Normal pedal hair growth. Skin temperature is warm to warm proximal to distally.

Orthopedic: Ankle and pedal joint range of motion (ROM) is within normal limits (WNL), without crepitation.

Studies: Negative noninvasive vascular studies. Negative X-rays.

Diagnosis: Deep Tissue Injury (DTI)

2. *Case study–Pressure*

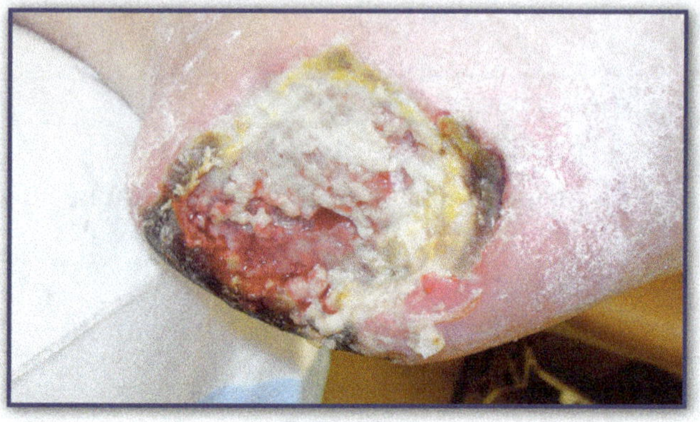

FIGURE 3.
Courtesy of Robert J. Snyder, DPM

History: This patient has been admitted to the intensive care unit for greater than six months. Patient has been intubated and sedated for an extended period of time, without proper heel offloading.

General: This patient is a 71-year-old male. Patient is on ventilator assist and is currently sedated.

Physical:
Dermatological: Full thickness ulcerative breakdown to the level of subcutaneous fat. Wound measures 3.1cm x 2.4cm x 0.2cm.

Neurological: Patient is unable to interact for protective threshold testing. Positive DTR testing. Negative superficial reflexive testing.

Vascular: Palpable pedal pulses, +2. Skin temperature warm to warm proximal to distal.

Orthopedic: Muscle strength testing, nonobtainable. Ankle and pedal joint ROM is WNL, without crepitation.

Studies: Negative noninvasive vascular studies. Periwound $tcpO_2$ 38mmHg.

Diagnosis: Left heel pressure ulceration, Stage 3.

B. PRoblem wounds—"R" Radiation

1. *Case study–Radiation*

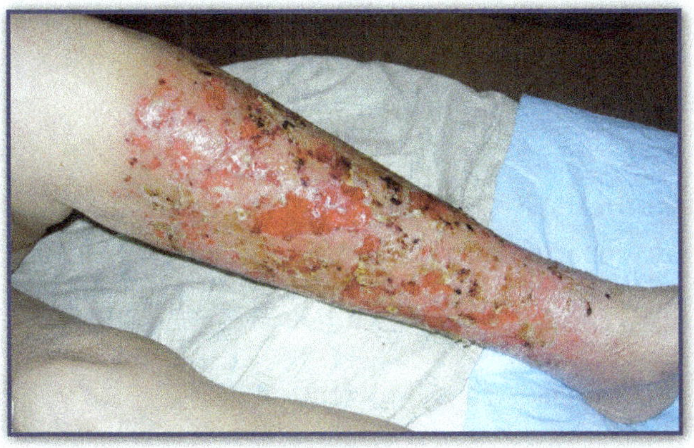

FIGURE 4.
Courtesy of Robert J. Snyder, DPM

History: This patient has a history of prolonged exposure to ionizing radiation. Patient presents to the hospital with multifocal ulcerations to the left leg.

General: This is a 46-year-old female in NAD with VSS.

Physical:
Dermatological: Multiple superficial ulcerations from ankle to knee, widespread and circumferential. With islands of necrosis intermittently between ulcerations.

Neurological: Protective and epicritic threshold intact. DTR testing positive.

Vascular: Palpable pedal pulses to DP and PT bilaterally +2.

Orthopedic: Ankle and pedal joint ROM are WNL.

Studies: Negative X-rays.

Diagnosis: Radiation burn.

C. PROblem wounds—"O" Oxygenation

1. *Case study–Oxygenation/perfusion/arterial/compromised STSG (split thickness skin graft)/flaps*

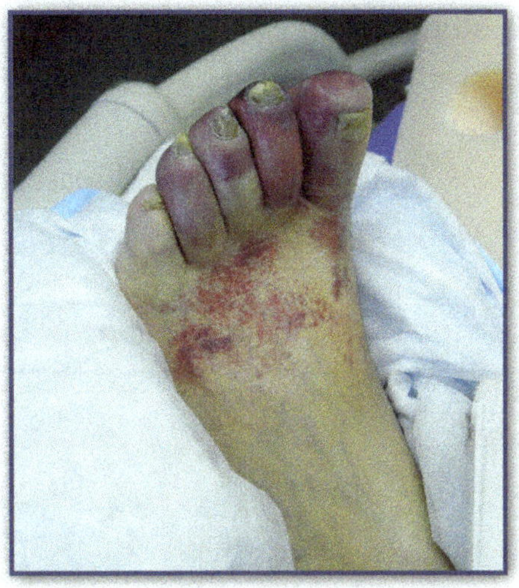

FIGURE 5.
Courtesy of Robert J. Snyder, DPM

History: This patient was admitted to the hospital for shortness of breath. Podiatry team subsequently consulted. Patient states that his toes have "always had a bit of color to them" but states the condition has been worsening over the past two years.

General: This patient is a 52-year-old male.

Physical:
Dermatological: Dermis intact. Left foot, digits 1-4 with circumferential lividity. Dorsal forefoot with patchy lividity.

Neurological: Protective and epicritic sensations intact to bilateral LE.

Vascular: Pedal pulses weakly palpable, +1. No pedal hair growth. Skin temperature is warm to cool, proximal to distal.

Orthopedic: Ankle and pedal joint ROM are WNL to bilateral LE. Muscle strength testing 5/5.

Studies: Irregular noninvasive vascular studies, monophasic waveforms. $TcpO_2 < 30mmHg$, TBI (toe brachial index) = 0.7. Angiogram shows stenosis along the anterior tibial artery, as well as the posterior tibial artery.

Diagnosis: Peripheral arterial disease (PAD), with associated low oxygen perfusion.

2. *Case study–Arterial ulceration*

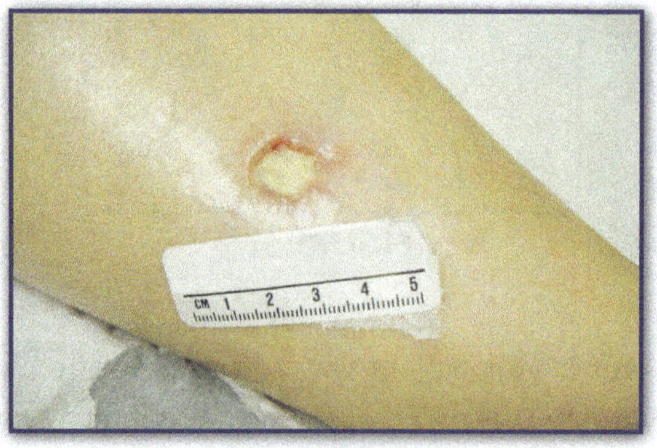

FIGURE 6.
Courtesy of Robert J. Snyder, DPM

History: This patient has a long history of tobacco smoking and a PMH of hypertension. Patient states that a wound developed on her right leg approximately two weeks prior to visiting the health clinic. States that she had a similar issue on the left leg last year.

General: This patient is a 47-year-old female in NAD and all VSS.

Physical:
Dermatological: Anterior right leg sub-dermal ulceration, well circumscribed. Wound bed 100% fibrotic.

Neurological: Protective and epicritic sensation intact. Positive DTR testing. Negative superficial reflexive testing.

Vascular: Pedal pulses weakly palpable +1, to the DP (dorsalis pedis) and PT (posterior tibial). Pedal hair growth is absent.

Orthopedic: All ankle and pedal joint ROM (range of motion) are WNL, without crepitation. Muscle strength testing 5/5.

Studies: ABI = 0.7 Biphasic waveforms detected on arterial ultrasound. Angiogram showed focal occlusion to the anterior tibial artery.

Diagnosis: Arterial ulceration.

3. *Case study–Dry gangrene*

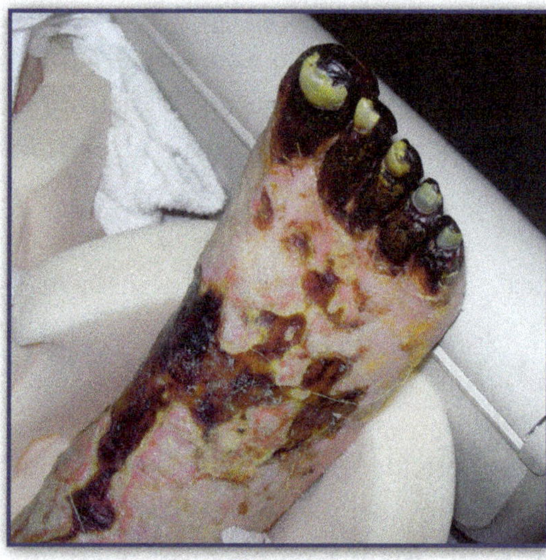

FIGURE 7.
Courtesy of Robert J. Snyder, DPM

History: This patient presents to the ER with necrotic digits 1-5 on the right foot. Patient admits to a history of tobacco smoking and alcohol abuse. Patient states that he has been living on the streets for the past two years and is currently taking no medication.

General: This patient is a 64-year-old male in NAD and VSS.

Physical:

Dermatological: Diffuse ischemic necrosis to the distal right LE. Digits 1-5 with clinical signs of gangrene.

Neurological: Protective and epicritic sensation are completely absent. Reflexive testing deferred due to patient's condition.

Vascular: Non-palpable pedal pulses. No pedal hair growth present. Skin temperature cool to cold, proximal to distal.

Orthopedic: Deferred due to patient's clinical condition.

Studies: Negative X-rays. Abnormal waveforms on arterial ultrasounds. Angiogram shows single vessel runoff to the peroneal artery.

Diagnosis: Dry gangrene.

D. PROBlem wounds—"B" Burns

1. *Case study–Burns*

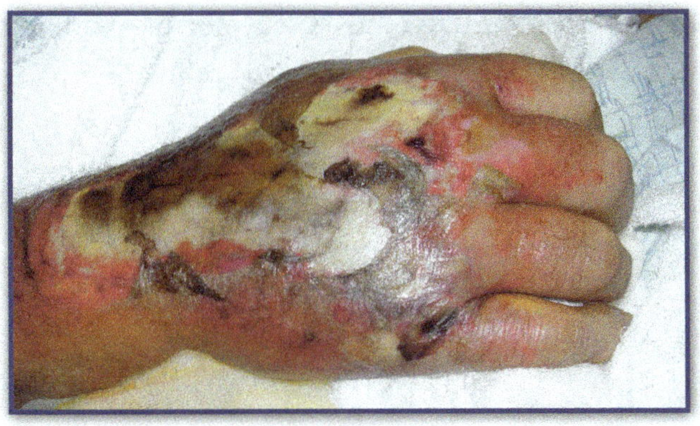

FIGURE 8.
Courtesy of Robert J. Snyder, DPM

History: Patient presents to the ED after an injury at work. Patient is employed as a chef and experienced an oil fire.

General: This patient is a 42-year-old male in NAD and VSS, experiencing pain 8/10.

Physical:

Dermatological: Full thickness burns on the dorsum of the hand and wrist, from the metacarpophalangeal joints to 3cm proximal to the wrist.

Neurological: In the acute setting, neurological testing was deferred.

Vascular: Palpable radial pulse, digital capillary refill time less than three seconds.

Orthopedic: Patient with intact motor function to all digits 1-5, full ROM. Further testing deferred due to pain.

Diagnosis: 3rd degree burn.

E. PROBLem wounds—"L" Lymphedema/venous

1. *Case study–Lymphedema/venous*

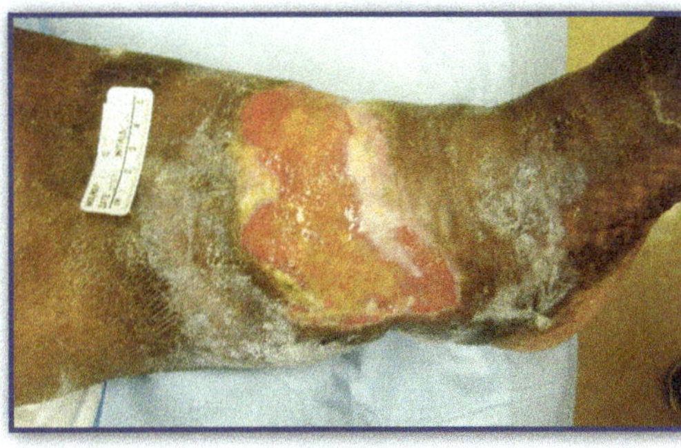

FIGURE 9.
Courtesy of Robert J. Snyder, DPM

History: This patient has a past medical history of diabetes mellitus Type II and morbid obesity. Patient presents to the wound care clinic with an anterior left leg wound. Patient states that the wound has been present for five months.

General: This patient is a 53-year-old male, in NAD and VSS.

Physical:

Dermatological: Wound present to the anterior leg, measuring 5.4cm x 13.6cm x 0.1cm.

Neurological: Protective and epicritic sensation are grossly impaired. Vibratory sensation testing reveals that the patient is below the normal range.

Vascular: Palpable pedal pulses +2, to both DP and PT. Skin temperature warm to warm, proximal to distal.

Orthopedic: Muscle strength testing is 5/5. Ankle and pedal joint ROM are limited and with crepitation. Patient has pain on both active and passive ROM.

Studies: Arterial ultrasound results within normal limits. Venous ultrasound with reflux, shows evidence of venous insufficiency.

Diagnosis: Venous ulcer.

2. *Case study–Lymphedema-related ulceration*

History: This patient presents to the wound care clinic with a family history of lymphedema. Her symptoms started four years prior to her consultation and consist of unilateral swelling and ulceration that goes through periods of healing and reopening.

General: This patient is a 47-year-old female in NAD and all VSS.

Physical:

Dermatological: Right lower extremity with diffuse nodule and plaques between the knee and ankle.

Neurological: Protective and epicritic sensation intact. All reflexive testing WNL.

Vascular: Palpable pedal pulses +2 to DP and PT bilaterally. Digital capillary refill time is less than three seconds. Pedal hair growth present.

Orthopedic: Ankle and pedal joint ROMs are limited in the hindfoot and midfoot, with crepitation in the forefoot. Patient's gait is WNL.

Studies: Arterial ultrasounds of bilateral lower extremities show triphasic waveforms. Venous ultrasounds without evidence of reflux.

Diagnosis: Lymphedema-related ulceration.

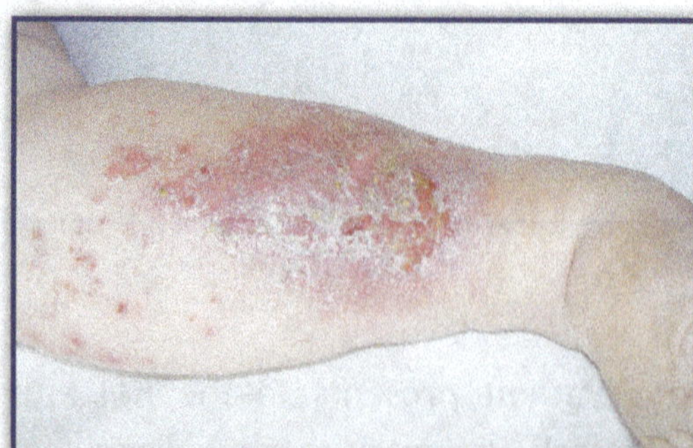

FIGURE 10.
Courtesy of Robert J. Snyder, DPM

F. PROBLEm wounds—"E" Edema

1. *Case study–Edema*

History: This patient presents to the wound care clinic with a history of alcohol abuse, tobacco use, and congestive heart failure. Patient states that her legs are prone to swelling.

General: This patient is a 48-year-old female in NAD and all VSS.

Physical:

Dermatological: Xerosis present to bilateral LE. Medial left leg wound measuring 0.8cm x 0.4cm x 0.2cm. Wound bed is 70% granular, 30% fibronecrotic.

Neurological: Protective and epicritic sensation are grossly intact. DTR are WNL. Superficial reflexive testing is negative.

Vascular: Palpable pedal pulses +2 to DP and PT. Pedal hair growth is scant, but present. Bilateral pitting edema +2

Orthopedic: Muscle strength testing is 5/5. Ankle and pedal joint ROM is WNL, without crepitation.

Studies: Arterial and venous ultrasounds are unremarkable.

Diagnosis: Edema.
(The physical strain the edema is placing on the integument is causing ulceration.)

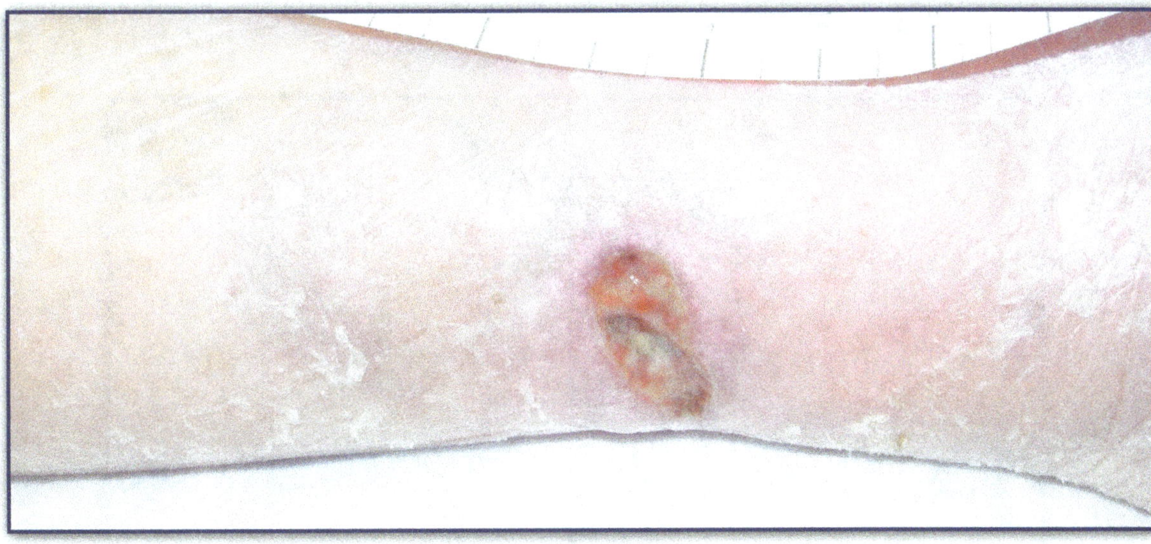

FIGURE 11.
Courtesy of Robert J. Snyder, DPM

G. PROBLEM wounds— "M" Medications

1. *Case study–Medications*

History: This patient has a medical history of HIV, and reports taking oral hydroxyurea in conjunction with his antiretroviral medication. Patient presents to the wound care clinic with an extensive wound on the right leg (left image). Patient instructed to discontinue his hydroxyurea medication and given routine wound care, wound diminishes in size only after two weeks (right image).

General: This patient is a 55-year-old male in NAD and all VSS.

Physical:

Dermatological: Initial presentation is with an anterior leg wound 11.4cm x 7.1 cm x 0.1cm. Wound bed is 80% fibrotic, 15% granular, and 5% necrotic.

Neurological: Protective and epicritic sensation are grossly intact. Superficial reflexive testing is WNL.

Vascular: Palpable pedal pulses +2 to the DP and PT. Pedal hair growth present.

Orthopedic: Gait analysis reveals guarded dorsiflexion motions. Ankle and pedal joint ROMs are WNL bilaterally.

Studies: Arterial and venous ultrasounds are unremarkable.

Diagnosis: Medication-induced wound.

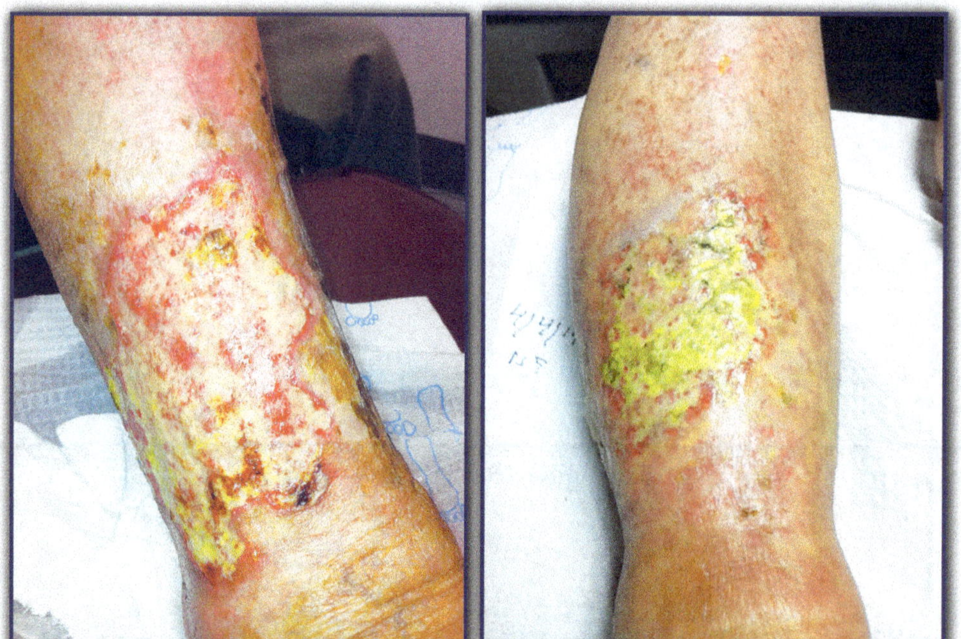

FIGURE 12.
Courtesy of Robert J. Snyder, DPM

H. PROBLEM Wounds— "W" Weird (psychosocial)

1. *Case study–Weird (psychosocial)*

History: This patient presents as a referral from a local psychiatric office. The patient does not have any other significant past medical history or comorbidities. The patient describes this particular wound as recurring. He states that the wound, "gets better . . . depending how I'm feeling."

General: This patient is a 60-year-old male.

Physical:

Dermatological: Posterior leg wound measuring 4.2cm x 3.0cm x 0.1cm. Wound is 50% granular and 50% fibrotic.

Neurological: Protective and epicritic sensations are intact and WNL. Superficial reflexive testing is negative. Positive DTR testing.

Vascular: Palpable pedal pulses +2 DP and PT. Pedal hair present. Skin temperature warm to warm, proximal to distal bilaterally.

Orthopedic: Ankle and pedal joint ROM are WNL, without crepitation.

Studies: Arterial and venous ultrasounds are unremarkable.

Diagnosis: Factitious wound (this particular patient was self-inflicting).

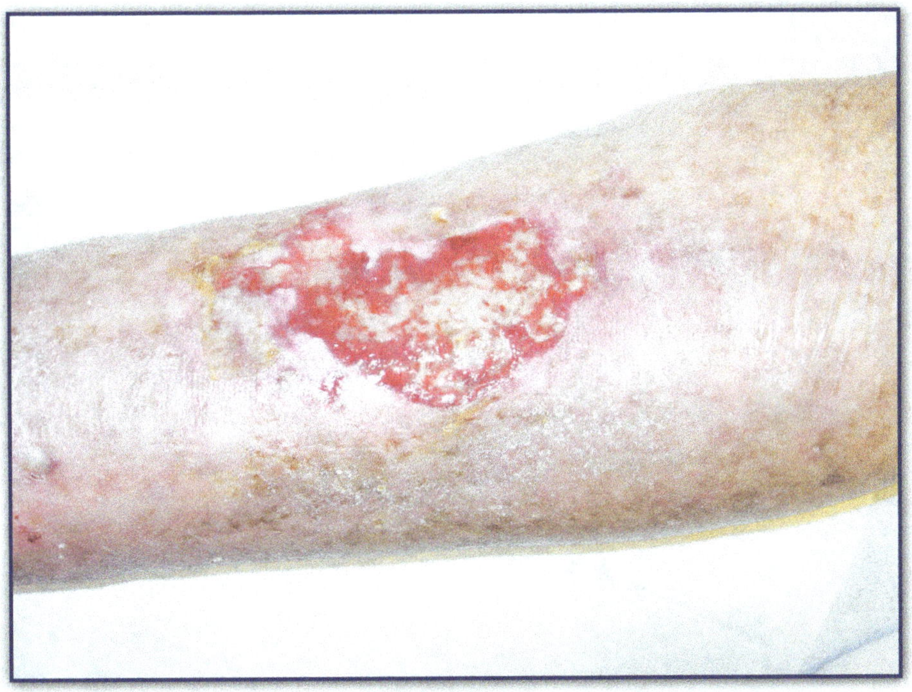

FIGURE 13.
Courtesy of Robert J. Snyder, DPM

I. PROBLEM WOunds—"O" Obesity

1. *Case study–Obesity*

History: This patient presents to the wound care clinic as a referral from a private practitioner who has been providing in office wound care for three months, without progress. Patient is morbidly obese with an HbA1c of 9.1% and a BMI of 36. Patient admits to a sedentary lifestyle and has poor nutritional behavior. When speaking with the previous provider, he describes the patient as "difficult." This patient has a documented history of noncompliance.

General: This is a 36-year-old female who is in NAD and with all VSS.

Physical:

Dermatological: Xerosis present to bilateral LE. Right lateral leg wound, measuring 3.2cm x 2.8cm x 0.2cm. Wound bed is 80% granular and 20% fibrotic. Skin color is pale, except for the peri-wound erythema.

Neurological: Protective and epicritic sensation are grossly impaired. Vibratory sensation, impaired. Sharp versus dull, impaired.

Vascular: Palpable pedal pulses 2+, DP and PT bilaterally. Digital capillary refill time is less than three seconds. Edema 2+.

Orthopedic: Severely limited ankle and pedal joint ROM, with crepitation and guarding from the patient.

Studies: Negative X-rays. Arterial and venous ultrasounds are unremarkable.

Diagnosis: Ulceration, secondary to obesity/diet/lifestyle.

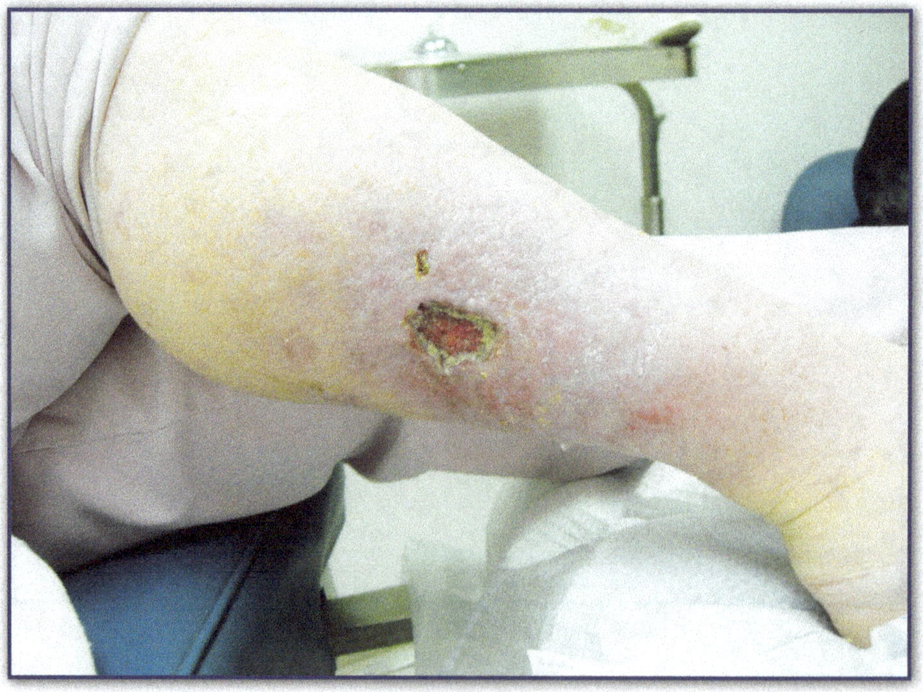

FIGURE 14.
Courtesy of Robert J. Snyder, DPM

J. PROBLEM WOUnds— "U" Unusual wounds

1. *Case study–Unusual wounds*

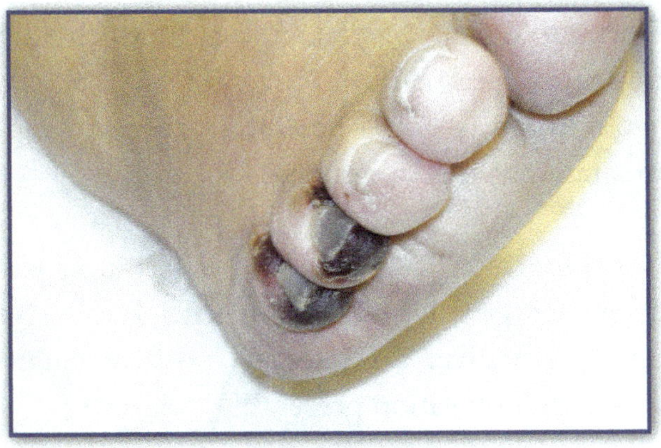

FIGURE 15.
Courtesy of Robert J. Snyder, DPM

History: This patient presents to the ER with two ischemic pedal digits. Patient with a history of spontaneous abortion less than one year prior.

General: This patient is a 27-year-old female patient in NAD and with all VSS.

Physical:
Dermatological: Dermis overlying the distal tufts and nailbeds of right 4th and 5th digits appear necrotic. All other dermatological findings in the right foot appear WNL.

Neurological: Protective and epicritic sensation intact to bilateral LE, with the exception of the lack of sensation to the distal tufts of digits 4 and 5. All other neurological findings are WNL.

Vascular: Palpable pedal pulses +2 to DP and PT. Right foot, digital capillary refill time to digits 1-3, less than three seconds. Right foot, digital capillary refill time to digits 4 and 5, undeterminable.

Orthopedic: All ankle and pedal joint ROM are WNL. Plantarflexion of digits still capable on command. Gait analysis deferred due to patient condition.

Studies: Arterial and venous ultrasound are unremarkable. Laboratory studies return with low platelet count. Additional lab testing for the presence of $\beta_2$glycoprotein antibodies as well as low levels of Protein S.

Diagnosis: Antiphospholipid Antibody Syndrome.

2. *Case study–Unusual wounds*

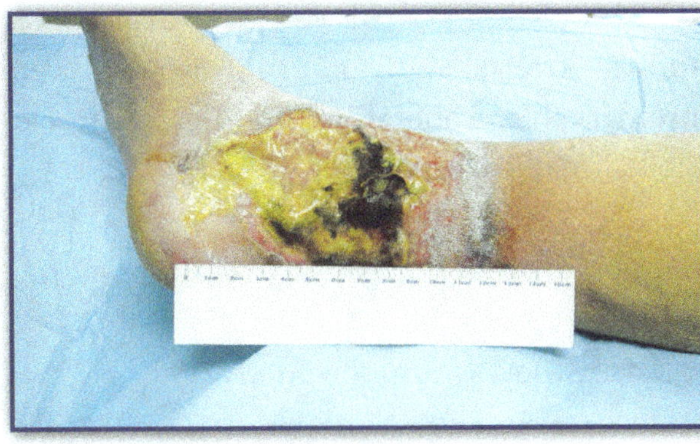

FIGURE 16.
Courtesy of Robert J. Snyder, DPM

History: This patient has a past medical history of Crohn's disease. Patient states that this wound on her right medial ankle started as what she assumed to be a bug bite. Patient exhibits severe pain on debridement. Wound demonstrates pathergy upon initial debridement.

General: This patient is a 43-year-old female in NAD and all VSS.

Physical:
Dermatological: Right medial ankle wound 8.1cm x 6.7cm x 0.2cm. Wound bed is 10% granular, 70% fibrotic, and 20% necrotic. Patient without telangiectasia.

Neurological: Protective and epicritic sensations are intact. DTR intact on the left, deferred on the right due to clinical condition. Sharp versus dull sensation intact to bilateral LE.

Vascular: Palpable pedal pulses +2 on DP and PT bilaterally. Digital capillary refill time is less than three seconds to digits 1-5 to bilateral feet. Skin temperature is warm to warm proximal to distal.

Orthopedic: Ankle and pedal joint ROM deferred on the right due to patient's clinical condition, left all ROM were WNL. Muscle strength testing to the left was 5/5.

Studies: Arterial and venous ultrasounds were unremarkable. Laboratory findings show elevated C-reactive protein.

Diagnosis: Pyoderma gangrenosum.

3. *Case study–Unusual wounds*

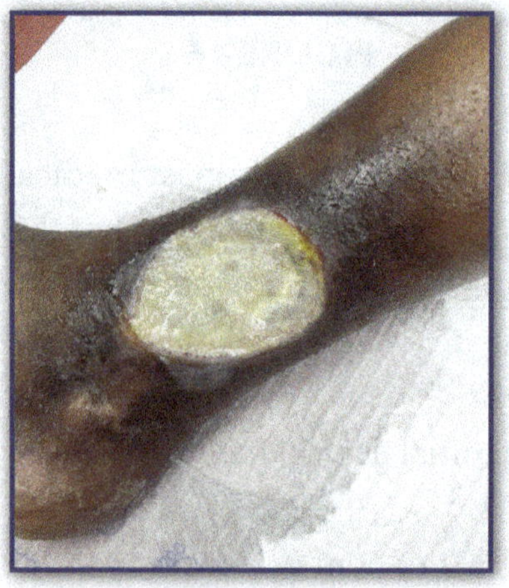

FIGURE 17.
Courtesy of Robert J. Snyder, DPM

History: This patient has a past medical history of sickle cell anemia, HgbSC. Patient has been dealing with this medial ankle wound for several years. This wound goes through phases of healing and reopening. Patient has undergone hyperbaric oxygen therapy as well as skin substitute grafting in the past.

General: This is a 51-year-old male patient in NAD and with all VSS

Physical:
Dermatological: Medial ankle wound, circular in shape, measuring 4.7cm x 4.6cm x 0.2cm. Wound bed is 100% fibrotic. Periwound pigmentation is hyperpigmented.

Neurological: Protective and epicritic sensations are grossly intact. Superficial reflexive testing negative. DTR testing positive. Sharp versus dull sensation present.

Vascular: Palpable pedal pulses +2, DP and PT bilaterally. Digital capillary refill time is less than three seconds to digits 1-5 bilaterally.

Orthopedic: Ankle and pedal joint ROM are WNL bilaterally. Muscle strength testing 5/5 bilaterally.

Studies: Arterial and venous ultrasounds are unremarkable. Negative X-rays.

Diagnosis: Sickle Cell ulceration.

K. PROBLEM WOUNds—"N" Nutrition and hydration

1. *Case study–Nutrition and hydration*

History: This patient is status post thyroid surgery. After surgery the patient was without appetite, refused meals, and refused enteral feeding tube. Patient also has previously diagnosed PAD. Over the course of two weeks, patient with rapidly advancing pedal wound formation.

General: This patient is an 88-year-old male in NAD and all VSS, but with hypotension 100/70.

Physical:
Dermatological: Multifocal pedal wounds of varying depths, some unstageable. Periwound erythema present

Neurological: Patient is not cooperative for neurological testing.

Vascular: Palpable pedal pulses to bilateral LE, DP and PT +2. Digital capillary refill time is less than four seconds.

Orthopedic: All ankle and pedal joint ROMs are limited with crepitation. Patient refuses to contribute to muscle strength testing.

Studies: Arterial and venous ultrasounds are unremarkable. Laboratory studies show of poor nutritional status, as well as dehydration.

Diagnosis: Wounds of a nutritional etiology.

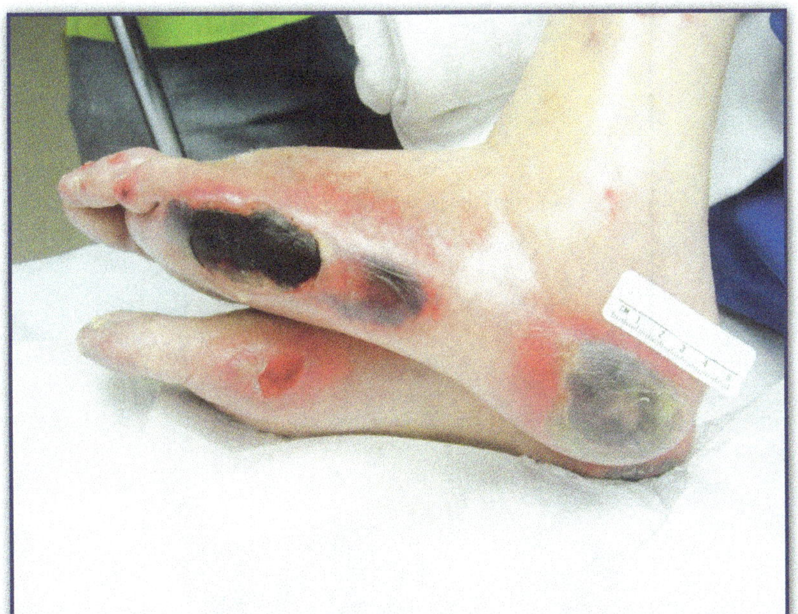

FIGURE 18.
Courtesy of Robert J. Snyder, DPM

L. PROBLEM WOUNDs— "D" Diabetes

1. *Case study–Diabetes*

History: This patient has a medical history of uncontrolled type II diabetes mellitus with associated peripheral neuropathy. She stepped on a needle without noticing while walking barefoot at home. The patient noticed drainage in her sock and proceeded to the primary care office which referred the case to podiatry.

General: This patient is a 54-year-old female in NAD, with all VSS

Physical:

Dermatological: Punctate ulceration, distal-lateral right forefoot. Ulcer is surrounded by hyperkeratotic tissue.

Neurological: Protective and epicritic sensation are impaired. Sharp versus dull sensation, impaired. Vibratory sensation, impaired. DTR intact.

Vascular: Bounding pedal pulses, DP and PT. Pedal hair growth absent.

Orthopedic: Ankle and pedal joint ROM are WNL, but with crepitation.

Studies: Arterial ultrasounds with biphasic waveforms. Venous ultrasounds, unremarkable. Laboratory findings of elevated white blood cell count. Positive probe to bone testing. X-rays are without signs of osteomyelitis. MRI shows signs of osteomyelitis to the distal 4th metatarsal.

Diagnosis: Diabetic foot ulcer.

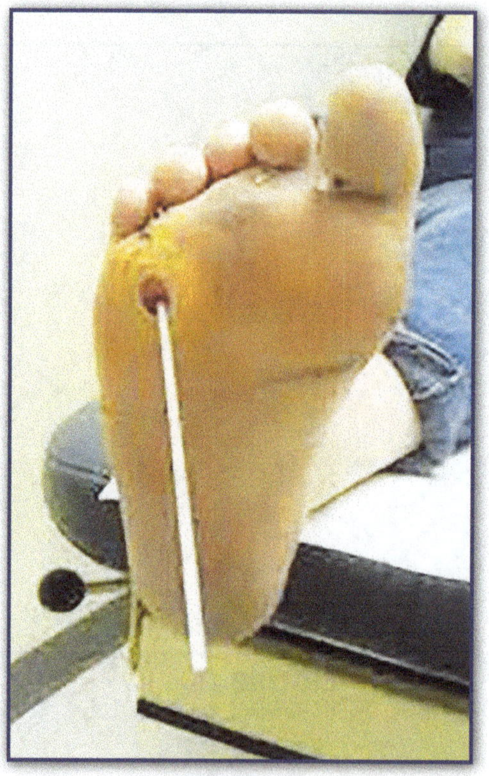

FIGURE 19.
Courtesy of Robert J. Snyder, DPM

M. PROBLEM WOUNDS—"S" Socioeconomic issues/surgical wounds

1. *Case study–Socioeconomic issues/surgical wounds*

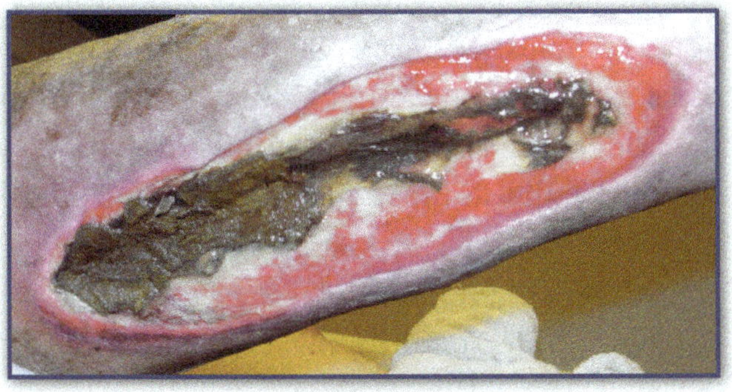

FIGURE 20.
Courtesy of Robert J. Snyder, DPM

History: This patient has a history of complete Achilles tendon rupture three months ago. The patient underwent open operative repair at that time. The patient admits at this time that he has been living on the streets. Patient also admits that he did not present for follow-up care due to financial concerns.

General: This patient is a 58-year-old male in NAD and all VSS.

Physical:
Dermatological: Posterior leg with full thickness ulceration down to the level of tendon. The wound bed is 40% necrotic, 35% granular, and 25% fibrotic.

Neurological: Protective and epicritic sensations are both grossly intact. DTR testing deferred. Superficial reflexive testing also deferred.

Vascular: Palpable pedal pulses +2 to DP and PT. Digital capillary refill time less than three seconds.

Orthopedic: This portion of the exam was deferred due to the patient's clinical condition.

Studies: Arterial and venous ultrasound, unremarkable. X-rays, negative.

Diagnosis: Surgical wound dehiscence

2. *Case study–Surgical flap dehiscence*

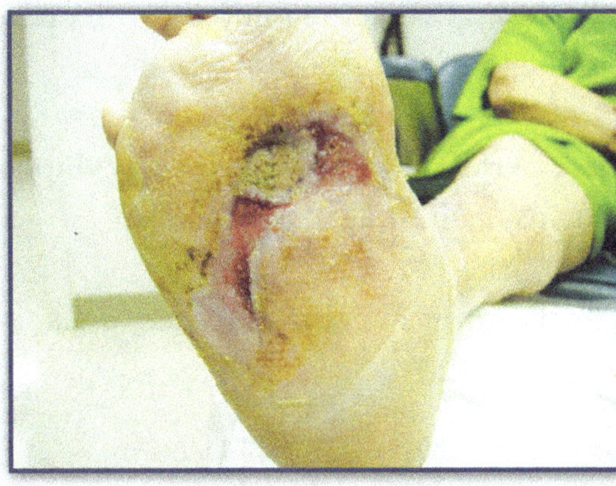

FIGURE 21.
Courtesy of Robert J. Snyder, DPM

History: This patient returns to the office. Three months prior to this visit, an in-office punch biopsy revealed squamous cell carcinoma. After excision of the carcinoma, a rotational flap procedure was performed. Unfortunately, the flap failed with necrosis at the surgical margins. Patient is a type II diabetic and is currently on hemodialysis.

General: Patient is a 61-year-old female, in NAD and all VSS.

Physical:
Dermatological: Surgical wound dehiscence on the plantar aspect of the right foot. Wound is semilunar. Wound base is 60% granular with a 40% fibrotic base located at the distal most aspect of the plantar wound.

Neurological: Protective and epicritic sensation grossly impaired. Sharp versus dull sensation absent. Vibratory sensation is at the upper limits of normal.

Vascular: Pedal pulses are palpable. Pedal hair absent. Skin temperature is warm to cool, proximal to distal.

Orthopedic: Patient with previous 4th digit amputation to the right foot. Ankle and pedal joint ROM limited at the midfoot, with crepitation in the forefoot.

Studies: Arterial ultrasounds show biphasic waveforms to all three major vessels.

Diagnosis: Surgical flap dehiscence.

Summary

We have discussed several factors that may contribute to wound formation. If a practitioner is diligent enough to trace back the source, every wound has a root cause. The root cause may be as complex as a systemic metabolic disease or as simple as a traumatic event. Identifying the underlying cause(s) of wound development should be the foundation for treatment planning. All wound care patients should receive a customized treatment plan based on wound etiology. Understanding the various pathways in which wounds may arise is key to successful wound care management. It is the duty of a practitioner to learn the appropriate therapies for each wound, in light of the wound's etiology.

Review questions

1. A 91-year-old female with Alzheimer's dementia who resides in a skill nursing facility with evidence of functional decline and a failure to thrive gradually develops wounds on her lower legs. Of the choices, which is the most likely etiology of the wounds?

    a. venous
    b. arterial
    c. edema
    d. nutrition

2. A 51-year-old quadriplegic has been wheelchair bound for one year since a motor vehicle accident with a full thickness ulcer developing over his right hip. Of the choices, which is the most likely etiology of the wounds?

    a. weird (psychosocial)
    b. pressure
    c. nutrition
    d. obesity

3. A 69-year-old female with a history of a myeloproliferative disorder was placed on hydroxyurea by her hematologist. The patient reports developing a wound to her lower leg without any known history of trauma. Of the choices, which is the most likely etiology of the wounds?

    a. venous
    b. diabetic
    c. medication
    d. unusual

4. A traumatic wound you have been following for two weeks appears to have a dry granular base with no evidence clinically or diagnostically of arterial insufficiency. What tenet of the Wound Bed Preparation Model needs attention?

    a. devitalized tissue
    b. infection
    c. moisture balance
    d. edge preparation

5. A physically healthy 23-year-old male with obsessive-compulsive disorder presents to you with a nonhealing wound to his right shin. The wound has had an irregular pattern with thickening of the margins without any histological evidence of malignancy from a biopsy performed by the referring physician. Of the choices, which is the most likely etiology of the wound?

    a. weird (psychosocial)
    b. socioeconomic
    c. radiation
    d. lymphedema

ANSWERS: 1) d
2) b
3) c
4) c
5) a

References

1. Jung K et al. Rapid identification of slow healing wounds. Wound Repair and Regen. 2015.
2. Mustoe TA, O'Shaughnessy K, Kloeters O. Chronic wound pathogenesis and current treatment strategies: a unifying hypothesis. Plast Reconstr Surg. 2006;117(7 Suppl):35S-41S.
3. Centers for Disease Control. Number (in millions) of civilian/noninstitutionalized persons with diagnosed diabetes, United States, 1980–2014. 2015.
4. Centers for Disease Control and Prevention (US). History of foot ulcer among persons with diabetes—United States, 2000-2002. MMWR Morb Mortal Wkly Rep. 2003;52(45):1098-102.
5. Bickley L, Szilagyi PG. Bates' guide to physical examination and history-taking. Lippincott Williams & Wilkins; 2012.
6. Wallace GF. Dermatologic causes of heel pain. Clin Podiatr Med Surg. 2010;27(3):407-416.
7. George SZ et al. Development of a review-of-systems screening tool for orthopaedic physical therapists: results from the optimal screening for prediction of referral and outcome (OSPRO) cohort. J Orthop Sports Phys Ther. 2015;45(7):512-526.
8. Petrilli CM et al. Understanding the role of physician attire on patient perceptions: a systematic review of the literature—targeting attire to improve likelihood of rapport (TAILOR) investigators. BMJ Open. 2015;5(1): e006578.
9. Cole SA, Bird J. The medical interview: the three function approach. Elsevier Health Sciences; 2013.
10. O'Toole JK et al. Resident confidence addressing social History: is it influenced by availability of social and legal resources? Clin Pediatr. 2012;51(7):625-631.
11. Woo KY. Trends in wound management. Adv Skin Wound Care. 2013;26(12):538-541.
12. Jarvis C. Physical examination and health assessment. Elsevier Health Sciences; 2015.
13. Sheehan P et al. Percent change in wound area of diabetic foot ulcers over a 4-week period is a robust predictor of complete healing in a 12-week prospective trial. Diabetes Care. 2003;26(6):1879-1882.
14. Snyder RJ, Fife C, Moore Z. Components and quality measures of DIME (devitalized tissue, infection/inflammation, moisture balance, and edge preparation) in wound care. Adv Skin Wound Care. 2016;29(5):205-215.

Additional resources

1. Greer N et al. Advanced wound care therapies for nonhealing diabetic, venous, and arterial ulcers: a systematic review. Ann Intern Med. 2013;159(8):532-542.
2. Snyder RJ et al. Macrophages: a review of their role in wound healing and their therapeutic use. Wound Repair Regen. 2016.
3. Smola H, Muceno G, inventors. Nutritional composition for wound healing. United States patent application US 14/464,257.
4. Clark R, editor. The molecular and cellular biology of wound repair. Springer Science & Business Media; 2013.
5. Tricco AC et al. A systematic review of cost-effectiveness analyses of complex wound interventions reveals optimal treatments for specific wound types. BMC Med. 2015;13(1):1.
6. Gottrup F. A specialized wound-healing center concept: importance of a multidisciplinary department structure and surgical treatment facilities in the treatment of chronic wounds. Am J Sur. 2004;187(5):S38-S43.
7. Wolcott RD et al. 7 types of wounds and infections. Microbiology of wounds. 2010. p. 219.
8. Abbott, CA et al. Multicenter study of the incidence of and predictive risk factors for diabetic neuropathic foot ulceration. Diabetes Care. 1998;21(7):1071-1075.
9. Lipsky, BA et al. 2012 Infectious Diseases Society of America clinical practice guideline for the diagnosis and treatment of diabetic foot infections. Clin Infect Dis. 2012;54(12):e132-e173.
10. Snyder RJ, Hanft JR. Diabetic foot ulcers—effects on quality of life, costs, and mortality and the role of standard wound care and advanced-care therapies in healing: a review. Ostomy Wound Manage. 2009;55(11):28-38.

Chapter 4
NUTRITIONAL ASSESSMENT AND MANAGEMENT

Elizabeth Friedrich, MPH, RDN, CSG, LDN, FAND

KEY CONCEPTS

1. Characteristics for identifying malnutrition (undernutrition) include insufficient energy intake, interpretation of weight loss, loss of subcutaneous fat, loss of muscle mass, localized or generalized fluid accumulation, and diminished functional status as measured by hand grip strength.

2. A comprehensive nutrition assessment always includes an evaluation of current diet and food, fluid, and supplement consumption to determine if an individual's intake meets his or her estimated needs to prevent skin breakdown and/or support wound healing.

3. Evidenced-based guidelines indicate that protein and calorie needs are increased in those at risk for, or those with, a pressure ulcer.

4. Nutrition recommendations for individuals at risk for, or those with, pressure ulcers, must be individualized based on a number of factors including comorbidities, food preferences, and socioeconomic status.

CONTENTS

Introduction

Nutrition is associated with both the prevention and treatment of pressure ulcers. Epidemiological data confirm the association of some nutrition factors, including weight loss, protein-calorie malnutrition, and dehydration with the incidence and prevalence of pressure ulcers.[1-2] Multivariate analysis of epidemiological data indicates that a poor nutritional status and variables that indicate potential for malnutrition (such as low body weight and poor food intake) are independent risk factors for pressure ulcer development.[3-5] Interestingly, although studies link undernutrition and malnutrition with pressure ulcer development, research indicates that nutrition therapy has small effects on prevention and treatment of pressure ulcers.[1] Strong research trials are needed to show the benefits of nutrition supplements over dietary interventions. Until more research is available, evidence suggests that screening for malnutrition, calculating resting energy expenditure and calorie needs, and monitoring nutrient intake are important to providing nutrition care.[2] Nutrition interventions can help correct undernutrition, dehydration, and weight loss, all underlying causes of pressure ulcers and potential causes of poor wound healing. Because many patients with wounds have comorbidities and other factors that can affect their nutritional status, clinical judgment is needed to develop a plan of nutrition care.

This chapter will outline the relationships between undernutrition, nutritional status, and wound healing and outline a systematic process of evaluating nutritional status. New guidelines for identification of malnutrition will be reviewed, and evidence-based recommendations for nutrition interventions with practical applications for nutrition care will be provided.

In 2014, the European Pressure Ulcer Advisory Panel (EPUAP), the National Pressure Ulcer Advisory Panel (NPUAP), and the Pan Pacific Pressure Ulcer Alliance released the *Prevention and Treatment of Pressure Ulcers: Clinical Practice Guidelines*. The evidence-based *Clinical Practice Guidelines* outline the importance of nutrition screening, assessment, care planning, and interventions to address undernutrition and prevent and treat pressure ulcers. They also categorize Strengths of Evidence and Strengths of Recommendations as outlined in Table 1. In most of the nutrition recommendations, but not all, Strength of Evidence is supported by indirect evidence rather than direct evidence. When appropriate, Strengths of Evidence and Strengths of Recommendations are mentioned throughout this chapter.

Registered dietitian nutritionists (RDNs) use the Academy of Nutrition and Dietetics (Academy) Nutrition Care Process to assess, diagnose, and follow up on residents at nutritional risk. RDNs incorporate the recommendations from the *Clinical Practice Guidelines* into the appropriate steps of the nutrition care process to develop a plan of nutrition care, as is outlined in Table 2. Information on the nutrition care process can be found at http://www.eatrightpro.org/resources/practice/nutrition-care-process.

I. Case study

Mr. Jones is an 87-year-old man who was admitted to a skilled nursing facility with a stage 2 pressure ulcer on his coccyx. His admission height was 72 inches, weight was 144 pounds, and body mass index was 19.5, which was within normal limits for his weight history. His diagnosis included type 2 diabetes mellitus, chronic obstructive pulmonary disease (COPD), and stage 3 chronic kidney disease. Medications included Levemir, Metformin, and Risperdal. He was admitted from the hospital on a low concentrated sweets (LCS) diet. His

TABLE 1. *Prevention and Treatment of Pressure Ulcers: Clinical Practice Guidelines* Strengths of evidence and strengths of recommendations [6]

STRENGTHS OF EVIDENCE

A. The recommendation is supported by direct scientific evidence from properly designed and implemented controlled trials on pressure ulcers in humans (or humans at risk for pressure ulcers), providing statistical results that consistently support the recommendation.

B. The recommendation is supported by direct scientific evidence from properly designed and implemented clinical series on pressure ulcers in humans (or humans at risk for pressure ulcers), providing statistical results that consistently support the recommendation.

C. The recommendation is supported by indirect evidence (i.e., studies in healthy humans, humans with other types of chronic wounds, animal models) and/or expert opinion.

STRENGTHS OF RECOMMENDATION

Strong Positive Recommendation: definitely do it

Weak Positive Recommendation: probably do it

No Specific Recommendation

Weak Negative Recommendation: probably don't do it

Strong Negative Recommendation: definitely don't do it

Reprinted with permission from NPUAP.

TABLE 2. The nutrition care process[7]

THE NUTRITION CARE PROCESS CONSISTS OF DISTINCT, INTERRELATED STEPS:

- **Nutrition Assessment:** The RDN collects and documents information such as food or nutrition-related history; biochemical data, medical tests and procedures; anthropometric measurements; nutrition-focused physical findings; and client history.
- **Diagnosis:** Data collected during the nutrition assessment guides the RDN in selection of the appropriate nutrition diagnosis (i.e., naming the specific problem).
- **Intervention:** The RDN then selects the nutrition intervention that will be directed to the root cause (or etiology) of the nutrition problem and aimed at alleviating the signs and symptoms of the diagnosis.
- **Monitoring/Evaluation:** The final step of the process is monitoring and evaluation, which the RDN uses to determine if the patient/client has achieved, or is making progress toward, the planned goals.

A1C was 7.5 and his blood sugars were usually 175-250. After one week in the facility, his pressure ulcer advanced to a stage 3 and he weighed 140 pounds. His documented meal intake was 25-50% of meals, but he drank at least 480 mL fluid per meal, sometimes much more.

The facility registered dietitian nutritionist completed a nutrition assessment and identified that Mr. Jones' protein and calorie intake was inadequate. She recommended that the LCS diet be discontinued and also recommended the addition of a multivitamin supplement and a high-protein, high-calorie oral nutrition supplement one time daily (HS). The patient's food preferences were revisited, and several foods Mr. Jones did not like were forwarded to the facility's kitchen.

Mr. Jones was weighed weekly, and the wound was evaluated weekly using the PUSH (Pressure Ulcer Scale for Healing) scale. After two weeks, his meal intake had not improved, his wound was not improving, and he had lost weight to 138 pounds. The registered dietitian nutritionist recommended supplements be increased to twice daily (BID). Over the next few weeks, he was closely monitored and began to eat more at meals, drink his supplements, and regain the weight he had lost to reach his baseline of 145. PUSH scores began to improve, and over several weeks, the wound progressed very slowly but never healed before he suffered cardiac arrest and died. His blood sugars and A1C remained elevated during his entire stay at the facility.

II. Pathway

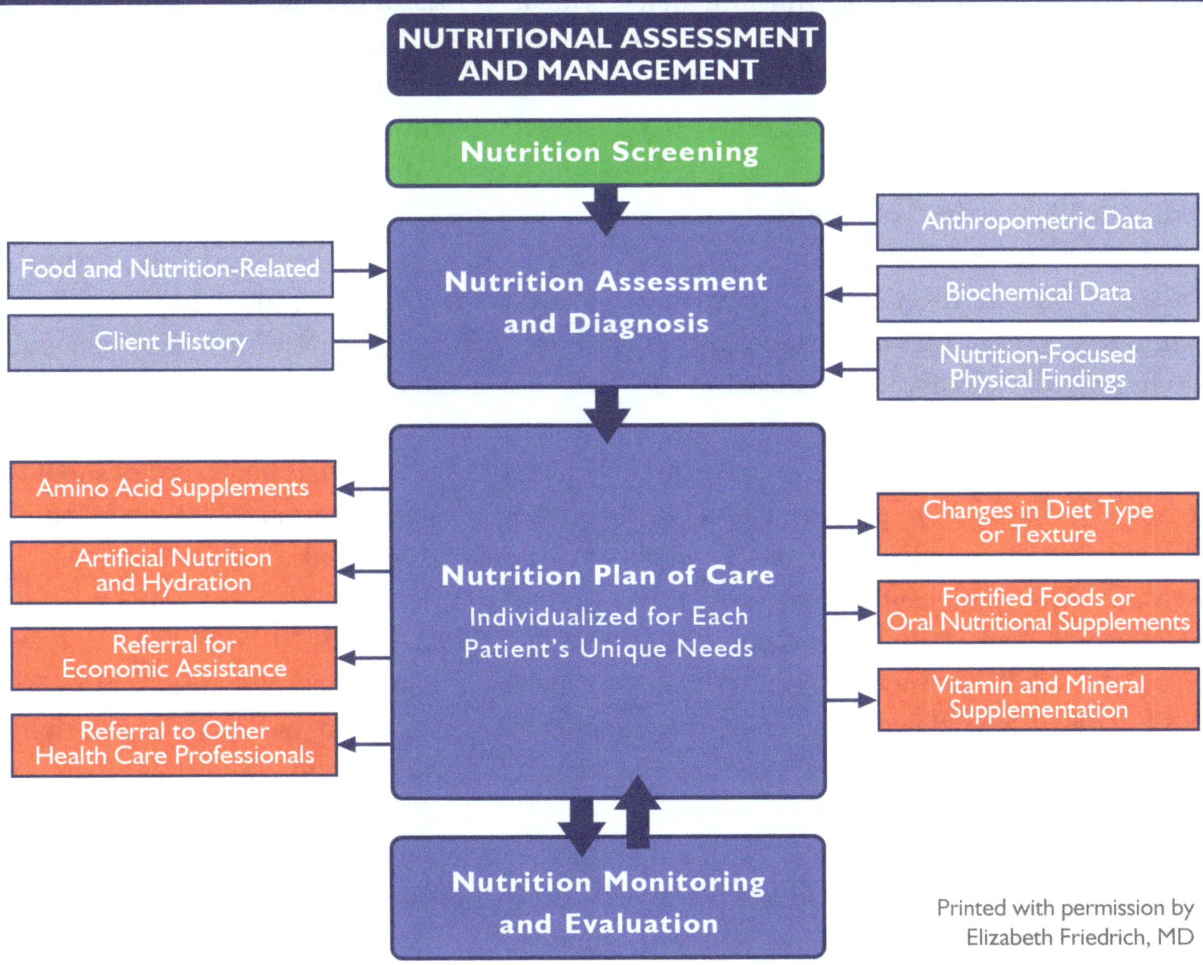

Printed with permission by Elizabeth Friedrich, MD

III. Overview of nutrition and wound healing

Most of the research investigating the relationship between nutrition and wound prevention and healing has focused on pressure ulcers rather than other types of wounds.[8] Because this knowledge has been inferred from management of pressure ulcers, it may not be relevant to the patient with other kinds of chronic wounds.[9]

It is clear that nutritional status is important to skin integrity. Nutrition and hydration are important to support tissue viability and repair for pressure ulcer healing.[10] Both inadequate nutritional intake and poor nutritional status have been shown to correlate with the development of pressure ulcers and pressure ulcer healing.[6] Malnutrition or nutrient deficiencies have been found to impair wound healing by affecting collagen synthesis, prolonging inflammation, decreasing phagocytosis, causing dysfunction of B and T cells, and decreasing the mechanical strength of the skin.[11-12] Unintentional weight loss, often associated with malnutrition, is associated with higher risks of infection, muscle wasting, decreased immune competence, and increased risks of infection,[13-14] potentially affecting wound healing. Malnutrition in combination with other comorbidities increases risk of pressure ulcer development.[15]

A well-nourished patient can become malnourished during a short period of time due to the increased metabolic needs of an injury or sepsis.[9] Any significant wound leads to a hypermetabolic and catabolic state, increasing nutritional needs[16] and increasing risk of muscle and body fat breakdown to meet increased energy requirements.[2] Pressure ulcers can lead to catabolism, which can result in increased inflammation and cachexia.[2]

The stress response to injury and/or protein energy malnutrition will affect wound healing.[16] If intake of calories is not adequate, protein stored in the body (such as in the muscle) will be used for energy, resulting in a loss of lean body mass (LBM). When this occurs, wound healing can be difficult or new wounds can develop.[16] If the stress response and protein energy malnutrition occurs simultaneously, wound healing can be difficult.[16] An adequate intake of protein, calories, vitamins, minerals, and fluids can help assure that the body has the nutrients needed both to support the body during periods of stress and to support healing of acute and chronic wounds.

IV. Nutrients needed to support wound healing

A. Energy

Energy (measured in the form of calories) is needed for the human body to function. Individuals at risk for malnutrition or pressure ulcer, or who have existing wounds, need additional calories to compensate for increased metabolic stress.[17] Energy is consumed in the form of protein, carbohydrates, and fat. Normally dietary carbohydrates and fat fuel the energy pathway, sparing protein for other roles.[10] Approximately 50% to 60% of total calorie intake should come from carbohydrates,[17] with a focus on nutrient-dense carbohydrates as outlined in Table 3. The remainder of calories should come from protein and fat. Enough total calories should be provided to prevent amino acids from being used to support calorie needs.[9]

B. Protein and amino acids

Protein is responsible for the synthesis of enzymes involved in healing, cell multiplication, and collagen and connective tissue synthesis.[10] It is essential for promoting positive nitrogen balance. When consumed in the diet, it is metabolized into amino acids and peptides, and under normal metabolic circumstances very small amounts are used for energy.[16] As has been previously stated, activation of the stress response, such as a wound or during starvation, will result in body protein being burned for fuel,[16] resulting in a change in the body composition and loss of lean body mass. Dietary protein is especially important in frail and older adults because of metabolic changes and loss of lean body mass associated with aging (sarcopenia) and reduced activity levels.[10] Good sources of protein are outlined in Table 3.

Amino acids are the building blocks of proteins. When the body is under stress, several amino acids (glutamine, cysteine, and arginine) become conditionally indispensable because body stores become depleted and demand increases.[17] Glutamine has direct immunological function and has anti-catabolic and anabolic properties.[16] Arginine has been shown to stimulate immune function and is used for a variety of components of healing,[16] including as a substrate for collagen and anti-oxidation through the formation of nitric oxide.[2] Growing moderate-quality evidence supports a positive effect of nutritional supplementation with additional protein, arginine, and micronutrients to

TABLE 3. Nutrient-dense foods that contain nutrients needed to support wound healing[26-31]

Nutrient	Dietary Sources
Carbohydrate	Carbohydrates include whole grains and enriched grains, fruits, and vegetables. Choose complex carbohydrates (as opposed to those containing sugar but few nutrients, such as sugar and sugar-sweetened foods and beverages) because they contain dietary fiber, vitamins, and minerals.
Protein	Meats, fish, poultry, eggs, legumes, nuts, seeds, soy products (soy beans, edamame, tofu, tempeh, textured vegetable protein), and dairy products (milk, yogurt, and cheese) are all good sources of protein. Lower-fat meat and/or dairy products contain fewer calories than their full-fat counterparts.
Fat	Many foods naturally contain fats, including many meats, eggs, and dairy foods. Other sources of fat include margarine, butter, salad dressings, vegetable oils, and many baked goods.
Fluid	Nutrient–dense fluids are suggested, including 100% fruit juices, milk, and beverages containing those ingredients. Some foods are high in fluid, including soups and stews and moist fruit like watermelon. Oral nutritional supplements are high in fluid.
Vitamin C	Good sources include citrus fruits and juices, fortified juices, tomatoes, strawberries, raspberries, blueberries, cranberries, cantaloupe, mango, papaya, watermelon, broccoli, brussels sprouts, cauliflower, green and red peppers, spinach, cabbage, turnip greens and other leafy greens, sweet and white potatoes, tomatoes and tomato juice, winter squash.
Vitamin A	Liver, fish oils, milk and eggs, fish, leafy green vegetables, orange and yellow vegetables, tomato products, fruits, and some vegetable oils are good sources of Vitamin A.
Vitamin E	Nuts, seeds, and vegetable oils, green leafy vegetables and fortified cereals are good sources of Vitamin E.
Zinc	Oysters, red meat, and poultry provide the majority of zinc in the American diet. Beans, nuts, certain types of seafood (such as crab and lobster), whole grains, fortified breakfast cereals, and dairy products also contain zinc.
Iron	Good sources include lean meat and seafood, nuts, beans, vegetables, and fortified grain products.

Reprinted from public domain, National Institute for Health.

promote pressure ulcer healing.[6] In a 12-week study in four nursing homes, rate of pressure ulcer healing was accelerated when a nutritional formula enhanced with protein, arginine, zinc, and vitamin C was consumed at least daily for eight weeks.[18] Other studies have had similar results.[19,20,21] According to Little,[2] the study quality in some studies is poor, and mixed formulations make it difficult to make firm conclusions regarding the exact substance leading to the improved outcomes. The *Prevention and Treatment of Pressure Ulcers: Clinical Practice Guidelines*[6] recommended oral nutritional supplements containing protein and/or supplemental arginine under certain circumstances, citing a weak positive recommendation, as will be outlined later in this chapter.

C. Fat and fat-soluble vitamins

Dietary fat is the most concentrated source of energy consumed in the diet and is a source of the fat-soluble vitamins A, D, E, and K. Sources of dietary fat are outlined in Table 3. Stored body fat provides a reserve source of energy if it is needed. Adequate fat, whether consumed or obtained from the fat stores in the body, is essential to healing of both acute and chronic wounds, to provide energy, and to provide a substrate for the roles of fat by-products in wound healing.[16] Immuno-nutrition that includes long-chain omega-3 fatty acids has been found to be cost effective in pressure ulcer prevention and treatment in critical care patients.[22] Research on specific fatty acid supplementation, the ratio of omega-6 to omega-3 fatty acids in the diet, and when to supplement in relation to wound healing progression is needed.[9]

D. Micronutrients

Micronutrients are essential for cellular function, and several have been connected with wound healing. Dietary sources of these micronutrients are outlined in Table 3. Vitamin A is responsible for epithelium maintenance and stimulates cellular differentiation. Vitamin A deficiency may result in delayed wound healing and increased susceptibility to infection, but limited research is available to support megadoses of vitamin A to support wound healing.[17] Vitamin C is essential for collagen synthesis and is an antioxidant.[6] A deficiency of vitamin C prolongs healing and contributes to reduced resistance to infection.[17] However, there is no evidence that supplementing vitamin C accelerates wound healing in patients who are not deficient in vitamin C.[1] B vitamins are needed for the production of energy from glucose, amino acids, and fat but do not appear to have a specific role in wound healing. Vitamin E is responsible for normal fat metabolism and collagen synthesis and is involved in immune function, but a deficiency does not appear to play an active role in wound healing.[23]

Zinc is a cofactor for collagen formation and has other roles in the body, including assisting in immune function and cell proliferation. Zinc deficiency has adverse effects on the healing process[16] and has been associated with delayed wound healing. The benefit of supplementing with zinc to improve wound healing has not been demonstrated.[1] High serum zinc levels may inhibit healing, impair phagocytosis, and interfere with copper metabolism.[17]

E. Fluid

Water constitutes about 60% of the adult body weight and serves many vital functions in the wound healing process, including aiding in hydration of wound sites and oxygen perfusion; acting as a solvent for vitamins and minerals, amino acids, glucose, and other small molecules; transporting vital materials to cells; and removing waste from cells.[17] Dehydration can contribute to poor wound healing, and poor hydration impairs skin turgor, leaving tissue vulnerable to new breakdown.[24] Individuals with draining wounds, diarrhea, vomiting, or increased perspiration may need additional fluids. Air-fluidized beds may increase fluid needs.[17] Fluid needs can be met by both liquids (including oral nutritional supplements) and foods consumed. Oral nutritional supplements and enteral feedings are usually 75% water,[6] and an estimated 19-27% of fluids are obtained through food.[25]

V. Nutrition screening and assessment

A. Nutrition screening

Nutrition screening is the process used to identify individuals who need a comprehensive nutrition assessment due to characteristics that put them at potential nutritional risk. According to the *Prevention and Treatment of Pressure Ulcers: Clinical Practice Guidelines*,[6] individuals at risk or with a pressure ulcer should be screened:

- at admission to a health-care setting;
- with each significant change in clinical condition; and
- when progress toward pressure ulcer closure is not observed (*Strength of Evidence = C, Strength of Recommendation = weak positive, probably do it).*

A valid and reliable nutrition screening tool should be used to determine nutritional risk (*Strength of Evidence = C, Strength of Recommendation = weak positive, probably do it*). Screening tools vary but are typically short questionnaires that evaluate weight history, food intake, and other factors that might contribute to undernutrition. A number of validated screening tools are available, including the Mini Nutritional Assessment (MNA), the Malnutrition Universal Screening Tool (MUST), the Malnutrition Screening Tool (MST), the Nutrition Risk Screening (NRS), the Short Nutritional Assessment Questionnaire (SNAQ), and the Subjective Global Assessment (SGA). Nutrition screening tools can be obtained online as outlined in Table 4.

When a screening tool triggers a risk for undernutrition or unintended weight loss, referral to a registered dietitian nutritionist (RDN) for nutrition assessment is recommended. Conditions that require nutrition assessment include the following:[17]

- Unintended weight loss: 5% in 30 days or 10% in 180 days;

TABLE 4. Validated nutrition screening tools available online

Mini Nutritional Assessment: http://www.mna-elderly.com/
Malnutrition Universal Screening Tool: http://www.bapen.org.uk/screening-and-must/must/introducing-must
Malnutrition Screening Tool: http://static.abbottnutrition.com/cms-prod/abbottnutrition.com/img/Malnutrition%20Screening%20Tool_FINAL.pdf
Nutrition Risk Screening: http://espen.info/documents/Screening.pdf
Short Nutritional Assessment Questionnaire: http://www.fightmalnutrition.eu/fileadmin/content/malnutrition/Screening_tools/SNAQ_Engels.pdf
Subjective Global Assessment: http://subjectiveglobalassessment.com/about-us

- Diseases and conditions including diabetes, malabsorption, dementia, chronic obstructive pulmonary disease (COPD), cancer, or renal disease;
- Immobility and/or inactivity, including hip fracture, spinal cord injury, or stroke;
- Chewing or swallowing problems resulting from stroke, Parkinson's disease, cerebral palsy, or other conditions;
- Decline in appetite, anorexia, poor food and/or fluid intake;
- Adverse effects of medications.

B. Nutrition assessment

A comprehensive assessment can be used to help identify nutrition diagnosis and areas for intervention and set the stage for developing a plan of care. The focus of nutrition assessment should be on evaluating energy intake, unintended weight change, and the effect of psychological stress or neuropsychological problems.[6] The *Prevention and Treatment of Pressure Ulcers: Clinical Practice Guidelines*[6] indicate that nutrition assessment should:

1. assess the weight status of each individual to determine weight history and identify significant weight loss (≥5% in 30 days or ≥10% in 180 days) (*Strength of Evidence = C, Strength of Recommendation = weak positive, probably do it*);
2. assess the individual's ability to eat independently (*Strength of Evidence = C, Strength of Recommendation = strong positive, definitely do it*); and
3. assess the adequacy of total nutrient intake (i.e., food, fluid, oral supplements, and enteral/parenteral feeds) (*Strength of Evidence = C, Strength of Recommendation = strong positive, definitely do it*).

C. Using nutrition assessment to identify protein energy malnutrition (PEM)

The term "malnutrition" (also known as undernutrition) has been used widely in conjunction with pressure ulcers. Adult undernutrition can result from inadequate intake and/or increased nutrient needs, impaired nutrient absorption or transport, and altered nutrient utilization.[32] Weight loss frequently occurs when a person is not adequately nourished. Individuals with malnutrition may present with inflammatory, hypermetabolic, and/or hypercatabolic conditions.

In the past decade, the clinical definition of malnutrition has changed.[32] Historically, laboratory tests (including low serum albumin and prealbumin levels) were used to identify undernutrition. Current research indicates that serum albumin and prealbumin increase or decrease because they are negative acute-phase reactants, falling in the presence of inflammation and rising when inflammation subsides,[10,32] not because of changes in nutrient intake. Serum albumin and preabumin may be useful in establishing an individual's overall prognosis but may not correlate well with clinical observation of nutritional status.[6,32-34]

As a result of the changing paradigm about serum proteins and malnutrition, the scientific community sought new ways to diagnosis malnutrition/undernutrition. In 2009, three etiology-based definitions of malnutrition were published:[35]

1. Starvation-related malnutrition (pure chronic starvation, anorexia nervosa)
2. Chronic disease-related malnutrition (organ failure, pancreatic cancer, rheumatoid arthritis, sarcopenic obesity)
3. Acute disease or injury-related malnutrition (major infection, burns, trauma, closed head injury)

In 2012 the Academy of Nutrition and Dietetics (Academy) and American Society of Parenteral and Enteral Nutrition (ASPEN) published a consensus statement recommending characteristics for the identification and documentation of adult malnutrition (undernutrition). Rather than using inflammatory biomarkers (albumin and prealbumin) for diagnosis of malnutrition, it is suggested that adult malnutrition be identified when two or more of the following criteria are present:[32]

1. **Insufficient energy intake.** Malnutrition is the result of inadequate food and nutrient intake or assimilation. Recent intake as compared to estimated needs is a criterion to determine malnutrition.

2. **Interpretation of weight loss.** Loss of weight is evaluated, considering comorbidities and hydration status. Weight should be measured regularly by medical providers for both community-dwelling adults and those residing in health care communities.

3. **Loss of subcutaneous fat.** This is identified by nutrition-focused physical assessment, such as orbital fat or fat overlying the ribs.

4. **Loss of muscle mass. This is i**dentified by nutrition-focused physical assessment when examining deltoids, scapula, quadriceps, and other muscle groups.

5. **Localized or generalized fluid accumulation.** This is identified by nutrition-focused physical assessment such as edema in the extremities or ascites. Edema may sometimes mask weight loss.

6. **Diminished functional status as measured by hand grip strength.** A dynamometer, used to measure hand grip strength, can indicate a loss of functional status.

It is recommended that clinicians, health-care facilities, and health-care communities incorporate these concepts into their assessment and diagnosis of malnutrition.[32]

VI. Components of a comprehensive nutrition assessment

A comprehensive nutrition assessment includes the following components:[7]

- **Food and nutrition-related history,** which provides information about an individual's eating habits, food preferences, food allergies or intolerances, intake, and use of oral nutrition supplements, herbal supplements, or vitamin and mineral supplements. Tracking of food and fluid intake using food diaries (community dwelling persons) or meal intake reporting (for those residing in health-care communities) is especially useful over time. Difficulty chewing or swallowing may also be identified, as may be a compromised ability to perform activities of daily living (ADLs) or instrumental activities of daily living (IADLs) that might affect food intake.

- **Biochemical data, medical tests, and procedures,** which can be useful to help identify nutrition problems and evaluate interventions. Medical tests or procedures might include gastric emptying time or resting metabolic rate. Routine biochemical testing often includes serum electrolytes, fasting blood sugar and A1C, renal function tests, and complete blood count (CBC). Undernutrition or malnutrition should not be diagnosed based on albumin and/or prealbumin; when these levels are low, they are indicators of morbidity and/or mortality but not of nutritional status.[32]

- **Anthropometric data,** such as height and weight, is used to estimate daily protein, calorie, and fluid needs and evaluate nutritional status over time. Serial weight measurements are important to help identify both insidious (slow) and significant weight loss. Significant unintended weight loss can be an indicator of dehydration or malnutrition and increases the risk of mortality. The Centers for Medicare and Medicaid Services defines significant weight loss as 5% of body weight in one month, 7.5% of body weight in three months, or 10% of body weight in six months.[36]

  Height and weight can be used to calculate body mass index (BMI). Individuals with a low BMI may be at increased risk for pressure ulcers.[37] Table 5 provides guidelines for interpretation of BMI. The formula to calculate BMI is weight (kg) / [height (m)]^2. Practitioners may find it easier to use a BMI calculator such as the one available at http://www.cdc.gov/healthyweight/assessing/bmi/adult_bmi/english_bmi_calculator/bmi_calculator.html. BMI will be calculated by entering height and weight when prompted.

TABLE 5. Interpreting BMI[38]

BMI	Weight Status
Below 18.5	Underweight
18.5-24.0	Normal or Healthy Weight
25.0-29.9	Overweight
30.0 and above	Obese

Reprinted from public domain.
Center for Disease Control and Prevention.

- **Nutrition-focused physical findings,** an assessment that includes vital signs; evaluation of condition of skin, hair, and nails; presence of edema; and presence of muscle wasting. Nutrition-focused physical assessment can be based on findings from a physical exam, patient interview, or the medical record review.[7] A nutrition-focused physical examination should evaluate overall appearance and include examination of the hair, skin, mouth, nails, abdomen, and extremities.[39] Physical condition can identify a number of medical problems such as dehydration (dry skin, cracked lips, poor skin turgor), deficiency of B vitamins (cheilosis, sore mouth, burning tongue), and other nutritional deficits. Traditionally, physicians, nurses, and other health-care providers perform physical assessment, but nutrition-focused physical assessment has been part of the dietetic curriculum since 1997,[40] and dietetics practitioners are incorporating it into their clinical practice.

- **Client history**, which can provide valuable information such as personal health and medical history, family history, treatments and complementary or alternative medicine use, and social history. If an individual is unable to provide information, it is useful to gather information from family members if possible.

A comprehensive nutrition assessment always includes an evaluation of current diet and food, fluid, and supplement consumption to determine if an individual's intake meets his or her estimated needs.

VII. Nutrition diagnosis

Nutrition and dietetic practitioners use nutrition assessment data to identify and label a patient's nutrition diagnosis. A nutrition diagnosis includes a PES (Problem, Etiology, Signs and Symptoms) statement to describe the problem, its root cause, and the assessment data that provide evidence for the nutrition diagnosis.[7] Standardized terminology has been developed and is categorized into three domains: intake, clinical, and behavioral.[7] Individuals with pressure ulcers could have any number of different nutrition diagnoses related to any of the three domains. One example of a nutrition diagnosis is *increased nutrient needs (protein and energy) related to increased demand for wound healing as evidenced by the presence of a stage 4 pressure ulcer.*

VIII. Nutrition intervention: using *Clinical Practice Guidelines* to estimate nutritional needs

Prevention and Treatment of Pressure Ulcers: Clinical Practice Guidelines recommends that an individualized care plan for individuals with or at risk of a pressure ulcer be developed (*Strength of Evidence = C, Strength of Recommendation = weak positive, probably do it*).[6] A registered dietitian nutritionist should be part of the interdisciplinary team that develops that plan of care based on the nutritional assessment.[7] The following guidelines for nutrient intake are adapted (with permission) from *Clinical Practice Guidelines*. The full guidelines can be accessed at http://international-pressure-ulcer-guidelines.myshopify.com/.

A. Energy intake

- Provide 30 to 35 kcal/kg body weight for adults at risk of a pressure ulcer who are assessed to be at risk of malnutrition (*Strength of Evidence = C, Strength of Recommendation = weak positive, probably do it*).
- Provide 30 to 35 kcal/kg body weight for adults with a pressure ulcer who are assessed to be at risk of malnutrition (*Strength of Evidence = C, Strength of Recommendation = weak positive, probably do it*).
- Adjust energy intake based on weight change or level or obesity. Adults who are underweight or obese or who have significant unintended weight loss may need additional energy intake (*Strength of Evidence = C, Strength of Recommendation = strong positive, definitely do it*).
- Revise and modify/liberalize dietary restrictions when limitations result in a decreased food and fluid intake, in consultation with a medical professional and managed by a registered dietitian nutritionist whenever possible. (*Strength of Evidence = C, Strength of Recommendation = weak positive, probably do it*).
- Offer fortified foods and/or high-calorie, high-protein oral nutritional supplements between meals if nutritional requirements cannot be achieved by dietary intake (*Strength of Evidence = B, Strength of Recommendation = strong positive, definitely do it*).

- Consider enteral or parenteral nutritional support when oral intake is inadequate, when consistent with the individual's goals of care (*Strength of Evidence = C, Strength of Recommendation = weak positive, probably do it*).

B. Protein intake

- Provide adequate protein for positive nitrogen balance for adults to be assessed at risk of a pressure ulcer (*Strength of Evidence = C, Strength of Recommendation = weak positive, probably do it*).
- Offer 1.25 to 1.5 grams of protein/kg body weight for adults at risk of a pressure ulcer who are assessed to be at risk of malnutrition when compatible with goals of care. Reassess as condition changes (*Strength of Evidence = C, Strength of Recommendation = weak positive, probably do it*).
- Provide adequate protein for positive nitrogen balance for adults with a pressure ulcer (*Strength of Evidence = B, Strength of Recommendation= weak positive, probably do it*).
- Offer 1.25 to 1.5 grams of protein/kg body weight daily for adults with an existing pressure ulcer who are assessed to be at risk for malnutrition, when compatible with goals of care. Reassess as condition changes (*Strength of Evidence = B, Strength of Recommendation = weak positive, probably do it*).
- Offer high-calorie, high-protein nutritional requirements in addition to the usual diet to adults with nutritional risk and pressure ulcer risk, if nutritional requirements cannot be achieved by dietary intake (*Strength of Evidence = A, Strength of Recommendation = weak positive, probably do it*).
- Assess renal function to ensure that high levels of protein are appropriate for the individual (*Strength of Evidence = C, Strength of Recommendation = strong positive, definitely do it*).
- Supplement with high protein, arginine, and micronutrients for adults with a pressure ulcer Category III or IV with multiple pressure ulcers when nutritional requirements cannot be met with traditional high-calorie and protein supplements (*Strength of Evidence = B, Strength of Recommendation = weak positive, probably do it*).

C. Hydration

- Provide and encourage adequate daily fluid intake for hydration for an individual assessed to be at risk of or with a pressure ulcer, consistent with comorbid conditions and goals (*Strength of Evidence = C, Strength of Recommendation = strong positive, definitely do it*).
- Monitor individuals for signs and symptoms of dehydration, including changes in weight, skin turgor, urine output, elevated serum sodium, and/or calculated serum osmolality (*Strength of Evidence = C, Strength of Recommendation = weak positive, probably do it*).
- Provide additional fluid for individuals with dehydration, elevated temperature, vomiting, profuse sweating, diarrhea, or heavily exuding wounds (*Strength of Evidence = C, Strength of Recommendation = strong positive, definitely do it*).

D. Vitamins and minerals

- Provide/encourage an individual assessed to be at risk of pressure ulcers to consume a balanced diet that includes good sources of vitamins and minerals *(Strength of Evidence = C, Strength of Recommendation = strong positive, definitely do it).*

- Provide/encourage an individual assessed to be at risk of a pressure ulcer to take vitamin and mineral supplements when dietary intake is poor or deficiencies are confirmed or suspected (*Strength of Evidence = C, Strength of Recommendation = weak positive, probably do it).*

- Provide/encourage an individual with a pressure ulcer to consume a balanced diet that includes good sources of vitamins and minerals (*Strength of Evidence = B, Strength of Recommendation = strong positive, probably do it)*

- Provide/encourage an individual with a pressure ulcer to take vitamin and mineral supplements when dietary intake is poor and/or deficiencies are confirmed or suspected (*Strength of Evidence = B, Strength of Recommendation = weak positive, probably do it).*

IX. Nutrition interventions for specific situations

A. Obesity

Overweight and obesity are defined by body mass index as outlined in Table 5. Obesity is associated with skin and tissue health problems and disease; however, precise causal relationships between obesity and pressure ulcer development are unclear.[7]

Estimating nutritional needs for obese individuals can be challenging. Currently there is limited evidence-based research to suggest one method of mathematical calculations for protein and fluids to meet the estimated needs for all obese individuals. There are no studies that specifically address the obese individual with pressure ulcers, so research is needed to define appropriate protein and calorie intake for these individuals.[41] Recommendations for estimating nutritional needs for the obese patient will continue to evolve as evidence-based research becomes available.

Calorie needs for healthy obese individuals are most accurately estimated by the Mifflin St. Joer equation,[42] but it is unclear if this formula provides adequate calories for those with wounds. Use of the NPUAP's recommendations of 30-35 kcal/kg body weight is suggested, but clinical judgment to determine calorie needs is necessary based on nutrition assessment, monitoring, and evaluation of wound healing. Goals of weight loss may need to be postponed or modified to ensure that adequate nutrients are provided for healing.[6]

B. Diabetes

Hyperglycemia and altered immune function may contribute to poor wound healing in patients with diabetes.[43-44] Appropriate nutrition intervention can help promote blood glucose control and simultaneously provide enough nutrients to support wound healing. According to the American Diabetes Association, there is no one-size-fits-all eating pattern for individuals with diabetes.[45] Nutrition intervention should promote and support healthful eating patterns, emphasizing a variety of nutrient-dense foods in appropriate portion sizes, in order to improve overall health; achieve and maintain body weight goals; attain individualized glycemic, blood pressure, and lipid goals; and delay or prevent complications of diabetes.[45] Individual nutrition needs should be based on personal and cultural preferences, health literacy, access to healthful foods, willingness and ability to make behavioral changes, and barriers to change.[45] An eating pattern that is consistent in carbohydrate intake (incorporating carbohydrates daily at each meal and snack) is recommended.[17]

Older adults who are functional and cognitively intact and have significant life expectancy may receive diabetes care with goals similar to those developed for younger adults.[45] Frail older adults with functional cognitive impairments and/or limited life expectancy may benefit from liberalized goals for glycemic control.[46] Hypoglycemia and hyperglycemia should be screened for and managed by adjusting glycemic targets and pharmacological interventions.

C. Chronic kidney disease (CKD)

The presence of kidney disease can complicate nutrition care of the individual with wounds. Comorbidities such as pressure ulcers and diabetes result in conflicting nutritional needs. Stage 3 or 4 CKD may require a restriction of calories, protein, potassium, sodium, and fluids that conflicts with the recommended increase in calorie and protein needs needed to support wound healing. Renal function should be assessed to determine if high levels of protein are appropriate.[6] Consultation with a registered dietitian nutritionist is essential when treating individuals with CKD and wounds so that priorities can be established and appropriate interventions put in place.

D. Enteral nutrition

When an individual is unwilling and/or unable to consume food and fluid orally, enteral nutrition may be considered. Enteral nutrition (tube feeding) is preferred over parenteral nutrition. The risks and benefits of tube feeding vary for each individual. Factors to consider before recommending tube feeding include the following:

- Does the individual have a living will or other advance directives on file indicating his or her wishes regarding tube feeding?
- Does the individual have religious beliefs that provide guidance for the initiation or withholding of tube feeding?
- From a medical standpoint, is the individual a candidate for tube feeding?
- Will the benefits of tube feeding outweigh the risks?
- Does the individual understand the risks and benefits of tube feeding?

Only a few recent studies have evaluated the effect of enteral nutrition on pressure ulcer prevention or treatment, and their results have been disappointing.[39] In one study of 49 long-term care patients, increasing protein intake with tube feeding had minimal effect on outcome.[47] An observational trial of long-term care residents hospitalized for a percutaneous endoscopic gastrostomy (PEG) placement found that residents with a pressure ulcer were 2.3 times more likely to develop a new pressure ulcer, and existing pressure ulcers were 30% less likely to heal.[48] A meta-analysis that reviewed high-quality research trials could not draw conclusions on the effect of enteral or parenteral nutrition on pressure ulcer prevention or treatment.[49]

E. End of life

When a patient is terminally ill, pressure ulcers may not be preventable and may be difficult to heal because of multiple comorbidities.[50] Several risk factors place the palliative care patient at increased risk for pressure ulcer development and poor healing, including undernutrition. Catabolism often occurs near the end of life and can result in weakness and weight loss.[50] Poor food and fluid intake is common and may occur weeks to months before death.[51] Near the end of life, maintaining nutrition and hydration is not always an achievable goal.[50] Because comfort is of utmost importance, goals of therapy should be directed at managing symptoms rather than reversing nutritional deficits.[52]

Near the end of life, oral feeding may be one of the few remaining pleasures for an individual. To help assure the best quality of life, favorite foods and fluids (whatever is tolerable or acceptable to each individual) should be provided at the appropriate textures and liquid consistencies for easiest consumption and swallowing safety. If an individual needs to be fed, food and fluids should be offered but not forced.

X. Translating evidence-based recommendations into a plan of care

A. Guidelines for healthy eating

To prevent and/or treat pressure ulcers, clinical recommendations of nutritional needs become food (and nutrients) available for consumption. Table 3 outlines nutrient-dense foods that are good sources of key nutrients to support wound healing. Food intake can be impacted by a variety of factors, including medical comorbidities, chewing or swallowing problems, ability to perform activities of daily living (ADLs), socioeconomic status, and food preferences and habits. As a result, nutrition interventions don't always follow a defined clinical pathway but must be tailored to meet the unique needs of each individual.

A 125-pound (57-kg) woman with stage 3 wounds has the following estimated needs (based on the *Clinical Practice Guidelines*):

- 1710-1995 kcal/day (30-35 kcal/kg)
- 71-86 grams of protein/day (1.25-1.5 g/kg), or 10- 12 ounces of meat per day (3 4-ounce servings)
- 1710-1995 mL fluid/day (30-35 mL/kg), or about 7-8 cups of fluid per day

The Dietary Guidelines for Americans (http://health.gov/dietaryguidelines/2015/guidelines/) and ChooseMyPlate (www.choosemyplate.gov) provide a good basis for a healthy eating pattern. The needs of many individuals with pressure ulcers, including the sample patient listed above, can be met through a healthy diet alone, assuming adequate food and fluid intake. ChooseMyPlate can serve as an excellent resource for both health care professionals and consumers. It recommends adults consume a variety of foods from each of the five food groups: lean meats and meat alternatives, low-fat dairy, fruits, vegetables, and grains. The graphic above outlines the basic eating pattern recommended by ChooseMyPlate.[53]

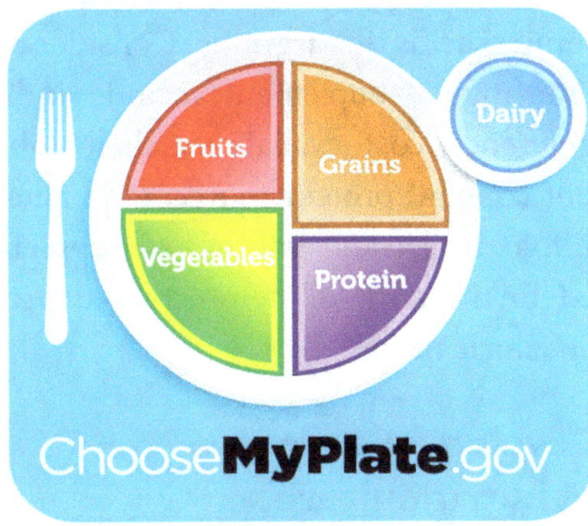

FIGURE 1.
Reprinted from public domain.
U.S. Department of Agriculture, www.choosemyplate.gov.

B. Using food and supplements to increase nutrients available

According to one study, a significant portion of residents at risk for pressure ulcers eat inadequately at meals.[54] When food and fluid is not well-consumed, or nutritional needs can't be met by meals and snacks alone, nutrition interventions are necessary. One way to increase the calorie and/or protein content of the diet is to fortify foods and/or beverages by adding full-fat dairy products, powdered milk, or extra sweeteners to foods that are commonly eaten. Whole milk, homemade milkshakes, and fortified cream soups can be an easy way to increase calories or protein for individuals who will consume those foods. A wide variety of commercial oral nutritional supplements (ONS) are also available in the form of beverages, bars, cookies, and pudding.

Although nutrition therapy has been found to have small effects on prevention and treatment of pressure ulcers,[1] oral nutritional supplementation with high levels of protein and calories has been associated with a reduction in pressure ulcer development compared to routine care[55] and with faster healing.[18] Commercial ONS can provide protein, calories, supplemental vitamins and minerals, and in some cases amino acids like arginine. Considerations for choosing a supplement include individual preference, cost, availability, shelf-stability, nutrient content, protein source, food allergies and intolerances, and volume of supplement needed to meet his or her increased protein and/or calorie needs.

C. Developing a plan of nutrition care

A plan of care should meet an individual's estimated needs, correct nutrition deficits, and support wound healing. Interventions might include but are not limited to the following:

- Individualizing the diet to increase food and/or fluid intake
- Discontinuing a therapeutic diet, especially if intake is poor
- Honoring food preferences
- Addressing food allergies and intolerances
- Assuring favorite foods are available and accessible
- Modifying food texture and fluid consistency if chewing or swallowing problems are affecting food or fluid intake
- Offering high-calorie, high-protein snacks a few times daily
- Offering several small meals daily, if appropriate
- Recommending targeted nutrition interventions as needed, including fortified foods and beverages or oral nutritional supplements, including those containing arginine
- Rotating the type of high-calorie, high-protein snacks or supplements given between meals to prevent flavor fatigue
- Recommending enteral nutrition, if appropriate and consistent with a patient's goals of care
- Providing or encouraging assistance with food shopping, preparation, or eating, as needed
- Improving access to food, especially if financial limitations affect nutritional status
- Providing referral to other health-care providers (such as a speech and language pathologist, occupational therapist, or dentist)
- Providing referral to sources of economic assistance, such as:
  —the Supplemental Nutrition Assistance Program (SNAP) (http://www.fns.usda.gov/snap/supplemental-nutrition-assistance-program-snap)

  —Congregate Nutrition Services and Home-Delivered Nutrition Services

(http://www.aoa.acl.gov/AoA_Programs/HPW/Nutrition_Services/)

—Commodity Supplemental Food Program (http://www.fns.usda.gov/csfp/commodity-supplemental-food-program-csfp

XI. Nutrition monitoring and evaluation

When an individual is at risk for or has a pressure ulcer, nutrition monitoring and evaluation are based on the nutrition diagnosis. Areas that are most relevant to pressure ulcer risk or treatment include weight and weight changes; laboratory tests (nitrogen balance, electrolytes, glucose); nutrient intake, quantity, and quality; wound stage/healing; and hydration status.[56] Based on periodic evaluation, the plan of nutrition care should be changed as necessary.

Summary

Weight loss, protein-calorie malnutrition, and dehydration are all risk factors for undernutrition. A systematic process of nutrition assessment, diagnosis, intervention, monitoring, and evaluation can have a positive effect on nutritional status and the prevention and/or treatment of pressure ulcers. Nutrition care should be individualized; there is not one nutrition clinical pathway for prevention and treatment of pressure ulcers that meets the needs of every individual.

Review questions

1. **Which of the following is not considered an indicator of potential malnutrition in a patient with a pressure ulcer?**

    a. Significant weight loss

    b. Low serum albumin level

    c. Poor intake of food over time

    d. Loss of muscle mass

2. **Patients with pressure ulcers usually need which of the following?**

    a. 1.25 to 1.5 grams of protein per kilogram of body weight

    b. 30-35 calories per kilogram of body weight

    c. Vitamin supplements if a deficiency is confirmed or suspected

    d. All of the above

    e. None of the above

3. **Nutrition assessment involves all of the following factors except:**

    a. Changing nutrition interventions as needed

    b. Evaluating weight status over time

    c. Determining ability to eat independently

    d. Observing adequacy of total nutrient intake

4. ***True/False.*** Evidence indicates that tube feeding usually improves outcomes in patients with stage 4 pressure ulcers.

5. **Which of the following statements about nutrition and wound healing is true?**

    a. Presence of a wound decreases metabolism so fewer calories are needed.

    b. Vitamin C and zinc supplements should be standard protocol to support wound healing.

    c. Most individuals with pressure ulcers will need an increase in calories and protein to help support wound healing.

    d. Fluid intake is not important to wound healing.

ANSWERS: 1) b
2) d
3) a
4) False
5) c

References

1. Thomas D. Role of nutrition in the treatment and prevention of pressure ulcers. Nutr Clin Pract. 2014 Aug;29(4):466-472.
2. Little MO. Nutrition and skin ulcers. Curr Opin Clin Nutr Metab Care. 2014 Jan;16(1):39-49.
3. Guenter P, Malyszek R, Bliss DZ, Steffe T, O'Hara D, Levan F, et al. Survey of nutritional status in newly hospitalized patients with stage III or stage IV pressure ulcers. Adv Skin Wound Care. 2000;14(4):164-168.
4. Mathus-Vliegen E. Nutritional status, nutrition, and pressure ulcers. Nutr Clin Pract. 2001;16:286-291.
5. Thomas DR, Verdery RB, Gardner L, Kant A, Lindsay J. A prospective study of outcome from previous protein-energy malnutrition in nursing home residents. JPEN J Parenter Enteral Nutr. 1991;15(4):400-404.
6. European Pressure Ulcer Advisory Panel; National Pressure Ulcer Advisory Panel; Pan Pacific Pressure Ulcer Alliance. Prevention and treatment of pressure ulcers: clinical practice guideline. Haesler E, editor. Perth (Australia): Cambridge Media; 2014.
7. Nutrition terminology reference manual (eNCPT): dietetics language for nutrition care [Internet]. [Chicago]: Academy of Nutrition and Dietetics [cited 2016 May 22]. Available from: https://ncpt.webauthor.com/.
8. Dorner B, Posthauer ME, Friedrich E. Nutritional assessment and support in relation to wound healing. In: Doughty DB, McNichol LL, editors. Wound, Ostomy and Continence Nurses Society core curriculum: wound management. [place unknown]: Wolters Kluwer; 2016. p. 89-106. Jointly published by the Wound, Ostomy and Continence Nurses Society.
9. Molnar JA, Underdown MJ, Clark WA. Nutrition and chronic wounds. Adv Wound Care. 2014;3(11):663-681.
10. Posthauer ME, Banks M, Dorner B, Schols J. The role of nutrition for pressure ulcer management: National Pressure Ulcer Advisory Panel, European Pressure Ulcer Advisory Panel, and Pan Pacific Pressure Ulcer Alliance white paper. Adv Skin Wound Care. 2015 April;28(4):175-188.
11. Wild T, Rahbarnia A, Kellner M, Sobotka L, Eberlein. Basics in nutrition and wound healing. Nutr. 2010 Sep;26(9):862-6.
12. Stechmiller JK. Understanding the role of nutrition and wound healing. Nutr Clin Pract. 2010;25(10):61-68.
13. Amarel FT, Matos LC, Tavares MM, Subtil A, Martins R, Sousa P. The economic impact of disease-related malnutrition at hospital admission. Clin Nutr. 2007;26:778-784.
14. Salva A, Coll-Planes L, Bruce S, Groot L, Andrieu S, Abellan G, et al. Nutritional assessment of residents in long-term care facilities (LTCFs): recommendations of the task force on nutrition and ageing of the IAGG European region and the IANA. J Nutr Health Aging. 2009;13:475-483.
15. Edsberg LE, Langemo D, Baharestani M, Postahauer ME, Goldberg M. Unavoidable pressure ulcer: state of the science and consensus outcomes. J Wound Ostomy Continence Nurs. 2014:41:313-334.
16. Demling RH. Nutrition, anabolism, and the wound healing process: an overview. Eplasty [Internet]. 2009 Feb 3 [cited 2016 May 3]:65-94. Available from: http://tinyurl.com/zd6mwdl
17. Posthauer ME, Dorner B. Nutrition and wound care. In: Baranoski S, Ayello EA. Wound care essentials: practice principles. [place unknown]: Wolters Kluwer; 2016. p. 227-250.

18. Cereda EA, Gini AM, Pedrolli C, Vanotti A. Disease-specific versus standard, nutritional support for the treatment of pressure ulcers in institutionalized older adults: a randomized controlled trial. J Am Geriatr Soc 2009;57(8):1395-1402.
19. von Anholt R, Sobotka L, Meijer E, Heyman H, Groen H, Topinkova E, et al. Specific nutritional support accelerates pressure ulcer healing and reduces wound care intensity in non-malnourished patients. Nutr. 2010;26(9):867-872.
20. Brewer S, Desneves K, Pearce LO, Mills K, Dunn L, Brown D et al. Effect of an arginine-containing nutritional supplement on pressure ulcer healing in community spinal patients. J Wound Care. 2010;19(7):311-316.
21. Leigh B, Desneves K, Rafferty J, Pearce L, King S, Woodward MC et al. The effect of different doses of an arginine-containing supplement on the healing of pressure ulcers. J Wound Care. 2012;21(3):150-6.
22. Theilla M. Nutrition support for wound healing in the intensive care unit patient. World Rev Nutr Diet. 2013;105:179-189.
23. Waldorf H, Fewekes J. Wound healing. Adv Dermatol. 1995;10:77-96.
24. Langemo DK. Palliative wound care. In: Baronski AS, Ayello EA, editors. Wound care essentials. [place unknown]: Wolters Kluwer; 2016. p. 543-561. Washington (DC): Institute of Medicine, National Academy of Sciences; 2004.
25. Dietary reference intakes for water, potassium, sodium, chloride, and sulfate. Washington (DC): Institute of Medicine, National Academy of Sciences; 2004.
26. Dietary guidelines for Americans 2015–2020 [Internet]. 8th ed. [Rockville (MD)]: Department of Health and Human Services (US), Office of Disease Prevention and Health Promotion; 2015 Dec [cited 2016 May 1]. Available from: http://health.gov/dietaryguidelines/2015/guidelines/. Jointly published by the Department of Agriculture (US).
27. Vitamin C fact sheet for health professionals [Internet]. [Washington (DC)]: Department of Health and Human Services (US), National Institutes of Health, Office of Dietary Supplements [Updated 2016 Feb 11; Cited 2016 May 5]. Available from: https://ods.od.nih.gov/factsheets/VitaminC-HealthProfessional/.
28. Vitamin A fact sheet for health professionals [Internet]. [Washington (DC)]: Department of Health and Human Services (US), National Institutes of Health, Office of Dietary Supplements [Updated 2016 Feb 11; Cited 2016 May 5]. Available from: https://ods.od.nih.gov/factsheets/VitaminA-HealthProfessional/.
29. Zinc fact sheet for health professionals [Internet]. [Washington (DC)]: Department of Health and Human Services (US), National Institutes of Health, Office of Dietary Supplements [Updated 2016 Feb 11; Cited 2016 May 5]. Available from: https://ods.od.nih.gov/factsheets/Zinc-HealthProfessional/.
30. Iron fact sheet for health professionals [Internet]. [Washington (DC)]: Department of Health and Human Services (US), National Institutes of Health, Office of Dietary Supplements [Updated 2016 Feb 11; Cited 2016 May 5]. Available from: https://ods.od.nih.gov/factsheets/Iron-HealthProfessional/.
31. Vitamin E fact sheet for health professionals [Internet]. [Washington (DC)]: Department of Health and Human Services (US), National Institutes of Health, Office of Dietary Supplements [updated 2016 Feb 11; cited 2016 May 5]. Available from: https://ods.od.nih.gov/factsheets/VitaminE-HealthProfessional/.

32. White JV, Guenter P, Jensen G, Malone A, Schofield M. Consensus statement of the Academy of Nutrition and Dietetics/American Society for Parenteral and Enteral Nutrition: characteristics recommended for the identification and documentation of adult malnutrition (undernutrition). J Acad Nutr Diet. 2012;112:730-738.

33. Covinsky KE, Covinsky MH, Palmer RM, Sehgal AR. Serum albumin concentration and clinical assessments of nutritional status in hospitalized older people: different sides of different coins? J Am Geriatr Soc. 2002;50(4):631-7.

34. Ferguson RP, O'Conner P, Crabtree B, Batchelor A, Mitchell J, Coppola D. Serum albumin and prealbumin as predictors of clinical outcomes in hospitalized elderly nursing home residents. J Am Geriatr Soc. 1993 May 4;41(5):545-9.

35. Jensen GL, Bistrian B, Roubenoff R, Heimburger DXC. Malnutrition syndromes: A conundrum vs. continuum. JPEN J Parenter Enteral Nutr. 2009;33(6):710-716.

36. State operations manual appendix PP—guidance to surveyors for long term care facilities (rev 149, 10-09-15) [Internet]. [Baltimore (MD)]: Centers for Medicare & Medicaid Services [cited 2016 May 12]. Available from: http://tinyurl.com/jpbepfm

37. Horn SD, Bender SA, Ferguson ML, et al. The National Pressure Ulcer Long-Term Care Study: pressure ulcer development in long-term care residents. J Am Geriatr Soc. 2004;52(3):359-367.

38. Centers for Disease Control and Prevention: CDC 24/7: saving lives, protecting people [Internet]. [Atlanta]: Centers for Disease Control and Prevention (US). About adult BMI [cited 2016 May 3]. Available from: http://www.cdc.gov/healthyweight/assessing/bmi/adult_bmi/index.html

39. Posthauer ME, Dorner B, Collins N. Nutrition: a critical component of wound healing. Adv Skin Wound Care. 2010;23:560-572.

40. Litchford MD. Nutrition-focused physical assessment: making clinical connections. Greensboro (NC): Case Software; 2012.

41. Dorner B, Posthauer ME, Thomas DR. The role of nutrition in the pressure ulcer treatment and prevention: National Pressure Ulcer Advisory Panel white paper. Adv Skin Wound Care. 2009;14(2):84-6.

42. Adult weight management guideline [Internet]. [Chicago]: Academy of Nutrition and Dietetics [cited 2016 May 3]. Available from: http://www.andeal.org/topic.cfm?menu=5276&cat=4690

43. Tsourdi E, Barythel A, Rietzsch H, Reichel A, Bornstein SR. Current aspects in the pathophysiology and treatment of chronic wounds in diabetes mellitus. Biomed Res Int [Internet]. 2013 [cited May 10, 2016]. Available from: http://tinyurl.com/gowvjmj

44. Lioupis C. Effects of diabetes mellitus on wound healing: an update. J Wound Care. 2005;14(2):84-86.

45. Cefalu WT, editor. American Diabetes Association standards of medical care in diabetes—2016. Diabetes Care. 2016 Jan;39(Suppl 1):S1-S119.

46. American Medical Directors Association. Diabetes management in the post-acute and long-term care setting clinical practice guideline. Columbia (MD): AMDA; 2015.

47. Pompeo M. Misconceptions about protein requirements for wound healing: results of a prospective study. Ostomy Wound Manage. 2007;53(8):30-44.

48. Teno JM, Gozalo P, Mitchell SL, et al. Feeding tubes and the prevention or healing of pressure ulcers. Arch Intern Med. 2012;172(9):697-701.

49. Langer G, Fink A. Nutritional interventions for preventing and treating pressure ulcers. Cochrane Database Syst Rev [Internet]. 2014 June 12 [cited 2016 May 2].

50. Langemo DK, Black J. Pressure ulcers in individuals receiving palliative care: A National Pressure Ulcer Advisory Panel White Paper. Adv Skin Wound Care. 2010 Feb; 59-72.

51. Gorecki C, Brown JM, Nelson EA, Briggs M, Schoonhoven L, Dealey C, et al. Impact of pressure ulcers on the quality of life in older patients; a systemic review. J Am Geriatr Soc. 2009;57:1175-183.

52. Dev R, Dalal S, Bruera E. Is there a role for parenteral nutrition or hydration at the end of life? Curr Opin Support Palliat Care. 2012;6:365-370.

53. ChooseMyPlate.gov [Internet]. [Alexandria (VA)]: Department of Agriculture (US); 2016 [cited May 4, 2016]. Available from: www.choosemyplate.gov

54. Roberts S, Chaboyer W, Desbrow B. Nutrition care-related practices and factors affecting nutritional intakes in hospital patients at risk of pressure ulcers. J Hum Nutr Diet. 2015 Aug;28(4):357-65.

55. Stratton RJ, Ek AC, Engfer M, Moore Z. Rigby R, Wolfe R, et al. Enteral nutritional support in prevention and treatment of pressure ulcers: a systematic review and meta-analysis. Ageing Res Rev. 2005;45(3):422-450.

56. Nutrition care manual [Internet]. [Chicago]: Academy of Nutrition and Dietetics (US) [cited 2016 May 3]. Available from: www.nutritioncaremanual.org

Chapter 5

WOUND ASSESSMENT

Robert J. Snyder, DPM, MSc, CWS
Joey K. Ead, MS
Cherison Cuffy, DPM, CWS

KEY CONCEPTS

1. An accurate wound assessment aids clinical decision making for management of wounds.
2. Because different wound classification systems emphasize different etiologic factors (e.g. ischemia, infection), integrating different classification systems may improve wound outcomes.
3. The implementation of any wound classification system improves both data collection and the quality of wound management.
4. The Society for Vascular Surgery (SVS) WIfI classification incorporates wound severity, ischemia, and foot infection, and better predicts lower-extremity amputation risk and morbidity.
5. A multidisciplinary team approach is particularly important in treating patients with chronic wounds.

CONTENTS

Introduction

Various theories have been proposed to explain why some wounds become chronic and nonhealing. Although the complete answer is not yet available, a great deal has been learned in recent years that sheds light on this phenomenon. First, there is markedly reduced mitogenic activity (new cell growth). Second, inflammation becomes chronic and does not progress. There are elevated levels of TNF-α and IL-1β. These molecules induce their own synthesis to set up a cycle of non-progressive inflammation, inhibit collagen formation, and decrease the production of protease inhibitors. Third, chronic wounds have elevated levels of proteases, which destroy growth factors and their receptors, and degrade important matrix proteins such as fibronectin and collagen. The resulting wound bed, lacking attachment sites for migration, is "unfriendly" to keratinocytes, leading to slow or absent wound closure. Fourth, fibroblasts in chronic wounds have been shown to be senescent, with decreased capacity to respond to growth factors and decreased capacity for proliferating. This is important because fibroblasts are the cells that produce collagen, fibronectin, and other matrix proteins to form the granulation tissue needed for wound closure. Accurate wound assessment helps in clinical decision making for management of wounds.

I. MEASURE: best practice for wound assessment

A consensus document by Keast et al.(1) reviewed clinically useful wound measurement approaches. This evidence-based document provided an overview of principles and practice regarding chronic wound assessment in a simple mnemonic format. The text articulated effective management of a nonhealing wound based upon:

- Complete history
- Detailed initial assessment
- Analysis of probable causes

A. Measure

Key measurement observations include length, width, depth, and area. These factors are critical parts of wound assessment and could have significant prognostic implications.(1) Measurements should always be done in the same way: Document in centimeters. The length is the measurement from head to toe; the width is taken perpendicular to length and the depth (at deepest point). Use the analogy of the face of a clock to document points both inside the wound bed and on the periwound skin (Figures 1 and 2). For example, the patient's head would be at 12 o'clock.

Aforementioned measurements should include the following parameters:(1)

- Document in centimeters

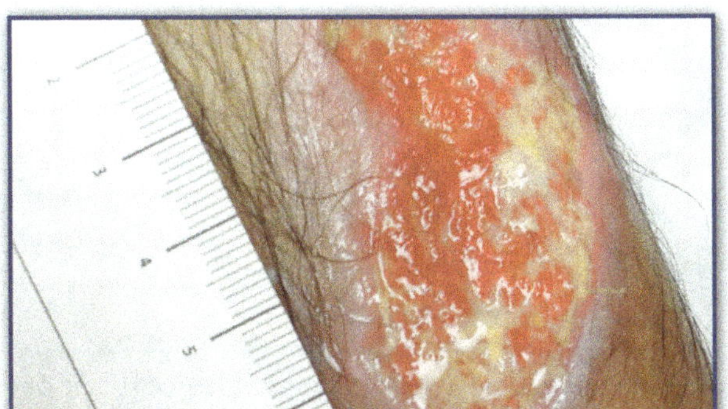

FIGURE 1. Length x Width
Courtesy of Caroline E. Fife, MD

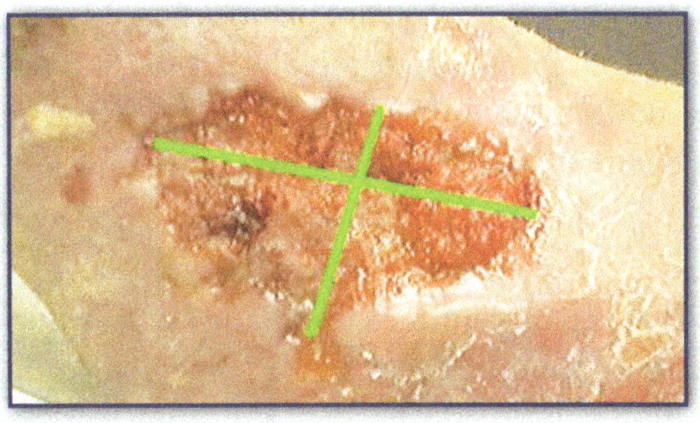

FIGURE 2. Wound Measurement Length x Width
Courtesy of Caroline E. Fife, MD

- Length (measurement head to toe)
- Width (perpendicular to length)
- Depth (at deepest point)
- Calculations of area and volume
- Tools:
  - Linear measuring ruler
  - Acetate wound tracings
  - Computerized planimetry
  - Digital photography

Issue of inter-rater reliability with ruler method of measurement

Ways to improve "measures" utilizing the ruler technique need to establish consistency.

- Better if only one person performs measures
- Repeat three times and take average value
- Use correct formulas for calculating surface area
- Avoid angles

Wound photographic grid films can provide valuable diagnostic measurements. In many clinical settings, both standard and Polaroid photography have been employed.[2] Griffin JE et al. found that the photographic and transparency methods provided equivalently reliable ulcer measurements.[2] Additionally, photographic methods in assessing wound surface areas in pressure ulcers provided reliable measurements. However, it should be noted that using this technique might not be feasible when dealing with wounds extending around a limb or various ulcers that present with extensive undermining.[2]

Tracing the wound edges onto a transparency and using a metric grid to count the number of square centimeters making up the wound is a commonly used but a time-consuming method. It should be noted that inaccuracies could arise from estimating partial squares.[1]

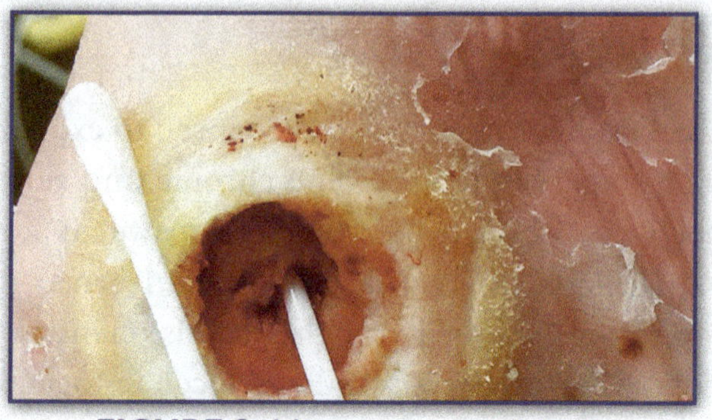

FIGURE 3. Measure size and depth (Shows probing) Courtesy of Caroline E. Fife, MD

- Insert tip of probe to greatest depth and measure perpendicular distance to wound edge
- 15% inter-rater variability seen in depth measurement by this technique

B. mEasure - Exudate[1,4]

Throughout the healing process, wound fluids contribute to the dynamic wound-healing cascade. Tissue regeneration may result from these intrinsic fluids due to various growth factors that help stimulate cellular migration, diminish necrotic tissue, and effectively manage the bacterial environment.

To objectively assess wound exudate, the wound care clinician should look at the exudate on the dressing that was applied, the kind of dressing that was applied to the wound, and the frequency of dressing changes required.

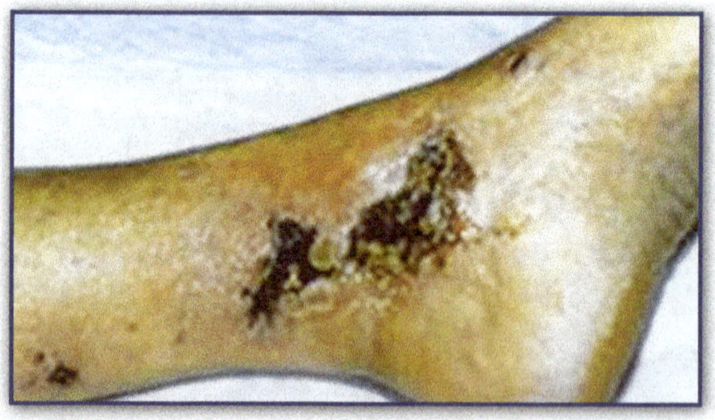

FIGURE 4a. Show no drainage. Desiccation: dry eschared tissue. No exudate present.
Courtesy of Caroline E. Fife, MD

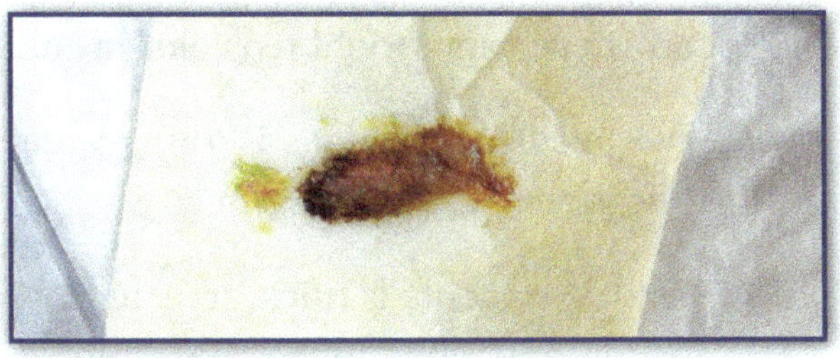

FIGURE 4b. Wound with small drainage seen on dressing Courtesy of Caroline E. Fife, MD

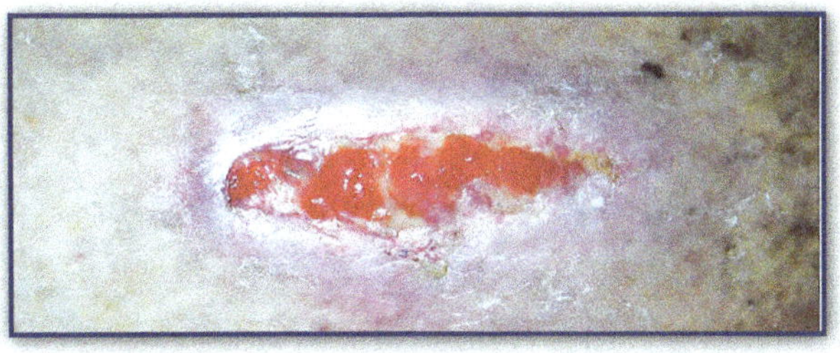

FIGURE 4c. Wound with small drainage Courtesy of Caroline E. Fife, MD

Although too little exudate results in a desiccated wound, excessive exudate complicates wound management. A copious exudate environment can collect and macerate wound edges. Common signs of an infection include: high levels of exudate or frank pus, redness/change in skin color, systemic fever, local inflammation or swelling, tenderness or warmth in the wound area, and a slow-healing wound. Moist wound healing requires keeping the wound bed moist but the periwound skin dry. Wound exudate should be assessed on the basis of quantity, quality, and odor.(1) Falanga et al. provided a guide to exudate volume quantification.(4)

Small exudate is defined as exudate which is fully controlled with nonabsorptive dressing and wear time is up to 7 days. Moderate exudate is defined as exudate which is controlled by using absorptive dressing for 2-3 days and Large exudate is defined as exudate which remains uncontrolled with absorptive dressings and wear time is less than one day.

Figures 5a, 5b: Moderate: Exudate controlled; absorptive dressings may be required

Figure 5c: Large (Copious): Exudate uncontrolled; absorptive dressings are required

Note: High exudate volume may have deleterious implications, including local infection or osteomyelitis.(1,4) A sudden increase in exudate should indicate to clinicians that there is an increased bacterial burden in the wound bed (even in the absence of typical signs of infection).(4)

In regard to describing exudate quality, the MEASURE system recommends using a protocol that entails a series of definitions.

1. Serous exudate is thin and watery and usually clear to yellow in color.
2. Sero-sanguineous exudate is thin and watery and pink to light red in color.

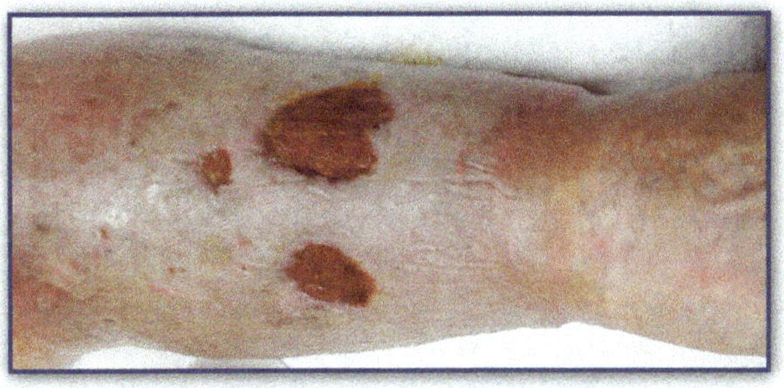

FIGURE 5a. Moderate exudate Courtesy of Caroline E. Fife, MD

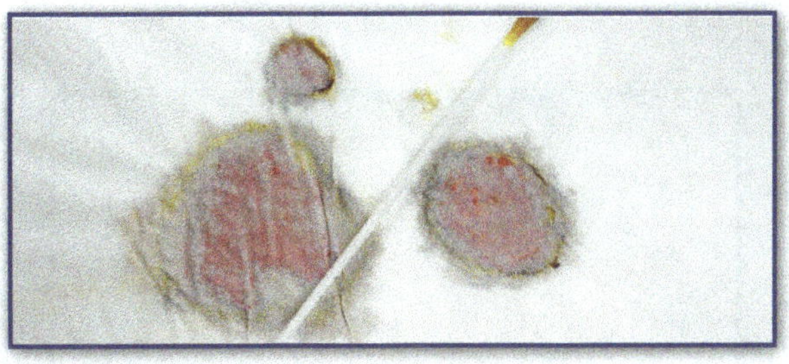

FIGURE 5b. Moderate exudate seen on dressing Courtesy of Caroline E. Fife, MD

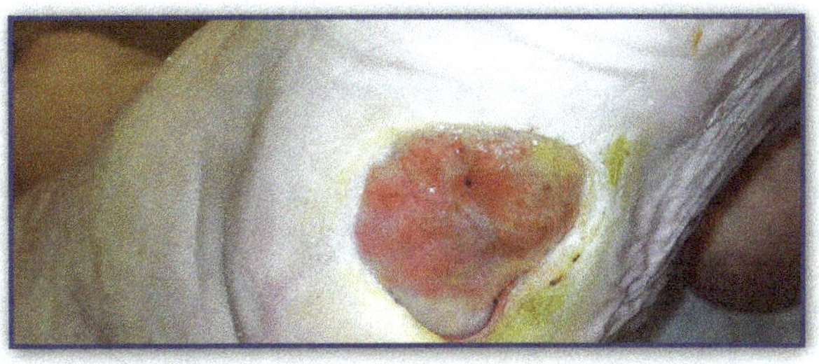

FIGURE 5c. Shows large exudate coming from wound Courtesy of Caroline E. Fife, MD

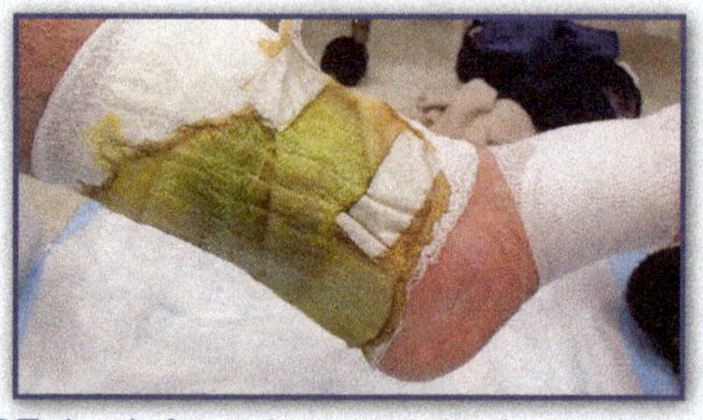

FIGURE 6a. Infected wound displaying large green drainage Courtesy of Caroline E. Fife, MD

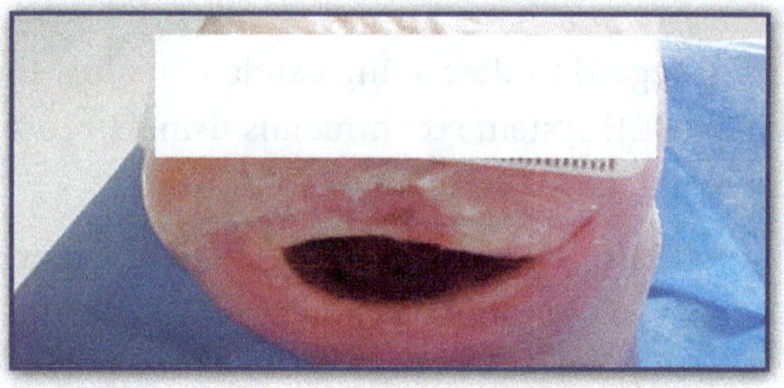

FIGURE 6b. Shows high exudate coming from wound causing maceration in periwound tissue Courtesy of Jayesh B. Shah, MD

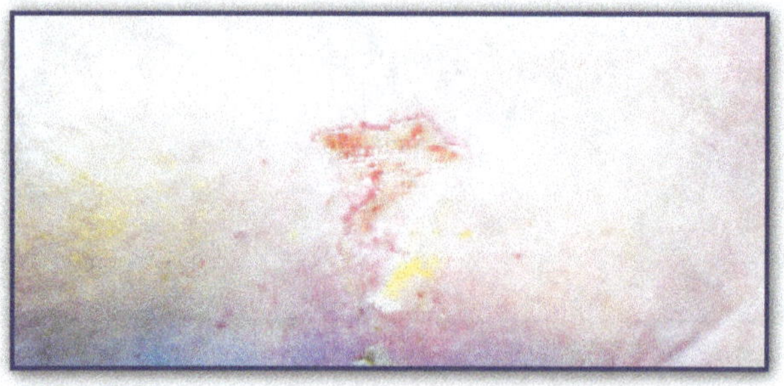

FIGURE 6c. Low exudate coming from wound Courtesy of Jayesh B. Shah, MD

3. Sanguineous exudate is frank blood in consistency and bright red color in color.
4. Sero-purulent exudate is thin, watery and white to cream in color.
5. Purulent exudate is thick, translucent to opaque, and white to cream in color.

Odor assessment is an integral part of the physical examination of wound environments; however descriptions can be subjective. Additionally, a standard terminology has not been universally adopted.[1,5] Transitions in the amount and type of odor could give important signs of the current status of the wound apparatus.[1,5] It should be noted that various types of dressings could affect wound odor. Anaerobes that proliferate in necrotic tissue commonly emit a distinctive foul odor.[1,5]

Van Rijswijk et al. proposed an odor assessment scale[5] on wounds with dressing in place as the following:

- No odor at close range
- Faint odor at close range
- Moderate odor in room
- Strong odor in room

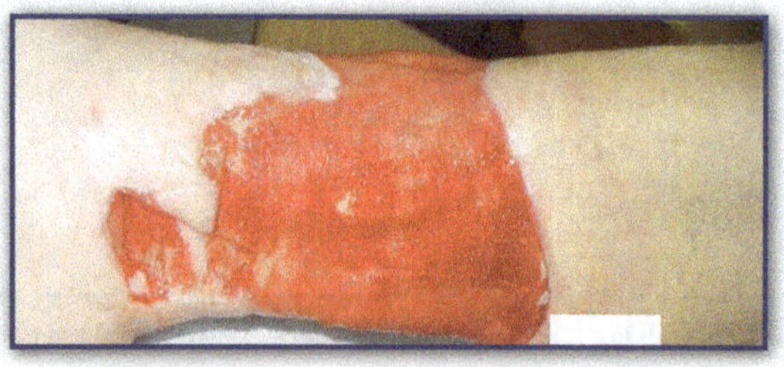

FIGURE 7a. meAsure: Appearance[1] Courtesy of Jayesh B. Shah, MD

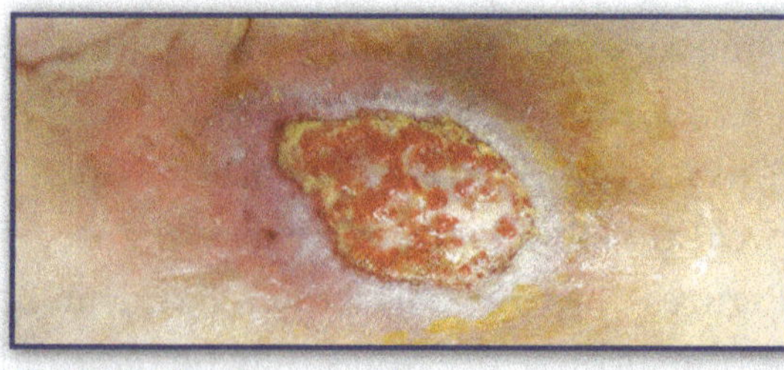

FIGURE 7b. Fibrin (yellow, firm—collagen and protein) Courtesy of Caroline E. Fife, MD

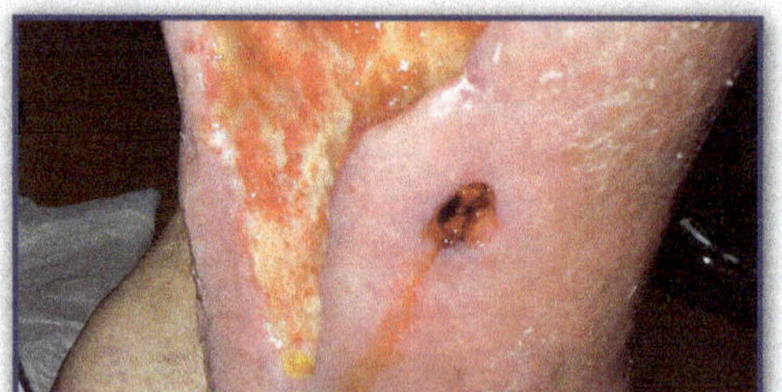

FIGURE 7c. Slough (yellow, gray, green) Courtesy Caroline Fife, MD

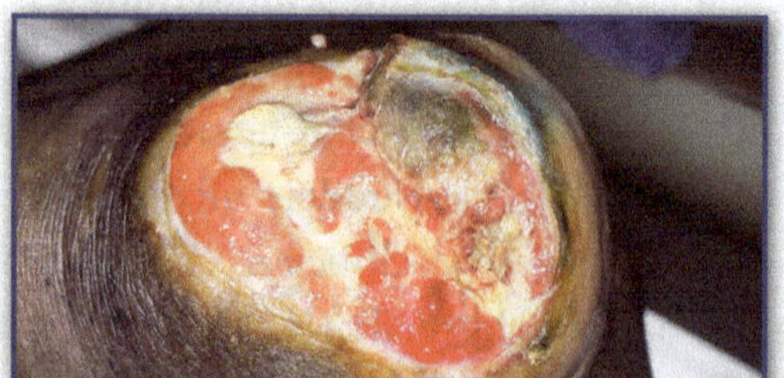

FIGURE 7d. Eschar—black, soft, wet, hard, or dry Courtesy of Caroline E. Fife, MD

C. meAsure - Appearance

Clinical assessment requires medical personnel to describe the texture and color of the wound bed.[1] The colors black, red, yellow, pink, and white are commonly used to describe the wound environment.[1] The distinct appearance of the wound bed could be attributed to a multitude of factors: necrosis, granulation tissue, exposed structures, fibrin, exudate, eschar, foreign body, inflammation, infection, and tunneling sinuses.[1]

Granulation is the formation of new dermal tissue to fill in deficits. Good granulation tissue is always red, firm, and pebbled. Hypergranulation, also known as proudflesh, extends over the epithelium and can interfere with epithelial migration. Hypergranulation, spongy granulation tissue, or friability may indicate bacterial, fungal, or viral infection. These scenarios may require debridement or cauterization with silver nitrate.

Fibrinous tissue in the wound bed is usually yellow and firm and might represent collagen in wound bed. Slough is usually yellow or gray and might represent necrotic fascia. Eschar is usually black and can be dry or wet.

Appearance: Eschar[1]

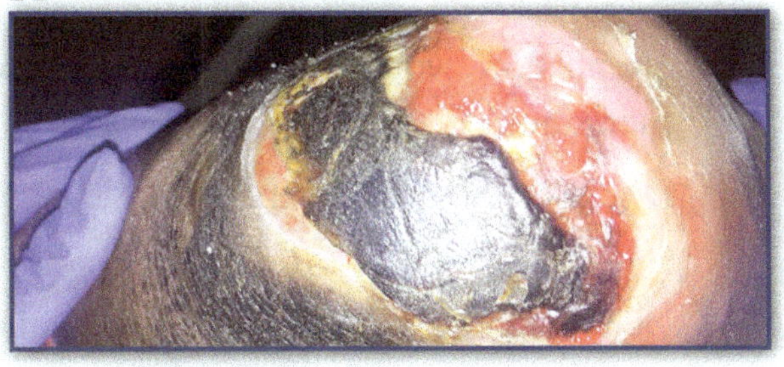

FIGURE 8a. Shows black eschar
Courtesy of Caroline E. Fife, MD

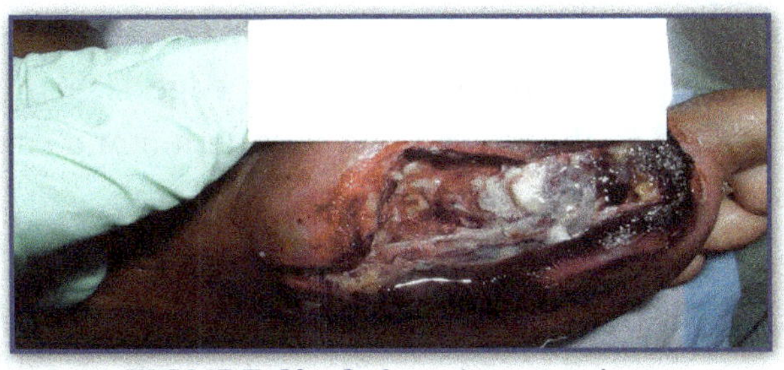

FIGURE 8b. Soft and wet eschar
Courtesy of Jayesh B. Shah, MD

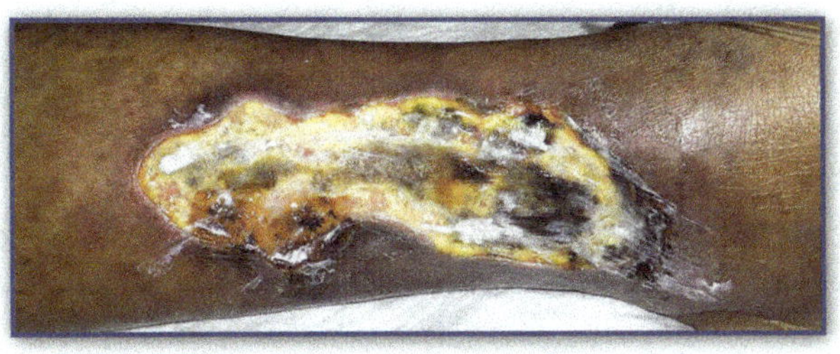

FIGURE 8c. Necrotic tissue from ischemia
Courtesy of Caroline E. Fife, MD

Appearance: Granulation and Epithealization[1]

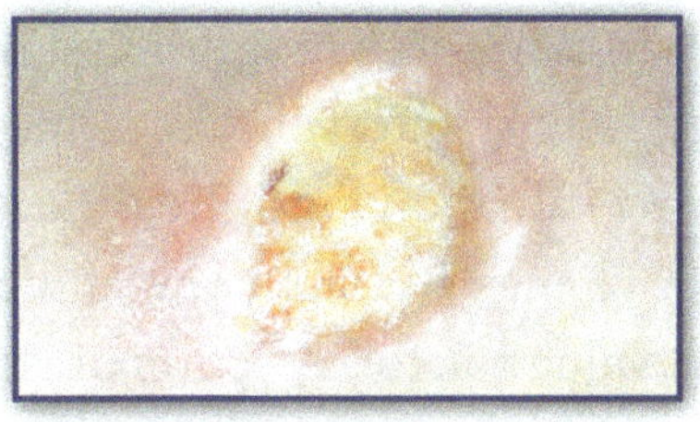

FIGURE 9a. Slough and fat
Courtesy of Caroline E. Fife, MD

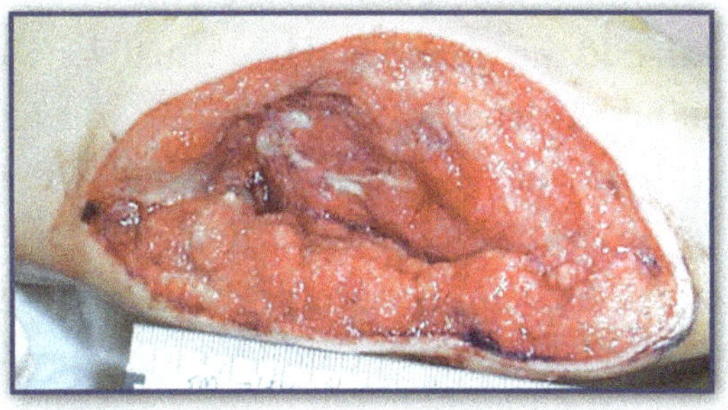

FIGURE 9b. Clean nongranulating tissue is deep pink or red and smooth (nongranular) or striated (when muscle fibers are exposed).
Courtesy of Caroline E. Fife, MD

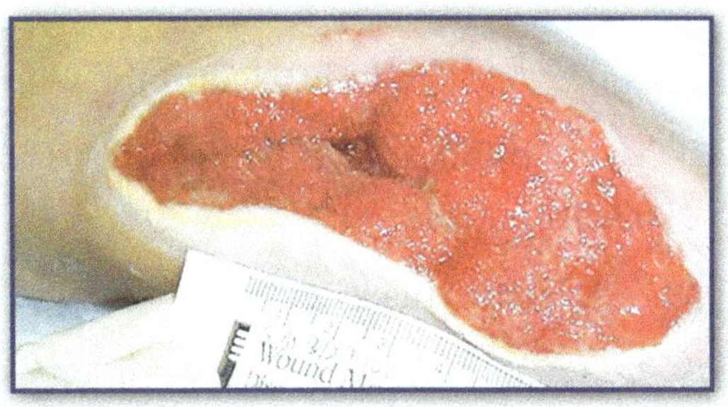

FIGURE 9c. Granulation tissue is typically deep pink or red and is characterized by an irregular granular surface that resembles raspberries.
Courtesy of Caroline E. Fife, MD

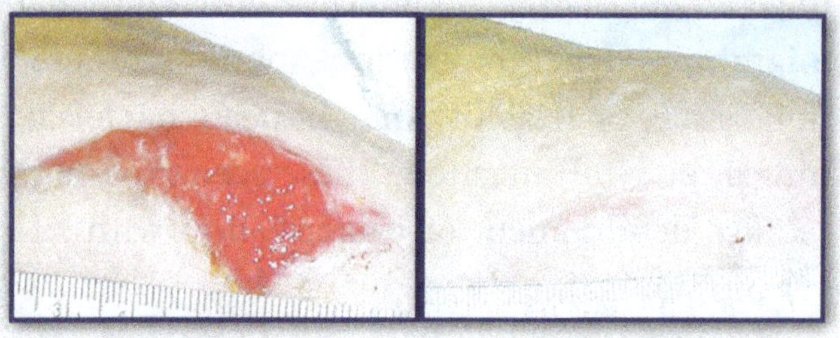

FIGURE 9d. **FIGURE 9e.**
(Left) New epithelial tissue is light pink or slightly lavender. (Right) New epithelial tissue migrates from the wound edges to gradually cover the granulation tissue.
Courtesy Caroline Fife, MD

D. meaSure - Suffering

The medical staff should evaluate pain by a standard grading scale in every patient at every visit.[1] It is important to monitor and reevaluate pain levels, adjust intervention strategies, and continue reevaluation and treatment adjustments.[1] A change in pain (worsening) should prompt reevaluation for infection or ischemia.[1]

E. measUre - Undermining[1]

Undermining is the space between the surrounding skin and the wound bed that usually involves a significant proportion of wound edges and may extend entirely around the wound. It usually involves subcutaneous fat necrosis and has more aerobic and anaerobic bacteria present than wounds that have no undermining present.

The space between the surrounding skin and the wound bed may include the following:

- Usually involves a significant proportion of wound edges
- May extend entirely around the wound
- May exhibit subcutaneous fat necrosis resulting from:
    1. Necrotizing infection
    2. Primary inflammatory etiology
    3. Friction, shearing

Wound documentation should include the following:

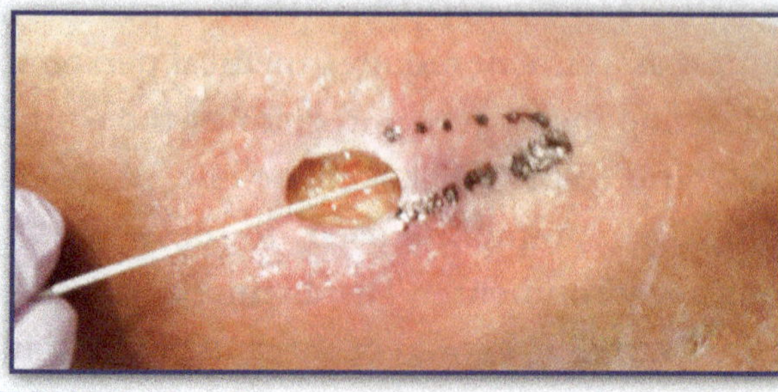

FIGURE 10a. Shows undermining with line drawn
Courtesy Caroline Fife, MD

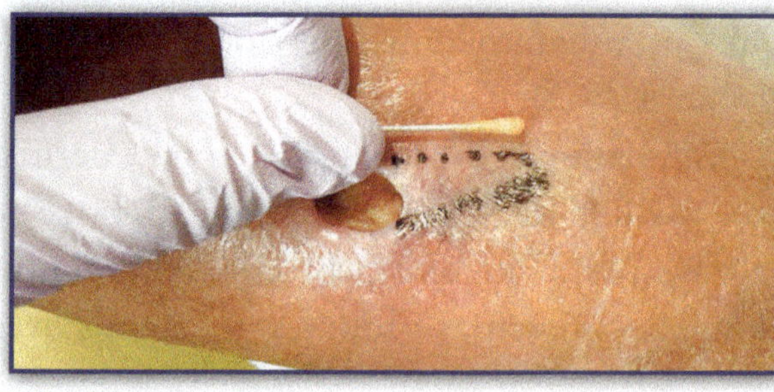

FIGURE 10b. Shows undermining with line drawn
Courtesy Caroline Fife, MD

- Number of wounds if there are more than one
- Direction of each wound, using face of clock
- Depth of each if there are more than one

Any indications of tunneling or sinus tracts are critical in the evaluation of chronic wounds.[1] This is because the healing process will stagnate unless the wound edge is firmly attached to the wound bed foundation and surrounding tissue.[1]

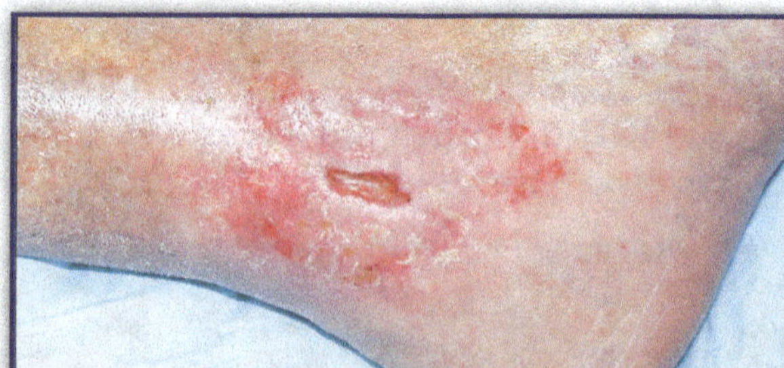

FIGURE 11. Epidermal margin: Nonadvancing because of undermining (necrosis also filling wound base). Courtesy Caroline Fife, MD © Best Publishing Company. *Wound Care Certification Study Guide 2nd edition*

F. measuRe - Re-evaluation

Too-frequent assessments may lead to inappropriate changes in treatment plan (not enough time for intervention to be effective). Infrequent assessments may miss early indicators of significant deterioration. Most wounds can be followed with a formal re-assessment every week, depending upon complexity of wound and care. Some wounds require much more frequent assessment if rapidly changing or high-risk.

G. measurE - Edge

Wound edge changes are a key indication of progress toward healing. Epithelial cells will not migrate across dry or necrotic tissue or undermining. Clinicians should assess the wound edges for signs of healing that are seen on the epithelial ridge and document the observed changes. Nutrition, oxygenation, and effective removal of necrotic tissue can enhance the epithelial ridge and promote keratinocyte migration.

Key factors to keep in mind when assessing the periwound environment should include induration, inflammation, pigmentation, edema, and maceration.[1] If unattached wound edges are present, they should be noted as undermining and treated accordingly. Induration is defined as firm swelling with or without erythema. By properly assessing the appearance of the ulcer shape, wound edge, and periwound environment, medical personnel will likely be able to pinpoint the wound etiology.[1]

H. MEASURE system takeaway

- Measure: The percentage of decrease in wound area in the first two to four weeks has been found to be a predictive of healing at 12 to 24 weeks.[1]
- Exudate: Use consistent and clear terminology, definitions, qualitative descriptions, and quantitative measures of wound exudate, such as those proposed by Falanga.[4]
- Appearance: Should include tissue type and a thorough description.
- Suffering: Intensity of pain should be measured using a validated pain instrument and reevaluated using the same instrument.
- Undermining: This aspect should be evaluated in every wound assessment, and the clock system is proposed as the standard approach to measuring this factor.
- Reevaluate: Most wounds can be followed with a formal re-assessment every week, depending upon complexity of wound and care.
- Edge: Evaluation of attachment or lack of attachment; observation of ulcer dimensions and edge alignment; and inspection of the condition of the periwound apparatus, noting especially induration, inflammation, and maceration.

II. Wound classification systems

The management and treatment of chronic wounds has evolved over the years. The etiology of a wound should be well understood before an intervention is initiated. A comprehensive assessment of the patient's overall health status and the identification of key systemic comorbidities will provide clinicians the proper framework to establish an etiology and develop a treatment plan. Alongside other pertinent health documentation, structured wound classification systems have provided clinicians the means to organize, record, and track the development of various wounds based on their pathologic features.

Although there are well-established wound classification systems directed at specific types of wounds, clinicians treat patients and not classification systems. Knowledge of the classification system does aid the clinician in making evidence-based decisions for usual care and perhaps in predicting patient outcomes. Each of the wound classification systems listed below provides a framework for implementing and assessing the effectiveness of the interventions necessary to heal a wound, salvage a limb, or preserve a life:

- Wagner grading for diabetic foot ulcers
- University of Texas at San Antonio (UTSA) for diabetic foot ulcers (Refer to Chapter 10: Diabetic Foot Ulcers)
- Infectious Disease Society of America Guidelines (IDSA) for diabetic foot infections and skin and soft tissue infections
- National Pressure Ulcer Advisory Panel (NPUAP) for pressure ulcers
- Payne Martin classification for skin tears
- CEAP Classification for chronic venous disorders
- Society for Vascular Surgery Wound, Ischemia and Foot Infection (WIfI)

A. Wagner ulcer classification

The Wagner classification system is one of the more widely used grading systems in the assessment of a diabetic foot ulcer (DFU). This scheme uses six wound grades (scored 0-5) to assess wound depth and the presence of infection-gangrene .The first four grades (0, 1, 2, and 3) are solely based on the physical depth of the DFU, while the last two grades (4 and 5) identify the loss of perfusion and the extent of gangrene in the foot. Grade 3 deep infection indicates forefoot gangrene, Grade 4 indicates forefoot gangrene, whereas Grade 5 refers to a complete foot gangrene. The superficial diabetic ulcer with a component of ischemia or infection is not accounted for in the Wagner grading system.[26]

TABLE 1. Photos according to Wagner Classification of diabetic foot wounds
Courtesy of Caroline E. Fife, MD

Figure 12a. Grade I	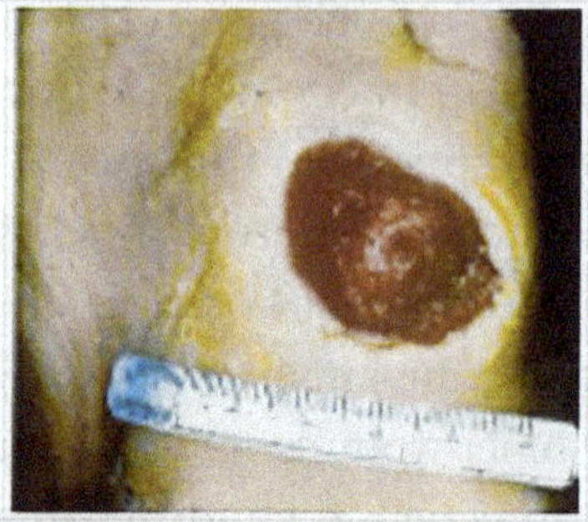
Figure 12b. Grade II	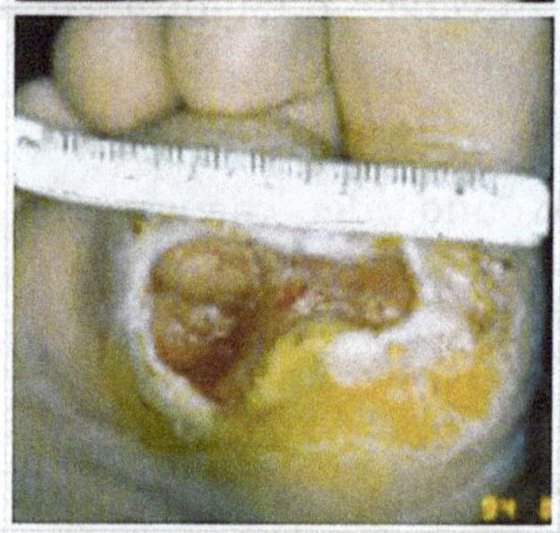
Figure 12c. Grade III	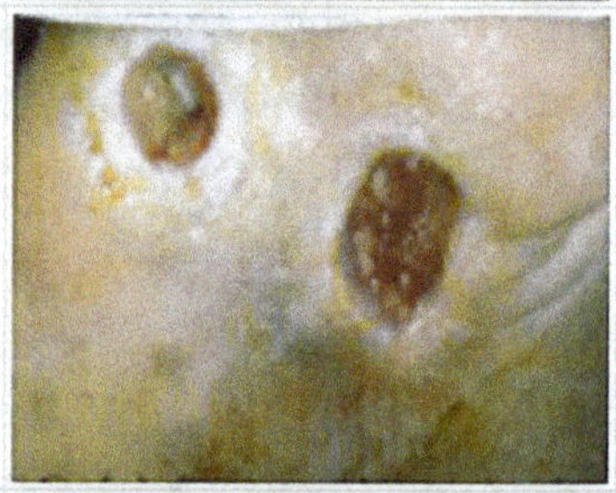
Figure 12d. Grade IV	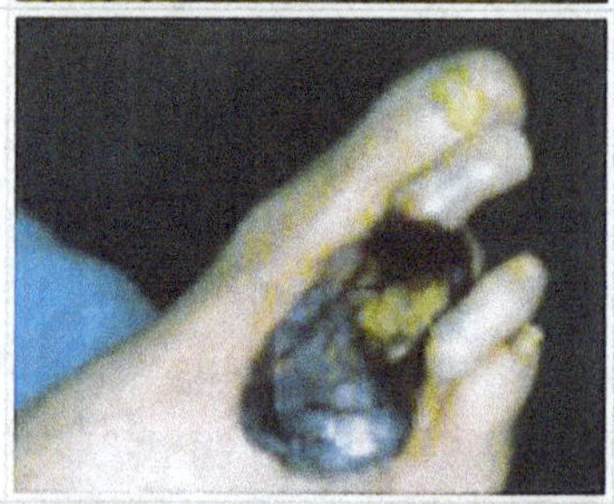
Figure 12e. Grade V	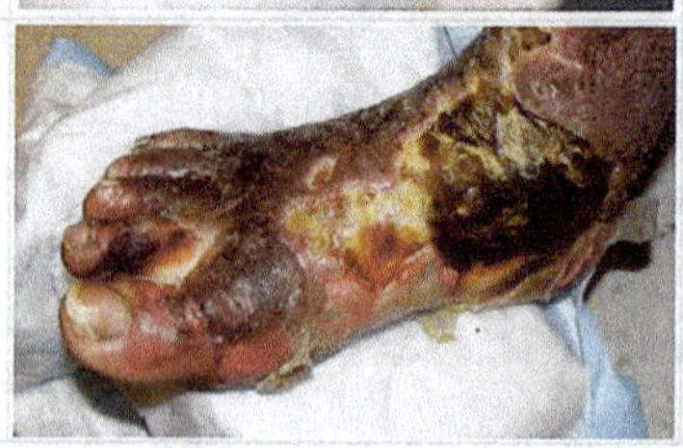

The American Diabetes Association (ADA) conducted a study comparing the Wagner and

University of Texas classification systems in predicting the clinical outcomes of diabetic foot ulcers. They found that Wagner Grades 4 and 5 did not add extra predictive power to the wound classification system.[6] The ambiguity of this classification system can lead to high risk of lower-limb amputation or prolonged wound healing. It is vital to understand whether the gangrene is a result of severe infection or a consequence of ischemia. Many clinicians using the Wagner scale combine Grades 4 and 5 ulcers when making clinical assessments.[6] Although this classification system is widely used in the clinical setting, it does not adequately address all the vital concerns dealing with diabetic foot ulcerations and infections.

B. University of Texas at San Antonio

The University of Texas at San Antonio (UTSA) system uses a matrix of grades (scored 0 to 3) and scales (scored A to D) to assess ulcer depth, along with the presence of wound infection and lower-extremity ischemia.[7] Regardless of the wound anatomic depth, this system integrates the identification of infection and vascular disease as independent factors.[7] The grades of the UTSA system are as follows: Grade 0 (pre- or post-ulcerative site that has healed), Grade 1 (superficial wound not involving tendon, capsule, or bone), Grade 2 (wound penetrating to tendon or capsule), and Grade 3 (wound penetrating bone or joint).[7] Within each wound grade there are four stages: clean wounds (Stage A), non-ischemic infected wounds (Stage B), ischemic non-infected wounds (Stage C), and ischemic infected wounds (Stage D).

As previously mentioned, a labeling of Grade 2 of the Wagner system will not alert clinicians to the presence of infection and ischemia, which can prolong wound healing and increase the risk of lower-limb amputation. Awareness of the presence of the aforementioned distinct pathological

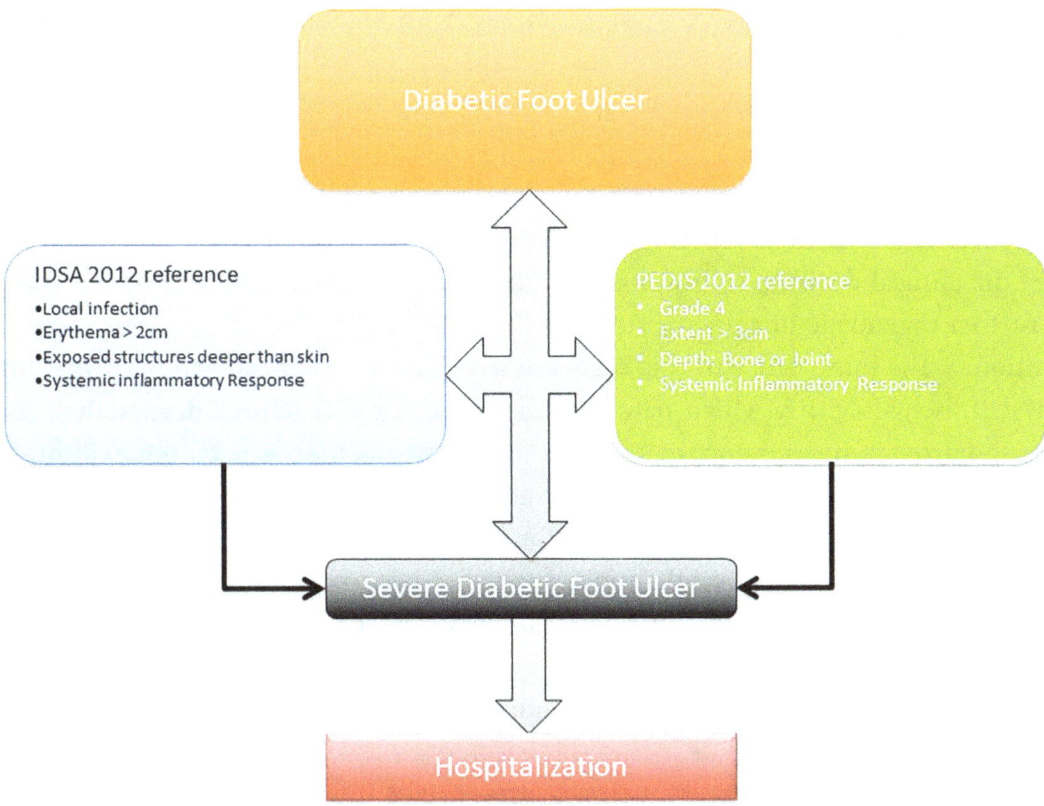

FIGURE 13.

features is critical to the successful management of the DFU. In contrast to the UTSA system, an infected ischemic ulcer that penetrates to tendon (Grade 2, Stage D, or, simply, Grade 2D) will be a Grade 2 of the Wagner system.[6-7] Incorporating the stage to grade framework significantly improved the descriptive and predictive power for DFU classification, especially for ulcers within the same grade.[6-7] By recognizing the presence of ischemia and infection separately as contributors to wound failure, the UTSA grading system does not account for the severity of these factors. Even though health- care providers more often utilize the Wagner system, the UTSA system has shown to be a better predictor of clinical outcome.[7] Please refer to Chapter 10: Diabetic Foot Ulcers for further information.

C. Infectious Disease Society of America (IDSA) and PEDIS classification systems

According to the Infectious Disease Society of America (IDSA), a robust multidisciplinary treatment of diabetic foot infections (DFI) can reduce amputations.[8] The IDSA classification provides the clinician with objective criteria to diagnose the severity of a diabetic foot infection and support the clinical decision to hospitalize or request further diagnostic imaging or surgical intervention.[8] The importance of this classification system helps identify which patients should be hospitalized in the presence of severe infection (Figure 14).[8] The majority of DFI lesions are poly-microbial with mainly aerobic gram-positive cocci (i.e. staphylococci the most causative organism).[8] Chronically infected wounds typically harbor aerobic gram-negative bacilli. Ischemic or necrotic wounds may be accompanied by anaerobic pathogens.[8] Based on their severity, DFIs that do not present clinical evidence of soft tissue or bone infection should not be treated with oral antibiotic therapy. However, clinically infected ulcers should undergo aerobic and anaerobic cultures using post-debridement specimens.[8] Obtaining a post-debridement specimen of tissue reduces potential contaminants and increases the probability of isolating the causative pathogen(s). See Chapter 10: Diabetic Foot Ulcers for more information.

The IDSA panel recommends that clinicians pay close attention to specific markers to detect infection beyond the classic signs of inflammation and purulent secretions such as:[8]

- Nonpurulent secretions
- Friable, discolored granulation tissue
- Undermining of wound edges
- Foul odor

The classic signs of infection (pain, erythema, swelling, leukocytosis) may be masked in the diabetic patient who may not exhibit a typical inflammatory response to infection.[9] As in the DFU, leukocytosis is also a poor indicator for determining the presence of acute osteomyelitis in the diabetic patient. The pathophysiology of osteomyelitis in the diabetic patient is the contiguous spread of a deep soft tissue infection through the cortex and into the bone marrow.[10] Clinicians are advised to use the probe-to-bone test (PTB) to establish whether the infection has spread to structures deeper than skin and subcutaneous tissues (e.g., bone, joint, tendon, muscle). Patients are at an increased risk of a DFU with a positive PTB test, an ulceration that has been present for more than 30 days, a history of recurring diabetic foot ulcers, peripheral arterial disease in the affected limb, renal insufficiency, loss of sensation, and walking barefoot.[8] The IDSA classification assesses the presence of infection defined by two or more classic findings of inflammation or purulence.[8]

Infections are then classified into mild (superficial and limited in size and depth), moderate (deeper or more extensive), or severe (accompanied by systemic signs or metabolic perturbations.)[8] Even though the UTSA classification system does classify the presence of infection, it does not include a specific grading scale or spectrum guideline. However, both the IDSA and UTSA classification systems could be utilized harmoniously for better clinical outcomes.

The IDSA incorporated a classification mechanism that assessed ulceration depth using perfusion, extent (size), depth, infection, and sensation classification (PEDIS).[3] The International Working Group on the Diabetic Foot developed the PEDIS classification system.[3] It is considered to be a semiquantitative grading scale that measures the severity of each category.[3] The PEDIS scale grades ulcers by depth and area using a grading scale of 0 through 3.

Twelve clinical signs of a localized wound infection were reported, which includes the classic signs of infection.[11] The additional criteria for wound infection were considered signs specific to secondary wounds.[11] The 12 clinical signs were developed after the investigation of a population with various wound types. The IDSA and PEDIS classification systems adequately assess the "classic" signs of infection; they fail to address scenarios when the diabetic patient presents an infected DFU with substantially diminished inflammatory responses. Studies have shown that the secondary signs specific to wounds are better indicators of infection in DFUs than the classic signs mentioned in the IDSA classification system.[12] It is vital that clinicians use these guidelines as a framework throughout the treatment process.

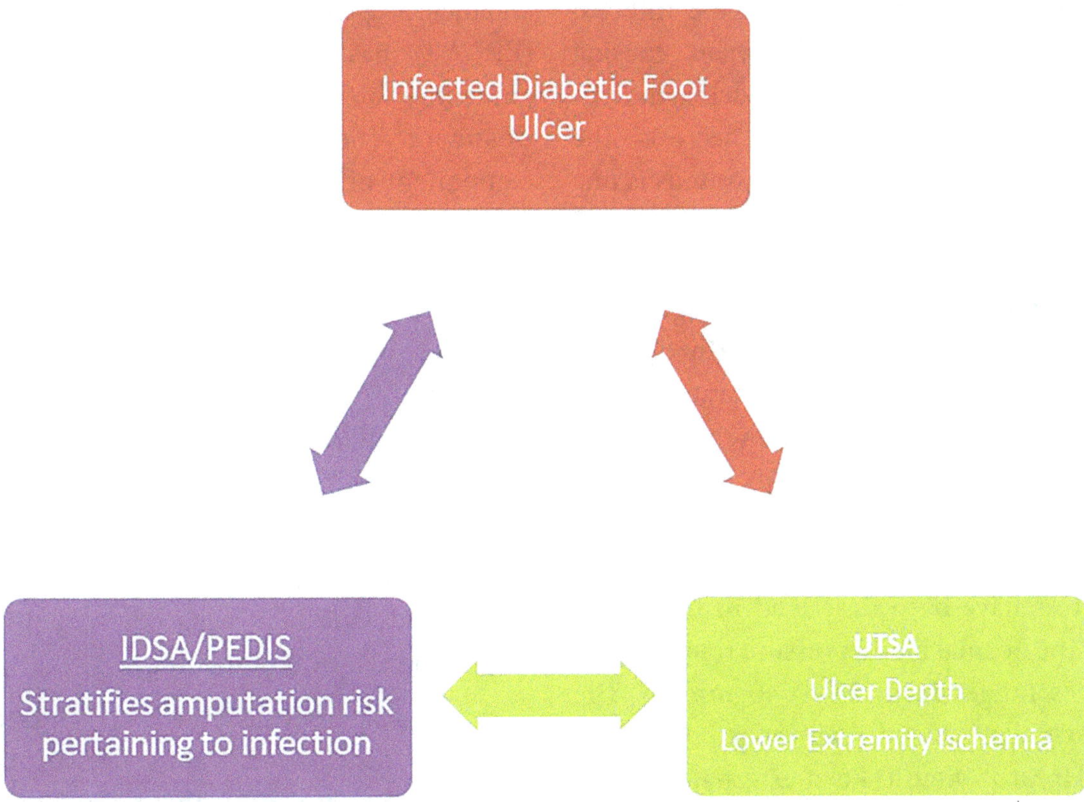

FIGURE 14. By integrating both the IDSA and UTSA classification systems, the clinician would be able to stratify amputation risk pertaining to infection and assess ulcer depth and lower extremity ischemia effectively.

D. National Pressure Ulcer Advisory Panel (NPUAP)

A pressure injury is a localized lesion to the skin tissue that typically arises over a bony prominence. They usually manifest in the lower extremity such as the sacrum, coccyx, ischial tuberosity, heels, and the medial/lateral malleoli. The specific localization of these wounds typically results in substantial pressure or a combination of shear force against the lesion. Shear force is a separation of the skin from underlying tissues. In patients who are partially sitting up at the bedside, this posture may result in their skin's sticking to the sheets, making them even more susceptible to pressure ulcerations. These instances may account for the number of sacral ulcers seen in hospitalized patients. Complete or partial obstruction of blood vessels due to friction or shear forces can diminish capillary perfusion to the site of the lesion. Obstruction of superficial blood vessels deprives the infected lesion of vital nutrients and oxygen, causing ischemia, hypoxia, mild to severe edema, inflammation, and in some cases tissue necrosis. The constant friction applied to these wounds is one of the main culprits of the stagnation of wound healing. Skin or tissues subjected to friction are more susceptible (pressure injury damage).

There is an inversely proportional relationship between pressure and duration. Low pressure over long periods of time can be just as deleterious as high amounts of pressure over shorter timeframes. A pressure injury can develop in two to six hours.(13) More than 100 risk factors have been described in the literature.(13) The normal blood pressure range within capillaries ranges from 20 to 40 mmHg. The average capillary blood pressure is considered 32 mmHg. It is vital to keep external pressure less than the aforementioned capillary pressure in order to prevent impairment to the microcirculatory system.(13) The Braden and Norton scales are two validated classification systems that have been used to identify patients at risk for pressure ulcers.(13) The Norton Scale scores five broad clinical categories: physical state, mental status, mobility, activity, and incontinence.(13) The Braden Scale evaluates six clinical categories: sensory perception, moisture, activity, mobility, nutrition, friction, and shear.(13) Patients with existing pressure ulcers are at high risk of forming new lesions, so it is paramount that all clinicians perform a risk assessment and utilize evidence-based protocols to address these conditions.

The National Pressure Ulcer Advisory Panel (NPUAP) has developed a common definition and classification system for pressure ulcers. This system is intended for the use of healthcare professionals who are involved in the care of patients with existing pressure ulcers. A four-year collaborative initiative between NPUAP and the European Pressure Ulcer Advisory Panel (EPUAP) has advanced the evidence-based guidelines on pressure ulcer prevention and treatment. The prevention guideline is a key component of this classification system. Refer to Chapter 11: Pressure Ulcers to review staging and updated recommendations by NPUAP.

When erythema is present around intact skin, the consensus NPUAP-EPUAP approach would be to implement the finger pressure or transparent disc method to assess whether the skin is blanchable or nonblanchable.

- Finger pressure method — a finger is pressed on the erythema for three seconds and blanching is assessed following removal of the finger.
- Transparent disk method — a transparent disk is used to apply pressure equally over an area of erythema, and blanching can be observed underneath the disk during its application.

Blanchable erythema is an erythematous lesion that becomes white when pressure is applied and reddens when pressure is relieved. Reactive hyperemia or inflammatory erythema with an intact capillary bed may induce blanchable erythema. In contrast, nonblanchable erythema maintains the red appearance in spite of pressure relief. It should be noted that non-blanchable erythema is indicative of structural damage to the capillary bed. A prospective cohort study of 109 individuals in an acute-care hospital found non-blanching erythema to be an independent predictor of category Stage 2 pressure ulcer development.[15]

As it is not always possible to identify erythema on darkly pigmented skin, localized heat, edema, and change in tissue consistency in relation to surrounding tissue (e.g., induration/hardness) are important indicators of early pressure damage to the skin in individuals of darker skin tone. When assessing these skin tones, it is recommended to use a natural light or halogen-fluorescent device, which gives an illusion of a bluish tint. This can help the

TABLE 2. Staging Comparison Table: Understanding differences in Wagner Classification for diabetic wounds and NPUAP Classification for pressure ulcers. Courtesy of Jayesh B. Shah, MD.

Depth	Diabetic Wagner Grading	NPUAP Pressure Ulcer	Others (i.e. venous, arterial, etc.)
No ulcer	Grade 0 Calluls/corn	Stage 1 Nonblanchable redness, DTI, deep injury, boggy, ischemic, no ulceration	N/A
Partial thickness; epidermal/ dermal loss	Grade 1 Shallow ulcer	Stage 2 Shallow ulceration, no slough	Partial thickness ulcer
Full thickness with fat layer exposed up to subq tissue	Grade 1 Shallow ulcer	Stage 3 Slough may be present	Full thickness with fat layer exposed
Full thickness up to bone; tendon and joint exposed; not infected	Grade 2 Deep ulcer	Stage 4 Ulcer with bone, tendon, and muscle exposed	Full thickness with muscle, tendon, or bone exposed
Full thickness with osteomyelitis; tendonitis or deep abscess	Grade 3 Deep ulcer with infection	Stage 4 Ulcer with tendon, bone, and muscle exposed with infection	Full thickness with muscle, tendon, or bone exposed with infection
Full thickness with gangrene	Grade 4 Localized gangrene, toe, toes, or heel Grade 5 Gangrene of complete or partial foot	Unstageable	Full thickness with necrosis

clinician find darker areas than the surrounding skin or identify taunt shiny indurated areas. Heat should be detected over an area of localized inflammation. Compromised skin region may have signs of non-pitting edema with or without color changes.

The NPUAP and EPUAP access the evidence as strongly positive that a wound covered with slough and eschar should be debrided although the evidence is level C. Also it should be noted that a stable eschar in an ischemic limb should not be debrided.

When clinical signs of infection are not present, the quantity of organisms (microbial load) is one of the better indicators of wound infection. The gold standard method for examining microbial bio burden is a quantitative culture of viable biopsied wound tissue.

E. Payne Martin Classification for skin tears

Skin tears are traumatic injuries that can result in partial or full separation of the outer layers of the skin. These tears may occur due to shearing and friction forces or a blunt trauma, causing the epidermis to separate from the dermis (partial-thickness wound) or both the epidermis and the dermis to separate from the underlying structures (full-thickness wound). Depending on the individual's age and medical status, skin tears can be significant and complex wounds; complications such as infection or compromised vascularity can increase morbidity or mortality risks.[16] Skin tears occur most commonly in the upper extremities.[16] Although nearly 70% to 80% of skin tears occur on the arms and hands, these wounds also may occur on other areas of the body.

Risk factors for skin tears include the following:[17]

- Age and gender
- History of previous skin tears
- Medications
- Poor nutrition – hydration
- Cognitive or sensory impairment
- Comorbidities
- Ecchymosis

Certain dressings that have adhesive properties should be removed carefully. Skin stripping is a potential problem for any person if the adhesive dressing or tape is removed in an aggressive manner.[16,17] There is currently no universally accepted classification system for the assessment of skin tears. However, the Payne Martin System provides classifications by severity using three categories and two sub-categories: A category 1 skin tear is skin tear without tissue loss; a category 2 skin tear is one with partial tissue loss (25% or less), and a category 3 is a skin tear with complete tissue loss.

F. CEAP Classification System – venous insufficiency

Venous leg ulcers can be largely attributed to venous or perforating valvular incompetence. When the valves are considered incompetent, blood backs into the distal veins during diastole. With loss of perforator valve function, the high intracompartmental venous pressure, which can approach 200 mmHg during active muscle contraction, results in distention of the saphenous system.[19] This pathologic condition causes a high-pressured spike within the superficial venous system, leading to venous hypertension.[19] Once veins become distended, the venous wall starts to disintegrate, often resulting in edema, hemosiderin formation, hyperpigmentation, lipodermatosclerosis, and prominent venous ulcers.[19] Sustained venous hypertension results in increased capillary permeability and the release of fibrinogen into the skin.[19] The weight of the column of blood due to the high intra-compartmental venous pressure consequently increases the pressure inside the capillary network. One current hypothesis explaining the pathogenesis of venous ulcers is the "fibrin cuff" theory. This theory stipulates that sustained venous hypertension causes distention of dermal capillary beds, which allows the plasma exudate to leak into the surrounding tissue apparatus.[19] Subsequently, fibrin accumulation down-regulates collagen synthesis, which eventually leads to the formation of peri-capillary "fibrin cuffs." [19] This manifestation impedes normal vessel function and inhibits cytokine proliferation, resulting in poor oxygen circulation and the stagnation of growth factors that help facilitate the distribution of vital nutrients. Patients with venous insufficiency commonly present an inverted Champagne-bottle look on the affected leg. It should be noted that the appearance of venous insufficiency could vary. Distention of the veins in the sub-dermal plexus results in varicosities.[19] When smaller subdermal capillary networks distend, they form telangiectasia, also known as "spider veins."

CEAP classification evaluates based on four categories:

C = clinical presentation (Class 1-6): C0 has no signs of venous disease; C1 has telangiectasia or reticular veins; C2 has varicose veins; C3 edema; C4 skin changes; C5 healed ulceration; C6 active ulceration.

E = etiologic basis: primary, secondary, congenital

A = anatomic distribution: superficial, deep, perforators

P = pathophysiolgic basis: reflux, obstruction, pathophysiology

Management of venous leg ulcers: clinical practice guidelines of the Society for Vascular Surgery and the American Venous Forum

The Society for Vascular Surgery (SVS) and the American Venous Forum (AVF) formed a guideline protocol for the management of venous leg ulcers in patients with lower-extremity venous disease. Clinical evaluation should always include serial venous leg ulcer wound measurements and documentation.[20] The committee recommends classifying patients with venous ulcers on the basis of a venous disease classification protocol, including clinical, etiology, anatomy, and pathophysiology also known as the CEAP Classification System.[20]

Routine cultures should not be taken on a regular basis if no clinical signs of infection are present. Venous leg ulcer management requires comprehensive clinical evaluation. The committee suggests that it is best practice to consistently maintain wound measurements and documents. For patients with suspected venous leg ulcers, the committee recommends utilizing the venous duplex ultrasound to evaluate symptoms,

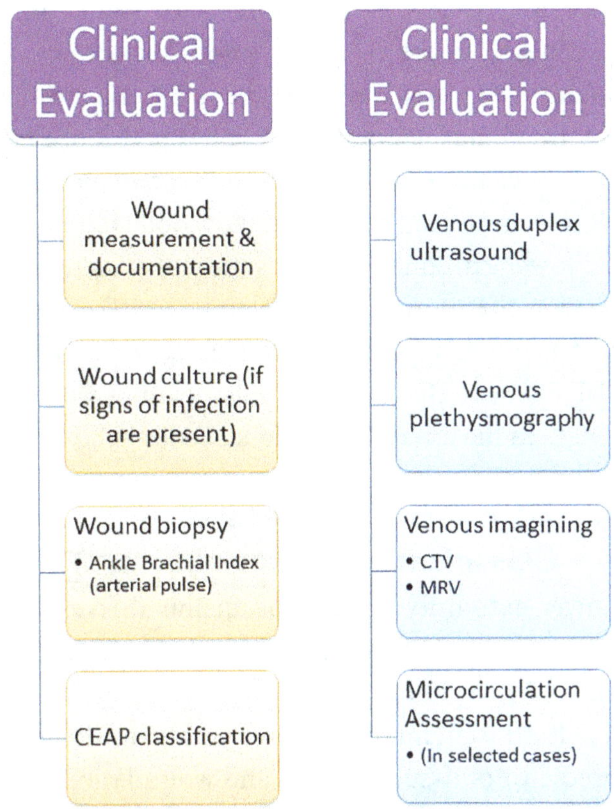

FIGURE 15. Clinical assessment of venous insufficiency should be comprehensive with a global perspective.[20]

including excessive varicosities, leg pain, and swelling.[20] In the event the venous duplex ultrasound does not provide adequate diagnostic information, the committee suggests the use of venous plethysomography.[20] This is a manometric test measuring changes in the blood volume of the lower extremity. There is sufficient evidence to support that an ankle-brachial index (ABI) should be taken to diagnose or exclude large-vessel arterial disease. This method will be discussed at length in the arterial ulcer classification sections.

G. Fontaine - Rutherford Classification (arterial ulcers)

Lower-extremity arterial perfusion thrives off homeostatic cardiac functionality. In the presence of peripheral arterial disease (PAD), critical limb ischemia has shown to be an integral predictor of tissue necrosis and wound morbidity. The Rutherford and Fontaine classifications originally used three broad categories to assess ischemic ulceration, gangrene, and rest pain. Refer to Chapter 10: Diabetic Foot Ulcers for further information on these classifications. It should be noted that even though this classification system is useful in identifying patients with increased risk of major limb amputation, it does not sufficiently determine the best therapy to apply to a diverse spectrum of patients.[21]

Robert B. Rutherford in 1986 made revisions to some of the categories by incorporating tissue loss and the degree of ischemic ulceration formation.[21] In 1997, Rutherford revised it again so that it now consists of four grades and seven categories.[21] The broad classifications of gangrene, ischemic ulceration, and rest pain help evaluate these clinical concerns pertaining to lower-limb ischemic wounds. However, the Rutherford and Fontaine classification systems needed to incorporate a more comprehensive system that includes a means to assess the presence of infection while stratifying the extent of tissue loss.

H. Society for Vascular Surgery Lower Extremity (SVSLE) Guidelines Committee – arterial ulcers

The Society for Vascular Surgery Lower Extremity Guidelines Committee formed a new classification system to take into account the changes in demographics over the past several decades, the increased incidence of diabetes mellitus in this population, and the advances in revascularization techniques.[22] Specifically, this system was developed to support clinicians in their management of patients whose comorbidities increase their risk of lower-extremity amputation. The three main risk factors stratified are: wound extent, ischemia, and foot infection (WIfi).

By assessing wound extent, ischemia, and foot infection, clinicians are able to use these key factors that need to be evaluated in predicting amputation risk.[22] Wounds are graded based on severity, 0 through 3 based on size and depth, and it notes whether there is any predictive ability possible to achieve and/or promote wound healing.[22]

If toe pressure (TP) and ankle brachial index (ABI) measurements result in different grades, TP will be the primary determinants of ischemia grade.[22] Critical limb ischemia (CLI) has been defined as the point where the lack of perfusion to the affected limb without revascularization would inevitably result in limb loss. A single cut-off point for CLI is no longer applicable in clinical practice.[22] Wound healing is governed by not only the severity of ischemia, but also other factors that should be taken into account, such as the extent, depth, and the severity of infection. The etiology of arterial disease can be attributed to systemic hypertension, diabetes, renal failure, vasculitis, and progressive atherosclerosis of peripheral vessels.[22] Arterial ulcers usually present a round "punched out" appearance with well-defined wound margins. They are usually found around the lateral malleolus, mid-tibia section, tips of toes (phalanges), or where there is distinct pressure from footwear or walking.

The Wound, Ostomy, and Continence Nurses Society (WOCN) constructed a multidisciplinary guideline for the management of wounds in patients with lower-extremity arterial disease.[24] The committee recommends a thorough assessment of the patient's health history to identify risk factors for lower-extremity arterial disease (LEAD).

It is imperative for clinicians to assess the characteristics of the arterial wound. Key features should include location, wound edges, exudate, and the presence or absence of necrotic nonviable tissue.[24] Initial examination should include a comprehensive, bilateral lower-extremity assessment that involves skin temperature, capillary refill, and venous refill and color changes.[24] When palpating pedal pulses, it should be noted that the presence of palpable pulses does not rule out LEAD.[24] The key risk factors for lower-extremity arterial disease (LEAD) are the following: dyslipidemia, renal insufficiency, tobacco use, diabetes, and hypertension.

To assess the level of ischemia the patient exhibits, an ABI should be conducted to measure

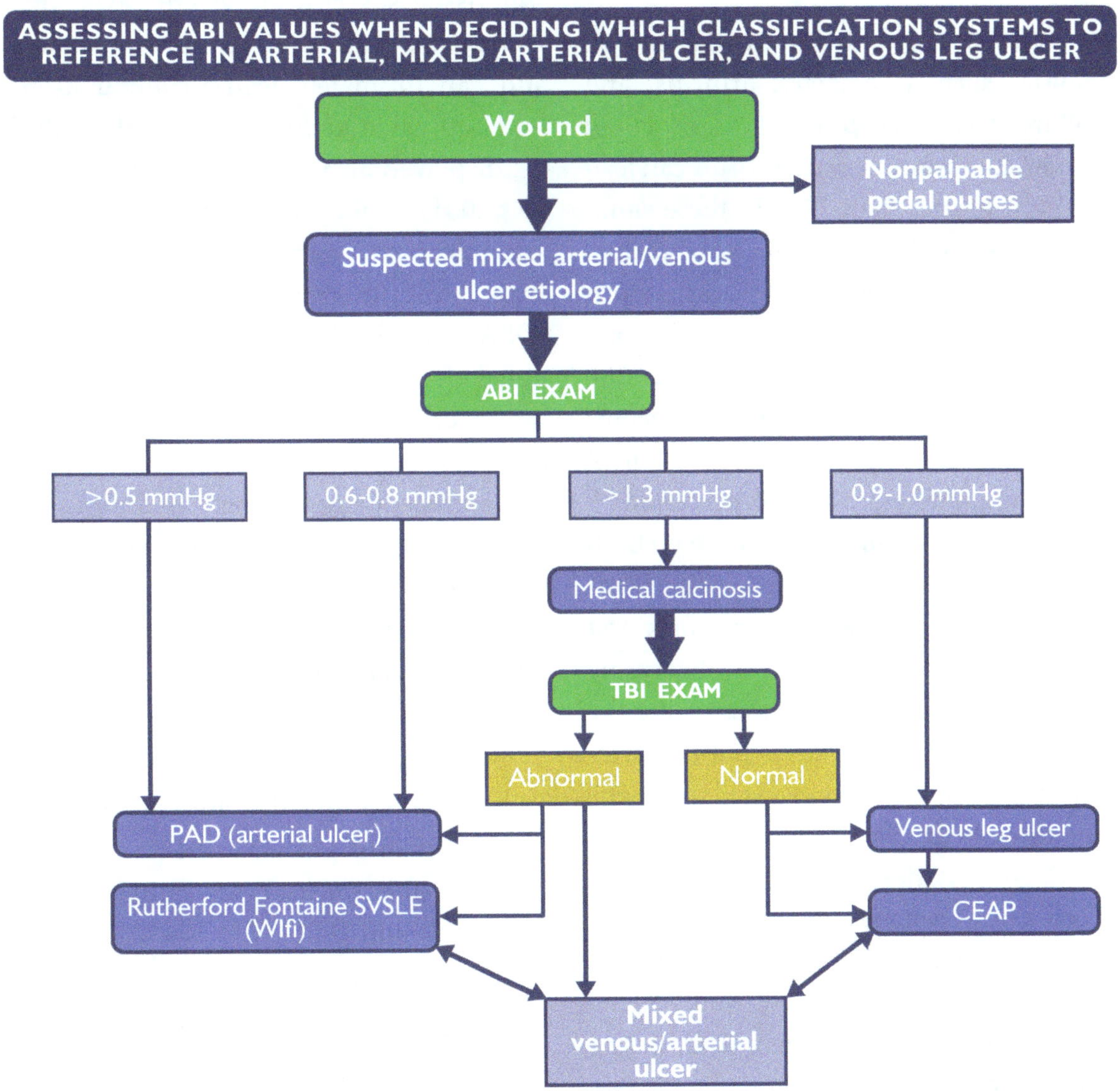

FIGURE 16.
Printed with permission by Robert J. Snyder, MD

arterial blood flow in both lower extremities. This is a noninvasive test to identify vascular disease by comparing systolic blood pressure in the ankle to the higher of the brachial systolic blood pressure.[22,24] The ABI values depict an estimation of central systolic blood pressure and should be analyzed to determine the appropriate treatment plan.[22,24]

- Normal ABI: 1.00
- ABI < 0.90: Borderline perfusion
- ABI range 0.6 -0.8: Severe ischemia
- ABI less than or equal to 0.5: Critical ischemia

It should be noted that in patients with comorbidities such as diabetes, arthritis, and renal failure ankle vessel calcification could result in non-compressible arteries. This can lead to an ABI test greater than 1.30. In these situations, clinicians should employ the toe-brachial index (Figure 16). Toe vessels are less susceptible to calcification. When a wound is not healing and the ABI is less than 0.90 and/or toe pressure is less than 30 mmHg, the committee recommends the transcutaneous oxygen measurement ($TcPO_2$) technique to assess tissue perfusion.[24] Neurosensory status should be evaluated on both feet for loss of protective sensation. The Semmes Weinstein monofilament, tuning fork and percussion hammer can be used to determine the neurosensory status.[22,24] In cases where the ABI range is between 0.8 and 1.0 mmHg, arterial occlusion is unlikely and can lead clinicians to utilize the CEAP Classification System and venous imaging studies to assess whether the wound could be of venous etiology.

Among patients with LEAD, the level of evidence differs somewhat for various methods of assessment; however, there is a Class I recommendation for ABI, arterial doppler or transcutaneous oximetry. There are task force consensus statements for monofilament testing for neuropathy and performing a complete history. There is good evidence and Class II recommendations for performing a toe-brachial index among patients with an ABI > 1.3, or, for patients who are surgical or endovascular candidates, using magnetic resonance angiography or multi-detector computed tomographic angiography.

Previous wound classification systems have in some ways disregarded infection and its threat to lower limbs. The SVS WIfI classification system incorporated the IDSA and PEDIS that takes into account both bone and soft tissue severity. In severe cases, infection is a major event that prompts hospitalization and can ultimately lead to amputation.[22] A longitudinal study of 1,666 people with diabetes displayed an increased risk for amputation ($p < .001$), higher-level amputation ($P < .001$), and lower-extremity related hospitalization ($P < .001$) with increasing infection based on the IDSA classification system.[22,25] It should be noted that patients who depict signs of infection in conjunction with ischemia are less likely to jumpstart the wound-healing cascade and are at high risk of amputation.

SVS Wifi Classification system includes the following: **W: Wound/Clinical category.** SVS grades for rest pain and wounds/tissue loss (ulcers and gangrene):

- Grade W0 is patient with no ulcer, no gangrene but has ischemic rest pain and has non-invasive assessment similiar to ischemia grade 3 (ABI < or = 0.39, ankle systolic pressure < 50 mmHg, $TcPO_2$ with <30 mmHg);
- Grade W1 is patient with small, shallow ulcer(s) on distal leg or foot, no exposed bone, unless limited to distal phalanx but no gangrene. Usually this patient has

minor tissue loss and they are salvageable with simple digital amputation (1 or 2 digits) or skin coverage;

- Grade W2 is patient with deeper ulcer with exposed bone, joint; or tendon, generally not involving the heel; shallow heel ulcer without calcaneal involvement or gangrenous changes mainly limited to digits. This patient has major tissue loss and they are salvageable with multiple (>3) digital amputations or standard TMA (transmetatarsal amputation) + or - skin coverage;
- Grade W3 is patient with extensive, deep ulcer involving forefoot and/or midfoot; deep, full thickness heel ulcer+ or - calcaneal involvement or shows extensive gangrene involving forefoot and /or midfoot; full thickness heel necrosis + or - calcaneal involvement. This patient has extensive tissue loss; salvageable only with a complex foot reconstruction or nontraditional TMA (Chopart or Lisfranc): flap coverage or complex wound management needed for large soft tissue defect.

Ischemia grades are based on noninvasive vascular assessment of ABI, ankle systolic pressure and $TcPO_2$. Ischemia Grade 0 has ABI > or = 0.80, Ankle systollic pressure > 100 mmHg and $TcPO_2$ > or + 60 mmHg. Ischemia Grade 1 has ABI of 0.6-0.79, ankle systolic pressure 70-100 mmHg, $TcPO_2$ 40 -59 mmHg. Ischemia Grade 2 has ABI 0.4-0.59, ankle systolic pressure 50-70 mmHg, $TcPO_2$ 30 -39 mmHg. Ischemia Grade 3 has ABI < or =0.39, ankle systolic pressure < 50 mmHg and $TcPO_2$ < 30 mmHg. Patient with diabetes should have $TcPO_2$ measurements because if arterial calcification precludes reliable ABI, then ischemia should be documented by $TcPO_2$, SPP, or PVR and in that scenario $TcPO_2$ is a primary determinant of ischemia grade.

Foot infection is assessed based on the IDSA and PEDIS classification systems.[22-23] A wound is considered uninfected (Grade 0) if there are no symptoms or signs of infection. A wound is considered to have a mild infection (Grade1) if at least two of the following clinical signs are present: 1) local swelling or induration, 2) erythema > 0.5 to <_cm around the ulcer, 3) local tenderness or pain, 4) local warmth, 5) purulent drainage. A wound is considered to have moderate infection (Grade 2) if there is local infection (as described above) with erythema > 2 cm, or involving structures deeper than skin and subcutaneous tissues (e.g., abscess, osteomyelitis, septic arthritis). Patients with Grade 2 infections do not have systemic inflammatory response signs (SIRS). If a patient has evidence of local infection with signs of SIRS, he/she is considered to have a (Grade 3) severe infection. Signs of SIRS are: 1) temperature > 38°C or < 36°C, 2) heart rate > 90 beats/min, 3) respiratory rate > 20 breaths/min, 4) PaCo2 < 32 mmHg.

Summary

An accurate wound assessment is important for managing wounds. The process outlined in this chapter defines essential steps to assess any problem wounds. The wound assessment information helps the wound care practitioner to develop an effective treatment plan. Ongoing wound assessment is necessary to monitor and evaluate response of the wound to treatment interventions. Evaluation of wound progress and healing requires analysis of qualitative and quantitative wound assessments. It is recommended that periodic wound assessment should be performed regularly, using the essential steps that are defined in this chapter. This chapter also describes various classification systems for different wound etiology that will enable readers to classify severity of the wounds.

Review questions

1. **Using the Wagner Classification System, what grade would be applied to a deep ulcer that penetrates to the tendon or joint capsule?**
    a. Grade 1
    b. Grade 2
    c. Grade 3
    d. Grade 4
    e. None of the above

2. **What is a key limitation to the Wagner Classification System?**
    a. Superficial diabetic ulcer with a component of ischemia or infection is not accounted in the Wagner Grading System.
    b. It is not a widely utilized classification system.
    c. Wagner Classification does not incorporate depth as a factor.
    d. Wagner Classification System does not incorporate infection/gangrene as a factor.
    e. None of the above

3. ***True/False.*** Secondary clinical signs of infection in the diabetic patient do NOT have any sort of predictive value.

4. ***True/False.*** Pressure may be a factor that could cause a skin tear, but the etiology of skin tears differs from that of pressure ulcers.

5. **What are the three main risk factors that are stratified in the updated Society for Vascular Surgery Lower Extremity (SVSLE) guideline in the management of arterial ulcers?**
    a. Wound extent, ischemia, foot infection
    b. HbA1c, infection, ischemia
    c. Pressure, shearing, friction
    d. Foul odor, friable discolored granulation tissue, undermining
    e. Local gangrene, erythema, systemic inflammatory response

ANSWERS: 1) b
2) a
3) False
4) True
5) a

References

1. Keast DH, Bowering CK, Evans AW, Mackean GL, Burrows C, D'Souza L. MEASURE: A proposed assessment framework for developing best practice recommendations for wound assessment. Wound Repair and Regeneration. 2004 Jun 7;12(s1):1-17.
2. Griffin JE et al. A comparison of photographic and transparency based methods for measuring wound surface area. Physical Therapy 1993;73:117-122..
3. Thawer HA, Houghton PE, Woodbury MG, Keast D, Campbell K. Computer-assisted and manual wound size measurement. Ostomy/wound management. 2002;48(10):46-53.
4. Falanga V. Classifications for wound bed preparation and stimulation of chronic wounds. Wound Rep Reg 2000;8:347–352.
5. Van Rijswijk L. Wound assessment and documentation. In: Krasner, DL, Rodeheaver, GT, Sibbald, RG, editors. Chronic wound care: a clinical source book for healthcare professionals. Wayne (PA): HMP Communications, 2001;3rd ed.:101–115.
6. Oyibo S, Jude E, Tarawneh I, Nguyen H, Harkless L, Boulton A. A comparison of two diabetic foot ulcer classification systems: the Wagner and the University of Texas wound classification systems. Diabetes Care. 2001;24(1):84-88.
7. Snyder RJ, Kirsner RS, Warriner 3rd RA, Lavery LA, Hanft JR, Sheehan P. Consensus recommendations on advancing the standard of care for treating neuropathic foot ulcers in patients with diabetes. Ostomy Wound Manage. 2010 Apr 1;56(4 Suppl):S1-24.
8. Lipsky B, Brandt A, Cornea P, Pile J, Peters E, Armstrong D et al. Executive summary: 2012 Infectious Diseases Society of America clinical practice guideline for the diagnosis and treatment of diabetic foot infections. Clinical Infectious Diseases. 2012;54(12):1679-1684.
9. Armstrong DG, Lavery LA, Sariaya M, Ashry H. Leukocytosis is a poor indicator of acute osteomyelitis of the foot in diabetes mellitus. J Foot Ankle Surg. 1996 Jul-Aug;35(4):280-283.
10. Pendsey SP. Understanding diabetic foot. International Journal of Diabetes in Developing Countries. 2010;30(2):75-79. DOI: 10.4103/0973-3930.62596.
11. Cutting KF, Harding KG. Criteria for identifying wound infection. Wound Care 1994;3(4):198–201.
12. Gardner SE, Hillis SL, Frantz RA. Clinical signs of infection in diabetic foot ulcers with high microbial load. Biological Research for Nursing. 2009;11(2):119-128. DOI:10.1177/1099800408326169.
13. Lyder CH, Ayello EA. Pressure ulcers: a patient safety issue. In: Hughes RG, editor. Patient Safety and Quality: An Evidence-Based Handbook for Nurses. Rockville (MD): Agency for Healthcare Research and Quality (US); 2008 Apr. Chapter 12. [Internet]. Available from: http://www.ncbi.nlm.nih.gov/books/NBK2650/.
14. Prevention and treatment of pressure ulcers: quick reference guide. National Pressure Ulcer Advisory Panel, European Pressure Ulcer Advisory Panel and Pan Pacific Pressure Injury Alliance. Emily Haesler, editor.Osborne Park(Australia): Cambridge Media;2014.
15. Nixon J, Cranny G, Bond S. Skin alterations of intact skin and risk factors associated with pressure ulcer development in surgical patients: a cohort study. Int J Nurs Stud. 2007 Jul;44(5):655-663. Epub 2006 Apr 24.
16. Baranoski S. Meeting the challenge of skin tears. Adv. Skin Wound Care 2005;18(2):74-75.
17. Stephen-Haynes J, Carville K. Skin tears made easy. Wounds International 2011;2(4). [Internet]. Available from http://www.woundsinternational.com.

18. LeBlanc K, Baranoski S. Skin tears: state of the science: consensus statements for the prevention, prediction, assessment, and treatment of skin tears. Adv. Skin Wound Care. 2011;24(9)(Supple 1):2-15.

19. Baranoski S, Ayello EA. Wound care essentials: practice principles. Philadelphia: Lippincott Williams & Wilkins; 2007; 2nd ed.:302-304.

20. O'Donnell TF Jr, Passman MA, Marston WA, Ennis WJ, Dalsing M, Kistner RL, Lurie F, Henke PK, Gloviczki ML, Eklöf BG, Stoughton J, Raju S, Shortell CK, Raffetto JD, Partsch H, Pounds LC, Cummings ME, Gillespie DL, McLafferty RB, Murad MH, Wakefield TW, Gloviczki P, Society for Vascular Surgery, American Venous Forum. Management of venous leg ulcers: clinical practice guidelines of the Society for Vascular Surgery and the American Venous Forum. J Vasc Surg. 2014 Aug;60(2 Suppl):3S-59S.

21. Rutherford RB, Baker JD, Ernst C et al. Recommended standards for reports dealing with lower extremity ischemia: revised version. J Vasc Surg 1997;26:517–538.

22. Mills JL, Conte MS, Armstrong DG, Pomposelli FB, Schanzer A, Sidawy AN, Andros G. Society for Vascular Surgery Lower Extremity Guidelines Committee. The Society for Vascular Surgery lower extremity threatened limb classification system: risk stratification based on wound, ischemia, and foot Infection (WIfI). Journal of vascular surgery. 2014 Jan 31;59(1):220-234.

23. Lew EJ, Giovinco NA, Armstrong DG. Clinical application of the Society for Vascular Surgery (SVS) lower extremity threatened limb classification system: risk stratification based on wound, ischemia, and foot infection (WIfI).

24. Wound, Ostomy and Continence Nurses Society (WOCN). Guideline for management of wounds in patients with lower-extremity arterial disease. Mount Laurel (NJ): Wound, Ostomy and Continence Nurses Society (WOCN); 2014:204 (WOCN clinical practice guideline series; no. 1).

25. Lavery L.A, Armstrong DG, Murdoch DP, Peters EJ, Lipsky BA. Validation of the Infectious Diseases Society of America's diabetic foot infection classification system. Clin Infect Dis.2007;44:562–565.

26. Wagner FW Jr. The dysvascular foot: a system for diagnosis and treatement. Foot Ankle. 1981; 2(2):64-122.

Chapter 6

WOUND BED PREPARATION

Kevin Y. Woo, RN, PhD, FAPWCA
Dimitri Beeckman, RN, PhD

KEY CONCEPTS

1. Chronic wounds are becoming more prevalent and complex, demanding an organized and systemic approach to wound caring.

2. The wound bed preparation paradigm is developed to help translate holistic wound care into practice.

3. Successful wound bed preparation is largely contingent upon whether the underlying pathologic process/comorbidities and patient-oriented concerns are sufficiently addressed prior to local wound care.

4. There are four essential components for wound bed preparation including debridement/devitalized tissue, control of infection (bioburden)/prolonged inflammation, maintaining an optimal moisture balance, and edge effect.

5. Advanced therapies (such as biological agents, skin substitutes, hyperbaric oxygen therapy, and negative-pressure wound therapy) may have a role in chronic wounds but only after debridement, infection, and moisture balance are addressed.

CONTENTS

Introduction

Chronic wounds are complex, requiring an organized and systematic approach to achieve the best patient outcome. Following the wound bed preparation paradigm, clinicians must first determine the wound etiologies and potential for healing. Patient-centered concerns should be evaluated to ensure treatment adherence. Local wound care involves debridement, infection/inflammation management, moisture balance, and edge effect.

I. Case study

Mr. Jones was a 55-year-old construction worker with a 7-year history of type 2 diabetes. He was overweight with a BMI of 27. His diet was poor, containing mostly fast food, due to his work schedule. He also smoked about 1 pack a day for the last 20 years. He did not have a lot of hobbies, but he enjoyed having a beer after work with his coworkers. He developed an ulcer on the plantar surface of his left hallux for three weeks. He presented himself to his family doctor with increased swelling to his left foot and increased redness around the ulcer. His doctor prescribed an antibiotic ointment for the lesion and told Mr. Jones to soak his foot twice a day. Mr. Jones developed a fever and was brought to the Emergency Department. On examination, his toe was black and exuded a pungent, thick drainage. Surgery was required to remove part of his foot. Could the amputation have been prevented? Was the wound management appropriate? What else should be considered other than local wound care? What does it mean when people say "Look at the whole patient not the hole on the patient"?

II. Wound bed preparation

The wound bed preparation paradigm (Figure 1) is developed to help translate holistic wound care into practice.[4-7] Central to the paradigm is a patient with a chronic wound. Optimal wound

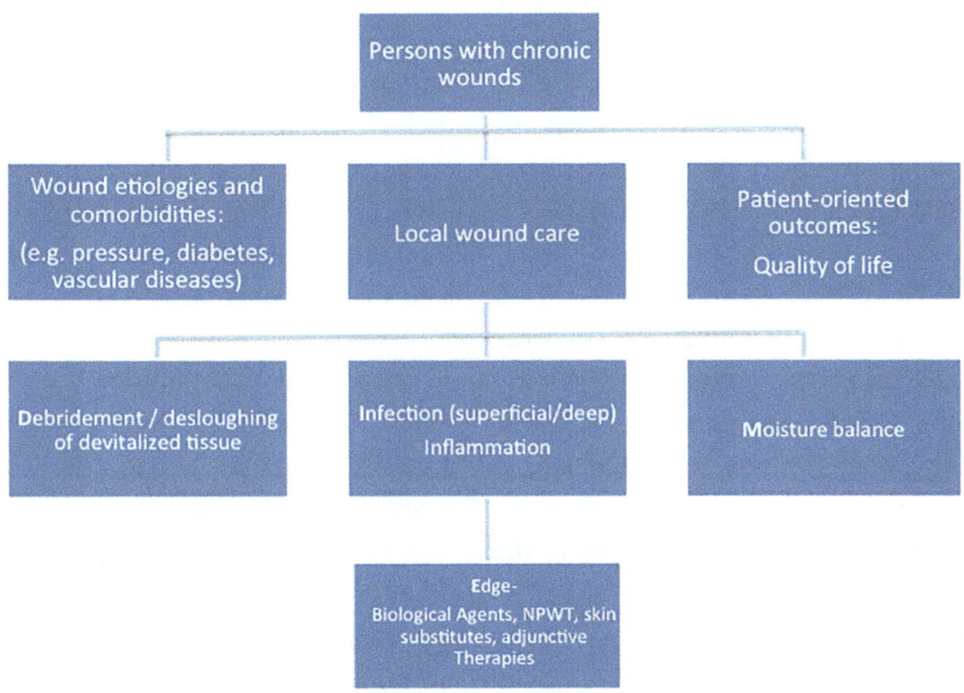

FIGURE 1. Wound bed preparation
Courtesy of Kevin Y. Woo, RN, PhD, FAPWCA

management will require i) meticulous assessment and treatment of the underlying cause, ii) understanding of patient's experience to identify meaningful patient-oriented outcomes, and iii) implementation of local wound care. There are four essential components for local wound care, including debridement or desloughing of devitalized tissue, control of infection (bioburden)/prolonged inflammation, maintenance of an optimal moisture balance, and treatment of stalled unhealthy wound edges (known as the edge effect). Successful wound bed preparation is largely contingent upon whether the underlying pathologic process/comorbidities and patient-oriented concerns are sufficiently addressed prior to local wound care.

III. Wound etiologies and comorbidities

Based on the predominant cause and pathophysiology of tissue damage, the three major types of chronic wounds are pressure ulcers, diabetic foot ulcers, and vascular leg ulcers (including venous, arterial, and mixed diseases). Although complete healing may seem to be the logical goal for most patients, certain wounds are difficult to heal because the underlying cause and comorbidities cannot be treated or corrected.(8)

A. Pressure injury

While the NPUAP has recommended that the term "pressure injury" be used instead of pressure ulcer, the "injury" term does not allow us to distinguish open lesions requiring dressings from deep tissue injuries, so for now we will use the term pressure injury to refer to the pathophysiological mechanism and "ulcer" to describe the lesion requiring treatment.

A pressure injury (PI) and/or pressure ulcer refers to localized cutaneous damage that is primarily caused by excessive or prolonged pressure or shear to the skin and contiguous underlying tissue.(9) There are five mechanisms or pathologic pathways responsible for the injury:

1. *Ischemia*

Ischemia is recognized as one of the primary etiological factors in pressure injury development. Pressure produces compressive forces between a surface, and bony prominence together with shear are two distinct but related mechanisms that reduce local blood flow, compromising nutrient/oxygen supply and producing high levels of metabolic waste products, calcium, and lactic acid inside the cell. Subsequent degradation of membrane phospholipids and increased cellular permeability give rise to intracellular edema and death.(10) However, ischemia alone does not fully explain why tissue injury can be produced by different pressure intensities within inconsistent duration of time. Dehydration, tissue mass (atrophy), as well as nutritional deficiency must also be taken into account to determine tissue tolerance for pressure and oxygen.

2. *Ischemic reperfusion injury*

Ischemic reperfusion injury is caused by reestablishment of blood flow and oxygen after ischemia generating reactive free oxygen radicals. Increased oxidative stress targets at the DNA interrupting normal cellular functions that can lead to tissue necrosis.(10)

3. *Direct cell deformation*

Mechanical load results in a variety of effects at a cellular level leading to strain on cell membrane, cell distortion (deformation), and cytoskeletal reorganization. The amount of tissue damage is directly correlated to the level of the deformation within minutes once the deformation threshold is exceeded.(11)

4. *Impaired lymphatic drainage*

Obstructed lymphatic drainage can contribute to pressure injury development due to the accumulation of anaerobic metabolic waste products.[10,12]

5. *Microclimate*

Microclimate refers to the environment at or near the skin surface that is influenced by the combined effect of skin temperature, humidity/moisture, and air movement.[9] Evidence to date suggests that extremes of skin temperature and/or humidity/skin moisture appear to increase the sensitivity of skin to the damaging effects of pressure, shear stresses, and friction. An increase of 1°C in skin temperature results in an increase of approximately 13% in tissue oxygen demand, making the skin more vulnerable to mechanical damage.[13] Excess moisture from incontinence, sweating, and wound exudation can cause skin maceration, weakening the connections between epidermal cells and collagen fibers. The interruption of normal barrier function increases skin permeability to irritants and pressure damages.

In a recent systematic review and meta-analysis, Beeckman and his colleagues[14] confirmed that individuals with bowel and bladder incontinence and related incontinence-associated dermatitis are five times more likely (95% CI 2.62-9.50) to develop PI than those who are continent. Overall, the extent and severity of tissue injury should also take into account tissue tolerance or the ability of the tissue to mitigate the damaging effect of pressure and related disruption to blood flow. Intrinsic factors that reflect the general conditions are linked to pressure injury but often omitted in routine evaluation. Some of these key factors may include specific disease comorbidities (e.g., cancer, stroke), poor nutritional intake, low Body Mass Index (BMI<18.5),[15] hypoproteinemia, low systolic blood pressure,[16] anemia,[17] contractures and prominent bony deformities, and vascular disease.[18] Despite advances in knowledge and treatment options, the prevalence of pressure ulcers remains high. According to a recent analysis of administrative data including 203,035 unique patients across the spectrum of health-care settings, the prevalence of pressure ulcers was approximately 13% between 2010 and 2013.[19] Of all long-term care residents with pressure ulcers, 72% exhibited more than one skin lesion. Optimal treatment of pressure injuries must include the "5 Rs," strategies to Redistribute pressure, Reduce shear, Remove moisture, Restore activity, and Replete nutritional status.

B. Diabetic foot ulcers

Individuals with diabetes are susceptible to immunodeficiency, neuropathy, and vasculopathy putting them at risk for developing complications in their lower extremities including intractable foot ulcerations.[6,20] The lifetime risk of developing a foot ulcer in people with diabetes is as high as 25%,[21] placing a significant burden on the person and the health-care system. Nonetheless, diabetic foot ulcers and associated complications are deemed highly preventable. In general, plantar pressure redistribution should be considered for all individuals with neurotrophic foot ulcers due to the loss of protective sensation.[22-23] The evidence for the use of total contact casting and irremovable cast walkers for the treatment of active diabetic foot ulcers is beyond refute. Therapeutic shoes and insoles are carefully selected to reduce recurrence.[6] Individuals with ischemic foot would warrant a thorough assessment by a vascular specialist to determine the most appropriate interventions based on the location, the involved angiosomes, and the extent of arterial compromise.[24] Blood glucose control should not be overlooked as an integral part of wound management. Hyperglycemia triggers a constellation of metabolic events leading to excessive production of advanced glycation end-products and overproduction of oxygen free radicals that can delay healing of foot.[21] It has been documented that every 1.0%-point increase in HbA1c could reduce the healing rate by 0.028 cm^2/day (95% CI: 0.003, 0.0054, p=0.027).[25]

C. Venous leg ulcers

Leg ulcers affect 1.5–5.0 per 1,000 in the adult population and 20 per 1000 in people aged over 80 years making this a common geriatric disease.[26] While chronic leg ulcers may involve an array of underlying pathologies including arterial, neuropathic, metabolic, hematological, infectious, malignant, and inflammatory diseases, venous insufficiency predominantly accounts for 70% of all cases.[27] Leg ulcers of venous origin are associated with a prolonged healing trajectory and frequent recurrence—up to 70% within the three months of healing.[28]

Increased venous pressure promotes extravasation and accumulation of white blood cells, growth factors, fibrin, and hemosiderin (ferritin and ferric iron from red blood cells) causing venous eczema, lipodermatosclerosis, edema, and eventually painful ulcers.[29] To treat the underlying cause, sustained compression therapy is considered the mainstay of treatment. In addition to the obvious benefits of edema reduction, external compression promotes venous blood flow velocity creating shear stress that signals endothelial cells to release nitric oxide.[30,31] Nitric oxide is a potent vasodilator that plays an important role in enhancing capillary perfusion tissue oxygenation.[31]

IV. Patient-oriented outcomes

Management of chronic wounds often requires comprehensive and lifelong behavioral modifications that may entail regular foot care, exercise, dietary changes, and smoking cessation. Patient orientation connotes shared decision making that is one of the determining factors associated with treatment adherence.[32] Emerging evidence highlights a need to shift the chronic disease-management paradigm away from traditional disease-centered care to focus on patient engagement and self-management. Patients with chronic wounds are labeled as "noncompliant" and blamed for allowing ulcers to develop due to their lack of self-control, willpower, and competence to make healthy choices.[33-34] Negative characteristics, stereotypes, or stigma can be disempowering. Through systematic provision of education and supportive interventions, the key objectives of chronic disease self-management is to help patients master skills of self-care, achieve a desired health goal, and experience the best possible quality of life. It is crucial that self-stigma be addressed in this population to avoid the vicious cycle of self-stigma, demoralization, and disengagement from disease management.[34]

Although the primary objective is often focused on healing of the wound, patients with various types of chronic wounds consistently relate pain to be of a higher management priority. In an international survey of over 2,018 people with chronic wounds, over 60% of the respondents reported the experience of pain "quite often" and "all the time."[35] Studies of patients with various chronic wound types validate the pervasiveness of pain that is described as intense, unrelenting, distressing, and often exacerbated at dressing change.[36-37] Even long after the ulcers are healed, people continue to conjure up vivid descriptions of the pain experiences. Among all the symptoms, pain has been described as the worst part of living with chronic wounds constituting significant level of stress.[38] Anticipation or negative expectation of discomfort has been shown to have an opposite effect causing amplification of pain, also known as nocebo hyperalgesia. In a study of 96

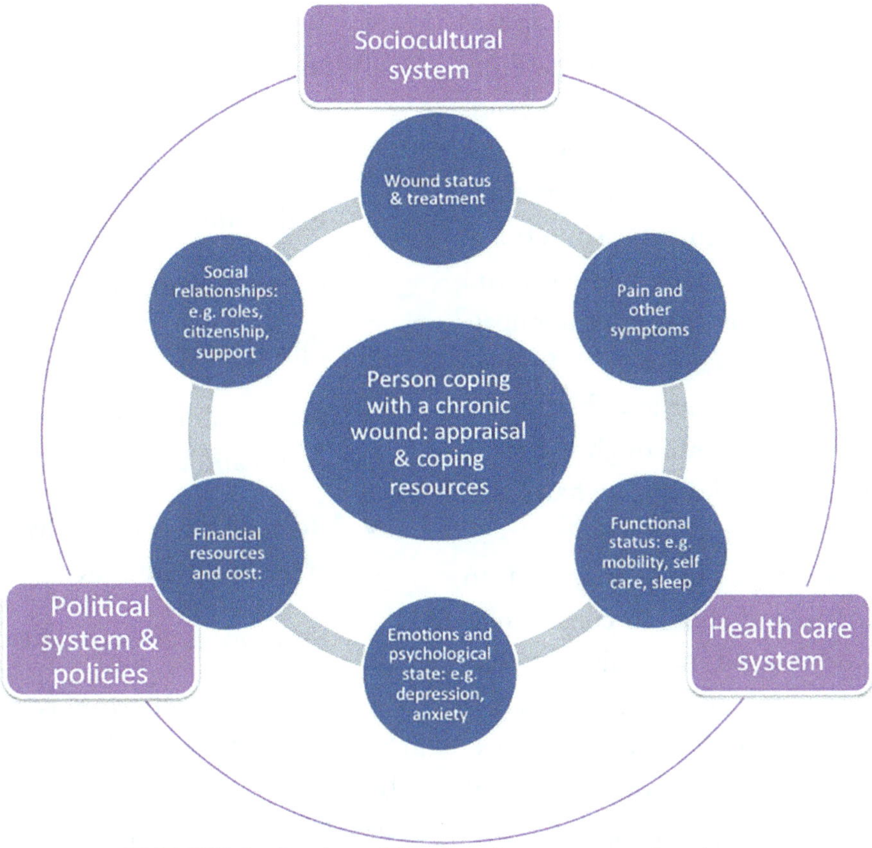

FIGURE 2. Quality of life for chronic wound patients
Courtesy of Kevin Y. Woo, RN, PhD, FAPWCA

patients with chronic wounds, Woo[39] reported that patients who experienced high levels of anxiety also reported high levels of anticipatory pain, leading to high levels of pain at dressing change. The result is a vicious cycle of pain, stress/anxiety, and worsening of pain.

Unremitting pain and increased psychological stress have been postulated to modulate wound healing through interplay between inflammatory and immune mechanisms. In a meta-analysis of 17 studies, Walburn et al.[40] validated the significant relationship between stress and wound healing; the higher the level of stress, the slower the healing process; r=–0.42 (95% CI=–0.51 to –0.32) (P<. 01). Pharmacotherapy should be individualized based on the type (nociceptive versus neuropathic) and severity of pain. In addition, there is a need to address psychosocial aspects of pain including anxiety and personal expectations as part of holistic pain management.[41] Inadequate information and misconceptions can have serious ramifications, hindering optimal pain management, evoking fear and anxiety. Emerging evidence lends support to psycho-educational and behavioral approaches to reduce anxiety and align expectations. Patient-oriented outcomes must be incorporated as an integral part of comprehensive wound management in order to promote comfort and dignity, relieve suffering, and improve quality of life (QoL) (Figure 2).

V. Local wound care

A. Debridement

Debridement and desloughing of devitalized tissue is a necessary step to prepare a clean wound bed and promote healing. The term debridement was initially introduced in the eighteenth century by French surgeons referring to the practice of making incisions into the skin and deep fascia to release pressure from localized swelling following war injuries.[42] Debridement in modern wound care involves various modalities to remove necrotic or devitalized tissue, hyperkeratotic epidermis, foreign debris, dysfunctional cells (cellular burden), bacteria sequestrum, and other undesirable materials that are incompatible with healing in the wound bed.[43] In general, necrotic tissues have been described in the form of eschar and slough. Although eschar is often depicted as the dark, desiccated, hard, and leathery tissue, it could also appear wet, soft, and spongy. Slough, on the other hand, tends to be stringy, mucinous, and slimy in consistency. Buildup of these devitalized materials that consist mainly of denatured protein activates the immune system contributing to an inflammatory response. Dead tissue also provides an ideal medium for the bacterial to proliferate.

Overall, the potential benefits of debridement may include the following:

- Reduction of bacterial burden and risk of infection
- Reduction of pain from excessive inflammation
- Removal of foreign materials and denatured protein that perpetuate an excessive inflammatory response
- Removal of senescent cells that lack normal cellular functions
- Evacuation and drainage of an abscess
- Elimination of the source of odor
- Proper determination of the wound depth and tissue types
- Restoration of a healthy wound base and edges for granulation
- Promotion of wound healing.[43]

However, not all wounds need and benefit from debridement. The decision to perform debridement should take into account whether complete wound closure is realistic and achievable (Table 1). Aggressive debridement is not recommended in non-healable wounds where causative factors that preclude healing cannot be addressed,[44] the most critical factor being compromised perfusion as often seen in diabetics and smokers. Under judicious deliberation, conservative debridement or desloughing—trimming

TABLE 1. Approaches to healable and nonhealable wounds

	Healable Wounds (healing)	Nonhealable Wounds (palliative)
Debridement	Aggressive and regular	Conservative Only for symptom management
Moisture Balance	Maintain moisture for healing	Keep dry Avoid moisture to decrease risk of infection
Infection	Topical antimicrobials for local wound infection Systemic antimicrobials for deep infection	Topical antiseptics, e.g., povidone iodine Systemic antimicrobials for deep infection

loose-hanging slough or fibrin to reduce necrotic mass and associated odor—may be appropriate. The goal of conservative debridement is to enhance quality of life and decrease the risk of infection, not to facilitate healing.[(44)] For healable wounds, different debridement methods have been used, and they are categorized broadly as sharp/surgical, mechanical (e.g., wet to dry dressing), ultrasonic, enzymatic, autolytic (endogenous enzymes from dressings), and biological (maggots).[(45-51)] Where appropriate, the choice of debridement method is dependent on the amount of necrotic tissue, urgency, infection risk, pain, resources or expertise available, and patient preference.

1. *Autolytic debridement*

Autolytic debridement involves creating a moist wound environment that augments the body's natural processes involving phagocytic cells and endogenous enzymes (matrix metalloproteinases) to remove non-viable tissue.[(46-47)] According to a Cochrane review of debridement in diabetic foot ulcers, hydrogel was related to faster healing rate compared with gauze dressings (relative risk [RR]=1·84; 95% confidence interval [CI]: 1·3–2·61).[(45)] However, autolytic debridement may take a long time to complete. Certain patients may not be able to produce noticeable inflammatory symptoms due to underlying condition and comorbidities including diabetes, poor nutritional status, advanced age, corticosteroid use, vascular disease, and immune deficiency.

2. *Surgical debridement*

Sharp surgical debridement involves the application of sharp instruments such as scissors, scalpel, and curette at the bedside—or in the operating room, when extensive debridement and subsequent blood loss is anticipated. Although the target of debridement is the necrotic area, it may be necessary to consider[(52)] removing viable tissues that overlay a tunnelling or undermining wound and unhealthy wound margins. However, this debridement method may not always be feasible due to pain, bleeding, potential cost, and lack of clinician expertise. One study[(53)] compared surgical debridement with conventional wound dressing in patients with diabetic foot ulcer, and the healing time was significantly shorter in the surgical group than in the conventional group (46.73 +/- 38.94 vs. 128.9 +/- 86.60 days; $P < .001$). Alternative options may include hydrosurgery and bipolar radiofrequency energy.[(46-47)]

3. *Mechanical debridement*

Mechanical debridement requires mechanical forces to remove or dislodge wound debris. Wet to dry dressing technique is probably one of the most common forms of mechanical debridement. As the wet (saline) dressing dries up, necrotic materials that are adhered to the structure of the dressing fabric are pulled and removed with force. This method of debridement is non-selective and may cause trauma and tissue damage.[(37)] Hydrotherapies such as whirlpool, pulsatile lavage, and irrigation systems are available, but warrant extra precautions to limit cross-contamination and aerosolizing bacteria droplets.[(47)]

Ultrasonic debridement devices offer a non-contact debridement method that is performed at a 5–15 mm distance from the wound surface.[(51)] Ultrasound wave is delivered to the wound in a saline medium generating two effects to the exposed tissue: (i) acoustic streaming (mechanical force that goes directly to the tissues) and (ii) cavitation (turbulence associated with implosion of vapor bubbles). In one randomized controlled trial, clinical outcomes were similar between ultrasound assisted wound debridement and surgical debridement.[(51)] Vigorous cleansing can be accomplished with monofilament fiber pads. While clinical experiences were promising, high-quality evidence remains elusive.

4. *Enzymatic and chemical debridement*

Enzymatic debridement adds exogenous agents such as proteolytic enzymes, including collagenase, streptokinase, streptodornase, Krill enzymes, trypsin-chymotrypsin, papain/urea, and plant enzymes (e.g., fig, pineapple) to accelerate the debridement process. Normal collagen is surrounded and protected by mucopolysaccharide sheaths from the activity of collagenase; collagenase is a water-soluble proteinase that selectively breaks down denatured collagen especially those that anchor necrotic tissue. According to a systematic review,(50) the authors included six randomized controlled trials that compare collagenase with a placebo ointment. Although meta-analysis was not possible due to the lack of consistent metrics for outcome measurement, five out of six trials reported more-rapid removal of necrotic tissue in wounds that were treated with collagenase.

5. *Biological debridement*

Maggot debridement therapy (MDT), also known as larval therapy or therapeutic myiasis, involves the inoculation of sterile fly larvae, usually the common green-bottle fly, Phaenicia (Lucilia) sericata and Phormia regina (black-bottle blowfly), in wounds to aid debridement and disinfection.(48-49) Larval secretions contain proteolytic enzymes, trypsin-like and chymotrypsin-like serine proteases, and a wide array of matrix metalloproteinases that only target at and break down necrotic tissue. Antimicrobial peptides and deoxyribonuclease in the secretions have also been demonstrated to exert antimicrobial effect and inhibit biofilm formation. In a systematic review of studies that evaluated MDT for chronic, infected wounds, data on healing rate from eight studies were pooled for analysis.(49) Results were in favor of MDT over control therapies (RR = 1.80; 95% CI 1.24–2.60). However, the negative perception had prohibited wider adoption of this therapy by patients and practitioners.

B. Infection

Recent advances in the understanding of wound infection pathogenesis have generated tremendous interest in biofilm and how it is related to wound healing.

When the bacterial burden reaches a critical threshold, increased levels of toxins and inflammatory cells induce local tissue damage (referred as critical colonization or biofilm infection) producing subtle clinical signs and symptoms. Bacteria organized into biofilm are well encapsulated and protected by extracellular polymeric substances (EPS) against host defenses.(54-55) It is a conservative estimation that 60% of chronic wounds have biofilm,(54) putting patients at risk for overt or deep wound infection.

The diagnosis of wound infection is complex taking into account a number of patient (host) factors, wound characteristics, and clinical presentations.(56) A tissue biopsy or aspirate of wound exudate is the gold standard to determine possible causative pathogens of a suspected deep wound infection.(56) As a rule of thumb, indiscriminate and routine wound cultures are not recommended for the diagnosis of wound infection (superficial or deep). Recognizing that all chronic wounds are colonized, a wound swab will always yield a positive culture that does not necessarily confirm or refute wound infection.(57-58) For the same reason, superficial wound swabs rarely identify the causative organisms when deep tissue infection is suspected. Therefore, culture results from a wound swab should be interpreted with caution. If a would culture is deemed appropriate, using the Levine technique had a sensitivity of 0.90, a specificity of 57%, and a positive predictive value and negative

U - unhealthy tissue	Increased surface area on wound bed covered by devitalized tissue and unhealthy granulation tissue (thin and friable, bleeds easily, dark red, dull or dusky discoloration, overgranulation, pocketing, and bridging)
P - poor healing	Stalled wound healing with no significant change in wound size or volume (approximately 10% in last 7 days)
P - pain	New or increased pain
E - exudate	Increased volume of exudate Change of consistency: viscous and thick exudate
R - reek	Presence of foul odor
L - larger in size	Sudden or unexplained increase in wound size or new areas of satellite breakdown
O - osseous tissue and/or deep structure	Wound that probes to bone or deep structures; crepitus may be present
W - warmth	Increased periwound temperature of more than 3° F compared to areas distant from the wound
E - edema	Increased edema or induration around the wound
R - redness	Redness of >2 cm beyond wound margin

TABLE 2. Clinical signs and symptoms of wound infection: UPPER and LOWER

predictive value of 0.77 and 0.91 respectively for chronic wound infections that were confirmed by tissue biopsy.(58)

Based on review of the literature, the proposed wound infection checklist (UPPER and LOWER checklist) describes two clusters of signs and symptoms that are associated with superficial/localized wound bioburden versus deep tissue infection (Table 2). The list of criteria to evaluate wound infection has been validated in previous studies.(59-60) There is no one individual sign or symptom that will accurately confirm the diagnosis of wound infection, but a combination of two or three of these possible signs should be sought for the diagnosis in each level. Collating three clinical signs reported the sensitivity and specificity for signs associated with critical colonization, reported as 73.3% and 80.5% respectively.(60) Patients who are immunocompromised may only present with a wound that is not healing or is worsening when an infection is present as other signs and symptoms may be suppressed.

There is no evidence to support the routine use of systemic antibiotics, and the relative benefits of systemic and topical antimicrobial treatments on wound healing remain unclear.(61) However, the lack of reliable evidence should not be construed as a disparagement against any of the agents.(61-62) Antimicrobial agents should only be used when bacterial burden becomes a clinical concern; a moist interactive dressing may replace dressings with active antimicrobial agents once bacterial burden is controlled. Systemic treatment is indicated for deep-skin and soft-tissue infections to avoid prolonged and excessive uses of systemic antibiotics that often lead to undesirable adverse effects (e.g., *Clostridium difficile* colitis) and promote emergence of resistant bacteria. Increased surface bacterial burden may be treated with topical antimicrobials, antibiotics, and antiseptics including povidone iodine, ethacridine lactate cadexomer iodine, gentian violet, lysozyme, silver dressings, honey, pine resin, polyhexanide, silver sulfadiazine, nitrofurazone with ethoxy-diaminoacridine peroxide-based preparations, chloramphenicol, framycetin, and mupirocin.[61-63]

Considering the recalcitrant nature of biofilm against commonly used antimicrobial agents, Wolcott et al.[64] demonstrated that sharp debridement is effective in physically disrupting the biofilm structure rendering bacteria more susceptible to antimicrobial treatment. In their study, the combination of sharp debridement and antibiotic treatment led to greater than a ninefold reduction in bacterial concentration compared with using antibiotic alone.

Prolonged and excessive inflammation is responsible for wound chronicity.

The imbalance between pro-inflammatory factors and inhibitory enzymes favors destruction of the extracellular matrix and growth factors, delaying cell proliferation, angiogenesis, and the formation of granulation tissue.[1] Systemic and topical anti-inflammatory agents have been used to correct the proteolytic environment in chronic wound milieu. Pentoxifylline is a xanthine derivative and a nonspecific inhibitor of cyclic adenosine monophosphate phosphodiesterases. The compound is anti-inflammatory and has the ability to improve the flexibility of red blood cells and blood viscosity.[65] In a meta-analysis, Jull reviewed twelve trials and concluded that pentoxifylline with and without compression is more effective than the placebo for wound healing.[66] Common gastrointestinal side effects may reduce treatment adherence. Flavonoids, such as escin, hydroxyethylrutoside,[67] and Daflon,[68] are synthetic and natural plant derivatives. Their anti-inflammatory property and potential to increase venous tone and reduce capillary permeability may attenuate symptoms associated with venous stasis disease (especially, sensation of leg heaviness and pain). Aspirin as a potent anti-inflammatory agent have been evaluated for the prevention of leg ulcer recurrence.[69] Collagen/oxidized regenerated cellulose dressing is an absorbent, open-pored, sterile, freeze-dried matrix that binds to and deactivates binding and inactivating excess-damaging proteases, both matrix metalloproteases (MMPs) and elastases in wound exudates. Nanocrystalline silver and manuka honey may also possess anti-inflammatory effects.[70] Other examples are doxycycline, aloe vera plant (anthracene hydroxyl active anti-inflammatory ingredient), Chinese medical herbs, recombinant human activated protein C (an anticoagulant with anti-inflammatory, cytoprotective, and angiogenic effects), and sulodexide (a glycosaminoglycan with antithrombotic, profibrinolytic, and anti-inflammatory effects). However, the paucity of high-quality evidence makes it impossible to draw definitive conclusions about the benefits and harms of these agents.

C. Moisture balance

The importance of moisture balance for wound repair is unequivocal. A moist wound environment promotes autolytic debridement, diffusion of growth factors, cell migration, and early epithelialization.[1-2] The choice of which type of advanced dressing to use is a clinical decision based largely on dressing features such as conformability, cushioning, ease of removal, and ability to minimize pain at the wound site and during dressing changes, all of which contribute to patient comfort; performance measures, such as ease of application, absorbency, wear time, barrier properties, and the ability to protect the periwound area and control wound odor; and of course, costs.[71] To handle and remove excess exudate from the wound, a plethora of absorbent dressings have been developed. According to previous meta-analyses of clinical trials, the relative effectiveness of dressings or topical treatments is inconclusive.[72-77] When drainage volume exceeds the fluid-handling capacity of dressing material, enzyme-rich and caustic exudate may spill over to wound margins causing maceration or tissue erosion and pain.[39] Maceration of the periwound skin typically presents as white, wrinkled, soggy tissue at the wound edge. High volume and viscous exudate is often associated with unpleasant and embarrassing odor, painful periwound maceration, increased infection risk, and exorbitant care cost due to frequent dressing changes.[14]

The major categories of dressings are foams, alginates, hydrofibers, hydrogels, hydrocolloids, and films.

- Foam dressings are designed to wick up a large volume of exudate with minimal lateral movement to prevent periwound skin maceration. The performance of various foam dressings can be affected by the type of contact layer, core material (e.g., polyurethane or polyvinyl alcohol), borders, and backing to determine their fluid-handling capacity and its water vapor transmission rate, leakage, peel force to remove dressing, and antimicrobial properties.[72]
- Alginate dressings are also capable of handling copious exudate, while the gelling effect of these materials will keep the wound base moist.[73] Alginates are derived from brown seaweed or kelp. Depending on the species and the origin of the calcium alginate (leaf or stem), they may have more gelling (high manuronic acid concentration) or a higher fiber strength (high galuronic acid concentration). The calcium component of the alginate may also trigger the coagulation cascade to facilitate hemostasis.
- Hydrofiber dressings consist of carboxymethyl cellulose and have a water-repelling (hydrophobic) component (methylcellulose) that gives this dressing its tensile strength and a water-absorbing (hydrophilic) component (carboxyl) that acts as a fluid lock. As the dressing absorbs fluid, the hydrofiber is converted into a gel consistency.[71]
- Hydrogel dressings are usually indicated for dry wounds. The major ingredient of hydrogels is water (70% to 90%) that donates moisture into the wound base. The backbone for a hydrogel may be a hydrocolloid, propylene glycol, sodium salt, collagen or other water binding substance.[71]
- Hydrocolloid dressings consist of a backing (often a film or polyurethane) with carboxymethyl cellulose, water absorptive components (such as gelatin and pectin), and an adhesive. Hydrocolloids are able to handle low to moderate amounts of fluid.
- Films are transparent, semiocclusive dressings with varying degrees of Moisture Vapor Transmission Rate (MVTR).[71]

D. Edge

The edge effect refers to epithelium that is failing to migrate across a firm and level granulation base despite adequate debridement, infection control and moisture balance.[1]

Based on results of in vitro studies, the normal functions of keratinocytes and fibroblasts to differentiate, migrate, and promote epithelialization are compromised due to overexpression of β-catenin and c-myc on the edge of chronic non-healing wounds.[78] Chronic wounds are notably hypoxic, with transcutaneous oxygen tensions ($TcPO_2$) measured from 5 to 20 mmHg, compared to control tissue values of 30 to 50 mmHg.[79] Temporary hypoxia after injury is a necessary trigger for the initial phases of wound healing, stimulating processes such as the release of growth factors and angiogenesis. However, chronic or prolonged periwound and wound bed hypoxia delays healing due to the imbalance between decreased oxygen delivery/availability and increased tissue demand during recovery from tissue injury.[80] Chronic low $TcPO_2$ and perfusion pressure may be associated with accumulation of necrotic tissue and poor formation of granulation tissue, and may contribute to the accumulation of harmful substances in the periwound microenvironment such as lactic acid (from hypoxia-induced anaerobic metabolism). Advanced therapies (such as biological agents, skin substitutes, hyperbaric oxygen therapy, and negative-pressure wound therapy) may have a role in chronic wounds but only after debridement, infection, and moisture balance are addressed.

Summary

Wound healing draws on art and science to treat wound etiologies, address patient-oriented outcomes, and select local treatment. The wound bed preparation paradigm is a simple model to illustrate the key components of wound care following a systematized approach. This comprehensive wound care paradigm helps guide the development of best practice to have a shared focus between cost effectiveness, evidence-based dressing selection, and individualized patient preference components such as comfort, ease of use, pain reduction, and conformability.

Review questions

1. **Which of the following is NOT associated with pressure injury development?**

    a. Lipodermatosclerosis
    b. Reperfusion injury
    c. Cell Deformation
    d. Microclimate
    e. Impaired lymphatic drainage

2. **Which of the following is NOT the purpose of debridement?**

    a. Reduction of biofilm
    b. Removal of foreign materials
    c. Removal of hyperkeratotic skin
    d. Removal of hypoxic wound bed
    e. Evacuation and drainage of an abscess
    f. Reduction of odor

3. ***True/False:*** Carboxymethyl cellulose dressings are derived from brown seaweed or kelp. They are selected for wound management because of their hemostatic property.

4. ***True/False:*** Aggressive debridement is not recommended for when the underlying cause and comorbidities cannot be treated or corrected:

5. Which of the **three** wound indicators are most likely related to wound infection in the deep or lower compartment?

    a. Foul odor, pruritus, clear exudate
    b. Lack of pain, erythema, size increase
    c. Probe to bone, erythema, increase in wound size
    d. Foul odor, friable discolored granulation tissue, scanty exudate
    e. Probe to bone, increased warmth, pink granulation tissue

ANSWERS: 1) b
2) d
3) False
4) True
5) c

References

1. Woo K, Ayello EA, Sibbald RG. The edge effect: current therapeutic options to advance the wound edge. Adv Skin Wound Care. 2007 Feb;20(2):99-117.
2. Velnar T, Bailey T, Smrkolj V. The wound healing process: an overview of the cellular and molecular mechanisms. J Int Med Res. 2009 Sep-Oct;37(5):1528-42.
3. Kantor J, Margolis DJ. Expected healing rates for chronic wounds. Wounds. 2000;12(6).
4. Sibbald RG, Goodman L, Woo KY, Krasner DL, Smart H, Tariq G, Ayello EA, Burrell RE, Keast DH, Mayer D, Norton L, Salcido RS. Special considerations in wound bed preparation 2011: an update©. Adv Skin Wound Care. 2011 Sep;24(9):415-36;
5. Snyder RJ, Fife C, Moore Z. Components and quality measures of DIME (devitalized tissue, infection/inflammation, moisture balance, and edge preparation) in wound care. Adv Skin Wound Care. 2016 May;29(5):205-15.
6. Woo KY, Botros M, Kuhnke J, Evans R, Alavi A. Best practices for the management of foot ulcers in people with diabetes. Adv Skin Wound Care. 2013 Nov;26(11):512-24
7. Shah JB. Correction of hypoxia—a critical element for wound bed preparation guidelines: TIMEO2 principle of wound bed preparation. J Am Col Certif Wound Spec. 2011 Jun;3(2):26-32.
8. Woo KY, Krasner DL, Kennedy B, Wardle D, Moir O. Palliative wound care management strategies for palliative patients and their circles of care. Adv Skin Wound Care. 2015 Mar;28(3):130-40;
9. European Pressure Ulcer Advisory Panel; National Pressure Ulcer Advisory Panel; Pan Pacific Pressure Injury Alliance. Prevention and treatment of pressure ulcers: clinical practice guideline. Haesler E, editor. Perth (Australia): Cambridge Media; 2014.
10. Coleman S, Nixon J, Keen J, Wilson L, McGinnis E, Dealey C, Stubbs N, Farrin A, Dowding D, Schols JM, Cuddigan J, Berlowitz D, Jude E, Vowden P, Schoonhoven L, Bader DL, Gefen A, Oomens CW, Nelson EA. A new pressure ulcer conceptual framework. J Adv Nurs. 2014 Oct;70(10):2222-34.
11. Reger SI, Ranganathan VK, Orsted HL, Ohura T, Gefen A. Shear and friction in context. In: International guidelines. Pressure ulcer prevention: pressure, shear, friction and microclimate in context. A consensus document. London: Wounds International; 2010. p. 11-18.
12. Takahashi M, Black J, Dealey C, Gefen A. Pressure in context. In: International guidelines. Pressure ulcer prevention: pressure, shear, friction and microclimate in context. A consensus document. London: Wounds International; 2010. p. 2-10.
13. Gefen A. Deep tissue injury from a bioengineering point of view. Ostomy Wound Manage. 2009;55(4):26-36.
14. Beeckman D, Van Lancker A, Van Hecke A, Verhaeghe S. A systematic review and meta-analysis of incontinence-associated dermatitis, incontinence, and moisture as risk factors for pressure ulcer development. Res Nurs Health. 2014 Jun;37(3):204-18.
15. Shahin ES, Meijers JM, Schols JM, Tannen A, Halfens RJ, Dassen T. The relationship between malnutrition parameters and pressure ulcers in hospitals and nursing homes. Nutrition. 2010 Sep;26(9):886-9.
16. Smith ME, Totten, A, Hickam DH, et al. Pressure ulcer treatment strategies: a systematic comparative effectiveness review. Ann Intern Med. 2013;159(1):39-50.
17. Keast DH, Fraser C. Treatment of chronic skin ulcers in individuals with anemia of chronic disease using recombinant human erythropoietin (EPO): a review of four cases. Ostomy Wound Manage. 2004 Oct;50(10):64-70.

18. Thomas Hess C. Checklist for factors affecting wound healing. Adv Skin Wound Care. 2011 Apr;24(4):192.

19. Woo KY, Sears K, Almost J, Wilson R, Whitehead M, VanDenKerkhof EG. Exploration of pressure ulcer and related skin problems across the spectrum of health care settings in Ontario using administrative data. Int Wound J. 2015 Nov 20. doi: 10.1111/iwj.12535.

20. Alavi A, Sibbald RG, Mayer D, Goodman L, Botros M, Armstrong DG, Woo K, Boeni T, Ayello EA, Kirsner RS. Diabetic foot ulcers: part I. Pathophysiology and prevention. J Am Acad Dermatol. 2014 Jan;70(1):1.e1-18.

21. Brem H, Sheehan P, Rosenberg H, Schneider JS, Boulton AJ. Evidence-based protocol for diabetic foot ulcers. Plast Reconstr Surg 2006;117(Suppl 7):193S-209S.

22. Alavi A, Sibbald RG, Mayer D, Goodman L, Botros M, Armstrong DG, Woo K, Boeni T, Ayello EA, Kirsner RS. Diabetic foot ulcers: part II. Management. J Am Acad Dermatol. 2014 Jan;70(1):21.e1-24.

23. Elraiyah T, Prutsky G, Domecq JP, Tsapas A, Nabhan M, Frykberg RG, Firwana B, Hasan R, Prokop LJ, Murad MH. A systematic review and meta-analysis of off-loading methods for diabetic foot ulcers. J Vasc Surg. 2016 Feb;63(2 Suppl):59S-68S.e1-2. doi: 10.1016/j.jvs.2015.10.006. Review.

24. de Oliveira AL, Moore Z. Treatment of the diabetic foot by offloading: a systematic review. J Wound Care. 2015 Dec;24(12):560, 562-70. doi: 10.12968/jowc.2015.24.12.560. Review

25. Christman AL, Selvin E, Margolis DJ, Lazarus GS, Garza LA. Hemoglobin A1c predicts healing rate in diabetic wounds. J Invest Dermatol. 2011 Oct;131(10):2121-7.

26. Labropoulos N, Wang ED, Lanier ST, Khan SU. Factors associated with poor healing and recurrence of venous ulceration. Plast Reconstr Surg. 2012;129(1):179-86.

27. Alavi A, Sibbald RG, Phillips TJ, Miller OF, Margolis DJ, Marston W, Woo K, Romanelli M, Kirsner RS. What's new: management of venous leg ulcers: approach to venous leg ulcers. J Am Acad Dermatol. 2016 Apr;74(4):627-40. doi: 10.1016/j.jaad.2014.10.048. Review.

28. Kantor J, Margolis DJ. A multicentre study of percentage change in venous leg ulcer area as a prognostic index of healing at 24 weeks. Br J Dermatol. 2000 May;142(5):960-4.

29. Woo KY, LeBlanc K, Livingston M. Management of venous stasis ulcers in the older adult. Curr Geriatr Rep. 2015;4:229-36.

30. Woo KY, Alavi A, Evans R, Despatis M, Allen J. New advances in compression therapy for venous leg ulcers. Surg Technol Int. 2013 Sep 30;23. pii: sti23/40.

31. Mayrovitz HN, Macdonald JM. Medical compression: effects on pulsatile leg blood flow. Int Angiol. 2010 Oct;29(5):436-41.

32. Anderson RM, Funnell MM. Compliance and adherence are dysfunctional concepts in diabetes care. Diabetes Educ. 2000;26:597-604.

33. Browne JL, Ventura A, Mosely K, Speight J. 'I call it the blame and shame disease': a qualitative study about perceptions of social stigma surrounding type 2 diabetes. BMJ Open. 2013 Nov 18;3(11):e003384.

34. Woo K. New initiative: online social support program for people with diabetes and foot ulcers. Diabet Foot Can. 2014;2:11-2.

35. Price PE, Fagervik-Morton H, Mudge EJ, Beele H, Ruiz JC, Nystrøm TH, Lindholm C, Maume S, Melby-Østergaard B, Peter Y, Romanelli M, Seppänen S, Serena TE, Sibbald G, Soriano JV, White W, Wollina U, Woo KY, Wyndham-White C, Harding KG. Dressing-related pain in patients with chronic wounds: an international patient perspective. Int Wound J. 2008 Jun;5(2):159-71.

36. Woo K, Sibbald G, Fogh K, et al. Assessment and management of persistent (chronic) and total wound pain. Int Wound J. 2008;5:205-15.

37. Upton D, Solowiej K, Hender C, Woo KY. Stress and pain associated with dressing change in patients with chronic wounds. J Wound Care. 2012;21:53-4.

38. Douglas V. Living with a chronic leg ulcer: an insight into patients' experiences and feelings. J Wound Care. 2001;10(9):355–360.

39. Woo KY. Unraveling nocebo effect: the mediating effect of anxiety between anticipation and pain at wound dressing change. J Clin Nurs. 2015 Jul;24(13-14):1975-84. doi: 10.1111/jocn.12858.

40. Walburn J, Vedhara K, Hankins M, Rixon L, Weinan J. Psychological stress and wound healing in human: systematic review and meta-analysis. J Psychocom Res. 2009;67:253-71.

41. Woo KY, Abbott LK, Librach L. Evidence-based approach to manage persistent wound-related pain. Curr Opin Support Palliat Care. 2013 Mar;7(1):86-94

42. Guthrie HC, Clasper JC. Historical origins & current concepts of wound debridement. J R Army Med Corps. 2011;157:130-2.

43. Elraiyah T, Domecq JP, Prutsky G, Tsapas A, Nabhan M, Frykberg RG, Hasan R, Firwana B, Prokop LJ, Murad MH. A systematic review and meta-analysis of debridement methods for chronic diabetic foot ulcers. J Vasc Surg. 2016 Feb;63(2 Suppl) 37S-45S.e1-2. doi: 10.1016/j.jvs.2015.10.002.

44. Woo KY, Krasner DL, Kennedy B, Wardle D, Moir O. Palliative wound care management strategies for palliative patients and their circles of care. Adv Skin Wound Care. 2015 Mar;28(3):130-40; quiz 140-2. doi: 10.1097/01.ASW.0000461116.13218.43.

45. Smith F, Dryburgh N, Donaldson J, Mitchell M. Debridement for surgical wounds. Cochrane Database Syst Rev. 2011;CD006214.

46. Gethin G, Cowman S, Kolbach DN. Debridement for venous leg ulcers. Cochrane Database Syst Rev. 2015. doi: 10.1002/14651858.cd008599.pub2

47. Hoppe IC, Granick MS. Debridement of chronic wounds. Clin Plast Surg. 2012;39(3):221-8.

48. Shi E, Shofler D. Maggot debridement therapy: a systematic review. Br J Community Nurs. 2014;19(Suppl 12):6-13. doi: 10.12968/bjcn.2014.19.sup12.s6

49. Sun X, Jiang K, Chen J, Wu L, Lu H, Wang A, Wang J. A systematic review of maggot debridement therapy for chronically infected wounds and ulcers. Int J Infect Dis. 2014;25:32-7.

50. Ramundo J, Gray M. Enzymatic wound debridement. J Wound Ostomy Continence Nurs. 2008;35(3):273-80.

51. Herberger K, Franzke N, Blome C, Kirsten N, Augustin M. Efficacy, tolerability and patient benefit of ultrasound-assisted wound treatment versus surgical debridement: a randomized clinical study. Dermatology. 2011;222(3):244-9.

52. O'Neill DK, Tsui SM, Ayello EA, Cuff G, Brem H. Anesthesia protocol for heel pressure ulcer debridement. Adv Skin Wound Care. 2012 May;25(5):209-19.

53. Piaggesi A, Schipani E, Campi F, Romanelli M, Baccetti F, Arvia C, Navalesi R. Conservative surgical approach versus non-surgical management for diabetic neuropathic foot ulcers: a randomized trial. Diabet Med. 1998 May;15(5):412-7.

54. James GA, Swogger E, Wolcott R, et al. Biofilms in chronic wounds. Wound Repair Regen. 2008;16(1):37-44.

55. Percival SL, Emanuel C, Cutting KF, Williams DW. Microbiology of the skin and the role of biofilms in infection. Int Wound J. 2012 Feb;9(1):14-32.

56. Woo KY, Alam T, Marin J. Topical antimicrobial toolkit for wound infection. Surg Technol Int. 2014 Nov;XXV:45-52.

57. Demetriou M, Papanas N, Panopoulou M, Papatheodorou K, Bounovas A, Maltezos E. Tissue and swab culture in diabetic foot infections: neuropathic versus neuroischemic ulcers. Int J Low Extrem Wounds. 2013 Jun;12(2):87-93.

58. Rondas AA, Schols JM, Halfens RJ, Stobberingh EE. Swab versus biopsy for the diagnosis of chronic infected wounds. Adv Skin Wound Care. 2013 May;26(5):211-9.

59. Woo KY, Coutts PM, Sibbald RG. A randomized controlled trial to evaluate an antimicrobial dressing with silver alginate powder for the management of chronic wounds exhibiting signs of critical colonization. Adv Skin Wound Care. 2012 Nov;25(11):503-8.

60. Woo KY, Sibbald RG. A cross-sectional validation study of using NERDS and STONEES to assess bacterial burden. Ostomy Wound Manage. 2009 Aug;55(8):40-8.

61. Norman G, Dumville JC, Moore ZE, Tanner J, Christie J, Goto S. Antibiotics and antiseptics for pressure ulcers. Cochrane Database Syst Rev. 2016 Apr 4; 4:CD011586. doi: 10.1002/14651858.CD011586.pub2.

62. O'Meara S, Al-Kurdi D, Ologun Y, Ovington LG, Martyn-St James M, Richardson R. Antibiotics and antiseptics for venous leg ulcers. Cochrane Database Syst Rev. 2014 Jan 10;(1): CD003557. doi: 10.1002/14651858.CD003557.pub5.

63. Percival SL, Cooper RA, Lipsky BA. Antimicrobial interventions for wounds. In: Percival SL, Cutting K, editors. Microbiology of wounds. CRC Press; 2010. p. 293-327.

64. Wolcott RD, Rumbaugh KP, James G, Schultz G, Phillips P, Yang Q, Watters C, Stewart PS, Dowd SE. Biofilm maturity studies indicate sharp debridement opens a time-dependent therapeutic window. J Wound Care. 2010 Aug;19(8):320-8.

65. Sloczynska K, Kozka M, Pekala E, Marchewka A, Marona H. In vitro effect of pentoxifylline and lisofylline on deformability and aggregation of red blood cells from healthy subjects and patients with chronic venous disease. Acta Biochim Pol. 2013;60(1):129-35.

66. Jull A, Waters J, Arroll B. Pentoxifylline for treatment of venous leg ulcers. A systematic review. Lancet. 2002;359:1550-4.

67. Aziz Z, Tang WL, Chong NJ, Tho LY.A systematic review of the efficacy and tolerability of hydroxyethylrutosides for improvement of the signs and symptoms of chronic venous insufficiency. J Clin Pharm Ther. 2015 Apr;40(2):177-85.

68. Rabe E, Agus GB, Roztocil K. Analysis of the effects of micronized purified flavonoid fraction versus placebo on symptoms and quality of life in patients suffering from chronic venous disease: from a prospective randomized trial. Int Angiol. 2015 May 14:1827-39.

69. Del Rio Sola ML, Antonio J, Fajardo G, Vaquero Puerta C. Influence of aspirin therapy in the ulcer associated with chronic venous insufficiency. Ann Vasc Surg. 2012;26(5):620-9.

70. Tsang KK, Kwong EW, Woo KY, To TS, Chung JW, Wong TK. The anti-inflammatory and antibacterial action of nanocrystalline silver and manuka honey on the molecular alternation of diabetic foot ulcer: a comprehensive literature review. Evid Based Complement Alternat Med. 2015;2015. doi: 10.1155/2015/218283.

71. Woo KY, Smith K. Wound dressing selection for pressure ulcers [Internet]. 2014. Available from: http://www.woundsource.com/files/wound_dressing_selection_for_pressure_ulcers.html

72. O'meara S, James MM. Foam dressings for venous leg ulcers. Cochrane Database Syst Rev. 2013. doi: 10.1002/14651858.cd009907.pub2

73. O'Meara S, Martyn-St James M, Adderley UJ. Alginate dressings for venous leg ulcers. Cochrane Database Syst Rev. 2015 Aug 19; 8:CD010182.

74. Dumville JC, Keogh SJ, Liu Z, Stubbs N, Walker RM, Fortnam M. Alginate dressings for treating pressure ulcers. Cochrane Database Syst Rev. 2015.

75. Dumville JC, Stubbs N, Keogh SJ, Walker RM, Liu Z. Hydrogel dressings for treating pressure ulcers. Cochrane Database Syst Rev.

76. Wu L, Norman G, Dumville JC, O'Meara S, Bell-Syer SE. Dressings for treating foot ulcers in people with diabetes: an overview of systematic reviews. Cochrane Database Syst Rev. 2015

77. Forster R, Pagnamenta F. Dressings and topical agents for arterial leg ulcers. Cochrane Database Syst Rev. 2015 Jun 29;6:CD001836.

78. Fadini GP, Albiero M, Menegazzo L, Boscaro E, Pagnin E, Iori E, Cosma C, Lapolla A, Pengo V, Stendardo M, Agostini C, Pelicci PG, Giorgio M, Avogaro A. The redox enzyme p66Shc contributes to diabetes and ischemia-induced delay in cutaneous wound healing. Diabetes. 2010 Sep;59(9):2306-14.

79. Rodriguez PG, Felix FN, Woodley DT, Shim EK. The role of oxygen in wound healing: a review of the literature. Dermatol Surg. 2008;34:1159-69.

80. Ruangsetakit C, Chinsakchai K, Mahawongkajit P, Wongwanit C, Mutirangura P. Transcutaneous oxygen tension: a useful predictor of ulcer healing in critical limb ischemia. J Wound Care. 2010;19(5):202-6.

Chapter 7

DRESSINGS IN WOUND CARE

Dot Weir, RN, CWON, CWS
Pamela Scarborough, PT, DPT, MS, CDE, CWS, CEEAA

KEY CONCEPTS

1. Moist wound healing practices are important for re-epithelialization, decreasing wound depth, and infection rates.

2. The dressing selection goes beyond simply choosing a product to cover the wound. Detailed assessments of the patient and wound should drive the components of goal-directed wound care.

3. Chronic wounds are dynamic, evolving as they progress toward closure or disintegrate to a worsened state. Therefore, the choice of dressings and treatments used for wound management must also change in tandem with the characteristics of the wound and the patient's condition.

4. When making decisions for treatment, one should consider whether the wound has healing potential, is more likely a maintenance wound, or evolved to a non-healable ulcer unable to garner the endogenous constituents needed for wound closure and healing.

5. Amount of drainage drives dressing decisions (i.e., moist wound=moisture maintenance dressings; dry wound=moisture donating dressings; highly exudating wounds=moisture absorbing dressings).

6. Malodorous wounds decrease a patient's health-related quality of life.

7. There is little evidence supporting the effectiveness of one dressing product over another, particularly within the same category of dressings.

CONTENTS

Introduction

Historical perspective on wound dressings

Wound care interventions have been recorded from ancient times. The oldest surviving writings describing wound care date back to 3000 BCE.[1] One 4,000-year-old Sumerian cuneiform clay tablet describes wound care for this era that included washing the wound in hot water and beer.[2] Egyptian papyrus recorded the use of honey and grease on lint (made from vegetable fiber) as a typical "plaster" for wounds.[2-3] Honey has been used for millennia as a component of wound care and is recorded in Egyptian and Indian writings as a treatment in these two diverse cultures long before the Christian era.[3] The Egyptians also wrote of wound care using copper, currently known to be toxic to bacteria.[3] The Greeks discussed cleansing the wound with boiled water, vinegar, and wine. Hippocrates (460-377 BCE) wrote about treating wounds with salves to promote suppuration of the wound. Ancient text written by Hippocrates referred to the removal of necrotic tissue and the importance of reducing inflammation.[2] The Romans described the "four cardinal signs of inflammation: rubor, tumor, calor, et dolor" (redness, swelling, heat, and pain) – assessment parameters we use in today's wound care. Different primitive peoples with diverse climates and availability of materials used – and still use in some cultures – substances from animals, vegetables, roots, herbs, and minerals for the treatment of wounds. Many of the lessons gleaned from ancient and primitive wound treatments have made their way into today's wound care practices. Think about our use of honey, aloe vera, cleansing practices, bandaging, nonadherent dressings, and use of antiseptics to prevent or treat infections. Across the millennia, these interventions are recorded in ancient writings as treatments appropriate for that era of medicine. Although ancient healers did not understand the science of wound healing from a cellular biology perspective, they used many of the same principles in their wound care as we do today.[1-2]

In the late 19th and 20th centuries, healthcare providers and manufacturing companies recognize the importance of infection control, necrotic tissue removal, and moisture balance. In 1886, Johnson & Johnson developed surgical wound dressings consisting of heated, sterilized absorbent cotton with a gauze overlay to prevent fibers from sticking to wounds.[4] Since then sterile wound dressings have become a standard of care in the treatment of surgical, acute, and chronic wounds. Henry Drysdale created Dakin's solution to wash British soldiers' wounds during World War 1.[5] French physician Auguste Lumiere introduced paraffin-impregnated gauze, and Drs. Allen and Koch introduced petrolatum gauze in 1942.[6] These were the first contemporary nonadherent dressings. George Odland, in 1958,[7] observed that blisters healed faster if kept intact, spurring other researchers, such as Walter Krawczyk[8] to investigate the benefits of moist wound healing further.

Dr. George Winter introduced our current understanding of moist wound healing practices in the early 1960s.[6-9] Dr. Winter's landmark study performed on live pigs demonstrated that the rate of epithelialization of acute wounds doubled when covered with a polyethylene film compared to wound healing under a dry scab.[9] Numerous studies followed, including those from Hinman and Maibach, validating Dr. Winter's finding in humans.[10] These studies demonstrated that occluding and maintaining moisture in the wound bed increased all phases of healing. Modern wound research literature demonstrates how important moist wound healing practices are for re-epithelialization, decreasing wound depth and infection rates.[6-10]

Although early modern evidence for the use of moisture-retentive dressings was performed on acute wounds, the results have been extrapolated to chronic nonhealing wounds.

I. Case study

Mr. AB is a 67-year-old male, retired airline pilot with a long history of lower extremity ulcers dating back at least 10 years with current wound open for five years. His past medical history includes type 2 diabetes, hypertension, pulmonary hypertension, antithrombin III deficiency, history of deep vein thrombosis and pulmonary embolus, resulting venous insufficiency and phlebolymphedema, coronary artery disease, obesity, and chronic anemia. Surgical history includes Greenfield filter placement, numerous ablative venous interventions, split-thickness skin graft to venous ulcers eight years earlier, with reopening of original wound three years later. His medications include metformin, omeprazole, allopurinol, warfarin, ferrous gluconate, K+ supplement, ASA, folic acid, a geriatric multivitamin formulation, atenolol, ranitidine, and simvastatin. Past treatments for his venous ulcers have included pretty much every possible dressing as well as short-stretch, long-stretch, multilayer wraps and a compression pump at home.

His initial presentation reveals large, almost circumferential venous ulcers with a large amount of serosanguinous exudate (Figures 1 and 2).

Based on his long history of the ulcers with numerous treatments used, it was recommended that an evaluation by a plastic surgeon be considered for skin grafting. The patient wanted to delay that and continue with dressings. Absorbent dressings such as calcium alginates and hydrofiber dressings were utilized with occasional periwound irritation. Superabsorbent dressings were utilized with better absorption of exudate with better protection of periwound skin. Multilayer compression was utilized the entire time.

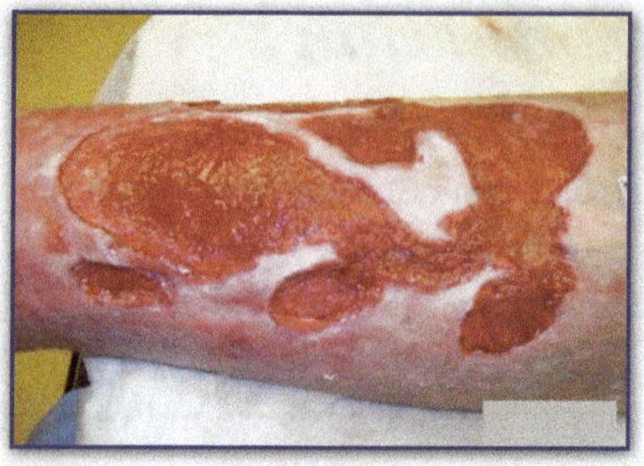

FIGURE 1.

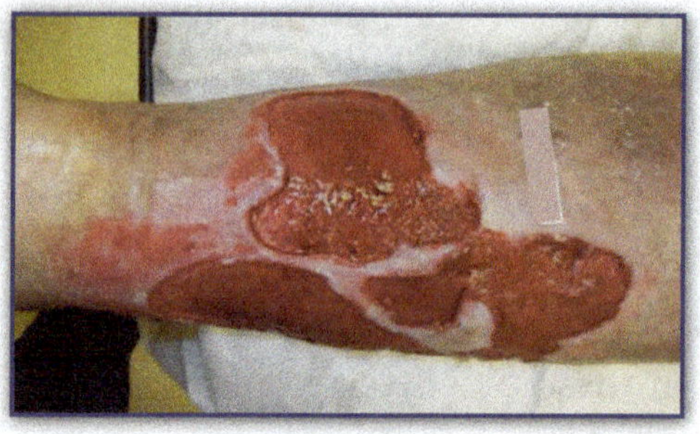

FIGURE 2.

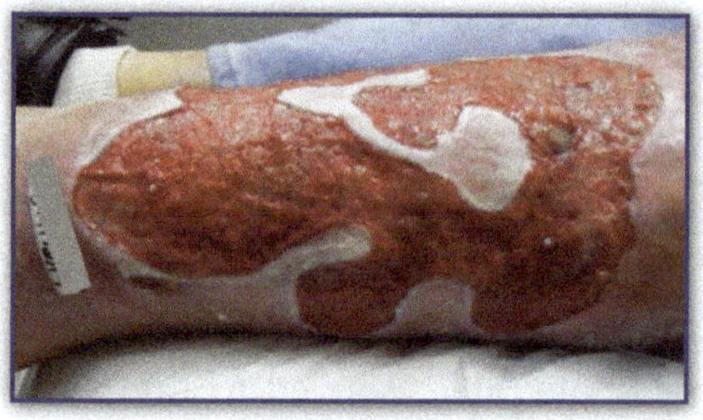

FIGURE 3.

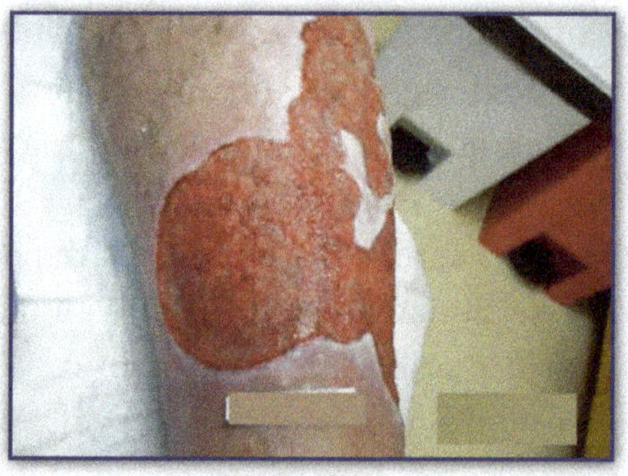

FIGURE 4.

After three more months (Figures 3 and 4), and marginal improvement in wound size, the patient agreed to a plastic surgery consult and a skin graft was planned.

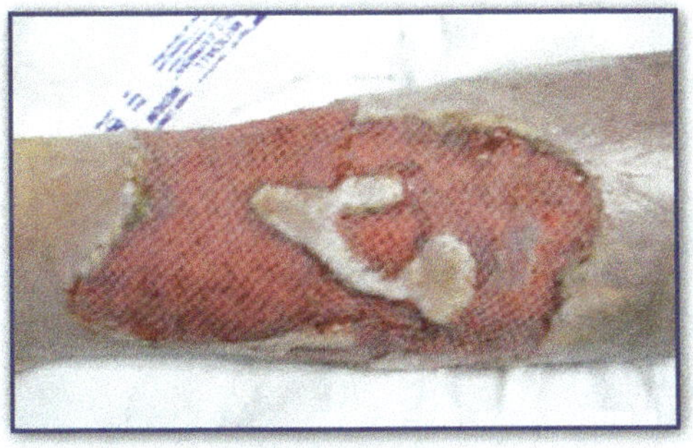

FIGURE 5.

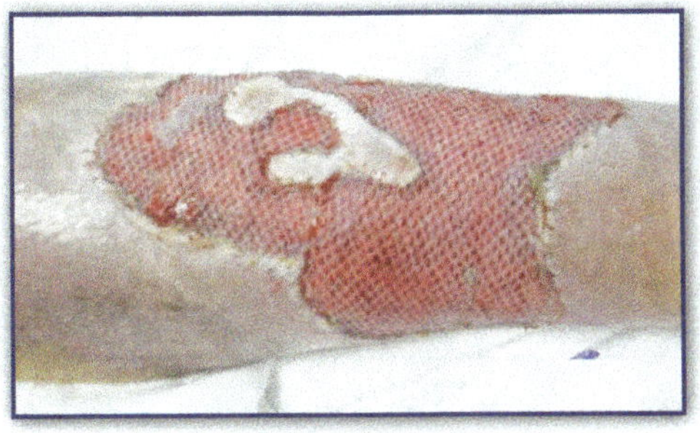

FIGURE 6.

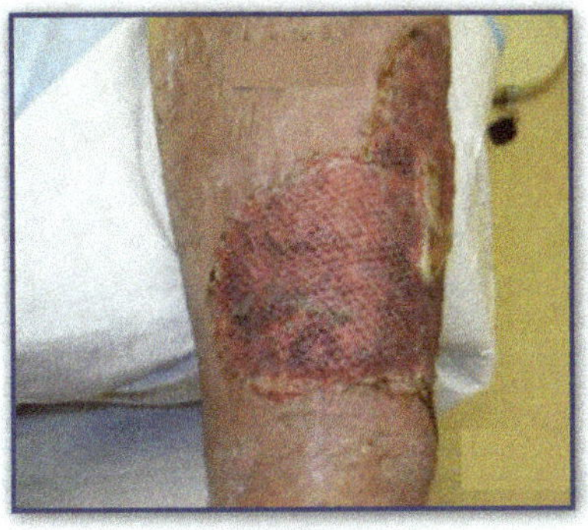

FIGURE 7.

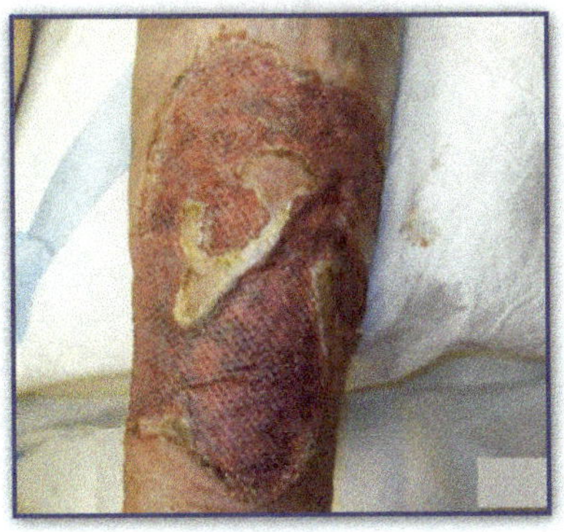

FIGURE 8.

A split-thickness skin graft was performed, and the graft was protected by a contact layer and bolstered down with a negative pressure wound therapy device.

The negative pressure bolster was removed the third postoperative day (Figures 5 and 6) at the insistence of the patient so he could go home.

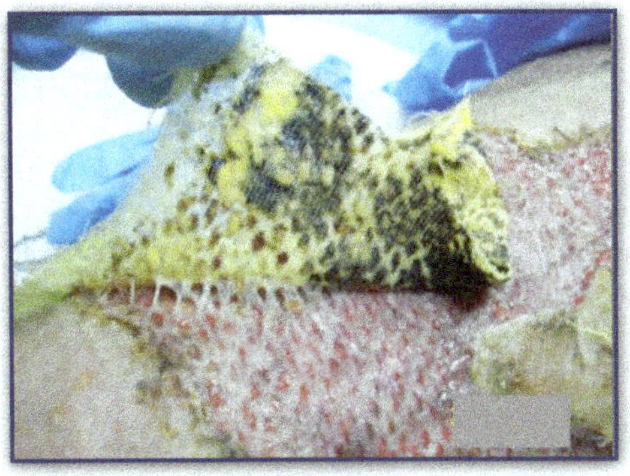

FIGURE 9.

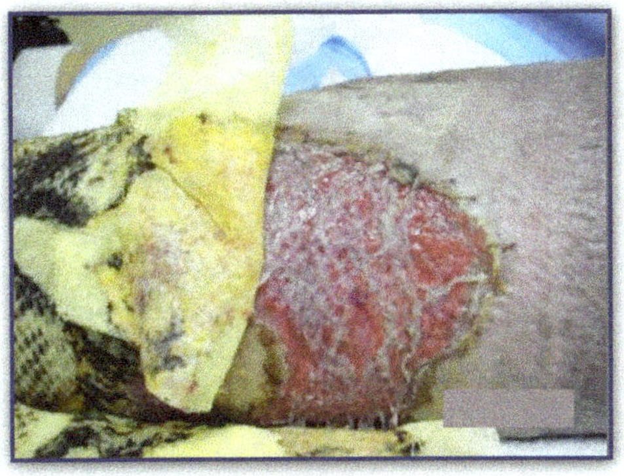

FIGURE 10.

The graft site was dressed with bismuth and petrolatum gauze, and the leg was compressed with a multi-layer wrap. The patient was to return to the outpatient wound center in one week for wound assessment and wrap change. At the visit to the wound center, the dressing was removed and the wound bed was a bit dusky in areas but the skin graft still remained intact (Figures 7 and 8). The same treatment was used, but the patient was instructed to return in three days to assess graft.

When the patient returned, the graft seemed to be lifting; it was unattached to the wound bed, with a small amount of dark green drainage (Figures 9 and 10).

At the 14th postoperative day, the graft seemed to be lying on top of the wound site but not attached (Figure 11), and by Day 17 the graft seemed nonexistent (Figure 12). Treatment continued with bismuth petrolatum gauze and dry gauze to bolster.

By the 20th postoperative day, the wound bed was clearly colonized, and green exudate and

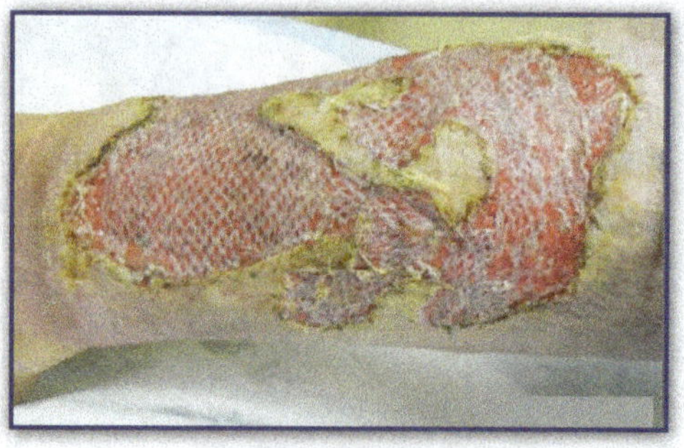

FIGURE 11.

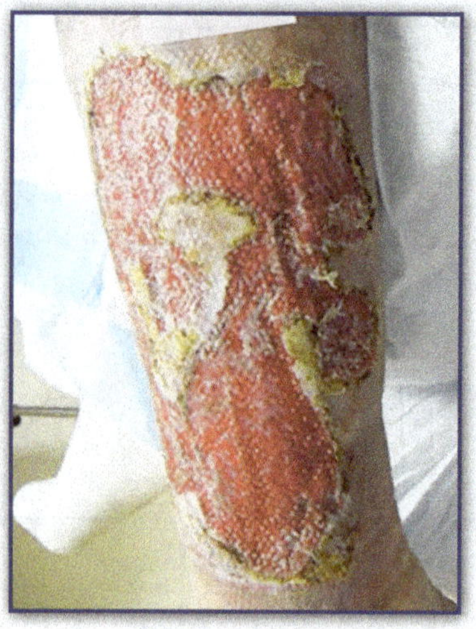

FIGURE 12.

surface debris were present (Figure 13). Treatment was changed to a nanocrystalline silver dressing fenestrated (Figure 14), and covered with a calcium alginate for absorption. Multilayer compression wrap continued, and the patient was treated with culture-driven oral antibiotics.

Three days later, the patient returned, now postoperative Day 23, with significant improvement in the drainage, as well as dramatically improved appearance to the wound bed, with areas of epithelialization noted (Figure 15). Continued with same plan of care with weekly compression wrap and dressing changes planned. One week later, wound still with moderate to large amount of exudate but wound bed continues to epithelialize (Figure 16).

Two weeks later, the wound was 100% epithelialized (Figure 17), treatment changed to thin silicone foam for protection, continued multilayer compression for two weeks when patient was measured and fit for compression stockings.

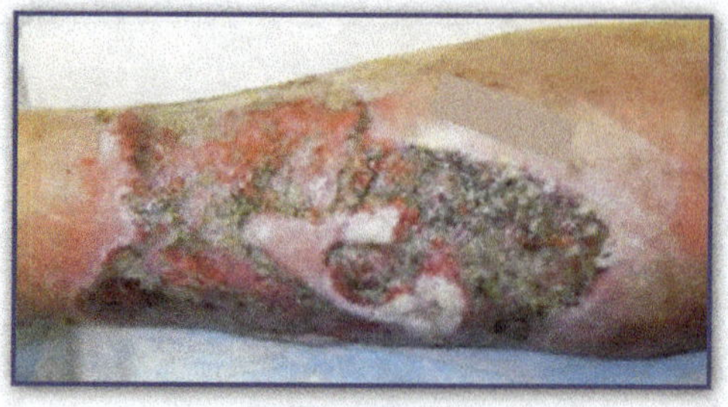

FIGURE 13.

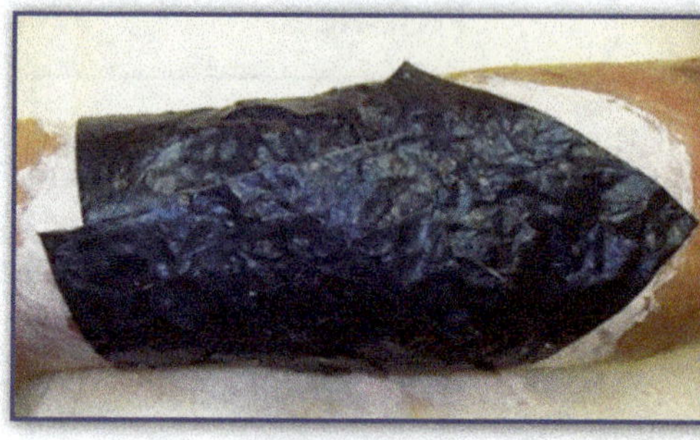

FIGURE 14.

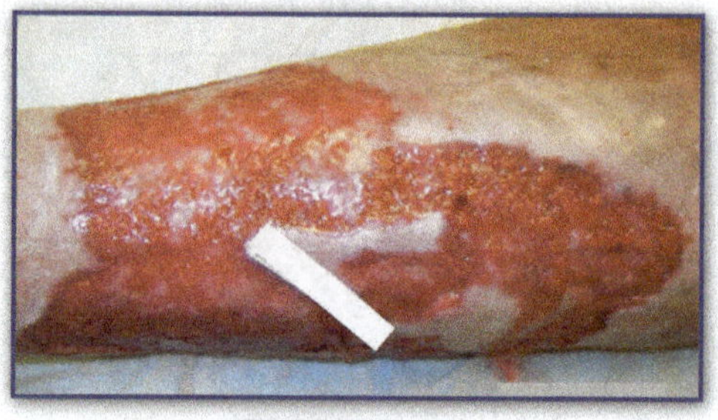

FIGURE 15.

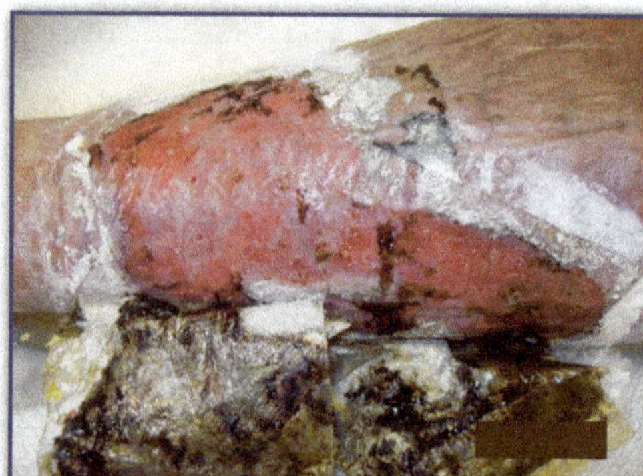

FIGURE 16.

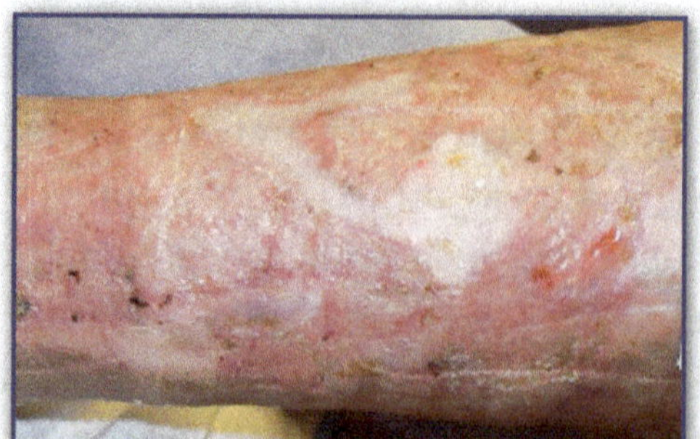

FIGURE 17.

II. Goal-directed wound care and dressing selection

Determining the best interventions, including dressing selection, for patients and their wounds requires looking at the situation holistically. Creating the treatment plan for a chronic wound is dependent upon many diverse patient, wound, economic, and social considerations. The dressing selection goes beyond simply choosing a product to cover the wound. Detailed assessments of the patient and wound should drive the components of goal-directed wound care. The health-care provider must determine the etiology of the wound, patient comorbidities that may impair the wound healing processes (e.g. diabetes and blood glucose levels), nutrition/hydration status, systemic and local tissue oxygenation, and patient/family concerns such as pain and odor issues. Each of these factors contributes to creating an individualized plan of care for choosing the most appropriate products and interventions.[11-18] (Figure 18)

A thorough wound assessment that looks at tissue types in the wound bed, infection/bioburden and chronic inflammation status, moisture/exudate issues, the edge effect, and the periwound status should be performed at regular intervals.[11,16,18-19] Please see Chapter 5: Wound Assessment for a review of the wound assessment parameters.

Chronic wounds are dynamic, evolving as they progress toward closure or disintegrate to a worsened state. Therefore, the choice of dressings and treatments used for wound management must also change in tandem with the characteristics of the wound and the patient's condition. It is uncommon for the initial wound care plan to remain the same throughout the healing processes. Clinicians should adapt treatments based upon ongoing assessments of the patient and the wound at regular intervals, so changes are made as the wound evolves.[13,17]

III. Overall purposes of wound dressings

Modern dressings have the ability to affect one or more aspects of the chronic wound environment. There are three broad purposes of wound

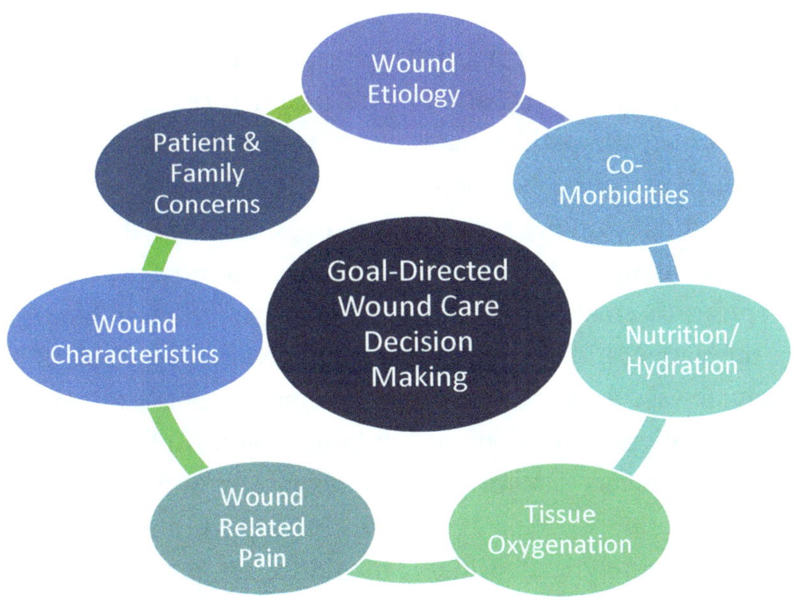

FIGURE 18.

dressings: 1) autolytic debridement, 2) moisture balance, and 3) addressing the bioburden and chronic inflammation. (Figure 19)

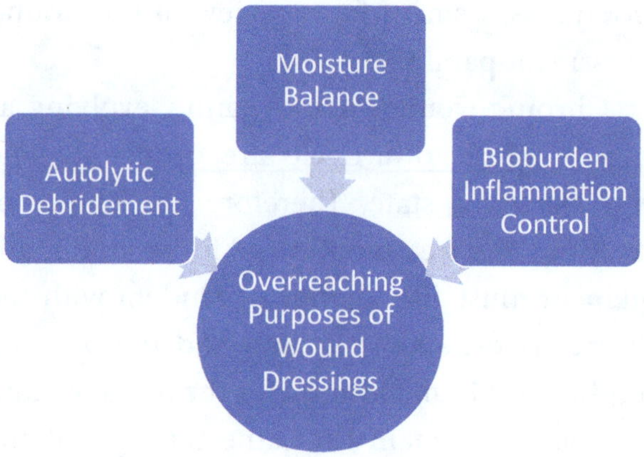

FIGURE 19.

Autolytic debridement is supported by the patient's overall immune system using the body's endogenous enzymes to debride necrotic tissue. Wound fluid contains these proteolytic enzymes and antimicrobial cells that enter during the inflammatory phase of wound healing to help clean the wound of necrotic tissue and bacteria.[20] One of the issues with our aging population is that the immune system often becomes depressed, particularly in older, frail individuals.[21] Also, patients with autoimmune diseases or those taking specific classes of medications such as corticosteroids will often have impaired wound healing. In such cases, the patient may require a different approach to wound care than the person with a functioning immune system (e.g. vitamin A for people taking high levels of steroids) when attempting to create a healing environment. When the patient's immune system is intact with adequate vascularity and oxygenation present, then autolytic debridement should take place when the correct category of dressing is applied to the wound.

Dressings that facilitate autolytic debridement include categories that create a moist wound environment such as hydrogels, hydrocolloids, transparent films, and alginates.[13] (See Chapter 6: Wound Bed Preparation for more information on autolytic debridement.)

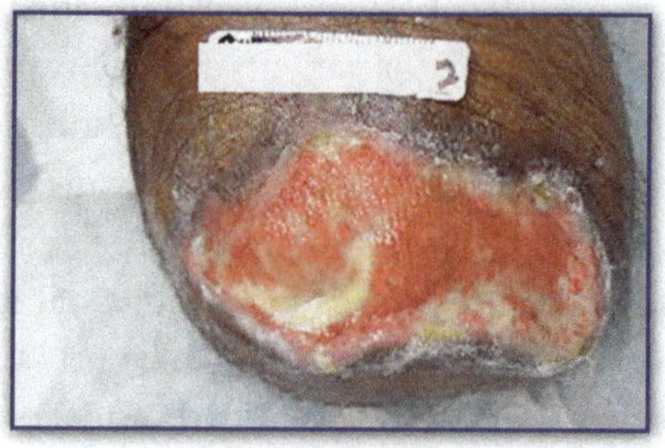

FIGURE 20.

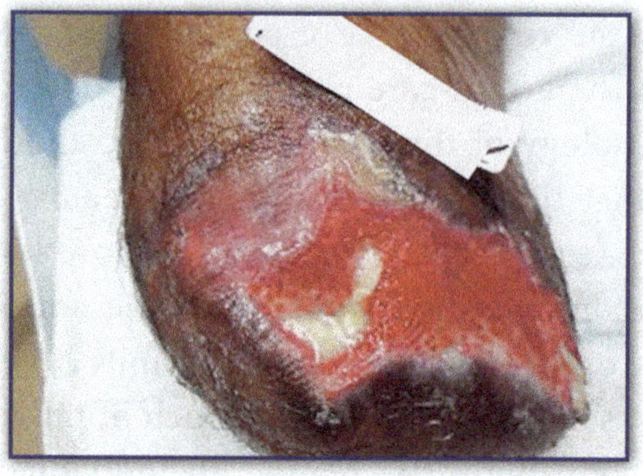

FIGURE 21. Wound with example of autolytic debridement following moist environment after one month

Moisture balance or a moist wound environment is the standard that most wound care clinicians strive to achieve. The literature supports that wounds are more likely to heal in a moist, clean, warm environment. A warm moist milieu enhances closure by promoting cellular activity responsible for new tissue growth.[8-13] Moisture balance in the wound bed is achieved by dressings that donate moisture or absorb excessive wound exudate.[12-16]

With bioburden/inflammation control, chronic wounds are described as being stalled in the inflammatory phase of wound healing, often exhibiting features of a high bacterial load and an overexpressed inflammatory response, both of which impair healing.[13-20] Clinicians must learn to address the pro-inflammatory environment in chronic wounds and recognize that a burgeoning bioburden is often a co-culprit, and then choose interventions addressing both issues. Please refer to the topical management wound bioburden section in this chapter for additional information on managing the bioburden.

IV. Decision making for dressing product selection

Dressing product selection is based on comprehensive assessments of the wound and the patient's overall physiology. Determining whether a person's body can support complete wound healing requires clinical skills and significant knowledge of the many barriers to healing, including which impediments can be influenced by the wound care team and which cannot. When making decisions for treatment, one should consider whether the wound has healing potential, is more likely maintenance wound, or has evolved to a nonhealable ulcer unable to garner the endogenous constituents needed for wound closure and healing.[12,16] For instance, a patient with end-stage cancer who has a Stage 4 infected pressure injury located on the sacrum may benefit from interventions aimed at pain and odor control, addressing the infection, support for activities of daily living, and other health-related quality-of-life issues addressed through a palliative care approach rather than aggressive debridement and advanced dressings looking at the end goal of wound closure.[16] In such a case, maintenance wound care would be more appropriate.

The advent of modern dressings in the 20th and 21st centuries has significantly enhanced wound care practices and improved outcomes for people with chronic wounds. However, deciding which product to use through the wound's trajectory toward healing, or in some cases deterioration, requires ongoing assessment of a multitude of factors that influence wound healing in addition to local considerations that drive dressing selection decisions. Another issue regarding dressings is that there is little evidence supporting the effectiveness of one dressing product over another, particularly within the same category of dressings, such as one company's hydrogel being better than another's.[16] However, with that said, it is important to learn how to choose the best dressing products in an attempt to create a functional wound environment capable of healing while addressing patient-centered concerns affecting the quality of life.[12,14]

A. Considerations for choosing dressings

Dressing selection can be a confusing process at first glance. In 2010 there were approximately 400 commercially available dressings.[22] Currently, in 2016, there are more than 700 different dressings on the market.[23] The combination of research providing clinicians with a better understanding of skin injuries and the chronic wound environment, and advances in the manufacturing of products that are safer and more compatible with the wound bed and periwound skin has created a dynamic, ever-growing industry. Some of the dressings available address a single function, whereas others are composites that have more than one purpose.[13]

Determining which dressing to use is influenced by a multitude of factors such as:

- Knowledge of the clinician choosing the dressing
- Dressing features such as moisture control, conformability and cushioning, ease and safety during removal, ability to minimize pain
- A facility's protocols
- Availability of dressing products
- Product cost considerations

TABLE 1. Dressings categorized by overall function

Dressing Function	Dressing Category
Maintain Moisture	Most advanced dressings; the exudate level drives dressing choice (excludes gauze)
Add Moisture	Hydrogels
Absorb Excessive Moisture	Foam Alginates Superabsorbent
Decrease Protease Levels	Collagen Collagen-ORC Absorptive dressings
Decrease Pain (during dressing changes)	Silicone dressings Contact layers
Protect Healthy/Fragile Wound Base Tissues	Nonadherent dressings
Decrease Odor	Charcoal impregnated, absorbent dressings that trap exudate and bioburden
Decrease Bacterial Load	Antimicrobial dressings

- The patients or caregiver's ability and commitment to support the wound healing process. For instance, if a diabetic patient is not willing to do his or her part to control blood glucose and is running glucose levels above 200mg/dL, then even the best wound care and dressings available may not be able to overcome the deleterious effects of significant hyperglycemia.[24-25]

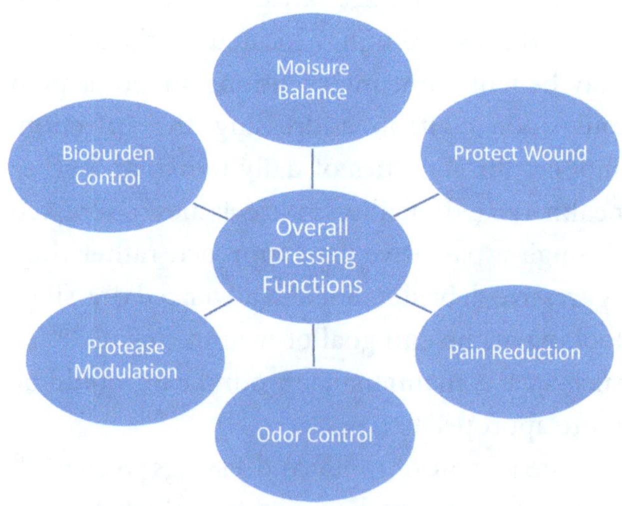

FIGURE 22. Dressing by product function

Dressings are designed to improve healing depending on specific properties of the product by affecting the local wound environment. Figure 22 lists the overall functions of dressings.

1. Moisture balance: Moisture balance is necessary to support all phases of wound repair.[12,14,16] If the wound is desiccated or dry, then a moisture donating dressing (e.g., a hydrogel) is needed. If the wound is highly exudating, then a primary dressing such as an absorbent wound filler (e.g. alginate or hydrofiber) may be needed to absorb excessive drainage to protect the wound base from the proinflammatory exudate while working in conjunction with a foam or superabsorbent secondary dressing that wicks the wound fluid up, trapping the harmful wound fluid with excessive proteases away from both the wound bed and periwound area while maintaining moisture balance at the wound bed-dressing interface.[13]

2. Protecting wound: The dressing should form a protective barrier against outside contaminants, including bacteria and incontinence. Dressings also function to protect the wound by mitigating the mechanical force of friction when the patient is actively moving or being moved (e.g., repositioning in bed or chair). Protecting the wound base is a primary objective when healthy or fragile granulation tissue is present. Nonadherent products such as silicone or petrolatum-impregnated dressings that maintain moisture and are nontraumatic to the tissue upon removal are recommended.[13]

3. Protease modulation: Chronic wounds are often described as being "stuck" in the inflammatory phase of wound healing in which growth factors and the proliferating cells responsible for healing (e.g. fibroblast, keratinocytes) are degraded by the excessive inflammatory cells (proteases) in the wound exudate.[11,13,26] Dressings are available to mitigate the harmful effects of this protease activity by absorbing and trapping protease-rich fluid in the dressings. In addition, the use of collagen products (dressings or particles) acts as a sacrificial substrate to harmful proteases, allowing native collagen and the cells responsible for healing to perform optimally.[13,26] Absorbing excessive exudate and the use of collagen products have been shown to be successful in changing the chronic wound milieu, thereby facilitating wound closure and subsequent healing.

4. Pain reduction: Pain has a negative impact on wound healing and the patient's quality of life.[27-33] Clinicians should assume all wounds are painful, even full-thickness lesions.[29] The World Union of Wound Healing Societies (WUWHS) describes three types of pain: background, incident, and procedural.[29] According to the WUWHS, background pain can be felt by the patient without undergoing any procedures, whereas incident pain, also known as breakthrough pain, can occur during any type of activity such as movement or repositioning the patient. Procedural pain happens from routine, basic procedures such as dressing changes.[29] Krasner[27-28] divides chronic wound pain into three similar categories: chronic, cyclical, and noncyclical wound-related pain. Within Krasner's conceptualization of the wound pain experience, chronic pain is described as continuous and is present without manipulation of the patient or the wound, with cyclic pain caused as a result of repeated treatments such as dressing changes, and noncyclic pain being defined as a single episode of pain that occurs sporadically, such as a single debridement procedure.[27-28] Literature supports dressing changes being the most frequent cause of reports of pain from patients as part of the chronic wound experience.[28-31] Using a pain intensity scale should be standard practice when working with chronic wound patients, including those who have minimal to moderate cognitive impairments.[27-34] The Wong-Baker FACES Pain Rating Scale[33] has been validated for use with patients with cognitive issues when the 0-10 numerical rating scale could not be used for these cognitively impaired patients.[34]

Clinicians should choose dressings that cause the least amount of pain and tissue trauma on application and removal. Petrolatum-impregnated and silicone dressings next to the wound base are purported to diminish pain during dressing changes and to be less traumatic to fragile granulation tissue or structures such as tendons upon removal.[17,35]

5. Odor control: Malodor is common in chronic wounds, specifically those that are have a bacterial colonization and necrotic tissue.[36-38] Foul-smelling wounds are known to lower health-related quality of life and to produce psychological stress and social isolation.[38] Malignant fungating wounds (MFW) are particularly known to have strong foul odors. Patients and clinicians have described wound odor as the worst part of these types of wounds.[38] Rating odor is a component of the wound assessment; however, each person has an individualized perspective on how things smell, making the odor assessment subjective for patients and clinicians. There is work on the horizon for assessing odor using technology such as a gas chromatography, termed the "electronic nose." How feasible this will be across the continuum of care remains to be seen.[36] Some clinician simply describe odor as minimal, moderate, or foul. In addition, there are several different scales that can be used to rate odor. Here are some odor-rating scales that have been referenced in the literature.[36]

- Baker and Haig method, scale from 1 to 4, where 1 is strong and 4 is no odor
- Overall evaluation scale, from 1 to 10, where 10 is excellent odor control
- Verbal rating scale of 1 to 4, where 1 is no odor and 4 is strong odor
- Verbal rating scale of strong (intolerable), moderate (noticeable), minimal (barely there), absent (no odor)
- Visual analogue scale from 1 to 10, where 1 is no odor and 10 is extremely strong odor.[36,38]

Treatments for malodorous wounds are aimed at debridement of devitalized tissue and addressing the bioburden.[36-38] Products that contribute to odor control include specialty dressings with odor-modifying compounds embedded as a component of the dressing. At times it is not feasible to eradicate the cause of wound odor, such as in patients on palliative care where aggressive debridement is not the best course of action. In such cases, odor-controlling dressings can help mitigate the quality-of-life issues associated with having a foul-smelling wound. Most fetid wound odors are associated with the wound's bioburden. The dressings, solutions, and products that reduce the bacterial load on the wound will assist in decreasing malodor.[36-38]

Steps to control odor include, but are not limited to:

- Regular, thorough wound cleansing
- Addressing the bioburden
- Debridement of devitalized tissue
- Topical metronidazole (addresses anaerobic bacteria and protozoal infections)
- Activated charcoal dressings
- External odor absorbers or maskers for the room (e.g. activated charcoal, kitty litter, vinegar, vanilla, coffee beans, potpourri, diffused essential oils).[15,36,38]

6. Protect periwound skin integrity: Choosing a dressing that will not damage the periwound area is a primary goal when selecting a product. Some patients, particularly at the extremes of age (i.e. neonates and elderly patients), often have fragile skin which is at higher risk for damage, such as denuding and skin tears when adhesives are used. Also, some people have skin sensitivities or allergies to adhesive products creating a challenging situation when deciding which adhesive the patient's skin can tolerate.

7. Bioburden control: All wounds have some level of a bioburden or bacterial load. Whether the bioburden reaches levels to have a deleterious effect on wound healing is dependent on several factors, including the host ability to garner the cells (neutrophils, macrophages) to fight the invading organism and the virulence of the polymicrobial (e.g., bacteria, yeast, fungi) invasion.[13,39] Dressings containing antimicrobial substances are readily available for treating wound bioburden topically. Please refer to the topical management of wound bioburden section in this chapter for more information on this topic.

B. Key local factors in dressing selection

Additional local factors to consider for choosing the most appropriate dressing product for a wound include the wound location, dimensions, exudate amount, wound bed tissue types, bacterial burden, wound-related pain, and periwound status.[13-17, 27-32]

1. Location: Location on the body influences how the dressing is to be secured.

- Trunk location: An adhesive is needed to secure the dressing, either a self-adherent dressing (e.g. polyurethane film), adhesive bordered dressings (e.g. adhesive bordered foam), or additional adhesive tape.
- Limb location: Several choices of securement are available when the wound is on a limb. Adhesive tape, gauze wrap, or tubular and netting products work for these areas of the body.

2. Wound dimensions: The length, width, and depth of the wound determine the size of dressing used to cover the wound, and when needed, fill the wound bed. If there is significant depth, undermining, or tunneling, a wound filler that is compatible with the needs of the wound bed is important to consider.

3. Exudate amount: Wound drainage is the primary consideration when choosing a dressing category. As mentioned previously, wound beds need to be moist, neither too dry nor too wet for cellular function to be optimal. A dry wound requires moisture donating dressings such as hydrogels, whereas a highly exudating, wet wounds need an absorbent dressing. Controlling exudate also protects the periwound area.

4. Wound bed tissues: Close scrutiny of the wound bed tissue will assist the clinician in choosing the appropriate dressing or dressing combinations. Is there healthy granulation tissue or viable structures such as tendons or bone that need to be protected? If so, then a dressing that keeps these tissues and structures moist and that is nonadherent upon removal so as not to cause damage should be used. What type of nonviable tissue is present, slough or eschar? The type of necrotic tissue in the wound bed will influence the mode of debridement (e.g. autolytic debridement, enzymatic, sharp) and which dressing will be needed after debridement.[16]

V. Gauze dressings

A. Wet-to-dry dressing changes

An understanding of the need for moist wound healing has been in evolution for 50-plus years. However, some clinicians still have not been exposed to this information and continue to use wet-to-dry, sometimes termed wet-to-moist, dressing changes, not understanding that this process is often a harmful practice for both the wound and patient.[13,17,31,40-43] Functionally, wet-to-dry dressings are considered a debridement method. However, should this technique be used, it is important to recognize there are very limited situations where it would be appropriate. One circumstance where wet-to-dry changes may be of benefit is for wounds that are 100% covered with soft slough.(43) The person performing the wet-to-dry technique should have the skill to recognize and understand that this dressing change should be stopped as soon as the slough is removed or when the healthy granulation tissue or structures such as muscle, tendon, or bone are exposed. It requires an attentive, well-trained clinician to use wet-to-dry technique appropriately. Because wet-to-dry is a non-selective method of debridement, it is impossible to control which tissues are removed from the wound bed during this dressing change, meaning nonviable and viable tissues may both be removed simultaneously.(13,17,31,40-42) In addition, it is almost impossible to ensure the dressing remains moist, as the evaporative processes cannot be controlled using woven gauze products. There have been studies looking at the prevalence of the use of wet-to-dry dressing changes. These studies validate that this technique is still being used frequently and inappropriately across the continuum of care.(13,41-43) Table 2 lists reasons for questioning the use of wet-to-dry dressing changes. Both the National Pressure Ulcer Advisory Panel (NPUAP) and the Centers for Medicare and Medicaid Services Guidance to Surveyors recommend limited use of wet-to-dry dressings because of the potential harm that may be caused to the wound and the patient.(15,43)

All of the above-mentioned issues should give health-care providers sufficient reasons for rethinking the use of gauze dressings, particularly wet-to-dry dressing changes, and guide the clinician to look at current wound care intervention and products to support their wound closure goals.

B. Impregnated gauze dressings

Impregnated gauze dressings are saturated with a solution, an emulsion, oil, or some other agent or compound.(17) Agents used include saline, oil, zinc salts, petrolatum, xeroform and scarlet red,

TABLE 2. Reasons to question the use of wet-to-dry dressings (13,15,17,40-42)

- The loose weave of the gauze does not provide thermoregulation, thereby diminishing cellular proliferation and movement, angiogenesis processes, and therefore granulation tissue formation due to the thermal cooling.
- The real potential for tearing out or damaging healthy granulation tissue or other structures exposed in full-thickness wounds due to this nonselective debridement method
- Can be painful to patient when removed dry
- Potential for cross-contamination due to dispersion of microbes into the air when removing the dressing
- Increased infection risk due to the open weave of gauze not providing a physical barrier to bacteria
- Prolonging the detrimental inflammatory environment due to an inability to absorb and trap the overabundant proteases away from the wound base
- Increased labor for the clinician
- Increased cost for the health-care system

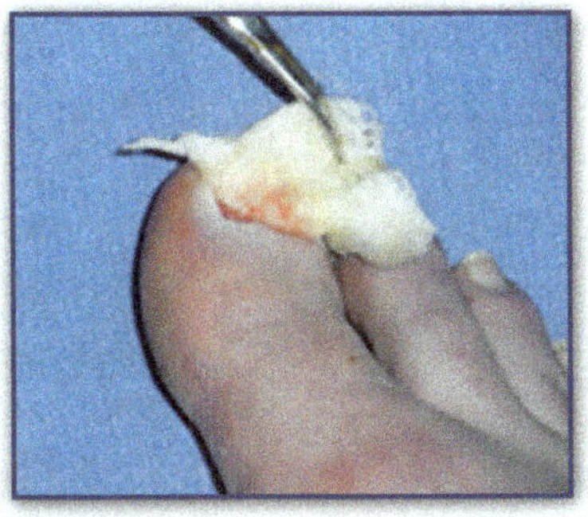

FIGURE 23. Wet to dry dressing adherent to wound bed

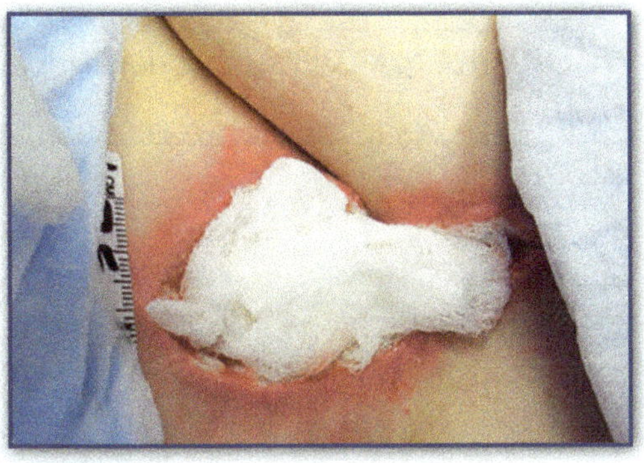

FIGURE 24. Moist gauze packed into wound

and other antimicrobial products such as acetic acid or Dakin's. Indications for use vary based on the compound. These dressings may be nonadherent, such as petrolatum-based products, and often require a secondary dressing to hold the impregnated dressing in place and work synergistically with the base compound in the dressing.

VI. Primary dressings

Primary dressings are therapeutic or protective coverings, which are applied with direct contact to the wound base or on skin lesions.[41] Primary dressings have three basic functions:

1. Address the wound bed moisture balance: add, maintain, or absorb moisture.
2. Affect the bioburden by being impregnated with an antimicrobial or have other functions that decrease the bacterial load such as the ability to draw the exudate and associated bacterial cells into the dressing.
3. Protect the wound bed, specifically to ensure the new granulation tissue or other viable structures such as tendons or muscles are not damaged during dressing changes.

VII. Secondary dressings

Secondary dressings have several functions.[41] Ask most clinicians what the purpose of a secondary dressing is they will tell you that it holds a primary dressing in place on the wound bed or assists with absorption in copiously exudating wounds. In addition to these two functions, secondary dressings support the protection of the wound bed and primary dressing from mechanical issues such as friction, provide thermoregulation (cells proliferate more readily in a warm environment), allow patients privacy when the wound is in a visible location on the body, and work synergistically with the therapeutic effects of the primary dressing.

An example of a primary and secondary dressing working synergistically together would be a silver alginate dressing on a wound with a high bioburden that is copiously draining and a bordered foam that covers the alginate. The silver alginate addresses the bacterial load and initial drainage while the secondary bordered foam holds both dressings in place, provides for thermoregulation, absorbs and wicks exudate that overwhelms the alginate away from the wound bed and periwound area, and protects the wound and primary dressing from mechanical forces such as friction and displacement when the patient is moving.

VIII. Protecting the periwound skin

While not dressings specifically, moisture barrier and skin protectants (also known as skin sealants and skin protectors) and adhesive removal products are often necessary and should be considered part of the dressing application and removal process.[13] Skin protectants should be used for anyone having an adhesive applied to the skin. Skin protectants and moisture barrier products are indicated for macerated periwound areas, incontinence on the skin, or excessive perspiration (e.g., intertriginous dermatitis).

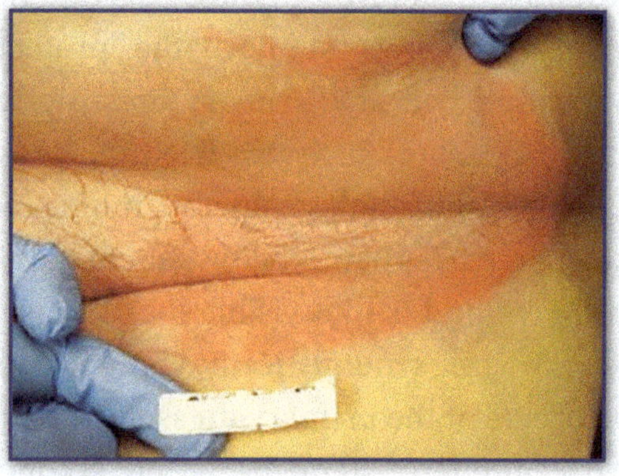

FIGURE 25. Intertriginous dermatitis

These conditions soften and irritate the skin, putting it at higher risk for mechanical damage from adhesive products. There is a relatively new term, medical-adhesive-related skin injury (MARSI),[44] describing skin injury caused by adhesives. The current definition of MARSI: "A medical adhesive-adhesive-related skin injury is an occurrence in which erythema and/or other manifestations of cutaneous abnormality (including, but not limited to, vesicle, bulla, erosion, or tear) persists 30 minutes or more after removal of the adhesive." [44]

Skin injury will occur from MARSI when the adhesive attachment is stronger than the epidermal/dermal attachment. Often MARSI damage is partial-thickness; however, in the

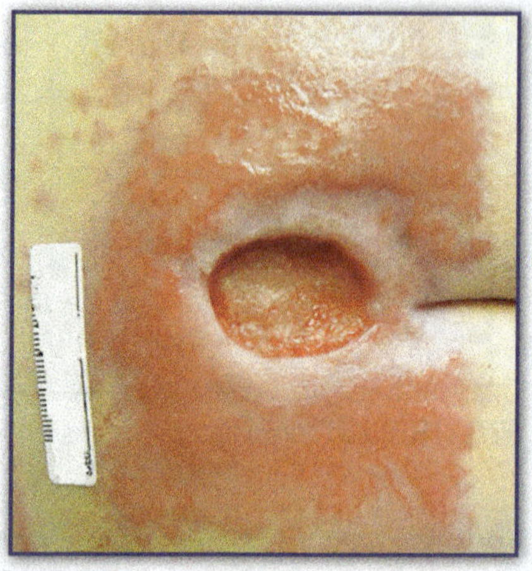

FIGURE 26. MARSI: Contact dermatitis

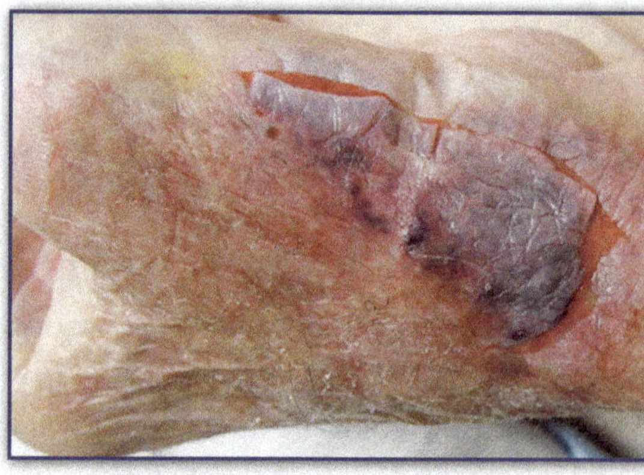

FIGURE 27. MARSI: Skin tear

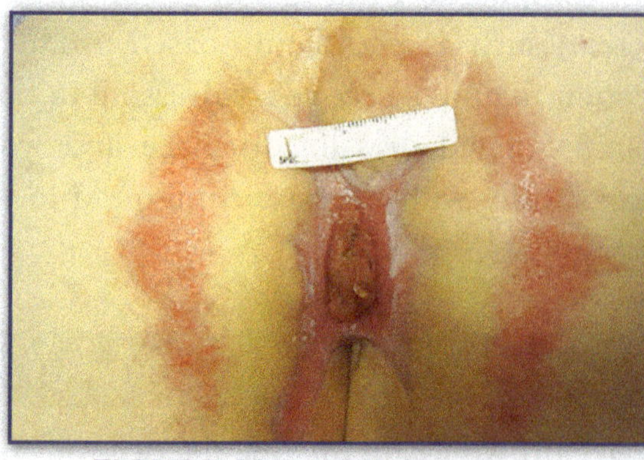

FIGURE 28. MARSI: Reaction to adhesive dressing border

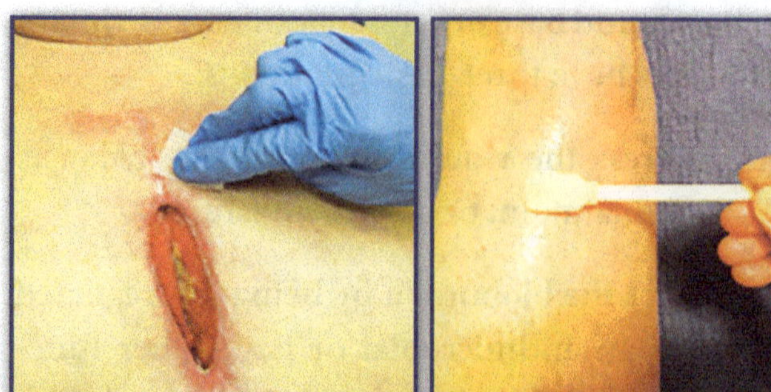

FIGURE 29. Barrier wipes being applied to skin

case of deep skin tear damage, these injuries can be full-thickness.[45]

Liquid skin protectants form a transparent coating on the surface of the skin. They are formulated to be wiped, sprayed, or painted on the skin.

When tapes or adhesive dressings are applied to this superficial coating, the skin is protected from moisture that softens and irritates the skin and from mechanical injuries such as dressing removals.[13]

Skin adhesive injuries happen across all age groups but are more prevalent at the extremes of age, the neonate and older individuals with fragile skin.[45] Use of skin protectant and liquid sealants enhances a patient's quality of life, contributes to patient safety, and supports lower health-care costs.[13,45]

IX. Dressing categories

A. Contact layer dressings

Contact layer dressings are single-layer, open-weave nets that perform as a low-adherence material, which is applied directly to the wound surface. They are constructed with nonadherent fabrics such a polyethylene and may be coated with an oil emulsion, silicone, or petrolatum to increase the non-adherence factor. This dressing category acts as a protective interface between the wound bed while allowing exudate to pass through the dressings into the secondary dressing or a negative pressure wound dressing.[13,41] Also contact layer dressings can be used over topical creams, ointments, and biologic products to protect the medication from the secondary dressing.

Clinical tips

- Cut to fit the wound or allow for overlap onto periwound area
- Not recommended for third-degree burns or dry wounds

B. Transparent film dressings

Transparent film dressings are thin, flexible polyurethane sheets with adhesive backing for self-adherence. They are impermeable to liquid, water, and bacteria but permeable to moisture vapor and atmospheric gases.[13,17,23,41] An advantage of this dressing category is that they allow visualization of the wound and surrounding skin. They also provide a moist, warm environment, which facilitates cellular process for wound healing, and promote autolytic debridement. They may be used over early skin changes such as Stage 1 pressure or suspected deep tissue injuries, allowing easy visualization of the site to determine whether these injuries are improving or degrading.[13,17,41] They can be used on primary-intention surgical sites, intravenous catheters, and areas exposed to friction. Films are often used as secondary dressings and are the dressing material used with most negative pressure wound therapy devices.[13] They are indicated for nondraining to minimally draining wounds. Standard film dressings are not

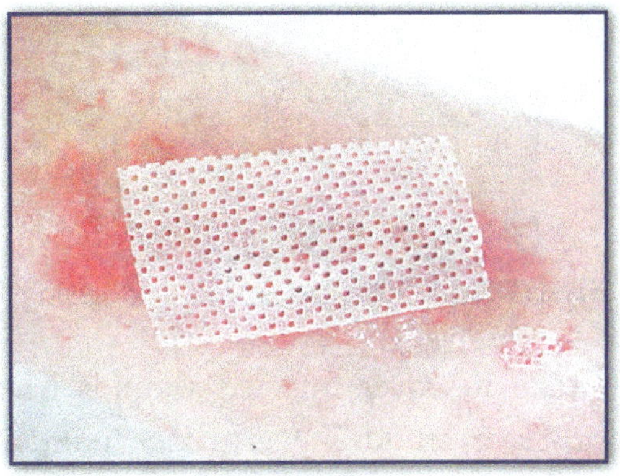

FIGURE 30.

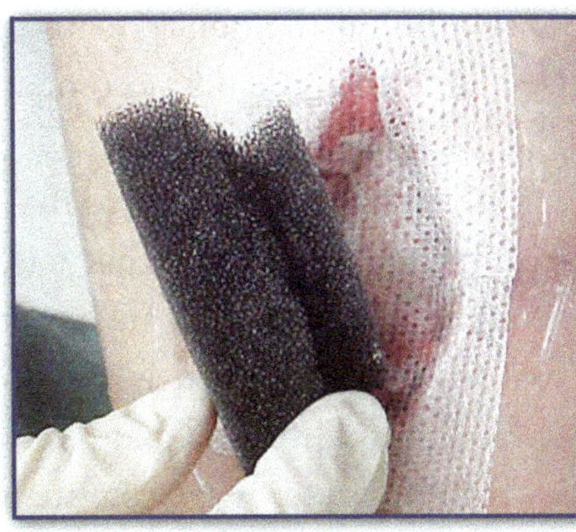

FIGURE 31.

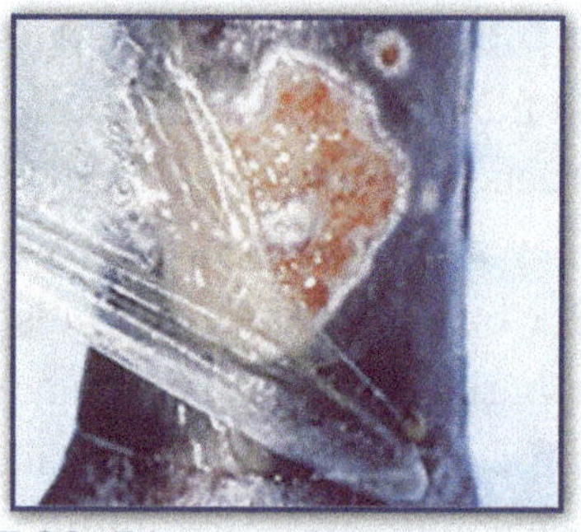

FIGURE 32. Film dressing over venous ulcer

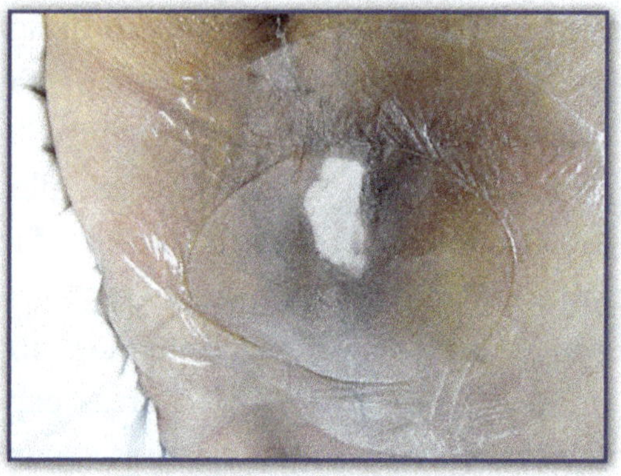

FIGURE 33. Film dressing incorporating acrylic layer

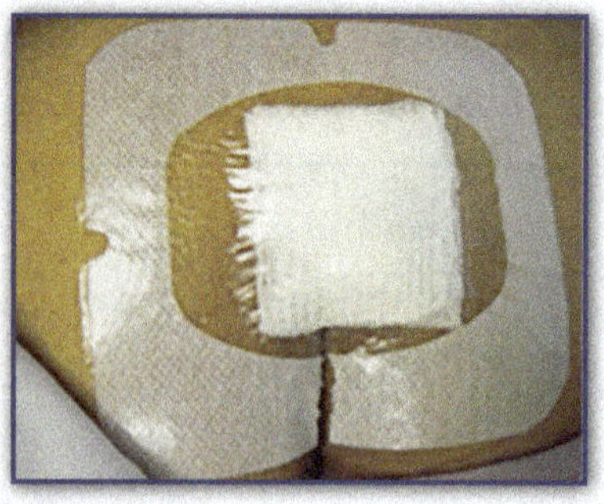

FIGURE 34. Film as secondary dressing

appropriate to cover infected wounds because bacteria have an ideal warm environment in which to multiply, creating a greater inflammatory response without the ability to control the increased exudate that usually accompanies an infection.[13,17]

There is a film dressing available that incorporates an acrylic polymer pad that has perforations allowing exudate to transfer through perforations into the pad and away from the wound surface.[13] Buildup of exudate beyond the vapor transfer rate will migrate out of the dressing area, causing maceration of the surrounding skin. When removing the dressing from fragile or macerated skin, take care to avoid mechanical stripping leading to denuding of the periwound area. When using this category of dressing, or any dressing with an adhesive, the use of a skin barrier should be used to protect the periwound skin,[13] as well as increase the adherence of the dressing.

C. Hydrogel dressings

Hydrogel dressing products come in three distinct forms: amorphous gels, three-dimensional sheets, and impregnated gauze. The primary purposes of hydrogel dressing products are to donate moisture to dry wound beds to assist with maintaining a moist healing environment and to soften necrotic tissue.[11-13,41] Hydrogels facilitate autolytic debridement in patients capable of garnering the enzymes for the autolytic debridement process. These dressings may contain other ingredients such as alginate to increase viscosity or to support small amounts of absorption, antimicrobial agents that address

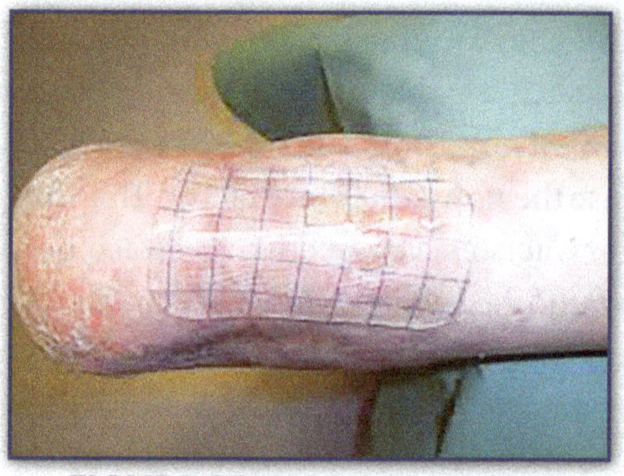

FIGURE 35. Solid sheet hydrogel

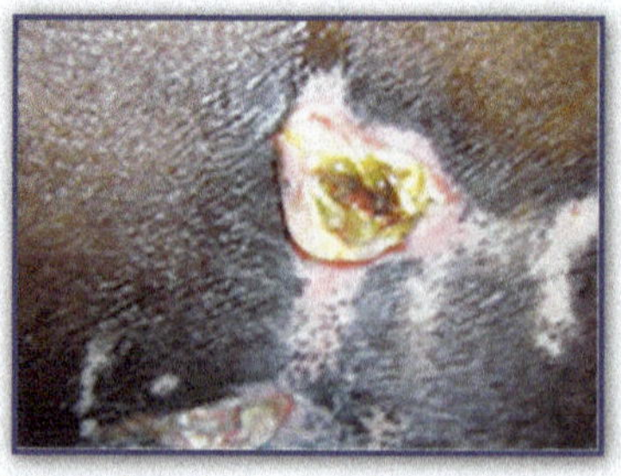

FIGURE 36. Amorphous hydrogel

FIGURE 37. Hydrogel-impregnated gauze

the bioburden, and growth factors or collagen to enhance wound healing.[13,41]

When using hydrogel products, it is important to protect the periwound skin from maceration with a protective moisture barrier or skin sealant. Hydrogels are indicated for many types of wounds, including partial and full-thickness wounds, pressure injuries, skin tears, radiation and partial-thickness burns, and vascular wounds.[17,41] Hydrogels are not indicated for moderately or copiously draining wounds.[13,17,41]

D. Hydrocolloid dressings

Hydrocolloid wound dressings are manufactured as wafers/sheets, powders, or pastes and are composed of gelatin, pectin, and carboxymethylcellulose.[13,17,46] The most common form of wafer or sheet is configured into three layers: an inner adhesive layer, a middle absorbent layer, and an outer semi-occlusive layer.[13,45] These wafer/sheet dressings are self-adhering and available with or without an adhesive border. Hydrocolloid dressings are available in a variety of shapes, sizes, and thicknesses and include products designed for specific anatomical areas such as the sacrum or heel.[13,17,41] Some products are thin or have tapered edges that make them less likely to wrinkle, ruck, or roll at the edges and may be semi-transparent, allowing visualization of the wound without the need to remove the dressing.[46] The hydrocolloid powders and pastes require a secondary dressing to hold then in place in the wound bed. Hydrocolloid dressings are indicated for partial- and full-thickness wounds with or without necrotic tissue.[23] Many hydrocolloids are occlusive, which supports anaerobic bacteria proliferations, and should be used with extreme care when an infection is suspected.[13]

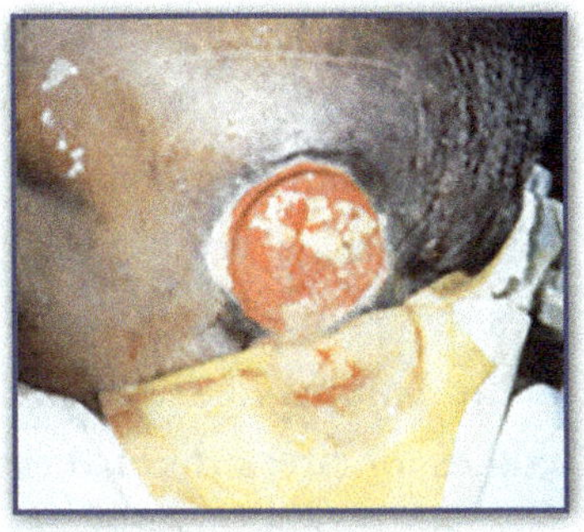

FIGURE 38. Hydrocolloid with normal gelling.

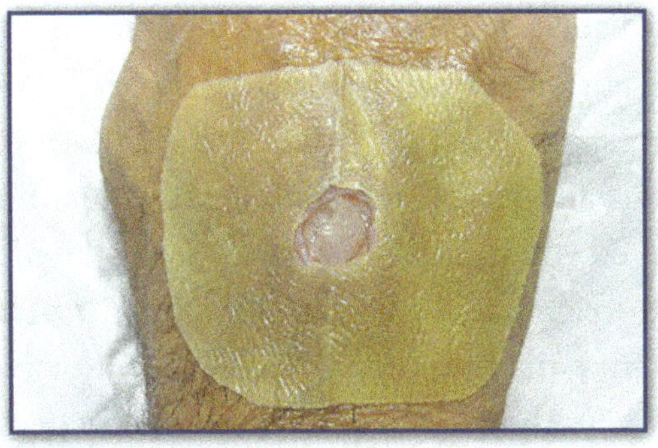

FIGURE 39. Hydrocolloid protecting periwound.

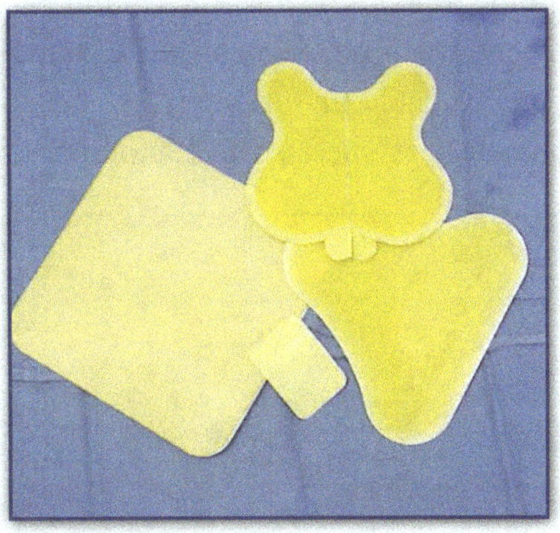

FIGURE 40. Multiple shapes of hydrocolloid dressings.

E. Absorbent dressings

Calcium alginate dressings

These dressings are derived from algae or kelp polysaccharides,[47] composed of calcium/sodium salts of alginic acid and mannuronic and guluronic acids. This category of dressing is indicated for moderately to heavily exudating wounds. They form a moist gel through a process of ion exchange with the wound exudate. Alginates are primary dressings placed in contact with the wound bed and are indicated for the etiologies of pressure, arterial, venous, diabetic ulcers, and postoperative and trauma wounds.[13,17,22,41,47] This dressing conforms to the wound surface, creating a moist wound environment, and can be used to tuck, pack, or fill uneven surfaces, tunnels, and undermining. Alginates support autolytic debridement and are painlessly removed when moist or can be remoistened with saline irrigation if they should dry out. In addition, they may be used to control minor bleeding.[13,41,47] Alginates require a secondary dressing to soak up drainage not absorbed by the alginate, to hold the dressing against the wound bed, and to protect the wound from outside contaminants. They are available in various sizes and conformations such as sheets, pads, and ropes.[13,41,47]

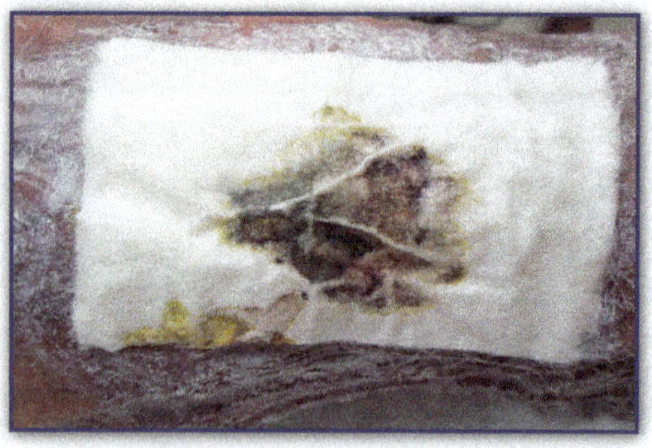

FIGURE 41. Calcium alginate with trapped exudate

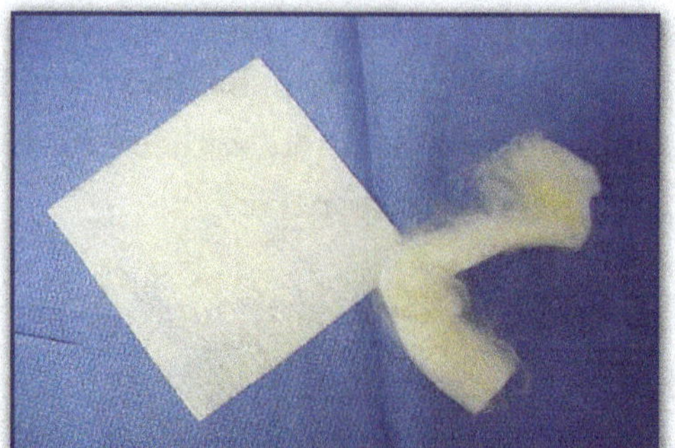

FIGURE 42. Example of sheet and rope calcium alginates

Alginate dressing are available with silver ions for addressing the bioburden.

Alginate dressings are contraindicated for:

- Dry wounds
- Wounds with minimal exudate
- Surgical implantations
- Allergies to any components of the dressing
- Third-degree burns

Gelling fiber dressings

Hydrofiber is constructed as a soft, sterile, nonwoven pad or ribbon dressing composed of sodium carboxymethylcellulose, which is incorporated in the form of a fleece held together by a needle-bonding process. This conformable material can absorb a large amount of wound fluid, such as exudate with bacteria.[48] The mechanisms of action include a hydrophobic (water-hating) component (methylcellulose) that gives this dressing its tensile strength and a hydrophilic (water-loving) component (carboxy)

FIGURE 43a. Hydrofiber sheet

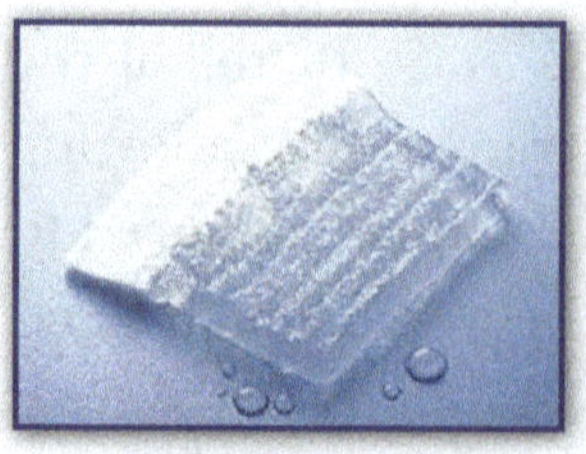

FIGURE 43b. Hydrofiber sheet gelled

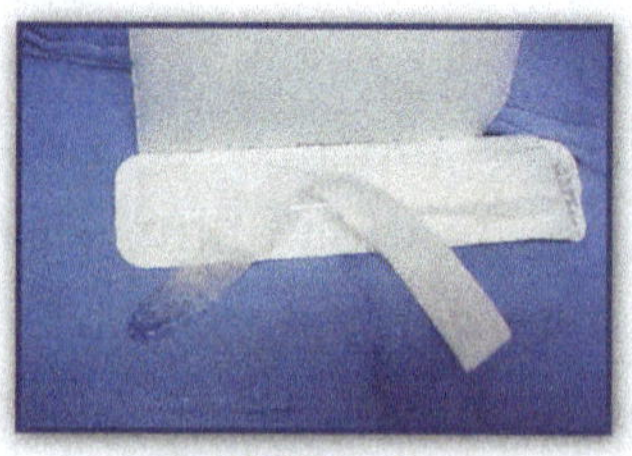

FIGURE 43c. Hydrofiber rope

that acts as a fluid lock.[12] Hydrofiber dressings are superabsorbent products capable of absorbing up to 30 times their weight, providing less risk of maceration because of their vertical fluid absorption properties.[12,48]

As the dressing absorbs fluid, the hydrofiber is converted into a gel consistency. When the hydrofiber is saturated, wound fluid strike-through will occur. These dressings require a secondary dressing to keep them in place because the addition of an adhesive will interfere with the fluid absorption properties of the dressing.[12] Hydrofibers are similar in structure to alginates and have some of the same properties but are technically a category in and of themselves due to their mechanism of action, composition, and features.[13] Hydrofibers have been proven to assist in reduction of MMPs and bacterial burden due to their highly absorptive properties.[16-17,47-48]

F. Foam dressings

Foam dressings are most commonly made of polyurethane with small, open cells capable of wicking drainage away from the wound through their hydrophilic properties, then holding exudate in the upper layers of the dressing to protect the wound bed from the detrimental proteases and the periwound skin from maceration. This dressing category is semi-occlusive, allowing for gas and vapor exchange. Foams are a very versatile category of dressings. Indications for use include:

- Absorbing moderate to copious amounts of fluids
- Used as prophylactic protection over bony prominences, particularly in areas at risk for friction
- Partial and full-thickness wounds
- Granulating or necrotic wound beds
- Use under compression
- Protecting skin tears

Foams often have a nonadherent contact layer, making them gentle on the wound bed during dressing removal. They may be bordered with an adhesive to hold the dressing in place, or they may be unbordered, without an adhesive, requiring tape to secure the dressing.[13,23,41] This category may function as a primary or secondary dressing and can be combined with topical treatments, including enzymatic debridement.[41]

Foams should not be used on stable dry eschar not appropriate for debridement, such as on ischemic limbs/heels, as the dressing may contribute to softening of the eschar, making it unstable and opening the area to bacteria infiltration and nonhealing due to lack of blood supply.[15,41] Foam dressings may have silver, PHMB, or other agents added to address the bioburden.[12-13]

G. Collagen dressings

Collagen, a major protein of the body, is necessary for wound healing. Collagen dressings are derived primarily from bovine, porcine, or ovine sources.[13,23,41] These dressing are available as sheets, gels, pads, particles, pastes, powders, or solutions and are indicated for partial- and full-thickness pressure ulcers, venous ulcers, donor sites, surgical wounds, vascular ulcers, diabetic ulcers, second-degree burns, abrasions, and traumatic wounds.[13,23,41,47] Collagen's primary functions in chronic wound healing include:

1. Attracting cells such as fibroblasts and keratinocytes at the wound site
2. Providing a temporary scaffolding to help guide and support the movement and growth of cells
3. Acting as a sacrificial substrate by binding with the excessive proteases (MMPs) found in chronic wounds that degrade the wound healing cells, cell receptors, growth factors,

and extracellular matrix, allowing the patient's native collagen to perform optimally.(13,23,41,49)

Collagen products should be placed on clean or granulation tissue in the wound bed, not on top of nonviable tissue. If it is placed over necrotic tissue, the clinician is wasting the collagen product, as the healthy cells in the wound bed needed for healing cannot interface with the collagen dressing due to the necrotic tissue covering the wound bed. Also, collagen products should not be used as an absorbent dressing because they are biodegradable, having minimal absorption, unless combined with an alginate. Collagen dressings require a secondary dressing to hold them in place and absorb excessive exudate. Most products have increased efficacy if moistened with normal saline unless adequate moisture is present in the wound via exudate.

Considerations for usage of collagen dressings include:

- Ensuring the patient is not allergic to the type of collagen from which the dressing is derived (i.e. bovine, porcine, ovine)
- Not using on full-thickness (third- and fourth-degree burns)
- Using a secondary dressing carefully in the presence of fragile periwound skin (e.g., neonates, elderly)
- Not using over necrotic tissue

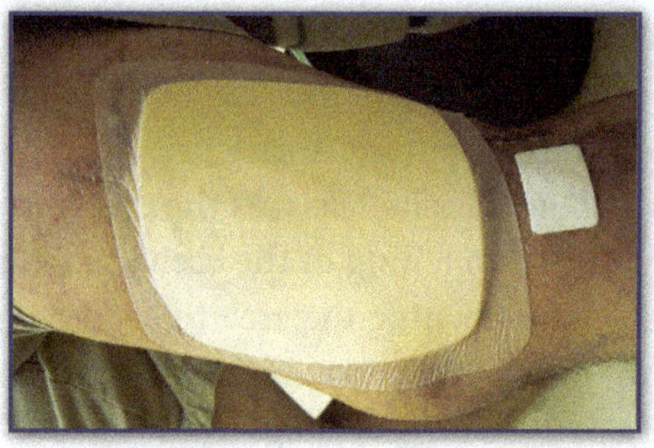

FIGURE 44a. Bordered foam

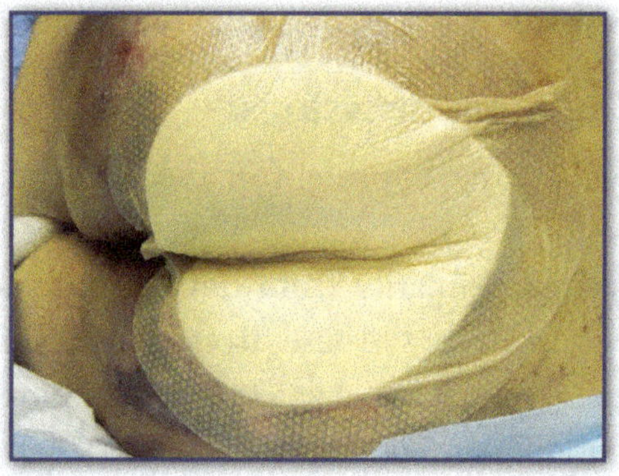

FIGURE 44b. Bordered foam, sacral shaped

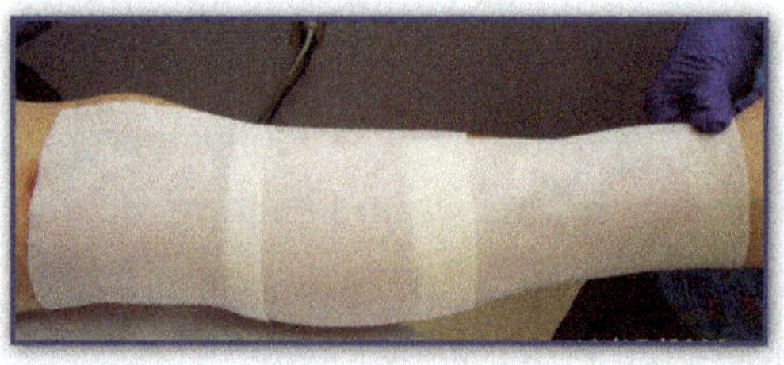

FIGURE 45a. Thin foam for skin protection

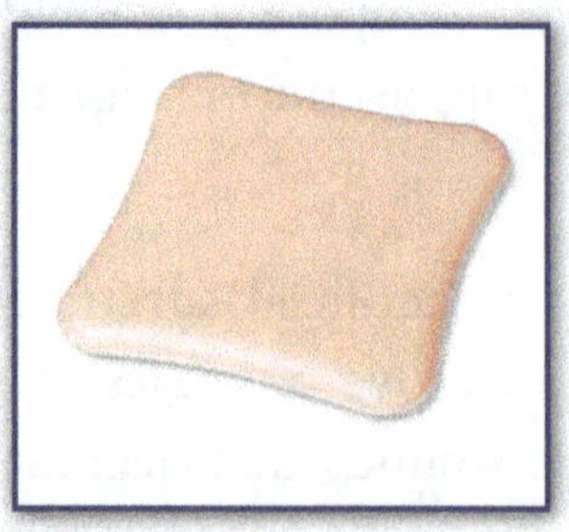

FIGURE 45b. Nonboarded foam

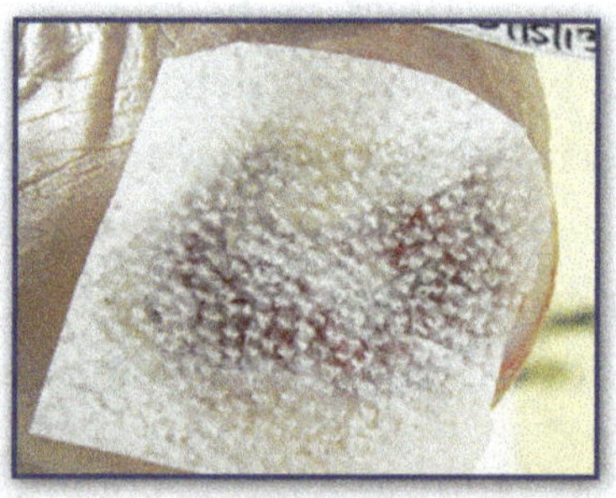

FIGURE 46.

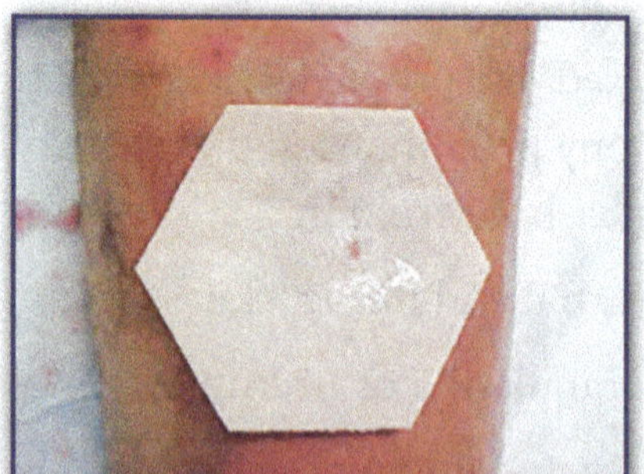

FIGURE 47. Collagen dressings

For optimal results with collagen products read the manufacturer's instructions.

H. Composite dressings

Composites are wound covers that combine different components or combinations of products into a single dressing to provide multiple functions.[13,23,41] Usually, they comprise multiple layers and incorporate a semi- or nonadherent pad that covers the wound. They may also include an adhesive border of nonwoven fabric tape or transparent film. Composite dressings can function as either a primary or a secondary dressing on a wide variety of wounds and may be used with topical medications.

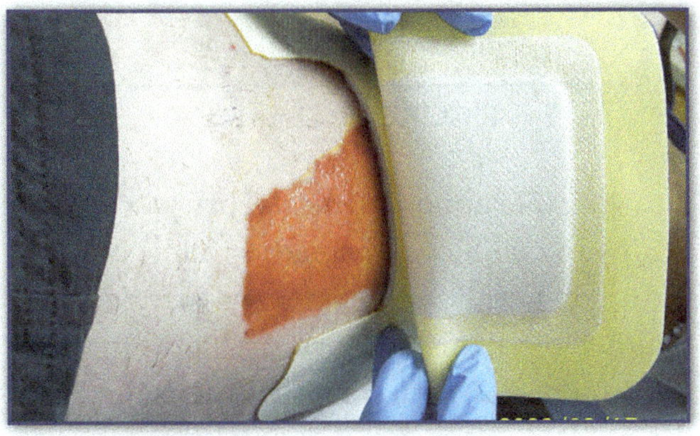

FIGURE 48. Composite dressing: absorbent and foam

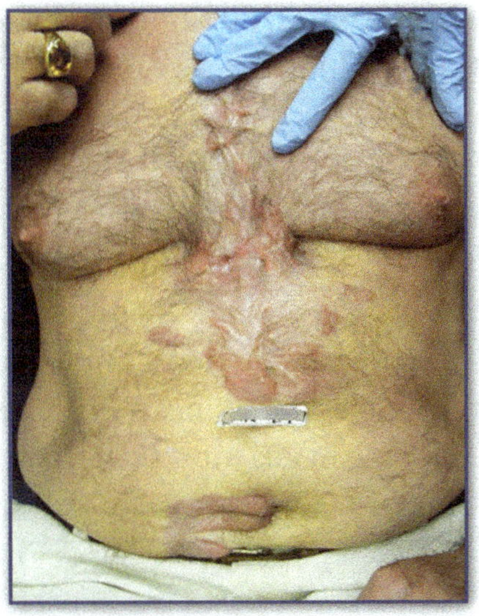

FIGURE 49. Keloid scar

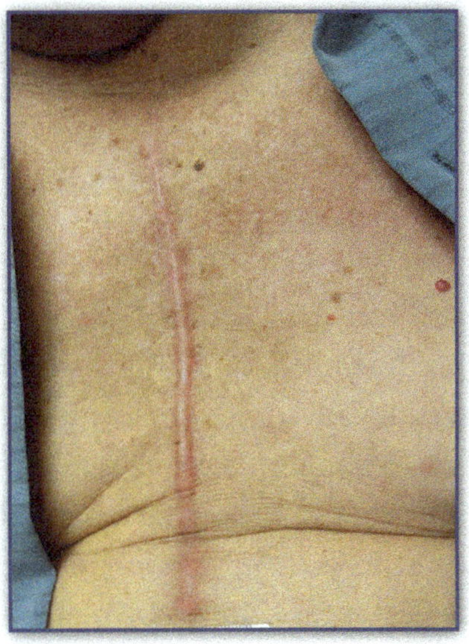

FIGURE 50. Hypertrophic scar

I. Silicone gel sheets

Silicone dressings are composed of cross-linked polymers reinforced or bonded to either a mesh or soft fabric.[22] This dressing category's primary purpose is to prevent or treat scar tissue, particularly hypertrophic and keloid scars.[22,35,50] Hypertrophic scars are purported to be caused by:

- Too much tension on sutures
- Poorly executed surgical closures
- Partial- and full-thickness burns
- Wound infections

These scars usually do not extend beyond the boundaries of the initial injury and may undergo partial spontaneous resolution. The second type of scar silicone gel sheets treat is termed keloid. People who acquire keloid scars are predisposed by their genetics due to both dominant and recessive genes.[50] The tissue of keloid scars extends beyond the borders of the original wound and usually does not spontaneously regress.

Greater than 50% of keloid scars recur after excision.[50] Both types of scars can have social and/or functional impacts on people.[50] Keloids scars are often the most troublesome, particularly if they are on exposed areas of the body such as the face or extend across a joint, causing contractures limiting range of motion.[50]

J. Diverse dressings that do not fit a particular category

Some dressings do not fit into a specific category. They may have more than one function, or the category description simply does not describe how these dressings work due to the unique mechanism of action.

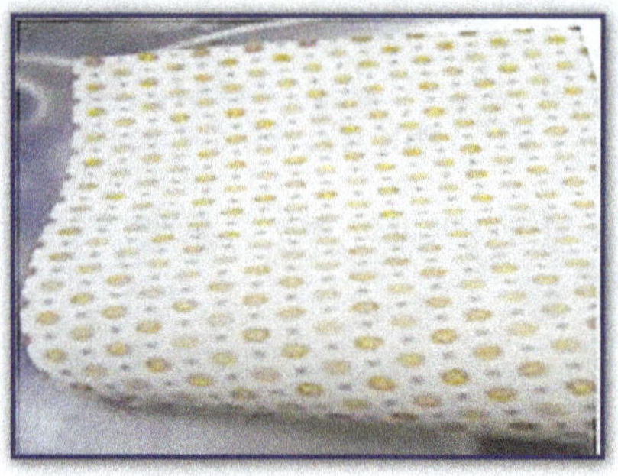

FIGURE 51. Procellera

Procellera (Vomaris Wound Care, Inc., Chandler, AZ) is the only antimicrobial wound dressing powered by advanced wireless microcurrent technology. This technology is designed to enhance the power of the body's natural electrical healing processes. Silver and zinc are applied on the device surface in a dot-matrix pattern, creating multiple microcell batteries. The microcurrents generated are designed to mimic the normal physiologic electric currents that are created in acute wounds. In chronic wounds, the body's normal electrical potentials at the wound site are damaged, contributing to the "stalled wound" condition. Procellera creates energy that drives the healing processes via the power of electricity for enhanced wound healing, mimicking the body's natural electrical processes.[51-52]

In the presence of moisture, which may come from wound exudate or exogenously applied saline or hydrogel; low-level microcurrents are generated at the device wound surface interface. These reactions occur without an external power source or accessories. Procellera antimicrobial dressing is indicated for partial- and full-thickness wounds such as pressure ulcers, venous ulcers, diabetic ulcers, burns, surgical incisions, donor and/or recipient graft sites. The dressing may be left in place for up to seven days; more frequent dressing changes may be needed with highly exudating wounds.[52]

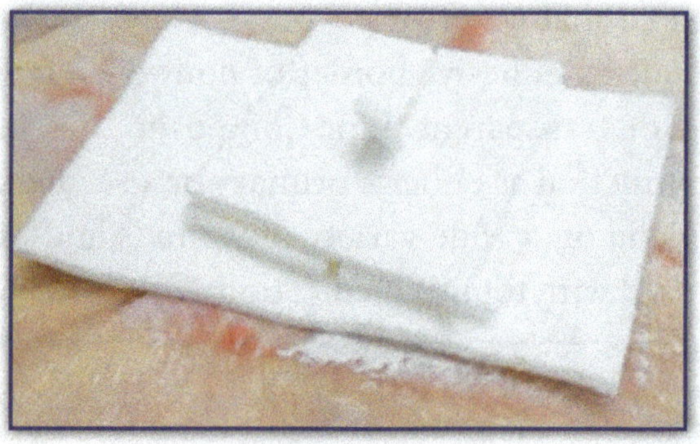

FIGURE 52. Drawtex

Drawtex (Steadmed Medical, Fort Worth, TX) is a hydroconductive primary wound dressing featuring LevaFiber technology that provides multiple mechanisms of action (MOA) to facilitate wound closure and subsequent healing. The three MOAs incorporated into this dressing include:

- A form of capillary wicking action that draws wound exudate and debris against the forces of gravity into material of the dressing
- A hydroconductive action controlled by Darcy's Law that defines the ability of fluid to move from wetter to drier regions against gravity (think about water being transported from tree roots to the leaves), and holds and transfers the exudate vertically and horizontally into the dressing
- An electrostatic action that occurs allowing the dressing to draw out relatively large amounts of exudate, devitalized

tissue, bacteria, and overabundant deleterious chemical mediators such as matrix metalloproteases (MMP)

The dressing actions, therefore, facilitate the removal of devitalized tissue, decrease excessive wound exudate, decrease bacterial levels, and remove harmful MMPs, thereby supporting a functional wound bed capable of supporting the endogenous wound healing processes. Drawtex is indicated for wounds with moderate to heavy exudate, burns, postoperative wounds, venous leg ulcers, pressure, diabetic foot, and Buruli ulcers, cavity wounds, complex surgical wounds, and tracheostomies (using Drawtex Tracheostomy Dressing).[13,23,53]

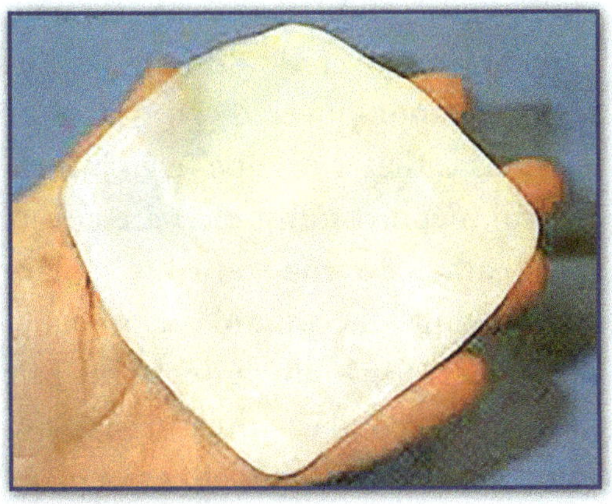

FIGURE 53. XCell cellulose wound dressing

XCell cellulose wound dressing provides optimum moisture balance required for wound healing. This dressing absorbs and/or donates moisture depending upon the wound exudate levels, mimicking the body's natural "blister" process for an optimal healing environment.[23] XCell is nonadherent to the wound surface, reducing pain and granulation tissue damage during dressing changes, and forms a protective barrier over the wound.[54]

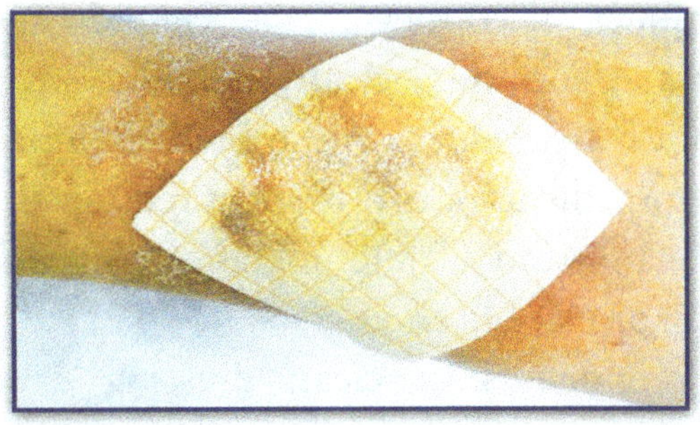

FIGURE 54. Enluxtra™ self-adaptive wound dressing

Enluxtra™ Self-Adaptive Wound Dressing (Osnovative Systems, Inc., Santa Clara, CA) is a self-regulating superabsorbent fiber dressing with adaptive absorbency and built-in adaptive hydration function.[13,23,55] The dressing material is designed to change its function according to the feedback from wound bed. The dressing dynamically balances the changes in the wound moisture environment, providing hydration or absorption depending on the real-time needs of the wound bed and periwound skin. Dry areas of the wound will stay properly hydrated with fluid being absorbed and locked in while protecting the periwound skin from maceration. The dressing is indicated for all wound types and all exudate levels. Enluxtra absorbs and locks drainage under compression, adjusts absorption to the amount of drainage, protects skin from maceration and desiccation, is nonadherent for nontraumatic removal, promotes autolytic debridement, and may be left in place for up to seven days.[55]

X. Dressing change practices

A. Clean technique dressing changes

Clean dressing changes are an acceptable practice for chronic wound care. Sterile dressing changes are impractical to perform in environments outside of the acute-care setting. Home-health, outpatient wound clinics, and long-term care primarily relies upon clean dressing change techniques. According to the Wound Ostomy Nurses Association, clean technique involves methods to reduce the overall number of microorganisms or to prevent or reduce the risk of transmission of microorganisms from one person or place to another.[56]

Components of clean dressing changes include:

- Creating a clean field on which to place the supplies needed for the dressing change process
- Meticulous hand hygiene (washing or use of alcohol/gel products) before, between each phase of the process, and after completion of the dressing change
- Use of clean gloves
- Using sterile instruments for processes such as debridement
- Applying sterile dressings
- Careful attention to the details of the process to prevent contamination of the supplies and materials being used[56]

B. Centers for Medicare and Medicaid Services (CMS) Surgical Dressing Policy[57]

In the United States, surgical dressings for chronic wounds are covered and will be reimbursed by CMS under traditional Medicare plans when specific criteria are met, such as:

- They are medically necessary for the treatment of a wound caused by or treated by a surgical procedure
- When debridement of a wound is medically necessary
- When a physician or other health-care professional, to the extent permissible, performs the surgical procedure or debridement under state law[57]

The Surgical Dressing Policy states that debridement of a wound may be any type of debridement, including but not limited to:

- Surgical (e.g., sharp instrument or laser)
- Mechanical (e.g., irrigation or wet-to-dry dressings)
- Chemical (e.g., topical application of enzymes)
- Autolytic (e.g., application of occlusive dressings to an open wound)

The Surgical Dressing Policy provides more directions for access to dressings using Medicare benefits by stating that dressings used for mechanical debridement, as secondary dressings over chemical debriding agents or to create a wound environment to allow for autolytic debridement are covered, although the agents themselves are non-covered. Dressings over a percutaneous catheter or tube (e.g., intravascular, epidural, nephrostomy, etc.) are covered as long as the catheter or tube remains in place and after removal until the wound is closed.

Surgical dressings include both primary dressings and secondary dressings. However, CMS has put utilization guidelines in place that must be adhered to when ordering for a patient. Your durable medical equipment (DME) company or health-care corporation that has an in-house DME department will be thoroughly up-to-date on how to access dressings through the patient's Medicare Part B benefits. Please refer to CMS Local Coverage Determination for the Surgical Dressing Policy guidance for more information.[57]

XI. Topical management of wound bioburden

As eloquently described in Chapter 6: Wound Bed Preparation, assessment of wound bioburden is an essential element in decision making for topical management. Careful attention to the factors that may place a patient at higher risk for infection including, but not limited to, nutritional status, glycemic control, blood flow, edema, and causative factors of the wound should be included in the decision making. Adoption of the principles of wound bed preparation implies a comprehensive program of care that prepares a wound to heal and involves the foundational elements of good wound care at every wound encounter: cleansing, debridement of necrotic or nonviable tissue with attention to wound edges, management and prevention of infection, and creation or maintenance of a moist wound bed.

Wound healing is generally not impaired simply due to the presence of bacteria on the wound surface; the impact of the microorganisms is determined by their number, their virulence, the bacterial "mix" (numbers and types of bacteria), and the host's resistance.[58] Wound clinicians frequently treat wounds that are infected and critically colonized with concerns of the potential presence of drug-resistant organisms and the potential to wipe out the "easy" bacteria and allowing the strong to survive. This is also true with the presence of bacterial biofilm (see Chapter 6: Wound Bed Preparation), with no systemic and few topical agents that can effectively eradicate biofilm. Recent focus on the impact that bacterial biofilm may have not only on our use of antimicrobial agents but the timing of that use heightens the importance of vigilant and repeated assessments, and respect for the impact that bacteria can have.[59] Wolcott et al. tested four different models, which showed that there was a 24-hour window of opportunity for use of a topical antibiotic agent postdebridement during which the biofilm population is most sensitive.[59] The Wound Healing Society Guidelines recommend that if wounds are appropriately debrided and there is still a suspicion of infection, and there is no evidence of epithelial migration from the margin despite adequate support (offloading the diabetic foot ulcer, compressing the leg with venous disease) and show no signs of improvement in two weeks, that the clinician should determine the type and level of infection in a debrided ulcer by tissue biopsy or by a validated quantitative swab technique.[60-61] If the clinician realizes that sudden changes in the previously healing wound may indicate an initial host response to rising bacterial loads, she/he can initiate topical measures to reduce the bacterial load, preventing continued replication and potential invasion into the deeper tissues.

A wide range of dressings to address local wound bioburden have become available over the years which at the same time can manage the other needs of the wound, such as absorbing exudate and balancing moisture while protecting the periwound skin, filling of space and wicking exudate from undermining and tunnels, and providing coverage, protection, and insulation.[62] The attributes of the ideal antimicrobial dressing have been described as one that:[63]

- Provides sustained antimicrobial activity
- Provides a moist wound healing environment
- Allows consistent delivery of the antimicrobial over the entire surface of the wound
- Allows monitoring of the wound with minimum interference

- Manages exudate, if problematic
- Is comfortable
- Is conformable
- Provides an effective microbial barrier
- Absorbs and retains bacteria
- Avoids wound trauma on removal

Dressing a wound involves attention to the assessed needs of the wound, as well as following accepted basic tenants of good wound care, which have already been addressed. This section will focus on those topical agents that directly address and impact wound bioburden: wound cleansing and disinfection, topical antibiotics, and antimicrobial wound dressings with the implied caveat that the entire patient condition should be taken into consideration and appropriate systemic therapy will be used when warranted.

A. Wound cleansing and disinfection

All wounds should be cleansed at each dressing change, before and after debridement, and in the event of contamination using a neutral, nonirritating, nontoxic solution, and routine cleansing should be accomplished with every effort to minimize chemical and/or mechanical trauma.[(60-61)] An exception to the requirement for routine cleansing may be the recent application of a skin graft or cellular tissue product, which should be left undisturbed; in this case the surrounding skin should be cleansed. The choice of solution or agent used, as well as the method of delivery, is driven by the condition and local factors in the wound. The literature abounds with references over many years and there has been much discussion related to the solutions used on the open wound and the perceived risks of cytotoxicity. Although definitive research is lacking, data against the use of antiseptics such as hydrogen peroxide, acetic acid (dilute vinegar solution), Dakin's solution (dilute bleach solution), and povidone iodine are based primarily on in vitro models demonstrating the toxicity of these agents to the viability of cells important to wound healing, such as fibroblasts, keratinocytes, and leukocytes. As a practical matter, the wound surface, the presence of necrotic or inflamed tissue and adherent exudates, the condition and hygiene of the patient, the location of the wound, and the potential for environmental or other contamination such as incontinence should drive the choice. Good practice evidence suggests use of a nontoxic cleaning solution in combination with a delivery device that will create sufficient mechanical force to remove the surface debris without injury to healthy tissue.[(15)] Topical antiseptics are antimicrobial agents that reduce the number of microorganisms and may be seen as an adjunct to infection control. Whereas antibiotics have a specific method of action, antiseptics utilize multiple targets to inhibit or kill organisms and have a larger spectrum of activity against bacteria, fungi, and viruses.[(64)] In choosing an appropriate wound cleanser, the clinician should consider the goals of cleaning based on a thorough assessment. Further consideration will be given to how the solution or cleanser may be used, whether to cleanse or irrigate the wound or leave it behind in a delivery vehicle such as gauze. While long-term exposure to tissues may be overwhelming to the cells, short duration of contact during cleaning may be beneficial in dealing with surface debris and contaminants from previous dressings being in place. One must always consider the risks and benefits in the use of a particular agent, as well as determine whether the goal is to achieve wound disinfection or wound cleansing. Newer antiseptic agents such as superoxide water solutions, dilute sodium hypochlorite, and hypochlorous acid can be advantageous in management of wounds with high bacterial loads because they can reduce microbes on the surface of the wound without causing injury to the host wound cells.

Commercially available wound cleansers contain surface active agents (surfactants) that break the bonds attaching contaminants and debris to the wound surface, allowing them to be rinsed away mechanically when the solution is sprayed or poured over the wound. The clinician should consider use of cleansing solutions with surfactants and/or antimicrobials for wounds with debris, confirmed infection, suspected infection, or suspected high levels of bacterial colonization.[15] Any potential toxicity of these cleansers should be weighed against the need for a more thorough removal of surface debris and contaminants based on the assessment of the wound. Normal saline is an effective agent for wound cleansing that will not interfere with wound healing when delivered with enough pressure to ensure adequate removal of surface debris. Pressures below 4 pounds per square inch (psi) are not sufficient to remove debris, and pressures exceeding 15 psi increase the risk that bacteria will be driven into the tissues.[64]

The use of potable water (tap water) for cleansing chronic wounds has been questioned many times and is more commonly used in community and home-care nursing because it is easily accessible, efficient, and cost-effective.[65-66] The decision to use tap water to cleanse wounds should take into account the quality of water, nature of wounds, and the patient's general condition, including the presence of comorbid conditions.[66] Recent guidelines suggest that most pressure ulcers can be cleansed with potable water (i.e., water suitable for drinking) or normal saline.[15] If the wound is going to be cleansed as part of the patient's personal shower, the decision should also take into account the location of the wound, water conditions in a geographic area, the patient's physical condition and immune system, and the overall hygienic advantage. Patients should be advised not to immerse an open wound into a tub.

The temperature of the wound cleansing solution and frequency of dressing change should also be considered. Neutrophil, fibroblast, and epithelial cell activity decreases when the wound bed temperature falls below 33°C (91.4°F).[67] Cleansing solutions should be used at body temperature, as it can take 40 minutes for a wound to return to normal temperature following cold cleansing (cleansing with room-temperature solutions), and around three hours for leukocyte activity to recover after irrigation with a cold (room-temperature) solution. The physiologic effects of hypothermia (e.g. vasoconstriction, depressed neutrophil activity, reduced ability of the cells to use oxygen free radicals to kill bacteria, and lower levels of collagen deposition) can result in impaired resistance to infection and delayed wound healing.[67-68]

B. Topical antibiotics

Antibiotics have decreased in popularity as first-line treatments for wound management secondary to the rise of bacterial resistance. While the specific mechanism of action varies from one antibiotic to another, they generally have one defined microbial target, which limits their effectiveness against multiple pathogens.[69] It is agreed that antibiotics should be avoided unless there is evidence of true clinical infection. In addition, some topical antibiotics should be avoided due to the risks of hypersensitivity reactions, super infections, and increased bacterial resistance.[70] This is not to say that antibiotics should be abandoned altogether; rather, they should be reserved for situations where advancing clinical infection is present, highly virulent organisms exist in the wound bed, or the host's immune response is severely compromised, such as in diabetic foot ulcer infections.

Possibly the most appropriate use of topical antibiotics is for infection prophylaxis in superficial skin wounds with high risk of infection, such as those that are likely to be contaminated (accidental wounds, lacerations, abrasions, and burns). Because all traumatic wounds should be considered contaminated, use of topical antibiotics is logical for these wounds to prevent wound infection.

C. Antimicrobial wound dressings

Clinicians face decision making related to the critically colonized and infected wound frequently, and given the increase in drug-resistant organisms, preventing progression to full tissue infection is a priority. Prompt reaction to often subtle changes that indicate an increasing bacterial load allows the clinician to intervene topically with dressing that will address the bacteria in the wound exudate and provide a barrier to further contamination to reduce the load and prevent further bacterial replication and potential invasion into the deeper tissue spaces.

The dressings that address local wound bioburden while managing the other needs of the wound, such as exudate, moisture balance, and protection of the periwound skin, wicking of tunnels and filling of wound space, coverage, protection, and insulation have increased over the years. Each antimicrobial dressing option provides unique but familiar mechanisms of action that address wound care needs. The attributes of the ideal antimicrobial dressing[71] have been described as one that:

- Provides sustained antimicrobial activity
- Provides a moist wound healing environment
- Allows consistent delivery of the antimicrobial over the entire surface of the wound
- Allows monitoring of the wound with minimum interference
- Manages exudate, if problematic
- Is comfortable
- Is conformable
- Provides an effective microbial barrier
- Absorbs and retains bacteria
- Avoids wound trauma on removal

The primary differentiating factor for the various dressings is the particular antimicrobial agent incorporated into the dressing. Antimicrobial agents are bound into or coated onto the dressing materials; they act as a barrier to outside contaminants in addition to interacting with wound exudate to further enhance the barrier effects and to reduce bacterial loads on the surface of the wound. Commonly used agents include silver, iodine, honey, polyhexamethylene biguanide (PHMB), and the pigments crystal violet and methylene blue. One other dressing that is included in this category but is technically not antimicrobial is a contact layer coated with dialkylcarbamoylchloride (DACC).

1. *Silver*

Silver has been used for centuries, with silver coins placed into vessels of water to prevent bacterial growth, and has historical documentation for medical uses dating back to AD 750. A renewed interest in the use of silver in topical antimicrobial dressings has resulted in multiple studies to assess its ability to reduce bacterial growth and the risk of wound infection, as an adjunct to systemic management of active infection, and to reduce the risk of hospital-acquired wound infections. This renewed interest is largely attributed to silver's bactericidal efficacy at low concentrations and its relatively limited toxicity to human cells. Silver has

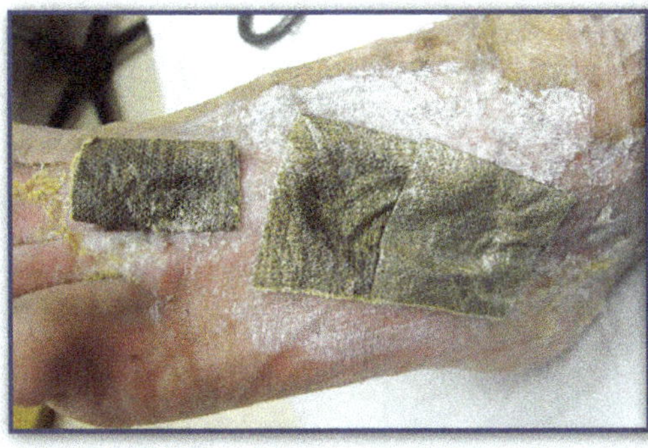

FIGURE 55a. Nanocrystalline silver

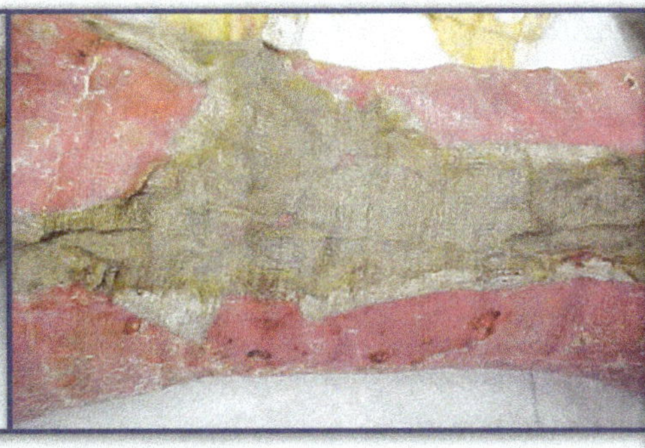

FIGURE 55b. Silver calcium alginate

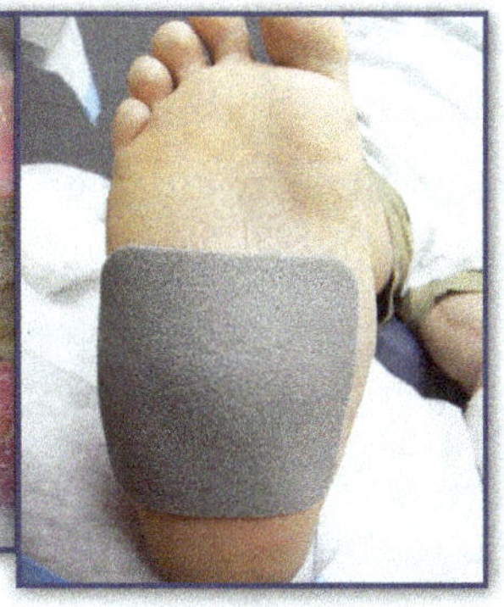

FIGURE 55c. Silver foam

proven antimicrobial activity, which includes antibiotic-resistant bacteria such as methicillin-resistant *S. aureus* (MRSA) and vancomycin-resistant enterococci (VRE).[72] Silver is now available in amorphous hydrogels, sheet hydrogels, alginates, hydrofibers, foams, silicones, contact layers, wound powders, ointments, negative pressure foams, and irrigation solutions (silver nitrate solutions). The choice of dressing for a particular wound is determined by the characteristics of the particular carrier dressing, the way silver is delivered to the wound bed, and the needs of the wound. Silver dressings work via one of two delivery systems: the silver may be donated via the exudate to the wound bed and may therefore kill organisms on the wound surface; or the silver may be retained in the dressing and may work by destroying bacteria contained in the exudate and absorb into the carrier dressing. In order for silver to realize its total bactericidal potential, there must be controlled and sustained release of silver over time that is sufficient to cause bacterial death but within a range that prevents tissue toxicity.[73] The ability of the dressing to conform, remain in place, and provide consistent coverage of the wound bed also contributes to antimicrobial effectiveness.[74-75]

Silver is biologically active when it is in soluble form, that is, as Ag+ or Ag0 clusters. Ag+ is the ionic form found in silver nitrate, silver sulfadiazine, and other ionic silver compounds. Ag0 is the uncharged form of metallic silver present in nanocrystalline silver products. Free silver cations have a potent antimicrobial effect that destroys microorganisms immediately by blocking cellular respiration and disrupting the function of bacterial cell membranes. Specifically, silver cations bind to tissue proteins, causing structural changes in the bacterial cell membranes that cause cell death. Silver cations also bind and denature bacterial DNA and RNA, thus inhibiting cell replication.[76]

Concerns related to the use of silver dressings revolve around the potential for development of resistance, the cellular toxicity, and the appropriate use of the right amount of silver at the right time. Percival et al.[77] looked at the prevalence of silver resistance in bacteria from diabetic foot ulcers and found that the incidence of silver-resistance genes from these ulcers is low and appears to be confined to an enteric bacterium, *Enterobacter cloacae,* which is not known to be a primary wound pathogen. No evidence of resistance genes in wound pathogens such as *S. aureus* and *P. aeruginosa* was found in this study. This study also found that the low proportion of wound bacteria that possess silver-resistance genes are killed when challenged with silver-containing wound dressings.[77]

The toxicity of silver in cells and tissues has been assessed. Silver dressings that have been shown to be cytotoxic in vitro within one day showed no cytotoxicity in vivo after one week, suggesting that in vitro cytotoxicity is more sensitive than in vivo because there is no means of reducing toxicity via blood circulation, tissue reservoir, metabolism, or by dilution effects.[78]

Every dressing category (films, foams, alginates, hydrofibers, gels, gauze, contact layers, and composites) is available with a silver component in one form or another. No data exist to strongly support one type of dressing over another based on their silver "dosage." Assurance of intimate contact with the wound bed has been shown to increase the success of the dressing by avoiding the formation of voids (dead space) where bacteria may flourish. The clinical result is the definitive test of the dressing (i.e., Does it work in practice?).[76] Continued discretion in the judicious use of silver, as well as all antimicrobial dressings, is required to mitigate potential further resistance patterns in common wound pathogens in the future.

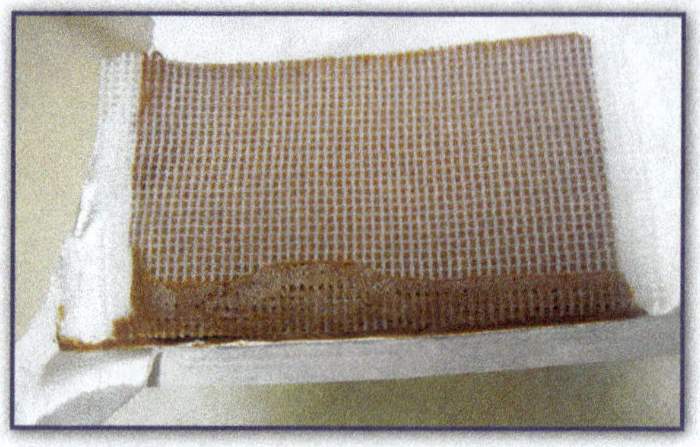

FIGURE 56a. Cadexomer iodine sheet

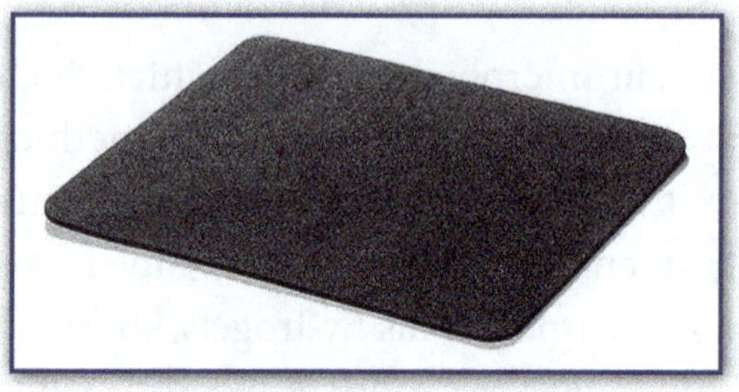

FIGURE 56b. Iodine foam

2. *Iodine*

Iodine as a disinfectant has been used for years, usually combined with a surfactant or povidone, which releases free iodine in solution. Povidone iodine has been used historically as a surgical scrub; iodophor in gauze packing has been used for packing wounds. Iodine has a broad spectrum of activity and works in many ways by disrupting cell walls and nuclei and facilitating oxidative killing of microorganisms and neutrophils.[79] It has been shown to be toxic at a cellular level in vitro.[80-82] The concern with toxicity and absorption of iodine has led to more judicious use in carriers that enable the slow release of the iodine into the wound exudate, thus reducing the bacterial load without the toxicity of the full-strength disinfectant.

The term cadexomer iodine describes a delivery system rather than an antimicrobial agent. In this novel delivery system, the iodine is contained within a cadexomer starch bead. As wound exudate is drawn up, it enters the cadexomer bead, causing its openings to swell and allowing a slow, sustained release of the iodine molecules maintaining a steady-state 0.9% concentration at the wound bed, providing a nontoxic level for healing wounds. Iodine is brown; iodide, which is the inactive form of iodine, is colorless. The dressing progresses from brown to colorless, indicating that the iodine has been used and as a signal to change the dressing. The dressing lasts for an average of 72 hours, depending on the amount of exudate, the size of the wound, and the amount of the dressing/gel used. Cadexomer iodine has also been shown to be effective against certain *S. aureus* in biofilm in vitro and in vivo.[82-83] Another novel delivery system for controlled release iodine is from a polyvinyl alcohol foam, again to prevent potential toxicity as well as provide sustained control and reformation of biofilm.[82-83]

3. *Honey*

The use of honey been documented as a treatment for open wounds for ages, having been mentioned in the Bible, the Koran, and the

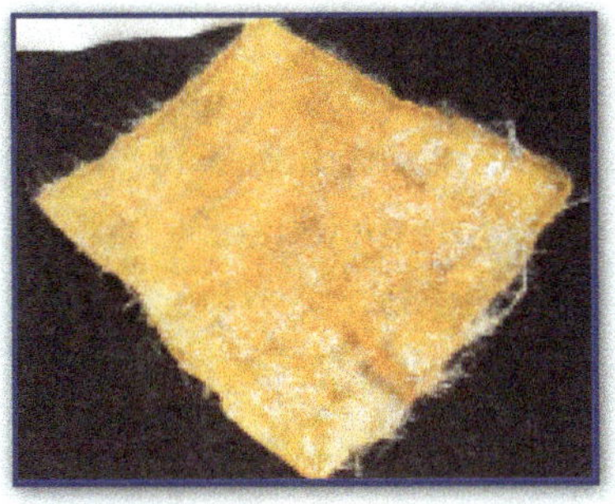

FIGURE 57a. Honey alginate
Courtesy of Jayesh B. Shah, MD

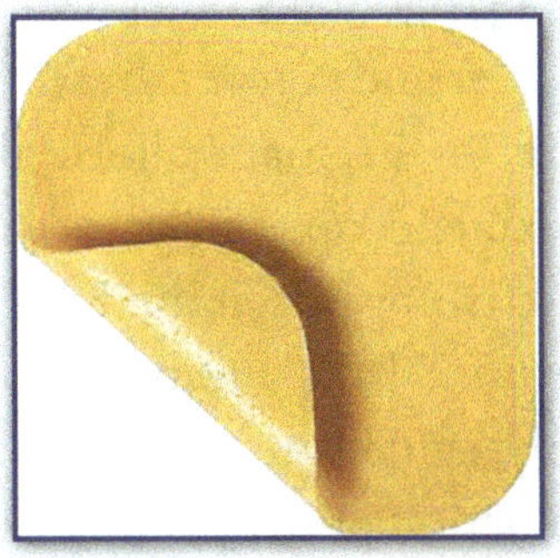

FIGURE 57b. Honey hydrocolloid.

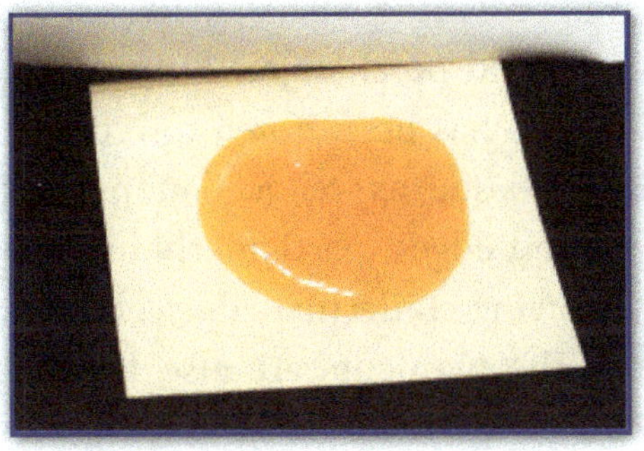

FIGURE 57c. Honey paste/gel
Courtesy of Jayesh B. Shah, MD

Torah. It was documented to be used in plasters by the Egyptians in 2,000 BC, was found documented in medical writings from 1392, and has experienced a renaissance in recent years as a topic of clinical and scientific research in wound healing.[84]

The form of medical-grade honey used today differs greatly from that of the natural or culinary versions. Tea plants, as well as leptospermum polygalifolium (jelly bush honey), have specific qualities related to their processing that affect the end product's bacterial count, pH, enzyme activity, and overall benefit in wound care. For example, while heat is used to prepare culinary honey for consumption, this invariably reduces the enzyme responsible for hydrogen peroxide production, whereas medical-grade honey's gamma radiation sterilization process allows it to retain its biologic activity.[85] The antimicrobial activity of honey has been related to the high sugar content and low water activity, creating an osmotic effect that dehydrates the bacteria and, along with the acidic pH of 3.2 to 4.5, inhibits bacterial growth. The fluid shift resulting from this osmotic effect also contributes to creating a moist wound healing environment and reduced pain on dressing removal due to decreased potential for desiccation and adherence to the wound surface. The presence of the glucose oxidase enzyme added by bees to the nectar that they collect results in the production of hydrogen peroxide, which, although known to be toxic as a rinse, is 1,000 times less toxic in honey. Honey dressings are available in an alginate, hydrocolloid, and paste form.[85-89]

4. *Polyhexamethylene biguanide*

Polyhexamethylene biguanide (PHMB) is a biocide that has been used for many years with no known resistance. It is used in a variety of products, including wound care dressings, contact lens cleaning solutions, perioperative cleansing products, and swimming pool cleaners.[90,91] The gauze sponges have also been used extensively as part of the dressing interface layer with numerous negative-pressure wound therapy devices. PHMB is a synthetic compound similar in structure to naturally occurring molecules produced by inflammatory cells to protect against infection. By attaching itself to the bacterial cell membrane, PHMB causes structural changes that kill the bacteria. Bacteria commonly protect themselves from resistance by pumping some antibiotics out of the cell using efflux pumps.[92-94] The structural changes caused by the PHMB prevent the bacteria from using their efflux pumps to pump out the biocide.[94] The incorporation of PHMB into dressings, including gauze sponges, gel dressings, foams, and biosynthesized cellulose wound dressings, has been shown to be an effective barrier to protect a wound from outside contamination as well as to have bactericidal activity on relevant bacteria absorbed into the dressing material. One study found that PHMB-impregnated foam showed a significant log reduction of pseudomonas aeruginosa within the wound, compared to standard gauze, and did not allow pseudomonas to colonize the PHMB-impregnated foam or change the normal wound milieu.[93] These results support one of the most common uses of PHMB by the wound care practitioner, which is as preventative barrier dressing against infection in high-risk individuals.[92] PHMB must come into direct contact with the bacterial organism. Therefore, once it is bound to a dressing material such as gauze, foam or alginate, it can only affect bacteria that have been absorbed into the dressing.[93] In the case of newer wound irrigations and solutions, time of exposure is the key determinant; at least 10 to 15 minutes of exposure is necessary to induce the most antimicrobial effect. [94] Therefore, clinicians utilizing PHMB in solution form should consider allowing the solution to dwell in the wound bed during the cleansing process, or provide the agent as a continuous irrigation such as through the use of negative-pressure wound therapy devices that instill or allow dwell time.[95]

5. *Methylene blue and gentian violet*

The pigments gentian violet and methylene blue have been used in medicine for more than 50 years as both laboratory stains[96] and antiseptics that have bacteriostatic properties on multiple clinically relevant bacteria, including resistant strains such as methicillin-resistant *S. aureus* (MRSA). They are available commercially bound within a polyvinyl (PVA) alcohol foam, which when hydrated becomes a soft, conformable wound filler and contact dressing. The open cell structure of the foam allows the removal of wound exudate up and into the dressing, where the active agents inhibit the growth of microorganisms. This unique uptake of exudate is visibly evident upon dressing removal, and the interaction of the exudate with the pigments will be noted to blanch out the color of the foam, providing visual evidence that the dressing should be changed.[97] In clinical use, the foam also has been noted to reduce hypergranulation tissue, as well as flatten out slightly rolled wound edges, particularly in venous leg ulcers, allowing epidermal edge cellular migration.[98-99] The pigments are also found bound within a polyurethane foam dressing designed for seven-day wear time.

6. *Dialkylcarbamoyl chloride (DACC)*

Microorganisms have the ability to attach to a denatured extracellular matrix through the interaction of their hydrophobic covering with

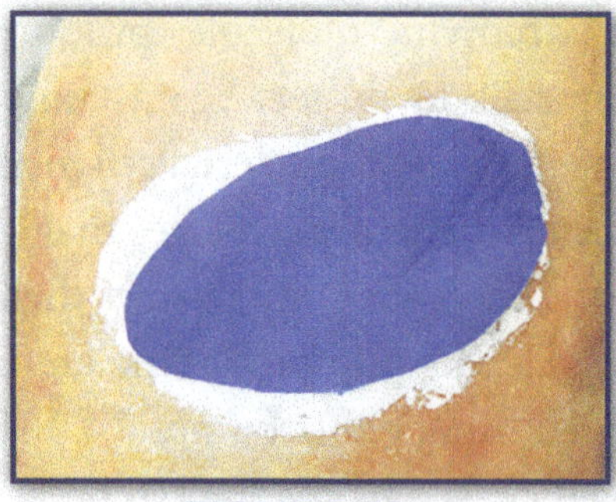

FIGURE 58a.
Pigmented foam dressing

FIGURE 58b.
Dressing covered with oil emulsion

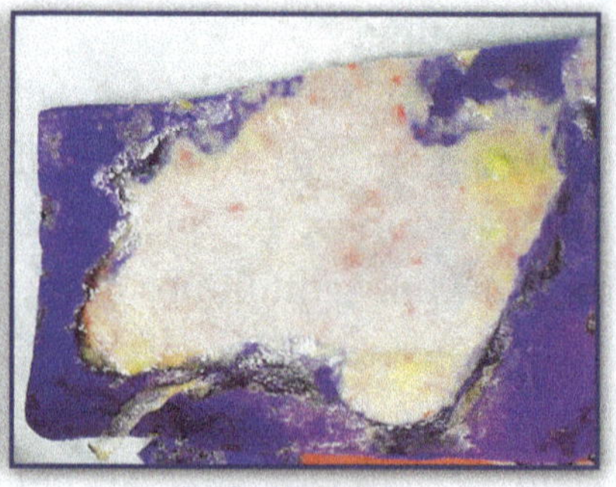

FIGURE 58c.
Dressing blanched out from exudate

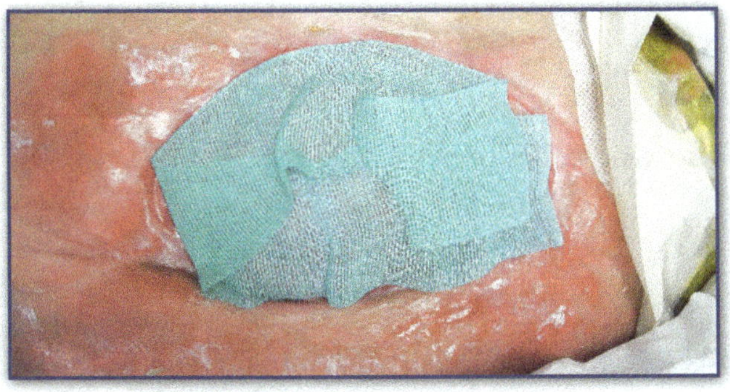

FIGURE 59. Dressing containing dialkylcarbamoyl chloride (DACC)

cell surface proteins in the collagen known as hydrophobins.[100] This method of surface attachment has been recently employed in the form of applying DACC, a naturally occurring hydrophobic fatty acid, to various dressing constructs in order to utilize the principles of hydrophobic binding and allow bandage fibers to stick to the hydrophobic covering of potential microbes in the wound bed.

Interestingly, dressings containing DACC, also known generically as pathogen-binding mesh, aren't technically antimicrobial. They have no chemical, pharmacological, or antimicrobial agents in the dressing. When bacteria are killed, endotoxins and cellular debris are released into the wound bed. This adds to the inflammatory response, risking the increase in an activation of MMPs.[101] To avoid these potentially disruptive insults to the wound environment, DACC-covered dressing fibers work instead to bind the microbes to the dressing, render them inactive, and then remove them whole. This concept of repetitive removal of microbes with each dressing change lowers the overall bacterial burden in the wound over time, in fact in-vitro testing shows that the bacteria begin to bind in about 30 seconds, and that the number of bacteria the dressing is capable of binding is more than would normally be found in an infected wound. Once the bacteria are bound, they become inactivated, their metabolism slows down, and they exhibit a decreased rate of replication and the formation of toxins slows down or stops completely.[101] The binding activity of the mesh requires moisture, so it must be moistened with saline or hydrogel for dry wounds.

Summary

Decision making related to the management of the patient with an open acute or chronic wound is complex because there are multiple factors to consider relative to supporting and treating the disease state that is the underlying cause of the wound, which have been well covered in this book. Once the patient-centered factors are addressed, the management of the actual wound is driven by the focused assessment of the wound for management of the moisture, the perceived condition of the wound environment for factors that can be balanced, and then the assessed presence of the bacterial load. Wound management is both a science and an art; attention to detail is essential, management based on evidence-based guidelines is the key driver, and the patient experience is critical in developing the best treatment plan. It is, though, the evaluation of the plan along the way and alterations based on the changing needs of the wound that enable the best decision making to put the wound on the optimal healing trajectory.

Review questions

1. **Primary dressings may function in all of the following capacities except:**

   a. Addressing wound bed moisture content

   b. Managing wound bioburden when impregnated with antimicrobial agents

   c. Protecting wound bed tissues or structures such as tendons from damage during dressing changes

   d. As a wound filler within the wound bed

   e. To secure absorbent wound packing in place

2. **A dressing category known to mitigate the harmful effects of excessive matrix metalloproteases (MMPs) on cells responsible for wound healing is:**

   a. Transparent film

   b. Gauze

   c. Collagen

   d. Hydrocolloid

   e. Hydrogel

3. ***True/False.*** Clean dressing changes (versus sterile dressings changes) are considered an acceptable practice in chronic wound care.

4. **Medical-adhesive related skin injuries (MARSI) include all of the following except:**

   a. Tension blisters

   b. Folliculitis

   c. Macerated periwound area

   d. Mechanical skin stripping

   e. Incontinence

5. ***True/False.*** Topical antimicrobial dressings have taken the place of antibiotic therapy for infected chronic wounds due to the emergence of antibiotic resistant organisms.

ANSWERS: 1) e
2) c
3) True
4) b
5) False

References

1. Teall EK. Medicine and doctoring in ancient Mesopotamia. Grand Valley Journal of History. 2014 (3).[Internet]. Available from: http://scholarworks.gvsu.edu/gvjh/vol3/iss1/2.
2. Forrest MD. Early history of wound treatment. Journal of the Royal Society of Medicine. 1982 Mar; 75. Centrallasarettet S-961 85 Boden, Sweden [cited 2016 July 27].
3. Shah JB. The history of wound care. J Am Col Certif Wound Spec. 2011 Sep; 3(3):65-66. [Internet]. 2012 Apr 9. [Cited 2016 July 27]. Available from: https://www.ncbi.nlm.nih.gov/pmc/articles/PMC3601883/
4. Hempstead CA, Worthington Jr, WE. Encyclopedia of 20th century technology. New York and London: Routledge; 2015.
5. King M. Our historical roots: Dr Richard Drysdale Dakins, DSc, and his solution. Journal of Wound, Ostomy & Continence Nursing, 2008 May/June; 35(3):289-292.
6. Demling RH, DeSanti L. The use of moist wound healing with infection control in the burn wound. [Internet]. [Cited 2016 July 27]. Available from: http://www.eplasty.com/images/PDF/MoistWoundHealing.pdf.
7. Orland GF. The fine structure of the interrelationship of cells in the human epidermis. J Biophys Biochem Cytol 1958 Sept 25; 4(5):529-538.
8. Krawczyk WS. A pattern of epidermal cell migration during wound healing. J Cell Biology. 1971;49:.247-263.
9. Winter GD. Formation of the scab and the rate of epithelization of superficial wounds in the skin of the young domestic pig. Nature. 1962 Jan 20:193-194.
10. Hinman CD, Mailbach HI. Effects of air exposure and occlusion on experimental human skin wounds. Nature. 1963:200:377.
11. Sibbald RG, Goodman L, Woo KY, Krasner DL, Smart H, Tariq G, Ayello EA, Burrell RE, Keast DH, Mayer D, Norton L, Salcido RS. Special considerations in wound bed preparation 2011: an update. Adv Skin Wound Care. 2011 Sep;24(9):415-436.
12. Krasner DL, Sibbald GR, Woo KY. Wound product dressing selection: A holistic, interprofessional patient-centered approach. [Internet]. A Kestral Wound Source White Paper. 2011 [cited 2016 Aug 6]. Available from: www.woundsource.com.
13. Weir D, Brindle T. Wound dressings. In: Hamm R,editor. Atlas of Wound Care. New York: McGraw-Hill; 2015; p. 337-378.
14. Woo KY, Smith K. Wound dressing selection for pressure ulcers. In: Wound Dressing Selection for Pressure Ulcers. [Internet]. [Cited 2016 Aug 6]. Available from: https://kestrelhealth.leadpages.co/pressure-ulcer-dressing-selection.
15. European Pressure Ulcer Advisory Panel; National Pressure Ulcer Advisory Panel; Pan Pacific Pressure Ulcer Alliance. Prevention and treatment of pressure ulcers: clinical practice guideline. Haesler E,editor. Perth (Australia): Cambridge Media; 2014.
16. Sibbald RG, Elliott JA, Ayello EA, Somayaji R Optimizing the moisture management tightrope with wound bed preparation. Advances in Skin & Wound Care 2015;28:466-476.
17. Sood A, Granick MS, Tomaselli NL. Wound dressings and comparative effectiveness data. Adv Wound Care. 2014 Aug 1; 3(8): 511-529.
18. European Wound Management Association Position Document: Wound bed preparation in practice. London: MEP Ltd., 2004.
19. Widgerow AD. Deconstructing the stalled wounds. Wounds 2012;24(3):58-60.

20. Simon PA. Skin Wound Healing. [Internet]. Medscape [cited 2016 Oct 24]. Available from: http://emedicine.medscape.com/article/884594-overview.

21. Larbi A, Rymkiewicz A, Low I, Binte N, et el. The immune system in the elderly: a fair fight against diseases? Aging Health. 2013;9:35-47.

22. WoundSource 2010 [Cited 2016 Oct 6]. Available from: http://www.woundsource.com/product-category/dressings. Accessed 06 Oct 2016.

23. Woundsource 2016 [Cited 2016 Oct 6]. Available from: http://www.woundsource.com/product-category/dressings. Accessed 06 Oct 2016.

24. Scarborough P, McGuire J. Diabetes and the diabetic foot. In: Hamm R, editor. Atlas of wound Care. New York: McGraw-Hill; 2015; p. 193-226.

25. Scarborough P. Diabetes and wound healing. In: Mculloch JM, Kloth LC, editors. Wound Healing: Evidence-Based Management. Philadelphia: FA Davis;2010; p. 231-247.

26. Cullen GD, Legerstee R, Harding KG, Schultz G. MMPa made easy. [Internet]. Wounds International. 2009; 1(1) [cited 2016 Sept 15]. Available from: www.woundsinternational.com.

27. Krasner D. The chronic wound pain experience: a conceptual model. Ostomy/Wound Management. 1995;41(3):20-9.

28. Woo KY, Krasner DL, Sibbald GR. Pain in people with chronic wounds: clinical strategies for decreasing pain and improving quality of life. In: Krasner DL,editor. Chronic Wound Care: The Essentials. Malvern, PA: HMP Communications, LLC; 2014; p. 111-122.

29. Principles of best practice: minimizing pain at wound dressing-related procedures. A consensus document. London: MEP Ltd, 2004.

30. Upton D, Hender C, Solowiej K, Woo K. Stress and pain associated with dressing change in patients with chronic wounds. J Wound Care. 2012b;22(2):53-61.

31. Hollinworth H. Pain at wound dressing-related procedures: a template for assessment. [Internet]. World Wide Wounds, 2005 Aug [cited 2016 Sept 28]. Available from: http://www.worldwidewounds.com/2005/august/Hollinworth/Framework-Assessing-Pain-Wound-Dressing-Related.html.

32. Dallam LE, Ayello EA, Woo KY, Sibbald GR. Pain management and wounds. In: Baranoski S, Ayello, EA. Wounds and Treatment in Wound Care Essentials Practice Principles. Wolters Kluwer, 2016, p. 281-306.

33. Wong-Baker FACES Pain Rating Scale. Wong-Baker FACES Foundation. [Cited 2016 Oct 25 with permission from http://www.WongBakerFACES.org. Originally published in Whaley & Wong's Nursing Care of Infants and Children. Elsevier Inc.

34. Kim E, Buschmann M. Reliability and validity of the faces pain scale with older adults. International Journal of Nursing Studies. 2006; 43(4):447-456.

35. Meuleneire F, Rucknagel H. Soft silicone dressings made easy. Wounds International. May 2013. [Internet]. [Cited 2016 Oct 1]. Available from: http://www.woundsinternational.com/made-easys/view/soft-silicones-made-easy.

36. Akhmetova A, Saliev T, Allan IU, Illsley MJ et al. A comprehensive review of topical odor-controlling treatment options for chronic wounds: A comprehensive review. [Internet]. JWOCN [cited 2016 Oct 10]. Available from: www.jwocnonline.com.

37. WoundSource. Wound odor. [Internet]. [Cited 2016 Oct 2]. Available from: http://www.woundsource.com/patientcondition/wound-odor.

38. Gethin G, McIntosh C, Probst S. Complementary and alternative therapies for management of odor in malignant fungating wounds: a critical review. Chronic Wound Care Management and Research. 2016 June 7. Accessed 22 Oct 2016.

39. Stotts NA. Bioburden Infection. In: Baranoski S, Ayello, EA, editors. Wound Care Essentials Practice Principles. Wolters Kluwer; 2016; p. 121-128.

40. Cowan LJ, Stechmiller J. Prevalence of wet-to-dry dressings in wound care. Adv. Skin Wound Care. 2009; 22(12):567-573

41. Baranoski S, Ayello, EA. Wounds and treatment in wound care essentials practice principles. Wolters Kluwer; 2016; p. 171-226.

42. Ovington, LG. Hanging wet-to-dry dressings out to dry. Advances in Skin & Wound Care; March/April 2002; 15(2):79-84.

43. Centers for Medicaid and Medicare Services. State Operations Manual Appendix PP–Guidance to Surveyors for Long Term Care Facilities. Rev 157, 2016 June 10.

44. McNichol L, Lund C, Rosen T, Gray M. Medical adhesives and patient safety: state of the science. Journal Wound Ostomy Continence Nursing. 2013;40(4):365-380.

45. LeBlanc K., Baranoski S, Langemo D, et al. State of the science: consensus statements for the prevention, prediction, assessment and treatment of skin tears. Advances in Skin & Wound Care. 2011;24(9):2.

46. Fletcher J, Mppre Z, Anderson I, Matsuzaki K. Pressure ulcers and hydrocolloids made easy. Wound International. 2011 Nov;2 (4).

47. Dabiri G, Damstetter E, Phillips T. Choosing a wound dressing based on common wound characteristics. Advances in Wound Care [Internet]. 2016;5(1):32–41 [cited 2016 Oct 24]. Available from: http://doi.org/10.1089/wound.2014.0586.

48. Queen D. Technology update: understanding Hydrofiber technology. Wounds International. 2010;1(5).

49. Galea E. Managing chronic/stalled arterial, venous and pressure ulcer with collagen and oxidized regenerated cellulose dressings. [Internet]. World Wide Wounds. 2014 July [cited 2016 Oct 24]. Available from: http://www.worldwidewounds.com/2015/August/Galea/wounds-galea.html.

50. Berman B, Amini S, Viera MH, Maderal AD. Silicone gel sheeting for preventing the development of hypertrophic and keloid scars and for treating existing hypertrophic and keloid scars. [Internet]. [Cited 2016 Oct 6]. Available from: http://www.cochrane.org/CD003826/WOUNDS_silicone-gel-sheeting-for-preventing-the-development-of-hypertrophic-and-keloid-scars-and-for-treating-existing-hypertrophic-and-keloid-scars. Accessed 2016 Oct 6.

51. Banerjee J, Ghatak P, Roy S, Khanna S, Sequin EK, Bellman K, Dickinson BC, Suri P, Subramaniam V, Chang CJ, Sen CK. Improvement of human keratinocyte migration by a redox active bioelectric dressing

52. http://procellera.com/procellera/technology [Cited 2016 Oct 23].

53. Steadmed. http://www.steadmed.com/ [Cited 2016 Oct 23].

54. https://www.medline.com/product/XCell-Wound-Dressings/Synthetic-Dressings/Z05-PF00210?question=xcell&index=P1&indexCount=1. [Cited 2016 Oct 23].

55. http://www.enluxtrawoundcare.com/ [Cited 2016 Oct 23].

56. Clean vs. sterile dressing technique for management of chronic wounds: a fact sheet. Journal of Wound, Ostomy & Continence Nursing. March/April 2012;39(25):S30-S34.

57. Local coverage determination (LCD): surgical dressings (L11460) [Internet]. [Cited 2016 Oct 31]. Available from: https://med.noridianmedicare.com/documents/2230715/2240927/surgical_dressings_lcd_2-4-11_-_10-31-13.pdf/1388f56b-f138-478b-836c-69af9348f3c7.

58. Cowan MK, Talaro KP. Infectious diseases affecting the skin and eyes. Microbiology: A Systems Approach. New York: McGraw-Hill; 2006:89-118.

59. Wolcott R, Rumbaugh K, James G, Schultz G, Phillips P, Yang Q, et al. Biofilm maturity studies indicate sharp debridement opens a time-dependent therapeutic window. J Wound Care. 2010;19(8):320–328.

60. Lavery LA, Davis KE. Berriman SJ, Braun L, Nichols A, Kim PJ, Margolis D, Peters EJ, Attinger C. WHS guidelines update: diabetic foot ulcer treatment guidelines. Wound Rep and Reg, 24:112–126. DOI: 10.1111/wrr.12391

61. Robson MC, Cooper DM, Aslam R, Gould LJ, Harding, KG, Margolis DJ, Ochs DE, Serena TE, Snyder RJ, Steed DL, Thomas DR, Wiersma-Bryant L. Guidelines for the treatment of venous ulcers. Wound Repair and Regeneration. 2006;14:649–662. DOI: 10.1111/j.1524-475X.2006.00174.x

62. Weir D, Schultz G. Assessment and management wound-related infections. In: Doughty DB, McNichol LL, editors. WOCN Core Curriculum: Wound Management. Philadelphia: Wolters Kluwer; 2015.

63. Maillard JY, Denyer SP. Focus on silver. EWMA Journal 2006;6:5-7.

64. Drosou A, Falabella A, Kirsner RS. Antiseptics on wounds: an area of controversy. Wounds 2003; 15.

65. Atiyeh BS, Dibo SA, Hayek SN. Wound cleansing, topical antiseptics and wound healing. Int Wound J 2009;6:420-430.

66. Fernandez R, Griffiths R, Ussia C. Water for wound cleansing. Art. No.: CD003861. 2008. Cochrane Database of Systematic Reviews.

67. Mcguiness W, Vella E, Harrison D. Influence of dressing changes on wound temperature. J Wound Care; 13:383-385.

68. Watret L, McClean A. Cleansing diabetic foot wounds: tap water or saline? Wounds International 2014; 5:1-5.

69. International Consensus Group. Appropriate use of silver dressings in wounds. An expert working group consensus. Wounds International 2012.

70. Lipsky BA, Hoey C. Topical antimicrobial therapy for treating chronic wounds. Clin Infect Dis 2009;49(10): 1541-1549.

71. Maillard JY, Denyer SP. Focus on silver. EWMA Journal 2006;6:5-7.

72. White RJ, Cutting KF. Critical colonization—the concept under scrutiny. Ostomy Wound Management 2006;52:50-6.

73. Cutting K, White R, Hoekstra H. Topical silver-impregnated dressings and the importance of the dressing technology. Int Wound J 2009;6(5):396-402.

74. An expert working group consensus. International Consensus. Appropriate use of silver dressings in wounds. An expert working group consensus. London: Wounds International, 2012.

75. Hamm R. Antibacterial dressings. In: Sen C, editor. Advances in Wound Care. New Rochelle, NY: Mary Ann Liebert, Inc.; 2010; p. 148-154.

76. Fong J, Wood F. Nanocrystalline silver dressings in wound management: a review. Int J Nanomedicine 2006;1(4):441-449.

77. Percival SL, Woods E, Nutekpor M, et al. Prevalence of silver resistance in bacteria isolated from diabetic foot ulcers and efficacy of solver-containing wound dressings. Ostomy Wound Manage. 2008;54:30-40

78. White R, Cutting K. Exploring the effects of silver in wound management—what is optimal? Wounds. 2006;18:307-314.

79. Cooper ML, Laxer JA, Hansbrough JF. The cytotoxic effects of commonly used topical antimicrobial agents on human fibroblasts and keratinocytes. J Trauma. 1991;31:775-782.

80. Lineaweaver W, Howard R, Soucy D et al. Topical antimicrobial toxicity. Arch Surg. 1985;120:267-270.

81. Lineaweaver W, McMorris S, Soucy D et al. Cellular and bacterial toxicities of topical antimicrobials. Plast Reconstr Surg. 1985;75:394-396.

82. Akiyama H, Oono T, Saito M et al. Assessment of cadexomer iodine against Staphylococcus aureus biofilm in vivo and in vitro using confocal laser scanning microscopy. J Dermatol. 2004;31:529-534.

83. http://www.woundsource.com/product/iodofoam [Cited 2016 Aug 28]. 84. Hage JJ et al. Honey-medicated dressing: transformation of an ancient remedy into modern therapy. Ann Plast Surg. 2003;50:143-148.

85. Pieper B. Honey-based dressings and wound care: an option for care in the United States. J Wound Ostomy Continence Nurs. 2009;36(1):60-66.

86. Eddy JJ, Gideonsen MD. Topical honey for diabetic foot ulcers (observations from practice). J Fam Pract. 2005;54:533-535.

87. Dunford C, Cooper R, Molan P et al. The use of honey in wound management. Nurs Stand. 2000; 15:63-.

88. Namias N. Honey in the management of infections. Surg Infect. 2003;4:219-226.8789.

88a. Molan PC. Potential of honey in the treatment of wounds and burns. Am J Clin Dermatol. 2001;2:13-19.

89. Lusby PE, Coombs A, Wilkinson JM. Honey: a potent agent for wound healing? J Wound Ostomy Continence Nurs. 2002;<AU31>:295-300.

90. Mulder GD, Cavorsi JP, Lee DK. Polyhexamethylene biguanide (PHMB): an addendum to current topical antimicrobials. Wounds. 2007;19:173-82.

91. Moore K, Gray D. Using PHMB antimicrobial to prevent wound infection. Wounds UK. 2007;3:96-102.

92. Cuttino C et al. Balancing a dynamic wound environment: multicenter experience with a novel antimicrobial foam dressing containing PHMB. Ostomy Wound Manage. 2009 March (suppl).

93. Cassinga A, Serralta V, Davis S, Orr R, Eaglstein W, Mertz PM. The effect of antimicrobial gauze dressing impregnated with 0.2-percent polyhexamethylene biguanide as a barrier to prevent Pseudomonas aeruginosa wound invasion. Wounds. 2010;14:169-176.

94. Barrett S, Battacharyya M, Butcher M, Enoch S, Fumarola S, Gray D. PHMB and its potential contribution to wound management. Wounds UK. 2010.

95. Butcher M. PHMB: an effective antimicrobial in wound bioburden management. British Journal Nursing. 2012;21:s16-s21.

96. https://labtestsonline.org/understanding/analytes/gram-stain/tab/test/ [Cited 2016 Oct 2].

97. Sibbald R, Ovington L, Goodman L, et al. Wound bed preparation 2014 update: management of critical colonization with a gentian violet and methylene blue absorbent antibacterial dressing and elevated levels of matrix metalloproteases with an ovine collagen extracellular matrix dressing. Advances in Skin and Wound Care: The International Journal of Prevention and Healing 3. Suppl 1 27 (2014):1-6.

98. Weir D, Blakely M. Case review of the clinical use of an antimicrobial PVA foam dressing. Poster Presentation: Clinical Symposium for Advances in Skin and Wound Care. September 9-11, 2011; Washington, D.C. Available from: www.hollisterwoundcare.com/files/pdfs/posters/HWC%20Weir%20Hydrofera%20Blue%20Poster.pdf

99. Doyle RJ. Contribution of the hydrophobic effect to microbial infection Microbes Infect. 2000 Apr; 2(4): 391-400.

100. Butcher M. Catch or kill. How DACC technology redefines antimicrobial management. Br J Comm Nurs .2011; supplement.

101. Ljungh A, Yanagisawa N, Wadström T. Using the principle of hydrophobic interaction to bind and remove wound bacteria. J Wound Care. 2006;15(4):175-180.

Chapter 8

EVIDENCE-BASED USE OF ADVANCED WOUND CARE MODALITIES IN CHRONIC WOUND PATIENTS

Jayesh B. Shah, MD
Caroline E. Fife, MD

KEY CONCEPTS

1. Advanced modalities range from cellular and/or tissue-based products to therapeutic procedures requiring specialized equipment.
2. Advanced therapeutics should not be provided in the absence of standard care interventions.
3. Advanced modalities are recommended with standard of care (SOC), if progress in healing is not made within 30 days for venous leg ulcers (VLUs) and diabetic foot ulcers (DFUs).

CONTENTS

Introduction

In recent years, there have been so many significant advances in the field of wound care that some terminologies in wound care treatment can be confusing. In this chapter, we will consider any product that is covered under Medicare's Surgical Dressing Policy to be a dressing, even though many of these products are highly sophisticated biomaterials. The more sophisticated materials are often referred to as "advanced dressings" (e.g. collagen) but they are not to be confused with advanced therapeutics or modalities.

Advanced wound care modalities have the potential to overcome specific barriers to healing, allowing this complex process to proceed along a more normal trajectory, thereby reducing the risk of infection and other serious complications.[1] Moreover, if used appropriately, advanced therapies can decrease the long-term costs associated with the care of chronic wounds.[1] Advanced modalities range from cellular and/or tissue-based products to therapeutic procedures requiring specialized equipment. This chapter attempts to review selected new advanced wound care modalities. Due to the number and rapid increase of both advanced dressings and advanced therapeutics, it is not possible to provide an exhaustive review. We have selected examples and included a few brand names for ease of identification since the generic classification of these materials is still under development. We have generally selected the earliest product marketed within a particular category but in no way wish to imply that the products we name are superior in any way to other currently available brands.

The Centers for Medicare and Medicaid Services (CMS) classify surgical and traumatic lesions as wounds, using the term ulcers to refer to lesions related to an underlying medical condition (e.g. diabetes). The terms "wound" and "ulcer" have important and distinct reimbursement implications. Although there is no English term that encompasses both concepts, we will use the term wound in its commonly understood meaning unless otherwise stated.

Given the rate at which new advanced therapeutics enter the market, it is inevitable that any textbook covering them will be obsolete by the time it is in print. It is also likely that entirely new categories of devices and drugs for wound healing that did not exist when this chapter was written will enter the market. The goal for the wound care clinician is to identify the barrier(s) to healing that any given therapy is meant to help overcome, and then utilize it when it makes sense in a particular patient. Unfortunately, when patients fail to make progress with wound healing, therapeutics may be selected via a process that more closely resembles "wheel of fortune" than a thoughtful analysis of the barriers to healing.

The other challenge for wound care clinicians will be to make the transition from volume to value in the use of advanced therapeutics. Currently, it can be argued that the ideal advanced therapeutic is the one that only works marginally well. If there were a product that could heal a wound on the first application, the current health-care system is not designed to encourage its use. However, as the outpatient payment system makes the shift to episode-based payment or a system that resembles outpatient diagnosis related groups, clinicians will be highly motivated to identify the most effective treatments at the lowest cost. This will likely result in increased use of modalities such as total contact casting, which is highly effective and low cost, but time-consuming to apply and poorly reimbursed currently. There will likely be fewer cellular product applications overall and a shift to products that providers have found to be the most effective with the fewest applications.

Similarly, providers will determine the fewest number of hyperbaric oxygen therapy treatments required to achieve a given outcome. It is unfortunate that for maladies as expensive as chronic wounds, no independent research funding exists to perform comparative effectiveness studies among the various cellular products, or indeed to identify the effectiveness of any of these products in real world patients, as opposed to the relatively healthy subjects enrolled in randomized, controlled trials. We are on the cusp of dramatic changes, which will certainly alter the way we utilize advanced therapeutics.

I. Case study

A 68-year-old male with a history of type 2 diabetes mellitus (DM), peripheral vascular disease (PVD), coronary artery disease (CAD), and diabetic retinopathy, presents to the wound care center with a necrotic wound on left medial ankle (Figure 1), which started as a blister in December.

Prior to the patient's visit to our wound care center, he was admitted for nine days at the University Hospital, where he was treated with antibiotics. The patient also had surgical debridement and vascular evaluation. He was recommended to undergo a below-knee amputation as he was found to have severe small vessel arterial disease not amenable to revascularization. When he refused amputation, he was discharged home under the care of his daughter along with skilled home nursing services.

His primary care physician referred him in February to the wound care center, where he underwent a second opinion by a vascular surgeon who confirmed that there were no revascularization options. Transcutaneous oximetry showed hypoxia with a good response to 100% oxygen, and an MRI was positive for osteomyelitis of the left medial malleolus. He underwent debridement of the osteomyelitic bone and Graftjacket placement by a podiatrist in the operating room (Figure 2). He was also started on intravenous (IV) antibiotics for six weeks and on HBO_2 therapy. At the next follow-up appointment, he showed failure of Graftjacket (Figure 3). His wound was not improving in spite of all advanced wound treatments, so he was once again recommended for below-knee amputation. The patient continued to refuse amputation.

A second opinion from a plastic surgeon was obtained. The plastic surgeon did a wide debridement of the wound with Integra placement (Figure 8.4). The patient also was started on negative pressure wound therapy and subsequently received a split thickness skin graft (STSG) (Figure 5) for wound closure while completing a total of 40 HBO_2 treatments. He had partial take of STSG (Figure 6) and continued to have a nonhealing wound (Figure 7). As he had refused below-knee amputation, he was placed on palliative wound care (Figure 8, Figure 9), which included local use of topical antibiotics daily and suppressive oral antibiotics as per ID specialist. The patient's wound completely healed after 14 months (Figure 10).

This case study addresses the use of multiple advanced wound modalities including more than one cellular based therapy, NPWT, and hyperbaric oxygen therapy, in addition to revascularization and IV antibiotics. Although this patient's wound completely healed after 14 months, the question that needs to be addressed is what is the evidence for using multiple advanced modalities? What is the cost benefit of multiple advanced modalities and continued care over long periods of time (e.g. years) for limb salvage? If the patient remains ambulatory and living independently, can we justify the cost?

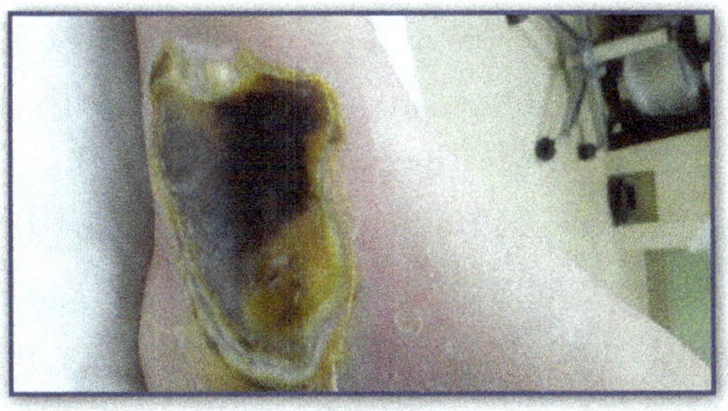

FIGURE 1.
68-year-old male with type 2 DM and history of CAD, PVD, and diabetic retinopathy presents to the wound care center with a necrotic wound on left medial ankle.

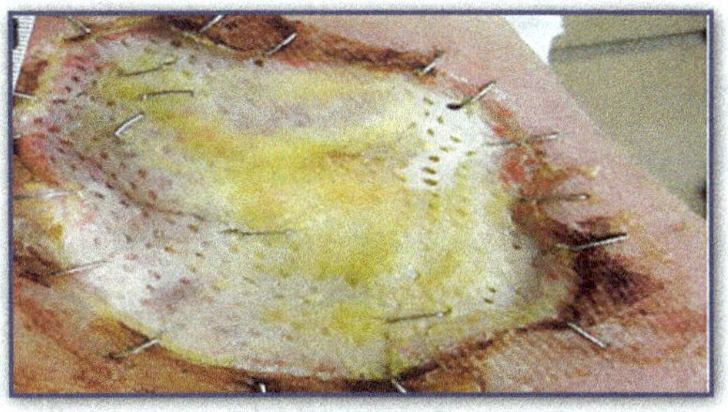

FIGURE 2.
Surgical debridement and application of Graftjacket

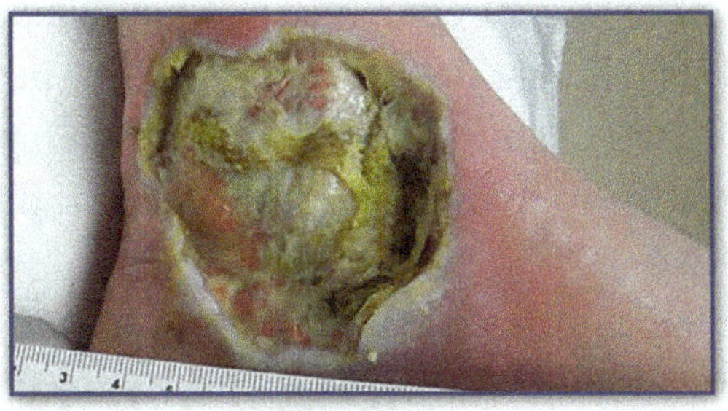

FIGURE 3.
Debridement was repeated as Graftjacket failed.

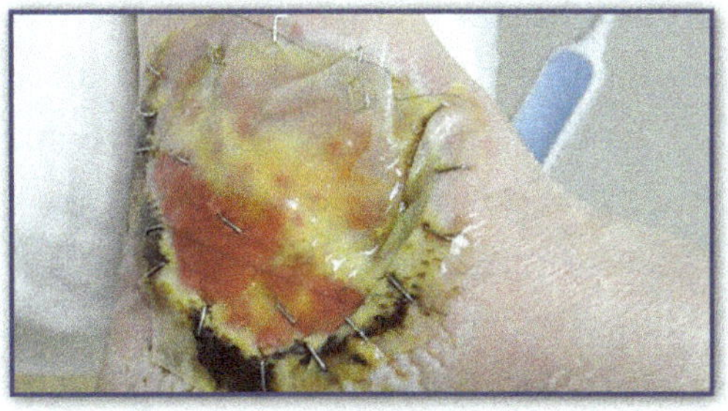

FIGURE 4.
Debridement and Integra placement

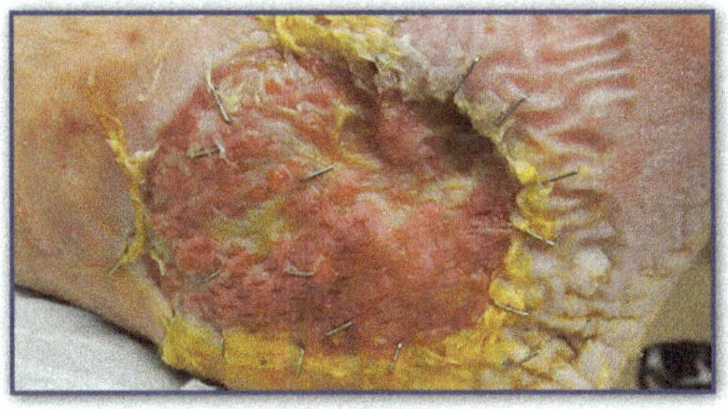

FIGURE 5.
Split thickness skin graft

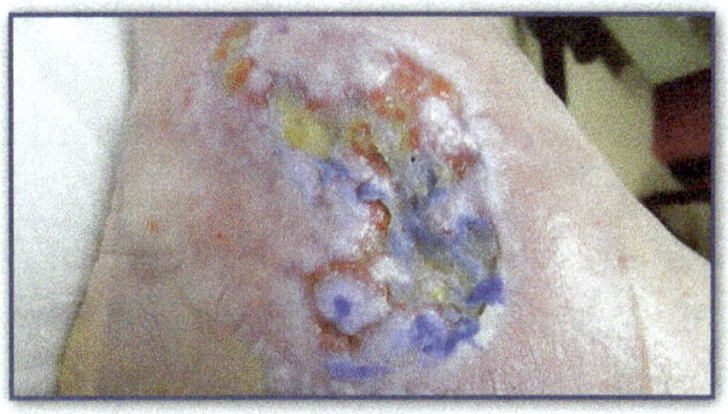

FIGURE 6.
Partial take of STSG - started on Hydrofera Blue

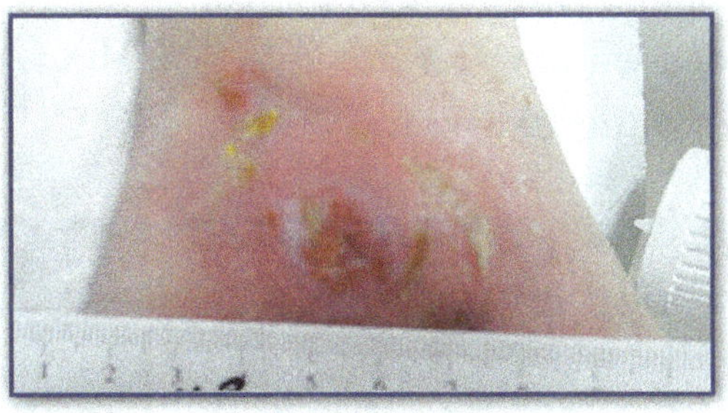

FIGURE 7.
Started on enzymatic debridement with Santyl and Hydrofera Blue

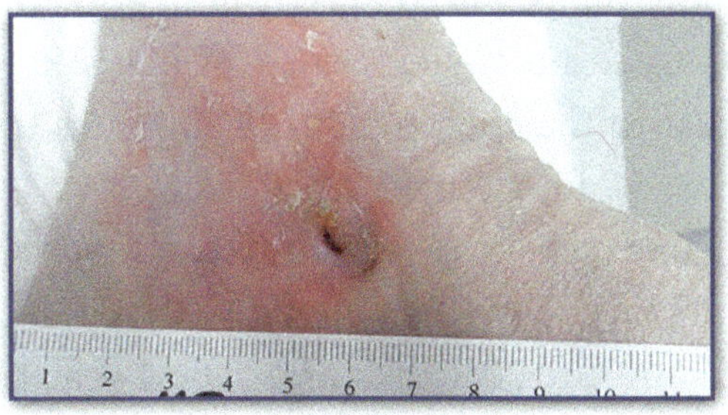

FIGURE 8.
Started on Bactroban daily

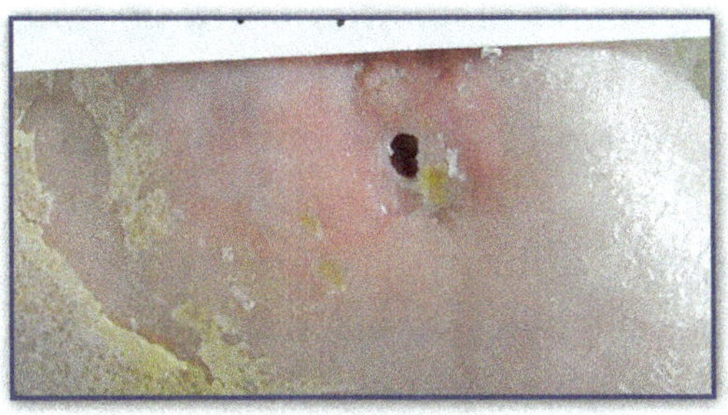

FIGURE 9.
Started on Bactroban daily

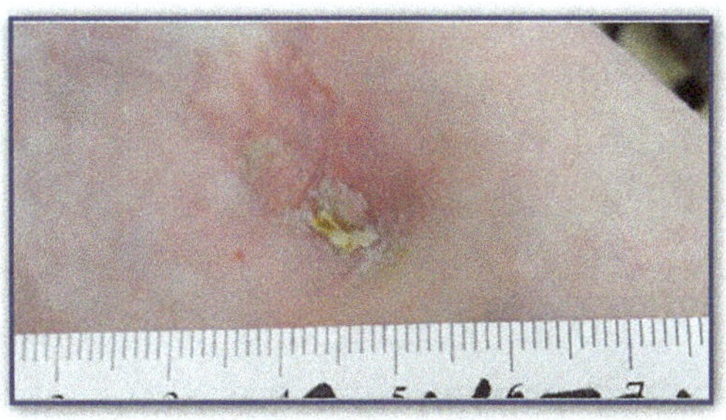

FIGURE 10.
Wound healed

II. When to use advanced wound modalities

There are differing opinions regarding when to use advanced wound modalities. Many believe that advanced wound modalities should only be used when a wound fails to heal with standard wound management over some period of time, while some believe that advanced therapies should be used immediately on wounds that are identified to be potentially difficult to heal.[2-6] Most insurance carriers have specific guidelines that govern when they will allow use of advanced wound modalities.

While standard of care (SOC) plays an important role in wound healing, standard care alone may be sufficient for only a small percentage of patients with hard-to-heal wounds.[7] Falanga and Sabolinski reported that only 20-40% of ulcers heal with standard compression therapy in venous stasis ulcer[8-9] while Cochrane review by O'Meara et al. found that only 30-75% of venous ulcers heal with standard compression therapy.[10] A meta-analysis by Margolis et al. revealed that less than 30% of the individuals with a DFU will heal within 20 weeks of commencing SOC.[11] This is in stark contrast to the spectacular healing rates touted by most wound centers on their websites, routinely in excess of 95%. Margolis also looked at prognostic factors associated with DFU healing failure for 20 weeks and found that ulcers greater than 2cm^2 had 47% likelihood of nonhealing. Ulcers with duration of more than two months have 45% likelihood of nonhealing. Patients with Wagner grade greater than 2 had 54% likelihood of nonhealing.[12] He also concluded that if a patient had ulcers with two of the above risk factors, then there was 62-70% likelihood of nonhealing and if all three risk factors were present, there was 81% likelihood of nonhealing.[12] The healing rates for VLUs range from 30-60% at 24 weeks and 70-85% by year one.[13-14] Sheehan concluded in his DFU trial that wounds that achieved less than 53% closure at week 4 have minimal chance of healing with conventional therapy in 12 weeks.[2]. The field of wound care would be better served if clinicians and clinics stopped reporting unrealistically high healing rates in their marketing materials and developed an honest system of outcome reporting. It is possible, if not likely, that a significant percentage of patients will require some type of advanced therapeutic modality to achieve complete healing if there is less than 50% of healing with standard wound management at four weeks.[2-3] Consensus statement of the American Diabetes Association[15] stated that any wound that remains unhealed after four weeks is cause for concern, as it is associated with worse outcomes, including amputation. Patients with unresolved ulcers are at risk of cellulitis, osteomyelitis and amputation, creating a cost-effective argument for advanced therapies in part based on avoidance of complications as well as a reduction in prolonged courses of ineffective treatments.

Adjunctive advanced modalities are recommended with SOC if progress in healing is not made within 30 days for VLUs and DFUs.[3,5-6]

III. Use of advanced wound modalities according to phases of wound healing

Case study depicting appropriate use of advanced wound modalities based on phases of wound healing.

The patient is a 74-year-old woman with poorly controlled, insulin-dependent diabetes, and rheumatoid arthritis on prednisone who developed an enlarging leg ulcer after minor trauma from hitting her leg on a coffee table (Figure 11). The wound had been present more than nine

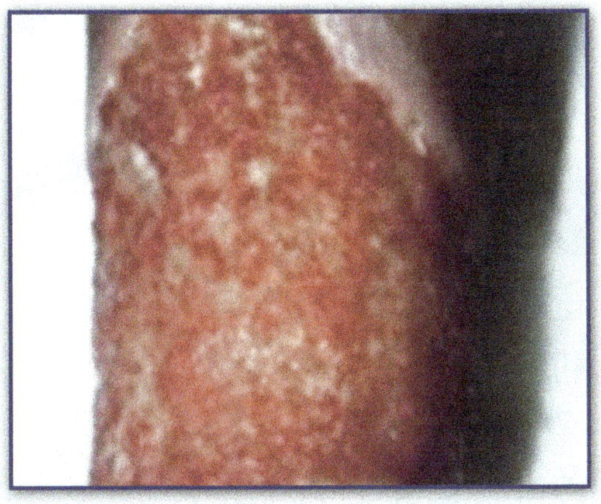

FIGURE 11. Leg ulcer not healing, secondary to diabetes and rheumatoid arthritis started because of trauma. Treated with debridement and topical antimicrobial dressings.

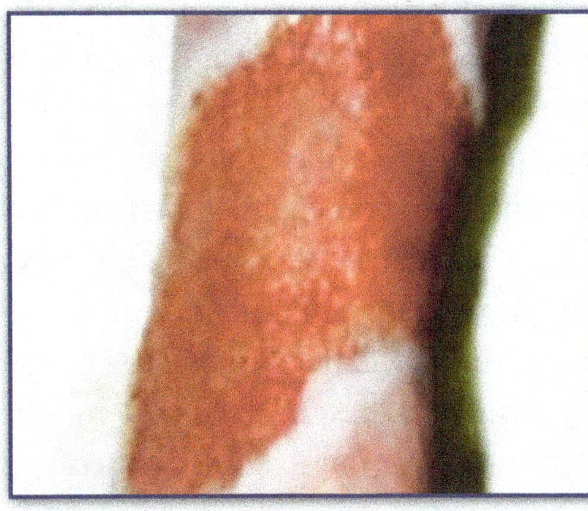

FIGURE 12. Leg ulcer after treatment with negative pressure therapy

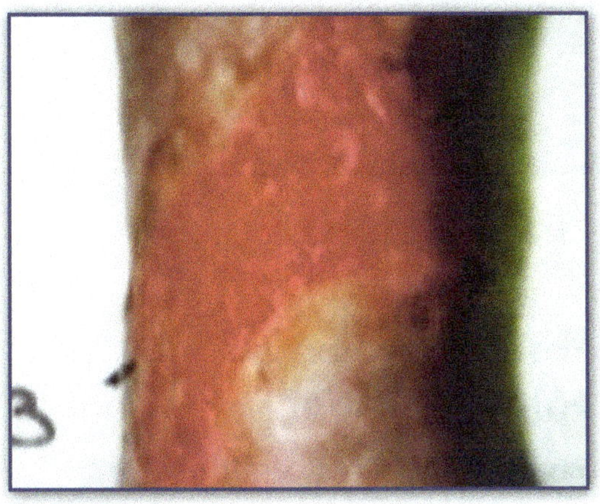

FIGURE 13. After wound bed preparation, wound ready for cellular based therapy.

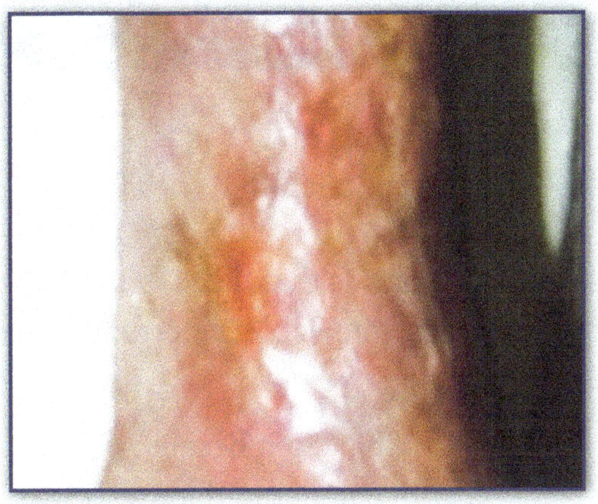

FIGURE 14. Wound epithelialized

months when she presented to the wound center. The biofilm was removed with debridement and topical antimicrobial dressings to control the inflammatory response, after which she underwent treatment with negative pressure wound therapy (NPWT) to facilitate vascular response (Figure 12). When the wound bed was completely granulated, she was treated with a cellular-based therapy to help facilitate cellular proliferation and epithelial migration (Figure 13). The wound closed completely with these interventions (Figure 14). This case exhibits the concept of selecting the advanced therapeutic that is needed to address the specific barrier to healing, which may be out-of-control inflammation or lack of vascular or cellular proliferation.

This case also exhibits an unfortunate reality regarding advanced therapeutics. The patients who most need these advanced treatments are the ones for whom payers may specifically decide not to cover treatment. Many Medicare administrative carriers (MACs) craft coverage policies for cellular products (for example) that mirror the prospective randomized, controlled trials (RCTs). Nearly all cellular product RCTs have excluded patients with autoimmune disease, on steroids, or with out-of-control diabetes. As a result, payers often deny the use of these products to the patients who most need them, using the irrefutable logic that the manufacturers have not demonstrated their effectiveness in such compromised hosts. This

Kafkaesque situation will likely only be rectified when the U.S. Food and Drug Administration allows real world data (RWD) to be used to supplement prospective trial data. It is vital that future studies of advanced therapeutics be more generalizable because as payment reform moves outpatient payment to bundled models or episodes of care, we will need to understand which products work the best in the fewest number of applications and in the sickest of patients.

IV. Phases of wound healing and recommended advanced wound modalities [16]

A. Vascular phase

1. Clotting phase
   a) For wounds that bleed excessively because of friable hypergranulation tissue
   b) Wound bleeding because patient is on anticoagulants (Figures 15, 16)
   c) Kaolin dressings
   d) Cellulose
   e) Calcium alginate
2. Vascular response
   a) Hyperbaric oxygen therapy
   b) Negative pressure wound therapy
   c) Platelet-rich plasma
   d) Collagen dressings (only used after granulation seen on wound)
   e) platelet-derived growth factor

B. Inflammatory phase

1. Debridement
2. Antimicrobial dressings (biofilm control)
3. Certain dressings that modulate MMPs
4. Antimicrobial dressings (biofilm control)
5. Anti-biofilm agents
6. Negative pressure wound therapy
7. Hyperbaric oxygen therapy

C. Proliferative phase and epithelialization

1. Epidermal bubble grafting
2. Collagen dressings
3. Regranex
4. Cellular and tissue based products
5. Hyperbaric oxygen therapy

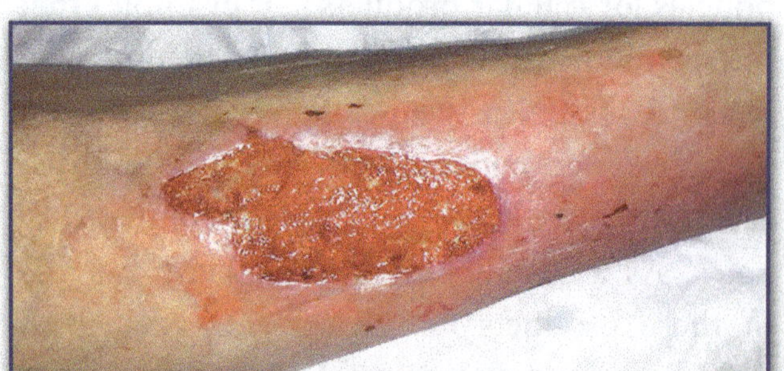

FIGURE 15. Bloody drainage from leg ulcer in a patient on anticoagulants

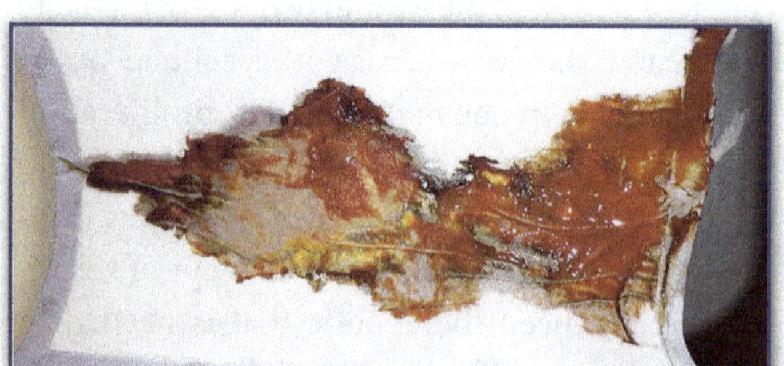

FIGURE 16. Bloody drainage from leg ulcer - dressing removed from patient who is on anticoagulants

V. Advanced wound modalities

A. Platelet-derived growth factors

Platelet-derived growth factor-BB

Growth factors are proteins that are primarily found in platelets and macrophages.[17-18] There are various types of growth factors, including epidermal growth factor (EGF), transforming growth factors (TGF), fibroblast growth factor (FGF), and vascular endothelial growth factors (VEGF).

The first FDA-approved recombinant human growth factor was REGRANEX Gel (becaplermin) 0.01% (rhPDGF-BB). It is synthesized by recombinant biotechnology using yeast cells genetically engineered to secrete rhPDGF-BB into medium. Prescription form that is available is active rhPDGF-BB.[17-19]

Mechanism of action

Platelet-derived growth factor works by the following mechanism:

- Activates endothelial cells and fibroblasts [19-21]
- Stimulates vascular proliferation, migration, and new blood vessel formation[19-21]
- Recruits smooth muscle cells and pericytes to stabilize newly formed vessels[19-21]

Indications

rhPDGF-BB (Regranex or Becalpermin) gel is indicated for the treatment of lower-extremity diabetic neuropathic ulcers that extend into the subcutaneous tissue or beyond and have an adequate blood supply.[19]

It is not indicated in wounds with exposed joint, tendon, or bone due to the limitations in the prospective trials.[19] (Clinical trials did not include any patients with wounds more severe than Wagner 1 and thus it is not recommended for use over bone and tendon; however, the mechanism of action of PDGF is not limited to superficial tissues.)

Evidence-based use

Review by Cochrane database shows that limited use of growth factor may help in healing of DFU.[22]

Contraindications[23]

i) Patients with known hypersensitivity to any component of the product

ii) Malignant wounds

iii) Black box warning for Regranex: Increased risk of cancer mortality in patients who use three or more tubes of the product[16]

Case study (Figures 17-19)

This 43-year-old black male developed full thickness tissue necrosis over the dorsal foot, probably due to necrobiosis lipoidica diabeticorum. His vascular supply was found to be reasonably good. After debridement he had exposed tendons. He was treated with becaplermin and completely closed the wound despite the exposure of nearly all the tendons of the foot. (Editor's note: Regranex is not clinically indicated for use on exposed tendons because, as is the case for nearly all prospective DFU trials, only relatively superficial ulcers were enrolled in the original trials. Nevertheless, as discussed in earlier chapters, PDGF plays a part in angiogenesis as well as epithelialization.)

B. Platelet-rich plasma

Platelet gels or releasates are prepared at the point of care for the patient. Platelet-rich plasma (PRP) is obtained by differential centrifugation of whole blood. Other components that are added to platelet-rich plasma are calcium gluconate, thrombin, and batroxobin.[17,24]

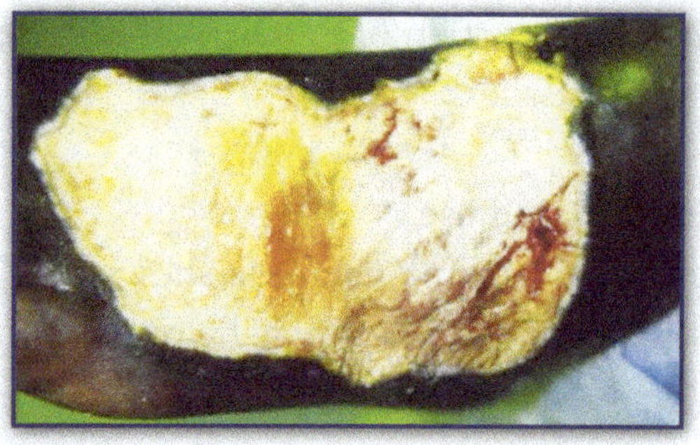

FIGURE 17. Necrobiosis lipoidica diabeticorum ulcer on foot s/q to debridement. Patient started on HBO_2 therapy.

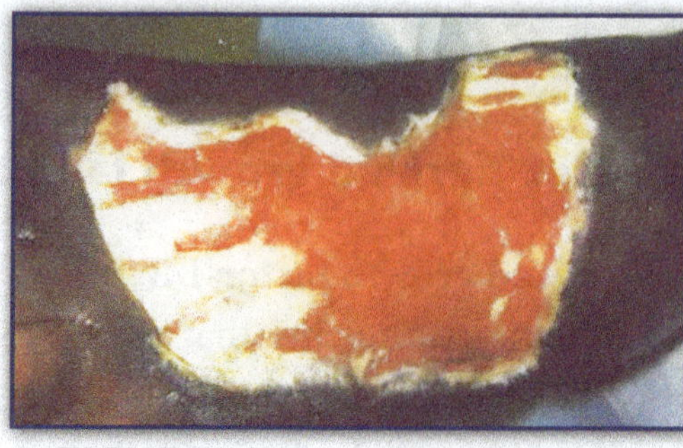

FIGURE 18. Foot ulcer s/q further debridement, foot ulcer with exposed tendons started on Regranex and continued on HBO_2 therapy.

Mechanism of action

Platelet-rich plasma has a plethora of growth factors (PDGF, VEGF, EGF, IGF-1, TGF-B), which induce signal transduction pathway that in turn regulates tissue regeneration cascade.[17,24]

Evidence-based use

Cochrane database concludes that PRP may improve healing of DFU-based on limited low-quality evidence from two small RCTs. Evidence is limited for healing in other types of wounds.[25]

Indications

Acute and chronic wounds of all etiology

Contraindications

Absolute contraindications

- Platelet dysfunction syndrome
- Critical thrombocytopenia
- Hemodynamic instability
- Septicemia
- Local infection at the site of the procedure

Relative Contraindications

- Consistent use of NSAIDs within 48 hours of procedure
- Systemic use of corticosteroids within two weeks

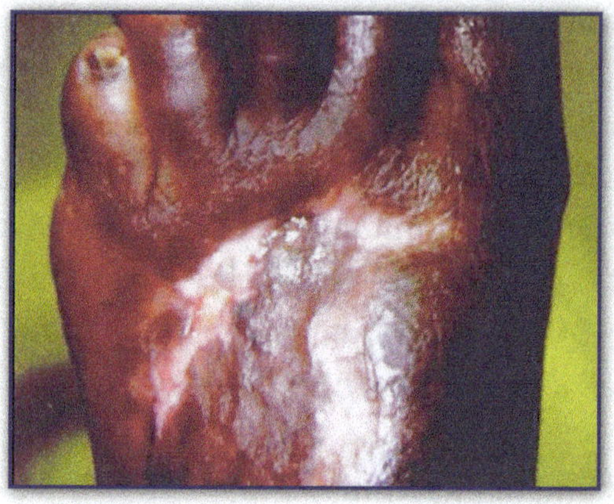

FIGURE 19. Wound epithelialized

- Tobacco use
- Recent fever or illness
- Cancer – especially hematopoietic or of bone
- HGB < 10 g/dl
- Platelet count < 105/ul

Case study (Figures 20-23)

A 73-year-old Caucasian male became a tetraplegic after a spinal cord infarction three years prior. He had multiple large pressure ulcers over the sacrum, ischium, hips, and heels. He was status post multiple hospitalizations, IV antibiotics, and topical wound dressings, as well as a diverting colostomy and suprapubic catheter. His nutrition was marginal, as he previously had lost weight, but with a normal albumin. He met criteria for enrollment in the Cytomedix pressure ulcer protocol CM001 under Coverage with Evidence Development (CED), and the sacral pressure ulcer, which had been present for one year, was enrolled in the trial. After two applications of Autologel (now called Aurix), the study was discontinued by the sponsor (now Nuo Therapeutics). However, the sponsor donated (at no charge to the patient) the kits he would have received had the trial continued. Donation of kits was the only option because, with that study closed, the CED process could not continue, and thus there was no mechanism by which to bill Medicare for the treatments. As a result, no data were collected for the purpose of the trial. He received 20 treatments over 24 weeks with almost complete closure of a sacral pressure that had been present without improvement for at least a year prior to treatment.

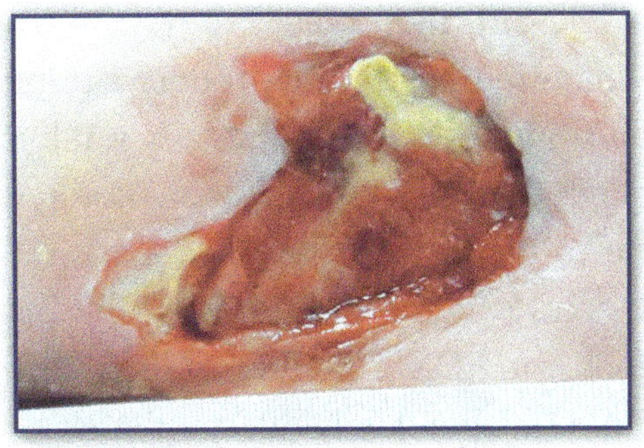

FIGURE 20. Stage 4 sacral pressure ulcer not healing for more than one year in patient with spinal cord injury and quadriplegia s/q to debridement started on platelet-rich plasma.

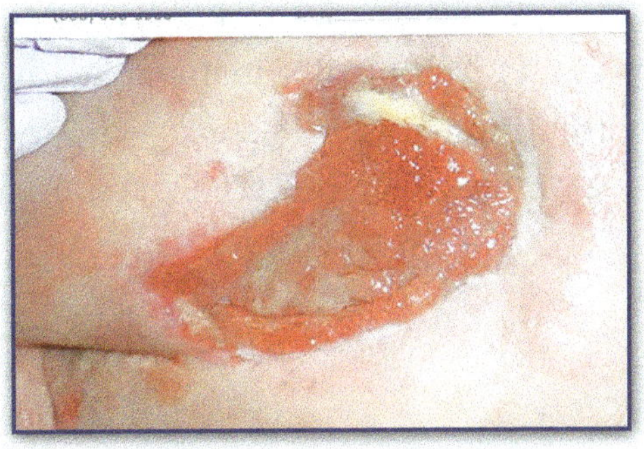

FIGURE 21. Sacral wound improving on platelet-rich plasma

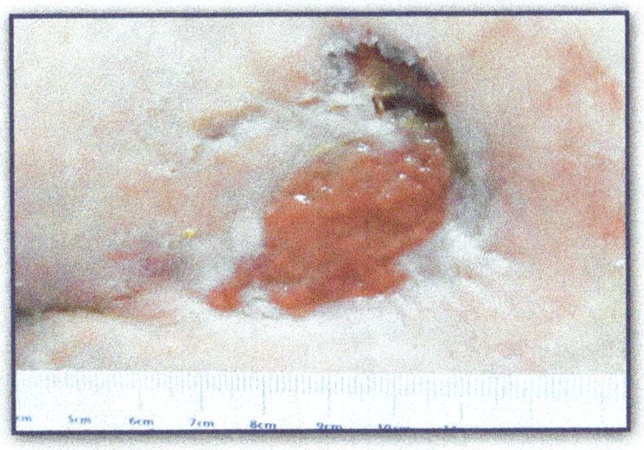

FIGURE 22. Wound with increased granulation tissue s/q to application of platelet-rich plasma

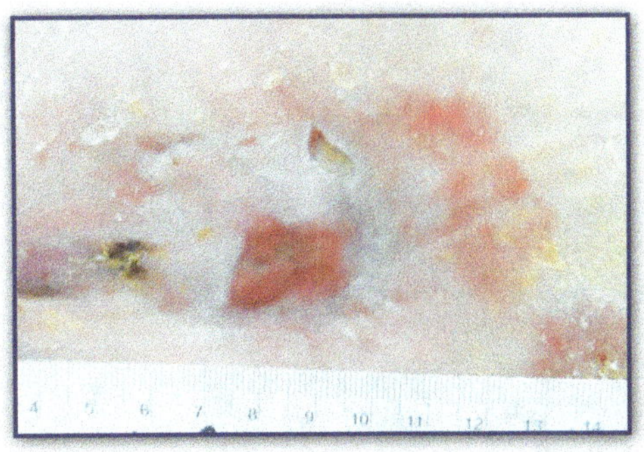

FIGURE 23. Sacral wound improving with platelet-rich plasma application

C. Cellular and tissue-based products (CTPs)

The terminology for these products is confusing. The same product may be referred to by any of the following terms: cellular wound dressing, interactive or biologically active wound dressing, cellular interactive wound dressing, biologic wound covering, allogeneic graft, human skin equivalent, engineered and bioengineered skin substitute, or cell-based therapeutic.[26] If the product contains living, allogeneic (same species) cells, then it is considered a human cell and it is regulated by the FDA Center for Biologics Evaluation and Research (CBER) Division of Cellular and Gene Therapies. If its mode of action is growth factors, then it is considered a biological CTP and is also regulated by CBER. If it is a physical material that interacts with tissue, it is a device and it is regulated by the Center for Devices and Radiological Health (CDRH). The Food and Drug Administration (FDA) continues to use the term human cells, tissues, and cellular and tissue-based products (HCT/Ps) for these diverse products; however, the term now accepted by the American Society for Testing Materials (ASTM) is cellular and/or tissue-based products (CTPs). While these regulatory pathways are complex and may seem irrelevant, they affect the type of research that is required before the product can be used clinically. Some products that lack randomized, controlled trial (RCT) data were not required to perform these studies prior to marketing due to the nature of the product and the pathway they took for FDA clearance.[26] Ironically, this may quite independently affect whether a payer decides to reimburse for the use of a product, since the ability to legally use a product does not mean that a payer will cover it.

The FDA sub-classifies HCT/Ps into three categories: 1) minimally manipulated/homologous use (human skin tissue such as Theraskin); 2) more than minimally manipulated/non-homologous use (e.g. Dermagraft or Apligraf); and 3) xenogeneic tissue (animal/non-human tissue, e.g. Oasis and Primatrix).

Mechanism of action

HCT/Ps have variable structure and cellular content. Some skin substitutes are cellular and some are acellular, but both induce influx of endogenous cells including fibroblasts, endothelial cells, macrophages, keratinocytes, and neutrophils into the wound bed.[27-29]

HCT/Ps function as sterile tissue grafts that are applied after wound bed preparation directly to the wound bed. After application, HCT/Ps integrate with the surrounding native tissues and stimulate angiogenesis, cell migration, and

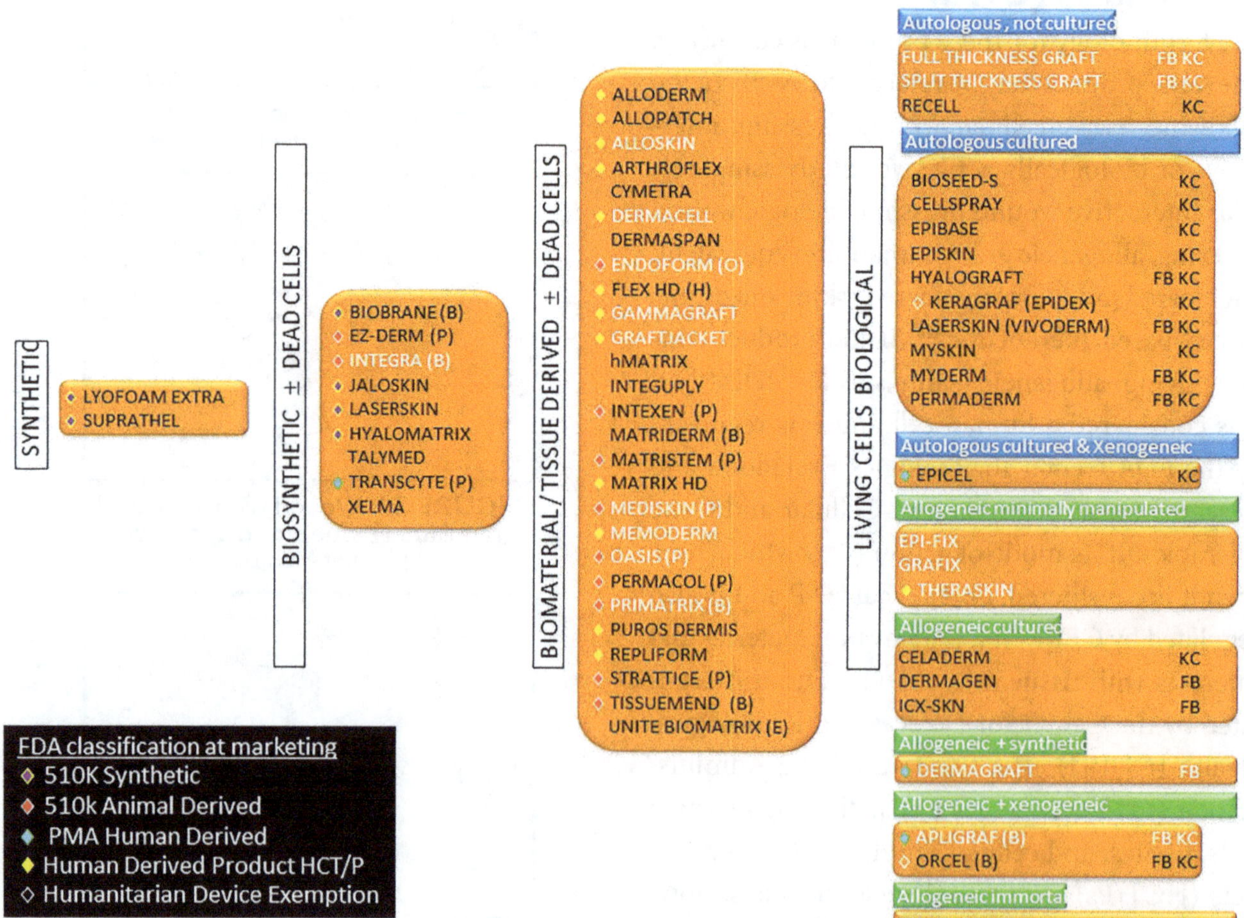

FIGURE 24.
Commonly used CTPs - Courtesy of Bert Slade, MD

epithelialization, resulting in accelerated wound healing.[27-29] HCT/Ps are slowly broken down and are replaced by native tissues to achieve complete reepithelialization.[27-29] HCT/Ps secrete a variety of cytokines and growth factors, which may alter the microenvironment of the wound and help with healing.[27-29]

Characteristics of Ideal HCT/Ps[17,27]

- Be able to develop rapid sustained adherence to wound surface
- Allow water vapor transmission
- Resist friction and shear stresses
- Prevent proliferation of bacteria
- Contain low antigenicity
- Be free of local and systemic toxicity

Kinds of HCT/Ps

- Biosynthetic
- Biomaterial
- Biological
  1) Autologous
  2) Allogeneic

Things to remember before application of skin replacement tissue:[17]

- Topical agents are safe to use with bioengineered tissue.
- Many antibiotic ointments are safe for use prior to application of bioengineered tissue. These prescriptions include, but are not limited to:

  1) Bacitracin zinc
  2) Gentamicin sulfate
  3) Neomycin sulfate
  4) Bactroban
  5) Silver sulfadiazine

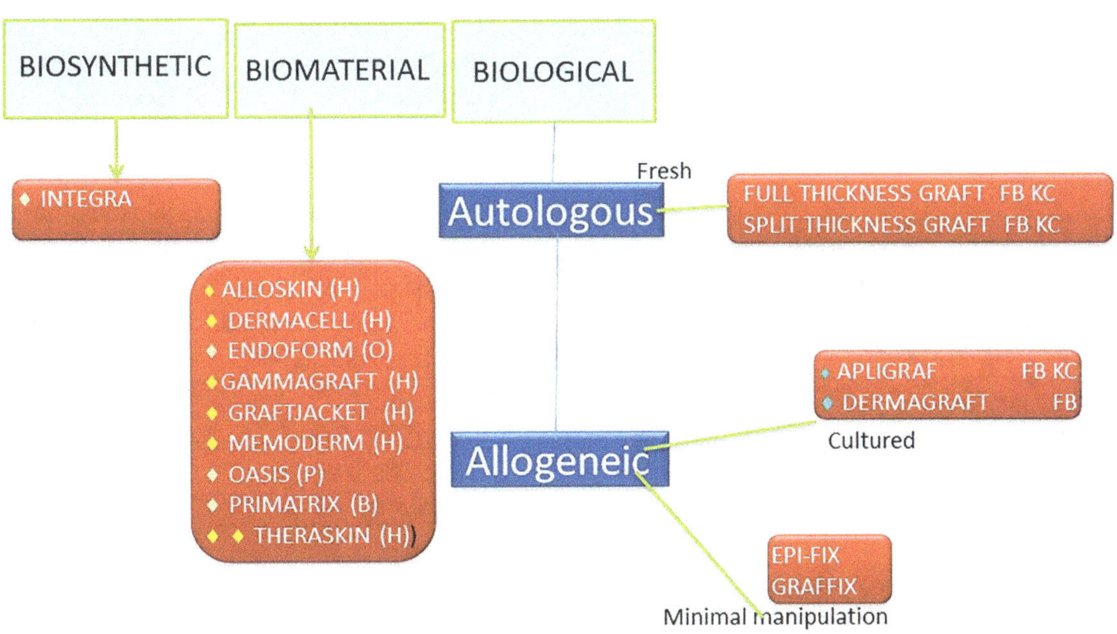

FIGURE 25.

CTP Classification - Courtesy of Bert Slade, MD

YELLOW = regulated as human-derived product HCT/P
BLUE = regulated as animal-derived product 510k
YELLOW MARGIN = regulated as synthetic product 510k
GREEN MARGIN = regulated as human-derived product PMA

TABLE 1. Classifications of CTPs (For more information, see reference[27])

Classification based on regulatory clearance requirements	Classification based on cells and tissue	Name of CTPs and skin substitutes	Composition	Indications
Synthetic				
	n/a	Suprathel	Acellular co-polymer based on DL-lactide containing Triethylenecarbonate and E- Caprolactone	Partial and full thickness burns Donor graft sites
Biosynthetic +/- Dead Cells				
	Dermal acellular	Integra	Bovine type 1 collagen and chondroitin - 6 sulfate with silicon covering.	Partial and full thickness wounds, pressure,venous, diabetic and chronic vascular ulcers
	Dermal acellular	Biobrane	Porcine collagen chemically bound to silicone/ nylon membrane	Temporary coverage of partial thickness burns and donor site wounds
	Dermal acellular	Tissue Tech	Combination of Hyalograft 3D and Laserskin	Chronic wounds and diabetic ulceration
	Dermal acellular	EZ- Derm	Acellular cross linked porcine-derived collagen dermal matrix	Temporary treatment of partial thickness burns
	Dermal cellular dermal grafts	Transcyte	Human neonatal foreskin fibroblasts grown on a nylon mesh and embedded in a silastic layer	Temporary wound coverage in partial and full thickness burns
Biomaterial/Tissue Derived +/- Dead Cells				
	Dermal acellular	Oasis	Decellullarized porcine jejunal submucosa	Pressure, venous, arteriovenous, and diabetic ulcers
	Dermal acelluar	Strattice	Decellularized porcine dermis processed and preserved in an aqueous phosphate buffered solution	Abdominal wall hernia repair,reconstructive breast surgery

TABLE 1. Continued

Classification based on regulatory clearance requirements	Classification based on cells and tissue	Name of CTPs and skin substitutes	Composition	Indications
	Dermal acelluar	Matriderm	Acellular scaffold made with bovine collagen types I,III,V,and elastin	Full and partial thickness burns
	Dermal acellular	Matristem	Porcine bladder derived single or multilayer extracellular matrix sheet	Partial and full thickness wounds, pressure, venous, diabetic, and chronic vascular ulcers
	Dermal acellular	Primatrix	Acellular collagen dermal tissue matrix derived from fetal bovine skin	Venous ulcers, diabetic ulcers, and burns
	Dermal acellular	Endoform*	Acellular extracellular matrix derived from sheep collagen	Venous, diabetic, pressure, and mix arteriovenous ulcers
	Dermal acellular	Puroply	Porcine derived purified native collagen matrix with the polyhexamethylene biguanide(PHMB)	All acute and chronic wounds of all types especially with suspected biofilm
Human Tissue				
	Dermal cellular composite graft	Theraskin	Human cadaveric allograft derived from split thickness skin graft containing donor fibroblast and keratinocytes	Diabetic and venous ulcers
	Dermal acellular	Graftjacket	Cadaveric human skin with epidermis and dermal cells removed	Diabetic and venous stasis ulcer
	Dermal cellular	Alloderm	Human allograft skin chemically treated to remove epidermis	Abdominal wall and hernia repair,breast reconstruction post-mastectomy
	Dermal acellular	Repliform	Acellular human dermal allograft collagen fibers are banded in omnidirectional patterns	Pelvic floor reconstruction

TABLE 1. Continued

Classification based on regulatory clearance requirements	Classification based on cells and tissue	Name of CTPs and skin substitutes	Composition	Indications
	Dermal acellular	Cymetra	A micronized particulate form of alloderm cadaveric acellular dermis	Refractory ulcers, wound filler, and soft tissue augmentation for cosmetic purposes
	Dermal cellular composite graft	GammaGraft	Gamma irradiated cadaveric allograft	Diabetic and venous stasis ulcer
Biologicals - living cells				
	Autologous grafts not cultured			
	Epidermis, dermis, and SQ tissue	Full thickness skin graft	Full thickness skin harvested from donor site	Open wound for skin coverage
	Epidermis and part of dermis	Split thickness skin graft	Split thickness skin harvested from donor site	Open wound for skin coverage
	Epidermis	Epidermal cellular autologous graft	Array of epidermal micrografts created at donor site from patient's own skin	Open wound for skin coverage
	Autologous cultured			
	Autologous keratinocytes	Epicel	Confluent autologous keratinocytes from skin biopsies delivered on a petroleum gauze backing	Full and partial thickness burns, venous ulcers, and diabetic ulcers
	Autologous keratinocytes	Epidex	Confluent autologous keratinocytes from hair follicles on a silicone membrane	Full and partial thickness burns, venous ulcers, and diabetic ulcers
	Autologous keratinocytes	Myskin	Cultured autologous keratinocytes seeded onto a silicone sheet treated with plasma polymer film	Partial thickness burns, donor graft sites, diabetic ulcers, and chronic wounds
	Autologous keratinocytes	Bioseed	Autologous oral mucosa cells in a fibrin glue matrix	Partial thickness burns, oral mucosa replacement, and venous ulcers

TABLE 1. Continued

Classification based on regulatory clearance requirements	Classification based on cells and tissue	Name of CTPs and skin substitutes	Composition	Indications
	Autologous keratinocytes	Cellspray	Preconfluent autologous keratinocytes delivered into a suspension for spray	Partial thickness burns
	Autologous keratinocytes	Celaderm	Living foreskin-derived allogenic keratinocytes	Venous ulcers
	Allogeneic + Xenogeneic			
	Dermal cellular composite graft	Apligraf	Composite bilayered product consisting of living keratinocytes and fibroblasts derived from neonatal human foreskin fibroblast in a bovine collagen.	Diabetic foot ulcers and venous ulcers
	Dermal cellular composite graft	OrCel	Bilayered absorbable bovine collagen sponge with matrix containing neonatal human fore-skin fibroblast	Venous, diabetic ulcers, skin graft donor sites, and mitten hand surgery for epider-molysis bullosa
	Allogeneic - Synthetic			
	Dermal cellular dermal grafts	Dermagraft	Cryopreserved allo-genic human neonatal foreskin fibroblast-de-rived bioabsorbable dermal matrix	Full thickness dia-betic foot ulcers Dystrophic epider-molysis bullosa
	Allogeneic - Minimal Manipulation			
	Placental membrane	Grafix	Cryopreserved pla-cental membrane comprised of an extracellular matrix rich in collagen, growth factors,fibroblasts,mes-enchymal stem cells, and epithelial cells	Acute and chronic wounds of all kinds

TABLE 1. Continued

Classification based on regulatory clearance requirements	Classification based on cells and tissue	Name of CTPs and skin substitutes	Composition	Indications
	Amnion and chorion	Epifix	Human amnion and chorion membranes that comprise the innermost layer of the placenta and line the amniotic cavity	Acute and chronic wounds of all kinds
	Amnion	Amniograft	Cryopreserved amniotic membrane	Acute and chronic wounds of all kinds
	Dermal cellular composite graft	Theraskin	Human cadaveric allograft derived from split thickness skin graft containing donor fibroblast and keratinocytes	Diabetic and venous ulcers

- Topical agents cytotoxic to skin replacement tissue[17]
  1) Avoid using cytotoxic topical agents immediately prior to or after application of skin replacement tissue. These prescriptions include, but are not limited to:
     - Chlorhexidine gluconate
     - Dakin's solution
     - Polymyxin/Nystatin
     - Mafenide acetate
     - Povidone-iodine solution
     - Scarlet red dressing
     - Tincoban
     - Zinc sulfate
  2) Note: If these agents are used prior to bioengineered tissue application, the wound bed must be thoroughly cleaned with saline before applying bioengineered tissue.

Contraindications

Skin replacement tissue is not recommended in:[17]

- Severe, uncontrolled diabetes mellitus or arterial disease
- A known sensitivity to the components of bioengineered tissue
- Clinically infected wound
- Wound with severe dermatitis
- Wound with unprepared wound bed

Conclusion

Although skin substitutes have a role to play in chronic wound management,[30-31] they are not a substitute for treatment of the underlying cause of the ulcer and standard wound management.[5-6,30-31] It is also important to do an appropriate wound bed preparation before application of skin substitutes. It is recommended to treat any suspected infection including biofilm before application of skin substitutes.[5-6,30]

Case study 1 (Figures 26-29)

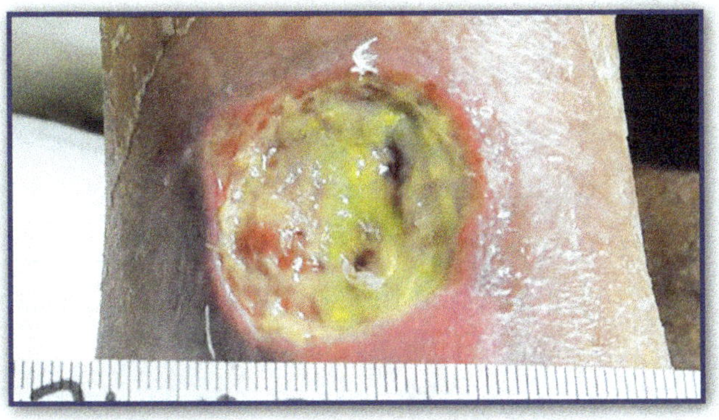

FIGURE 26. 52-year-old female with history of lupus on immunosuppressants with vasculitic ulcer

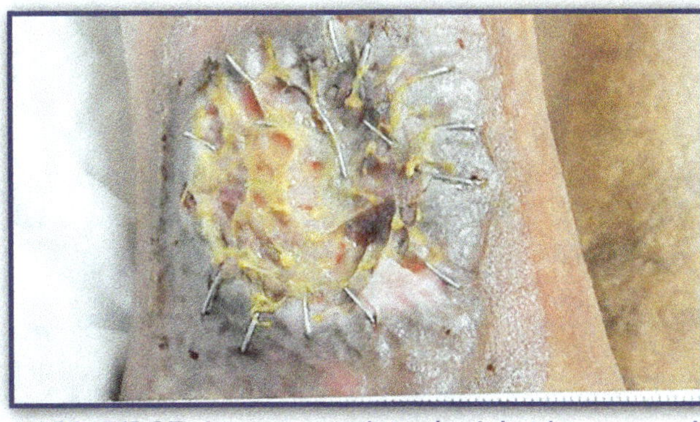

FIGURE 27. Lupus vasculitis s/q debridement and STSG with non-take

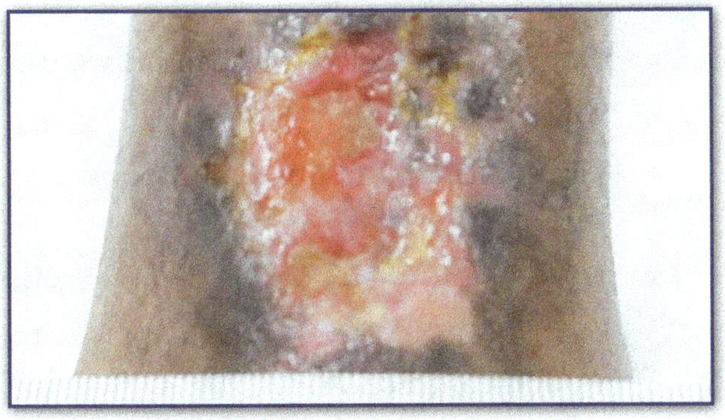

FIGURE 28. Lupus vasculitis ulcer s/q application of TheraSkin

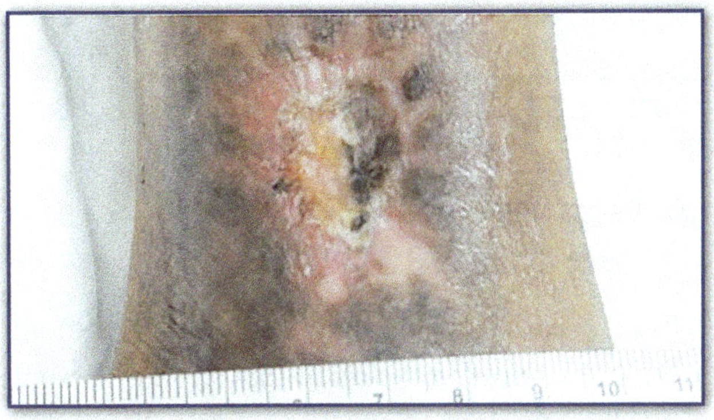

FIGURE 29. Lupus vasculitis ulcer patient epithelialized after eight weeks of TheraSkin application

Case study 2 (Figures 30-35)

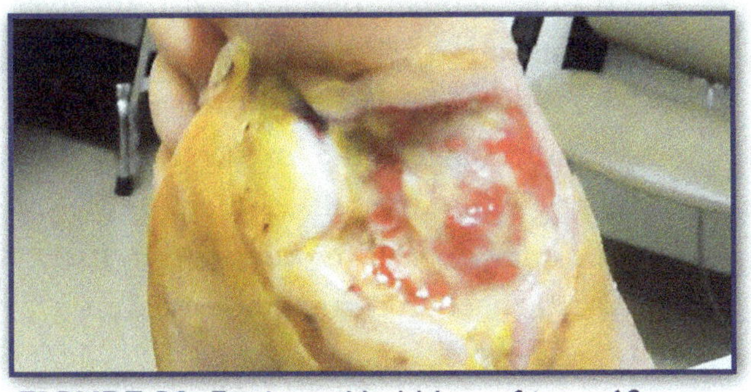

FIGURE 30. Epidermal bubble grafting—60-year-old diabetic male with infected neuroischemic diabetic foot ulcer; initial presentation

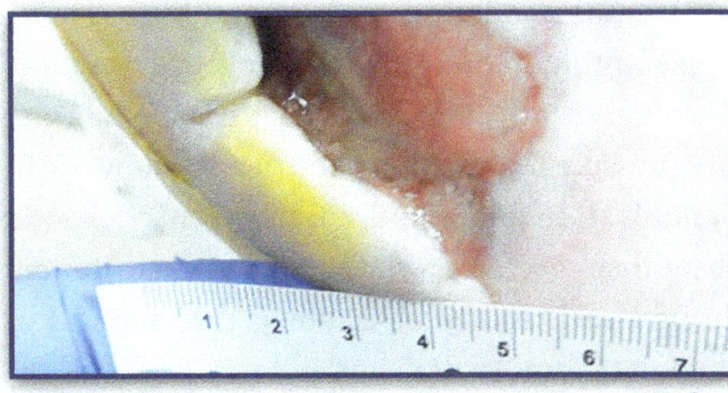

FIGURE 31. S/q debridement, antibiotics, HBO_2 six weeks after initial presentation

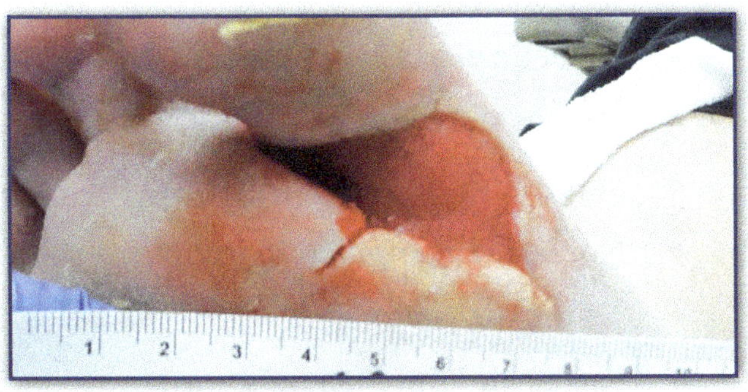

FIGURE 32. Acticoat x two weeks to decrease bacterial bioburden

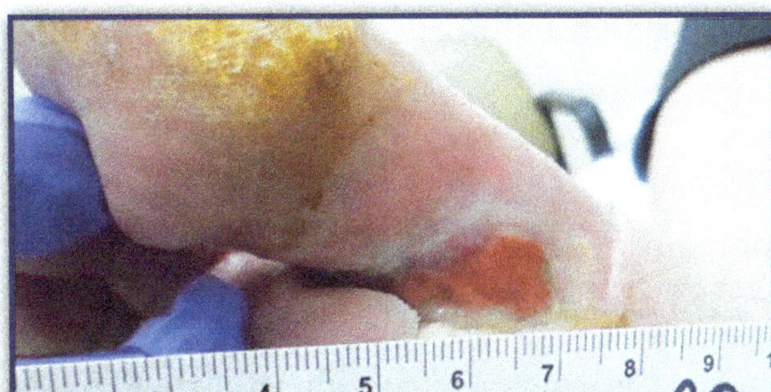

FIGURE 33. One week after epidermal bubble skin grafting application

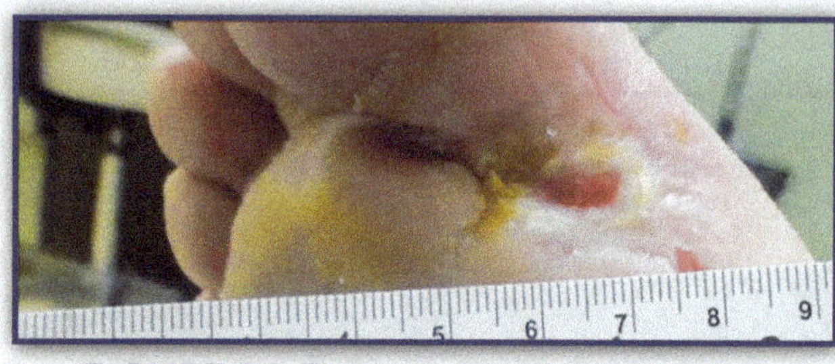

FIGURE 34. Three weeks after epidermal bubble skin grafting

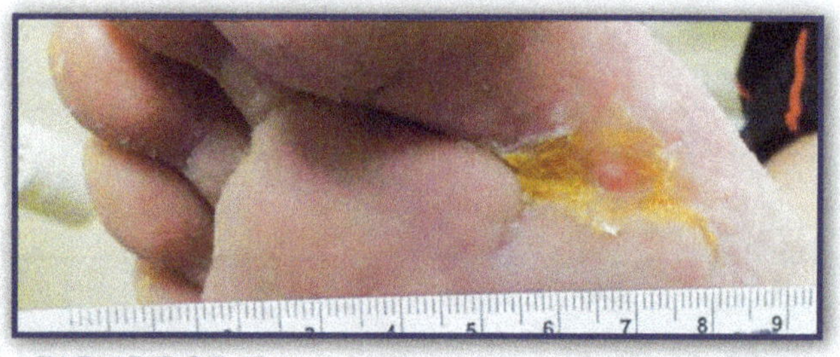

FIGURE 35. Four weeks after epidermal bubble skin grafting

D. Negative pressure wound therapy (NPWT)

NPWT was first used as an adjunct treatment for open wounds in the early 1990s.[32] At present NPWT is standard of care for a variety of wound types.[33-34] NPWT systems consist of a negative pressure pump unit that provides suction and in some cases also irrigation, a wound filler (foam, gauze, antimicrobial gauze dressing, hydrocolloid dressing, or other dressing) that transfers negative pressure to the wound bed. It also allows flow of fluids from the wound, a transparent occlusive sheet that covers the wound filler and creates an airtight seal, and flexible tubing that allows for suction to remove drainage and wound debris.[35] All existing negative pressure systems have regulated suction and tubing, but they differ in type of dressing used and amount of suction delivered.[35]

Mechanism of action of NPWT

Negative pressure therapy works by several mechanisms, including:

- Providing a moist healing environment[35-37]
- Clearing matrix metallo-proteinases (MMPs), which creates better biochemistry for wound healing[35-37]
- Mechanical distraction, which stimulates mitosis[35-37]
- Converting an uncontrolled open wound to a controlled closed wound[35-37]
- Controlling edema [35-37]
- Removing excess interstitial fluid to decrease the intercellular diffusion distance[36-37]
- Improving blood flow[35-37]
- Conflicting data suggest that it may reduce bacterial colonization[35]
- Sequestering excess MMPs and wound exudation[35-37]
- Augmenting local functional blood perfusion[35-37]
- Causing microstrain (releasing growth factors) and macro strain (helping with wound contraction)[35-37]
- Fibroblasts produce growth factors in response to deformity (i.e. suction)[35-37]
- The mechanism of action also involves perturbation of integrin bridges between the cells with subsequent release of second messengers, the expression of early genes within the cells, protein synthesis, and angiogenesis to produce the characteristic beefy red granulation tissue.[35-37]

Indications[33-35]

- Pressure ulcers
- Diabetic ulcers
- Venous stasis ulcers
- Surgical wounds
- Nonhealing amputation wounds
- Traumatic wounds
- Partial and full thickness burns
- Necrotizing fasciitis s/q fasciotomy

- Compartment syndrome s/q fasciotomy
- Meshed grafts and flaps
- Over CTPs and skin substitutes
- Full thickness wound with tendon and bone exposed
- Wounds associated with arterial insufficiency with caution
- Clean closed incisions and skin grafts/flaps

Contraindications for NPWT[17,33-35]

- Malignancy in the wound
- Untreated osteomyelitis
- Non-enteric and unexplored fistula
- Necrotic tissue with eschar
- Exposed blood vessels and organs

Precautions with NPWT [17,33-35]

- Patients with bleeding disorder
- Patients on anticoagulants
- Patients with low platelet count
- Nonenteric and unexplored fistula
- Needs special precautions and specialized technique to dress wounds with tendon and bone exposed
- Patient with arterial insufficiency can get worsening of ischemia
- Putting drape in patients with skin condition
- Needs special training to do dressing in patients with abdominal fistula and wound to isolate fistula before putting negative pressure therapy.

See Tables 3 and 4.

TABLE 2. Kinds of NPWT (For more information, see reference[35])

Classified based on energy source used	Kinds of negative pressure wound therapy
Electrical and Battery-powered	V.A.C. Ulta and V.A.C. Instill V.A.C. Via ACTIV.A.C. V.A.C. Freedom V.A.C. ATS and INFOV.A.C ABThera Prevena extriCARE (Portable) PRO-II and PRO-II (Portable) SVED (Portable) Invia Liberty Medela XLRB(Portable), Advanced PMS-800 and PMS-800V RENASYS EZ PLUS PICO Venturi Avanti
Electrical	Eugenex Advanced NPWT System
Battery-powered	XLRB (Portable)
Mechanical (spring-powered)	SnaP Wound Care System

Evidence-based conclusion

Indications for the use of negative pressure wound therapy are broadening as listed in the indication list in this chapter. Cochrane review of database shows that evidence for effectiveness of NPWT remains uncertain in spite of widespread clinical use for most indications.[42-47] Several randomized trials show effectiveness of negative pressure wound therapy in comparison to standard therapy in several wound types.[48-51] Clinically in author's opinion, this therapy has shown clinical benefits of improved granulation tissue and faster healing in every wound type.

TABLE 3. Recommended guidelines for modes of delivery and pressure for treating different wound types. (For more information, see references.[35,38-40])

Modes	Pressure recommendation	Advantages	Disadvantages
Continuous	Usually between 80 -125mmHg for most wounds	Allow for continuous removal of fluid collection which is excellent for heavily exudative wounds	Slower granulation tissue formation compared to intermitttent mode
	Lower pressure recommended for arterial wounds		
	Lower pressure recommended for painful wounds	Provides better stability of wound dressings	
	Lower pressure recommended for abdominal wounds because of presence of pressure receptors in abdomen	Less pain because of one compression cycle	
Intermittent	100 -125 mmHg for 5 min and 2 min off	Increase amount of mechanical stimulation may help with increase granulation tissue compared to continuous therapy	Accumulation of wound exudate during off cycle which might cause pooling, leading to leaks and periwound maceration
	Lower pressures for arterial and painful wounds		
			Potential for increase pain
		Cyclic compression may be better for patients with arterial wounds	Less stability of wound dressings
Variable	Only allowed in selected units; pressure setting is between 10 -125mmHg depending on type of the wound and patient comfort	Provides benefit of intermittent therapy to stimulate more granulation tissue; at same time allows removal of exudate on continuous basis to prevent leaks and maceration	
		Decreases pain during compression and intermittent therapy	

TABLE 3. Continued

Modes	Pressure recommendation	Advantages	Disadvantages
Instillation	100 -125mmHg pressure for 5 min and 2 min instillation	Allows for instillation of normal saline or topical solutions with negative pressure therapy	May increase chance of leaks and periwound maceration
	Lower pressures for arterial wound		
		May allow for better removal of detrimental wound fluids	

TABLE 4. Recommended guidelines for different filler dressings with negative pressure wound therapy. (For more information, see reference.[41])

Kind of filler dressing	Advantages	Disadvantages	Examples of negative pressure therapy system
Black Foam (Black reticulated open cell polyurethane foam)	Increase granulation tissue formation faster than gauze dressing due to increase tissue deformation	Overgrowth of granulaton tissue into the foam causing painful removal of foam dressings	ACTIV.A.C., Invia Liberty, V.A.C. Freedom, RENASYS EZ PLUS, V.A.C. ATS and INFOV.A.C.
	Compressibility of foam helps in wound contraction	Small pieces can break off and may cause complications (i.e. complications secondary to retained foam)	
	Works well for both deep and shallow wounds		
	Tends to produce thicker, less dense, and less organized granulation tissue compared to foam dressing	Time consuming to cut the foam to size of the wound	
Silver foam (Black reticulated open cell polyurethane foam with silver ions)	Same as above but has silver ions for antimicrobial properties	same as above	ACTIV.A.C., Invia Liberty, V.A.C. Freedom, RENASYS EZ PLUS,V.A.C. ATS and INFOV.A.C.
White foam	Does not adhere so best for tunnels, sinus tracts or undermining	Slower granulation tissue formation compared to black foam	ACTIV.A.C., Invia Liberty, V.A.C. Freedom, RENASYS EZ PLUS,V.A.C. ATS and INFOV.A.C.

TABLE 4. Continued

Kind of filler dressing	Advantages	Disadvantages	Examples of negative pressure therapy system
Polyvinyalcohal foam	Less painful on removal	Decrease negative pressure at the sensor site	
	Less likely to produce overgrowth of granulation tissue		
Green polyurethane foam	Used in some devices	Cannot visualize green drainage	Medela XLRB (Portable), Advanced
	Allows for easy visualization of any active bleeding		
Bio-dome (Multilayer polyester and silicone elastomer)	Less granulation inflitration	Not easily available	Eugenex Advanced NPWT System
	Less pain during removal of dressing		
	Large pore dressing encourages fast granulation tissue		
Antimicrobial gauze dressing	Less expensive	Produces less granulation tissue formation	PRO-II and PRO-II (Portable)
	Some antimicrobial dressing may contain polyhexamethylene biguanide which may help with bioburden control	Produces less contraction compared to black foam	Invia Liberty
		Gauze fibers might shed in the wounds	PMS-800 and PMS-800V
	Less pain	Absorbs less exudate	RENASYS EZ PLUS
	Easier to apply and molds well into contours		
Hydrocolloid based dressing	Better for shallow wounds with less drainage	Absorbs less exudate	SnaP Wound Care System
	Excellent for ambulatory patients	Cannot be used in heavily exudative wounds	
	Lightweight and easy to carry		
Seven-day stick-on dressing	Excellent for sugical incision wound immediately post surgery	Cannot absorb lot of exudate	Prevena
		Incision line cannot be visualized for clinical signs of infection or dehisence	PICO

TABLE 4. Continued

Kind of filler dressing	Advantages	Disadvantages	Examples of negative pressure therapy system
Irrigation system with black and white foam dressings	Helps with irrigation of wound while providing negative pressure therapy	Expensive compared to other negative pressure system	V.A.C. Ulta and V.A.C. Instill

Case study (Figures 36-43)

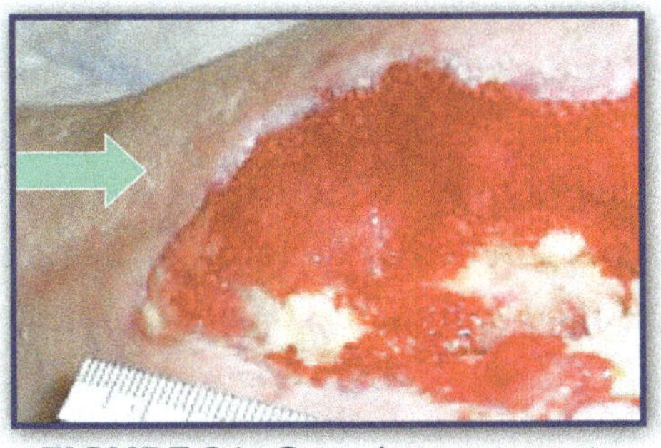

FIGURE 36. Granulation tissue in response to NPWT

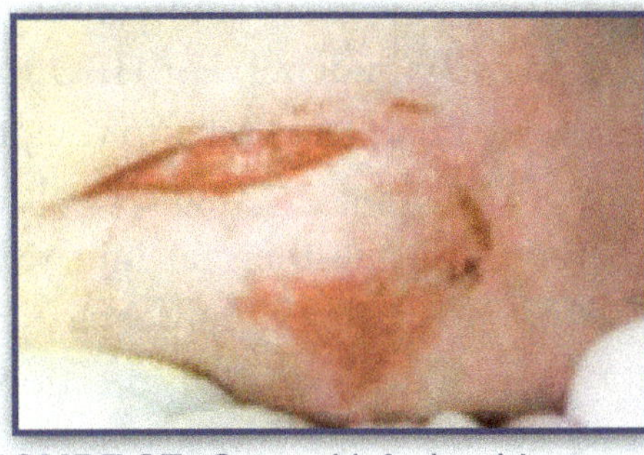

FIGURE 37. Original left shoulder wound

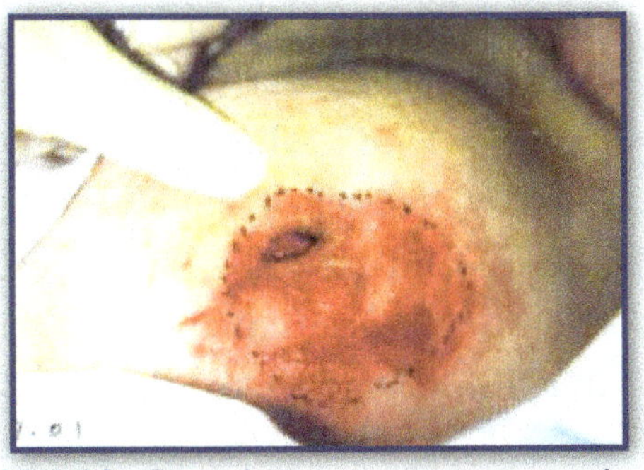

FIGURE 38. Granulation tissue growing through skin from improperly applied NPWT sponge (note smaller original wound). This demonstrates the powerful effect of NPWT to stimulate angiogenesis.

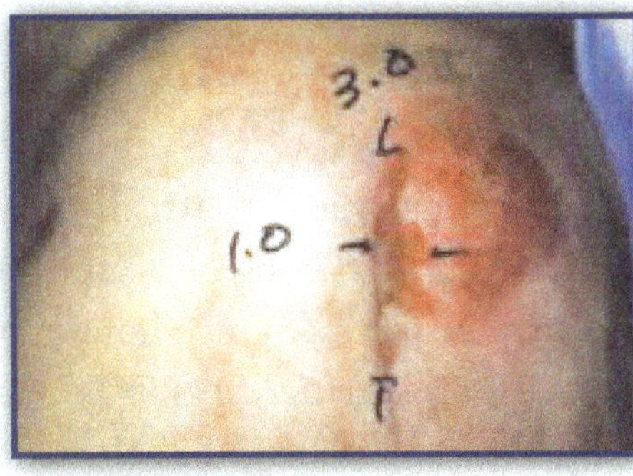

FIGURE 39. Periwound skin healing after NPWT sponge was discontinued

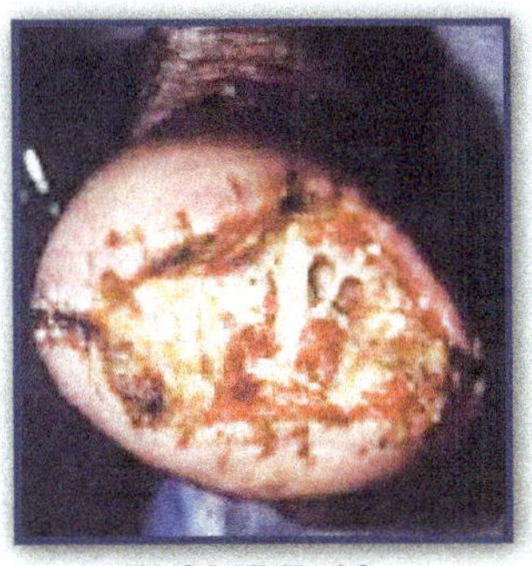

FIGURE 40. Failed transmetatarsal amputation

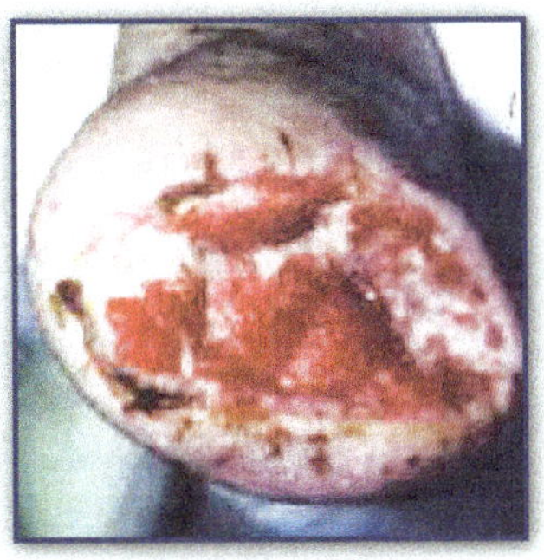

FIGURE 41. Wound after two weeks of NPWT

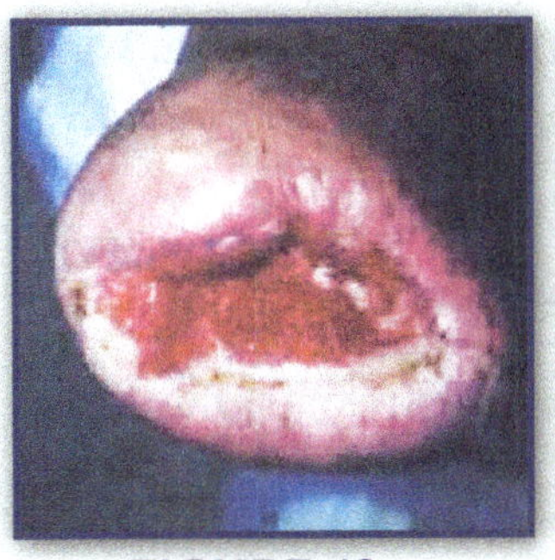

FIGURE 42. Wound after four weeks of NPWT

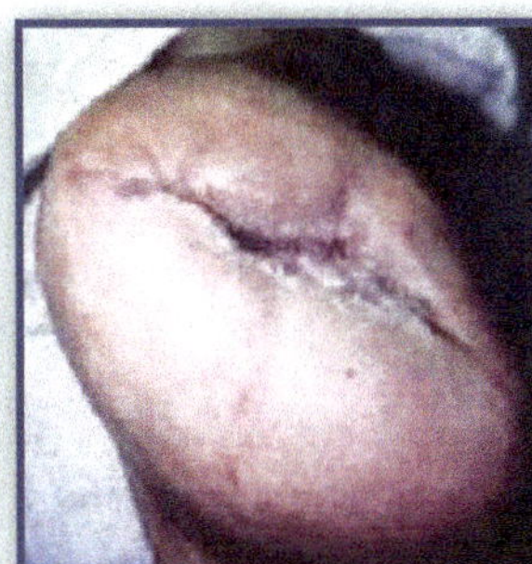

FIGURE 43. Wound after eight weeks of NPWT

E. Hyperbaric oxygen therapy

In 1960, Dutch Professor Ita Boerema, a cardiac surgeon, published a landmark article titled, "Life Without Blood," in which he described anaesthetized pigs being sustained without injury by breathing hyperbaric oxygen in the absence of circulating hemoglobin (Hgb 0.5%).[52] Hyperbaric oxygen therapy is defined as administration of 100% oxygen under increased atmospheric pressure of at least 1.4 ATA and above.[53] This chapter discusses use of HBO_2 therapy in diabetic wounds and compromised skin grafts and flap in detail. For HBO therapy in radiation wounds, please refer to Chapter 17: The Effects of Radiation on Wound Healing. For HBO_2 therapy in acute thermal injury, please refer to Chapter 18: Practical Approach to Burns. For HBO_2 therapy in clostridial infections and necrotizing soft tissue infections, please refer to Chapter 15: Approach to Commonly Misdiagnosed Ulcers and Atypical Ulcers.

Mechanism of action

Oxygen transport occurs by two mechanisms: chemical binding to hemoglobin and physical dissolution in plasma. Once hemoglobin is saturated with oxygen, increases in FiO_2 can be affected only by the plasma dissolved oxygen fraction. As the pO_2 increases, the amount of O_2 physically dissolved in plasma increases in a linear fashion.[54] The role of oxygen in wound healing is well defined. It helps in several ways, including the following:

- enhanced WBC killing[55]
- inhibition of toxin formation [55-57]
- inactivation of toxins (clostridium perfringens)[57]
- bacteriostatic[55-57]
- antibiotic transport across cell wall[58]
- collagen cross-linking[59]
- angiogenesis[60-65].

Recent work from Thom et al. shows HBO_2 therapy exerts its effects largely through controlled and brief increases in reactive oxygen species (ROS) and reactive nitrogen species (RNS).[66] The increase in ROS and RNS raises the levels of growth factors and the levels of growth factor receptors. It also mobilizes the stem/progenitor cells from the bone marrow and reduces integrin function. These changes reduce the pathologic neutrophil adhesion causing changes in monocyte chemokine synthesis, hemoxygenase-1, heat shock proteins, and hypoxia-inducible factor-1, ultimately leading to reduction of pathologic inflammation.[66]

1. *Correction of hypoxia*

Local oxygen tensions in wound are approximately half the values observed in normal, non-wounded tissue.[67-71] Hypoxia correlates with impaired wound healing.[67-71] Hypoxia has been defined in a consensus statement from the 2007 Undersea and Hyperbaric Medical Society Workshop on Transcutaneous Oximetry ($PtcO_2$) in Clinical Practice as follows[70]:

Hypoxia definition

- Hypoxia is defined as $PtcO_2 < 40$ mmHg (respiring air).
- Normal extremities reach $PtcO_2 > 100$ mmHg (respiring O_2).
- Critical limb ischemia usually has $PtcO_2$ < 30mmHg.
- Amputation healing unlikely at $PtcO_2$ < 40mmHg or if $PtcO_2$ rise on O_2 is <10 mmHg.
- After revascularization, healing usually occurs if $PtcO_2$ increases to > 40 mmHg (increase might be delayed).

- $PtcO_2$ obtained while breathing normobaric air can identify patients who will not heal spontaneously.

$PtcO_2$ as a predictor of wound healing in diabetic foot wounds

- $PtcO_2$ < 20 mmHg indicated 39-fold increased risk of early healing failure.[67]
- Multicenter study of diabetic wounds showed relationship between in-chamber $PtcO_2$ and HBO_2 success.[68]

It showed the following:

(i) As in-chamber $PtcO_2$ increases, likelihood of success from HBO_2 increases;

(ii) Overall 75.6% of diabetic foot ulcers improved after HBO_2;

(iii) Best discriminator of success or failure was in chamber $PtcO_2$ during HBO_2 > 200 mm Hg.[68]

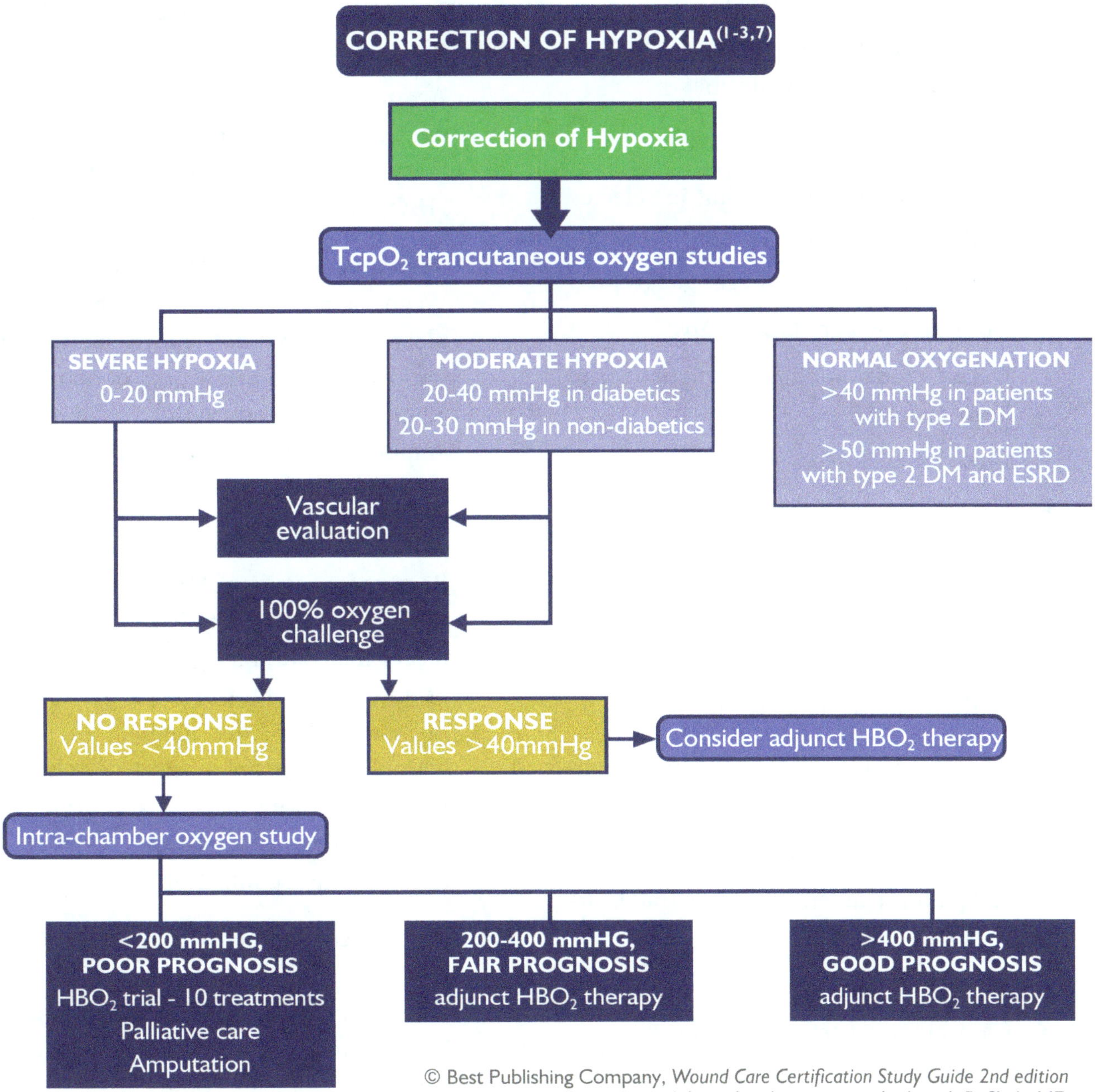

- Cohort study showed that a reliable test is combination of 1 ATA air and oxygen $PtcO_2$. Mean values simultaneously taken at the same anatomic level (TC-air > 0 mm Hg; TC-O_2 > 35 mm Hg; TC % rise > 50%) were more reliable than single air values in predicting healing outcome.[70]

Indications[53,69]

Wound related indications[53]

- Acute thermal burn injury
- Acute traumatic ischemia
  - (i) Crush injury
  - (ii) Compartment syndrome
- Arterial insufficiencies:
  - (i) Enhancement of healing in selected problem wounds
- Clostridial myositis and gas gangrene
- Compromised grafts and flaps
- Delayed radiation injury (soft tissue and bony necrosis)
- Intracranial abscess
- Necrotizing soft tissue infections
- Osteomyelitis (refractory)

Non-wound indications[53]

- Air or gas embolism
- Carbon monoxide poisoning
  - (i) Carbon monoxide poisoning complicated by cyanide poisoning
- Decompression sickness
- Idiopathic sudden sensorineural hearing loss
- Severe anemia
- Central retinal artery occlusion

Every medical treatment requires a risk/benefit analysis. Whether any risk is acceptable depends on the severity of the problem for which the patient is undergoing treatment, the likelihood of experiencing that side effect, and the consequence of the side effect.

2. Evidence-based recommendations

HBO_2 therapy in diabetic wounds

HBO_2 is an expensive modality but is cost-effective for the limb and life threatening problem of infected diabetic foot ulcers.[74]

UHMS published clinical practice guidelines for diabetic wounds in 2015[74] which recommends:

1. Against using HBO_2 therapy for Wagner Grade 2 or lower diabetic foot ulcers (very low-level evidence in support of HBO_2, conditional recommendation).
2. Recommends using HBO_2 therapy for Wagner Grade 3 or higher diabetic foot ulcers that have not shown significant improvement after 30 days of standard wound care to reduce the risk of major amputation and incomplete healing (moderate-level evidence, conditional recommendation).
3. Recommends using HBO_2 therapy for Wagner Grade 3 or higher diabetic foot ulcers that had a surgical debridement of an infected foot (e.g. partial toe or ray amputation; debridement of ulcer with underlying bursa, cicatrix or bone; foot amputation; incision and drainage [I&D] of deep space abscess; or necrotizing soft tissue infection).
4. Recommends adding acute postoperative HBO_2 therapy to the standard of care to reduce the risk of major amputation and incomplete healing (moderate-level evidence, conditional recommendation).

TABLE 5. Risk/benefit analysis of possible side effects in patients receiving HBO_2 therapy [53,73]

Possible side effect from HBO_2 therapy	Reported frequency in routine practice	Potential outcome of this side effect	Examples of factors which might increase risk of this side effect	Examples of conditions that might justify the increased risk of HBO_2 therapy (NOTE: The hyperbaric physician should assess.)
Otic barotrauma	Common (~10% of patients)	Worst case is impaired hearing long term (rare) Most common is temporary discomfort due to otic effusion	History of radiation to the neck; active upper respiratory infection; chronic sinusitis; history of ear surgery	Soft tissue radiation damage affecting patient quality of life; chronic nonhealing wounds
Central nervous system oxygen toxicity	~1:400-1:20,000 treatments	Grand mal seizure No long-term effects reported	High fever; disulfiram (theoretical); steroids; electrolyte disturbances	Chronic wounds; soft tissue radiation injuries; failing flaps, all emergency indications such as CO poisoning and DCI
Pulmonary oxygen toxicity	Not seen in routine treatments; may occur in patients treated with US Navy TT6 for severe decompression sickness	Usually transient pain with deep inspiration which resolves spontaneously after HBO_2 therapy within hours; could be fatal if HBO_2 therapy is given repeatedly to a patient requiring high FIO_2 between treatments	History of doxyrubicin use; history of bleomycin use	Chronic wounds; soft tissue radiation injuries; failing flaps; all emergency indications such as CO poisoning and DCI
Pulmonary barotrauma	Exceedingly rare	Lung collapse requiring a chest tube; death or arterial gas embolism are possible	Asthma, chronic obstructive pulmonary disease; thoracic surgery (small risk of trapped air in scarred tissue)	Limb and life threatening indications
Arterial gas embolism (likely due to pulmonary barotrauma)	Fewer than six cases reported	Severe neurological injury is possible; death is possible		Limb and life threatening indications

TABLE 5. Continued

Possible side effect from HBO_2 therapy	Reported frequency in routine practice	Potential outcome of this side effect	Examples of factors which might increase risk of this side effect	Examples of conditions that might justify the increased risk of HBO_2 therapy (NOTE: The hyperbaric physician should assess.)
Flash pulmonary edema	Occasionally reported	Death is possible but acute respiratory distress requiring intubation or ICU admission are likely	Extremely low ejection fraction; severe aortic stenosis; rarely in patients with diastolic dysfunction	Limb and life threatening indications; chronic wounds; soft tissue radiation injuries; failing flaps; all emergency indications such as CO poisoning and DCI
Anxiety attack	Occasionally reported	Termination of treatment, but usually no serious side effects; pretreatment with anxiolytics may be necessary	History of claustrophobia	Limb and life threating indications; chronic wounds; soft tissue radiation injuries; failing flaps; all emergency indications such as CO poisoning and DCI

Case study (Figures 44-46)

A 68-year-old male with severe peripheral arterial disease, diabetes, and large, nonhealing high above the knee amputation stump for the past four months (the open lesion is on his left inner thigh near the groin). His periwound transcutaneous oximetry values are 1 and 2mmHg and periwound ischemia is apparent in Figure 44. He is not a candidate for further revascularization.

He underwent 14 hyperbaric oxygen therapy treatments and NPWT was initiated. NPWT was continued for a total of eight weeks at which time there was a fully granulated wound (Figure 45). Moist wound care was continued until closure.

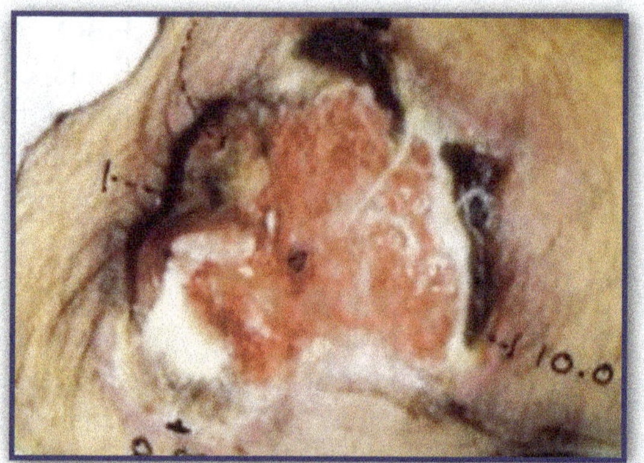

FIGURE 44.

HBO_2 therapy in compromised skin grafts/flaps

The FDA includes the treatment of jeopardized flaps and grafts in its list of indications for the use of HBO_2 therapy. The benefit of HBO_2 therapy in such circumstances (including re-implantation after long periods of warm ischemia) was once thought limited to enhancing tissue oxygen

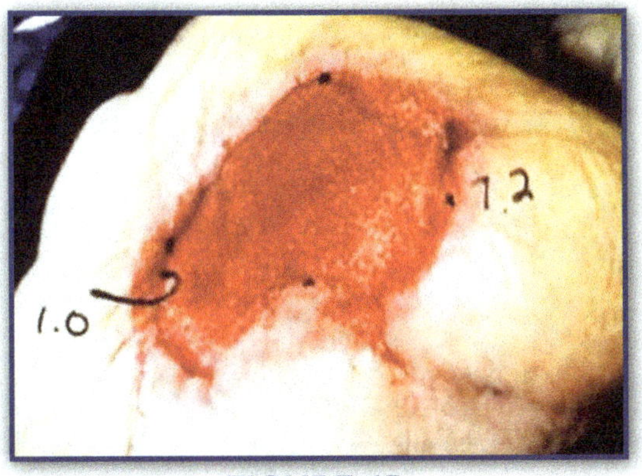

FIGURE 45.

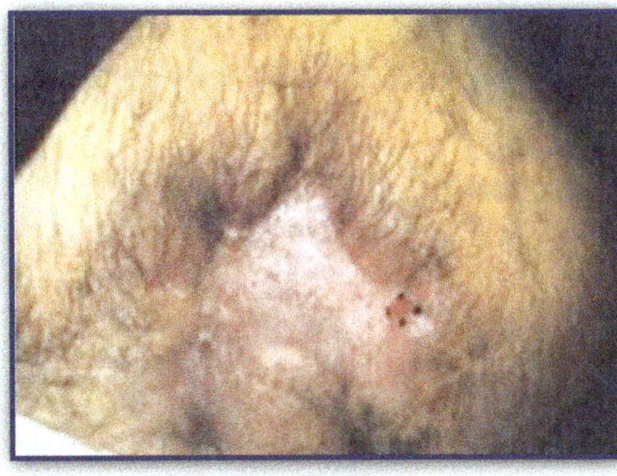

FIGURE 46.

levels. Figure 46 taken during a study performed in 1977 shows the effect of HBO_2 therapy on an ischemic full thickness skin flap model. Flap loss was approximately 75% in untreated animals (example below) and 25% in animals treated with HBO_2 therapy (example top). The effect was presumed primarily due to the increase in oxygen diffusion distance resulting from HBO_2. Since those early days, as a result of the elegant work of Zamboni, Thom, Piantidosi, and others, it is now understood that HBO_2 therapy induces oxidative stress with controlled production of reactive oxygen and nitrogen species that activate various beneficial cellular processes.

The three most relevant biochemical mechanisms are:

1. the production of growth factors (VEGF, HIF-1, PDGF)
2. mobilization of bone-marrow derived stem/progenitor cells (CD34)
3. the reduction of neutrophil adhesion (modification of integrin beta-2)[75-76]. It should be emphasized that the primary role of HBO_2 therapy is not the treatment of venous congestion. Leech therapy can be a useful adjunct in such cases. Venous engorgement and ischemia reperfusion can coexist.

Figure 47 is a 12-year-old girl whose right index finger was bitten off by a dog and re-implanted after a prolonged warm ischemia time. Venous engorgement was treated with leeches and she was given HBO_2 therapy for ischemia reperfusion (IR) with salvage of the re-implanted finger and good subsequent function (Figure 48). It should be noted that the optimal time to use HBO_2 therapy for IR is early, long before visible tissue necrosis has occurred, although it can be difficult to determine tissue viability.

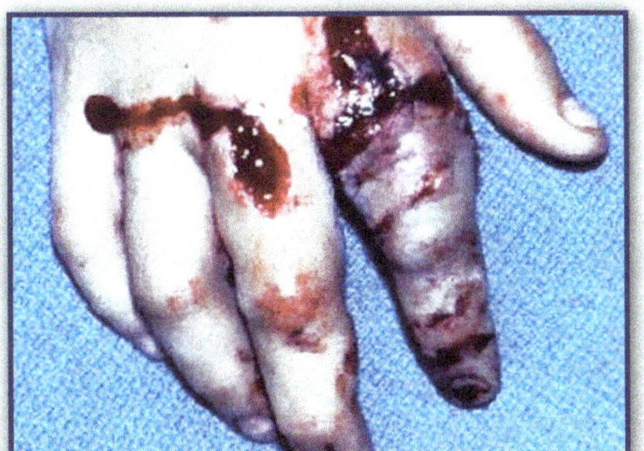

FIGURE 47.
Courtesy of Caroline E. Fife, MD

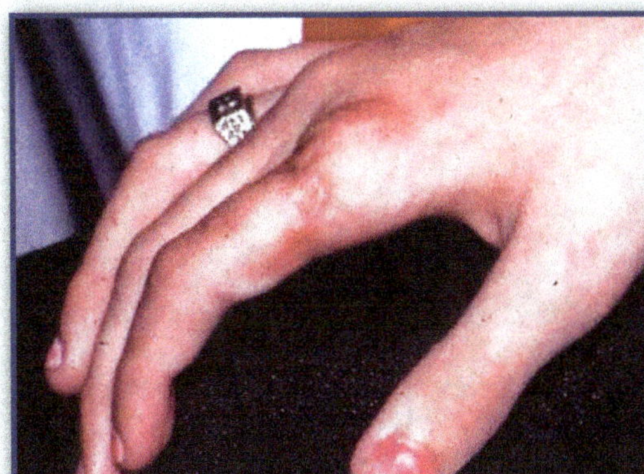

FIGURE 48.
Courtesy of Caroline E. Fife, MD

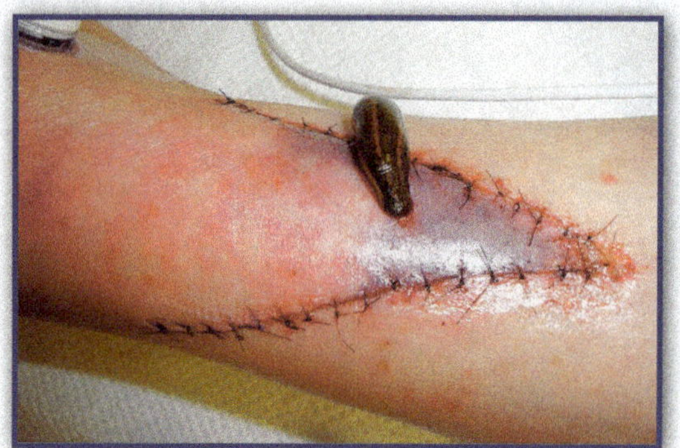

FIGURE 49.
Courtesy of Caroline E. Fife, MD

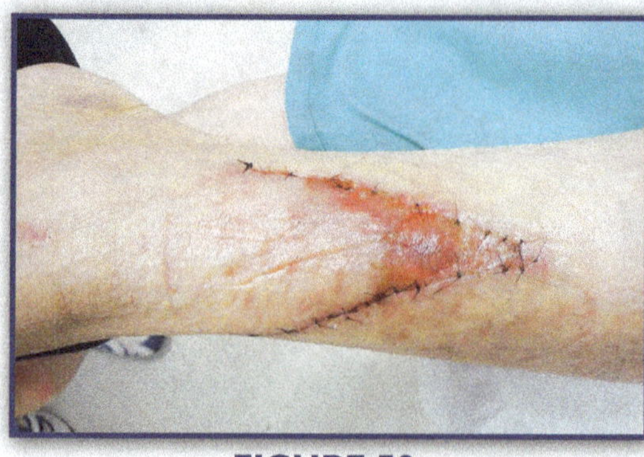

FIGURE 50.
Courtesy of Caroline E. Fife, MD

Figure 49 shows a 68-year-old woman with rheumatoid arthritis on low-dose prednisone who fell and cut her anterior shin resulting in a long, full thickness flap with an ischemic apex. Note the edema and venous engorgement of the most distal area of the flap. Transcutaneous oximetry confirmed periwound ischemia. Leeches were used to decongest the venous engorgement and daily HBO_2 was initiated.

Figure 50 shows the leg after six daily treatments of HBO_2; Figure 51 shows the leg four weeks later. She did have some tissue loss at the most distal portion of the flap, but the majority of the flap survived.

Unfortunately, at the time of this writing, the implementation of the ICD-10 coding system has negatively impacted the clinical use of HBO_2; therapy for ischemic flaps. Jeopardized grafts and flaps were a combined concept in the ICD-9 diagnosis coding system but are separated under ICD-10. The crosswalk to ICD-10 endorsed by CMS encompasses only jeopardized skin grafts and excludes the various ICD-10 flap codes. Thus, with the advent of ICD-10, jeopardized flaps have effectively become an uncovered indication for HBO_2; therapy, even though there has been no formal change in coverage policy. This problem has yet to be rectified or even acknowledged by CMS. Nevertheless, the mitigation of ischemia reperfusion injury by HBO_2 therapy may represent a vital adjunctive treatment for flaps and one for which there is currently no other equally effective option.

Figure 52 shows a pig model of full thickness ischemic flap. Flaps are raised and then sutured in place. Animal above was treated with

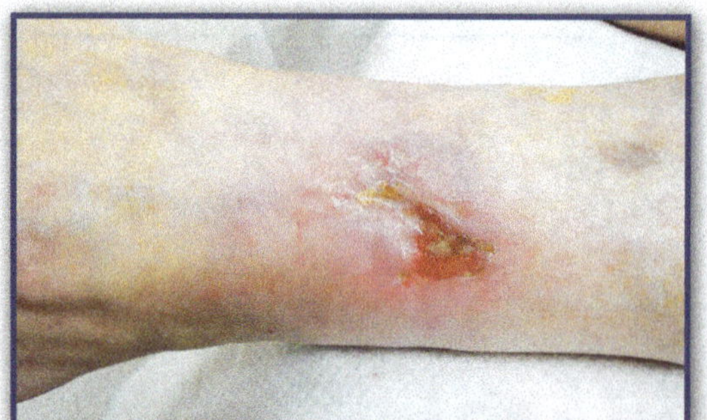

FIGURE 51.
Courtesy of Caroline E. Fife, MD

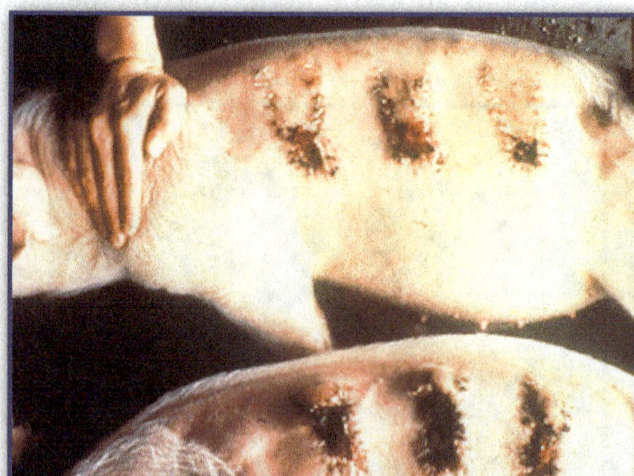

FIGURE 52.
Photo taken in 1977. Courtesy of Texas A&M Hyperbaric Laboratory, W.P Fife, PhD and Caroline E. Fife, MD.

HBO_2 and experienced only about 25% flap loss compared to animal below, which had about 75% flap loss. The photo was taken in 1977 in the Texas A&M Hyperbaric Laboratory. At the time, the salutary effect of HBO_2 on ischemic flaps was thought primarily due to improvement in tissue oxygen levels due to the increase in oxygen diffusion distance.

Summary

For the management of chronic wounds, if conventional therapy has not been successful within 4 weeks, alternative therapies should be considered.[2,75] The initial rate of healing during the first 4 weeks can predict whether ulcers are likely to heal by 24 weeks. If initial healing rate is < 0.1 cm/wk at the 4-week interval, then advanced therapy should be considered.[2,77] Ulcers with a poor prognosis should be treated with a more advanced therapy. Rapid identification of patients who are unlikely to respond to conventional care will allow for earlier interventions with advanced therapies. Key challenge with advanced modalities in wound care is to find a safe and efficient product that is economically viable with the trend shifting from volume-based wound care to value-based wound care. It is important for wound care providers to start thinking about the cost. What is the value of your good outcome? The question of whether we can deliver the same outcome at a lower cost needs to be answered. Can we lower the cost of healing wounds by using some of the advanced wound modalities, which can heal wounds faster and more quickly, decreasing the overall cost and burden to the healthcare system?

Review questions

1. **The supplemental metal needed by enzyme systems with regards to wound healing is**

    a. iron

    b. silver

    c. zinc

    d. copper

2. **The only growth factor currently available commercially for use in nonhealing wounds is**

    a. PDGF

    b. VEGF

    c. TGF-B

    d. KGF

3. **All of the following statements are mechanisms by which hyperbaric oxygen therapy can be of benefit except:**

    a. stimulating angiogenesis

    b. correction of hypoxia

    c. mobilization of stem cells from bone marrow

    d. activating growth factors receptors

    e. inhibiting bacterial growth

    f. decreasing collagen cross-linking

4. **All of the following statements are mechanisms by which negative pressure therapy can be of benefit except:**

    a. microstrain

    b. macrostrain

    c. autolytic debridement

    d. mechanical debridement

    e. increased local perfusion

    f. correction of hypoxia

    g. promotion of moist wound healing

    h. reduction of edema and interstitial fluid

5. **In which of the following scenario you will discontinue use of negative pressure wound therapy (NPWT)?**

    a. The wound size has decreased by 60%.

    b. The wound is more than 60% granulated.

    c. The wound shows evidence of bleeding that does not stop with pressure.

    d. The wound has tendon exposed.

ANSWERS: 1) c
2) a
3) f
4) f
5) c

References

1. Sen CK, Gordillo GM, Roy S, et al. Human skin wounds: A major and snowballing threat to public health and the economy. Wound repair and regeneration: official publication of the Wound Healing Society [and] the European Tissue Repair Society. 2009;17(6):763-771.
2. Sheehan P. Jones P, Caselli A, et al. Percent change in wound area of diabetic foot ulcers over a 4-week period is a robust predictor of complete healing in a 12-week prospective trial. Diabetes Care. 2003;26(6):1879-82.
3. Association for the Advancement of Wound Care (AAWC). AAWC venous ulcer guideline. Malvern (PA): 2010.
4. Steed DL, Attinger C, Colaizzi T, et al. Guidelines for the treatment of diabetic ulcers. Wound Repair Regen. 2006;14(6):680-692.
5. Sibbald RG, et al. Special considerations in wound bed preparation 2011: an update. Wound Healing Southern Africa. 2011;4(2):55-72.
6. Woo K, Ayello EA, Sibbald RG. The edge effect: current therapeutic options to advance the wound edge. Adv Skin Wound Care. 2007; 20(2):99-117.
7. Margolis DJ, Allen-Taylor L, Hoffstad O, Berlin JA. Healing diabetic neuropathic foot ulcers: are we getting better? Diabet Med. 2005;22:172-176.
8. Falanga V, Sabolinski M. A bilayered living skin construct (Apligraf®) accelerates complete closure of hard-to-heal venous ulcers. Wound Repair Regen. 1999;7:201-7.
9. Falanga V, Sabolinski ML. Prognostic factors for healing of venous ulcers. Wounds. 2000;12(5 Suppl A):42A-46A.
10. O'Meara S, et al. Compression for venous leg ulcers. http://onlinelibrary.wiley.com/doi/10.1002/14651858.CD000265.pub3/pdf/
11. Margolis D, Kantor J, Berlin J. Healing of neuropathic ulcers receiving standard treatment: a meta-analysis. Diabetes Care. 1999;22(5):692-694.
12. Kantor J, Margolis DJ. Efficacy and prognostic value of simple wound measurements. Arch Dermatol. 1998;134:1571-1574.
13. Kantor J, Margolis DJ. A multicenter study of percentage change in venous leg ulcer area as a prognostic index of healing at 24 weeks. Br J Dermatol. 2000;142:960-964.
14. Margolis DJ, Berlin JA, Strom BL. Risk factors associated with the failure of a venous leg ulcer to heal. Arch Dermatol. 1999;135:920-926.
15. American Diabetic Association Consensus Statement: Diabetes Care: 22(8):13541360, April 1999.
16. Ennis WJ, Lee C, Meneses P. A biochemical approach to wound healing through the use of modalities. Clin Dermatol. 2007;25:63-72.
17. Fife CE, Shah JB. Wound bed preparation & advanced technologies for wound healing. In: Shah JB et al, Wound Care Certification Study Guide, 2nd edition. North Palm Beach, Florida: Best Publishing Company; 2016; p.97-112.
18. Barrientos S, Stojadinovic O, Golinko MS, Brem H, Tomic-Canic M. Growth factors and cytokines in wound healing. WWR. 2008;16:585–601.
19. Steed DL, the Diabetic Ulcer Study Group. Clinical evaluation of recombinant human platelet-derived growth factor for the treatment of lower extremity diabetic ulcers. J Vasc Surg. 1995;21(1):71-81.
20. Schultz GS, Wysocki A. Interactions between extracellular matrix and growth factors in wound healing. Wound Repair Regen. 2009;17(2):153-62.

21. Heldin CH, Westermark B. Mechanism of action and in vivo role of platelet-derived growth factor. Physiol Rev. 1999;79:1283-1316.

22. Martí-Carvajal AJ, Gluud C, Nicola S, Simancas-Racines D, Reveiz L, Oliva P, Cedeño-Taborda J. Growth factors for treating diabetic foot ulcers. Cochrane Database of Systematic Reviews 2015, Issue 10. Art. No.: CD008548. DOI: 10.1002/14651858.CD008548.pub2

23. Wieman TJ, Smiell JM, Su Y. Efficacy and safety of a topical gel formulation of recombinant human platelet-derived growth factor-BB (becaplermin) in patients with chronic neuropathic diabetic ulcers. Diabetes Care. 1998;21:822-827.

24. Lacci KM, Dardik A. Platelet-rich plasma: support for its use in wound healing. Yale J Biol Med. 2010;83(1):1–9.

25. Martinez-Zapata M, Martí-Carvajal AJ, Solà I, Expósito J, Bolíbar I, Rodríguez L, Garcia J, Zaror C. Autologous platelet-rich plasma for treating chronic wounds. Cochrane Database of Systematic Reviews 2016, Issue 5. Art. No.: CD006899. DOI: 10.1002/14651858.CD006899.pub3

26. Carter MJ, Fife CE, Walker D, Thomson B. Estimating the applicability of wound-care randomized controlled trials to general wound care populations by estimating the percentage of individuals excluded from a typical wound care population in such trials. Adv Skin Wound Care. 2009; 22:316-24.

27. Greaves NS, Iqbal SA, Baguneid M, Bayat A. The role of skin substitutes in the management of chronic cutaneous wounds. Wound Repair and Regeneration. 2013;21(2):194-210.

28. Brem H, Young J, Tomic-Canic M, et al. Clinical efficacy and mechanism of bilayered living human skin equivalent (HSE) in treatment of diabetic foot ulcers. Surg Technol Int. 2003;11:23-31.

29. Ronfard V, William T. Development of cell-based therapy for wounds. In: Sen CK, Advances in Wound Care. Mary Ann Liebert, Inc. Publishing Company. 2010;1:412-418.

30. Schultz GS, Sibbald RG, Falanga V, et al. Wound bed preparation: a systematic approach to wound management. Wound Repair Regen. 2003. Suppl 1:S1-28.

31. Santema TB, Poyck PPC, Ubbink DT. Skin grafting and tissue replacement for treating foot ulcers in people with diabetes. Cochrane Database of Systematic Reviews 2016, Issue 2. Art. No.: CD011255. DOI: 10.1002/14651858.CD011255.pub2.

32. Nanwell PE. Topical negative pressure therapy in wound care. J Wound care. 1999:8(2):79-84

33. Banwell PE, Musgrave M. Topical negative pressure therapy: mechanisms and indication. Int. Wound J. 2004;1(2):95-106.

34. Bovill E, Banwell PE, Teot L, et al. Topical negative pressure therapy: a review of its role and guidelines for its use in the management of acute wounds. Int. Wound J. 2008;5(4):511-529.

35. Gibbs KA, Hamm RL. Negative pressure wound therapy. In: Hamm RL. Text and atlas of wound diagnosis and treatment. McGraw Hill Education Publishing Company; 2015;p.401-422.

36. Glass GE, Nanchahal J. The methodology of negative pressure wound therapy: separating fact from fiction. J Plast Reconstruc Anesthet Surg. 2012;65(8):989-1001.

37. Orgill DP, Manders EK, Sumpio BE, et al. The mechanisms of action of vacuum assisted closure: more to learn. Surgery. 2009;146:40-51.

38. Borgquist O, Ingemansson R, Malmsjo M. Wound edge microvascular blood flow during negative pressure wound therapy examining the effects of pressures from -10 to -175mm Hg. Plast Reconstruct Surge. 2010:125(2):502-509.

39. Borgquist O,Ingemansson R, Malmsjo M. The effect of intermittent and variable negative pressure wound therapy on wound edge microvascular blood flow. Ostomy Wound Manage. 2010:56(3):60-67.

40. Malmsjo M, Gustafsson L, Lindstedt S, Gesslein B, Ingemansson R. The effects of variable, intermittent, and continuous negative pressure wound therapy, using foam, or gauze, on wound contraction, granulation tissue formation, and ingrowth into the wound fillet. Eplasty. 2012;11:42-54.

41. Tuncel U, Turan A, Bayrktar MA, Aydin U, Erkorkmaz U. Clinical experience with the use of gauze-based negative pressure wound therapy. Wounds. 2012;24(8):227-233.

42. Dumville JC, Webster J, Evans D, Land L. Negative pressure wound therapy for treating pressure ulcers. Cochrane Database of Systematic Reviews 2015, Issue 5. Art. No.: CD011334. DOI: 10.1002/14651858. CD011334.pub2

43. Dumville JC, Munson C, Christie J. Negative pressure wound therapy for partial-thickness burns. Cochrane Database of Systematic Reviews 2014, Issue 12. Art. No.: CD006215. DOI: 10.1002/14651858.CD006215.pub4

44. Dumville JC, Land L, Evans D, Peinemann F. Negative pressure wound therapy for treating leg ulcers. Cochrane Database of Systematic Reviews 2015, Issue 7. Art. No.: CD011354. DOI: 10.1002/14651858.CD011354.pub2

45. Dumville JC, Hinchliffe RJ, Cullum N, Game F, Stubbs N, Sweeting M, Peinemann F. Negative pressure wound therapy for treating foot wounds in people with diabetes mellitus. Cochrane Database of Systematic Reviews 2013, Issue 10. Art. No.: CD010318. DOI: 10.1002/14651858.CD010318.pub

46. Webster J, Scuffham P, Stankiewicz M, Chaboyer WP. Negative pressure wound therapy for skin grafts and surgical wounds healing by primary intention. Cochrane Database of Systematic Reviews 2014, Issue 10. Art. No.: CD009261. DOI: 10.1002/14651858.CD009261.pub3

47. Dumville JC, Owens GL, Crosbie EJ, Peinemann F, Liu Z. Negative pressure wound therapy for treating surgical wounds healing by secondary intention. Cochrane Database of Systematic Reviews 2015, Issue 6. Art. No.: CD011278. DOI: 10.1002/14651858. CD011278.pub2

48. Joseph E, et al. A prospective randomized trial of vacuum assisted closure versus standard therapy of chronic nonhealing wounds. WOUNDS. 2000; 12(3):60-67.

49. Armstrong DG, Lavery LA. Negative pressure wound therapy after partial diabetic foot amputation: a multicenter, randomized controlled trial. Lancet. 2005;366:1704-1710.

50. Vuerstaek JDD, Vainas T, Wuite J, Nelemans P, Neumann MH, Veraart CJM. State-of-the-art treatment of chronic leg ulcers: a randomized controlled trial comparing vacuum assisted closure (VAC) with modern wound dressings. J Vasc Surg. 2006;44:1029-38.

51. Wanner MB, Schwarzl F, Strub B, Zaech GA, Pierer G. Vacuum-assisted wound closure for cheaper and more comfortable healing of pressure sores: a prospective study. Scand J Plast Reconstr Surg Hand Surg. 2003; 37:28-33.

52. Boerema, I, Meyne NG, Brummelkamp WK, Bouma S, Mensch MH, Kamermans, F, Stern Hanf M, Van Aalderen W. Life without blood. J Cardiovasc Surg. 1960;1:133-146.

53. Rios PE, Hall YP,Shah JB. Hyperbaric oxygen therapy. In: Shah JB et al, Wound Care Certification Study Guide, 2nd edition. North Palm Beach, Florida: Best Publishing Company. 2016; p.231-240.

54. Saltzman HA. Rational normobaric and hyperbaric oxygen therapy. Ann Intern Med. 1967;67:843-852.

55. Knighton DR, Halliday B, Hunt TK. Oxygen as an antibiotic: the effect of inspired oxygen on infection. Arch Surg. 1984;119:199-20.

56. Kenward MA, Alcock SR, McKay IC. Effect of hyperbaric oxyhelium gas on response of bacteria to antimicrobial agents in vitro. Antimicrob Agents Chemother. 1984;26:833-836.

57. Gill AL, Bell CN. Hyperbaric oxygen: its uses, mechanisms of action and outcomes. Q J Med. 2004;97:385–95.

58. Mader JT. Phagocytic killing and hyperbaric oxygen: antibacterial mechanisms. HBO Rev. 1981;2:37-49.

59. Hunt TK, Pai MP. The effect of varying ambient oxygen tensions on wound metabolism and collagen synthesis. Surg Gynecol Obstet. 1972;135:561-567.

60. Knighton DR, Hunt TK, Scheuenstuhl H, Halliday BJ, Werb Z, Banda MJ. Oxygen tension regulates the expression of angiogenesis factor by macrophages. Science. 1983;221:1283-1285.

61. Jensen JA, Hunt TK, Scheuenstuhl H, Banda MJ. Effect of lactate, pyruvate and pH on secretion of angiogenesis and mitogenesis factors by macrophages. Lab Invest. 1986;54:574-8.

62. Asano T, Kaneko E, Shinozaki S, Imai Y, Shibayama M, Chiba T, et al. Hyperbaric oxygen induces basic fibroblast growth factor and hepatocyte growth factor expression, and enhances blood perfusion and muscle regeneration in mouse ischemic hind limbs. Circ J. 2007;71:405-11.

63. Kant TS, Gorti GK, Quan SY, Ho M, Koch RJ. Effect of hyperbaric oxygen on the growth factor profile of fibroblasts. Arc Facial Plast Surg. 2004: 6:31-35.

64. Sheikh AY, Gibson JJ, Rollins MD, Hopf HW, Hussain Z, Hunt TK. Effect of hyperoxia on vascular endothelial growth factor levels in a wound model. Arch Surg. 2000;135:1293-1297.

65. Bonomo SR, Davidson JD, Tyrone JW et al. Enhancement of wound healing by hyperbaric oxygen and transforming growth factor beta3 in a new chronic wound model in aged rabbits. Arch Surg. 2000;135:1148-1153.

66. Thom SR, Bhopale VM, Velazquez OC, Goldstein Lj, Thom LH, Buerk DG, Stem cell mobilization by hyperbaric oxygen. American Journal of Physiology – Heart and Circulatory Physiology. 2006; 290(4): H1378-H1386.

67. Pecoraro RE, Ahroni J, Boyko E, et al. Chronology and determinants of tissue repair in diabetic lower-extremity ulcers. Diabetes. 1991;40:1305-1313.

68. Fife CE, Buyukcakir C, Otto GH, et al. The predictive value of transcutaneous oxygen tension measurement in diabetic lower extremity ulcers treated with hyperbaric oxygen therapy: a retrospective analysis of 1144 patients. Wound Repair Regen. 2002;10:198-207.

69. Fife CE. Hyperbaric oxygen therapy applications in wound care. In: Sheffield PJ, Fife CE, editors. Wound Care Practice. 2nd ed. North Palm Beach, Florida: Best Publishing Company; 2007;p.947-980.

70. Sheffield PJ, Dietz D, Posey KI, et al. [Abstract] Mean PtcO2 values as an outcome predictor in hyperbaric oxygen treatment of hypoxic wounds. Undersea Hyperb Med. 2008;35(4):27.

71. Fife CE, Smart DR, Sheffield PJ, et al. Transcutaneous oximetry in clinical practice: consensus statements from an expert panel based on evidence. Undersea Hyperb Med. 2009;36(1):43-53.

72. Rollins MD, Gibson JJ, Hunt TK, Hopf HW. Wound oxygen levels during hyperbaric oxygen treatment in healings wounds. Undersea Hyperb Med 2006; 33:17-25.

73. Sheffield PJ, Sheffield JC. Complication rates for hyperbaric oxygen therapy patients and their attendants: a 22-year analysis. Proceedings of the Fourteenth International Congress on Hyperbaric Medicine. 2003:312-318.

74. Huang E T, Mansouri J, M. Hassan Murrad et al. A clinical practice guideline for the use of hyperbaric oxygen therapy in treatment of diabetic foot ulcers. UHM. 2015;. 42(3):205-212.

75. Thom SR. Oxidative stress is fundamental to hyperbaric oxygen therapy. J Appl Physiol. 2009;. 106:988-995.

76. Thom SR. Hyperbaric oxygen: its mechanisms and efficacy. Plast Reconstr Surg. 2011; 127(Suppl 1):131S–141S.

77. Robson MC, Hill DP, Woodske ME, et al. Wound healing trajectories as predictors of effectiveness of therapeutic agents. Arch Surg. 2000; 135:773-777.

Chapter 9

PLASTIC SURGERY APPROACH TO WOUND MANAGEMENT AND CLOSURE

Regina M. Fearmonti, MD

KEY CONCEPTS

1. Identify wounds that need surgical closure, and involve your surgeon early. This will help to expedite wound optimization, better prepare the wound and patient for definitive closure, and prevent delay.

2. Venous congestion is the most common cause of flap failure. Early recognition can salvage a threatened flap.

3. Pressure ulcers recur in chronically debilitated patients and those with spinal cord injuries. A "burn no bridges" approach is necessary for flap design in order to preserve options for future closure. If factors predisposing to ulcer development cannot be modified (pre- and postoperatively), surgical closure should not be performed.

CONTENTS

Introduction

Complex and full-thickness wounds, or those requiring replacement of soft tissue, obliteration of dead space, or coverage of exposed bone, tendon, nerves, blood vessels, grafts, implants, hardware, or other vital structures (e.g., brain, pericardium, lung) present a challenge to the wound care team and reconstructive surgeon alike. These wounds present as the result of a trauma, a surgical wound dehiscence, or an extirpative procedure for a malignancy. They are referred to a wound care center at various stages of healing for aid in closure. Some require urgent coverage; others require optimization of the factors leading to their development prior to any attempt at reoperation for definitive closure. Discerning the difference is sometimes difficult. Here we discuss identification and management of these difficult wounds and present basic concepts of surgical wound management and closure.

I. Case study

GM is a 42-year-old male and 20-pack-a-year smoker with osteopetrosis who sustained a 20-foot fall from a construction scaffold. He sustained an open fracture of his left tibia that was treated with open reduction internal fixation. He underwent adjuvant hyperbaric oxygen therapy in a wound clinic for delayed healing at his wound edges and eventual wound dehiscence. Negative-pressure wound therapy was initiated, and the patient was taken back to the operating room for removal of the plate due to nonunion. Serial debridements and bony curretages were performed in the operating room, and smoking cessation was achieved. The patient received a six-week course of culture-specific intravenous antibiotic therapy under the consult of an infectious disease specialist. The distal tibial wound was ultimately closed with a free latissimus flap and skin graft.

II. Types of wounds requiring surgical intervention

Wounds that fail to progress through inflammatory (days 1–6), fibroproliferative (days 4–21), and remodeling (21 days to 1 year) phases of wound healing present to a wound care center as stalled wounds.[(1)] Diagnosis and correction of various metabolic, immunologic, infectious, vascular, and endocrine etiologies as well as judicious use of hyperbaric oxygen therapy and advanced wound care dressings often lead to closure by secondary intention. This relies on the wound healing by its own cellular contraction and epithelialization. This is in contrast to an acute surgical wound, which is closed within hours of creation by primary intention or direct reapproximation of wound edges. Delayed primary closure involves converting a subacute or chronic wound to an acute wound by surgical excision and sharp debridement, allowing it to be closed and heal comparably to primary closure. Stalled wounds often benefit from conversion to an acute phase through surgical debridement.

Chronic wounds with ongoing contamination, exposure to pressure or frictional trauma, active infection, or foreign bodies, even if able to be closed, have a high incidence of dehiscence and recurrence. Treatments should be implemented to decrease the bacterial inoculum in the wound to below $1x10^5$ when possible, and subsequent coverage with a vascularized muscle flap may further decrease the bacterial load and lead to sustained wound closure.[(2)] In cases of osteomyelitis, serial operative debridement to ensure removal of all infected bone can be performed. Culture-specific antibiotics are requisite in the perioperative period to successfully

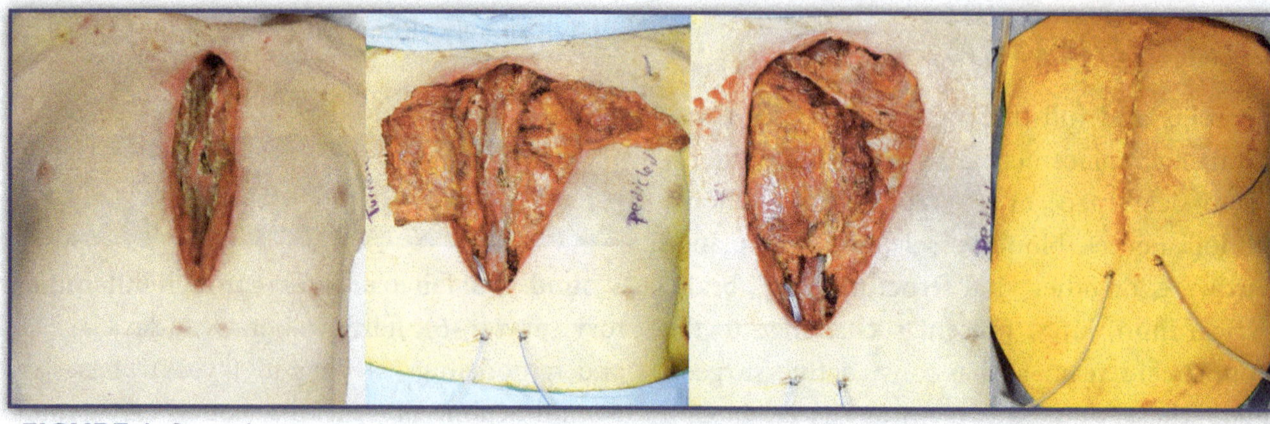

FIGURE 1. Sternal wound dehiscence following a bypass. Left to right: following debridement, and with elevated right pectoralis turnover and left pedicled pectoralis myofascial flaps. Flaps placed over sternal defect and to fill dead space, followed by delayed skin closure.

eradicate the chronic infection. Coverage by a flap (regional or free) should then be planned concomitant with the final debridement. Flap coverage leads to obliteration of the space left by the resected bone by vascularized, healthy tissue as well as stable wound coverage (Figure 1).

Nonhealing wounds associated with vascular insufficiency often require extremity amputation when salvage measures fail. If revascularization does salvage an extremity, the restored macroscopic blood flow may still not provide sufficient microvascular perfusion to heal a large wound. Flap coverage, which carries with it its own tissue and microcirculation, is often still necessary.

Radiation induces chronic, irreparable injury to the affected tissue. These wounds do not respond to local wound care as regenerative abilities have been compromised. Treatment requires wide debridement of necrotic soft tissue and bone where possible, which often exposes vital structures. Local and regional flaps are often not feasible if they are harvested from the zone of radiation injury. Microvascular free flaps are often required to provide vascular coverage, though even these present a challenge, as recipient vessels are also damaged by radiation. Likewise, the radiated wound periphery where the flap is inset may experience delayed healing and dehiscence along the flap margin. These are some of the most difficult wounds to treat. Figure 2 illustrates an algorithm for closure of complex wounds.

III. Wound optimization and management

There are a multitude of factors that complicate wound healing. Those characteristics that make patients less-than-ideal surgical candidates are also the very factors that contribute to surgical complications and wound dehiscence. Ideally, a surgical candidate should be optimized prior to any elective surgical intervention. Patients may present for urgent or even emergent surgery, however, following trauma, an open fracture, or an acute vascular or cardiopulmonary event. These patients are at risk for wound breakdown in the postoperative period, and when dehiscence does occur, they present challenges to the wound care team. In patients with an active malignancy, on chemotherapy, with some inherited conditions, or with history of radiation exposure, the inciting morbidity cannot be corrected. We shift focus from correcting to optimizing them for a definitive stage of closure or reconstruction.

Genetic factors that complicate healing include abnormalities in collagen and elastin

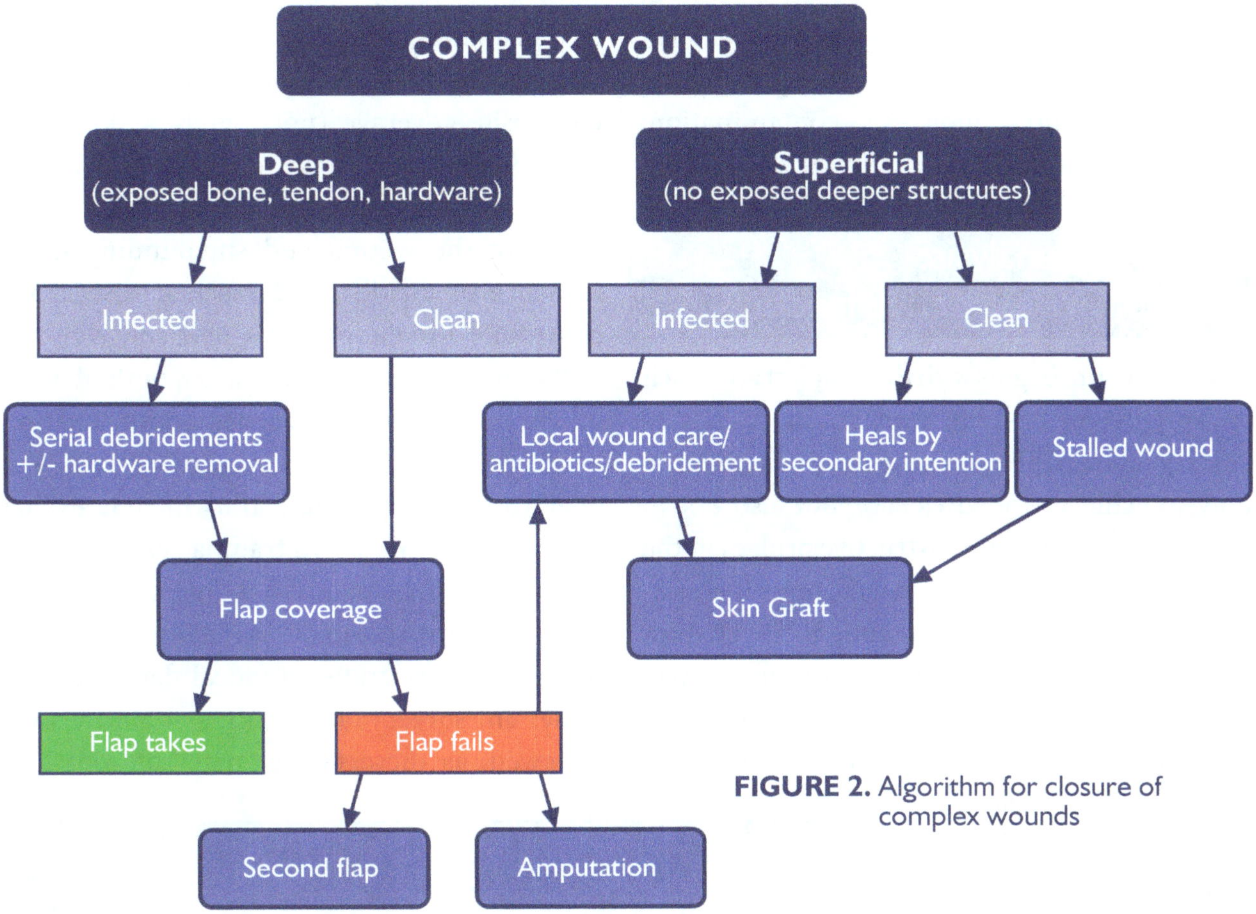

FIGURE 2. Algorithm for closure of complex wounds

production and breakdown. Patients may present with systemic problems (aneurysms) and slow healing. Examples include pseudoxanthoma elasticum (increased collagen breakdown), cutis hyperelastica (Ehlers-Danlos syndrome), progeria, Werner's syndrome, and epidermolysis bullosa.

In contrast, active smokers or poorly managed diabetics present an opportunity to remove those factors that contributed to the wound complication. Those factors that *can* be corrected *should* be corrected in the perioperative phase. Acute exposure to nicotine (active smokers and exposure to secondhand smoke) incites norepinephrine-induced skin vasoconstriction and impairment of endothelium-dependent skin vasorelaxation, which at a critical level can lead to wound dehiscence or flap epidermolysis in an already compromised wound bed. Smoking irreversibly increases the risk of flap necrosis up to eight weeks after preoperative cessation[(3)] Smoking cessation for a minimum of eight weeks preoperative and eight weeks postoperative allows the return of the wound environment to a more favorable state. Other correctible factors include nutritional deficiencies such as caloric and protein malnutrition and vitamin deficiencies; supplements typically only help when deficiencies exist.

Other drug use, including steroids, antineoplastic agents, and anti-inflammatory medications can also be adjusted or halted. Consultation with the patient's rheumatologist or medical oncologist may determine safety in initiating a break from those drugs that are halting the healing process or interruption in administration in the perioperative period. Local wound factors can also be targeted, such as oxygen delivery to tissue, vascular inflow and outflow, infection, moisture, contamination, and free radicals.

IV. Defect analysis: the reconstructive ladder

Wound closure begins with the simplest approach and progresses to more complex modalities as efficacy dictates. The goal of each approach is not only to achieve wound closure, but also not to burn any proverbial reconstructive bridges in the event wound dehiscence or recurrence necessitates further operative intervention. The goals of surgical reconstruction are preservation and restoration of form and function while minimizing morbidity and avoiding creation of a secondary wound defect. Replacing "like with like" often leads to an aesthetically and functionally superior result in the end. The optimal reconstructive option can be determined through a systematic analysis of wound type, defect size and thickness, medical and functional status of the patient, and available reconstructive options.

Wound defect evaluation should include analysis of wound surface area after adequate debridement as well as those components missing or exposed in the defect, e.g., skin, mucosa, subcutaneous tissue, muscle, nerve, artery, vein, cartilage, or bone. A full-thickness defect will require obliteration of dead space with the chosen reconstructive option. Likewise, neurovascular structures, vascular anastomoses, bone, and hardware or prostheses require durable, composite coverage (not merely a skin graft) for protection and to prevent exposure. Reconstructive choice also hinges on the vascular status of the wound and surrounding tissue. Presence of unaddressed vascular disease can contribute to venous stasis and congestion as well as inadequate arterial inflow, both of which hinder healing by secondary intention and limit local and regional flap coverage options. Preoperative workup should thus include evaluation of zone of injury in trauma cases to ensure adequate debridement of nonviable tissue as well as ensure an intact regional microcirculation to support grafts and local flaps. Previous radiation, surgery, and trauma should also be reviewed, as these factors may rule out local

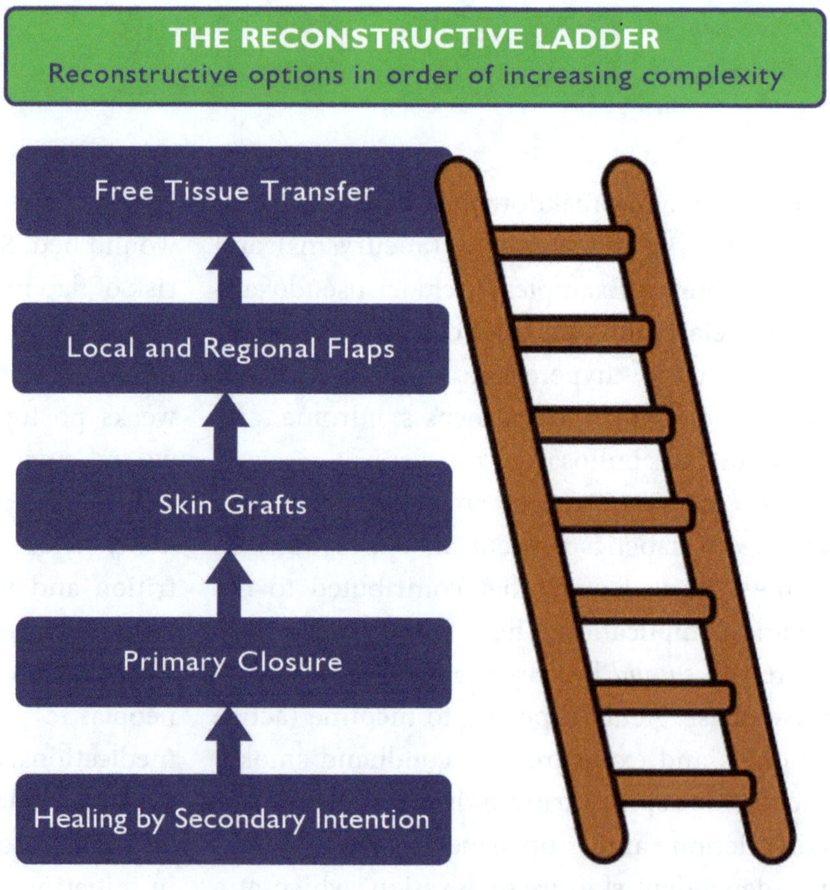
THE RECONSTRUCTIVE LADDER
Reconstructive options in order of increasing complexity
Free Tissue Transfer
Local and Regional Flaps
Skin Grafts
Primary Closure
Healing by Secondary Intention

FIGURE 3. The reconstructive ladder

coverage options. In addition, flap coverage often involves sacrifice of certain muscles or muscle groups. The resultant impact will be tolerated very differently in a paraplegic versus an athlete. Functional status, lifestyle, and rehabilitative capacity of the patient require consideration. Complex reconstruction, with a complex and often lengthy recovery, may not be the best option in a patient with limited life expectancy, end-stage cancer or organ failure, or cognitive dysfunction.

Healing by secondary intention comprises the first rung of the reconstructive ladder. This is facilitated by use of advanced wound dressings, splinting for immobilization, negative-pressure wound therapy, and adjunctive hyperbaric oxygen therapy. When a wound cannot or will not close on its own in a timely fashion, primary closure can be attempted. Basic principles involve adequate tissue mobilization to allow for tension-free closure, obliteration of dead space, and adequate drainage, as well as care to create well-vascularized flaps to advance over the wound defect. In cases where a wound bed has fully granulated and only epithelium is required, both full- and split-thickness skin grafts can be placed over the defect for coverage. Full-thickness coverage is needed when neurovascular structures, bone, tendon, or hardware lie at the base of the wound. Local flaps recruit tissue from an adjacent area to cover a wound, whereas free flaps recruit tissue from remote locations. Figure 3 depicts the logical progression up the reconstructive ladder and provides a framework for closure based on wound type.

V. Skin grafts

For wounds that cannot be closed primarily, skin grafts are the next option for wound closure. A skin graft is an autologous graft, meaning the graft recipient is also the donor. It consists of epidermis with some papillary dermis (split-thickness skin graft) or the entire layer of dermis (full-thickness skin graft). The dermis contains epithelial appendages (sebaceous glands, hair follicles, sweat glands with sympathetic innervation). Full-thickness skin grafts thus may maintain the ability to produce sweat and grow hair and may even regain sensation.

Grafts are completely devascularized and rely on vascularization from the bed into which they are placed. All grafts contract immediately upon harvest from the donor site (primary contracture) and again after revascularization in their final recipient site (secondary contracture). The more dermis a graft contains, the more contraction that is observed. A full-thickness skin graft contracts more on initial harvest (primary contracture) due to recoil of the elastin contained in

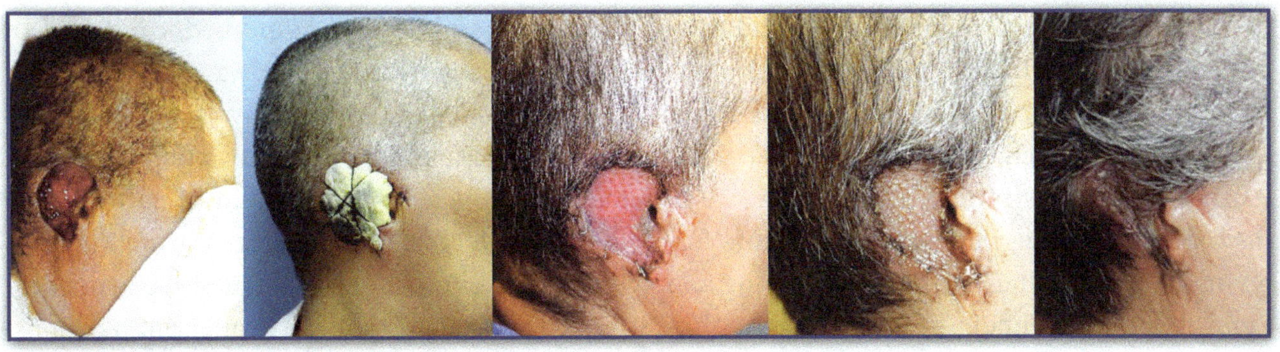

Two weeks postoperative Four weeks postoperative Two months postoperative

FIGURE 4. Left: total right ear defect following resection of cutaneous malignancy. Defect repaired with meshed split-thickness skin graft secured with a tie-on Xeroform bolster. Left to right: note progressive secondary contraction of the graft and persistent "cobblestoned" appearance of meshed interstices.

its dermal elements, yet less upon healing (secondary contracture) than a split-thickness skin graft. The thinner the split-thickness skin graft, the greater the secondary contracture as a result of myofibroblast activity (Figure 4). This can result in hypertrophic scarring, with this process demonstrated in granulating wounds left to heal secondarily, which exhibit the greatest degree of contracture. Split-thickness skin grafts are typically .0125 inches in thickness, but this can be adjusted based upon dermal quality and needs. Grafts can be meshed or applied as sheet grafts. Meshing allows expansion, drainage, and increased surface area of coverage. Sheet grafts lack those advantages, but heal without the irregular, cobblestone appearance, which is an advantage in cosmetically sensitive recipient areas like the face.

Graft "take" relies on vascular ingrowth for nutrient supply. Skin grafts will not take on exposed bone or tendon devoid of their respective periosteum or peritenon. Burring down of exposed bone in the case of cranial reconstruction to bleeding periosteum, however, may support grafting. Close coaptation of the graft to its recipient bed is essential. Seroma or hematoma formation under a graft will compromise survival. Likewise, shear forces, dessication, or too moist of a recipient bed environment can lead to graft loss. Proper environment can be maintained with use of a petroleum-impregnated tie-on bolster or negative pressure wound therapy. In regard to the skin graft donor site, the lateral thigh, buttock, and scalp are ideal donor sites that can be reharvested following epithelialization, which typically occurs within 7–10 days. These less conspicuous sites are more forgiving for the resultant pathologic scarring and hypo-/hyperpigmentation that can occur. They heal best with the application of a semiocclusive dressing (Xeroform, Adaptic, Tegaderm) that prevents dessication and decreases pain. Full-thickness skin graft donor sites contain the entire donor site dermis and leave exposed subcutaneous tissue at the base. They are closed primarily. Optimal harvest sites include the preauricular region, upper eyelid (as part of a blepharoplasty), hypothenar eminence of the hand, lower abdomen, and antecubital fossa.

Principles of skin grafts can be applied to the use of allografts and skin substitutes for temporary wound coverage. In the event a skin graft fails to take, in the absence of infection a failed graft may remain on a wound and protect the recipient bed from dessication and trauma until definitive closure can be achieved. Human allografts (cadaveric) and xenografts (porcine, bovine) become vascularized but are rejected by the recipient after two weeks. By the same mechanism, they protect and temporize the wound until comorbidities can be corrected.

VI. Local and regional flaps

A "flap," unlike a graft, carries with it its own blood supply and is used when the recipient bed lacks vascularity to nurture a graft. Flaps are needed to cover vital structures, reconstruct full-thickness defects, and provide bulk over bony prominences. Flaps may contain skin only, skin and fascia (adipofascial), muscle (myofascial), muscle and skin (myocutaneous), and bone (osseous), and, through carrying well vascularized tissue to the wound bed, can be used to cover vital structures, hardware, or even control infection. Muscle flaps have superior bacterial clearance and offer a viable option to salvage hardware when removal would impart significant morbidity (e.g., spinal instrumentation).[2]

A skin flap consists of skin and subcutaneous tissue that maintains its attachment to its donor site by a vascular bridge. These thin flaps are often used for podiatric defects without exposed bone or joint and for facial defects resulting from Mohs

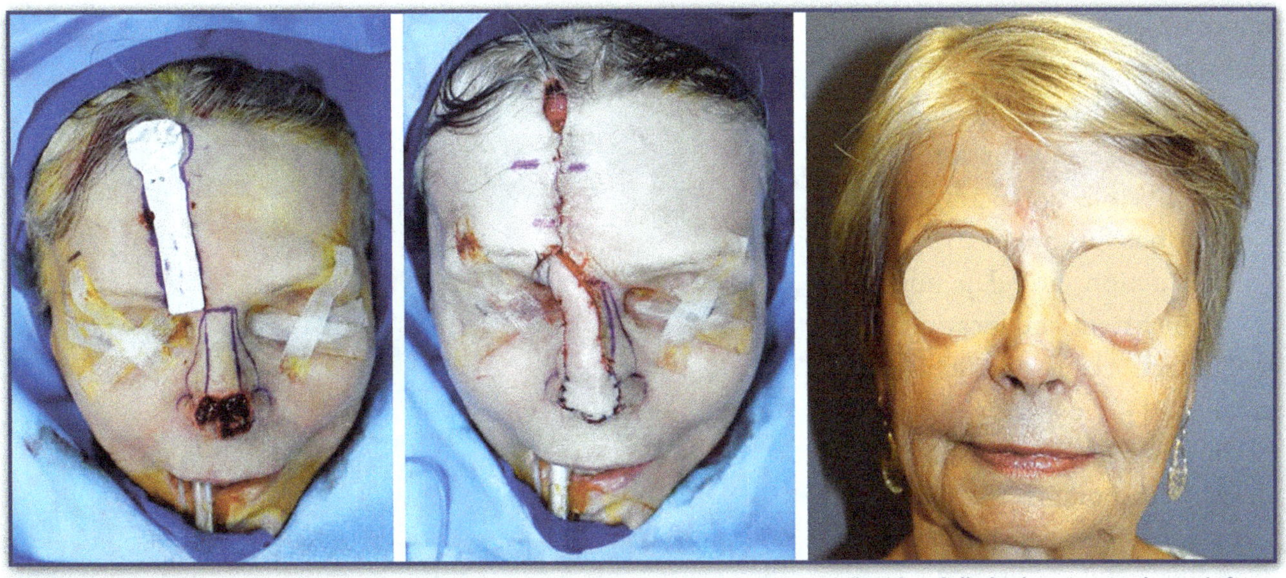

FIGURE 5. Delay phenomenon. Left: design for paramedian forehead flap for full-thickness nasal tip defect. Middle: blood supply from right supratrochlear artery is left intact for delay phenomenon; flap will be divided in three weeks and inset. This allows time for choke vessels to open to optimize venous outflow from flap. Right: final appearance at three months postoperative. Distal donor site on forehead healed by secondary intention.

surgery. These local flaps are either rotational (rotate around a pivot point) or advancement (moved directly into the defect) in their design. Their donor sites can be closed primarily by direct closure, with a skin graft, or with a second flap. Rotational flaps create a standing cone deformity (a "dogear") around their pivot pint; it is important to avoid pressure at this site, and debulking should not be attempted, as this is the flap's blood supply. The most distal tip of both rotational and advancement flaps carries that skin that is furthest from its blood supply. It is this tissue that is inset over the wound and most critical to closure. We often employ a "delay phenomenon" by staging flap elevation from its donor site and ultimate inset into the recipient wound bed. This creates an ischemia in the flap that recruits the opening of "choke vessels" that are normally closed, thus rerouting blood flow to the ischemic portion of the flap and even triggering angiogenesis.[4] The flap is then inset and donor defect closed in a separate procedure, approximately three weeks later. The paramedian forehead flap illustrates the augmentation of flap inflow and outflow by the delay phenomenon (Figure 5).

Too tight of an inset or closure may also contribute to venous congestion and ischemia at the flap tip. Struggling flaps may exhibit epidermolysis at this area, which may evolve into blistering and dehiscence. Close monitoring of the flap in the postoperative period by the surgeon aids in early identification of a problem. Hyperbaric oxygen therapy and suture/staple removal to remove tension from the flap may halt these processes in local flaps.

The most common regional, or pedicled, flaps, used to reconstruct trunk defects include the pectoralis major and the latissimus dorsi flap. Both can be taken as muscle-only flaps or with a skin paddle. The pectoralis major receives its blood supply from internal mammary artery perforators, which allow it to be transferred as a turnover flap, and in cases where a coronary bypass has sacrificed that vessel, it can be transferred on the thoracromial artery as a pedicled flap. Both have application in the closure of sternal wounds as well as proximal upper extremity and neck defects (Figure 1, Figure 6). The latissimus dorsi flap is based upon the thoracodorsal artery and vein, and its long pedicle (up to 15 cm) makes it an optimal flap for use in coverage of upper extremity wounds as well as in breast reconstruction and chest wall coverage (Figure 7).

Options for lower extremity reconstruction are dependent upon the extent and location of the defect. Local muscle flaps are useful in covering defects in the proximal or mid-third of the leg. The medial gastrocnemius flap offers robust coverage of wounds of the proximal tibia (Figure 8). It is usually harvested as a myofascial flap (no skin paddle) to allow primary closure of the donor defect, and it is covered with a skin graft. For defects of the knee, it can be harvested with the lateral gastrocnemius flap to provide more lateral coverage.

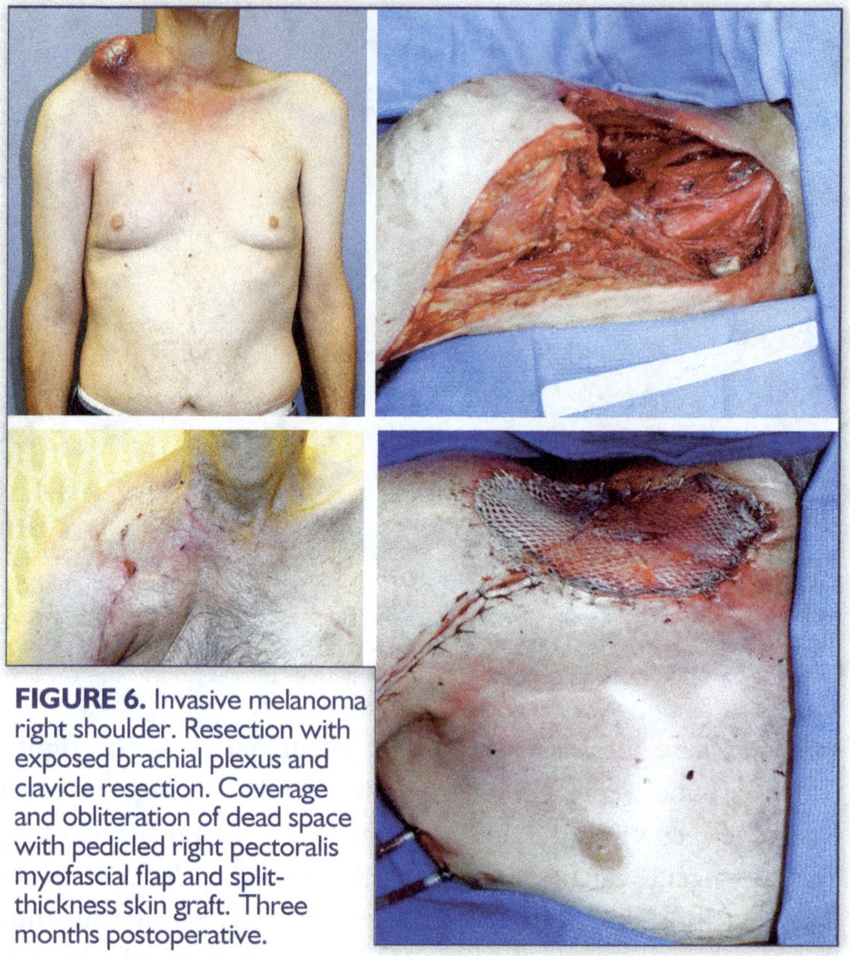

FIGURE 6. Invasive melanoma right shoulder. Resection with exposed brachial plexus and clavicle resection. Coverage and obliteration of dead space with pedicled right pectoralis myofascial flap and split-thickness skin graft. Three months postoperative.

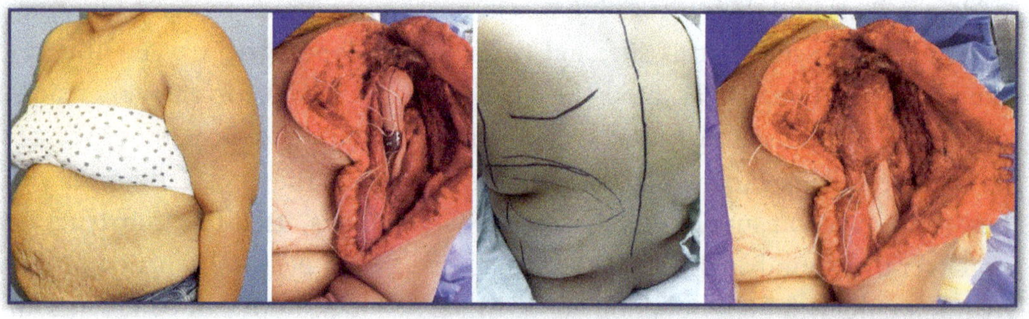

FIGURE 7. Left humeral osteosarcoma. Left to right: Humerus resected and prosthesis in place. Design for left pedicled latissimus dorsi flap myofascial to cover hardware. Flap tunneled into defect to cover hardware and obliterate dead space.

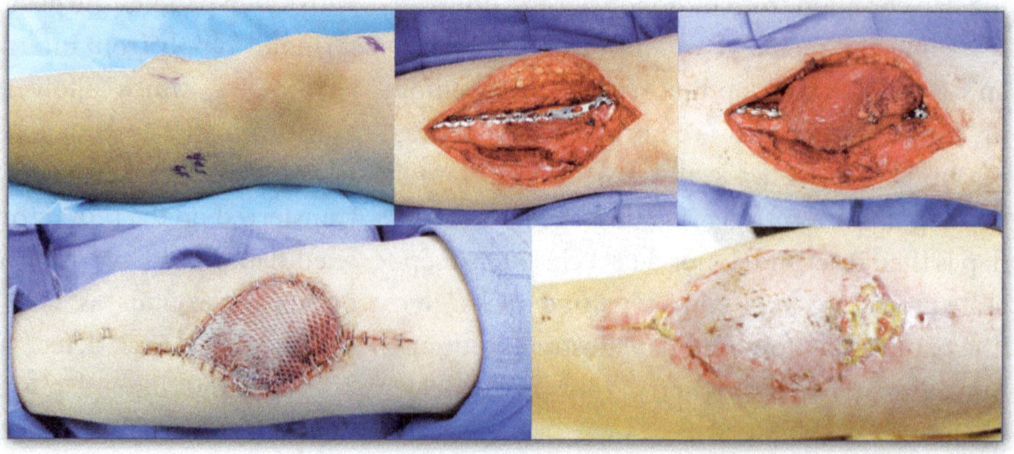

FIGURE 8. Left tibial osteosarcoma. Left to right: Resected and allograft with hardware in place. Covered with medial gastrocnemius myofascial flap and split-thickness skin graft. Three weeks postoperative.

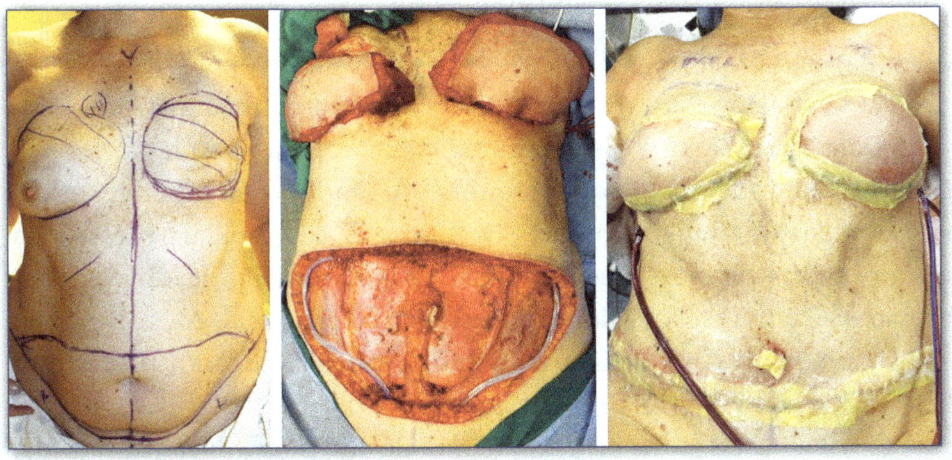

FIGURE 9. Left: design for free TRAM flap for bilateral breast reconstruction. Middle: flaps elevated and tacked in place. Right: closure of abdominal donor site and flap inset.

VII. Distant flaps

In the current era of microvascular proficiency, and with advances in flap monitoring, free-flap reconstruction is no longer a last resort but rather a reliable method of full-thickness wound coverage and even limb salvage. Whereas local and regional flaps are helpful in closing cutaneous defects, more complex wounds often involve more complex methods of closure. Unlike regional pedicled flaps with a limited arc of rotation due to their attachment to their blood supply, free tissue transfer allows tissue and its vascular leash to be carried to any site of the body with a patent recipient artery and vein. At the site, arteries are sewn, or anastomosed, to arteries and veins are anastomosed to veins to restore flap inflow and outflow, respectively, using a 9-0 nylon suture or smaller. The flap is then inset into the defect. Wounds of the distal third of the tibia, some foot defects, and head and neck defects have deficient or no local options for closure. In addition, a larger flap carrying more tissue than available locally is often needed. The transverse rectus abdominis myocutaneous flap and the muscle- and fascial-sparing deep inferior epigastric perforator flap carry an entire hemiabdomen based upon the superior epigastric vessels (as a pedicled flap) or the inferior epigastric vessels (as a free flap). It is a large flap that can be harvested for complete chest wall coverage as well as for breast reconstruction, and the donor site can be closed primarily (Figure 9). The latissimus dorsi can also be harvested as a free flap for use in both total scalp and lower extremity reconstruction.

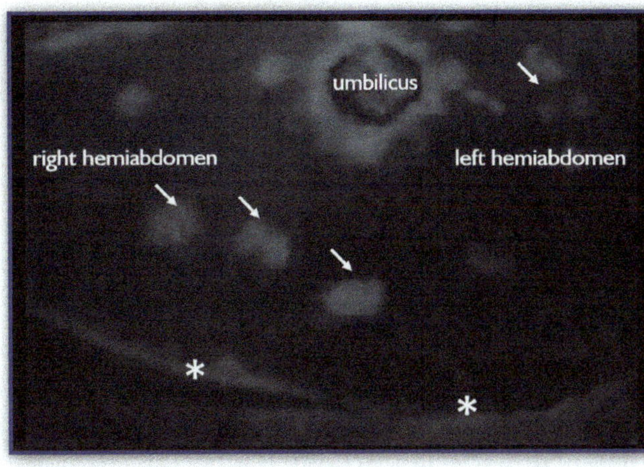

FIGURE 10. Intraoperative indocyanine green angiography in the free TRAM harvest from previous patient detailing location of arterial perforators (arrows) and bleeding edge of flap periphery (asterisks). This helps with intraoperative decision making on what vessels to base the flap, and, after inset, what portions of the flap to trim. Note the position of the umbilicus for reference.

Flap survival postoperatively hinges on maintenance of a moist environment along the flap edges, avoidance of local hypothermia, early detection and correction of venous congestion or arterial inflow obstruction, avoidance of pressure on the flap tissues, and protection of the microanatomoses. Patients undergoing free-flap reconstruction often have bulky dressings or splints placed to offload or immobilize the tissues and prevent any disruption of the delicate vascular anastomoses. These dressings often have a window for flap monitoring, which may include an implantable Doppler probe placed across the microanastamosis, an external skin paddle that can be assessed with a pencil Doppler probe and evaluated for any visible signs of congestion, or a transcutaneous oximeter. All of these devices help to detect early flap compromise, which often presents as venous congestion. Preoperative and even intraoperative angiography is now used to ensure the presence of suitable recipient vessels for free tissue transfer. Fluorescein, and now indocyanine green angiography, can be applied to ensure adequate microcirculation all the way out to the flap edges (Figure 10). Similar indocyanine-based technologies are becoming available in wound clinics to assess tissue inflow and outflow and are being studied to measure response to interventions.

Whereas removing tension on a local flap may help with flap ischemia, any signs or congestion or ischemia in a free flap mandates operative evaluation and often exploration. (Further information on hyperbaric oxygen therapy in skin grafts and flaps can be found in Chapter 8: Evidence-Based Use of Advanced Wound Care Modalities in Chronic Wound Patients.)

Early surgical exploration can often salvage a threatened, congested flap, and patients are often placed on postoperative anticoagulation if clot is detected intraoperatively. In the event a flap cannot be salvaged, patients often undergo a second free flap for coverage after a hematologic workup ensues to rule out a hypercoagulable state and correct any conditions that may have contributed to flap failure. Negative-pressure wound therapy and wound care assists in managing the interim defect.

VIII. Pressure ulcers

Pressure ulcers are best defined as tissue injuries resulting from unrelieved pressure on a bony prominence and occur when external compressive forces exceed capillary pressure in the soft tissue (12–32 mmHg), leading to capillary congestion and ischemia. A cone-shaped pattern of injury is observed, with the highest pressure, and hence the greatest injury, tracking deep to the muscle and bone, in contrast to the more visible, circumferential cutaneous wound. Supine patients present with sacral, scalp, shoulder, and heel ulcers, wheelchair-bound patients appreciate ischial ulcers, and trochanteric ulcers develop in patients who lie in a lateral position (especially in those with hip contractures). Aside from constant pressure at the site, other factors playing a role in ulcer formation include poor nutrition, incontinence with exposure to moisture and feces, dementia, friction, and shear forces from bed sheets and lifts. Flaps fail under the same conditions in which ulcers originate – from untreated infections, ongoing soilage, poor nutrition, and ongoing trauma from patient bathing and transport. The dictum that the best time to operate on a pressure ulcer is when the ulcer is improving holds true, as it is evidence that outside factors have been adequately addressed, and the site is now optimized for surgical closure.

Following adequate ulcer staging, patient optimization, and correction of all modifiable factors, a comprehensive and patient-specific strategy should be developed, and this must include postoperative placement and care. When developing a surgical plan, one must keep in mind that every flap surgery burns a bridge for subsequent future surgeries. Ulcers recur in spinal cord injury patients, and as the first flap is usually the most optimal flap, every measure should be employed to ensure its take and survival.

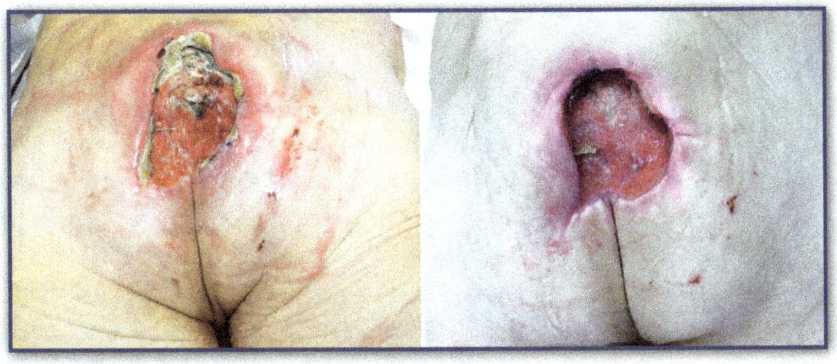

FIGURE 11. Stage IV sacral pressure ulcer before debridement and exhibiting periwound maceration (left) and after debridement, partial sacrectomy, and negative-pressure wound therapy (right). This wound is now optimized for flap closure.

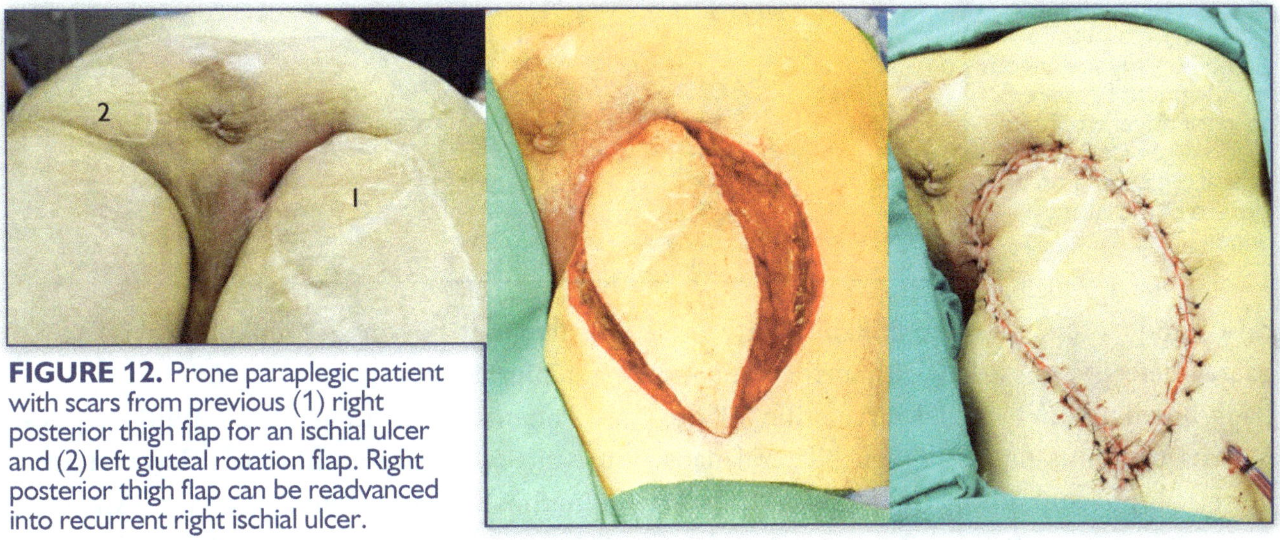

FIGURE 12. Prone paraplegic patient with scars from previous (1) right posterior thigh flap for an ischial ulcer and (2) left gluteal rotation flap. Right posterior thigh flap can be readvanced into recurrent right ischial ulcer.

Debridement is performed in the operating room, and, as in cases of osteomyelitis, is often staged to allow a second (and third) look to ensure excision of all nonviable tissue and bone. Quantitative tissue cultures are obtained to guide perioperative antibiotic coverage. Ostectomy, or removal of the underlying bony prominence, is performed judiciously to prevent skeletal instability and redistribution of pressure points. Wound dressings or negative-pressure wound therapy can be applied to assist with granulation, yet adhesive dressings and tape must not contribute to further breakdown of the periwound (Figure 11).

As ulcers result from tissue ischemia and loss, primary closure is not an option. Primary closure and skin grafts do not obliterate a dead space, cannot be performed without undue tension, and will not adequately pad a bony prominence. Closure strategy is influenced by ulcer location as well as scars from previous surgeries performed. Flap design should allow ulcer coverage and not prevent the use of other flaps in the future. In addition, incisions should be designed so as to not traverse bony prominences. Local fasciocutaneous and myocutaneous flaps bring vascularized tissue and coverage to the site and are the most common flaps employed. Myocutanous flaps provide more padding than fascial flaps and are the best option for larger, deeper ulcers, yet they cause greater donor site deformity and may relay functional compromise in ambulatory patients.

Ischial ulcers can be closed with medially, laterally, and posteriorly based thigh flaps and gluteal flaps (Figure 12). The inferior gluteal myocutaneous flap employs only the inferior aspect of the gluteus maximus based on the inferior gluteal artery and offers less debilitation to ambulatory patients, especially when

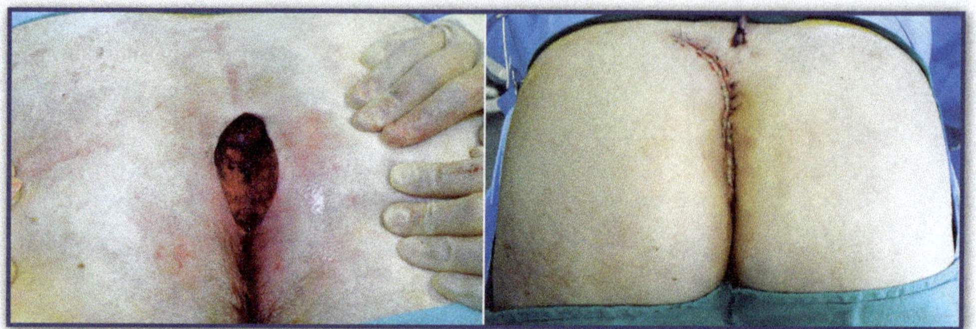

FIGURE 13. Left gluteal rotation flap

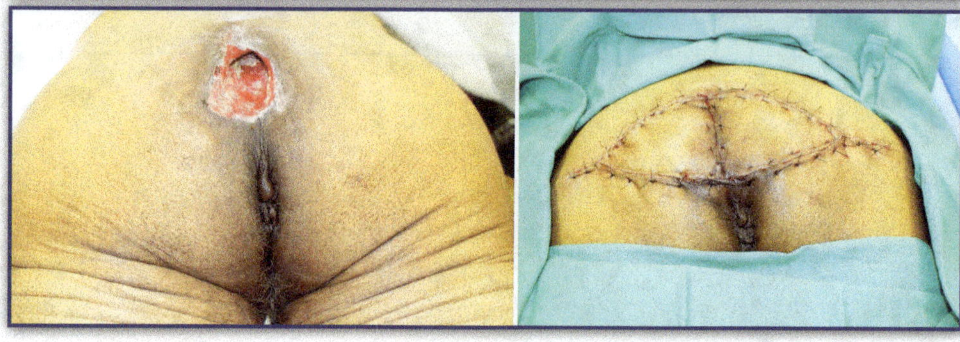

FIGURE 14. Left, a Stage IV sacral pressure ulcer. Right, bilateral gluteal V-Y myocutaneous advancement flaps are used for coverage. Note tension-free closure at gluteal crease and primary closure of the lateral donor sites.

raised and closed as a rotation flap (Figure 13). Sacral defects are closed with myocutaneous flaps based upon the dual circulation of the gluteus maximus muscle. Often bilateral flaps are employed and advanced in a V-Y fashion ("V"-shaped flap, with donor site closed as a "Y") to allow for tension-free closure (Figure 14). When unavailable, lumbosacral flaps based on lumbosacral perforating vessels can be used to close more superficial ulcers. Trochanteric ulcers are best treated with a tensor fascia lata (TFL) flap. Harvested with the L1-L3 nerve roots and the lateral femoral cutaneous nerve, this flap may be sensate in patients with spinal cord injuries below L3.

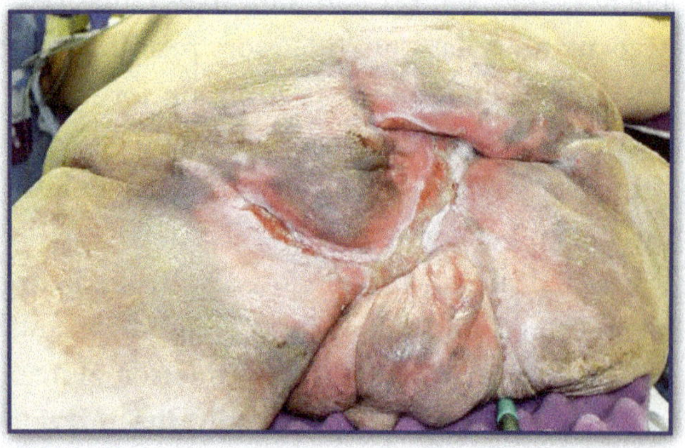

FIGURE 15. Failed right total thigh (fillet) flap in a paraplegic patient with recurrent Stage IV bilateral ischial and sacral pressure ulcers. Note periwound maceration and previous donor site scars.

Patients presenting with multiple pressure ulcers, especially those who have endured numerous prior procedures, may have exhausted all local options. Pelvectomies and fillet flaps, in which the femur is removed to create a total thigh flap to close a defect, may be the best options (Figure 15). This again emphasizes the need to correct all predisposing factors in the preoperative period (social issues, placement issues, behavioral issues, contractures) before any surgical treatment is offered for closure of an otherwise clean, stable wound.

IX. Postoperative care

Postoperative care should be performed by the operating surgeon, who is familiar with the procedure performed, can assess graft and flap take or viability, and has knowledge of the location of flap blood supply as well as what lies deep to any surgical drain or vacuum-assisted closure device. The surgeon's involvement in the postoperative care helps in achieving the most optimal outcome. The *first* operation performed for closure is often the *best* operation, using the optimal flap and best donor site. Any dehiscences or flap/graft losses that mandate operative revisions burn a major reconstructive bridge. Likewise, careful postoperative monitoring and identification of a struggling graft or flap can allow early intervention and possible salvage.

Nutrition and medical, psychological, and rehabilitative care should continue in the postoperative period. Low air-loss mattresses should be employed to alleviate pressure on all flaps and donor sites. Absorptive, nonocclusive dressings are employed to prevent maceration, and splints are used in extremities as needed to protect the flap. Drains placed intraoperatively should be well secured, monitored, and ultimately removed by the operating surgeon. Culture-specific antibiotic therapy should be implemented under the guidance of an infectious disease specialist. Continued multidisciplinary care can minimize wound dehiscence and graft/flap loss and decrease the acuity of those surgical wounds that present to wound care centers and for hospital readmission.

Summary

Management of complex wounds requires proper and timely analysis of the defect and a team-based approach. An acute wound subjected to environment factors detrimental to healing should have these factors addressed and corrected prior to definitive plans for coverage, if possible. An acute wound that fails to respond to these interventions or threatens the patient's life or limb may benefit from urgent surgical intervention in anticipation of a challenging postoperative course and increased recurrence rate. A chronic wound similarly commands correct diagnosis, recognition, and correction of its contributing factors before closure. Collaboration of the wound care team with a plastic and reconstructive surgeon is paramount to practicing the "burn no bridges" approach and may expedite wound closure and lower hospital readmission rates.

Review questions

1. **Regarding the reconstructive ladder, the simplest, first-line option for wound closure is:**

    a. healing by secondary intention
    b. a split-thickness skin graft
    c. a local pedicled flap
    d. free tissue transfer
    e. a full-thickness skin graft

2. ***True/False.*** The presence of more dermal elements in a skin graft translates into more graft contraction.

3. **On postoperative Day 3, a patient who underwent a free flap for wound coverage presents to wound clinic, and exam reveals the flap to have a mottled appearance consistent with venous congestion (yet with dopplerable arterial signals present). The most appropriate first treatment is:**

    a. administer hyperbaric oxygen therapy STAT
    b. apply nitropaste and other topical venous dilators
    c. debride the nonviable flap and commence negative-pressure wound therapy
    d. start oral antibiotic therapy.
    e. call the plastic surgeon STAT; this patient needs to return to the operating room for exploration

4. ***True/False.*** A graft, unlike a flap, carries with it its own blood supply and does not rely on the recipient wound bed for vascular ingrowth.

5. ***True/False.*** Debridement and primary closure should be attempted as a first-line closure option for all pressure ulcers.

ANSWERS: 1) a
2) True
3) e
4) False
5) False

References

1. Goldman R. Growth factor and chronic wound healing: past, present, and future. Adv Skin Wound Care. 2004;17:24-5.
2. Mathes S, Alpert B, Chang N. Use of the muscle flap in chronic osteomyelitis: experimental and clinical correlation. Plast Reconstr Surg. 1982;69:815.
3. Manchio JV, Litchfield CR, Sati S, et al. Duration of smoking cessation and its impact on skin flap survival. Plast Reconstr Surg. 2009;124(4):1105-17.
4. Dhar SC, Taylor GI. The delay phenomenon: the story unfolds. Plast Reconstr Surg. 1999;104(7):2079-91.

Section 3

PATHOPHYSIOLOGY, DIAGNOSIS, AND MANAGEMENT OF SPECIAL WOUND PATIENTS

Editor - Kelly Johnson-Arbor, MD, FACEP, FUHM, FACMT

Chapter 10
DIABETIC FOOT ULCERS

Javier La Fontaine, DPM, MS
Suzanne Van Asten, MD
Lawrence Lavery, DPM, MPH

KEY CONCEPTS

1. Epidemiology
   a) Diabetes is the single most common underlying cause of lower-extremity amputation in the United States.
   b) The risk of lower-extremity amputation in diabetics is 15 to 46 times higher than in nondiabetic patients.
   c) After the initial amputation, the risk of re-amputation or amputation of the contralateral extremity is also high.
   d) The five-year survival rate after a lower-extremity amputation ranges from 41% to 70%.
2. Contributory factors to diabetic foot ulcers (DFUs)
   a) The majority of studies suggest that a diabetic foot ulcer most likely develops in patients with poorly controlled blood sugar.
   b) The etiology of ulcerations in diabetes is associated with the presence of peripheral sensory neuropathy and repetitive trauma due to normal walking activities to areas on the foot that are subject to moderate or high pressures and shear.
   c) The three types of ulcerations are neuropathic, neuro-ischemic, and ischemic.
   d) Neuropathy is one of the most common risk factors for lower-extremity complications.
   e) A decreased ABI also increases the patient's risk for complications in wound healing.

3. Diagnostic considerations

   a) Patients with diabetes can have a unique pattern of atherosclerosis, causing vascular calcifications that limit the effectiveness of the ABI (Monckeberg's sclerosis).

   b) Home temperature evaluation demonstrated a 3- to 10-fold reduction in re-ulceration compared to standard prevention practices.

   c) Toe-brachial index values less than 0.7 are usually considered diagnostic for lower-extremity PAD.

   d) Infections must be diagnosed clinically rather than microbiologically.

   e) Most patients with a diabetic foot infection (DFI) have diminished signs of a local inflammatory response and may not have fever or high WBC count.

   f) The gold standard for diagnosing osteomyelitis is bone biopsy and culture.

   g) MRI has been suggested as the modality of choice in determining the extent of infection.

4. Treatment

   a) Offloading therapy is a key part of the treatment plan for diabetic foot ulcers.

   b) Use of a TCC is considered the gold standard for offloading the foot.

   c) Higher healing rates have been observed in patients who have had more frequent debridement.

   d) The long-term outcome of this "prophylactic" surgery in high-risk diabetic patients (Risk Group 3) were uniformly good with approximately 96% remaining ulcer free at a mean of three years follow-up.

   e) Lengthening the Achilles tendon is indicated when short Achilles tendon limits ankle joint dorsiflexion.

   f) Education message to patients is to inspect their feet, to avoid going barefoot, avoid hot surfaces, avoid hot water, and seek professional foot care on a regular basis.

CONTENTS

Introduction

There are approximately 26 million people in the U.S. who have diabetes mellitus (DM), which is the eighth leading cause of death in this country.[133] It is estimated more than 640 million people will have diabetes worldwide in 2040. About 50% of patients with uncontrolled DM would develop diabetic polyneuropathy or diabetic peripheral neuropathy due to the damage of their nerve fibers, which significantly affects their activities of daily living. Diabetic foot ulcer is the leading cause for nontraumatic lower extremity amputation, accounting for 70,000 cases annually. In addition, diabetic foot ulcer patients have a low survival prognosis, with a 3-year cumulative mortality rate of 28%, and rates among amputated patients approaching 50%. These wounds often require extensive healing time and are associated with increased risk for infections and other sequelae that can result in severe and costly outcomes.

I. Case study

A 72-year-old Caucasian male with DM has had an ulceration of his right foot for 10 weeks. He had a transmetatarsal amputation six years ago secondary to a foot infection. Past medical history includes uncontrolled type 2 DM for 16 years (A1c= 8.5), depression, and smoking. He had absent protective sensation, palpable pulses, and noninvasive studies revealed ankle-brachial index = 0.78. After six weeks of treatment with standard of care strategies, the wound showed no evidence of healing even though the patient was compliant with the plan of care. Treatment included offloading, debridement, enzymatic debridement, and moist wound care. Offloading treatments included total contact cast, removable cast boot, and half (wedge) shoe. The patient underwent an Achilles tendon lengthening because of limited ankle range of motion, decreasing forefoot pressure. Adequate DM control and offloading also played a role in achieving healing. The wound progressed to complete healing after tendon lengthening. (See Figures 1-5.)

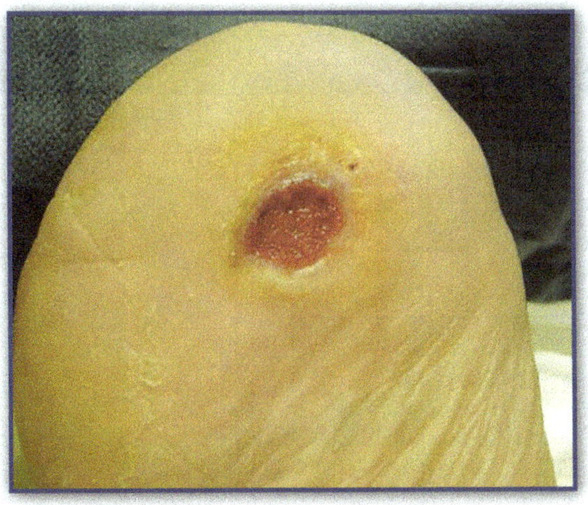

FIGURE 1. 2.5cm x 2.0cm x 0.3cm
Arterial Doppler demonstrating on the right calf a normal pulse volume recording (PVR) with dicrotic notch, and an abnormal PVR (bowed and blunted) in left metatarsal region, and an abnormal toe-brachial index (TBI) of 0.39

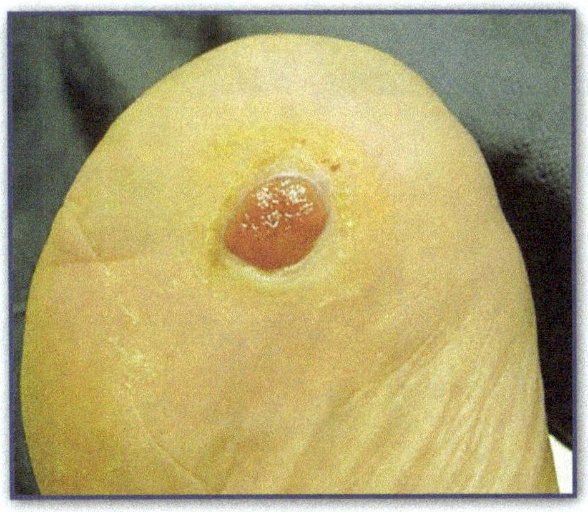

FIGURE 2.
2.0cm x 1.5cm x 0.2cm—Februrary 1, 2012

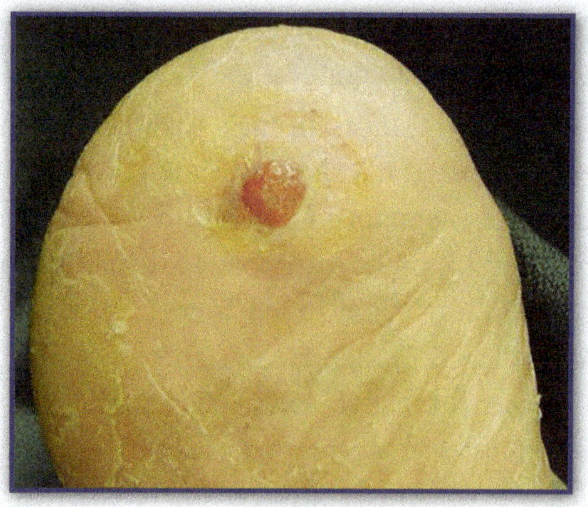

FIGURE 3.
1.2cm x 1.0cm x 0.2cm—Februrary 8, 2012

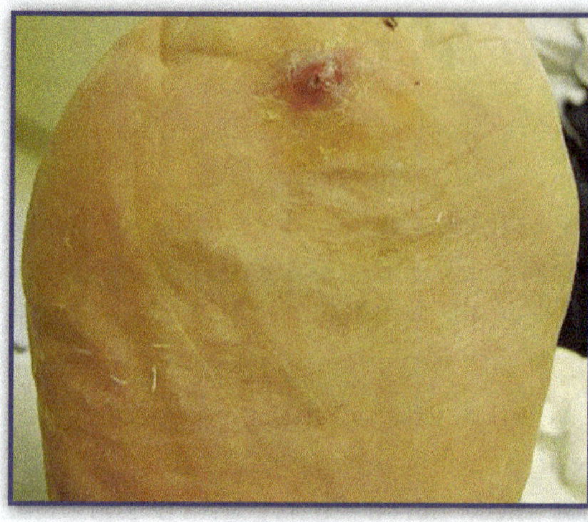

FIGURE 4.
0.4cm x 0.2cm x 0.1cm—Februrary 22, 2012

CASE STUDY

- 72-year-old male, with ulcer present for 12 weeks
- PMH: uncontrolled DM, depression, smoking, h/o of TMA
- Palpable pulses (DP, PT)
- ABI=0.78
- Various dressing changes daily
- Offloading: TCC, CAM walker

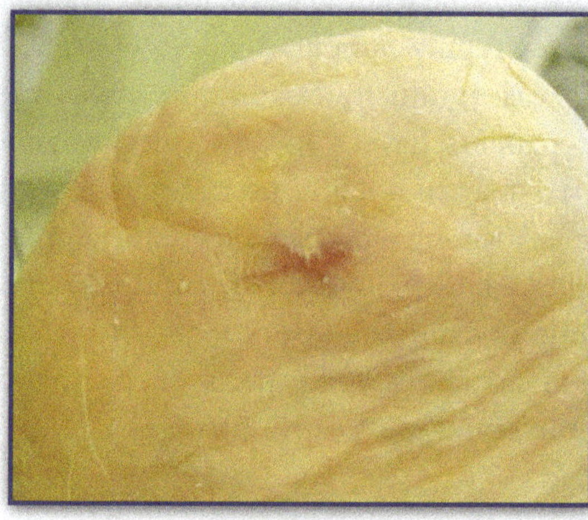

FIGURE 5.
Wound healed—March 1, 2012

II. Pathways

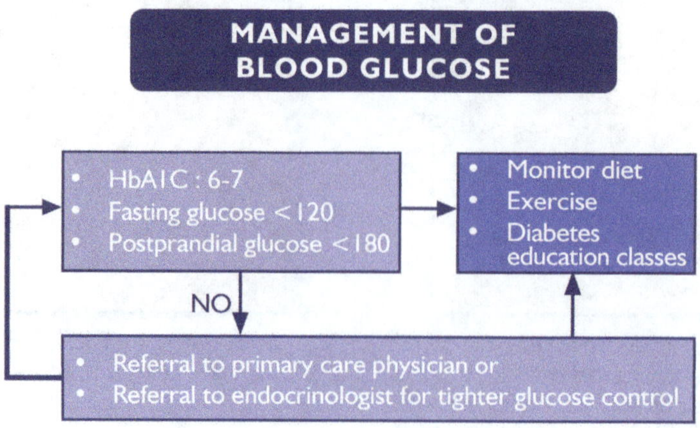

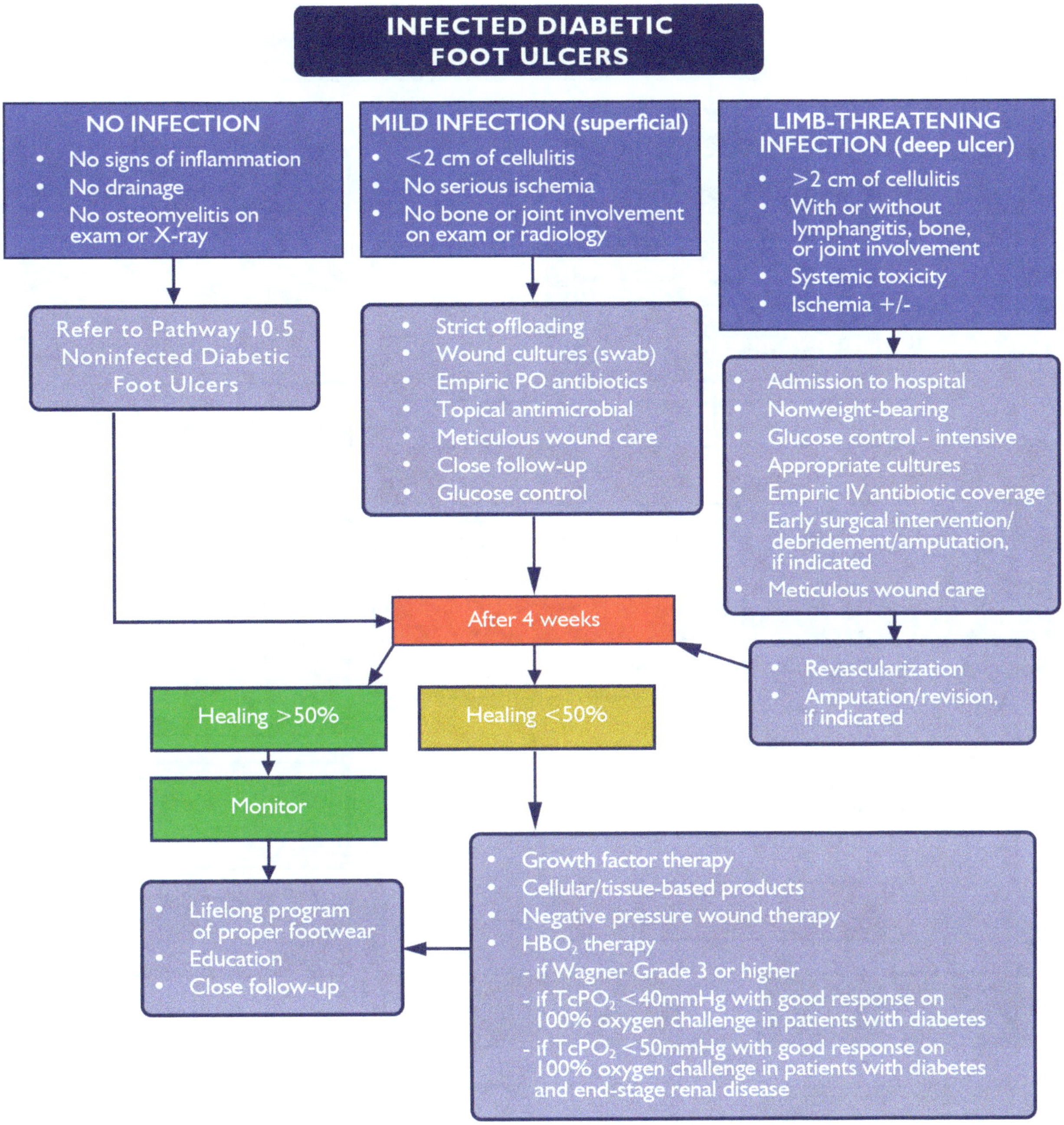
INFECTED DIABETIC FOOT ULCERS
NO INFECTION
No signs of inflammation
No drainage
No osteomyelitis on exam or X-ray
MILD INFECTION (superficial)
<2 cm of cellulitis
No serious ischemia
No bone or joint involvement on exam or radiology
LIMB-THREATENING INFECTION (deep ulcer)
>2 cm of cellulitis
With or without lymphangitis, bone, or joint involvement
Systemic toxicity
Ischemia +/-
Refer to Pathway 10.5 Noninfected Diabetic Foot Ulcers
Strict offloading
Wound cultures (swab)
Empiric PO antibiotics
Topical antimicrobial
Meticulous wound care
Close follow-up
Glucose control
Admission to hospital
Nonweight-bearing
Glucose control - intensive
Appropriate cultures
Empiric IV antibiotic coverage
Early surgical intervention/ debridement/amputation, if indicated
Meticulous wound care
After 4 weeks
Revascularization
Amputation/revision, if indicated
Healing >50%
Healing <50%
Monitor
Lifelong program of proper footwear
Education
Close follow-up
Growth factor therapy
Cellular/tissue-based products
Negative pressure wound therapy
HBO$_2$ therapy
- if Wagner Grade 3 or higher
- if TcPO$_2$ <40mmHg with good response on 100% oxygen challenge in patients with diabetes
- if TcPO$_2$ <50mmHg with good response on 100% oxygen challenge in patients with diabetes and end-stage renal disease

NONINFECTED DIABETIC FOOT WOUNDS

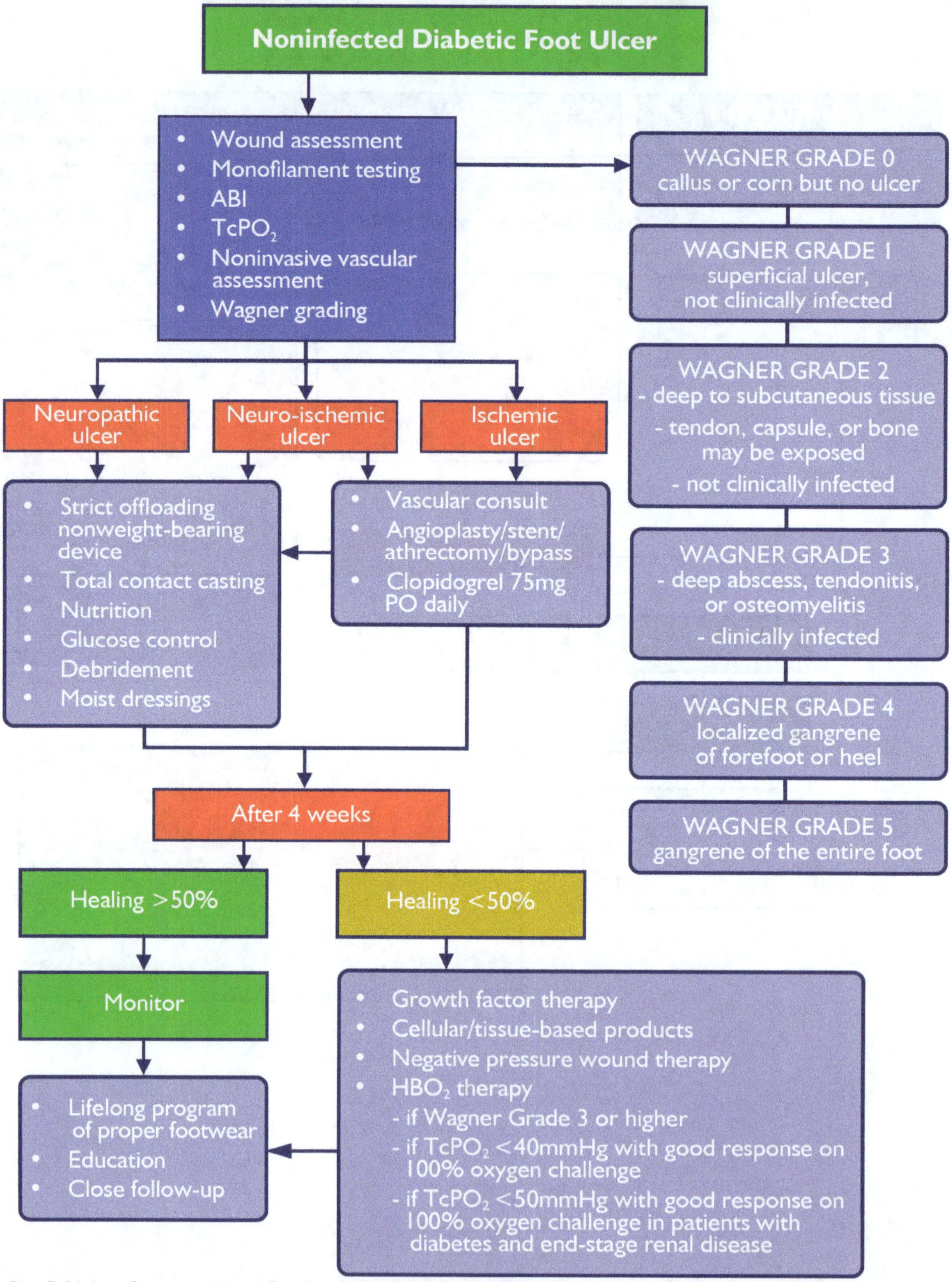

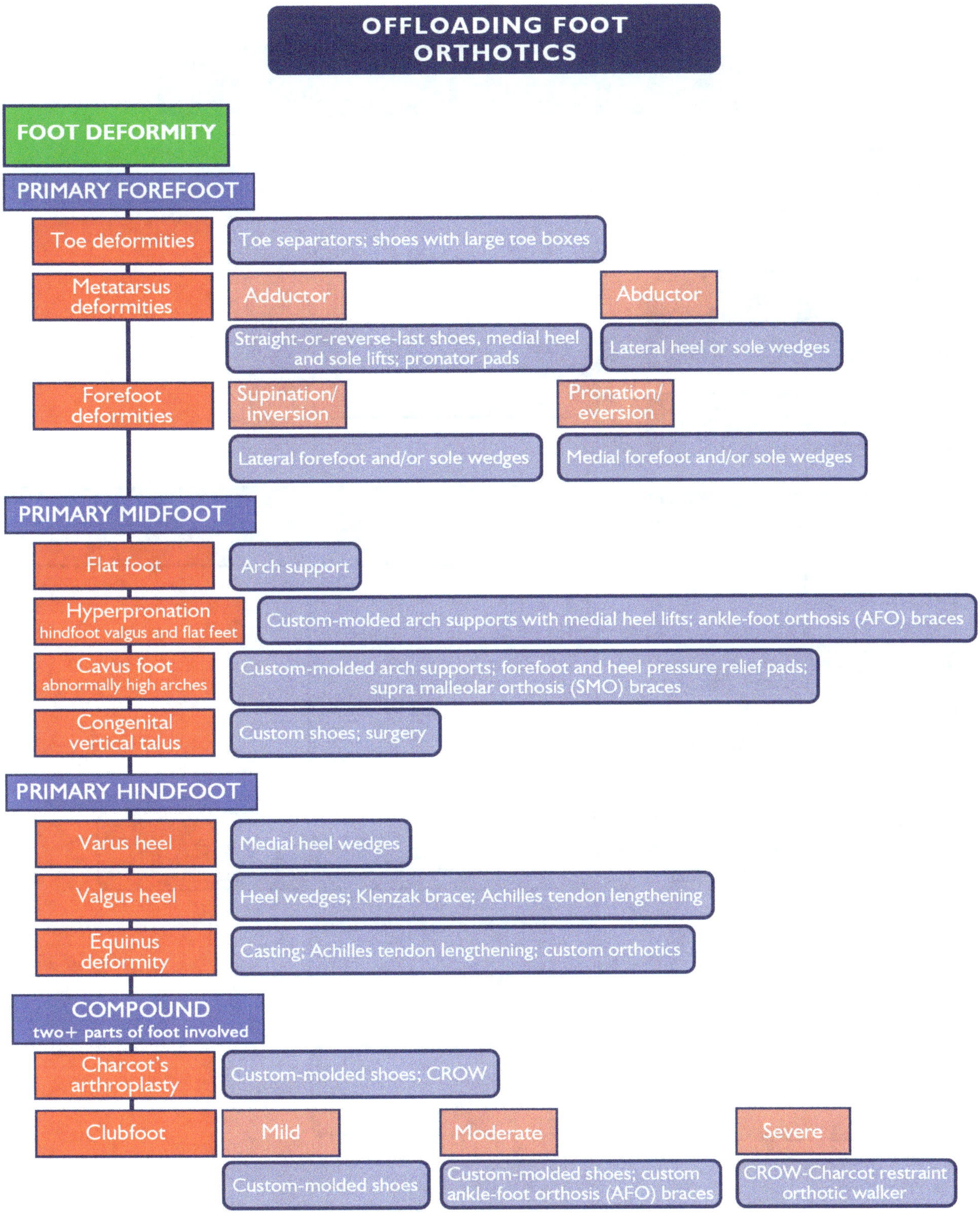
OFFLOADING FOOT ORTHOTICS
FOOT DEFORMITY
PRIMARY FOREFOOT
Toe deformities
Toe separators; shoes with large toe boxes
Metatarsus deformities
Adductor
Straight-or-reverse-last shoes, medial heel and sole lifts; pronator pads
Abductor
Lateral heel or sole wedges
Forefoot deformities
Supination/ inversion
Lateral forefoot and/or sole wedges
Pronation/ eversion
Medial forefoot and/or sole wedges
PRIMARY MIDFOOT
Flat foot
Arch support
Hyperpronation hindfoot valgus and flat feet
Custom-molded arch supports with medial heel lifts; ankle-foot orthosis (AFO) braces
Cavus foot abnormally high arches
Custom-molded arch supports; forefoot and heel pressure relief pads; supra malleolar orthosis (SMO) braces
Congenital vertical talus
Custom shoes; surgery
PRIMARY HINDFOOT
Varus heel
Medial heel wedges
Valgus heel
Heel wedges; Klenzak brace; Achilles tendon lengthening
Equinus deformity
Casting; Achilles tendon lengthening; custom orthotics
COMPOUND two+ parts of foot involved
Charcot's arthroplasty
Custom-molded shoes; CROW
Clubfoot
Mild
Custom-molded shoes
Moderate
Custom-molded shoes; custom ankle-foot orthosis (AFO) braces
Severe
CROW-Charcot restraint orthotic walker

PRESCRIPTION OFFLOADING SHOE ADJUSTMENTS(4)

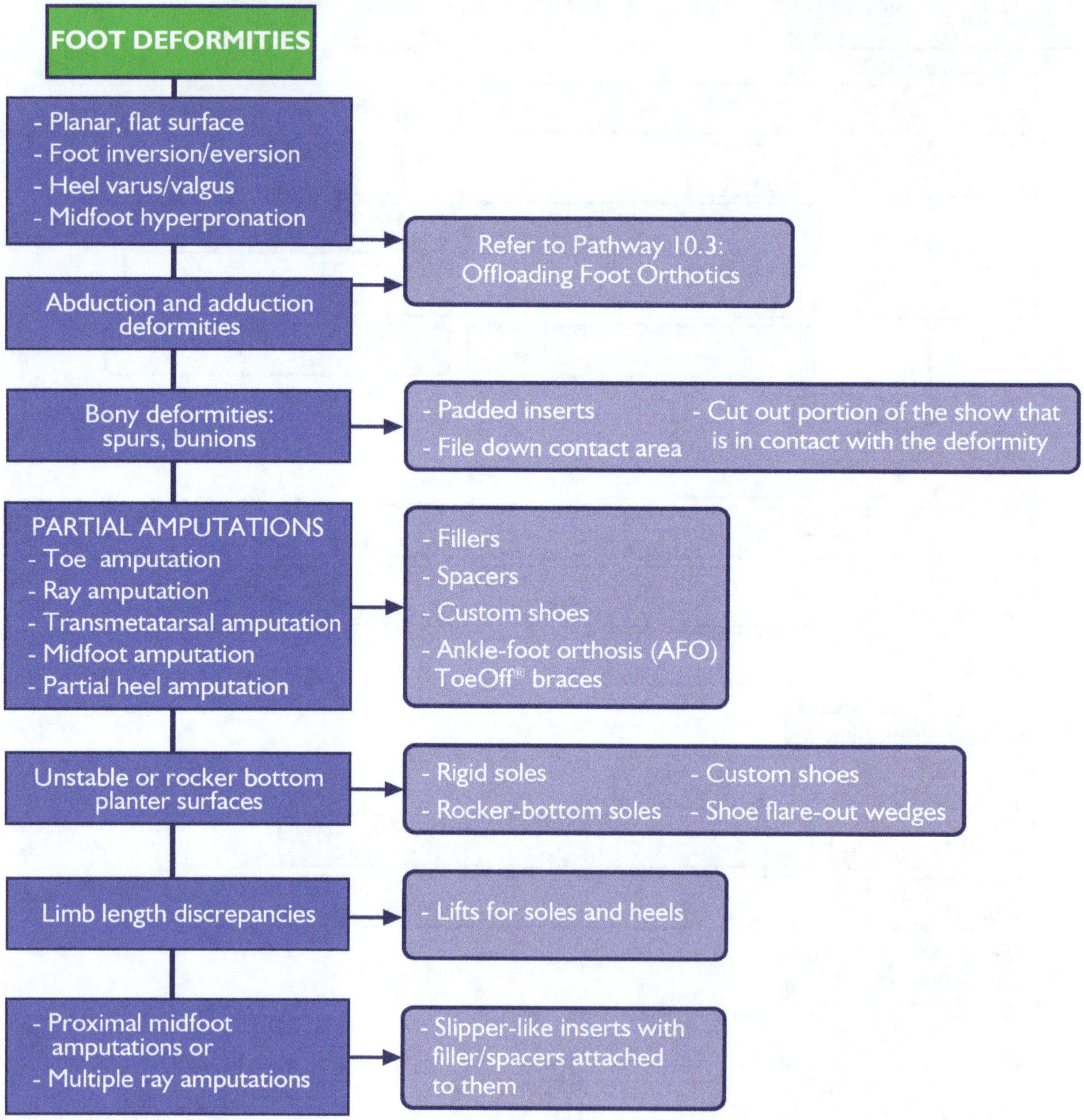

III. Epidemiology of foot ulcers

Diabetes mellitus is a significant health-care problem worldwide. The incidence of diabetes has increased 48% since 1980, with a 70% increase in patients under the age of 40. However, of the 29.1 million Americans who have diabetes, only 21.0 million are diagnosed, leaving more than one-fourth unaware they have the disease. African Americans, Hispanics, Native Americans, and Asian Americans have the highest prevalence of diabetes mellitus.[1]

The American Diabetes Association (ADA) defines diabetes as "a disease in which the body doesn't produce or properly use insulin." Between 90% and 95% of Americans have type 2 diabetes, making it the most common form of the disease in the United States.[2] The failure to diagnose this type of patient population results in progressive morbidity and mortality, with severe insulin resistance existing for years before the onset of hyperglycemia.

Diabetes is the single most common underlying cause of lower-extremity amputation in the United States. Foot problems are one of the most common complications of diabetes that lead to hospitalization.[3] Indeed, admissions for foot complications account for 20% to 25% of all hospital days for patients with diabetes.[4] In the United States, approximately 120,000 non-traumatic lower-extremity amputations are performed each year, with 45% to 83% of these amputations involving patients with diabetes.[5] The risk of lower-extremity amputation in diabetics is 15 to 46 times higher than in nondiabetic patients.[3,6] The incidence of lower-extremity amputation is 1.5 times higher in Hispanics and 2.1 times higher in blacks compared with non-Hispanic whites.

After the initial amputation, the risk of re-amputation or amputation of the contralateral extremity is also high: 9% to 17% of patients will experience a second amputation within the same year,[6-7] and 25% to 68% will have an amputation of the contralateral extremity within three to five years.[8,9] The 5-year survival rate after a lower-extremity amputation ranges from 41% to 70%.[10] Diabetes is a contributing factor in 75% to 83% of all amputations among African Americans, Hispanics, and Native Americans.[6,10]

IV. Pathophysiology

Diabetes affects sensory, motor, and autonomic nerve function. Sensory neuropathy contributes to an inability to perceive injury to the foot.[3] Sensory neuropathy or loss of protective sensation represents a level of sensory loss where patients cannot recognize a foot injury. Perhaps the strongest and easiest risk factor to identify is the presence of a previous ulceration or amputation, which indicates the potential for recurrence due to a high susceptibility profile, scar formation, or biomechanical abnormalities. The underlying pathology usually is not reversible, and most disease processes affecting the diabetic foot will continue to worsen over time. Three primary pathways or mechanisms of injury have been identified in the development of foot ulcers. These include wounds that result from ill-fitting shoes (low-pressure injuries that are associated with prolonged or constant pressure), ulcers on weight-bearing areas (repetitive moderate pressure and shear forces on the sole), and penetrating injuries from puncture wounds or other traumatic events (high-pressure injuries with a single exposure of direct pressure).[11]

V. Importance of the management of blood glucose in a diabetic patient

See Management of Blood Glucose Pathway. Because the increased mortality in patients with diabetic foot ulcers cannot fully be explained by all the known cardiovascular risk factors, the importance of the management of blood glucose has been investigated more frequently over the last couple of years. Metabolic control and the role of hypoglycemia appear to be important factors in the disease process of these patients. The majority of studies suggest that a diabetic foot ulcer most likely develops in patients with poorly controlled blood sugar.[12,13] A recent retrospective study of 873 patients[14] admitted to the hospital with diabetic foot ulcers reported a mean A1c of 9.51%. Although 92% of the enrolled patients were under treatment to decrease their blood sugar, only 14.4% were well regulated. These results underline the poor management of blood glucose in patients at risk for developing foot ulcers. In 2013, Fagher et al.[15] designed a longitudinal prospective study to evaluate the impact of different HbA1c levels and QTc prolongation on all-cause mortality in patients with diabetic foot ulcers. Two hundred fourteen patients were followed up and grouped into three HbA1c groups: HbA1c<7.5% [<58mmol/mol], HbA1c 7.5-8.9% [58-74mmol/mol and >8.9% [>74mmol/mol]. At eight years follow-up, 70.6% of patients died, and an A1c of <7.5% was associated with increased mortality. Also, an A1c of <7.5% and Qtc prolongation had the highest mortality in 8 years (92.1%). An optimal management of blood glucose in this high-risk population will decrease the ulceration risk and increase survival rates.

VI. Evaluating a diabetic foot ulcer patient

The etiology of ulcerations in diabetes is associated with the presence of peripheral sensory neuropathy and repetitive trauma due to normal walking activities to areas on the foot that are subject to moderate or high pressures and shear.[16] Pressure sites on the sole of the foot are often associated with limited joint mobility of the foot or ankle or structure deformities such as hammertoes and hallux valgus deformity. This commonly exceeds the soft tissue's ability to absorb and dissipate the repetitive forces of ambulation, resulting in full-thickness ulceration.

The wound assessment should be comprehensive as any other part of the body. The wound should be measured in length, width, and depth if possible. Documentation of type of drainage and odor must be noticed. There are three types of ulceration the health-care professional will encounter: neuropathic, neuro-ischemic, and ischemic (Figure 1). The neuropathic ulcer is painless with hyperkeratotic rim and red granular base. Maceration is usually present underneath the hyperkeratosis. It occurs in a location where there is increased pressure, commonly in the plantar aspect of the foot. The neuro-ischemic is the most difficult ulcer to treat in the foot. It has characteristics of the neuropathic ulcer, but microvascular disease makes this ulcer a challenge to heal. Often, noninvasive arterial studies demonstrate mild macrovascular disease. The appearance of the foot is consistent with signs of vascular disease as well as severe neuropathy. The wound base is pink in color mixed with a fibrinous type tissue, which recurs even with sharp debridement. Finally, the ischemic ulcer has a yellowish or grayish base with margins that bleed for a short period of time. This sign is deceptive, as the clinician may believe that the wound is well perfused. It is usually painful since the patient may present with rest pain as well. Vascular consultation is imperative for the treatment of this type of wound.

VII. Neuropathy assessment

Diabetes affects sensory, motor, and autonomic nerve function. In patients with sensory neuropathy, pain is defective. Sensory neuropathy contributes to an inability to perceive injury to the foot due to what is commonly referred to as loss of protective sensation (LOPS).[3] LOPS represents the threshold of sensory loss where patients do not perceive an injury to the foot.

Motor neuropathy contributes to wasting of the intrinsic muscles of the foot; muscle imbalance; structural foot deformity, such as claw toes, and metatarsophalangeal joints subluxation along with limited joint mobility. Autonomic neuropathy causes shunting of blood[17] and impaired sweat function, which leads to dry, scaly skin that can easily fissure. The combined effect of these neuropathies results in a foot with structural deformity and biomechanical faults; dry, poorly hydrated integument; and an inability to respond to pain and repetitive injury.

A. Monofilament testing

Neuropathy is one of the most common risk factors for lower-extremity complications.[3] Several screening methods can be used to identify sensory neuropathy, which include a systematic clinical examination, vibration perception threshold (VPT) testing with a biothesiometer, and pressure assessment with Semmes-Weinstein monofilaments.[18] Although these methods are noninvasive and have good sensitivity and specificity to identify patients with loss of protective sensation,[19] Semmes-Weinstein monofilaments in particular may present several problems. Semmes-Weinstein monofilaments should be purchased from a vendor that sells calibrated instruments because considerable variability exists among different brands of monofilament.[20] Booth and Young found that some brands of monofilaments buckled at 8 g of force rather than at the 10 g for which they were designated.[19,21] In addition, the material properties of the monofilament wear out after repetitive testing. Young and colleagues[22] found that after 500 cycles of testing (or the equivalent of testing 10 sites on each foot for 25 patients), there was an average reduction of 1.2 g of testing force. A worn-out monofilament may result in patients' being diagnosed as having sensory neuropathy with loss of protective sensation when they are not at risk.

B. Vibration perception testing

VPT testing is a quantitative evaluation that measures large myelinated nerve function. It is less prone to inter-operator variation than are monofilaments, and it does not need to be replaced to continue providing accurate results. The VPT Meter is a handheld device with a rubber head that is applied to a bony prominence, such as the medial aspect of the first metatarsal head or the tip of the great toe. The unit contains a linear scale that displays the applied voltage, ranging from 0 to 100 V. The amplitude is then slowly increased until the patient can feel the vibration. The inability to feel greater than 25 V is indicative of LOPS and puts the patient at risk for ulceration and amputation.

A systematic clinical examination can be an effective way to diagnose neuropathy and identify high-risk patients. Abbott et al. used a modification of the neuropathy disability score to evaluate a large cohort of patients (n = 9,710) with diabetes.[3] The neuropathy disability score evaluates vibration with a 128-Hz tuning fork, pinprick, hot-cold perception, and Achilles deep tendon reflex. The deep tendon reflex is scored 0 if it is normal, 1 if reinforcement is required, and 2 if it is absent. The other tests are scored 0 for normal and 1 for abnormal. Each foot is scored, for a possible high score of 10. Abbott showed that high neuropathy disability scores (>6) were associated with a higher ulcer incidence.

C. Temperature testing

Temperature assessment has been used in clinical practice to diagnose neuropathy and soft tissue injury in patients with neuropathy, and it has been used as a tool for self-assessment and monitoring. Clinicians have used temperature assessment to evaluate foot ulcers and Charcot neuroarthropathy. The rationale to use temperature as part of a daily foot assessment is that temperatures could provide an objective measurement of tissue injury. A change in skin temperature could be used to identify tissue that is inflamed. It is a similar thought process as described in the National Pressure Ulcer Advisory Panel ulcer classification. A Stage 1 pressure ulcer is recognized as having signs of tissue injury before there is a break in the epithelium. It can be characterized by changes in temperature, color, or texture of the skin.

There are three randomized clinical studies[23-25] that compare standard prevention therapies consisting of therapeutic shoes and insoles, regular foot care by a podiatrist and a standard, foot-specific education to temperature home monitoring intervention in addition to standard care. All three studies demonstrated a 3- to 10-fold reduction in re-ulceration when patients used home temperature evaluation compared to standard prevention practices. All three studies used a similar approach. Patients used an infrared thermometer to record the temperatures from 10 sites on the foot and then compare temperatures at corresponding anatomic sites on the right and left feet to see whether there was >4 degree Fahrenheit difference. This temperature difference was used to define a high temperature that was felt to be associated with soft tissue injury that could lead to ulceration. Patients were to reduce their activity by 50% until temperatures normalized. If they did not return to a normal range in a set time frame, they called the study coordinator to be seen by the study physician.

VIII. Evaluating foot deformity in diabetic patients

In patients with neuropathy, ulcerations typically develop as a result of repetitive pressure and shear on the sole of the foot or from shoe pressure on the top or sides of the foot; however, no specific level of pressure has been determined to be abnormal or pathologic.[20] Diabetes alters biomechanics in patients with preexisting structural and functional foot deformities. Motor neuropathy is thought to contribute to atrophy and weakness of the intrinsic muscles of the foot. This leads to what has been called the "intrinsic minus foot," which describes wasting of the small (intrinsic) muscles that originate in the foot (Figure 4).

Metatarsal ulcers can develop when digital deformities severely contract. The lesser digits contract and dislocate dorsally, resulting in a claw toe deformity and a strong plantar flexor force at the metatarsophalangeal joints. As the toes contract and the metatarsophalangeal joints dislocate, retrograde forces push the metatarsal heads plantarly.[21] Therefore, three areas are subject to excessive pressure: the distal tip of the toes, dorsal aspect of the lesser digits, and the metatarsal heads, which in the presence of loss of protective sensation, can lead to ulceration.[26] Limited mobility of the ankle and metatarsophalangeal joints has been associated with soft tissue glycosylation involving the gastro-soleus-Achilles complex and periarticular tissues.[27] Limited motion of the ankle, subtalar, and metatarsophalangeal joints has been associated with high pressures in the forefoot. Often patients with an intrinsic minus foot will appear to have a high arch; however, this is not a congenital deformity but rather is due to atrophy of the abductor hallucis muscle belly on the medial side of the foot. A profound example of musculoskeletal abnormality of the diabetic foot is represented by Charcot neuroarthropathy, which is characterized by fracture, subluxation, and/or dislocation of joints in the foot or ankle. These structural deformities typically cause plantar bony deformities resulting in areas of high pressure leading to ulceration.

IX. Noninvasive vascular assessment

Peripheral arterial disease is a clinical diagnosis that can usually be assessed with noninvasive inexpensive methods. First, all peripheral pulses of the lower extremity should be manually palpated: femoral, popliteal, dorsalis pedis, and posterior tibial arteries. When any of these are difficult to palpate, a ratio between the systolic pressure in the ankle divided by the systolic pressure of the brachial artery should be obtained (ankle brachial index, ABI). The systolic pressure of the dorsalis pedis and the posterior tibial artery of each leg, as well as the systolic pressure of brachial artery in each arm, should be obtained and the higher pressure in the leg should be divided by the higher of the two brachial pressures. An ABI of less than 0.9 is an independent risk factor for cardiovascular events, including death.[(28)] A decreased ABI also increases the patient's risk for complications in wound healing; however, several authors have reported successful wound healing rates approaching 90% if the ABI is greater than 0.45.[(29-30)] These results were more recently reproduced with an ABI equal to or greater than 0.5 in patients with diabetes.[(31)] However, caution must be taken in patients with ABI between 0.5 and 0.9 as this range indicates peripheral vascular disease, and should be treated, if indicated, in patients having elective foot surgery.

Patients with diabetes can have a unique pattern of atherosclerosis that causes vascular calcifications that limit the effectiveness of the ABI (Monckeberg's sclerosis) (Figure 5). An ABI greater than 1.4 is suspect of this condition and these patients may be at greater risk for cardiovascular events.[(28)] In this instance pulse volume recordings, skin perfusion pressure, and transcutaneous oxygen tensions are valuable noninvasive exams.[(19,32-33)] If peripheral vascular disease is detected, a consult with a vascular surgeon should be given for a more thorough cardiovascular work-up and treatment. A noninvasive vascular exam can often result in normal large vessel perfusion and significant microvascular disease. These patients have a greater risk for a complicated healing course and should be advised of this increased risk and referred to vascular surgery. Also, pertinent medical history should be gathered in relation to cardiovascular disease. Patients with history of coronary artery disease, stroke, and smoking may have significant peripheral vascular disease, and further vascular evaluation is warranted. A complete evaluation of the wound is essential to formulate a treatment plan. Assessment of the contralateral limb should be done as well to screen and compare pathology.

A. Ankle-brachial index measurements

Patients with vascular disorders can usually be assured that an accurate anatomic diagnosis will be made with modern noninvasive vascular diagnostic techniques (e.g., ankle- and toe-brachial indices, segmental pressure measurements, pulse volume recordings, duplex ultrasound imaging, Doppler waveform analysis, and exercise testing). These tests will usually provide adequate information for creation of a therapeutic plan. When required, these physiological and anatomic data can be supplemented by use of MRA and CTA and selective use of invasive aortic and lower-extremity angiographic techniques. The noninvasive vascular laboratory provides a powerful set of tools that can objectively assess the status of lower-extremity arterial disease and facilitate the creation of a therapeutic plan. The ABI is a measurement that provides objective data that serves as the standard for the diagnosis of lower-extremity PAD in field epidemiological surveys, in vascular laboratories, and in office practice. The ABI offers prognostic data that are useful to predict limb survival, wound healing, and patient survival. The ABI can be used either as a screening tool for lower-extremity PAD or to monitor the efficacy of therapeutic interventions. The ABI is performed by measuring the systolic blood pressure from both brachial arteries and from both the dorsalis pedis and posterior tibial arteries after the patient has been at rest in the supine position for 10 minutes. Optimal recordings are obtained with blood pressure cuffs that are appropriately sized to the patient's lower calf (immediately above the ankle), and systolic pressures are recorded with a handheld 5- or 10-mHz Doppler instrument. In normal individuals, there should be a minimal (less than 12 mmHg) interarm systolic pressure gradient during a routine examination.

The ABI may not be accurate in individuals in whom systolic blood pressure cannot be abolished by inflation of an air-filled blood pressure cuff. The incidence of noncompressablearteries is highest in diabetics and elderly patients; in these individuals, it may be impossible to abolish the systolic pressure signal despite cuff inflation to pressures in excess of 200 mmHg. Despite the artifactual high systolic pressure, these individuals may have arterial disease, and cardiovascular event rates have been noted to be increased in one population that was characterized by a high prevalence of diabetes and other risk factors.(34) This application of the ABI to office practice has been supported by the American Diabetes Association consensus statement that suggested that the ABI be performed in all individuals with diabetes who are 50 and older, in diabetic individuals younger than 50 who have other atherosclerosis risk factors, and in individuals with diabetes of more than 10 years' duration.(35)

B. Toe-brachial index measurements

Many individuals with long-standing diabetes, elderly patients, and individuals who require dialysis for end-stage renal disease may have noncompressable leg arterial segments due to medial calcification. This may preclude accurate assessment of either the ABI or segmental pressure measurements in a subset of these patient cohorts. Such noncompressable arteries are suggested when the ABI is greater than 1.3 or when there is an abnormal augmentation in a measured lower extremity systolic pressure beyond the normal physiological amplification of systolic pressure from the heart to the limb arterial segment (usually greater than 20 mmHg or 20% higher than the brachial systolic pressure). In such individuals, diagnostic information to establish the lower extremity PAD diagnosis can be obtained by the measurement of toe systolic pressure and calculation of the toe-brachial index, and toe-brachial index values less than 0.7 are usually considered diagnostic for lower-extremity PAD.(36-37) The toe pressure measurement remains a sensitive diagnostic test in such patients because digital arteries are usually spared the calcinosis that alters compressibility of more proximal arteries. This test is performed by placement of a small occlusive cuff on the proximal portion of the great or second toe, with the return of toe pulsatility (which represents the systolic perfusion pressure) assessed by use of a plethysmographic detection device.

C. Pulse volume recordings

Measurement of these cyclical volume changes can be documented by a plethysmographic technique to provide qualitative or quantitative data regarding the adequacy of limb perfusion in patients with lower extremity PAD. Pulse volume recordings provide a method to evaluate the arterial pressure waveform profile via the use of either a pneumoplethysmograph or a mercury-in-silastic strain gauge. Both of these devices can be applied in a segmental manner from the thigh to the ankle to assess the change in limb volume between diastole and systole. When such data are recorded on chart paper, the magnitude of the pulse volume provides an index of large-vessel patency and correlates with blood flow. The prognostic value of PVR tracings in predicting risk of amputation has also been evaluated in a small patient cohort with diabetes before and after renal transplantation. Makisalo et al. studied 129 consecutive diabetic (n equals 34) and nondiabetic (n equals 95) renal transplantation patients and measured the predictive value of clinical factors (e.g., pretransplant lower extremity PAD and claudication) and noninvasive vascular perfusion measurements (ABI, toe-brachial index, and PVRs) on lower-limb amputations, renal allograft survival, and patient survival during a five-year period of follow-up.[37] A low PVR amplitude (below 5 mm) was observed before transplantation in 82% of the diabetic patients and 36% of the nondiabetic patients. During the five-year follow-up period, abnormal toe-brachial index and PVR values (and diabetes) at the time of transplantation were the greatest predictors for proximal foot amputations. In summary, the presence of a low pulse volume serves as a measurable hallmark that correlates with other signs of limb jeopardy and an adverse prognosis. In summary, the PVR technique is useful as an initial diagnostic test for patients with suspected lower-extremity PAD and to assess limb perfusion after revascularization procedures, and it can predict risk of CLI and amputation. Pulse volume recordings can provide a tool to evaluate small-vessel disease when applied to the feet. They are also useful in individuals with noncompressablevessels in whom ABIs and segmental pressures are spuriously elevated. Although PVRs are useful and cost-effective, especially as a screening tool in office practices or vascular laboratories, other noninvasive techniques can provide more quantitative perfusion data and better arterial anatomic lower extremity PAD localization.

Many societal guidelines are in agreement that arterial screening should be performed on patients with diabetic foot ulcers. However, there is no consensus on the ideal way to accomplish this. A variety of methods exist, all of which are acceptable and each of which has various advantages and disadvantages with regard to sensitivity, specificity, cost of equipment, training required, and the time it takes to perform them. ABI, TBI and pulse volume recordings might be considered anatomical assessments of the pressure head (or pressure wave) in specific named arteries and thus the macro circulation. Another approach is to evaluate the micro circulation by measuring tissue perfusion or oxygenation, which are more physiological measurements.

D. $TcPO_2$, SPP, and hyperspectral imaging

Transcutaneous oxygen tension ($TcPO_2$) assessment is a noninvasive technique for the investigation of arterial occlusive disease in the legs. It measures the partial pressure of oxygen that diffuses to the skin after a heated thermistor is applied, allowing objective quantification of the degree of limb ischemia.[40] The device consists of a heating element and a sensor attached to the skin via a gas permeable membrane in contact with an electrolyte solution. Although the results are reported in mmHg, in this case, the measurement refers to the partial pressure of gas, analogous to an arterial blood gas. $TcPO_2$ can be a challenging test to perform consistently and reliably due to the number of factors that can affect the sensor and the results. However, 15 studies (with a total of 1,137 patients) have demonstrated that $TcPO_2$ provides better overall predictive capability for healing than arterial dopplers or ABI measurements. Many factors other than ischemia can result in low $TcPO_2$ values (e.g. edema, infection, hypotension). Thus, using $TcPO_2$ as a screen for arterial disease requires either a leg elevation or drop test (to assess for positional change in $TcPO_2$) or an oxygen challenge test (to see if values improve dramatically when breathing 100% oxygen). Regional transcutaneous oximetry has been shown to be more accurate than ankle-brachial index assessment and toe blood pressure measurement for the diagnosis of arterial occlusive disease in diabetic patients.(41) Evidence-based guidance for interpreting $TcPO_2$ values have been published in a consensus document but there is still much misunderstanding about how to use $TcPO_2$.(130)

Skin perfusion pressure (SPP) is the measurement of the capillary opening pressure after release of occlusion. While similar to blood pressure, the laser device senses the first blood cells entering the capillaries, sometimes referred to as the capillary opening pressure. This measurement is also in mmHg but in this case, it is a unit of pressure like to blood pressure. SPP technology has a number of advantages over $TcPO_2$ in that it is not affected by vessel calcification, is less affected by edema, can be used on the plantar foot and the digits, is not affected by callus or thickened skin, and no calibration of the machine is required. Lo and colleagues compared SPP and $TcPO_2$ in terms of ability to predict healing outcome in 100 patients with lower extremity wounds. A threshold of <30 mmHg was selected as the cutoff below which the test was considered significantly abnormal and indicative of a wound unlikely to heal. SPP alone successfully predicted outcome in 87% of the patients compared to $TcPO_2$ at a rate of 64% ($P< 0.0002$). Skin perfusion pressure was more sensitive in its ability to predict wound healing relative to $TcPO_2$ (99% vs. 66%).(131)

SPP is also highly reliable in the prediction of healing after amputation, and it can be used to diagnose limb ischemia and thus select patients who need further vascular testing. In addition to the uses above, SPP testing may be useful for planning foot and ankle surgery and ensuring that the patient can tolerate compression therapy for venous ulcers.

Hyperspectral imaging (HSI) is a method for determining oxygenated (OxyHgb) and deoxygenated hemoglobin (DeOxyHgb) levels in the superficial microcirculation of the skin using differential reflectance spectroscopy of light.(38) In other words, this test is measuring oxygen saturation of hemoglobin. Previous studies on HSI methods have found hemoglobin measurements to correlate with changes in skin perfusion differences in the microcirculation of the foot between diabetic patients and healthy individuals.(39) Hyperspectral imaging (HSI) may be utilized during surgery to visualize tissue oxygenation as the percentage of oxyhemoglobin without touching the patient, using visible light and in real time. No data are available to assess the reliability of HSI in screening for arterial disease or in predicting wound healing or amputation level. Further studies are needed.

The important lesson is for clinicians to select a method or methods of noninvasive arterial screening that they are able to use reliably and implement consistently. Appropriate noninvasive vascular screening can reduce unnecessary amputations and help clinicians make better use of advanced technology, thus saving money, limbs and lives.

X. Evaluating diabetic foot infections

See Infected Diabetic Foot Ulcers Pathway. Infection is defined as the pathologic presence of bacteria in a site or wound that is supported by the body's response to inflammation.[42] Knowing that all skin wounds contain microorganisms, infections must be diagnosed clinically rather than microbiologically. Unfortunately, most patients with a diabetic foot infection (DFI) have diminished signs of a local inflammatory response, possibly due to peripheral neuropathy or ischemia. Systemic signs of toxicity are also uncommon in diabetic foot infections. Most patients are afebrile without elevated white blood cell count, sedimentation rate, or C-reactive protein and report no pain. If any of these symptoms are present, then a severe infection most likely is present.[43] Once there is a suspicion of infection based on clinical diagnosis infection, tissue cultures can be obtained to determine the causative agent. At this time a treatment plan should be implemented. Generally, the treatment option will be dependent upon the infection severity. Assessing the severity of the infection helps to determine the need for hospitalization, the potential necessity and timing of surgery, and the likelihood of amputation. As a general rule, mild infections can be treated with oral antibiotics in the outpatient setting, whereas moderate and severe infections will usually require intravenous antibiotic therapy and hospitalization.[44]

Commonly, patients with a DFI present with laboratory results such as white blood cell count within normal limits. More often than not, it does not exclude the fact that a diabetic person is infected. It has been suggested that patient with longstanding diabetes may not mount an effective immunological response to invading pathogens.[43] For example, Armstrong found that 82% of the patients with diabetic foot osteomyelitis had normal oral temperatures.[45-46]

In DFI involving the soft tissues, most of ancillary studies are not helpful.[47-48] However, suspicion of osteomyelitis may warrant additional evaluation with imaging. Initial imaging should include weight-bearing plain radiographs to assess for fractures or dislocations, foreign bodies, subcutaneous emphysema, and associated degenerative changes. CT or MRI can be used to further evaluate the bony architecture. With either of these advanced imaging techniques, consideration must be given to the patient's renal function before administration of contrast material. Nuclear medicine studies, including technetium tc-99m and indiumin-111-labeled leukocyte scans can be used in the setting of equivocal findings or relative contraindications to other imaging techniques.

A. Classifications of diabetic foot infections

Most of the classification systems previously reported in medical literature have primarily focused on the depth of the ulceration and fail to comment on a patient's infection and arterial supply. Traditionally, the Wagner's classification is the most commonly used classification. It is simple, as it uses a grade system from 0 to 5. However, the classification is cumbersome as the earliest stages in the classification describes ulcer depth (Grade 0-2), transition to infection (Grade 3), and then to gangrene (Grade 4-5).

Despite the obvious limitations of the Wagner grading system, the Centers for Medicare and Medicaid Services (CMS) uses it to define Medicare coverage policy for certain advanced therapeutics (e.g. hyperbaric oxygen therapy), and many clinical trials use it to establish inclusion and exclusion criteria for research. Clarity regarding the definition of each grade remains important. They are as follows:

- Wagner Grade 1 lesion: superficial ulcer without penetration to deeper layers of issue
- Wagner Grade 2 lesion: can reach tendon, joint capsule or bone
- Wagner Grade 3: deep ulcer with osteomyelitis, abscess or tenosynovitis (pyarthrosis)
- Wagner Grade 4: gangrene of some portion of the toes or forefoot
- Wagner Grade 5: gangrene of the entire foot.

Guidance documents from various Medicare carriers have suggested that in order to substantiate the presence of a Wagner Grade 3 lesion with an abscess, the medical record should note some fluid release (however small) during any of the following:

- Surgical debridement or incision OR
- Documenting moderate to large growth of appropriately acquired cultures from the deep structures of the foot OR
- Via radiographic evidence of osteomyelitis.

The University of Texas Classification has the capability of not only staging the wound, but also risk stratifying the patient including infection (Table 1).[49] Once the diagnosis of diabetic foot infections has been made, it is helpful to classify the infection by its severity to delineate a proper treatment plan. The Infectious Diseases Society of America and the International Working Group for the Diabetic Foot have suggested and validated a classification and grading system whereby such infections may be labeled mild, moderate, or severe based on clinical findings and the patient's systemic health status. This scale has been validated in a prospective observational study.[44,50] When applied to 1,666 patients with foot ulceration, there was a significant increase in rates of hospitalization and lower-extremity amputation with increased severity of the infection. These classification systems have now been widely accepted. Gibbons et.al. described a classification system to distinguish between the clinical presentations of mild, moderate, and severe infections and recommending treatment for each situation.[51]

TABLE 1: University of Texas Wound Classification

Stage	Grade 0	Grade I	Grade II	Grade III
A	Pre- or post ulcerative lesion completely epithelialized	Superficial wound, not involving tendon, capsule, or bone	Wound penetrating to tendon or capsule	Wound penetrating to bone or joint
B	Infected	Infected	Infected	Infected
C	Ischemic	Ischemic	Ischemic	Ischemic
D	Infected and ischemic	Infected and ischemic	Infected and ischemic	Infected and ischemic

Adapted and reprinted with permission. Lavery LA, Armstrong DG, Harkless LB. Classification of diabetic foot wounds. J Foot Ankle Surg. 1996 Nov-Dec;35(6):528-531.

TABLE 2: Classification of diabetic foot infection

Clinical manifestations of infection	Infection Severity	PEDIS grade
Wound lacking purulence or any manifestations of inflammation	Uninfected	1
Presence of: 2 manifestations of inflammation (purulence, or erythema, pain, tenderness, warmth, or induration), erythema extending 2 cm around the ulcer, and superficial skin/subcutaneous infection; no other local complications or systemic illness.	Mild	2
Infection (as above) in a patient who is systemically well and metabolically stable but which has: 1 of the following characteristics: cellulitis extending 12 cm, lymphangitic streaking, or deep soft-tissue infection	Moderate	3
Infection in a patient with systemic toxicity or metabolic instability	Severe	4

Adapted and reprinted with permission from IDSA guidelines. Lipsky BA, Berendt AR, Deery HG, Embil JM, Joseph WS, Karchmer AW, et al. Diagnosis and treatment of diabetic foot infections. Clin Infect Dis. 2004 Oct 1;39(7):885-910.

B. Medical therapy of diabetic foot infections

Based on the results of the available studies, no single drug or combination of agents appears to be superior to any others.[51-52] The U.S. Food and Drug Administration (FDA) has approved three antibiotics (ertapenem, linezolid, and piperacillin-tazobactam), specifically for the treatment of "complicated skin and skin structure infections including DFI," but not for any accompanying osteomyelitis. Whenever possible, clean biopsy and culture should be obtained to determine the appropriate organism-specific therapy. For ulcers with gross evidence of infection, the initial empiric regimen must take into account the severity of infection and likely etiologic agents. Empiric broad-spectrum antibiotic therapy should be reserved for severe infections and should be narrowed based on culture results and antibiotic susceptibility data. In a systematic review by Peters et.al., 12 studies comparing different antibiotic regimens in the management of skin and soft-tissue infection, none reported a better response with any particular regimen. Of seven studies that compared antibiotic regimens in patients with infection involving both soft tissue and bone, one reported a better clinical outcome in those treated with cefoxitin compared with ampicillin/sulbactam. The author concluded that no published data support the superiority of any particular route of delivery of systemic antibiotics or clarify the optimal duration of antibiotic therapy in either soft-tissue infection or osteomyelitis. Therefore, further studies are necessary in answering the questions above.[53] Once the decision is made that surgical intervention is necessary for infection control, the surgeon should follow a systematic approach. This approach includes: incision, inspection, debridement, culture, irrigation, hemostasis, and post-operative care. A systematic approach for deep abscess is helpful to plan an appropriate treatment: decompression, drainage, debridement, and drugs. Decompression could be done at the bedside or in the operating room. It is important to perform this initial procedure to avoid increased pressure within the foot compartment, thus gangrenous extension occur.

C. Diabetic foot osteomyelitis

Contiguous osteomyelitis with vascular involvement, most often involving diabetics, is a commonly observed form of osteomyelitis that exemplifies the challenges in diagnosis and treatment of chronic bone infections. In one study, the majority of diabetic foot ulcers (68%) had an underlying osteomyelitis that was infrequently (32%) diagnosed clinically.[54] They also found that all patients with ulcers that exposed bone had osteomyelitis.[54] Palpation of bone in the infected foot ulcer of a diabetic patient has 66% sensitivity and 85% specificity, and is a reasonable initial assessment tool.[55] Diagnostic imaging presents a particular challenge in the neuropathic foot,[56] even with MRI.[57] Indeed, in one decision and cost-effectiveness analysis,[56] it was suggested that noninvasive testing adds significant expense to the treatment of diabetic patients with pedal osteomyelitis and may offer little improvement in outcome. The gold standard for diagnosing osteomyelitis is bone biopsy and culture. Most literature suggests that ulcer swabs correlate poorly with tissue specimens in this population,[58] although there is debate as to whether treatment based on bone biopsy results will improve the clinical outcome and prognosis compared with broad-spectrum empirical treatment or treatment based on swab culture results.[58-59] The treatment studies for contiguous osteomyelitis with vascular involvement are of a similar quality to those for osteomyelitis in general.[60] In fact, they are often one and the same, with diabetics not infrequently representing the larger cohort of patients in these trials. Despite these limitations in evidence, the Infectious Diseases Society of America has published a guideline for the diagnosis and treatment of diabetic foot infections.[44] They state that highly bioavailable oral antibiotics can be used in some cases of osteomyelitis, and that at least four to six weeks of therapy is required, and probably longer if infected bone remains.[44]

The diagnosis and management of osteomyelitis (OM) remains a controversial subject despite many years of research. Although surgical management has been the mainstay of a successful treatment, long-term intravenous (IV) antibiotics have been used even when the bone has been removed. The evidence of long-term antibiotics once infected bone is removed is poor.[60-61] The success of long-term antibiotics has been demonstrated in acute OM, and in other parts of the body such vertebral OM, long bones OM. In 1970, Waldvogel et al.[62] recommended that hematogenous OM be treated with high-dose antibiotics for at least four weeks. The rationale was that hematogenous OM represented a septic metastasis, and that penicillin penetration of bone required high doses of antibiotics. They supported this recommendation by describing the outcomes of patients who had received intensive (four weeks or longer) or limited therapy and, incidentally, noted that surgery was not necessarily required. However, for chronic OM, they noted that the outcome of therapy was similar in patients who received intensive and limited antimicrobial treatment, but a pattern of prolonged therapy for chronic OM emerged.[62]

Some clinicians consider selecting a specific antimicrobial based on its reported penetration into bone. Data related to bone penetration come from animal studies in which the bone and serum concentrations of antibiotics used to treat experimentally infected rats or rabbits are measured. These studies generally demonstrate excellent bone penetration by rifampin[63-64] and clindamycin,[65] with good penetration by fluoroquinolones[63] and low bone concentrations achieved by cefazolin.[64-65] Human pharmacokinetic studies are largely performed in the setting of surgical prophylaxis for joint arthroplasty. From several studies,[66-67] it appears that beta-lactams penetrate to a lesser extent into uninfected bone than clindamycin. However, Darley and MacGowan[68] suggest caution in interpreting the results of such bone penetration studies in humans. They note that the methodology has not been standardized, assay procedures may affect results considerably, healthy bone may not reflect pharmacokinetics in infected bone, penetration into cortical and medullary bone differs, and that blood contamination may not have been accounted for.

XI. Imaging of the diabetic foot

Diagnostic imaging has long played a major role in the investigation of suspected osteomyelitis. When interpreting the literature on performance characteristics of different radiographic tests, it is important to remember that osteomyelitis is a heterogeneous condition, and to be clear on what clinical entity the particular modality is assessing (e.g. acute or chronic osteomyelitis, presence or absence of neuropathic changes). In a similar vein, it is critical that any individual patient's imaging results be interpreted in light of the clinical situation, considering what patient-specific features may interfere with the test's reported sensitivity and specificity.

Computed tomography (CT) and magnetic resonance imaging (MRI) have become popular diagnostic methods, in part because of their high anatomical resolution. CT identifies areas of necrotic bone, soft-tissue infection and altered marrow density due to osteomyelitis.[65] However, altered marrow density can also be seen with neoplasms, hemorrhage, fractures, or irradiation.[69] In the one small study that met Termaat et al.'s criteria,[70] CT had a sensitivity of 67% (95% CI 24 to 94) and specificity of 50% (92% CI 3 to 97) in the diagnosis of chronic osteomyelitis of the spine. Where CT can play an important role is in delineating the extent of necrotic bone, thereby guiding debridement.[69] In the meta-analysis (five eligible studies), MRI had a sensitivity (84%) in the same range as that of a bone scans, with somewhat better specificity (60%, 95% CI 38 to 78). MRI has been suggested as the modality of choice in determining the extent of infection.[69] Despite being a relatively new technique, there were four studies on positron emission tomography (PET) in the meta-analysis.[70] PET had a sensitivity of 96% (95% CI 88 to 99), which was higher than all other modalities. The specificity of PET was lower at 91% (95% CI 81 to 95), but this was still an improvement over all other imaging types. Based on this meta-analysis, PET scanning has the highest diagnostic accuracy for confirming or excluding the presence of chronic osteomyelitis.[70] Unfortunately, PET is of limited availability in most health-care facilities.

In the diabetic population, an accurate diagnosis of diabetic foot osteomyelitis (DFO) is essential to institute appropriate therapy and to avoid unnecessary treatment of patients that do not have a bone infection. The Infectious Disease Society of America (IDSA) guidelines recommend MRI to diagnose DFO, although they acknowledge that bone biopsy for pathology and microbiology is the gold standard. MRI is considered to be the best imaging technique for the early diagnosis of DFO with a pooled sensitivity of 0.90 (CI 0.82-0.95), a specificity of 0.79 (CI 0.62-0.91) and a diagnostic odds ratio of 24.4. Unfortunately, MRI has often been reported to have low specificity and positive predictive value when noninfectious changes are present, especially in patients with previous foot surgery, trauma, or Charcot neuroarthropathy.

Among the different types of nuclear imaging techniques, the three-phase bone scan might be one of the most sensitive to diagnose osteomyelitis (90%). Unfortunately, it also suffers from a high rate of false positive results in cases of degenerative or reparative changes in the bone unrelated to infection. In addition, nuclear medicine studies have poor resolution, and the specific site and extent of infection in the foot is often difficult to visualize. A new hybrid imaging technology - 99mTc-WBC SPECT/CT - combines radiolabeled white blood cells and high-resolution X-ray Computed Tomography. This technique has the advantage of the three-dimensional CT scan, which improves the assessment of the WBC intensity and the extent of infection into bone. Also, by grading the WBC intensity, a physiologic response of local tissue can be seen and declining intensity might be used as a prognostic tool predicting success of treatment. So far only a few studies have evaluated the diagnostic accuracy and prognostic value of this new technique. It is our hypothesis that the accuracy of hybrid image 99mTc labeled WBC SPECT/CT for diagnosing diabetic foot osteomyelitis is superior to MRI.

Given the less-than-perfect performance characteristics, the role of diagnostic imaging should be viewed as confirming the presumed clinical diagnosis and providing information regarding the exact site and extent of infection.(69) Thus, no technique can absolutely confirm or exclude the diagnosis.

XII. Management of noninfected diabetic foot ulcer

See Noninfected Diabetic Foot Wounds Pathway, Offloading Foot Orthotics Pathway, and Prescription Offloading Shoe Adjustments Pathway. Reduction of pressure and shear forces on the foot may be the single most important yet most often neglected aspect of neuropathic ulcer treatment. Offloading therapy is a key part of the treatment plan for diabetic foot ulcers. The goal is to reduce the pressure at the ulcer site and keep the patient ambulatory.(71-72) Several methods are available to protect the foot from abnormal pressure. Offloading strategies must be tailored to the age, strength, activity, and home environment of the patient. In general, however, more restrictive offloading approaches will result in less activity and better wound healing. Education is critical to improve compliance with offloading. The patient must understand that the wound is a result of repetitive pressure and that every unprotected step is literally tearing the wound apart.

A. Total contact cast (TCC)

Use of a TCC is considered the gold standard for offloading the foot. TCCs reduce pressure at the ulcer site while still allowing the patient to be ambulatory.(73) A skilled clinician or technician is required to apply the molded plaster cast to ensure a proper fit. A TCC is a modification of a traditional fracture cast that uses minimal cast padding and includes a covering to protect the toes. The cast is molded to the contour of the foot and leg so that no movement is possible within the cast. TCCs are generally changed every one to two weeks but may need to be replaced more frequently in patients with edema or other concerns.

A TCC is one of the most effective ways of treating plantar neuropathic foot ulcers. Numerous studies(74-77) have shown that TCCs can heal ulcers in six to eight weeks. In descriptive and randomized clinical trials, the proportion of wounds that heal with TCCs is consistently much higher than those using topical growth factors, bioengineered tissue, or special dressings.(78-79)

One of the main advantages of using a TCC is that it forces patient compliance with offloading. The ulcer is protected with every step the patient takes. Using a TCC to facilitate wound healing is analogous to using a cast to heal a fracture - in both cases, healing is facilitated by rest and immobilization. The TCC reduces the patient's activity level, decreases stride length and cadence, and significantly reduces pressure at the ulcer site.(73,75) The main disadvantages for patients are the same as their complaints with a fracture cast – a cast is heavy and hot and makes bathing, walking, and sleeping difficult.

B. Removable cast walkers

The effectiveness of removable cast walkers to reduce pressure at ulcer sites has been shown in several studies to be comparable to that of TCCs.[73,75] Many practitioners consider removable cast walkers to be their preferred offloading device because they are less time-consuming and easier to apply than TCCs and patients more readily accept them. Wounds can be inspected regularly and treated with advanced wound care products such as growth factors, electrical stimulation, and other biologically active dressings. Also, the wound and limb can be inspected frequently.

Additional advantages of removable walking boots (as compared with TCCs) are that they are relatively inexpensive, the protective insole can be easily replaced if it shows signs of wear, no special training is required for correct and safe application, and they can be easily removed to assess and debride the wound as appropriate.[80] It's also possible to modify removable walkers into nonremovable devices by securing the walker with cast material or a nonremovable cable tie; this is known as an instant TCC. If patients can't remove the walker, the element of forced compliance that makes the TCC attractive is maintained and the outcomes for healing improve to the levels seen with the TCC.[81-82]

No single offloading device is appropriate for every patient. McGuire[83] has suggested a transitional approach to healing and maturing the diabetic foot ulcer that uses the instant TCC for initial pressure management and transitioning to removable devices and shoe-based platforms before the patient is ready for definitive footwear.

In a randomized controlled trial, Armstrong et al.[80] compared the effectiveness of TCCs, removable cast walkers, and half-shoes in healing neuropathic foot ulcerations in individuals with diabetes. The percentage of healing at 12 weeks was 89.5% for the TCC, 65.0% for the cast walker and 58.3% for the half-shoe. When the cast walker is made nonremovable (iTCC), the difference between the TCC and cast walker effectively disappears.[84]

C. Healing sandals and half-shoes

A number of healing sandals and half-shoes or wedged shoes are available to reduce pressure on the forefoot. These sandals and shoes are useful for patients who can't tolerate a TCC or for those who need a transitional device after removal of a TCC while they are awaiting custom-made therapeutic shoes and insoles.

Surgical shoes with a rocker sole design are preferable to the flat design for postoperative use. Royce Medical has a healing sandal that utilizes the Active Hex insole, described above, and can be used as a transitional device after closing the wound. The OrthoWedge by Darco products was originally designed to protect the forefoot after elective surgery. This shoe has a sole that's wedged at a 10-degree dorsiflexion angle, effectively removing pressure from the forefoot area. However, these types of shoes are not well accepted by patients because they are difficult to walk in, they typically cause pain of the contralateral extremity, and they are not safe for use in patients with postural instability. Also, many people with diabetes have equinus and cannot tolerate the negative heel position created by the shoe. Further, suspension of the heel during ambulation increases pressure on the forefoot and stresses the midfoot, a common site for collapse in the diabetic Charcot foot. In a randomized clinical trial that compared TCCs with healing sandals and removable cast boots, patients in the healing sandal group were less compliant and used the device during walking significantly less than did subjects in the TCC group.[85]

D. Ankle-foot orthoses

Custom-made ankle-foot orthoses can be used for lower-extremity pathology, including Charcot fractures, tendon injuries, and neuropathic ulcers. The Charcot Restraint Orthotic Walker, for example, initially was used to treat patients with neuropathic fractures. It provides protection to the neuropathic foot and aids in controlling lower-extremity edema. This device looks like a ski boot; it has a rigid polypropylene shell with a rocker bottom sole.

The primary drawback to custom-made devices is that they typically cost more than $1,000. If the structure of the foot changes or local edema resolves, the device can no longer be used. Since a number of less expensive, off-the-shelf products are now available to treat neuropathic wounds, custom ankle-foot orthoses are used less commonly. Off-the-shelf devices should be replaced at regular intervals because the materials in the insoles will lose their effectiveness over time.

E. Debridement

Sharp debridement of the ulcer removes devitalized tissue, reduces the bacterial load of the wound, eliminates proteases from the wound bed, and provides a bleeding wound bed. A diabetic ulcer typically has a thick rim of keratinized tissue surrounding it. Debridement must remove the callus and devitalized tissue, so that a clean wound edge is created and all edge pressure from the callus is removed. Enzymatic or autolytic debridement may be an option if sharp debridement is not possible or if the patient has PAD.(86) Ongoing debridement is imperative throughout the healing process.(87) Indeed, higher healing rates have been observed in patients who have had more frequent debridement. In addition, in a post-hoc evaluation from the becaplermin gel pivotal trial, Steed reported a higher proportion of healed wounds in both the treatment and placebo study groups when wound debridement was performed more frequently.(88)

It is important to acknowledge that not all forms of sharp debridement are the same. Sharp debridement performed in the clinic has significant limitations that may result in insufficient removal of devitalized tissue and pathogens. The inability to control significant bleeding, pain control, and the nonsterility of the environment in which it is performed limit aggressive debridement. Operating room debridement eliminates these barriers. An evolution in thought for the treatment of chronic wounds should include "excisional debridement."(89) This technique describes the excision of the entirety of the wound and its perimeter much like the approach to a soft-tissue tumor. Further, in the operating room setting, after this type of debridement is performed, a definitive closure or graft can be placed.

Maggot therapy consists of the topical application of medical-grade, sterile, growth-arrested fly larvae. Sherman reported a significant reduction in necrotic tissue with maggot therapy as compared with conventional wound therapy with complete removal of all necrotic tissue after four weeks.(90) Maggots are applied onto the wound surface and are housed in a breathable mesh cage about the wound site for two to three days at a time. The maggots digest and degrade infected and necrotic tissue continuously without affecting healthy tissue.

Ultrasound debridement imparts sound energy to the wound site. The two types of ultrasound are contact and noncontact. As the name indicates, the contact ultrasound is in direct contact with the wound surface while the noncontact ultrasound transmits sound energy through a saline medium. Beyond removal of nonviable tissue, ultrasound energy can penetrate to deeper layers of the wound surface, thereby potentially disrupting biofilm. Seth et al. reported in a rabbit ear wound biofilm model that ultrasound significantly reduced biofilm inflammatory cytokine production.[91] Robust human studies are still needed to fully understand the impact of this technology.

XIII. Surgical approach to managing the diabetic foot

The rationale for surgical intervention is to correct the structural deformity and/or increase motion and interrupt the causal pathway to foot ulceration. Surgical treatment of the diabetic foot can be classified in one of four groups: elective, prophylactic, curative, and emergent. This supports the premise that there may be opportunities to intervene in the pathway to deformity, ulceration, and infection before amputation becomes the only surgical option. The probability of obtaining and maintaining a healed, functional foot after surgical intervention is difficult to determine for patients with diabetes because they have greater complication rates than age-matched, nondiabetic patients. However, a patient recently diagnosed with diabetes or who has controlled the disease since diagnosis may have normal or near normal healing parameters. On the other hand, patients with chronically elevated blood glucose, peripheral neuropathy, peripheral vascular disease, pedal deformities, or end-stage renal disease and those whose duration of diabetes is greater than 10 years, which correlates with high prevalence of said comorbidities, have greater risk of complications.[92]

The surgeon must consider and discuss the risks and benefits of treatment with the patient. First, the risk of a chronic open wound must be discussed. The patient should understand the incidence of soft-tissue and bone infection, and foot or leg amputation is high. More than 50% of foot ulcers are treated for infection and 20% develop osteomyelitis.[33,93-94] In cohort studies of patients with foot wounds, 56% of patients develop infections and 6% to 15% of foot ulcers end in amputation.[95-96] Adequate assessment of the patient's neurovascular status and medical condition will give the surgeon an opportunity to discuss their individual risk of surgically treating his or her condition. Several authors have reported the results of planned surgical procedures to heal foot ulcers. These studies suggest a relatively low infection rate (4.4%-40%), while 40% is quite high it did not differ from the nonoperative group, which had a 38% infection rate. Even with a relatively high infection rate 91%- 96% of the wounds went on to heal and only 2.4%-6.6% of those surgically treated had recurrence of the ulcer.[33,97-98]

TABLE 3: Classification of different types of surgery in the diabetic foot

Class 1 ELECTIVE	To relief of PAINFUL deformity	Ex: bunion, hammertoe
Class 2 PROPHYLACTIC	To prevent ulcer formation	Ex: no active ulcer (or has healed ulcer) but has potential to occur/reoccur
Class 3 CURATIVE	To cure active ulcer	Ex: Keller arthroplasty, exostectomy
Class 4 EMERGENT	ACUTE limb/foot salvage	Ex: Deep plantar space infection

Adapted and reprinted with permission. Armstrong DG, Frykberg RG. Classifying diabetic foot surgery: toward a rational definition. Diabet Med. 2003 Apr;20(4):329-331.

Armstrong et al.[98] retrospectively examined 31 diabetics and 33 nondiabetic patients who underwent a single lesser digit arthroplasty for hammertoe deformity. This would be considered "prophylactic" surgery.[99] They further divided the diabetic group into Risk Group 2 (peripheral neuropathy and deformity) and Risk Group 3 (peripheral neuropathy, deformity, and history of ulcer).[98,100] They examined postoperative infection rates and dehiscence rates with an average follow-up of three years. Their results showed there was no significant difference in overall complications between diabetic and nondiabetic patients with this procedure, but there was a significantly higher risk of postoperative infection in patients who had a previous history of neuropathic ulcers. The long-term outcome of this "prophylactic" surgery in high-risk diabetic patients (Risk Group 3) were uniformly good with approximately 96% remaining ulcer free at a mean of three years follow-up.[98]

The overall goal of surgical care is to reduce the long-term risk for ulceration by preserving motion and reducing abnormal pressure and shear forces. Understanding pathologic structural and biomechanical abnormalities is essential to plan appropriate surgical procedures. Both static and dynamic components of the deformities must be evaluated. We will now discuss clinical evaluation of specific pathologic deformities by anatomic location and the evidence-based procedures currently used to correct these deformities. Procedures to correct biomechanically foot deformities can be divided in forefoot and rear foot procedures. Although many procedures can be attempted, several have enough medical evidence to support their use. Greater than 50% of plantar foot ulcers occur either on the hallux or the first metatarsal head.[49,101]

A. Forefoot procedures

Distal tip ulcers of the hallux usually occurs because of a flexion deformity at the interphalangeal joint causing excessive stress.[32] This deformity should be evaluated and classified as either rigid (unable to manually reduce the deformity) or flexible (manually reducible). A flexible deformity can be treated with a flexor tenotomy.[102] Rigid deformities can be addressed with an interphalangeal joint arthroplasty.[97]

Hallux rigidus and hallux valgus can present individually or combined; both lead to imbalances of forces about the first metatarsal phalangeal joint and hallux. Structural deformity and limited joint mobility of the first metatarsophalangeal joint is often associated with ulcers under the metatarsal head and interphalangeal joint of the great toe. Arthroplasty of the base of the proximal phalanx of the great toe (Keller arthroplasty) is the most common procedure described. The surgical options to heal and prevent recurrence include arthroplasty of the interphalangeal joint of the great toe, metatarsophalangeal joint arthroplasty, or metatarsophalangeal joint arthroplasty with implant (total or hemi-implant). Total and hemi implants are avoided in this patient population because the ulceration causes increased risk of infection with retained implants. Armstrong found that performing an arthroplasty of the first metatarsophalangeal joint resulted in a faster healing time, fewer recurrent ulcers, and no increase in infection rate for patients with plantar interphalangeal joint ulcers of the hallux.[33]

Lin reported that 14 or 14 recalcitrant plantar hallux wounds healed in 23 days or less after resecting the base of the proximal phalanx of the hallux and offloading in a total contact cast compared to 15 randomly selected controls. All of the controls healed in an average of 47 days with total contact cast immobilization. All of the surgical candidates had toe-brachial indices of at least 0.65 and initially failed 40 days of total contact cast therapy before surgery. There were no recurrences or other complications 26 weeks after surgery.[103]

Toe deformities are common in people who have had diabetes for more than 10 years.[104-105] They are thought to develop in some cases because of motor neuropathy that first affects the intrinsic muscles in the foot (intrinsic minus foot) (Figure 4). One of the functions of the intrinsic muscles is to stabilize the toes against the metatarsals. Thus, weak intrinsic muscles allow the long flexors and extensors to become imbalanced causing toe contractures. This type of deformity may cause pathologic pressure on the distal aspect of the toe when weight-bearing, dorsal aspect of the head of the proximal phalanx from rubbing the toe box in shoe gear, and plantar aspect of the corresponding metatarsal head from ground force when weight bearing.

Ulcers of the toes are usually associated with structural deformity.[106] In many cases, toe ulcers are associated with a high rate of recurrence.[33,107] The definitions of toe deformities should facilitate discussion of the level and severity of pathology; however, considerable ambiguity exists in the literature regarding the exact definitions.[108,109] A hammertoe deformity is a dorsal contracture (extension) of the proximal phalanx at the metatarsophalangeal joint and plantar contracture (flexion) of the middle phalanx at the proximal interphalangeal joint. A claw toe deformity is a dorsal contracture (extension) of the proximal phalanx at the metatarsophalangeal joint and plantar contractures (flexion) at both the proximal and distal interphalangeal joints. If the long flexor tendon becomes overpowering, flexion deformity at the DIPJ level can occur, placing the normally distal-facing end of the toe plantar-ward, bearing weight when standing and walking. The distal tip of the toe has very little fat pad to absorb the shock and shear of standing, walking, and running. The increased pressure on this skin results in excessive hyperkeratotic build-up, which exacerbates the pathologic pressure on the distal toe.

Kearney et al. retrospectively reviewed a cohort of 48 patients with 58 FHL tenotomy procedures with diabetes related neuropathic ulceration at the tip of the toe.[110] Almost all ulcerations healed (98.3%) at approximately five weeks. However, 12.1% had a recurrence of ulceration at the same site at a mean time of 13.9 months. They concluded that flexor tenotomy is a safe, simple procedure, which can enhance patients' healing potential with very little risk. Tamir retrospectively assessed the results of flexor tenotomy and hyperextension of rigid joint (osteoclasis) in 34 toes (14 patients with diabetes). Twenty-four (71%) digits had a concomitant ulceration at the time of tenotomy. The other digits had a claw toe deformity and had the tenotomy performed prophylactically. Three of the ulcerations had osteomyelitic changes of the tuft of the distal phalanx on radiographs. These ulcerations healed in eight weeks; all of the other ulcers healed in three weeks. They concluded that this procedure is effective for healing wounds penetrating to bone with osteomyelitis (with appropriate antibiotic therapy), but the wound healing will be prolonged.[104] When there is a rigid deformity that cannot be manually reduced, resecting the head of the phalanx is usually necessary. The procedure can be performed at the proximal or distal interphalangeal joint, depending on where the deformity lies. If there is accompanying soft-tissue contracture at the metatarsophalangeal joint, additional procedures may be required to reduce these deformities. Kim reported results of a cohort of patients with diabetes with ulcers and osteomyelitis. Kim reviewed 72 lesser toe arthroplasties performed because of ulceration and underlying osteomyelitis. He removed devitalized tissue and infected bone, and 79% of the toes went on to complete healing in 32 days.[111]

Metatarsal head ulcers are very common in the diabetic foot. This is likely due to focal plantar pressure from a prominent/deformed metatarsal. Concomitantly, ankle joint equinus could be contributing to these local deformities in the forefoot. The causes of such ulcers are often due to the following deformities: hammertoe, hallux valgus, forefoot arthropathy, soft tissue atrophy, compensated or uncompensated forefoot varus or valgus.[112-113] Often these deformities are rigid. Blume conducted at retrospective study of 67 diabetic patients that had peripheral neuropathy and an ulcer without osteomyelitis. All patients underwent a single-stage osseous procedure (arthroplasty, exostectomy, phalangectomy, planing, etc.) of the forefoot, midfoot, or rearfoot with primary closure with local flaps. Ultimately, 97% of the ulcers healed after surgery and 96% were healed 20 weeks after surgery. The most common complications were wound dehiscence (18%), infection (12%), skin slough (9%), and fracture/Charcot collapse (6%). They report a low rate of transfer or recurrence 11.9% (8/67) after at least 22 months of follow-up.[114]

The surgeon can elect to excise a single metatarsal head or all metatarsal heads to prevent recurrence. Rosenblum excised 22 metatarsal heads, performed 15 metatarsal osteotomies, and five panmetatarsal head resections in 42 feet that had recently undergone lower extremity revascularization procedures (aortobifemoral bypass [1], bypass to the popliteal [8], tibial/peroneal [20], dorsalis pedis/plantar artery [13]. Eighty-three percent [35/42] healed primarily and maintained an ulcer-free foot and patent bypass grafts during the 21-month follow-up period. Two patients (5%) required a revision of the original foot surgery to heal, and three patients (7%) experienced transfer lesions and had a secondary procedure to obtain an ulcer-free foot. One patient required a below-knee amputation secondary to a thrombosed graft and ischemia, and one patient died six months after foot surgery and before his ulcer had healed. Ultimately, 40 (95%) went on to heal with no recurrence in the follow-up period.[115] Giurini retrospectively analyzed 34 panmetatarsal head resections in patients with diabetes and a forefoot ulcer.[116] Thirty-two feet healed primarily, one healed slowly with secondary intention, and one had a recurrent ulcer. Ultimately, 97% of the ulcers healed and remained ulcer free for an average of 20.9 months.

B. Rear foot procedures

Ankle joint equinus (reduced dorsiflexion) has been associated with high pressures on the plantar aspect of the foot and increased risk of foot ulceration in persons with diabetes. For instance, diabetic patients with equinus were three times more likely to have elevated foot pressures compared to diabetic patients without equinus.[26,117] Grant noted a disorganized structure of the Achilles tendon in patients with diabetes compared to persons without diabetes using electron microscopy. He identified increased packing density of collagen fibrils, decreases in fibrillar diameter, and abnormal fibril morphology.[27] If this same process occurs in humans with diabetes, advanced glycation end products could shorten and stiffen the Achilles tendon. In gait this would reduce the time of heel strike and subsequently increase the duration of midfoot and forefoot loading and increase peak foot pressures in the forefoot.

To address this deformity in patients with recalcitrant forefoot ulcers, several authors have surgically lengthened the Achilles tendon. Several approaches can be used to lengthen the

Achilles tendon: endoscopic or open gastrocnemius recession, Z lengthening of the Achilles tendon, and percutaneous Achilles tendon lengthening (ATL). Lengthening the Achilles tendon is indicated when short Achilles tendon limits ankle joint dorsiflexion. Ankle joint motion is measured with the long axis of the goniometer along the fibula and the fifth metatarsal bone. The patient should be supine with the knee extended. The subtalar joint should be in neutral position, and the foot should be dorsiflexed on the lower leg.

Holstein stressed the importance of evaluating the severity of sensory neuropathy, particularly of the heel pad before proceeding with an ATL. He defined complete anesthesia of the heel as the inability to feel the 10-gram monofilament, or a sharp or dull instrument firmly applied to the heel and suggested an ATL is contraindicated in such patients. He came to this conclusion because 47% of his patients that met the criteria of complete anesthesia developed heel ulcers postoperatively.[118] Mueller and colleagues performed the only randomized clinical trial assessing the effectiveness of ATL versus a total-contact cast control in healing diabetic foot ulcers.[117] The criterion for surgery was ankle dorsiflexion less than 5 degrees, recurrent or non-healing Wagner Grade 2 ulceration, palpable ankle pulse, and neuropathy. All of the ATL patients healed in an average of 58 ± 47 days and 88% healed in a mean time of 41 ± 28 days in the total contact cast group. Average ankle joint dorsiflexion increased 15.2 degrees with the knee extended in the ATL group and patients maintained this motion at their seven-month follow-up visit. There was no change in ankle range of motion in subjects treated with casting. However, an ATL is not without its complications. In addition to the completely neuropathic patients mentioned above, Holstein reported that 18% of patients with more than 10 degrees of ankle dorsiflexion after surgery developed a heel ulcer.[118] Barry and Mueller report heel ulcers in 16% and 13% of patients after undergoing an Achilles tendon lengthening procedure.[117,119] Decreasing the strength of the ankle joint plantar flexors effectively reduces the pressure on the forefoot and redistributes the pressure to the heel, which may cause an ulcer on the heel.

XIV. Adjunctive therapies for diabetic foot ulcers

Electrical stimulation to treat wounds has been evaluated in pressure ulcers, venous stasis ulcers, vascular ulcers, and diabetic foot wounds. The majority of trials with electrical stimulation and wound healing show a significant improvement in wound area reduction or wound healing compared to standard of care or sham therapy.[120-121] Although there is a substantial body of work that supports the effectiveness of electrical stimulation in wound healing, most clinicians have a poor understanding of the technology and its potential applications in patients with diabetes. The application of transcutaneous electrical nerve stimulation (TENS) to improve skin perfusion and venous flow in diabetic patients is reported frequently.[121-122] When the human skin becomes hypoxic and releases cytokines, the expression of vascular endothelial growth factor (VEGF) is increased. Electrical stimulation initiates the release of stored VEGF followed by an increase in gene expression of VEGF. Daily electrical stimulation might allow secretion of VEGF to remain above basal levels throughout the healing process. Another advantage of electrical stimulation might be the bacteriostatic effect in infected ulcers as described in several experimental studies.[123]

Hyperbaric oxygen therapy (HBO_2 therapy) is another adjunctive therapy used for difficult wounds to heal. HBO_2 exerts its effects largely through controlled and brief increases in reactive oxygen species (ROS) and reactive nitrogen species (RNS). The increase in ROS and RNS leads to increased levels of a number of wound growth factors as well as growth factor receptors, mobilization of stem/progenitor cells from the bone marrow, reduced integrin function and thus reduced pathologic neutrophil adhesion, and changes in monocyte chemokine synthesis and changes in hemoxygenase-1, heat shock proteins and hypoxia-inducible factor-1 that reduce pathologic inflammation.[(124)] Several studies[(125)] with stringent selection criteria have demonstrated a beneficial effect on the healing of chronic ulcers. Over a 15-year period, there are 10 published evidence-based studies that have been directed to the effectiveness of HBO_2treatment and diabetic foot ulcers. Although the clinical trials show positive responses when $HBO_2$is used as an adjunctive therapy, different designs criteria could be highlighted such as, population chosen, type of intervention used, treatment pressure, outcomes, surgical endpoints, and study protocols. However, the addition of HBO_2 as an adjunctive therapy has shown consistently positive results. High-quality trials with a health economic analysis and large patient populations are further needed to evaluate this adjunctive therapy.

Negative pressure wound therapy (NPWT) utilizes the local application of subatmospheric pressure to stimulate healing and provide a granular wound base for graft acceptance. Since the development of next generation devices, this adjunctive therapy has been more widely adopted with more reliable mechanisms and greater portability. NPWT with instillation allows for programmed cycles of a solution at the same time as subatmospheric pressure. Especially in the case of an infected foot ulcer, the application of an antimicrobial solution directly to the wound bed seems ideal. However, the ideal type of solution, the duration of therapy, and the dosing need to be further evaluated before this adjunctive therapy can be fully implemented in clinical practice.

XV. Education of patients with diabetic foot ulcers

The diabetic foot is wrapped in mythology and misinformation for patients, their families, and clinicians. Education is a key component to get the patient and family to participate in the prevention process. By itself, education is unlikely to be effective. The high-risk patient needs to have education as one of the primary layers of prevention, but other elements such as therapeutic shoes and insoles, professional foot care, and systemic disease modification must be included. It is difficult to evaluate education as a single intervention in a randomized clinical trial unless the other aspects of care are standardized. Several studies to evaluate diabetic foot education incorporate standard prevention strategies; however, many do not specify the availability of these services or how they were provided.[(126-127)]

There are three randomized clinical studies that evaluate clinical outcomes with an education intervention.[(127,129)] Most studies evaluate a change in patient knowledge as the primary outcome. It is unclear whether better knowledge translates into sustained changes in behavior and a reduction in ulcers, infections, or amputations. Understanding the disease process is not enough. The diabetic foot is a mechanical problem more than a medical problem. If the abnormal biomechanics of the foot are not addressed, the high-risk patient's understanding of the disease process alone will be insufficient to prevent repetitive ulcers, infections, and amputations. Usually, the educational message to patients is to inspect their feet, to avoid going barefoot, to avoid hot surfaces and hot water, and to seek professional foot care on a regular basis. These instructions are not practical or effective for most high-risk patients. Many patients are obese with poor vision and limited mobility of their backs, hips, knees, and ankles. Most patients are unable to provide any meaningful self-inspection.[6] Because of obesity or limited joint range of motion, they cannot physically position themselves to see the bottoms of their feet. As a consequence of poor vision, they cannot see the bottoms of their feet or recognize subtle changes that identify tissue damage. For instance, in a study by Lavery and colleagues, 48% of study patients had impaired vision and 41% lacked the flexibility to adequately position the foot so it could be examined.[6] Locking-Cusolito et al. evaluated similar criteria in a dialysis population and found that 25% of study patients had impaired vision and 45% lacked flexibility to correctly position the lower extremity so it could be visualized.[6,130] Perhaps a more rational approach would be to assess the skills of the patient, and if he or she is unable to see the top and bottom of the foot, someone else in the family could help with this type of assessment.

If patients have good vision and can position themselves to see their feet, they still may not be able to identify any changes that are meaningful. The early changes in the skin before an ulcer develops are too subtle for a patient or caregiver to recognize. However, they may be able to identify an ulcer as soon as it develops. Lavery and colleagues reported the results of a randomized clinical study where the control group received therapeutic shoes and insoles, education and regular foot care. Patients were instructed to contact the study nurse if they identified any abnormalities during visual inspection. A list of local signs they should look for was provided such as changes in color, temperature, or swelling. An ulcer had already developed in the vast majority of cases (97%) by the time the patients saw something that was "abnormal."[23] Visual changes and self-inspection may not be effective for most patients to prevent foot ulcers, if warning signs are too subtle to see.[24]

Lincoln randomized 172 patients with newly healed DFUs to receive usual care or one-to-one education. Patients who received the "education intervention" participated in a single session. Lincoln reported that subjects in the education group demonstrated improved knowledge compared to the control group. However, clinical outcomes were no different. There was no difference in foot ulcers or amputations among the treatment groups. The incidence of foot ulcers at six and 12 months was 30% and 41% in the education group and 21% and 41% in the control group.[128]

Litzelman et al. randomized 395 patients with diabetes to be assigned to either an education and prevention program or the standard care they would normally receive. The education-intervention group received foot education, telephone follow-up calls, and reminders to their primary care providers to do diabetic foot examinations. Patients who received "community standard care" were more likely to develop a foot ulcer, not perform recommended self-care practices, or have their feet examined by their primary care physician (education group 68%, standard of care group 28%).[127]

XVI. Foot amputations

Toe amputations, ray resections, and transmetatarsal amputations are highly functional amputations that require minimal prosthetic/orthotic intervention. Accommodative shoes with custom insoles, arch supports, and toe fillers are usually adequate and protect and/or help to relieve pressure on the foot. More active individuals with a transmetatarsal amputation may benefit from orthotic modifications that better substitute for the lost anterior foot lever arm. Options include the addition of carbon fiber or spring steel sole shanks, rocker soles, or short ankle foot orthosis.

Partial foot amputations at the tarsal-metatarsal and transtarsal levels (e.g. Lisfranc, Chopart) are relatively uncommon and have historically been associated with equinovarus contracture of the hindfoot, increasing the likelihood of skin breakdown over the plantar surface of the foot. However, improved surgical techniques that include Achilles tendon lengthening/resection and anterior tibialis and peroneus tendon transfers have reduced equinovarus deformities to result in a functional and useful amputation level. Prosthetic/orthotic devices for the individual with a proximal partial foot amputation need to supply medial-lateral stabilization of the hindfoot and substitute for the lost forefoot lever. Options include: 1) an extra-depth shoe with toe filler, steel shank and rocker bottom modifications; 2) custom posterior leaf-spring ankle foot orthosis with toe filler; or 3) a custom prosthetic foot with a self-suspending rear opening split socket. A major advantage of all partial foot amputations is the ability to be fully end bearing, allowing ambulation without any devices.

Summary

Diabetic foot ulcer care is a challenging problem for any health-care professional. As the population continues to age, the incidence of diabetes will continue to increase. Strong prevention programs are essential to reduce the number of foot ulcers. Ideally, a team approach will be the infrastructure for prevention and adequate treatment of these wounds. As demonstrated in this chapter, there are numerous techniques and strategies that can be used to manage foot ulcers. Offloading and regular debridement are the basic foundation to heal the wounds when infection and vascular disease have been addressed. Clinicians can choose among many products available to offload the diabetic foot. Adjunctive therapies along with debridement, offloading, and appropriate dressings can be critical in salvaging the diabetic limb.

Review questions

1. **The most important single independent risk factor for ulceration is:**

    a. peripheral vascular disease
    b. neuropathy
    c. foot deformity
    d. history of prior amputations

2. **The Semmes-Weinstein test is used to assess:**

    a. blood flow to the feet
    b. protective sensation of the feet
    c. pressure on the feet
    d. temperature of the feet

3. **The following are treatments that are considered standard of care for foot ulcers with adequate blood flow except:**

    a. debridement
    b. offloading
    c. antibiotics
    d. glucose control

4. **The most important treatment to heal a plantar foot ulcer is:**

    a. moisturizer
    b. offloading
    c. collagenase
    d. swab culture

5. **When foot ulcers continue to recur and obvious deformity exists, the best option is:**

    a. casting
    b. diabetic shoe
    c. surgical correction
    d. dressing changes and hope it never gets infected

6. Sometimes palpable pulses are unreliable in the diabetic patient because:

a. loss of protective sensation

b. of the diabetes

c. Mockenberg's sclerosis

d. lack of pedal hair

ANSWERS: 1) b
2) b
3) c
4) b
5) c
6) c

References

1. Danaei G, Finucane MM, Lu Y, Singh GM, Cowan MJ, Paciorek CJ, et al. National, regional, and global trends in fasting plasma glucose and diabetes prevalence since 1980: systematic analysis of health examination surveys and epidemiological studies with 370 country-years and 2.7 million participants. Lancet. 2011 Jul 2;378(9785):31-40. PubMed PMID: 21705069.
2. Lavery LA, Armstrong DG, Harkless LB. Classification of diabetic foot wounds. J Foot Ankle Surg. 1996 Nov-Dec;35(6):528-531. PubMed PMID: 8986890.
3. Abbott CA, Carrington AL, Ashe H, Bath S, Every LC, Griffiths J, et al. The North-West Diabetes Foot Care Study: incidence of, and risk factors for, new diabetic foot ulceration in a community-based patient cohort. Diabet Med. 2002 May;19(5):377-384. PubMed PMID: 12027925.
4. Lavery LA, van Houtum WH, Ashry HR, Armstrong DG, Pugh JA. Diabetes-related lower-extremity amputations disproportionately affect blacks and Mexican Americans. Southern Medical Journal. 1999 Jun;92(6):593-9. PubMed PMID: 10372853.
5. Lavery LA, Peters EJ, Armstrong DG. What are the most effective interventions in preventing diabetic foot ulcers? Int Wound J. 2008 Jun;5(3):425-33. PubMed PMID: 18593392.
6. Lavery LA, Armstrong DG, Vela SA, Quebedeaux TL, Fleischli JG. Practical criteria for screening patients at high risk for diabetic foot ulceration. Arch Intern Med. 1998 Jan 26;158(2):157-162. PubMed PMID: 9448554. Epub 1998/02/04. eng.
7. Calhoun JH, Overgaard KA, Stevens CM, Dowling JP, Mader JT. Diabetic foot ulcers and infections: current concepts. Advances in skin & wound care. 2002 Jan-Feb;15(1):31-42; quiz 4-5. PubMed PMID: 11905449.
8. Lavery LA, Peters EJ, Williams JR, Murdoch DP, Hudson A, Lavery DC. Reevaluating the way we classify the diabetic foot: restructuring the diabetic foot risk classification system of the International Working Group on the Diabetic Foot. Diabetes Care. 2008 Jan;31(1):154-6. PubMed PMID: 17934155. Epub 2007/10/16. eng.
9. Levin M. Diabetic foot wounds: pathogenesis and management. Advances in Wound Care: the Journal for Prevention and Healing. 1997 Mar-Apr;10(2):24-30. PubMed PMID: 9204808.
10. Wunderlich RP, Armstrong DG, Husain K, Lavery LA. Defining loss of protective sensation in the diabetic foot. Advances in Wound Care : the Journal for Prevention and Healing. 1998 May-Jun;11(3):123-128. PubMed PMID: 9729943.
11. Booth J, Young MJ. Differences in the performance of commercially available 10-g monofilaments. Diabetes Care. 2000 Jul;23(7):984-8. PubMed PMID: 10895851.
12. Nather A, Bee CS, Huak CY, Chew JL, Lin CB, Neo S, et al. Epidemiology of diabetic foot problems and predictive factors for limb loss. J Diabetes Complications. 2008 Mar-Apr;22(2):77-82. PubMed PMID: 18280436.
13. Shojaiefard A, Khorgami Z, Larijani B. Independent risk factors for amputation in diabetic foot. International Journal of Diabetes in Developing Countries. 2008 Apr;28(2):32-37. PubMed PMID: 19902045. Pubmed Central PMCID: 2772008.
14. Madanchi N, Tabatabaei-Malazy O, Pajouhi M, Heshmat R, Larijani B, Mohajeri-Tehrani MR. Who are diabetic foot patients? A descriptive study on 873 patients. Journal of Diabetes and Metabolic Disorders. 2013;12:36. PubMed PMID: 23826947. Pubmed Central PMCID: 3708818.

15. Fagher K, Londahl M. The impact of metabolic control and QTc prolongation on all-cause mortality in patients with type 2 diabetes and foot ulcers. Diabetologia. 2013 May;56(5):1140-1147. PubMed PMID: 23404446.

16. Pecoraro RE, Reiber GE, Burgess EM. Pathways to diabetic limb amputation. Basis for prevention. Diabetes Care. 1990 May;13(5):513-521. PubMed PMID: 2351029.

17. Tooke JE, Brash PD. Microvascular aspects of diabetic foot disease. Diabet Med. 1996;13 Suppl 1:S26-9. PubMed PMID: 8741825.

18. LoGerfo FW, Misare BD. Current management of the diabetic foot. Advances in surgery. 1996;30:417-426. PubMed PMID: 8960346.

19. Hirsch AT, Haskal ZJ, Hertzer NR, Bakal CW, Creager MA, Halperin JL, et al. ACC/AHA 2005 guidelines for the management of patients with peripheral arterial disease (lower extremity, renal, mesenteric, and abdominal aortic): executive summary a collaborative report from the American Association for Vascular Surgery/Society for Vascular Surgery, Society for Cardiovascular Angiography and Interventions, Society for Vascular Medicine and Biology, Society of Interventional Radiology, and the ACC/AHA Task Force on Practice Guidelines (Writing Committee to Develop Guidelines for the Management of Patients With Peripheral Arterial Disease) endorsed by the American Association of Cardiovascular and Pulmonary Rehabilitation; National Heart, Lung, and Blood Institute; Society for Vascular Nursing; TransAtlantic Inter-Society Consensus; and Vascular Disease Foundation. J Am Coll Cardiol. 2006 Mar 21;47(6):1239-1312. PubMed PMID: 16545667.

20. Catanzariti AR, Haverstock BD, Grossman JP, Mendicino RW. Offloading techniques in the treatment of diabetic plantar neuropathic foot ulceration. Advances in Wound Care: the Journal for Prevention and Healing. 1999 Nov-Dec;12(9):452-458. PubMed PMID: 10687557.

21. Lavery L, Gazewood JD. Assessing the feet of patients with diabetes. The Journal of Family Practice. 2000 Nov;49(11 Suppl):S9-16. PubMed PMID: 11093554.

22. Yong R, Karas TJ, Smith KD, Petrov O. The durability of the Semmes-Weinstein 5.07 monofilament. J Foot Ankle Surg. 2000 Jan-Feb;39(1):34-8. PubMed PMID: 10658948.

23. Lavery LA, Higgins KR, Lanctot DR, Constantinides GP, Zamorano RG, Armstrong DG, et al. Home monitoring of foot skin temperatures to prevent ulceration. Diabetes Care. 2004 Nov;27(11):2642-7. PubMed PMID: 15504999. Epub 2004/10/27. eng.

24. Lavery LA, Higgins KR, Lanctot DR, Constantinides GP, Zamorano RG, Athanasiou KA, et al. Preventing diabetic foot ulcer recurrence in high-risk patients: use of temperature monitoring as a self-assessment tool. Diabetes Care. 2007 Jan;30(1):14-20. PubMed PMID: 17192326.

25. Armstrong DG, Holtz-Neiderer K, Wendel C, Mohler MJ, Kimbriel HR, Lavery LA. Skin temperature monitoring reduces the risk for diabetic foot ulceration in high-risk patients. The American Journal of Medicine. 2007 Dec;120(12):1042-1046. PubMed PMID: 18060924. Epub 2007/12/07. eng.

26. Lavery LA, Armstrong DG, Boulton AJ, Diabetex Research G. Ankle equinus deformity and its relationship to high plantar pressure in a large population with diabetes mellitus. J Am Podiatr Med Assoc. 2002 Oct;92(9):479-482. PubMed PMID: 12381796.

27. Grant WP, Sullivan R, Sonenshine DE, Adam M, Slusser JH, Carson KA, et al. Electron microscopic investigation of the effects of diabetes mellitus on the Achilles tendon. J Foot Ankle Surg. 1997 Jul-Aug;36(4):272-8; discussion 330. PubMed PMID: 9298442.
28. Fowkes FG, Murray GD, Butcher I, Heald CL, Lee RJ, Chambless LE, et al. Ankle brachial index combined with Framingham Risk Score to predict cardiovascular events and mortality: a meta-analysis. JAMA. 2008 Jul 9;300(2):197-208. PubMed PMID: 18612117. Epub 2008/07/10. eng.
29. Dickhaut SC, DeLee JC, Page CP. Nutritional status: importance in predicting wound-healing after amputation. J Bone Joint Surg Am. 1984 Jan;66(1):71-5. PubMed PMID: 6690446. Epub 1984/01/01. eng.
30. Wagner FW, Jr. Amputations of the foot and ankle. Current status. Clin Orthop Relat Res. 1977 Jan-Feb(122):62-9. PubMed PMID: 837621. Epub 1977/01/01. eng.
31. Pinzur MS, Stuck RM, Sage R, Hunt N, Rabinovich Z. Syme ankle disarticulation in patients with diabetes. J Bone Joint Surg Am. 2003 Sep;85-A(9):1667-1672. PubMed PMID: 12954823. Epub 2003/09/05. eng.
32. Boffeli TJ, Bean JK, Natwick JR. Biomechanical abnormalities and ulcers of the great toe in patients with diabetes. J Foot Ankle Surg. 2002 Nov-Dec;41(6):359-364. PubMed PMID: 12500786. Epub 2002/12/26. eng.
33. Armstrong DG, Lavery LA, Vazquez JR, Short B, Kimbriel HR, Nixon BP, et al. Clinical efficacy of the first metatarsophalangeal joint arthroplasty as a curative procedure for hallux interphalangeal joint wounds in patients with diabetes. Diabetes Care. 2003 Dec;26(12):3284-3287. PubMed PMID: 14633815. Epub 2003/11/25. eng.
34. Resnick HE, Lindsay RS, McDermott MM, Devereux RB, Jones KL, Fabsitz RR, et al. Relationship of high and low ankle brachial index to all-cause and cardiovascular disease mortality: the strong heart study. Circulation. 2004 Feb 17;109(6):733-739. PubMed PMID: 14970108.
35. American Diabetes A. Peripheral arterial disease in people with diabetes. Diabetes Care. 2003 Dec;26(12):3333-3341. PubMed PMID: 14633825.
36. Carter SA, Tate RB. The value of toe pulse waves in determination of risks for limb amputation and death in patients with peripheral arterial disease and skin ulcers or gangrene. J Vasc Surg. 2001 Apr;33(4):708-714. PubMed PMID: 11296321.
37. Brooks B, Dean R, Patel S, Wu B, Molyneaux L, Yue DK. TBI or not TBI: that is the question. Is it better to measure toe pressure than ankle pressure in diabetic patients? Diabet Med. 2001 Jul;18(7):528-532. PubMed PMID: 11553180.
38. Zuzak KJ, Schaeberle MD, Gladwin MT, Cannon RO, 3rd, Levin IW. Noninvasive determination of spatially resolved and time-resolved tissue perfusion in humans during nitric oxide inhibition and inhalation by use of a visible-reflectance hyperspectral imaging technique. Circulation. 2001 Dec 11;104(24):2905-2910. PubMed PMID: 11739304.
39. Khaodhiar L, Dinh T, Schomacker KT, Panasyuk SV, Freeman JE, Lew R, et al. The use of medical hyperspectral technology to evaluate microcirculatory changes in diabetic foot ulcers and to predict clinical outcomes. Diabetes Care. 2007 Apr;30(4):903-10. PubMed PMID: 17303790.
40. Quigley FG, Faris IB. Transcutaneous oxygen tension measurements in the assessment of limb ischaemia. Clinical physiology. 1991 Jul;11(4):315-320. PubMed PMID: 1914435.

41. Kalani M, Brismar K, Fagrell B, Ostergren J, Jorneskog G. Transcutaneous oxygen tension and toe blood pressure as predictors for outcome of diabetic foot ulcers. Diabetes Care. 1999 Jan;22(1):147-151. PubMed PMID: 10333917.

42. Joseph WS, Lipsky BA. Medical therapy of diabetic foot infections. J Vasc Surg. 2010 Sep;52(3 Suppl):67S-71S. PubMed PMID: 20804935. Epub 2010/09/10. eng.

43. Eneroth M, Apelqvist J, Stenstrom A. Clinical characteristics and outcome in 223 diabetic patients with deep foot infections. Foot Ankle Int. 1997 Nov;18(11):716-722. PubMed PMID: 9391817. Epub 1997/12/10. eng.

44. Lipsky BA, Berendt AR, Deery HG, Embil JM, Joseph WS, Karchmer AW, et al. Diagnosis and treatment of diabetic foot infections. Clin Infect Dis. 2004 Oct 1;39(7):885-910. PubMed PMID: 15472838. Epub 2004/10/09. eng.

45. Kaleta JL, Fleischli JW, Reilly CH. The diagnosis of osteomyelitis in diabetes using erythrocyte sedimentation rate: a pilot study. J Am Podiatr Med Assoc. 2001 Oct;91(9):445-50. PubMed PMID: 11679625. Epub 2001/10/27. eng.

46. Armstrong DG, Lavery LA, Sariaya M, Ashry H. Leukocytosis is a poor indicator of acute osteomyelitis of the foot in diabetes mellitus. J Foot Ankle Surg. 1996 Jul-Aug;35(4):280-3. PubMed PMID: 8872749. Epub 1996/07/01. eng.

47. Jay PR, Michelson JD, Mizel MS, Magid D, Le T. Efficacy of three-phase bone scans in evaluating diabetic foot ulcers. Foot Ankle Int. 1999 Jun;20(6):347-355. PubMed PMID: 10395336. Epub 1999/07/08. eng.

48. Ledermann HP, Schweitzer ME, Morrison WB. Nonenhancing tissue on MR imaging of pedal infection: characterization of necrotic tissue and associated limitations for diagnosis of osteomyelitis and abscess. AJR. 2002 Jan;178(1):215-22. PubMed PMID: 11756124. Epub 2002/01/05. eng.

49. Armstrong DG, Lavery LA, Harkless LB. Validation of a diabetic wound classification system. The contribution of depth, infection, and ischemia to risk of amputation. Diabetes Care. 1998 May;21(5):855-859. PubMed PMID: 9589255. Epub 1998/05/20. eng.

50. Lavery LA, Armstrong DG, Murdoch DP, Peters EJ, Lipsky BA. Validation of the Infectious Diseases Society of America's diabetic foot infection classification system. Clin Infect Dis. 2007 Feb 15;44(4):562-565. PubMed PMID: 17243061. Epub 2007/01/24. eng.

51. Vardakas KZ, Horianopoulou M, Falagas ME. Factors associated with treatment failure in patients with diabetic foot infections: An analysis of data from randomized controlled trials. Diabetes Res Clin Pract. 2008 Jun;80(3):344-51. PubMed PMID: 18291550. Epub 2008/02/23. eng.

52. Lipsky BA. Evidence-based antibiotic therapy of diabetic foot infections. FEMS immunology and medical microbiology. 1999 Dec;26(3-4):267-276. PubMed PMID: 10575138. Epub 1999/11/27. eng.

53. Peters EJ, Lipsky BA, Berendt AR, Embil JM, Lavery LA, Senneville E, et al. A systematic review of the effectiveness of interventions in the management of infection in the diabetic foot. Diabetes Metab Res Rev. 2012 Feb;28 Suppl 1:142-62. PubMed PMID: 22271738.

54. Newman LG, Waller J, Palestro CJ, Schwartz M, Klein MJ, Hermann G, et al. Unsuspected osteomyelitis in diabetic foot ulcers. Diagnosis and monitoring by leukocyte scanning with indium in 111 oxyquinoline. JAMA. 1991 Sep 4;266(9):1246-51. PubMed PMID: 1908030.

55. Grayson ML, Gibbons GW, Balogh K, Levin E, Karchmer AW. Probing to bone in infected pedal ulcers. A clinical sign of underlying osteomyelitis in diabetic patients. JAMA. 1995 Mar 1;273(9):721-723. PubMed PMID: 7853630.

56. Eckman MH, Greenfield S, Mackey WC, Wong JB, Kaplan S, Sullivan L, et al. Foot infections in diabetic patients. Decision and cost-effectiveness analyses. JAMA. 1995 Mar 1;273(9):712-720. PubMed PMID: 7853629.

57. Ahmadi ME, Morrison WB, Carrino JA, Schweitzer ME, Raikin SM, Ledermann HP. Neuropathic arthropathy of the foot with and without superimposed osteomyelitis: MR imaging characteristics. Radiology. 2006 Feb;238(2):622-631. PubMed PMID: 16436821.

58. Senneville E, Melliez H, Beltrand E, Legout L, Valette M, Cazaubiel M, et al. Culture of percutaneous bone biopsy specimens for diagnosis of diabetic foot osteomyelitis: concordance with ulcer swab cultures. Clin Infect Dis. 2006 Jan 1;42(1):57-62. PubMed PMID: 16323092.

59. Embil JM, Trepman E. Microbiological evaluation of diabetic foot osteomyelitis. Clin Infect Dis. 2006 Jan 1;42(1):63-65. PubMed PMID: 16323093.

60. Stengel D, Bauwens K, Sehouli J, Ekkernkamp A, Porzsolt F. Systematic review and meta-analysis of antibiotic therapy for bone and joint infections. The Lancet Infectious diseases. 2001 Oct;1(3):175-188. PubMed PMID: 11871494.

61. Lazzarini L, Lipsky BA, Mader JT. Antibiotic treatment of osteomyelitis: what have we learned from 30 years of clinical trials? International journal of infectious diseases : IJID : official publication of the International Society for Infectious Diseases. 2005 May;9(3):127-138. PubMed PMID: 15840453.

62. Waldvogel FA, Medoff G, Swartz MN. Osteomyelitis: a review of clinical features, therapeutic considerations and unusual aspects. N Engl J Med. 1970 Jan 22;282(4):198-206. PubMed PMID: 4902833.

63. Dworkin R, Modin G, Kunz S, Rich R, Zak O, Sande M. Comparative efficacies of ciprofloxacin, pefloxacin, and vancomycin in combination with rifampin in a rat model of methicillin-resistant Staphylococcus aureus chronic osteomyelitis. Antimicrobial agents and chemotherapy. 1990 Jun;34(6):1014-1016. PubMed PMID: 2393259. Pubmed Central PMCID: 171748.

64. Norden CW. Experimental chronic staphylococcal osteomyelitis in rabbits: treatment with rifampin alone and in combination with other antimicrobial agents. Reviews of infectious diseases. 1983 Jul-Aug;5 Suppl 3:S491-4. PubMed PMID: 6635438.

65. Mader JT, Adams K, Morrison L. Comparative evaluation of cefazolin and clindamycin in the treatment of experimental Staphylococcus aureus osteomyelitis in rabbits. Antimicrobial agents and chemotherapy. 1989 Oct;33(10):1760-1764. PubMed PMID: 2589843. Pubmed Central PMCID: 172751.

66. Nicholas P, Meyers BR, Levy RN, Hirschman SZ. Concentration of clindamycin in human bone. Antimicrobial agents and chemotherapy. 1975 Aug;8(2):220-221. PubMed PMID: 1180546. Pubmed Central PMCID: 429291.

67. Smilack JD, Flittie WH, Williams TW, Jr. Bone concentrations of antimicrobial agents after parenteral administration. Antimicrobial agents and chemotherapy. 1976 Jan;9(1):169-171. PubMed PMID: 1259390. Pubmed Central PMCID: 429494.

68. Darley ES, MacGowan AP. Antibiotic treatment of gram-positive bone and joint infections. The Journal of antimicrobial chemotherapy. 2004 Jun;53(6):928-935. PubMed PMID: 15117932.

69. Pineda C, Vargas A, Rodriguez AV. Imaging of osteomyelitis: current concepts. Infectious disease clinics of North America. 2006 Dec;20(4):789-825. PubMed PMID: 17118291.

70. Termaat MF, Raijmakers PG, Scholten HJ, Bakker FC, Patka P, Haarman HJ. The accuracy of diagnostic imaging for the assessment of chronic osteomyelitis: a systematic review and meta-analysis. J Bone Joint Surg Am. 2005 Nov;87(11):2464-2471. PubMed PMID: 16264122.

71. Frykberg RG. A summary of guidelines for managing the diabetic foot. Advances in skin & wound care. 2005 May;18(4):209-214. PubMed PMID: 15920373.

72. Lavery LA, Vela SA, Lavery DC, Quebedeaux TL. Total contact casts: pressure reduction at ulcer sites and the effect on the contralateral foot. Archives of physical medicine and rehabilitation. 1997 Nov;78(11):1268-1271. PubMed PMID: 9365359.

73. Lavery LA, Vela SA, Lavery DC, Quebedeaux TL. Reducing dynamic foot pressures in high-risk diabetic subjects with foot ulcerations. A comparison of treatments. Diabetes Care. 1996 Aug;19(8):818-821. PubMed PMID: 8842597.

74. Lavery LA, Armstrong DG, Walker SC. Healing rates of diabetic foot ulcers associated with midfoot fracture due to Charcot's arthropathy. Diabet Med. 1997 Jan;14(1):46-49. PubMed PMID: 9017353.

75. Armstrong DG, Nguyen HC, Lavery LA, van Schie CH, Boulton AJ, Harkless LB. Offloading the diabetic foot wound: a randomized clinical trial. Diabetes Care. 2001 Jun;24(6):1019-1022. PubMed PMID: 11375363.

76. Sinacore DR. Total contact casting for diabetic neuropathic ulcers. Phys Ther. 1996 Mar;76(3):296-301. PubMed PMID: 8602415.

77. Caputo GM, Ulbrecht JS, Cavanagh PR. The total contact cast: a method for treating neuropathic diabetic ulcers. American family physician. 1997 Feb 1;55(2):605-611, 15-6. PubMed PMID: 9054227.

78. Veves A, Falanga V, Armstrong DG, Sabolinski ML, Apligraf Diabetic Foot Ulcer S. Graftskin, a human skin equivalent, is effective in the management of noninfected neuropathic diabetic foot ulcers: a prospective randomized multicenter clinical trial. Diabetes Care. 2001 Feb;24(2):290-295. PubMed PMID: 11213881.

79. Veves A, Sheehan P, Pham HT. A randomized, controlled trial of Promogran (a collagen/oxidized regenerated cellulose dressing) vs standard treatment in the management of diabetic foot ulcers. Arch Surg. 2002 Jul;137(7):822-827. PubMed PMID: 12093340.

80. Armstrong DG, Lavery LA, Wu S, Boulton AJ. Evaluation of removable and irremovable cast walkers in the healing of diabetic foot wounds: a randomized controlled trial. Diabetes Care. 2005 Mar;28(3):551-554. PubMed PMID: 15735186.

81. McGuire JB. Pressure redistribution strategies for the diabetic or at-risk foot: Part II. Advances in skin & wound care. 2006 Jun;19(5):270-277; quiz 7-9. PubMed PMID: 16732073.

82. Sibbald RG, Woo K, Ayello EA. Increased bacterial burden and infection: the story of NERDS and STONES. Advances in Skin & Wound Care. 2006 Oct;19(8):447-461; quiz 61-3. PubMed PMID: 17008815.

83. McGuire J. Transitional offloading: an evidence-based approach to pressure redistribution in the diabetic foot. Advances in Kkin & Wound Care. 2010 Apr;23(4):175-88; quiz 89-90. PubMed PMID: 20299844.

84. Katz IA, Harlan A, Miranda-Palma B, Prieto-Sanchez L, Armstrong DG, Bowker JH, et al. A randomized trial of two irremovable offloading devices in the management of plantar neuropathic diabetic foot ulcers. Diabetes Care. 2005 Mar;28(3):555-559. PubMed PMID: 15735187.

85. Myerson M, Papa J, Eaton K, Wilson K. The total-contact cast for management of neuropathic plantar ulceration of the foot. J Bone Joint Surg Am. 1992 Feb;74(2):261-269. PubMed PMID: 1311710.

86. Mulder GD. Evaluating and managing the diabetic foot: an overview. Advances in Skin & Wound Care. 2000 Jan-Feb;13(1):33-36. PubMed PMID: 11061708.

87. Steed DL, Donohoe D, Webster MW, Lindsley L. Effect of extensive debridement and treatment on the healing of diabetic foot ulcers. Diabetic Ulcer Study Group. Journal of the American College of Surgeons. 1996 Jul;183(1):61-64. PubMed PMID: 8673309.

88. Steed DL. Becaplermin: a viewpoint by David L. Steed. BioDrugs : clinical immunotherapeutics, biopharmaceuticals and gene therapy. 1999 May;11(5):366. PubMed PMID: 18031147.

89. Cornell RS, Meyr AJ, Steinberg JS, Attinger CE. Debridement of the noninfected wound. J Am Podiatr Med Assoc. 2010 Sep-Oct;100(5):353-359. PubMed PMID: 20847349.

90. Sherman RA. Maggot therapy for treating diabetic foot ulcers unresponsive to conventional therapy. Diabetes Care. 2003 Feb;26(2):446-451. PubMed PMID: 12547878.

91. Seth AK, Nguyen KT, Geringer MR, Hong SJ, Leung KP, Mustoe TA, et al. Noncontact, low-frequency ultrasound as an effective therapy against Pseudomonas aeruginosa-infected biofilm wounds. Wound repair and regeneration: official publication of the Wound Healing Society [and] the European Tissue Repair Society. 2013 Mar-Apr;21(2):266-274. PubMed PMID: 23421692.

92. The effect of intensive treatment of diabetes on the development and progression of long-term complications in insulin-dependent diabetes mellitus. The Diabetes Control and Complications Trial Research Group. N Engl J Med. 1993 Sep 30;329(14):977-986. PubMed PMID: 8366922.

93. Lavery LA, Armstrong DG, Wunderlich RP, Mohler MJ, Wendel CS, Lipsky BA. Risk factors for foot infections in individuals with diabetes. Diabetes Care. 2006 Jun;29(6):1288-1293. PubMed PMID: 16732010.

94. Lavery LA, Harkless LB, Ashry HR, Felder-Johnson K. Infected puncture wounds in adults with diabetes: risk factors for osteomyelitis. J Foot Ankle Surg. 1994 Nov-Dec;33(6):561-566. PubMed PMID: 7894402. Epub 1994/11/01. eng.

95. Winkley K, Stahl D, Chalder T, Edmonds ME, Ismail K. Risk factors associated with adverse outcomes in a population-based prospective cohort study of people with their first diabetic foot ulcer. J Diabetes Complications. 2007 Nov-Dec;21(6):341-349. PubMed PMID: 17967704. Epub 2007/10/31. eng.

96. Jeffcoate WJ, Chipchase SY, Ince P, Game FL. Assessing the outcome of the management of diabetic foot ulcers using ulcer-related and person-related measures. Diabetes Care. 2006 Aug;29(8):1784-1787. PubMed PMID: 16873780. Epub 2006/07/29. eng.

97. Rosenblum BI, Giurini JM, Chrzan JS, Habershaw GM. Preventing loss of the great toe with the hallux interphalangeal joint arthroplasty. J Foot Ankle Surg. 1994 Nov-Dec;33(6):557-560. PubMed PMID: 7894401. Epub 1994/11/01. eng.

98. Armstrong DG, Lavery LA, Stern S, Harkless LB. Is prophylactic diabetic foot surgery dangerous? J Foot Ankle Surg. 1996 Nov-Dec;35(6):585-589. PubMed PMID: 8986899. Epub 1996/11/01. eng.

99. Armstrong DG, Frykberg RG. Classifying diabetic foot surgery: toward a rational definition. Diabet Med. 2003 Apr;20(4):329-331. PubMed PMID: 12675649. Epub 2003/04/05. eng.

100. Armstrong DG, Lavery LA, Harkless LB. Treatment-based classification system for assessment and care of diabetic feet. J Am Podiatr Med Assoc. 1996 Jul;86(7):311-316. PubMed PMID: 8757481. Epub 1996/07/01. eng.

101. Birke JA, Sims DS. Plantar sensory threshold in the ulcerative foot. Lepr Rev. 1986 Sep;57(3):261-267. PubMed PMID: 3784758. Epub 1986/09/01. eng.

102. Laborde JM. Neuropathic toe ulcers treated with toe flexor tenotomies. Foot Ankle Int. 2007 Nov;28(11):1160-1164. PubMed PMID: 18021584. Epub 2007/11/21. eng.

103. Lin SS, Lee TH, Wapner KL. Plantar forefoot ulceration with equinus deformity of the ankle in diabetic patients: the effect of tendo-Achilles lengthening and total contact casting. Orthopedics. 1996 May;19(5):465-475. PubMed PMID: 8727341. Epub 1996/05/01. eng.

104. Tamir E, McLaren AM, Gadgil A, Daniels TR. Outpatient percutaneous flexor tenotomies for management of diabetic claw toe deformities with ulcers: a preliminary report. Can J Surg. 2008 Feb;51(1):41-44. PubMed PMID: 18248704. Pubmed Central PMCID: 2386314. Epub 2008/02/06. eng.

105. Singh N, Armstrong DG, Lipsky BA. Preventing foot ulcers in patients with diabetes. JAMA. 2005 Jan 12;293(2):217-228. PubMed PMID: 15644549. Epub 2005/01/13. eng.

106. Leung PC. Diabetic foot ulcers--a comprehensive review. Surgeon. 2007 Aug;5(4):219-231. PubMed PMID: 17849958. Epub 2007/09/14. eng.

107. Dargis V, Pantelejeva O, Jonushaite A, Vileikyte L, Boulton AJ. Benefits of a multidisciplinary approach in the management of recurrent diabetic foot ulceration in Lithuania: a prospective study. Diabetes Care. 1999 Sep;22(9):1428-1431. PubMed PMID: 10480504. Epub 1999/09/10. eng.

108. Padanilam TG. The flexible hammer toe flexor-to-extensor transfer. Foot and Ankle Clinics. 1998 June;3(2):259-267. English.

109. Schrier JC, Verheyen CC, Louwerens JW. Definitions of hammer toe and claw toe: an evaluation of the literature. J Am Podiatr Med Assoc. 2009 May-Jun;99(3):194-197. PubMed PMID: 19448169. Epub 2009/05/19. eng.

110. Kearney TP, Hunt NA, Lavery LA. Safety and effectiveness of flexor tenotomies to heal toe ulcers in persons with diabetes. Diabetes Res Clin Pract. 2010 Sep;89(3):224-226. PubMed PMID: 20580458. Epub 2010/06/29. eng.

111. Kim JY, Kim TW, Park YE, Lee YJ. Modified resection arthroplasty for infected non-healing ulcers with toe deformity in diabetic patients. Foot Ankle Int. 2008 May;29(5):493-497. PubMed PMID: 18510902. Epub 2008/05/31. eng.

112. Mueller MJ, Hastings M, Commean PK, Smith KE, Pilgram TK, Robertson D, et al. Forefoot structural predictors of plantar pressures during walking in people with diabetes and peripheral neuropathy. J Biomech. 2003 Jul;36(7):1009-1017. PubMed PMID: 12757810. Epub 2003/05/22. eng.

113. Mueller MJ, Minor SD, Diamond JE, Blair VP, 3rd. Relationship of foot deformity to ulcer location in patients with diabetes mellitus. Phys Ther. 1990 Jun;70(6):356-362. PubMed PMID: 2345779. Epub 1990/06/01. eng.

114. Blume PA, Paragas LK, Sumpio BE, Attinger CE. Single-stage surgical treatment of noninfected diabetic foot ulcers. Plast Reconstr Surg. 2002 Feb;109(2):601-609. PubMed PMID: 11818842. Epub 2002/01/31. eng.

115. Rosenblum BI, Pomposelli FB, Jr., Giurini JM, Gibbons GW, Freeman DV, Chrzan JS, et al. Maximizing foot salvage by a combined approach to foot ischemia and neuropathic ulceration in patients with diabetes. A 5-year experience. Diabetes Care. 1994 Sep;17(9):983-987. PubMed PMID: 7988319. Epub 1994/09/01. eng.

116. Giurini JM, Basile P, Chrzan JS, Habershaw GM, Rosenblum BI. Panmetatarsal head resection. A viable alternative to the transmetatarsal amputation. J Am Podiatr Med Assoc. 1993 Feb;83(2):101-107. PubMed PMID: 8478794. Epub 1993/02/01. eng.

117. Mueller MJ, Sinacore DR, Hastings MK, Strube MJ, Johnson JE. Effect of Achilles tendon lengthening on neuropathic plantar ulcers. A randomized clinical trial. J Bone Joint Surg Am. 2003 Aug;85-A(8):1436-1445. PubMed PMID: 12925622. Epub 2003/08/20. eng.

118. Holstein P, Lohmann M, Bitsch M, Jorgensen B. Achilles tendon lengthening, the panacea for plantar forefoot ulceration? Diabetes Metab Res Rev. 2004 May-Jun;20 Suppl 1:S37-40. PubMed PMID: 15150812. Epub 2004/05/20. eng.

119. Barry DC, Sabacinski KA, Habershaw GM, Giurini JM, Chrzan JS. Tendo Achillis procedures for chronic ulcerations in diabetic patients with transmetatarsal amputations. J Am Podiatr Med Assoc. 1993 Feb;83(2):96-100. PubMed PMID: 8478802. Epub 1993/02/01. eng.

120. Szuminsky NJ, Albers AC, Unger P, Eddy JG. Effect of narrow, pulsed high voltages on bacterial viability. Phys Ther. 1994 Jul;74(7):660-667. PubMed PMID: 8016198.

121. Peters EJ, Armstrong DG, Wunderlich RP, Bosma J, Stacpoole-Shea S, Lavery LA. The benefit of electrical stimulation to enhance perfusion in persons with diabetes mellitus. J Foot Ankle Surg. 1998 Sep-Oct;37(5):396-400; discussion 47-8. PubMed PMID: 9798171.

122. Gilcreast DM, Stotts NA, Froelicher ES, Baker LL, Moss KM. Effect of electrical stimulation on foot skin perfusion in persons with or at risk for diabetic foot ulcers. Wound repair and regeneration: official publication of the Wound Healing Society [and] the European Tissue Repair Society. 1998 Sep-Oct;6(5):434-441. PubMed PMID: 9844163.

123. Kincaid CB, Lavoie KH. Inhibition of bacterial growth in vitro following stimulation with high voltage, monophasic, pulsed current. Phys Ther. 1989 Aug;69(8):651-655. PubMed PMID: 2501804.

124. Thom SR. Hyperbaric oxygen: its mechanisms and efficacy. Plast Reconstr Surg. 2011 Jan;127 Suppl 1:131S-141S. Review. PMID: 21200283; PMCID: PMC3058327.

125. Londahl M, Katzman P, Nilsson A, Hammarlund C. Hyperbaric oxygen therapy facilitates healing of chronic foot ulcers in patients with diabetes. Diabetes Care. 2010 May;33(5):998-1003. PubMed PMID: 20427683. Pubmed Central PMCID: 2858204.

126. Donohoe ME, Fletton JA, Hook A, Powell R, Robinson I, Stead JW, et al. Improving foot care for people with diabetes mellitus--a randomized controlled trial of an integrated care approach. Diabet Med. 2000 Aug;17(8):581-587. PubMed PMID: 11073179. Epub 2000/11/10. eng.

127. Litzelman DK, Slemenda CW, Langefeld CD, Hays LM, Welch MA, Bild DE, et al. Reduction of lower extremity clinical abnormalities in patients with non-insulin-dependent diabetes mellitus. A randomized, controlled trial. Ann Intern Med. 1993 Jul 1;119(1):36-41. PubMed PMID: 8498761. Epub 1993/07/01. eng.

128. Lincoln NB, Radford KA, Game FL, Jeffcoate WJ. Education for secondary prevention of foot ulcers in people with diabetes: a randomised controlled trial. Diabetologia. 2008 Nov;51(11):1954-1961. PubMed PMID: 18758747. Epub 2008/09/02. eng.

129. Malone JM, Snyder M, Anderson G, Bernhard VM, Holloway GA, Jr., Bunt TJ. Prevention of amputation by diabetic education. American journal of surgery. 1989 Dec;158(6):520-523; discussion 3-4. PubMed PMID: 2589581. Epub 1989/12/01. eng.

130. Locking-Cusolito H, Harwood L, Wilson B, Burgess K, Elliot M, Gallo K, et al. Prevalence of risk factors predisposing to foot problems in patients on hemodialysis. Nephrol Nurs J. 2005 Jul-Aug;32(4):373-384. PubMed PMID: 16180779. Epub 2005/09/27. eng.

131. Fife CE, Smart DR, Sheffield PJ, Hopf HW, Hawkins G, Clarke D. Transcutaneous oximetry in clinical practice: consensus statements from an expert panel based on evidence. Undersea Hyperb Med. 2009; 36(1):43-53.

132. Lo T, Sample R, Moore P, Gold P. Prediction of wound healing outcome using skin perfusion pressure and transcutaneous oximetry: a single-center experience in 100 patients. Wounds 2009; 21(11);310-316.

133. Centers for Disease Control. National diabetes fact sheet: national estimates and general information on diabetes and prediabetes in the United States. Centers for Disease Control and Prevention Publication. 2011.

Chapter 11
PRESSURE ULCERS

Aimee D. Garcia, MD, CWS, FACCWS

KEY CONCEPTS

1. The two most common groups that develop pressure ulcers are the elderly and individuals with spinal cord injuries.
2. Intrinsic factors contributing to pressure ulcer development are those inherent to the patient, including medical conditions, age, functional status, and nutrition.
3. Extrinsic factors contributing to pressure ulcer development include pressure, friction, shear, and moisture.
4. The most-validated pressure ulcer risk assessment tool is the Braden Scale.
5. Management of a pressure ulcer begins with pressure redistribution, as this is the primary factor that caused development of the wound.
6. Immobility is one of the main risk factors for pressure ulcer development.
7. Incontinence is a major factor in the moisture-associated risk for pressure ulcer development.
8. Nutritional assessment is another clinical component that requires clinical assessment in pressure ulcer patients.
9. Surgical procedures may include debridement, deep cultures, or lap procedures.

CONTENTS

Introduction and epidemiology

Pressure ulcers continue to be a significant health-care issue in the United States and around the world. The two most common groups that develop pressure ulcers are the elderly and individuals with spinal cord injuries. The main risk factor in both of these populations is immobility. An estimated 2.5 million patients are treated for pressure ulcers in the acute-care setting yearly.(1-2) The cost of pressure ulcers to the health-care system in the United States ranges from $9.1–11.6 billion per year. As per Medicare data from 2007, treatment of a pressure ulcer added an additional $43,180 in cost to a hospital stay.(3) The additional cost includes additional hospital days, dressings, nursing time, and therapeutic modalities, such as negative pressure therapy or electrical stimulation therapy. If the patient experiences complications from pressure ulcers, additional costs might include IV antibiotic therapy, surgical debridement, and more complex treatments such as diverting colostomy or rotational flaps to promote wound healing. In addition, patients who develop pressure ulcers during hospitalizations are more likely to require long-term care placement as opposed to going home, adding additional cost to the health-care system. The development of a single pressure ulcer can increase the length of stay in the hospital five-fold.(4)

Despite the advances in technologies, dressings, and support surfaces, the prevalence and incidence of pressure ulcers has not significantly decreased in the last 20 years. Although the average life expectancy has increased, we have not significantly impacted functional status or chronic medical conditions; therefore these conditions continue to plague individuals into their older years.(5) As of 2012, 11.5% of the world's population was over the age of 60.(6) Given the global aging population, it is estimated that 20% of the population will be over the age of 65 by the year 2030, with the fastest-growing segment of the population being individuals over the age of 80.(7) Seventy percent of pressure ulcers occur in individuals over the age of 70, which is by far the largest group in which pressure ulcer occurs.(4) In the spinal cord injury population, it is expected that 25%–40% of individuals will develop a pressure ulcer in their lifetime.(8)

I. Pathophysiology

The National Pressure Ulcer Advisory Panel has changed the terminology for pressure ulcer staging by removing the word "ulcer" and replacing it with "injury." The NPUAP definition of a pressure injury as revised in April 2016 now reads:

"A pressure injury is localized damage to the skin and/or underlying soft tissue usually over a bony prominence or related to a medical or other device. The injury can present as intact skin or an open ulcer and may be painful. The injury occurs as a result of intense and/or prolonged pressure or pressure in combination with shear. The tolerance of soft tissue for pressure and shear may also be affected by microclimate, nutrition, perfusion, comorbidities and condition of the soft tissue."(9)

Since the term "injury" is now used by the NPUAP to denote both changes in skin color which are not yet open ulcers as well as open ulcers requiring some sort of dressing, in this chapter we will use the term "ulcer" to designate open skin lesions. The amount of time and the amount of pressure can vary among individuals, but it is well documented that pressures above 32 mmHg will cause capillary collapse. The amount of time is dependent on the amount of pressure. The more pressure is placed on a specific area of tissue, the less time necessary to lead to tissue necrosis.[10-11]

Contributing factors to the development of pressure ulcers include both intrinsic and extrinsic factors. Intrinsic factors are those inherent to the patient, including medical conditions, age, functional status and nutrition.[12] In addition, a history of previous pressure ulcers would also be a consideration. These factors cause changes to the skin that may predispose the patient to skin breakdown. The more comorbidities a patient has, the more significance it may have on skin integrity. For example, if a patient has a history of congestive heart failure, end stage renal disease on dialysis, incontinence secondary to diuretics, hypotension due to dialysis, limited mobility from being short of breath, and that patient also requires dialysis three times a week which will impact mobility, fluid status and potentially blood pressure, the cumulative effect of these various factors will increase that individual's risk for the development of a pressure ulcer. It is therefore important to take a holistic view of the patient when assessing risk factors.

Extrinsic factors include pressure, friction, shear, and moisture. Pressure is the major risk factor for pressure ulcers. The main cause is immobility, although there can be pressure from external sources such as medical devices as well. Poor mobility may be secondary to underlying comorbidities such as cerebrovascular accident, spinal cord injury or progressive neurologic disorders, or advanced age leading to functional decline. When assessing the patient's risk from mobility, it is important to look not only at the patient's ability to transfer and ambulate, but at bed mobility as well. Patients with limited bed mobility in the home environment still need to be repositioned frequently by caregivers if they cannot make shifts in body positioning. Friction is defined as the force when two objects rub against each other. In patients at risk for pressure ulcers, friction can cause additional damage to the skin. Some examples commonly noted are patients using their heels to push themselves up in the bed or patients who are dragged across the sheets instead of being lifted. In both these scenarios, friction can lead to superficial damage to the epidermis or blisters when fluid enters the space between the epidermis and dermis. Preventive strategies would be the use of trapezes to allow the patient to use his or her upper body for mobility, use of offloading boots to prevent use of heels for pushing up in the bed, and appropriate turning strategies to prevent dragging patients instead of lifting them with draw sheets. Shear force occurs when the head of the bed is elevated above 30 degrees, and the patient begins to slide down the mattress. The blood vessels in the sacral area are sheared by the opposing forces and can lead to skin breakdown in the sacral/coccyx area. In some clinical situations, the clinician has no choice but to elevate the head of the bed due to underlying medical issues. In these scenarios, prevention strategies such as sacral dressings to minimize tension on the tissue might be utilized. Moisture is another extrinsic factor in the development of pressure ulcers. Moisture can occur from numerous sources including urinary and bowel incontinence, wound drainage, obesity, and excessive sweating. When the skin is exposed to excess moisture, it leads to maceration of the tissue. This makes the skin friable and more susceptible to damage from friction and shear forces.

II. Pathway

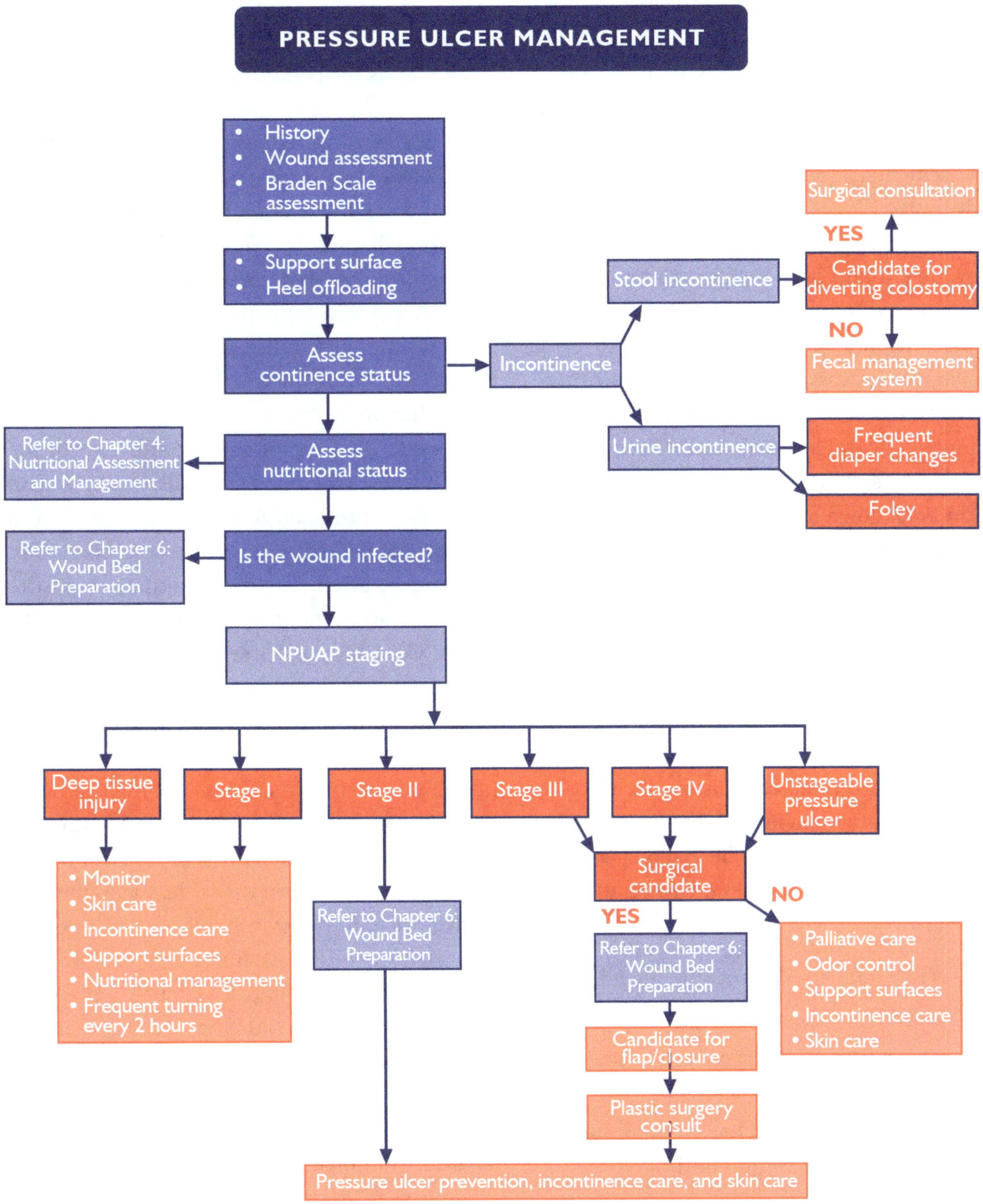
PRESSURE ULCER MANAGEMENT
• History
• Wound assessment
• Braden Scale assessment
• Support surface
• Heel offloading
Assess continence status
Incontinence
Stool incontinence
Candidate for diverting colostomy
YES
Surgical consultation
NO
Fecal management system
Urine incontinence
Frequent diaper changes
Foley
Assess nutritional status
Refer to Chapter 4: Nutritional Assessment and Management
Is the wound infected?
Refer to Chapter 6: Wound Bed Preparation
NPUAP staging
Deep tissue injury
Stage I
Stage II
Stage III
Stage IV
Unstageable pressure ulcer
• Monitor
• Skin care
• Incontinence care
• Support surfaces
• Nutritional management
• Frequent turning every 2 hours
Refer to Chapter 6: Wound Bed Preparation
Surgical candidate
YES
NO
Refer to Chapter 6: Wound Bed Preparation
Candidate for flap/closure
Plastic surgery consult
• Palliative care
• Odor control
• Support surfaces
• Incontinence care
• Skin care
Pressure ulcer prevention, incontinence care, and skin care

III. Case study: evaluation of the pressure ulcer patient

See Pressure Ulcer Management Pathway. Mrs. S is an 88-year-old female who lives in an assisted-living facility. The patient has multiple medical problems including a history of cerebrovascular accident, hypertension, diabetes mellitus, and early dementia. The staff at the assisted-living facility noted Mrs. S had not been seen in the dining room in the past 24 hours. Upon entering her room, they found Mrs. S sitting in her recliner. She was noted to be very confused and lethargic and had incontinence episodes. 911 was called, and the patient was sent to the emergency room. Upon evaluation, she was noted to have a urinary tract infection and be dehydrated. On evaluation of the patient's skin, she was noted to have an area of skin breakdown on the sacrum measuring 3.5 x 2.5 cm, partial thickness with no noted necrotic tissue. There is minimal serous drainage, no odor, and no surrounding erythema.

When the clinical team evaluates a patient, a wound-care history needs to be performed. In the same way that a comprehensive history is obtained to find out the background of any clinical problem, a wound-care history incorporates many elements to gain insight into the wound.[13] Some questions that might be asked specifically in the case of a pressure ulcer include the following items:

- How long has the pressure ulcer been present?
- What treatments have been implemented for wound healing?
- What comorbidities are present that might impact wound healing?
- Has the patient had previous pressure ulcers, and if so, where? What stage?
- Has there been a change in functional status?
- Is the patient able to offload?
- Are there any preventive devices currently being used, such as a wheelchair cushion or specialty support surface?
- Does the patient have any social support?

After a comprehensive history has been completed, there needs to be a comprehensive wound assessment done of the wound. Please refer to Chapter 5: Wound Assessment. The patient also needs to have a risk assessment done. A risk-assessment tool does not replace clinical judgment, but it does give the wound-care team a basis on which to implement protocols for prevention. Risk assessment should be done at the time of initial evaluation of the patient and at scheduled intervals, depending on the facility's protocol. A new assessment should also be completed when there is a change in clinical condition. The most-validated pressure ulcer risk assessment tool is the Braden Scale. Other validated risk-assessment tools include the Norton and the Waterloo scales. The Braden Scale contains six domains to determine risk: sensory perception, activity, mobility, moisture, nutrition, and friction/shear. The highest number that can be achieved is 23.[14] A patient is considered at risk when the score is 18 or below. The lower the score on the scale, the higher the clinical risk for pressure ulcer development. The Norton Scale has five domains: physical condition, mental condition, activity, mobility, and incontinence. A score of 14 or less denotes clinical risk.[15] The Waterloo Scale was developed in 1987 and is used mostly in Europe. It looks at the BMI, continence, skin type, mobility, age, and nutrition. In addition, it takes into account special conditions such as tissue malnutrition, surgery or trauma, medications, and neurologic deficit.[16] Whatever risk-assessment tool is used at the clinical site, the health-care

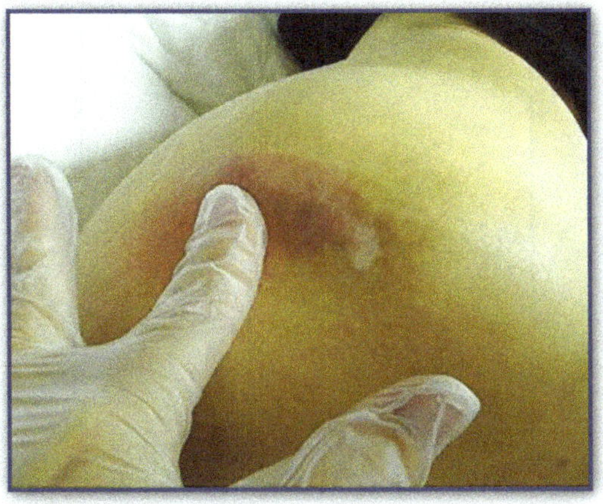

FIGURE 1. Redness on right buttock; checking for blanching
Courtesy of Caroline E. Fife, MD

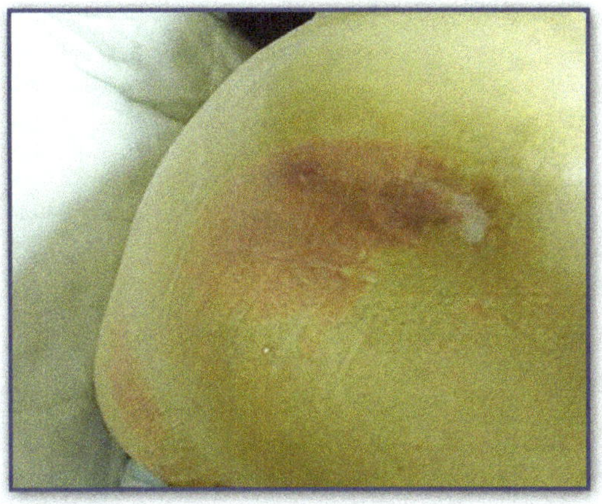

FIGURE 2. Nonblanchable redness on right buttocks; NPUAP Stage 1 Pressure Injury
Courtesy of Caroline E. Fife, MD

providers need to understand the elements and levels of risk associated with the different tiers. There are elements, such as underlying clinical diagnoses, that are not included in these scales, so the clinician needs to make a comprehensive assessment of the patient's risk in addition to the risk-assessment tool.

Staging of the wound is the next step in management. Many health-care settings have developed protocols based on the staging of pressure ulcers. There are six stages of pressure ulcers as defined by the National Pressure Ulcer Advisory Panel, and as per the 2016 NPUAP consensus conference they are defined as the following:(9)

STAGE I. Pressure injury: non-blanchable erythema of intact skin

The skin is intact with a localized area of non-blanchable erythema, which may appear differently in darkly pigmented skin. Presence of blanchable erythema or changes in sensation, temperature, or firmness may precede visual changes. Color changes do not include purple or maroon discoloration; these may indicate deep tissue pressure injury. Since the ICD-10 coding system continues to use the term "ulcer", we will use that term for this chapter.

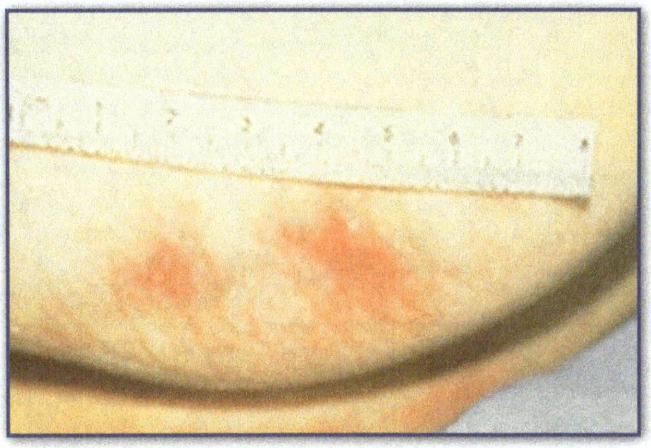

FIGURE 3. NPUAP: Stage I Pressure Injury Left buttock - intact skin with nonblanchable redness on buttock. Courtesy of Caroline E. Fife, MD

STAGE II. Pressure Injury: partial-thickness skin loss with exposed dermis

The wound bed is viable, pink or red, moist, and may also present as an intact or ruptured serum-filled blister. Adipose (fat) is not visible and deeper tissues are not visible. Granulation tissue, slough, and eschar are not present. These injuries commonly result from adverse microclimate and shear in the skin over the pelvis and shear in the heel. This stage should not be used to describe moisture associated skin damage (MASD) including incontinence associated dermatitis (IAD), intertriginous dermatitis (ITD), medical adhesive related skin injury, or traumatic wounds (skin tears, burns, abrasions).

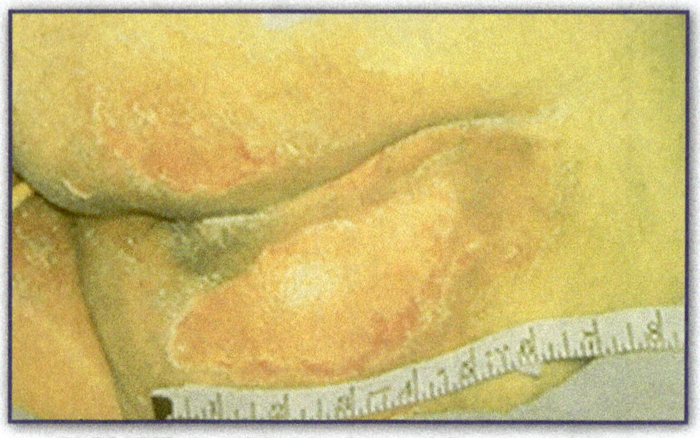

FIGURE 4. NPUAP -Stage II Pressure Ulcer Both buttocks - partial thickness loss of dermis presenting as a shallow open ulcer
Courtesy of Caroline E. Fife, MD

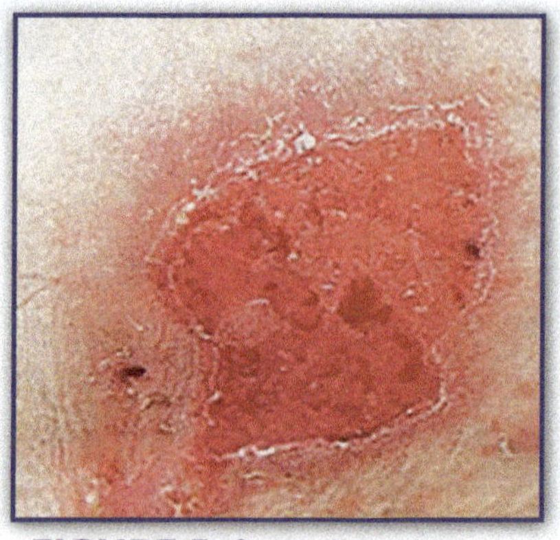

FIGURE 5. Stage II on sacrum
Courtesy of Caroline E. Fife, MD

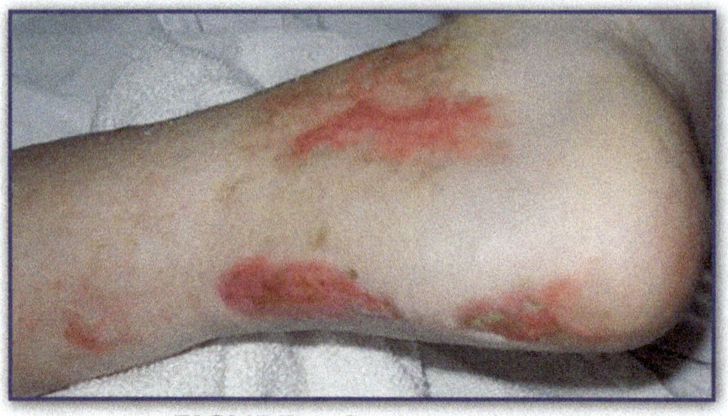

FIGURE 6. Stage II on heel
Courtesy of Caroline E. Fife, MD

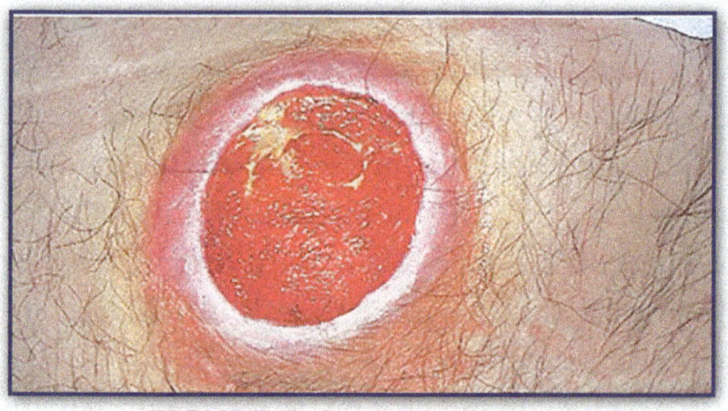

FIGURE 7. Stage III on sacrum
Courtesy of Caroline E. Fife, MD

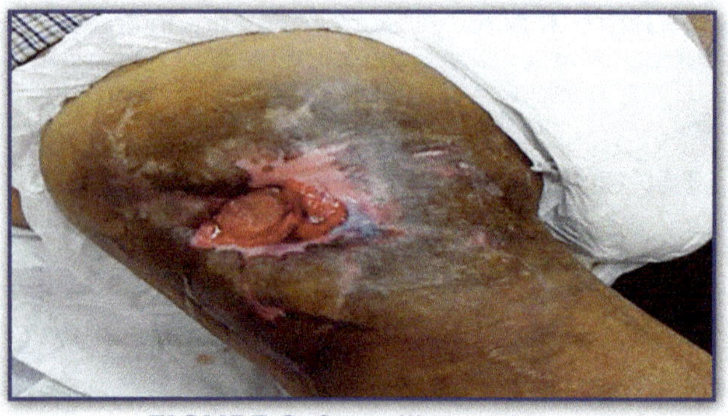

FIGURE 8. Stage III on ischium
Courtesy of Caroline E. Fife, MD

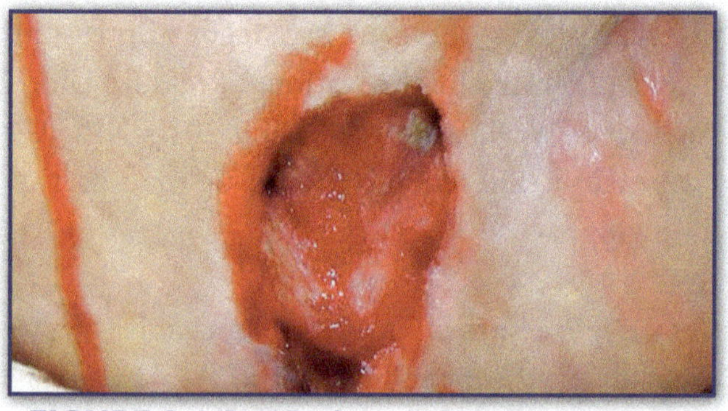

FIGURE 9. NPUAP - Stage III Pressure Ulcer - full thickness tissue loss; sacrum - subcutaneous fat may be visible but bone, tendon, or muscle is not exposed.
Courtesy of Jayesh B. Shah, MD

STAGE III. Pressure injury: full-thickness skin loss

Full-thickness loss of skin, in which adipose (fat) is visible in the ulcer and granulation tissue and epibole (rolled wound edges) are often present. Slough and/or eschar may be visible. The depth of tissue damage varies by anatomical location; areas of significant adiposity can develop deep wounds. Undermining and tunneling may occur. Fascia, muscle, tendon, ligament, cartilage, and/or bone are not exposed. If slough or eschar obscures the extent of tissue loss this is an unstageable pressure injury.

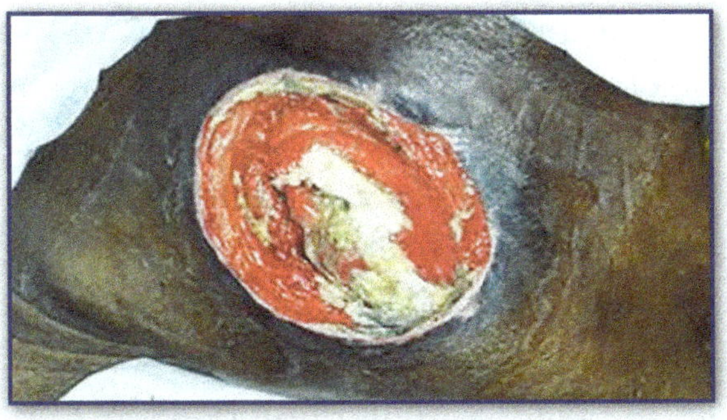

FIGURE 10. Stage IV on ischium
Courtesy of Caroline E. Fife, MD

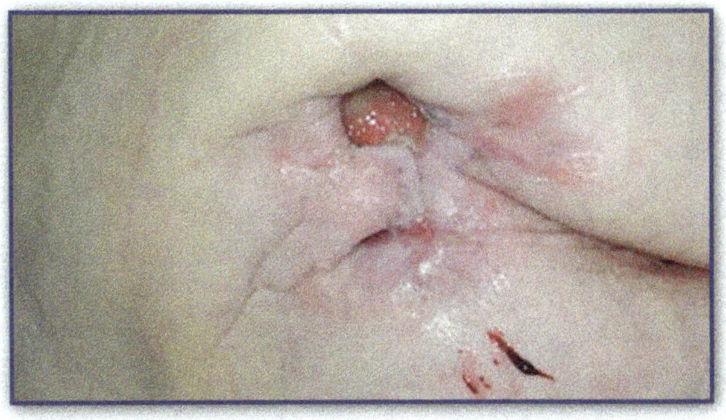

FIGURE 11. Stage IV on sacrum and coccyx.
Courtesy of Caroline E. Fife, MD

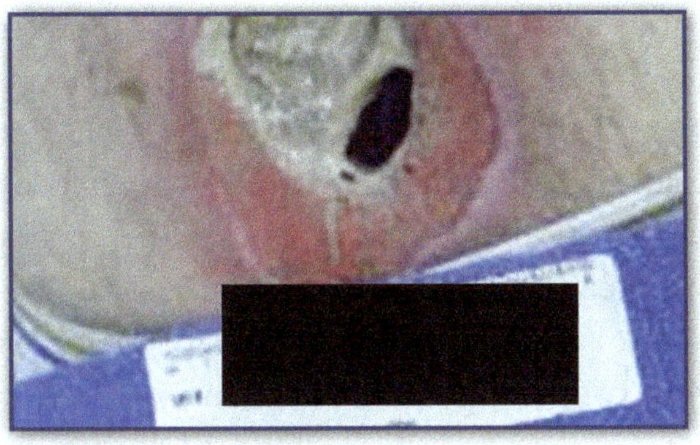

FIGURE 12. Unstageble Pressure Ulcer Full - thickness tissue; left buttock - loss with exposed bone, tendon, or muscle.
Courtesy of Jayesh B. Shah, MD

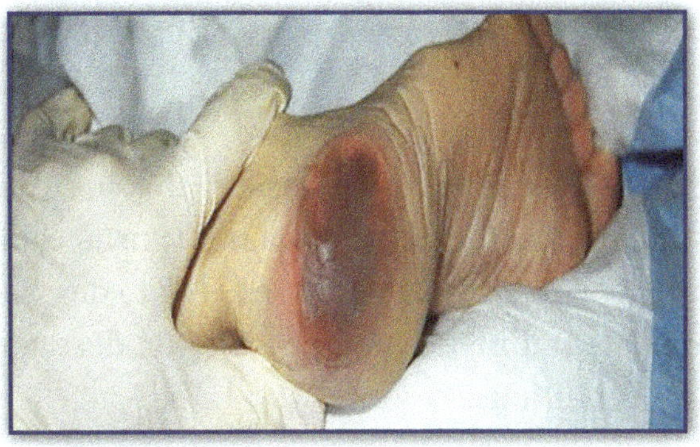

FIGURE 13. Deep tissue injury of heel.
Courtesy of Caroline E. Fife, MD

STAGE IV. Pressure Injury: full-thickness skin and tissue loss

Full-thickness skin and tissue loss with exposed or directly palpable fascia, muscle, tendon, ligament, cartilage, or bone in the ulcer can occur. Slough and/or eschar may be visible. Epibole (rolled edges), undermining and/or tunneling often occur. Depth varies by anatomical location. If slough or eschar obscures the extent of tissue loss this is an unstageable pressure injury.

Unstageable pressure injury: obscured full-thickness skin and tissue loss

Full-thickness skin and tissue loss occurs, in which the extent of tissue damage within the ulcer cannot be confirmed because it is obscured by slough or eschar. If slough or eschar is removed, a Stage 3 or Stage 4 pressure injury will be revealed. Stable eschar (i.e. dry, adherent, intact without erythema or fluctuance) on the heel or ischemic limb should not be softened or removed.

Deep tissue pressure injury (DTPI): persistent nonblanchable deep red, maroon or purple discoloration

Intact or nonintact skin occurs with localized area of persistent nonblanchable deep red, maroon, purple discoloration or epidermal separation revealing a dark wound bed or blood filled blister. Pain and temperature change often precede skin color changes. Discoloration may appear differently in darkly pigmented skin. This injury results from intense and/or prolonged pressure and shear forces at the bone-muscle interface. The injury may evolve rapidly to reveal the actual extent of tissue damage and subsequent ulceration, or may resolve without tissue loss. If necrotic tissue, subcutaneous tissue, granulation tissue, fascia, muscle or other

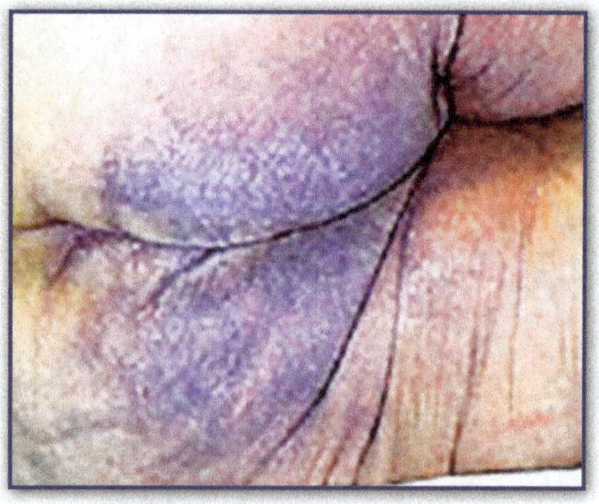

FIGURE 14. Deep tissue injury of bilateral buttocks
Courtesy of Caroline E. Fife, MD

underlying structures are visible, this indicates a full thickness pressure injury (unstageable, Stage 3 or Stage 4). Do not use DTPI to describe vascular, traumatic, neuropathic, or dermatologic conditions.

Two additional definitions related to pressure ulcer include the following:

Medical device related pressure injury
This describes an etiology. Medical device related pressure injuries result from the use of devices designed and applied for diagnostic or therapeutic purposes. The resultant pressure injury generally conforms to the pattern or shape of the device. The injury should be staged using the staging system.

Mucosal membrane pressure injury
Mucosal membrane pressure injury is found on mucous membranes with a history of a medical device in use at the location of the injury. Due to the anatomy of the tissue, these injuries cannot be staged.

If the provider is unsure how to stage the pressure ulcer or is unsure that the wound is a pressure ulcer, it is better to describe the wound clinically than to assign a diagnosis or stage. Many regulatory bodies such as Centers for Medicare & Medicaid Services (CMS) will withhold payment or penalize health-care systems for development or worsening of pressure ulcers. If a wound that is not a pressure ulcer is described as such, or if a wound is incorrectly staged, the facility can face fines that are not justified. If there is any doubt, it behooves the provider to obtain a wound history and describe the wound per the assessment as outlined in Chapter 5: Wound Assessment and to obtain a wound-care consult for assessment of the site.

After risk assessment and staging have been performed, the clinician needs to determine how best to offload the patient. A turning regimen needs to be developed as part of routine, overall care. The current standard of turning every two hours was based entirely on animal data. Until recently, this "standard of care" had never been subjected to a prospective, randomized, controlled study in humans.

A recent study by Bergstrom et al. demonstrated in a prospective trial that even among patients at high risk for pressure ulcers, according to the Braden Scale, the patients did not have an increased incidence of ulcer formation if they were turned every four hours rather than every two hours.[17] This study has profound implications for clinical care and supports the findings of Defloor et al. that pressure ulcer formation is lowest among patients turned every four hours.[18] However, there are patients for whom turning every two hours is insufficient to prevent pressure ulcer formation; therefore, clinical judgement is required when turning schedules are recommended on a given patient.

Given that incontinence is a major factor in the moisture-associated risk for pressure ulcer development, it should be part of the clinical evaluation of the patient to assess their level of incontinence. For urinary incontinence, scheduled voiding methods can be used to help the patient remain dry. Use of a Foley catheter may be indicated if risk of wound contamination is high, but there needs to be a clear understanding that an indwelling Foley catheter will increase the patient's risk of urinary tract infection. With fecal incontinence, management may be easier. The patient can be put on a bowel regimen to regulate the bowel movements, which makes perineal care easier to control. In patients with loose stools or diarrhea, use of a fecal containment system may be appropriate. When there is high risk of fecal contamination to the wound bed, the clinical team may consider a diverting colostomy to bypass the rectum until the pressure ulcer is healed.

The evaluation of nutrition is another clinical component that requires clinical assessment. In the geriatric population, nutritional compromise is common. Appetite decreases as individuals age, but in addition, factors such as dentition, poor health conditions, medications, or lack of access to food can put patients at nutritional risk. Patients with underlying malignancy or significant weight loss, regardless of age, are also at risk for nutritional compromise that can impact the skin and increase the risk for pressure-ulcer development or poor wound healing. Health-care providers used the prealbumin or albumin levels as markers of underlying nutrition. These markers may be helpful to assess overall clinical prognosis, but they do not necessarily correlate well with clinical assessment of nutritional status. The NPUAP white paper on nutrition indicates that these markers are not good markers of nutrition as they are affected by many underlying clinical conditions.[19] A study by Langkamp-Henken and colleagues concluded that use of a mini-nutritional screening tool was superior to use of visceral protein screening in determining at-risk patients.[20] Obtaining a nutritional consult early in the evaluation of an at-risk patient is a good clinical practice to address underlying nutritional risk at the beginning of the clinical course and potentially impact nutrition to decrease risk or increase wound healing.

IV. Managing infection in a pressure ulcer patient

Infection can be an issue when dealing with pressure ulcers, especially when the area of breakdown is in the buttocks/perineal area. In this region, there is a high risk of contamination of the wound bed if the patient is incontinent of bowel and bladder. It is important to understand that every pressure ulcer is colonized with bacteria, since our skin and the environment are colonized with bacteria. This does not mean a wound is infected. The gold standard of assessment of a potentially infected wound is tissue biopsy for quantitative culture. With this technique, a sample of tissue is obtained and cultured for growth of bacteria so that the number of bacterial colonies can be reported in relation to grams of tissue. Quantitative cultures allow a clinician to determine whether the bacteria present in a wound are merely colonizing agents or are likely to represent an infection requiring treatment.

A superficial swab of the wound will only grow the organisms that are on the surface of the wound, and not necessarily the organism that is actually causing clinical infection, if present. If a superficial swab is the only method available for quantitative analysis, the Levine method should be utilized. Areas of necrotic tissue or slough should be avoided and the deepest part of the wound selected. Before culture by the Levine technique, it is recommended to clean the wound with normal saline. Once the wound is cleaned, the swab is applied to a clean area (1 cm^2 area) in the deepest section for 30 seconds. That sample is then sent for analysis.[21]

The levels of infection of a wound are defined

as colonization, critical colonization, and cellulitis. Colonization is bacteria in the wound bed, but not to a level where the bacteria are negatively affecting wound healing. Every wound is colonized, but not every wound is infected. Critical colonization is when bacteria have reached a level where they are now affecting the wound bed and inhibiting healing. This is defined as 1 x 10^5 bacteria. Depending on the time frame the wound has been open, different types of bacteria are more likely to be present. For wounds present less than one month, gram-positive organisms will be more prevalent. For wounds present greater than one month, or if the patient has medical conditions that make him or her immunocompromised, the clinician should also consider gram-negative and anaerobic organisms. At this point, there are no systemic signs of infection, although local signs such as change in the quality of the tissue in the wound, increased drainage, pain, friable granulation tissue, and odor may be present. Critical colonization may also be noted when a clean wound is not showing signs of healing within a 14-day period despite appropriate wound care.[22] It is important to note that when critical colonization is present, systemic antibiotic therapy is not indicated. Treatment of the critical colonization should be done at the level of the wound with a topical antimicrobial or antiseptic agent. Antimicrobial agents for wounds include topical antibiotics, manuka honey, cadexomer iodine, and silver dressings. Antiseptic agents include povidone iodine, chlorhexidine, acetic acid, and sodium hypochlorite. The provider should become familiar with the products available in his or her health-care setting. These agents should only be used for a limited time to decrease bacterial load and achieve bacterial balance in the wound, at which time treatment should be changed to moist wound healing. Topical antibiotic use is becoming increasingly common for wounds that have moderate or high bacterial loads. A more aggressive stage of infection is cellulitis. It is defined as a soft-tissue infection where bacteria has now invaded the deeper tissue and is causing tissue necrosis and clinical signs and symptoms of infection, which include edema, erythema, pain, and odor. At this level, systemic antibiotic therapy with oral or intravenous agents is indicated. A deeper infection should also be considered any time a wound probes to bone. If bone is visible or palpable, a work-up for osteomyelitis may be appropriate depending on the plans for surgical debridement and/or closure. In some cases, the infected bone can be removed at the time of surgery and/or debridement, or a bone biopsy may be obtained for definitive treatment. Thus, an extensive work up for osteomyelitis prior to a planned surgical procedure may not be appropriate.

V. Plastic surgery approach in management of a pressure ulcer

If a pressure ulcer is full thickness or affecting quality of life, surgical intervention might be indicated for management. Prior to pursuit of surgical intervention, the clinician needs to manage the underlying factors that may affect healing. Factors such as nutritional maximization, management of underlying infection, and pressure redistribution must be managed, or the likelihood of postoperative complications will increase. If there is significant fecal soiling occurring in the wound bed, a diverting colostomy may be indicated. Referral to a general or plastic surgeon will depend on what type of surgical intervention is required. If excisional debridement of a pressure ulcer is needed, general surgery is appropriate, but if a surgical flap procedure is warranted, a plastic surgery consult is required. The decision to pursue a specific surgical intervention is going to be dependent on the surgeon's level of expertise and his or her preference.[23] Surgical procedures may include debridement, deep cultures, or flap procedures. When a surgical debridement is performed, the surgeon will remove all devitalized and nonhealing tissue from the wound bed. This may include subcutaneous tissue, fat, muscle, or bone. Removal of necrotic tissue will decrease bacterial load in the wound bed and facilitate wound healing. At this point, the surgeon can choose to heal the wound via secondary intention, or he or she will consider primary closure with a flap. Factors the surgeon will consider prior to determination of what procedure he or she will pursue will be location of the pressure ulcer and the size and the depth of the wound. The most commonly used flaps in the treatment of pressure ulcers are musculocutaneous and fasciocutaneous flaps, as these surgical interventions provide vascularized tissue for coverage of the defect. A posterior lateral thigh V-Y procedure is also indicated for pressure ulcer management. There has been no study that has compared the effectiveness of myocutaneous flaps versus fasciocutaneous flaps.

The decision to pursue surgical intervention is not without inherent risk. A review of the literature of all of the previously mentioned flaps performed for ischial pressure sores found an overall complication rate ranging from 0% to 80% and a recurrence rate from 0% to 33.3%.[24] The most-common complication after a flap surgery is suture line dehiscence.[25] If the patient has surgical resection of bone prior to flap surgery, the incidence of dehiscence increases. Hospitalized patients who develop pressure ulcers tend to have multiple underlying comorbidities including osteomyelitis and are at increased risk for death.[26]

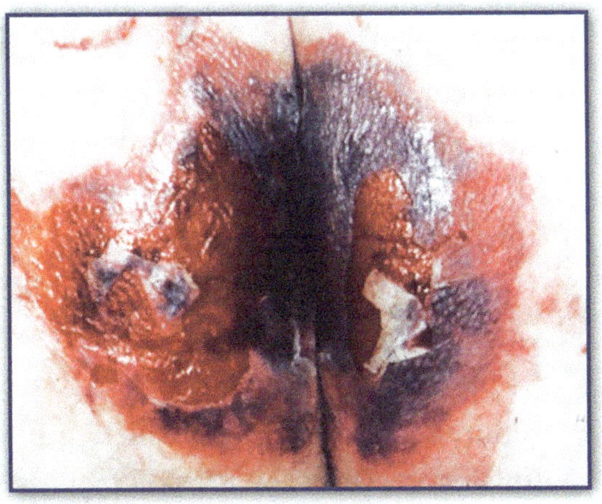

FIGURE 15. Deep tissue injury of both gluteal regions
Courtesy of Caroline E. Fife, MD

VI. Support surfaces for patients with pressure ulcers

See Pathway 11. Management of a pressure ulcer begins with pressure redistribution, as this is the primary factor that caused development of the wound. A Cochrane analysis of 52 randomized trials reported that patients at high risk for pressure ulcers should have a specialized support surface as opposed to a standard hospital mattress.[27] The first step is evaluation of the patient's functional status. Is the patient bedbound, or does he or she spend the majority of time in a chair? Pressure redistribution should be considered for both settings. For the wheelchair, the patient should be referred to occupational or physical therapy for evaluation. Wheelchair cushions should be ordered for all patients who spend significant time in a wheelchair, since the seat upholstery is not designed to offer support.[28] The therapist will assess seating balance and will determine what type of seating surface is most appropriate. The four basic categories of cushions include foam, air, viscous fluid, and elastomeric cushions. The therapist will choose the correct type of cushion depending on patient's functional status, ability to transfer, continence status, and seating balance.

The choice of mattress support surface is going to depend on whether the patient has a pressure ulcer or not. If the patient has no open wounds, most payers will not cover the cost for a preventive support surface unless the patient is completely immobile in the bed or has partial mobility and skin breakdown. Many facilities have purchased their own pressure redistribution surfaces for prevention, and if the facility has these support surfaces, a static air, gel, or foam mattress can be used for prevention. As per CMS, the categories for ordering of a pressure redistribution surface are as follows:[29]

- **Group 1** - Support surfaces are generally designed to either replace a standard hospital or home mattress or as an overlay placed on top of a standard hospital or home mattress. Products in this category include mattresses, pressure pads, and mattress overlays (foam, air, water, or gel).
- **Group 2** - Support surfaces are generally designed to either replace a standard hospital or home mattress or as an overlay placed on top of a standard hospital or home mattress. Products in this category include powered air flotation beds, powered pressure reducing air mattresses, and non-powered advanced pressure reducing mattresses.
- **Group 3** - Support surfaces are complete bed systems, known as air-fluidized beds, which use the circulation of filtered air through silicone beads.

CMS and most payers will only cover the cost of a support surface with appropriate documentation of clinical need. The patient has to meet certain criteria for each type of mattress. CMS requirements are outlined below:[29]

- **Group 1** - A Group 1 support surface is covered if the patient is completely immobile. Otherwise, he or she must be partially immobile, or have any stage pressure ulcer and demonstrate one of the following conditions: impaired nutritional status, incontinence, altered sensory perception, or compromised circulatory status. A physician order must be obtained prior to delivery of the equipment and should be kept on file by the supplier.
- **Group 2** - A Group 2 support surface is covered if the patient has a Stage II pressure sore located on the trunk or pelvis, has been on a comprehensive pressure sore treatment program (which has included the use of an appropriate Group 1 support surface for at least one month), and has sores which have worsened or remained the same over the past month. A Group 2 support surface is also covered if the patient has large or multiple Stage III or IV pressure sores on the trunk or pelvis, or if he or she has had a recent myocutaneous flap or skin graft for a pressure sore on the trunk or pelvis and has been on a Group 2 or 3 support surface.
- **Group 3** – A Group 3 support surface is covered if the patient has a Stage III or Stage IV pressure ulcer, is bedridden or chair-bound, would be institutionalized without the use of the Group 3 support surface, the patient is under the close supervision of the patient's treating physician, at least one month of conservative treatment has been administered (including the use of a Group 2 support surface), a caregiver is available and willing to assist with patient care, and all other alternative equipment has been considered and ruled out.

The other situation in which a Group 3 surface would be utilized would be in a patient who had a post-flap procedure or a patient in which multiple turning surfaces are affected by pressure ulcers, therefore limiting the ability of the patient to be turned and repositioned.

In 2015, McNichol et al. created an evidence-based and consensus-based algorithm to help clarify the selection of specialty support surfaces.[30] A group of clinical experts convened to look at systematic reviews and publications related to support surfaces. When evaluating a patient for a support surface, a multitude of factors should be considered. Some of the factors include the patient's weight, rehab potential, level of pain, and whether the patient has any contraindications to being on a support surface. The type of support surface used in the past for prevention and treatment of pressure ulcers is also a consideration. Once a support surface is selected, the clinician must implement a turning and repositioning schedule, as a specialty support surface will not decrease pressures below capillary closing pressure and pressure necrosis can still occur. The only category of specialty support surface on which a patient does not have to be turned and repositioned is a high-air-loss mattress. The other aspect noted by the consensus panel is that for the support surface to effectively offload the patient, it must be in good working order and must be used appropriately by the clinical staff to achieve maximum benefit.

VII. Preventing recurrence of pressure ulcers

The majority of publications on recurrence of pressure ulcers are focused on the spinal cord injury population. Studies have shown a recurrence rate of 31% to 79%. Some of the characteristics associated with a higher recurrence rate in this population include male, younger patients, African American ethnicity, residence in a nursing home, and a history of previous pressure ulcer surgery.[31] In the elderly population, clinical evidence supports the fact that a patient who has developed a pressure ulcer in the past is usually at high risk for further development of pressure ulcers unless the factors leading to development are modified.

Full-thickness pressures heal with scar tissue. A Stage 1 pressure ulcer heals with offloading. There is never a break in the skin, therefore no re-epithelialization or scar tissue formation occurs. A Stage 2 pressure ulcer is partial thickness and therefore heals with re-epithelialization. In Stage 3 or Stage 4 pressure ulcers, healing of the pressure ulcer occurs with laying down of scar tissue as these injuries are full thickness and involve the subcutaneous tissue. Based on the wound-healing cascade, the time frame for remodeling can be up to 1.5 years. The tensile strength of the scar tissue is at maximum 70%–80% of the surrounding tissue; therefore the patient is always going to be more susceptible to having recurrence of a pressure ulcer at that site.[32] Once a patient is identified as having a history of a healed, full-thickness pressure ulcer in an area, it is important to be especially vigilant. This includes monitoring of the patient's skin closely, maintaining moisture balance, and attenuating underlying internal and external risk factors. Maintenance of moisture balance may include use of moisture-barrier creams to protect the skin from excessive moisture, such as bowel or bladder incontinence. If the skin is excessively dry, use of emollients to keep the skin hydrated are utilized to prevent cracks and fissures in the skin.

Prevention requires the use of proper equipment to minimize the risk of recurrence. As discussed previously, a correct pressure redistribution cushion for a wheelchair is necessary if the patient spends many hours a day up in a chair. Other types of seating surfaces also need to be considered, such as Gerichairs. If a patient is spending multiple hours a day on this type of seating surface, the patient needs to be turned and repositioned, and pressure needs to be offloaded if the patient is at risk for pressure ulcers. In terms of a prevention surface for the bed, there is no current CMS payment source for prevention unless the patient is completely immobile. Use of Group 1 support surfaces are usually adequate for prevention of pressure ulcers. For heel pressure ulcers, prevention includes floating the heels with pillows and use of offloading boots. If the patient is in a wheelchair, use of appropriate footwear to prevent excessive pressure from the footrests is required. The patient's skin should be assessed on a daily basis and during routine clinical care.

Given that immobility is one of the main risk factors for pressure-ulcer development, improvement of activity and mobility will decrease risk of pressure-ulcer recurrence. Referral of a patient to physical and occupational therapy, if appropriate, can improve strength, balance, and mobility. The individual will then need to maintain that level of activity to prevent losing any forward progress. Nutritional assessment and maximization should be achieved. The use of prophylactic dressings might also be considered. As per the NPUAP clinical practice guidelines, there were four studies that demonstrated a reduction in the occurrence of pressure ulcers with polyurethane foam dressing applied to at-risk anatomical locations. These clinical trials included patients that were critically ill and immobile patients in critical care setting.[33]

Summary

Pressure ulcers continue to be a significant and costly clinical condition. As a health-care system, we need to utilize consistent protocols to identify and minimize the risk of pressure ulcer development. Although there is no way to eliminate the risk of pressure ulcers completely, we can continue to develop clinical strategies to attenuate the impact to patient care and quality of life.

Review questions

1. **What stage would you call a partial-thickness area of skin breakdown on the sacrum?**

    a. Stage I

    b. Stage II

    c. Stage III

    d. unstageable

2. **A patient in a long-term care facility is noted to have a pressure ulcer on the left trochanter with 30% necrotic tissue. The patient has a history of a stroke and is immobile. What type of support surface is most appropriate?**

    a. The patient does not qualify for a support surface.

    b. a viscoelastic foam mattress

    c. a low-air-loss mattress

    d. a high-air-loss mattress

ANSWERS: 1) b
2) c

References

1. Reddy M, Gill SS, Rochon PA. Preventing pressure ulcers: a systematic review. JAMA. 2006;296:974.
2. Lyder CH. Pressure ulcer prevention and management. JAMA. 2003;289:223
3. Agency for Healthcare Research and Quality [Internet]. Rockville (MD): Department of Health and Human Services (US). Preventing pressure ulcers in hospitals. Available from: http://www.ahrq.gov/professionals/systems/hospital/pressureulcertoolkit/putool1.html
4. Allman RM. Pressure ulcers among the elderly. N Engl J Med. 1989;320:850-3.
5. Cassel CK. Successful aging: how increased life expectancy and medical advances are changing geriatric care. Geriatrics. 2001;56:35-40.
6. United Nations Population Fund (UNFPA) Ageing in the 21st Century: A Celebration and A Challenge. 2012.
7. U.S. Census Bureau. Population Projections Program, Population Division, U.S. Census Bureau. Washington, DC. 2000.
8. Kirshblum S, Gonzalez P, Cuccurullo S. Spinal cord injuries. In: Cuccurullo S, editor. (ed.) Physical medicine and rehabilitation board review. New York: Demos Medical Publishing; 2004. p. 545–48.
9. National Pressure Ulcer Advisory Panel [Internet]. [Washington (DC)]: National Pressure Ulcer Advisory Panel. NPUAP pressure injury stages. Available from: http://www.npuap.org/resources/educational-and-clinical-resources/npuap-pressure-ulcer-stages/
10. Kosiak M. Etiology of decubitus ulcers. Arch Phys Med Rehabil. 1961;42:19-29.
11. Reswick JB, Rogers JE. Experience at Rancho Los Amigos Hospital with devices and techniques that prevent pressure sores. In: Kenedi RM, Cowden JM, editors. Bedsore biomechanics. 1st ed. The Macmillan Press; 1976: p. 301-10.
12. Magalhães MG, Gragnani A, Veiga DF, Blanes L, Galhardo VA, Kállas H, Juliano Y, Ferreira. Risk factors for pressure ulcers in hospitalized elderly without significant cognitive impairment. Wounds. 2007 Jan;19(1):20-4.
13. Stotts NA, Sparacino PSA. Assessing the patient with a wound as the basis for home care wound management. Home Healthc Nurse. 2005 Feb;23(2):82-92.
14. Bergstrom N, Braden BJ, Laguzza A, Holman V. The Braden Scale for predicting pressure sore risk. Nurs Res. 1987; 36(4): 205-10.
15. Norton D, Exton-Smith AN, McLaren R. An investigation of geriatric nursing problems in hospital. London: National Corporation for the Care of Old People; 1962.
16. Waterlow J. Pressure sores: a risk assessment card. Nurs Times. 1985;81:24-7.
17. Bergstrom N, Horn SD, Rapp MP, Stern A, Barrett R, Watkiss M. Turning for ulcer reduction: a multisite randomized clinical trial in nursing homes. J Am Geriatr Soc. 2013 Oct;61(10):1705-13.
18. Defloor T, De Bacquer D, Grypdonck MHF. The effect of various combinations of turning and pressure reducing devices on the incidence of pressure ulcers. Int J Nurs Stud. 2005;42:37–46.
19. Dorner B, Posthauer ME, Thomas D. The role of nutrition in pressure ulcer prevention and treatment: National Pressure Ulcer Advisory Panel white paper [Internet]. [Washington (DC)]: National Pressure Ulcer Advisory Panel; 2009. Available from: http://www.npuap.org/wp-content/uploads/2012/03/Nutrition-White-Paper-Website-Version.pdf

20. Langkamp-Henken B, Hudgens J, Stechmiller JK, Herrlinger-Garcia KA. Mini nutritional assessment and screening scores are associated with nutritional indicators in elderly. J Am Diet Assoc. 2005 Oct;105(10):1590-96.

21. Rondas AA, Schols JM, Halfens RJ, Stobberingh EE. Swab versus biopsy for the diagnosis of chronic infected wounds. Adv Skin Wound Care. 2013;26:211-19.

22. Sibbald RG, Woo K, Ayello EA. Increased bacterial burden and infection: the story of NERDS and STONES. Adv Skin Wound Care. 2006;19(8):447-61; quiz 462-3.

23. Linder RM, Morris D. The surgical management of pressure ulcers: a systematic approach based on staging. Decubitus. 1990;3:32-8.

24. Tchanque-Fossuo C, Kuzon WM Jr. An evidence-based approach to pressure sores. Plast Reconstr Surg. 2011;127(2):932-9.

25. Schryvers OI, Stranc MF, Nance PW. Surgical treatment of pressure ulcers: 20-year experience. Arch Phys Med Rehabil. 2000;81:1556-62.

26. Schiffman J, Golinko MS, Yan A, Flattau A, Tomic-Canic M, Brem H. Operative debridement of pressure ulcers. World J Surg. 2009;33:1396–1402.

27. McInnes E, Cullum N. Support surfaces for pressure ulcer prevention. Cochrane Database Syst Rev. 2010;12:CD009490.

28. Garcia A, Sprigle S. Pressure ulcers. In: Hamm R, editor. Text and atlas of wound diagnosis and treatment. New York: McGraw Hill; 2015.

29. Medicare policy regarding pressure reducing support surfaces—JA1014 [Internet]. Baltimore (MD): Center for Medicare & Medicaid Services. Available from: https://www.cms.gov/Medicare/Medicare-Contracting/ContractorLearningResources/downloads/JA1014.pdf

30. McNichol L, Watts C, Mackey D, Beitz JM, Gray M. Identifying the right surface for the right patient at the right time: generation and content validation of an algorithm for support surface selection. J Wound Ostomy Continence Nurs. 2015;42(1):19-37.

31. Bates-Jensen BM, Guihan M, Garber SL, Chin AS, Burns SP. Characteristics of recurrent pressure ulcers in veterans with spinal cord injury. J Spinal Cord Med. 2009 Feb;32(1):34–42.

32. Flanagan, M. Improving accuracy of wound measurement in clinical practice. Ostomy Wound Manage. 2003;49(10):28-40.

33. National Pressure Ulcer Advisory Panel; European Pressure Ulcer Advisory Panel; Pan Pacific Pressure Injury Alliance. Prevention and treatment of pressure ulcers: clinical practice guideline. Haesler, E editor. Cambridge Media: Perth (Australia); 2014.

Additional resources

1. Allman R, Good PD, Burst N, Bartolucci AA, Thomas DR. Pressure ulcer, hospital complications, and disease severity: implications of hospital costs and length of stay. Adv Wound Care. 1999;12(1):22-30.
2. National Pressure Ulcer Advisory Panel [Internet]. Washington DC: National Pressure Ulcer Advisory Panel. Available from: www.npuap.org.
3. Levine SM, Sinno S, Levine JP, Saadeh PB. An evidence-based approach to the surgical management of pressure ulcers. Ann Plast Surg. 2012 Oct;69:482-4.
4. Becker H. The distally based gluteus maximus muscle flap. Plast Reconstr Surg. 1979;63:653-656.
5. Kroll SS, Rosenfield L. Perforator-based flaps for low posterior midline defects. Plast Reconstr Surg. 1988;81:561-566.
6. Park C, Park BY. Fasciocutaneous V-Y advancement flap for repair of sacral defects. Ann Plast Surg. 1988;21:23-26.
7. Brown G. Long-term outcomes of full-thickness pressure ulcers: healing and mortality. Ostomy Wound Manage. 2003;49:42–50.

Chapter 12

VENOUS INSUFFICIENCY ULCER

Samih Bittar, MD
John Fish, MD
Fedor Lurie, MD, PhD

KEY CONCEPTS

1. Venous ulcers (VUs) are the most common chronic wound in the lower extremity and account for 70% of all leg ulcers.
2. Four pathological processes causing venous stasis and ulceration are reflux, obstruction, muscle pump dysfunction, and inflammation.
3. CEAP is an acronym for clinical, etiology, anatomy, pathophysiology and is developed to standardize reporting and treatment of diverse manifestations of chronic venous disorders.
4. An ankle brachial index (ABI) should be performed on all patients with leg ulcers as a screening test for peripheral artery disease (PAD).
5. Venous duplex ultrasound provides diagnostic clues for reflux disease, post-thrombotic syndrome, and chronic venous stenosis.
6. Strong 1A recommendation is assigned for the role of surgery or ablation of incompetent superficial veins to decrease recurrence of venous ulcers.
7. Endovenous thermal ablation is recommended over open surgery (stripping) for incompetent saphenous veins because of reduced convalescence and less surgical pain.(1B)
8. The guidelines recommend compression as the primary therapeutic modality for healing venous ulcers.
9. Compression is recommended as an adjuvant treatment to superficial vein ablation for the prevention of ulcer recurrence.
10. Pentoxifylline or micronized purified flavonoid fraction, if available, in combina-tion with compression is recommended to accelerate healing of venous ulcers.

CONTENTS

Introduction

There are several reasons venous leg ulcers (VLUs) have a special place in the wound care practice. They are the second most common type of chronic wound among wound care patients. Like many other chronic wounds, it is a preventable condition. They develop in patients who remained untreated for their venous disease for many years. However, after the first occurrence, VLU changes the natural history of venous disease and is likely to recur in at least half of the patients. Most VLUs respond well to conservative therapy, but such treatment does not prevent their recurrence. Patients with VLUs frequently have other vascular diseases that affect healing and impact the choice of therapy. This is why early diagnosis and correction of underlying vascular conditions is essential, even though it may not significantly affect the initial healing of the ulcer.

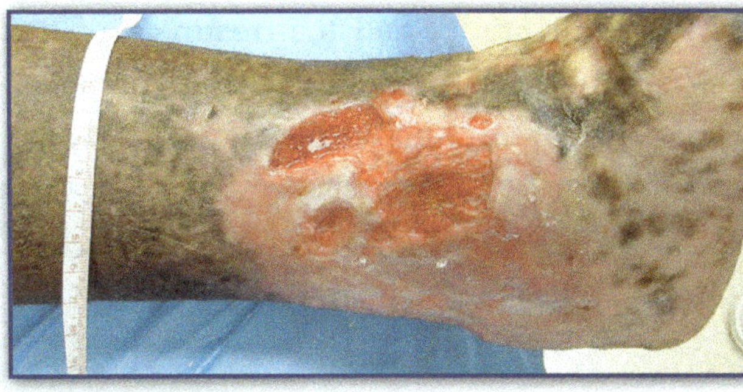

FIGURE 1. Venous stasis ulcer on left leg on initial presentation

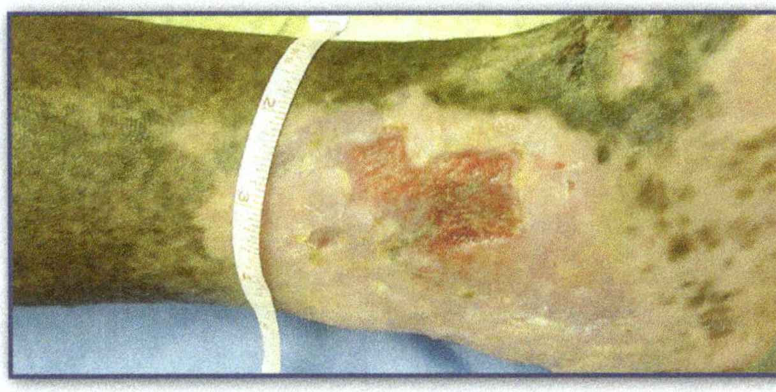

FIGURE 2. Venous stasis ulcer s/q to compression therapy

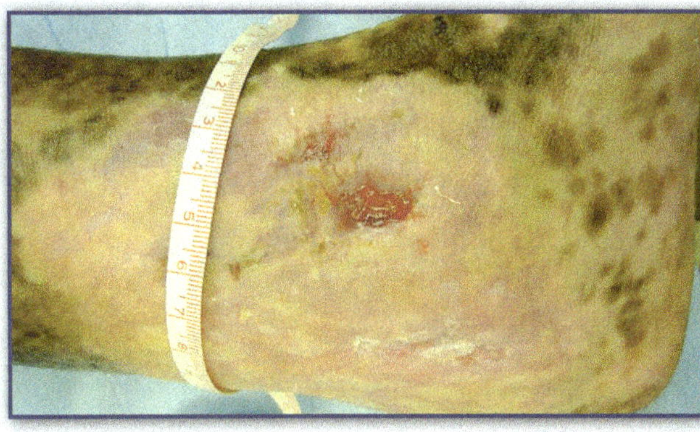

FIGURE 3. Venous stasis ulcer s/q to GSV ablation and compression therapy

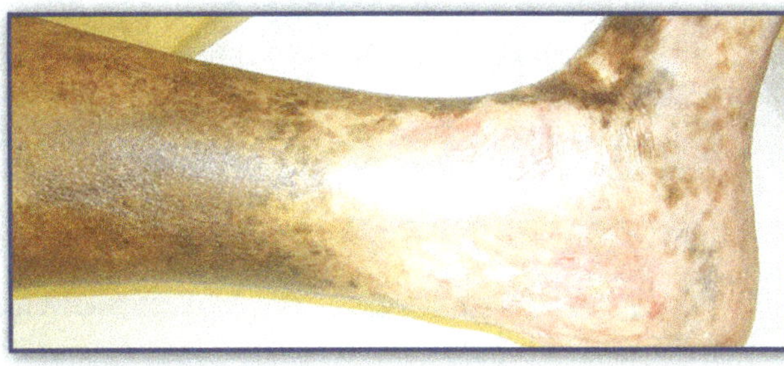

FIGURE 4. Epithealilized venous stasis ulcer on follow-up

I. Case study

Mr. SN is a 63-year-old maintenance worker who has a history of multiple recurrent ulcers in his left medial ankle area. He has no leg swelling and no varicose veins but has a history of acutely developed significant swelling of left leg 15 years ago. He does not have a history of diabetes. He was prescribed compression stocking multiple times but never wore them. He usually comes to the wound clinic with a new ulcer and disappears after the wound heals. He does not have a primary care provider (see Figure 1).

On examination, the pedal pulses are palpable in the right foot but not in the left foot. Because of these findings, the ABI was obtained and was 0.9 on the right and 0.7 on the left.

Venous duplex was obtained and showed post-thrombotic changes in left distal femoral vein (synechia and wall thickening), and reflux in left great saphenous vein from the saphenofemoral junction to ankle. Vascular consultant recommended ablation of the left GSV to prevent future recurrences and possibly to facilitate the healing. A month later with weekly Unna boot applications, the ulcer showed some improvement (see Figure 2), and the treatment of the GSV was performed. Two weeks later the ulcer showed significant improvement (see Figure 3), and a month later it was completely healed. Patient came for a follow-up at 6 and 12 months. He refuses to use any form of compression therapy, but the ulcer did not recur (see Figure 4).

II. Pathways

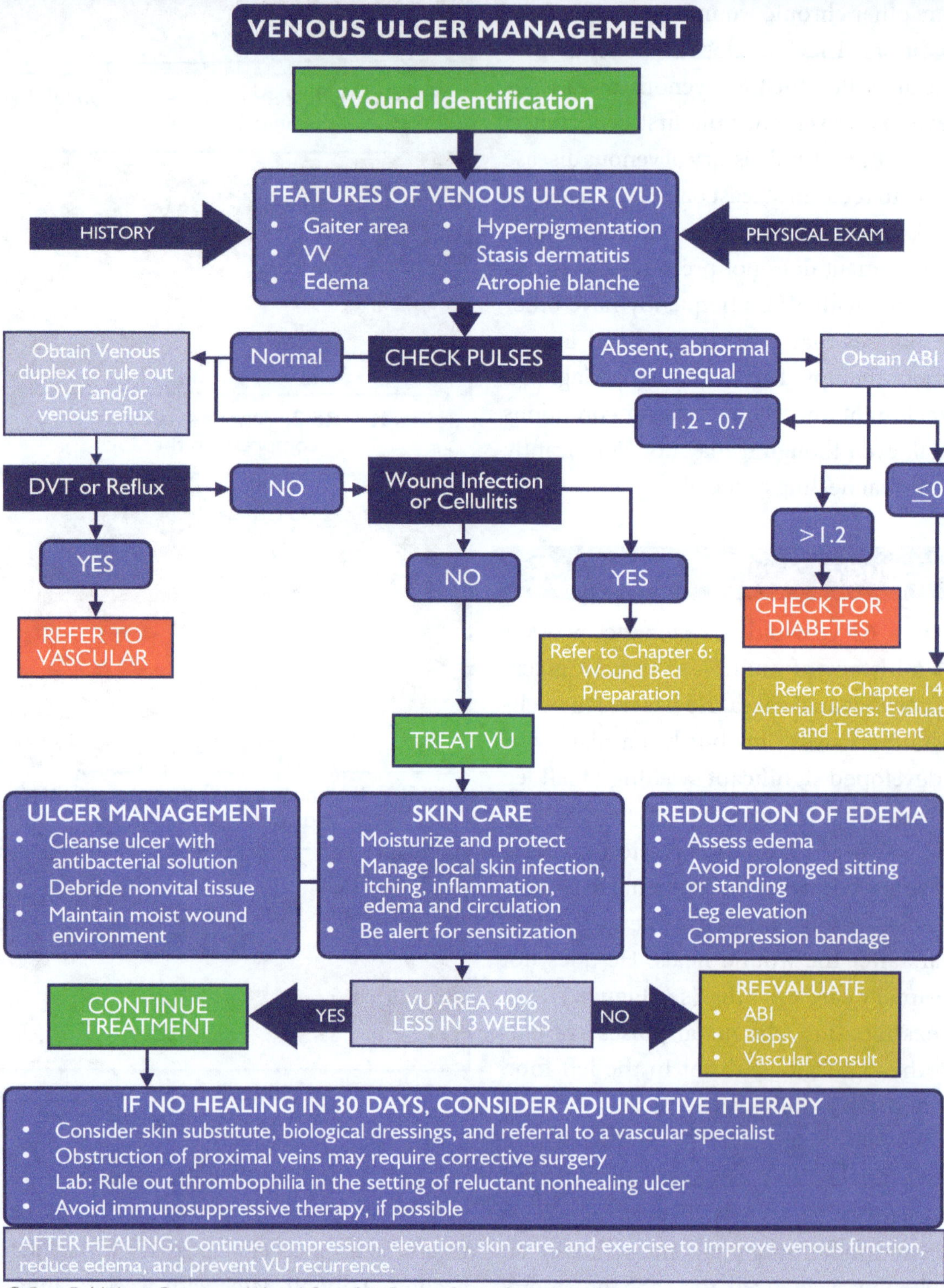

© Best Publishing Company, *Wound Care Certification Study Guide 2nd edition*
Modified with permission by Jayesh B. Shah, MD

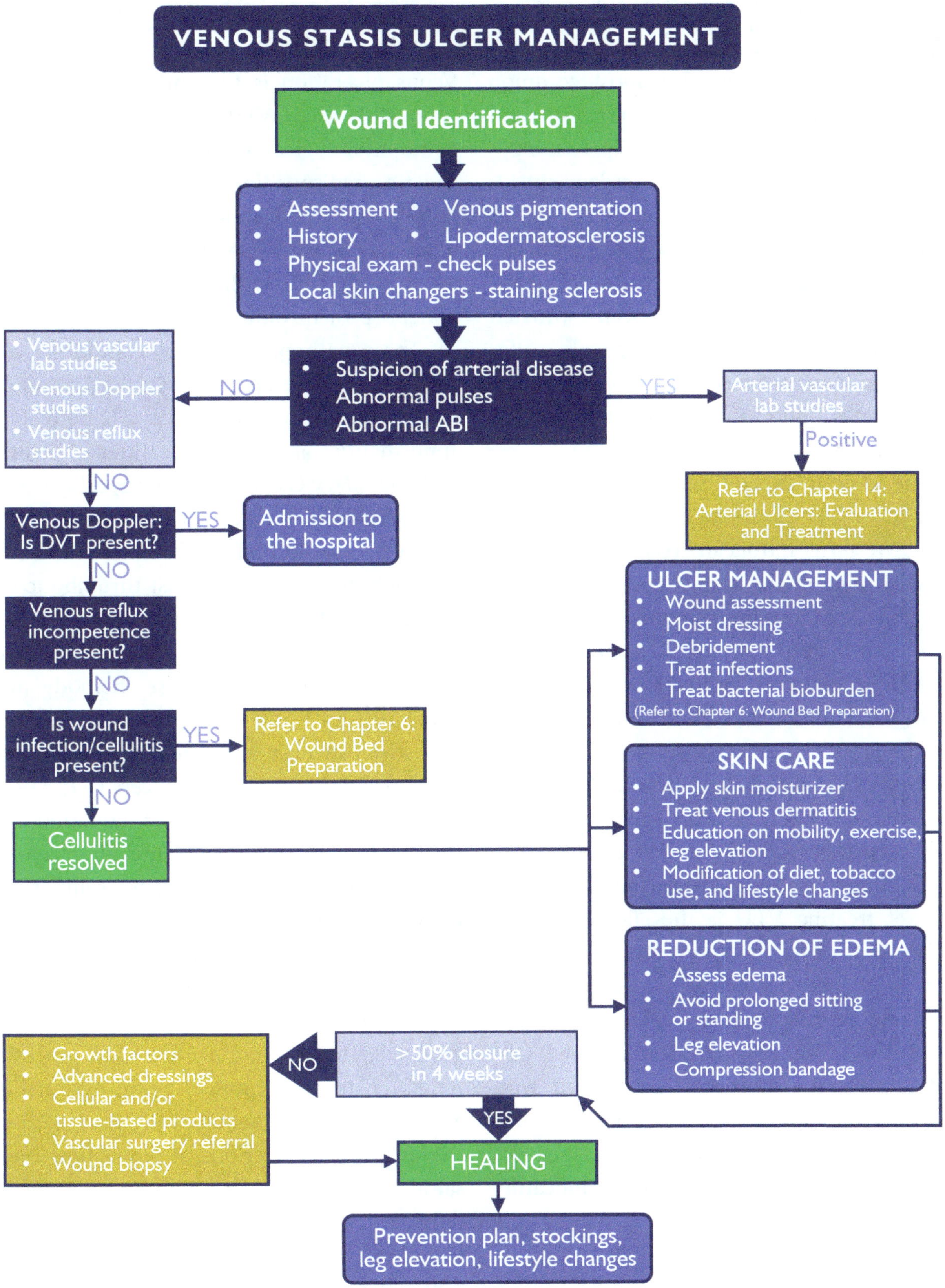

Modified with permission by Jayesh B. Shah, MD

III. Epidemiology and economic impact of venous stasis ulcer

Venous ulcers (VUs) are the most common chronic wound in the lower extremity and account for 70% of all leg ulcers. Epidemiological studies demonstrated VU prevalence in 1% of the population of Western countries. Venous leg ulcer (VLU) prevalence increased with age; thus it is much higher in the portion of population age 40 and older. It has been estimated that approximately 2.5 million people suffer from chronic venous insufficiency (CVI) in the United States, and of those about 20% develop venous ulcers.

The overall expenditure related to VLU approaches 1% of the health-care budget of some Western European countries. In the United Kingdom the annual cost is estimated to approach 600 million pounds per year. In the United States, it is estimated that $2.5 billion will be spent on the treatment of VLUs in more than 6 million patients or about $2500 per month per patient. A recent study on the cost of treating VLUs in Germany demonstrated that mean cost was 9569 Euros/patient/year and 92% of this expenditure was related to direct costs.

The most important determinant of the costs of treating VLU is the effectiveness of initial treatment and prevention of recurrences. Delayed healing is associated with a three-fold increase in cost. Patients who experienced recurrence incurred double the cost of treatment. In contrast, VLU treated with surgical intervention of the superficial venous system did not increase total cost over patients receiving best medical therapy but significantly reduced recurrence rates.[(1)]

IV. Pathophysiology of venous stasis ulcers

Venus ulceration is the end stage of chronic venous disease (CVD) and a result of complex pathophysiological events that include some genetic predisposition, inflammation, changes in vein wall, and abnormal venous hemodynamics. The vast majority of venous ulcers occur in patients with either primary or secondary (post-thrombotic) diseases.

These pathophysiological conditions contribute to the development of an ulcer, chronicity of the wound, and recurrences. Hemodynamic abnormalities are essential features of primary and secondary CVD. Reflux in superficial veins is a signature of primary CVD. Deep vein reflux can be present in both of these conditions, but obstruction is specific to post-thrombotic disease and nonthrombotic central vein compression commonly referred to as the May-Thurner lesion. Persistence of these hemodynamic abnormalities leads to progression of the disease and, through a cascade of events, some patients develop venous leg ulcers (VLUs). The process linking hemodynamic alteration with progression to ulceration includes changes in the microcirculation causing cellular and molecular mechanisms involving inflammation, proteolytic activity, and fibrosis.

Despite the complexity of pathophysiology, clinically relevant mechanisms can be grouped into just four pathological processes: reflux, obstruction, muscle pump dysfunction, and inflammation. Venous valve incompetence causes prolonged periods of blood flow reversal in veins (reflux). The clinical importance of reflux depends on its severity and anatomical distribution. Deep vein obstruction can cause elevation of venous pressure, especially if iliofemoral venous segments are obstructed. Distal venous obstruction is less severe but in some cases may also be associated with venous ulcers.

Dysfunction of the muscle pump can contribute to hemodynamic abnormalities, especially in the limbs with severe lipodermatoesclerosis that limits ankle mobility.

In most of the limbs with VUs, these mechanisms are correctable and need to be addressed as early in the disease process as possible. They can be identified by proper examination and vascular testing, justifying the inclusion of these steps in the initial management of patients with VUs.

V. Evaluating patient with venous stasis ulcer

See pathways on previous page. Prior to treatment, it is essential to confirm the diagnosis of VLU and differentiate the types of lower-extremity ulcers that requiring treatment. Clinical evaluation starts with a review of health history to identify risk factors for chronic venous disease (CVD) (i.e. family history, pregnancy, older age, thrombophilia, systemic inflammation, obesity, and venous thromboembolism (VTE).

Clinical examination of the lower limbs should include inspection (telangiectasia, varicosity, edema, skin discoloration, corona phlebectatica, lipodermatoesclerosis, ulcer), palpation (cord, varicosity, tenderness, induration, reflux, pulses, thrill, groin or abdominal masses), auscultation (bruit), and examination of ankle mobility.[2] Patients should be asked about symptoms of CVD, which may include tingling, aching, burning, pain, muscle cramps, swelling, sensations of throbbing or heaviness, itching skin, restless legs, leg tiredness, and fatigue. Note that pain may be variable from mild to severe, and all CVD symptoms worsen with prolonged leg dependency and are relieved by leg elevation.

Physical examination of the lower extremities should assess functional ability and determine perfusion status by assessing skin temperature, capillary refill, venous refill, color changes, and presence of paresthesias. It is also crucial to palpate both dorsalis pedis and posterior tibial pulses of each lower extremity. Venous ulcers can exist in the presence of mixed arterial/venous pathology. However, treatment of only the CVD will not succeed when significant arterial disease is present (See Table 1).

TABLE 1. "Classic" vascular ulcers

	Arterial	Venous	Neuropathic	Mixed
Localization	Toes, foot, pressure points, bony prominences	Medial leg and ankle	Lat/med forefoot sole: metatarsal heads	Lat/med leg
Skin color	Dependent rubor	Hyperpigmented	Pale	Hyperpigmented
Skin temp	↓↓	↑	Normal	↓
Ulcer border	Sharp, smooth, round	Irregular	Callous, undermined	Variable
Ulcer base	Fibrotic, necrotic, pink granulation	Red granulation weeping	Need to debride deep, tracking	Fibrotic, smooth
Pain	Yes	Variable	Little→none	Variable
Sensation	Normal	Normal	↓↓	↓
Reflexes	Normal to ↓	Normal	↓↓	Normal

A. Ankle brachial index

An ankle brachial index (ABI) should be performed on all patients with leg ulcers as a screening test for evaluation of peripheral artery disease (PAD). The ABI is the ratio of the systolic blood pressure (SBP) measured at the ankle (highest of the dorsalis pedis and posterior tibialis) to that measured at the brachial artery (highest one). Any ABI less than 0.9 suggests some degree of vascular disease, and compression therapy is usually considered to be contraindicated with an ABI<0.7. An ABI of >0.8 is most likely consistent with perfusion status adequate for wound healing.

In elderly patients, patients with diabetes mellitus, or patients with an ABI>1.2 (falsely elevated ABI due to arterial medial calcinosis), a toe brachial index (TBI) of >0.6 or a transcutaneous oxygen partial pressure of >30 mmHg in the region of the ulcer may help to suggest an adequate arterial flow.

B. Venous duplex ultrasound

Venous duplex ultrasound is beneficial for management of every patient with VLU. Venous duplex ultrasound provides diagnostic clues for reflux disease, post-thrombotic syndrome, and chronic venous stenosis. It provides therapeutic guidance for possible endovenous ablation, angioplasty, and surgical corrective procedure of a stenosis or obstruction. It is important that a vascular lab to which VLU patients are referred has a separate protocol for the assessment of venous insufficiency apart from standard venous duplex used for the assessment of thrombosis. The latter is not indicated for VLU patients, while the former helps to determine if invasive treatment is indicated to prevent ulcer recurrence.[3]

It is recommended to obtain a venous duplex ultrasound in every patient with VLU. A combination of gray scale image, color duplex, and doppler is used. It provides anatomic and physiologic data helping to confirm a venous etiology for the leg ulcer, and it is the most reliable noninvasive test to diagnose anatomical and hemodynamic abnormalities and to detect reflux in any venous segment in either the superficial or deep system.

Venous duplex ultrasound provides diagnostic clues for reflux disease, post-thrombotic syndrome, and chronic venous stenosis. It is also used for therapeutic guidance for possible endogenous ablation, angioplasty, and surgical corrective procedure of a stenosis or obstruction. In most vascular labs there is a separate protocol for the assessment of venous insufficiency that is necessary for VLUs apart from "standard" venous duplex used for the assessment of thrombosis.

C. Air plethysmography

Air plethysmography (APG) is another noninvasive testing modality to evaluate the patient for CVI. It provides physiological information about the presence of obstruction, venous reflux, or calf muscle pump failure. APG should be used selectively for the noninvasive evaluation of the venous system in patients with simple varicose veins *(CEAP Class C2) and in patients with advanced CVD if duplex scanning does not provide definitive information on pathophysiology *(CEAP Class C3-C6).

* *The CEAP Classification was developed to standardize reporting and treatment of diverse manifestations of chronic venous disorders and allow uniform diagnosis. CEAP is an acronym for clinical, etiology, anatomy, pathophysiology. For details please see Chapter 5: Wound Assessment.*

D. Venography

Contrast-enhanced venography is still considered the gold standard for deep vein thrombosis (DVT) diagnosis. For the diagnosis of DVT, ascending venography is performed in selected patients, such as patients with a non-diagnostic duplex ultrasound examination for whom a duplex examination is not technically feasible or patients with a high clinical suspicion for DVT but with a negative duplex examination. It is also performed as an adjunct during venous thrombolysis and angioplasty. While in the evaluation of valvular insufficiency prior to stripping or ligation of superficial varicose veins, descending venography is used.

Venography is also used for venous mapping prior to or following a surgical interventional procedure, for the evaluation of venous stenosis or venous hypertension and venous malformations.

E. Biopsy and differential diagnosis

Apparent venous ulcers that have been open continuously without signs of healing for three months or that do not demonstrate any response to treatment after six weeks should be biopsied for histological diagnosis.

Apparent venous ulcers that are excessively painful and progressively increase in size after debridement and/or despite treatment should be considered for other diagnoses such as pyoderma gangrenosum, IgA monoclonal gammopathies, Wegener's granulomatosis, cutaneous chronic granulomatous disease, and mycobacterial or fungal etiologies. This suspicion should be especially high if the ulcer is darker in color, has blue/purple borders, or if the patient has a systemic disease such as Crohn's disease, ulcerative colitis, rheumatoid arthritis, collagen vascular diseases, leukemia, or immunosuppression. In such patients, a wound biopsy may be indicated.

Patients presenting with an apparent venous ulcer and who are suspected of having sickle cell disease should have a sickle cell prep and a hemoglobin electrophoresis.

Leg ulcers that worsen in size and symptoms despite treatment or do not show any improvement over four weeks of treatment should raise suspicion that the ulcer etiology is not venous in origin or that the therapy needs to be re-evaluated. At this point, specific cultures for mycobacteria and/or fungi are useful, as biopsies for histology.

VI. Role of different venous procedures in venous stasis ulcer patient

The role of venous procedures in the management of the venous stasis ulcer is in evolution but has been solidified for prevention with the ESCHAR (effect of surgery and compression on healing and recurrence) study originally published in 2004 with four-year data that was subsequently published in 2007.[3] This multicenter prospective trial randomized 500 patients classified as CEAP 5-6 venous disease to saphenous stripping with or without phlebectomy along with compression versus compression therapy alone. Ulcer recurrence was demonstrated to be significantly less in all three distinct reflux presentations: (a) those with isolated superficial reflux, (b) those with superficial and segmental deep reflux, and (c) those with both superficial and total deep reflux. Overall ulcer recurrence at four years was 56% in the conservative group and 31% in the surgical group. Ulcer healing rates remained unchanged between the two major groups. Because of the significant reduction in both ulcer recurrence and ulcer free time in all different reflux presentations, it was surmised that the presence of deep valvular reflux should not be considered a contraindication to superficial venous surgery. This study supports a shift toward vein surgery for the reduction of venous insufficiency ulcer recurrence, irrespective of the type of reflux.

The Society for Vascular Surgery (SVS) and the American Venous Forum (AVF) published clinical practice guidelines for the treatment of varicose veins associated with chronic venous disease in 2011.[4]

They assigned a strong 1A recommendation for the role of surgery or ablation of incompetent superficial veins to decrease recurrence of venous ulcers. Furthermore, endovenous thermal ablation was recommended over open surgery (stripping) for incompetent saphenous veins because of reduced convalescence and less surgical pain (1B).

A. Thermal ablation of superficial veins

Thermal ablation procedures utilize thermal energy delivered through specialized catheter systems utilizing either radiofrequency ablation (RFA) or endovenous laser ablation (EVLA) generators to obliterate trucal or perforator veins with the great saphenous vein as the most frequent target. The mechanism targets either the endothelium (water) or red blood cells to damage the vein and iatrogenically cause thrombosis, eventual fibrosis, and reabsorption. Both treatment modalities are performed with minimal sedation in outpatient treatment centers with tumescent anesthesia and are associated with lower morbidity and greater efficacy than traditional saphenous stripping surgery.

Venous stasis ulcers that persist or have not reduced in area by at least 30-50% despite the best adequate standard wound care and the judicious use of compression for four weeks should also be considered for advanced therapies. This is supported by mostly retrospective data and expert opinion including a consensus panel summary for the venous leg ulcer published by the Veterans Administration.[5-8] A retrospective analysis of 86 patients with venous leg ulcers published in 2013 was conducted to compare conventional (compression) treatment to those treated with conventional plus minimally invasive procedures (a heterogenous group comprised of thermal ablation, ultrasound-guided foam sclerotherapy, phlebectomy, high ligation and conventional sclerotherapy).[9] Patients who were treated with intervention were found to have a significantly greater percentage of ulcer healing per week than those treated with compression alone and overall one-year healing without recurrence was 65% in the intervention group versus only 36% in the compression-only group (P=0.004).

B. Chemical ablation of superficial veins

Venous sclerotherapy has been utilized for decades with various sclerosing agents as an adjunctive treatment for chronic venous insufficiency. It is indicated for a variety of conditions ranging from spider telangiectasias to moderate-sized varicose veins and vascular malformations. It is particularly useful in eliminating bleeding varices (usually less than 4 mm) and small venous blebs in the lower gaiter region where ambulatory venous pressures can become extremely high. There are two FDA-approved agents available in the United States to be administered intravenously as liquid only: sodium tetradecyl sulfate (STS) and polidocanol, used at various concentrations depending on the caliber of the veins being injected. Care must be taken with higher concentrations, however, since these are associated with increased incidence of irritation, thrombosis, and even the iatrogenic development of new skin ulcers.

Treatment of larger-diameter veins often requires ultrasound guidance and foaming of the solution using air, CO_2, nitrogen, or a combination of gases and was regarded as off-label use of the FDA-approved label for sclerosants. The foamed sclerosant has a much longer dwell time in the vein prior to systemic washout and dilution, thus enabling the effective treatment of larger caliber veins with safer and lower concentrations of STS or polidocanol. The foam can be delivered into truncal veins with or without ultrasound guidance and has even proven effective for perforator management. A recent prospective randomized trial comparing foamed polidocanol and surgery for active ulcer management showed no difference in ulcer healing, QOL/clinical outcome scores, and complications.[10]

Ultrasound-guided foam sclerotherapy for the great saphenous vein has been utilized as an effective alternative to more conventional saphenous surgery for several years. It is sometimes combined with high saphenous ligation but was shown in a prospective study to have only an 80% short-term closure rate, requiring secondary foam injections. A newer delivery system of polidocanol 1% foam in a bi-canister is now available in the United States and other countries for treatment of the great saphenous vein and its tributaries (Varithena, Provensis Ltd, UK). The VANISH (VAsopressin versus Norepinephrine as Initial therapy in Septic sHock) trials showed 80-86% treatment success at two months and in the FDA label of 1,333 patients treated with Varithena proximal DVT occurred in 1.7% of patients.[11]

C. Nonthermal nontumescent venous ablation

Two recently developed technologies do not require thermal energy or tumescent anesthesia and are known as nonthermal nontumescent ablations. Mechanical occlusion chemically assisted ablation (MOCA) ablation is the first nonthermal, nontumescent procedure integrated into clinical practice. It has been in use since 2009 and in over 60,000 cases worldwide. MOCA uses a rotating wire-tipped catheter that agitates and destroys vessel intima as it delivers sclerosant to fully close the vessel.

The VenaSeal closure system and procedure (Medtronic, U.S.) uses a proprietary formulation of cyanoacrylate adhesive delivered endovenously to close the vein. It was approved by the FDA in February 2015.

Both nonthermal nontumescent modalities demonstrated vein ablation rates similar to thermal ablations and have obvious advantages such as elimination of a need for injecting large volumes of anesthetics and less patient discomfort during treatment. More importantly, they eliminate risk of nerve damage and are suited to treat saphenous veins below knee.[12-13]

D. Ablation of perforating veins

Incompetent perforator veins have commonly been implicated as a cause for focal venous hypertension and subsequent lower leg venous ulcers, particularly in the medial gaiter region. This is often thought to lead to ascending reflux with secondary superficial valvular dysfunction. Perforator veins are regarded as incompetent when their diameter exceeds 3.5 mm and/or reflux of >500 msec is demonstrated with duplex ultrasound.

The most recent AVF/SVS guidelines provide more specific indications for treating limbs with C4b – C6 disease.[2] These guidelines include the following statements:

- In a patient with a venous leg ulcer (C6) and incompetent superficial veins that have reflux to the ulcer bed in addition to pathologic perforating veins (outward flow of >500 msec duration, with a diameter of >3.5mm) located beneath or associated with the ulcer bed, we suggest ablation of both the incompetent superficial veins and perforator veins in addition to standard compressive therapy to aid in ulcer healing and prevent recurrence. [GRADE -2; LEVEL OF EVIDENCE -C]

- In a patient with skin changes suggestive of an impending venous ulcer (C4b) or healed venous ulcer (C5) and incompetent superficial veins that have reflux to the ulcer bed in addition to pathologic perforating veins (outward flow of >500 msec duration, with a diameter of >3.5mm) located beneath or associated with the healed ulcer bed, we suggest ablation of the incompetent superficial veins to prevent the development or recurrence of a venous leg ulcer. (GRADE -2; LEVEL OF EVIDENCE -C) Treatment of the incompetent perforating veins can be performed simultaneously with correction of axial reflux or can be staged with re-evaluation of perforator veins for persistent incompetence after correction of axial reflux. [GRADE -2; LEVEL OF EVIDENCE -C]
- In a patient with isolated pathologic perforator veins (outward flow of >500 msec duration, with a diameter of >3.5mm) located beneath or associated with the healed (C5) or active ulcer (C6) bed regardless of the status of the deep veins, we suggest ablation of the pathologic perforating veins in addition to standard compression therapy to aid in venous ulcer healing and to prevent recurrence. [GRADE -2; LEVEL OF EVIDENCE -C]

Ligation of perforator veins has long been held as a sound surgical principle, but the traditional Linton procedure and its modifications were often plagued by morbidity and wound complications. In addition to this, the offending vein may lie directly deep to an ulcerated area, thereby precluding open dissection and ligation under direct surveillance by the surgeon. Subfascial endoscopic perforator surgery (SEPS), therefore, emerged in the 1990s as a means to ligate incompetent perforator veins by gaining access from a remote site with a specialized endoscope that is distant from ulceration, inflammation and lipodermatoesclerosis. Several studies and a systematic review demonstrated that ulcer healing rate after SEPS is close to 90% and two-year recurrence rate less than 15%.

Contemporary percutaneous endovenous therapies combine the precision of a surgical approach with the minimal invasiveness of an injection. Patients can ambulate immediately after such treatment, and experience minimal postoperative pain. Endovenous options gradually replaced all surgical procedures of perforator treatment to the point when the evidence-based guidelines make Grade 1 recommendation to treat perforating veins by percutaneous techniques over open venous perforator surgery to eliminate the need for incisions in areas of compromised skin.[2]

VII. Wound management in patients with venous stasis ulcer

Medical treatment

The guidelines suggest:

1. Venoactive drugs (diosmin, hesperidin, rutosides, sulodexide, micronized purified flavonoid fraction, or horse chestnut seed extract [aescin]) for patients with pain and swelling due to CVD, in countries where these drugs are available.

2. Pentoxifylline or micronized purified flavonoid fraction, if available, in combination with compression, to accelerate healing of venous ulcers.

Compression Treatment

The guidelines recommend compression as the primary therapeutic modality for healing venous ulcers and recommend compression as an adjuvant treatment to superficial vein ablation for the prevention of ulcer recurrence.

Venous ulcers of the lower extremity are a chronic long-term problem. Recurrence rates are as high as 70%. Therefore, long-term maintenance must be addressed even for healed ulcers. Patients with healed or surgically repaired venous ulcers should use compression stockings indefinitely when their legs are dependent. Most treatments do not eliminate the underlying increased ambulatory venous pressure (venous hypertension), so a degree of compression is necessary long term. Exercises to increase calf muscle pump function have been demonstrated to be helpful in long-term maintenance and venous ulcer prevention.

Nutrition must be adequate to provide sufficient protein to support the growth of granulation tissue.

Wounds will heal in an environment that is adequately oxygenated. Oxygen delivery to a wound will be impaired if tissue perfusion is inadequate. Dehydration and factors that increase sympathetic tone such as cold, stress, or pain will all decrease tissue perfusion. Cigarette smoking decreases tissue oxygen by decreasing NO release. For optimal tissue perfusion, these factors must be eliminated or minimized.

Initial debridement is required to remove the obvious necrotic tissue, excessive bacterial burden, and cellular burden of dead and senescent cells. Maintenance debridement is needed to maintain the appearance and readiness of the wound bed for healing. The health-care provider can choose from a number of debridement methods including sharp, enzymatic, mechanical, biological, or autolytic. More than one debridement method may be appropriate. Sharp debridement is often the most advantageous.

Necrotic tissue, excessive bacterial burden, senescent cells, and cellular debris can all inhibit wound healing. Wounds should be cleansed initially and at each dressing change using a neutral, nonirritating, nontoxic solution. Routine wound cleansing should be accomplished with a minimum of chemical and/or mechanical trauma.

A moist wound environment physiologically favors cell migration and matrix formation while accelerating healing of wounds by promoting autolytic debridement. Moist wound healing also reduces pain. Dry dressings, except over intact skin, are considered injurious and can cause desiccation of the wound.

Use clinical judgment to select a wound dressing that facilitates continued moisture. Select a dressing that will manage the wound exudate and protect the peri-ulcer skin. Periwound maceration and continuous contact with wound exudate can enlarge the wound and impede healing.

VIII. Preventing recurrence of venous stasis ulcers

The most challenging aspect of care for patients with venous ulcers is the transition from wound care settings to primary care settings. It is still a widespread view among primary care providers that the treatment stops when the wound is healed. Several avenues are available to overcome this barrier.

Patient education is probably the most important way to ensure that treatment continues and the risk of recurrence is properly addressed. Patient adherence to treatment such as compression therapy is known to be low. Part of this non-compliance is due to the lack of systematic effort to educate the patients (and their primary care providers) about the importance of such treatment.

If the pathological condition that caused the ulcer is not corrected, the recurrence rate is at its maximum. This is why proper evaluation of patients at the initial presentation is so important. If correctible hemodynamic abnormalities are identified, they should be treated even before the ulcer has healed. This is the best time to ensure high compliance with such treatment, thus most effectively preventing recurrence.

Finally, lifestyle modification is the most cost-effective way to prevent ulcer recurrence. Weight loss and regular physical activity may significantly decrease the risk of recurrence.

Summary

In summary, the clinical management of patients with VLUs in addition to the fastest and most functionally achievable healing should be aimed at the diagnosis of underlying vascular abnormalities and correction of them in order to decrease recurrence rate.

Review questions

1. **Which is the most appropriate management of a patient with venous ulcer who has no palpable pedal pulses?**

   a. order an ultrasound test to rule out DVT
   b. avoid any type of compression therapy
   c. use the Unna wrap without applying any pressure
   d. check ankle-brachial index (ABI)
   e. prescribe Class 2 compression stockings

2. **What is the most appropriate diagnostic test for a patient with a chronic ulcer in medial malleolus area?**

   a. clinical examination is sufficient
   b. ultrasound scan to rule out DVT
   c. duplex ultrasound scan for venous insufficiency (reflux study)
   d. venography
   e. ankle-brachial index (ABI)

3. ***True/False.*** Leg ulcer that worsens in size despite treatment for six weeks should be biopsied for histological diagnosis.

4. ***True/False.*** Initial treatment of venous ulcer does not require compression therapy.

5. **What is the natural history in cases when the saphenous vein reflux remains untreated after the ulcer healed?**

   a. Patients who continue using compression stockings are unlikely to have recurrent ulcers.
   b. Symptoms of venous disease improve in the majority of patients after the ulcer healed.
   c. Saphenous reflux does not affect the natural history after ulcer healed.
   d. More than 40% of the patients will have a recurrent ulcer.
   e. Patient may be at a higher risk for DVT.

ANSWERS: 1) d
2) c
3) True
4) False
5) d

References

1. Ma H, Rosen NA, Lafrati MD, O'Donnell TF. The real costs of treating venous ulcers in a contemporary vascular practice. Journal of Vascular Surgery: Venous and Lymphatic Disorders 2013; 1(1):105.
2. O'Donnell TF, Jr., Passman MA. Clinical practice guidelines of the Society for Vascular Surgery (SVS) and the American Venous Forum (AVF): Management of venous leg ulcers. Introduction. J Vasc Surg 2014;60(2 Suppl):1S-2S.
3. Gohel MS, Barwell JR, Earnshaw JJ, Heather BP, Mitchell DC, Whyman MR, Poskitt KR. Randomized clinical trial of compression plus surgery versus compression alone in chronic venous ulceration (ESCHAR study)—haemodynamic and anatomical changes. Br J Surg. 2005;92(3):291-297.
4. Gloviczki P, Comerota AJ, Dalsing MC, Eklof BG, Gillespie DL, Gloviczki ML, et al. The care of patients with varicose veins and associated chronic venous diseases: clinical practice guidelines of the Society for Vascular Surgery and the American Venous Forum. J Vasc Surg 2011;53(5 Suppl):2S-48S.
5. Andersen CR, Aung BJ, Chandy RM, Doucette M, Garcia M, Garoufalis MG. Improving the Standard of Care for Treating Venous Leg Ulcers within the Veterans Administration. Wounds 2012; 24(4)(suppl):1-8.
6. Phillips TJ, Machado F, Trout R, Porter J, Olin J, Falanga V. Prognostic indicators in venous ulcers. J Am Acad Dermatol 2000; 43(4):627-630.
7. Cardinal M, Eisenbud DE, Phillips T, Harding K. Early healing rates and wound area measurements are reliable predictors of later complete wound closure. Wound Repair Regen 2008;16(1):19-22.
8. Kantor J, Margolis DJ. A multicentre study of percentage change in venous leg ulcer area as a prognostic index of healing at 24 weeks. Br J Dermatol 2000;142(5):960-964.
9. Alden PB, Lips EM, Zimmerman KP, Garberich RF, Rizvi AZ, Tretinyak AS, et al. Chronic venous ulcer: minimally invasive treatment of superficial axial and perforator vein reflux speeds healing and reduces recurrence. Ann Vasc Surg 2013;27(1):75-83.
10. Campos W, Jr., Torres IO, da Silva ES, Casella IB, Puech-Leao P. A prospective randomized study comparing polidocanol foam sclerotherapy with surgical treatment of patients with primary chronic venous insufficiency and ulcer. Ann Vasc Surg 2015;29(6):1128-1135.
11. Todd KL 3rd, Wright DI; VANISH-2 Investigator Group. The VANISH-2 study: a randomized, blinded, multicenter study to evaluate the efficacy and safety of polidocanol endovenous microfoam 0.5% and 1.0% compared with placebo for the treatment of saphenofemoral junction incompetence. Phlebology. 2014;29(9):608-618.
12. van Eekeren RRJP, Boersma D, Holewijn S, Werson DAB, de Vries JP, Reijnen MMJP. Mechanochemical endovenous ablation for the treatment of great saphenous vein insufficiency. Journal of Vascular Surgery: Venous and Lymphatic Disorders 2014;2(3):282-288.
13. Morrison N, Gibson K, McEnroe S, Goldman M, King T, Weiss R, et al. Randomized trial comparing cyanoacrylate embolization and radiofrequency ablation for incompetent great saphenous veins (VeClose). Journal of Vascular Surgery 2015;61(4):985-994.

Chapter 13
LYMPHEDEMA

Heather Hettrick, PT, PhD, CWS, CLT-LANA, CLWT
Robyn Bjork, MPT, CWS, CLT-LANA, CLWT

KEY CONCEPTS

1. Lymphedema is a vascular disorder that is either due to congenital malformations of the lymphatic system (primary etiology) or related to an insult or injury to the lymphatic system (secondary etiology) such as surgery, trauma, radiation, malignancies, or infections.
2. Secondary lymphedema is more prevalent than primary lymphedema.
3. On a global scale, the leading cause of lymphedema in the world is due to lymphatic filariasis, a parasitic form of lymphedema spread through mosquitoes.
4. Cellulitis is common in patients with lymphedema and may require recurrent hospitalizations.
5. A positive Stemmer's sign is a simple clinical finding that yields a definitive diagnosis of lymphedema.
6. Lymphoscintigraphy is accurate for detecting abnormalities of the lymphatic system in the extremities and shows slow or absent lymph flow and areas of reflux (backflow).
7. Complete decongestive therapy (CDT) is considered the standard of care for lymphedema management.
8. Surgery for lymphedema is not curative but may help manage severe cases.
9. Multilayered lymphedema bandaging (MLLB) is composed of multiple layers of short-stretch bandages, along with hygienic lining and padding materials, to create graduated compression with high containment.
10. All patients need to be transitioned into compression garments for lifelong maintenance management of lymphedema.
11. Intermittent pneumatic compression (IPC) devices, or lymphedema pumps, may be considered adjunctive to effectively manage lymphedema.

CONTENTS

Introduction

This chapter will provide the health-care practitioner with a comprehensive overview of lymphedema pathophysiology, examination, and intervention strategies to improve early recognition and diagnosis of the disease. A case study will accompany the chapter providing context for the health-care practitioner as relevant topics are presented. Known as a hidden epidemic, lymphedema can lead to a spectrum of mild to severe complications ranging from integumentary dysfunction to severe functional limitations. Although there is no cure, lymphedema can be successfully managed. The key is to recognize the disease so proper management can be rendered.

I. Case study

A 61-year-old Caucasian female, 5'2" tall and 349 pounds, reports a 12-year history of lymphedema and failed medical treatment since 2004. She is married and has a supportive spouse. She reports no history of congestive heart failure or kidney disease and has never been diagnosed with chronic venous insufficiency (CVI), although she states she has not seen a phlebologist and has never had an ankle-brachial index (ABI) study. She has a negative history of deep vein thrombosis (DVT) confirmed by previous duplex ultrasound (Figure 1).

The patient reports the problem began 12 years ago with swelling, cracking, and weeping of the right foot. She was diagnosed with lymphedema by her primary care physician and treated with diuretics (Lasix) for six months and oral antibiotics for a few months, combined with limb elevation and bed rest. The edema subsided enough to resolve the skin issues, but gradually the right foot and leg increased in size. One year later, she developed cellulitis in

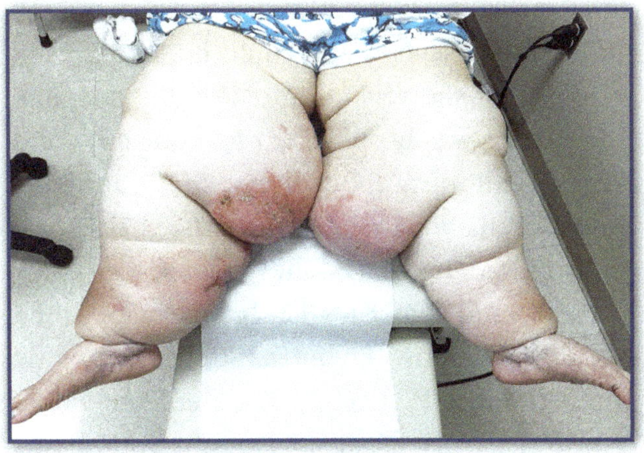

FIGURE 1. Case study
Courtesy of Robyn Bjork, MPT, CWS, CLT-LANA, CLWT

the right leg, ankle to mid-calf. She was treated with oral antibiotics for six weeks, leg elevation, and bed rest. Following the cellulitis, the patient wore a larger shoe size and was unable to go back to her regular shoe size thereafter.

Approximately 15 months after the bout of cellulitis, two ulcers developed on the right calf. She was treated with an Unna boot one to two times per week for six months to heal the ulcers. However, two months later, the right foot and leg started swelling again and started weeping, and the left foot started to swell too. Despite rest and elevation, as advised by her physician, the edema slowly progressed.

After researching local lymphedema treatment options, the patient's primary care physician referred her to a certified lymphedema therapist for outpatient treatment two times per week for two weeks, then one time per week for a total of eight weeks. She received manual lymphatic drainage therapy but was only bandaged to the knees and was discharged without long-term compression garments as soon as the skin weeping resolved.

Eight months later, the legs swelled significantly and were leaking copious amounts of fluid. The patient placed a towel under her legs to absorb the draining fluid. Acute cellulitis rapidly progressed. Her legs became red, swollen, and cracked open; she rated her pain as 9/10 (0=none, 10=severe) and could no longer walk by the time she was admitted to the hospital. The patient was hospitalized for four days and treated with intravenous therapy (IV) antibiotics and Unna boot bandaging to the knees bilaterally. After discharge, she was referred back to the wound center for 12–16 weeks for Unna boot applications. An intermittent pneumatic compression (IPC) pump was recommended. Due to lack of Medicaid coverage, the pump was not received until after one was donated to her a year later. She then started IPC pump treatment one hour per day for two weeks, followed by one hour two times per day thereafter. The patient reported she had a full leg sleeve, but it barely fit above the knee, and she could not get good closure of the sleeve above the knee.

After using the pump for four months, the patient started developing lobes on inside of her right knee, and the ulcer recurred on her right calf. She returned to the wound center for one time per week for six weeks for Unna boot treatments. The edematous lobes on the inside of both knees progressively got larger at every weekly visit. The patient stopped using the IPC pump. Her wound healed, and she was discharged from the wound center without further recommendations. The lobes on the medial aspect of her knees continued to slowly enlarge; she used emollients to keep the skin hydrated.

Toward the end of 2013, the patient sought out a new certified lymphedema therapist and received authorization from Medicaid for eight weeks of treatment; no wounds were present at this time. She received education, handouts, and an average of only 20 minutes of MLDT per session, with no compression therapy. The patient reported there were no results.

By 2015, the lymphedematous lobes on her medial knees had increased in size to a circumference of ~113 cm around each knee and lobe and weighed approximately 15–20 pounds on the right and 10–15 pounds on the left. In March of 2015, lymphorrhea developed in the apex of the lobes, denuding the skin and causing painful partial-thickness wounds. She traveled 1.5 hours from her home to see a certified wound specialist physician who successfully treated the wounds. Her need for comprehensive CDT was identified, but the patient did not have access to appropriate care, due to lack of comprehensive services being available and financial constraints.

In October of 2015, she suffered yet another bout of cellulitis, was treated with oral antibiotics for six weeks, and remained on a low-dose antibiotic therapy for another six months. Currently, the patient complains of tremendous strain on her knee joints from the weight of the lobes, severely limited mobility, pain rated 10/10 in her knees, and decreased sensation from her waist to her ankles bilaterally. Even though she has severe osteoarthritis, she is not a candidate for total knee replacements due to high risks associated with the chronic lymphedema. She is currently taking oxycodone/acetaminophen one pill, four times per day. Her social life is markedly limited due to the lymphedema.

II. Epidemiology and economic impact of lymphedema and integumentary dysfunction on lymphedema patients

Lymphedema is a chronic, incurable disease that can be readily managed with the appropriate interventions. Lymphedema is a vascular disorder that is either due to congenital malformations of the lymphatic system (primary etiology) or related to an insult or injury to the lymphatic system (secondary etiology) such as surgery, trauma, radiation, malignancies, or infections.

The clinical course of lymphedema involves a progressive swelling of the limb or areas affected due to a mechanical insufficiency of the lymphatic system. Over time, this protein-rich fluid burden may lead to various integumentary complications ranging from fibrosis and hyperkeratosis to weeping skin with or without ulceration.

The challenge is to appreciate the magnitude of those affected by both lymphedema and integumentary dysfunction. Even though various forms of lymphedema worldwide affect millions, the existing literature fails to fully define the population-based prevalence, health outcomes, and treatment costs of this disorder. This information is even harder to obtain or quantify for lymphedema patients with associated integumentary complications.

Although evidence-based best-practice guidelines have been outlined in consensus documents, lymphedema is a relatively underrecognized condition in both medical and public domains. The reasons for this include a lack of public awareness of the condition, insufficient education and knowledge among health-care providers regarding its etiology and management, and limited reimbursement coverage to support lymphedema care models.[1] This is further compounded by the fact that patients with integumentary dysfunction are also faced with the same limitations. Although highly interrelated, lymphedema and integumentary dysfunction have traditionally been taught, researched, and even managed separately. Only recently has progress been made addressing the interdependent nature of these conditions.

A rough population prevalence rate for chronic nonhealing wounds in the United States is 2% of the general population;[2] this translates to roughly 7 million individuals. A conservative estimate of the cost of caring for chronic wounds exceeds $50 billion per year.[3-5] The majority of chronic nonhealing wounds involve peripheral vascular disease (arterial and venous insufficiency). Estimated prevalence reports of chronic venous insufficiency vary geographically (highest reports in Western countries) and range from <1% to 40% in females and from <1% to 17% in males.[6] To gain perspective, in patients with advanced chronic venous disease, 20%–30% will have associated lymphatic dysfunction believed to be related to overload from the fluid burden, damage from venous hypertension, and repeated infections (cellulitis).[7-9]

With respect to lymphedema, it is estimated that 3–5 million people in the United States alone suffer from this disease, yet it is likely that estimate is not truly reflective as many remain undiagnosed and/or underreported. More data is available on lymphedema secondary to various forms of cancer. The overall risk for lymphedema for all cancers is reported to be 15.5%.[10] Specifically, lymphedema is reported to occur in up to 49% of breast, 20% of gynecologic, 16% of melanoma, 10% of genitourinary, and 6% of head and neck cancer patients after lymph node dissection and/or radiotherapy. Additionally, 10% of patients who receive isolated axillary sentinel lymph node biopsy report subjective symptoms of lymphedema.[10-17] On a global scale, the leading cause of lymphedema in the world is due to lymphatic filariasis, a parasitic form of lymphedema spread through mosquitoes. Over 1.2 billion people are at risk for contracting lymphatic filariasis (LF), which is 1 of 13 neglected tropical diseases and 1 of only 6 infectious diseases considered eliminable by the World Health Assembly. This disfiguring and debilitating disease affects over 120 million people in 83 countries.

III. Starling's law and ultrafiltration

In order to understand the pathophysiology of lymphedema and its potential impact in wound healing, one must first understand the integration and fluid dynamics of the arterial, venous, and lymphatic vasculature. Ernest Henry Starling (1866–1927) discovered that under normal conditions, the average blood capillary pressure (BCP) and colloid osmotic pressure (COP) of the blood plasma proteins are equal. Blood capillary pressure in the arterial end of the capillary is higher (29 mmHg) than the COP (25 mmHg), resulting in fluid leaking through the capillary membrane into the interstitium. In contrast, the BCP in the venous end of the capillary is lower (14 mmHg) than COP of the plasma proteins (25 mmHg), resulting in fluid being reabsorbed back into the blood capillaries. This results in a steady "stream" of 20 liters of nutrient-rich fluid bathing cells each day.[18]

In the presence of inflammation, congestive heart failure, venous disease, or kidney disease, for example, the blood capillary hydrostatic pressure exceeds colloid osmotic pressure of plasma proteins. This results in ultrafiltration of fluid from the blood capillary into the tissues. In the presence of ultrafiltration, the lymphatic system must maintain fluid balance by increasing the uptake of interstitial fluid as lymph, or the tissues will swell. Conversely, lymphatic vessels that are congested or obstructed will result in back pressure in the lymphatic system and insufficient drainage of fluid from the tissues. The ensuing pathological changes and clinical presentation are related to the composition of that accumulating lymph fluid, or lymphatic load.

IV. Composition of lymph and the lymphatic load

Plasma is the colorless, watery, nutrient-rich fluid component of the blood that leaks into the interstitial space to bathe and nourish the cells. Once plasma enters the interstitial space, it is called "interstitial fluid." This same fluid comprises the serous drainage from a wound. When this fluid enters a lymphatic capillary, it is then called lymph. As lymph flows through the lymphatic system, it becomes thicker as water content is reduced and eventually becomes milky in appearance from the absorption of fat from the gut.

Each day, 50% (75–100/day) of proteins circulating in the plasma of the blood leak out into the interstitial space and are recovered by the lymphatic capillaries.[19] This includes albumins, small plasma proteins that make up ~55% of all plasma proteins by weight and maintain osmotic balance described by Starling. It also includes globulins, large plasma proteins that make up ~38% of all plasma proteins by weight and act as carriers for other molecules, as well as fibrinogen, a very large protein that makes up ~7% of all plasma proteins by weight and is important in blood clotting.[20]

Large plasma proteins are too big to reenter the blood capillary, and small plasma proteins cannot go "uphill" back into an area of higher pressure and concentration within the blood capillaries. The primary task of the lymph vascular system is to handle this lymphatic protein load.[21]

By definition, lymphatic loads are those substances that must leave the location where they are formed and can only do so via the lymphatic system.[21] Lymphatic loads include more than just blood proteins. Other components of lymph include by-products of wound healing, dead and senescent cells, immune cells, such as lymphocytes, macrophages, and Langerhans's cells, proteases, hyaluronic acid, cytokines, chemokines, and growth factors, such as VEGF, tumor necrosis factor alpha, and Interleukin-1.[19]

V. Pathophysiology

Proteins trapped in the tissues result in a high protein edema, or lymphedema. These excess proteins increase COP, and their strong affinity to pull and hold fluid in the tissue results in increasing lymphedema. Further, the "flow" of nutrients and removal of waste products is disrupted, and the diffusion distance for nutrients to reach cells of the skin is increased. As the lymphatic system becomes more congested, bicuspid valves and the small contractile units (lymphangions) in the lymphatic vessels can become insufficient, leading to mechanical failure secondary to the dynamic fluid overload.

As flow slows, white blood cell migration toward regional lymph nodes is impaired, compromising the immune function of the lymphatic system to respond to mounting bioburden in wounds. Further, the accumulation of protein in the tissue provides ample "food" for bacteria to thrive. Consequently, cellulitis is common in this patient population, and recurrent hospitalizations pose a significant cost burden to our health-care system.

In addition to the propensity to retain fluid in the tissues, trapped proteins break down, inducing a pathohistological state of chronic inflammation.[21] Like butter becoming rancid, free radicals trapped in the tissues denature proteins and oxidize cell membranes. Monocytes are attracted to the area and differentiate into macrophages. These macrophages take in proteins through pinocytosis and digest them, which activates the macrophages to release cytokines, such as Interleukin-1, which in turn activates fibroblasts.[21] The fibroblasts are stimulated to produce excess collagen. Excess collagen formation causes connective tissue proliferation and fibrosis resulting in the thickened, fibrotic skin and wart-like projections seen in lymphedema. Additionally, some fibroblasts differentiate into adipocytes. The clinical presentation results in enlargement of the body part with thickened, fibrotic dermis and subcutaneous tissues and significant skin changes.

Although poorly studied, given the composition of lymph, it is easy to extrapolate the potential negative effects on wound healing. Some of the consequences of lymphedema in the tissues may include a stagnant wound milieu, impaired immune response to bioburden and infection, decreased oxygenation and nutrition to the wound bed, accumulation of dead and senescent cells, higher concentration of proteases, and chronic inflammation surrounding the wound. Consequently, treatment for lymphedema must address the lymphatic load. The watery component of edema can be squeezed back into the venous system through compression therapy and result in rapid reduction of limb size. However, removal of watery components of the fluid in this way relatively increases the concentration of the lymphatic load in the tissues and can accelerate the pathohistological process, worsening the condition long-term. Manual lymphatic drainage therapy facilitates redundant and alternate, unaffected pathways to reduce the lymphatic load in the tissues. It is used in tandem with compression to achieve physiologically safe lymphedema reduction long-term. Over time, the tissues can return to a more normalized physiological state.

VI. Examination and differential diagnosis

There are two main classifications of lymphedema, primary and secondary. Primary lymphedema is caused by developmental abnormalities of the lymphatic system, such as incomplete development of lymph vessels, reduced number or absent lymphatic structures, enlarged and incompetent vessels, or fibrosis of lymph vessels and nodes. Congenital lymphedema occurs within first two years of life, lymphedema praecox before age 35, and lymphedema tarda after age 35.[18]

Secondary lymphedema is more prevalent than primary lymphedema. There are a number of risk factors that can contribute to the development of secondary lymphedema. Classification of causes include trauma and tissue damage, malignant disease, venous disease, infection, inflammation, endocrine disease, immobility and dependency, and factitious or self-mutilation practices.[22] Risk factors that can lead to secondary lymphedema include but are not limited to breast, head and neck, uterine, and prostate cancer, chronic venous insufficiency, DVT, thrombophlebitis, vein stripping or harvesting, hysterectomy, orthopedic surgery, obesity, cellulitis and wound infections, chronic wounds, orthopedic injuries, burns, scarring, immobility from advancing age or hemiparesis, congestive heart failure, and renal insufficiency.[22] Factors that complicate the care of a patient with lymphedema include peripheral arterial disease, obesity, diabetes, neuropathy, limited mobility and strength, difficulties with activities of daily living, financial constraints, depression, social isolation, lack of family support for long-term management, and other psychosocial factors.

Between 2012 and 2050, the United States will experience considerable growth in its older population. In 2050, the population aged 65 and over is projected to be 83.7 million, almost double its estimated population of 43.1 million in 2012.[23] With this rise, we can expect to see more medically complex patients with multiple comorbidities contributing to higher risks of developing secondary lymphedema. Because of this, it is important that clinicians recognize risk factors and the early signs and symptoms of lymphedema and implement early intervention practices.

VII. Lymphedema staging

The current staging system for lymphedema is rudimentary at best. Further work is needed to create a lymphedema severity score that will provide a better assessment of the complexities of each patient. The International Society of Lymphology (ISL) lymphedema staging system follows below:

Stage 0: This is the latency stage. Risk factors and comorbidities are present. Swelling is not yet evident despite impaired lymph transport. There are subtle changes in tissue fluid/composition and changes in subjective symptoms. Stage 0 may exist months or years before overt edema occurs (Stages 1–3).

Stage 1: This stage represents an early accumulation of fluid relatively high in protein content which subsides with limb elevation. Pitting may occur. An increase in various proliferating cells may also be seen.

Stage 2: In this stage, limb elevation alone rarely reduces tissue swelling, and pitting is manifest. Late in Stage 2, the limb may or may not pit as excess fat and fibrosis develops. Limb elevation alone rarely reduces swelling.

Stage 3: This stage encompasses lymphostatic elephantiasis where pitting can be absent and trophic skin changes such as papillomatosis and hyperkeratosis are present. Further deposition of fat and fibrosis and warty overgrowths has developed.[24]

The ISL staging system does not reflect lymphedema severity in terms of volume of the limb. For example, within Stage 3, one patient may have severe skin changes, massive enlargement

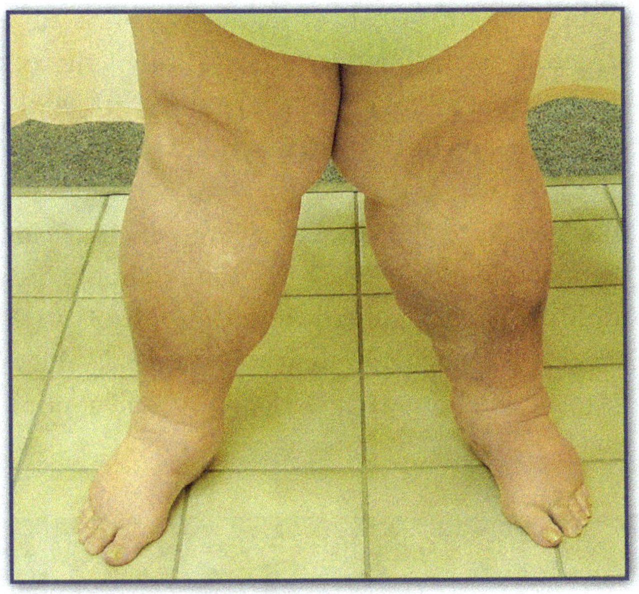

FIGURE 2. Stage 3
Courtesy of Robyn Bjork, MPT, CWS, CLT-LANA, CLWT

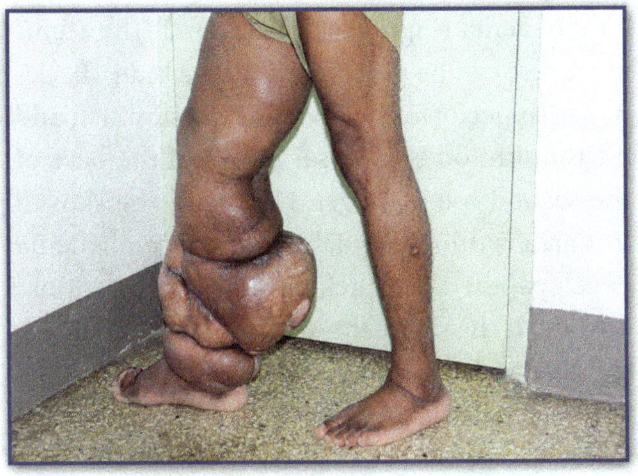

FIGURE 3. Stage 3 due to LF
Courtesy of Robyn Bjork, MPT, CWS, CLT-LANA, CLWT

of the extremity, and large, overhanging lobes of hardened, fibrotic tissue. This patient may require many months of intensive treatment and more than one staff member to treat the limb, and fitting for long-term compression can be complex. In contrast, another patient may have minimal increase in limb size but with focal areas of advanced skin changes, resulting in classification of the lymphedema as Stage 3.

Within each Stage 0–3, the severity of lymphedema can also be graded according to percent volume difference between limbs. Minimal = <20% volume increase; moderate = 20%–40% volume increase; and severe = >40% volume increase.[18] However, this can be calculated if only one arm or leg is affected and is difficult to objectively measure in other areas of the body.

Relevance to case study

This patient (Figure 4, Figure 5, Figure 6) presents with Stage 3 secondary lymphedema with lymphostatic elephantiasis of the medial aspect of both knees. Risk factors contributing to the development of her lymphedema are slow progression of underlying lipedema and CVI, osteoarthritis of both knees with repeated steroid injections, recurrent courses of Unna boot applications with compression stopping just below the knee, lack of adequate compression therapy long-term, and recurrent bouts of cellulitis.

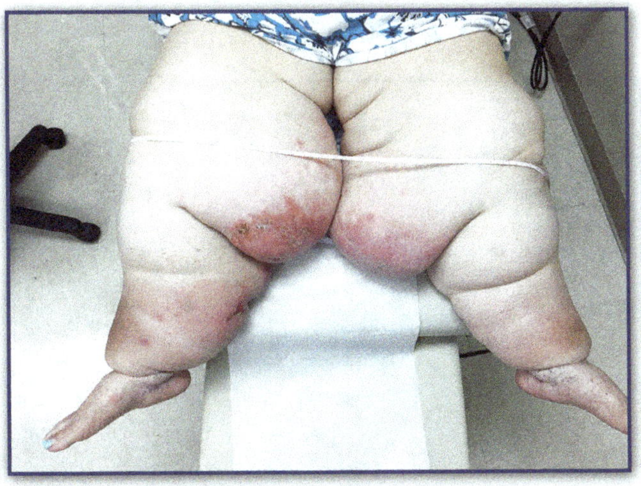

FIGURE 4. Case study Stage 3
Courtesy of Robyn Bjork, MPT, CWS, CLT-LANA, CLWT

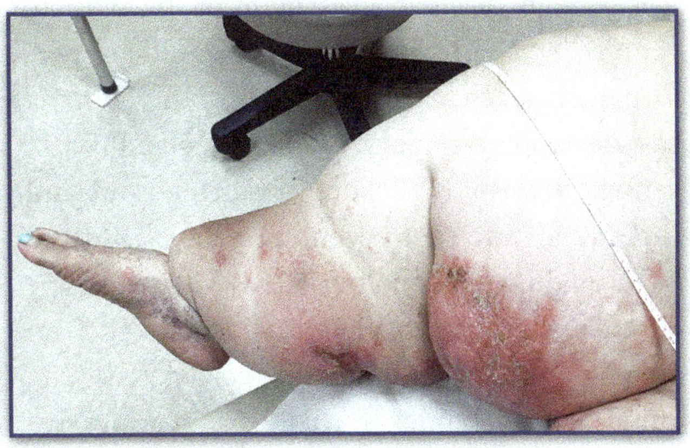

FIGURE 5. Case study left leg
Courtesy of Robyn Bjork, MPT, CWS, CLT-LANA, CLWT

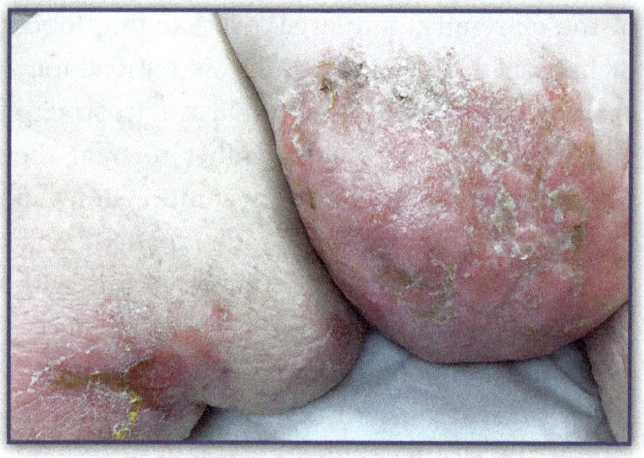

FIGURE 6. Case study skin issues
Courtesy of Robyn Bjork, MPT, CWS, CLT-LANA, CLWT

VIII. History and physical exam

A history and physical examination by a healthcare provider who has experience with diagnosis and treatment of lymphedema is important for all patients with chronic swelling. The National Lymphedema Network Medical Advisory Committee recommends the history include age of onset; location(s) of swelling, pain and other symptoms; medications that can cause swelling; the course of progression of the swelling; factors associated with swelling onset such as cancer, injury, or infection; and family history of lymphedema.

IX. Vascular assessment

A thorough vascular assessment of the arterial, venous, and lymphatic system should be performed in each patient. Because lymphedema can develop secondary to, or concurrent with, venous disease, DVT should be ruled out and superficial and deep venous reflux assessed by a qualified phlebologist. As with any type of edema requiring compression therapy, an arterial assessment must be performed. The ankle-brachial index (ABI) is a noninvasive vascular screening test to identify large-vessel peripheral arterial disease by comparing the systolic blood pressures in the posterior tibial and dorsalis pedis arteries to the higher of the brachial systolic blood pressures, which is the best estimate of central systolic blood pressure.(25) ABI measurements with pocket Doppler and vascular laboratory equipment yield comparable results.(26) ABI results should be uniformly reported with noncompressible values defined as greater than 1.40, normal values 1.00 to 1.40, borderline 0.91 to 0.99, and abnormal 0.90 or less.(27)

X. Stemmer's sign

A positive Stemmer's sign is a simple clinical finding that yields a definitive diagnosis of lymphedema (Figure 7, Figure 8).(28) The Stemmer's test can be performed in less than 10 seconds. To perform the Stemmer's test, pinch and lift the skin on the dorsal aspect of the base of the second toe or finger. Normally, the skin in this area is thin and pliable, but as lymphedema develops, the skin thickens and becomes more fibrotic. If the skin cannot be pinched and lifted, the test yields a positive Stemmer's sign. The Stemmer's sign is never falsely positive and considered accurate to diagnose lymphedema of the extremities.(21) Conversely, when the skin at the base of the second toe or finger can be pinched and lifted, the Stemmer's sign is

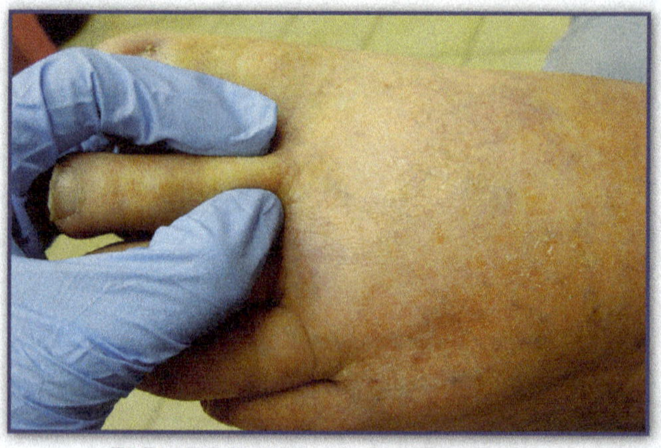

FIGURE 7. Positive Stemmer signs
Courtesy of Robyn Bjork, MPT, CWS, CLT-LANA, CLWT

negative (Figure 9, Figure 10). A negative Stemmer's sign may be falsely negative and does not exclude lymphedema.[21] The Stemmer's sign can also be performed at other locations, such as periwound tissues, to determine more focal areas of lymphedema.

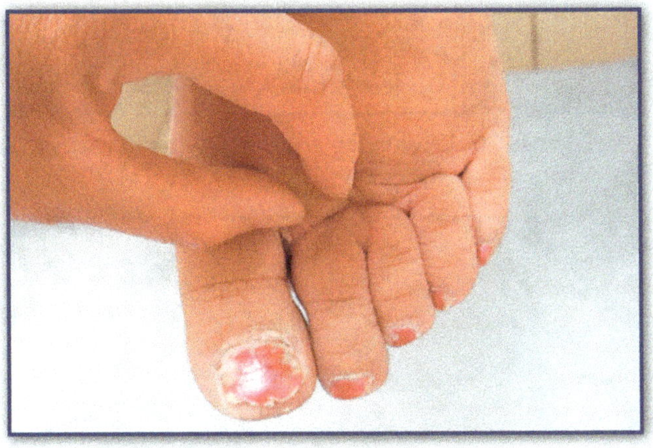

FIGURE 8. Positive Stemmer signs
Courtesy of Robyn Bjork, MPT, CWS, CLT-LANA, CLWT

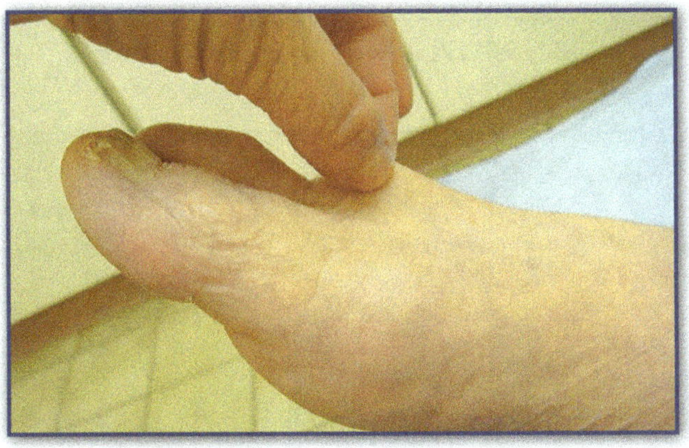

FIGURE 9. Negative Stemmer signs
Courtesy of Robyn Bjork, MPT, CWS, CLT-LANA, CLWT

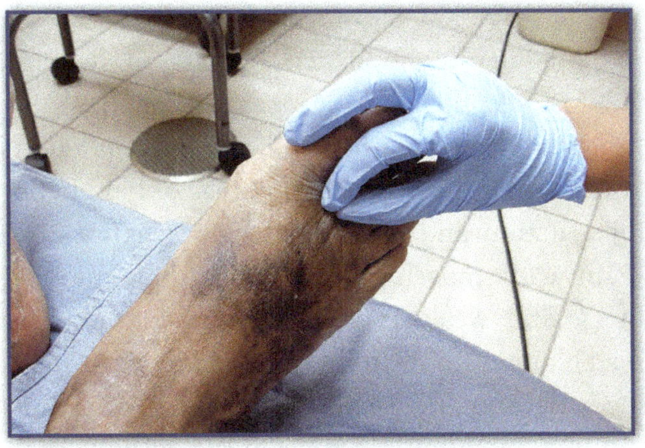

FIGURE 10. Negative Stemmer signs
Courtesy of Robyn Bjork, MPT, CWS, CLT-LANA, CLWT

XI. Clinical features

Other distinguishing clinical features of lymphedema are papillomatosis and hyperkeratosis.[22,29] Papillomatosis presents as lumpy, bumpy, cobblestone-appearing skin or fibrotic wartlike projections (Figure 11, Figure 12, Figure 13). Hyperkeratosis is scaly, brown or grey patches of overproliferated keratin layers (Figure 14, Figure 15, Figure 16, Figure 17). Lymphedema of the extremities is usually asymmetrical, with a distal to proximal progression, and can present with deep creases and folds, fibrotic tissue, loss of limb contours, and square or sausage-shaped toes (Figure 18). The onset of nonmalignant

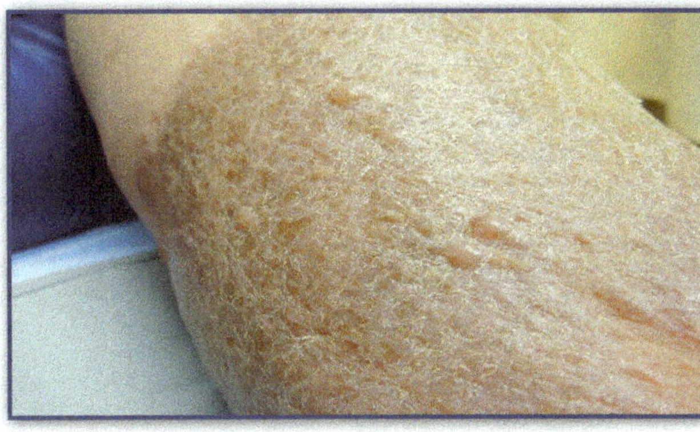

FIGURE 11. Typical papillomatosis
Courtesy of Robyn Bjork, MPT, CWS, CLT-LANA, CLWT

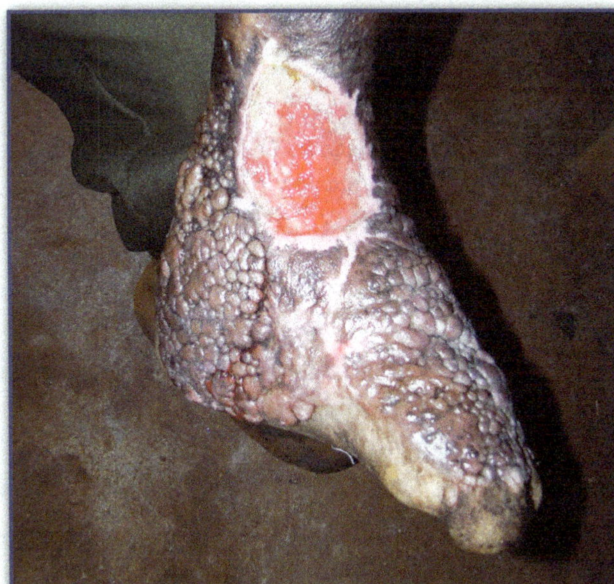

FIGURE 12. Significant foot papillomatosis
Courtesy of Robyn Bjork, MPT, CWS, CLT-LANA, CLWT

lymphedema is slow, developing and worsening over many years, if untreated (Figure 19). It is typically not painful, although lymphorrhea with skin denudement can lead to painful partial-thickness wounds, and the patient may suffer from painful, recurrent bouts of cellulitis.

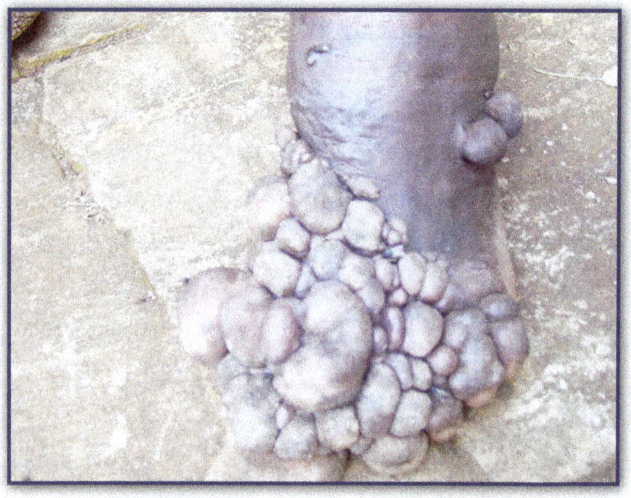

FIGURE 13. Severe papillomatosis
Courtesy of Robyn Bjork, MPT, CWS, CLT-LANA, CLWT

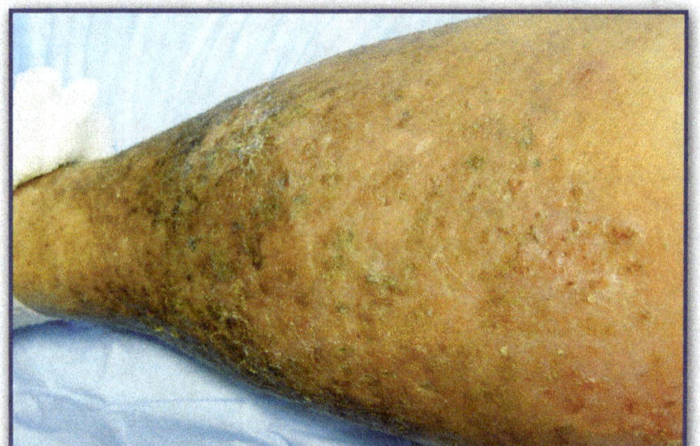

FIGURE 14. Hyperkeratosis and hemosiderin staining
Courtesy of Robyn Bjork, MPT, CWS, CLT-LANA, CLWT

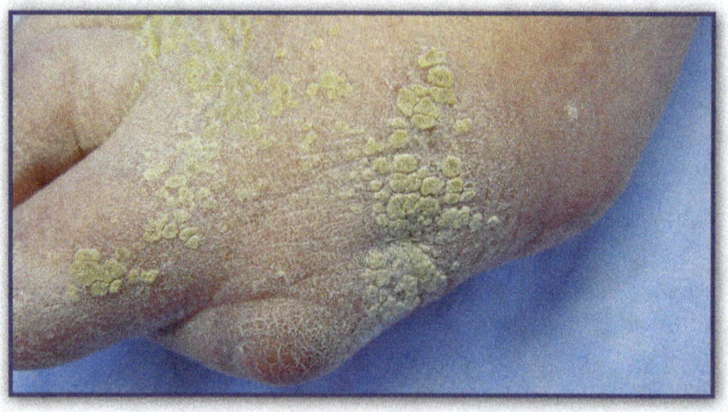

FIGURE 15. Foot hyperkeratosis
Courtesy of Robyn Bjork, MPT, CWS, CLT-LANA, CLWT

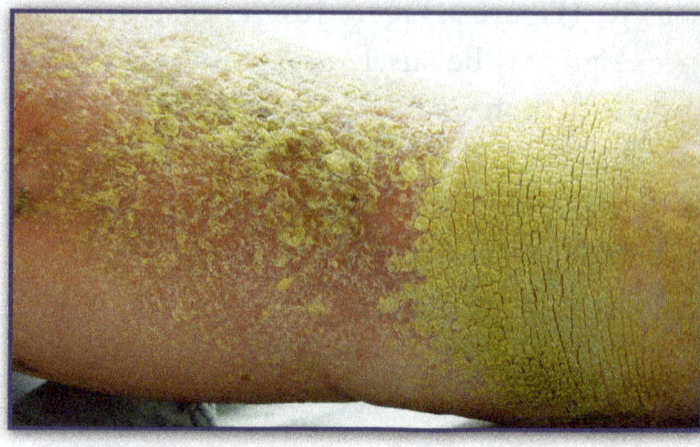

FIGURE 16. Lower leg and heel hyperkeratosis
Courtesy of Robyn Bjork, MPT, CWS, CLT-LANA, CLWT

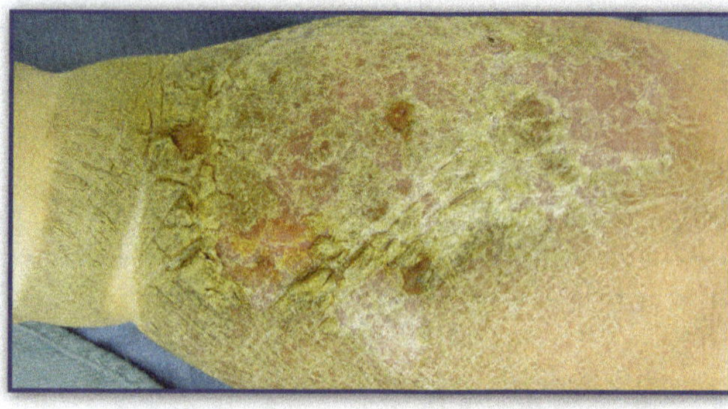

FIGURE 17. Lower leg hyperkeratosis
Courtesy of Robyn Bjork, MPT, CWS, CLT-LANA, CLWT

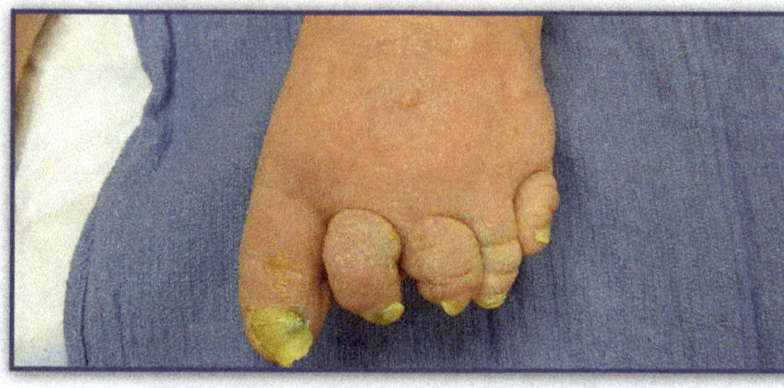

FIGURE 18. Sausage-shaped toes
Courtesy of Robyn Bjork, MPT, CWS, CLT-LANA, CLWT

Malignant lymphedema refers to lymphedema secondary to cancer. In contrast to nonmalignant lymphedema, the onset is rapid and may start proximally in areas of lymphatic obstruction and progress distally (Figure 20). Pain with muscle guarding, tingling, numbness, and weakness may be present. Masses or enlarged nodes may be palpable. Skin may become inflamed and distended. Fungating tumors, radiation ulcers or burns, or angiosarcomas may also develop.

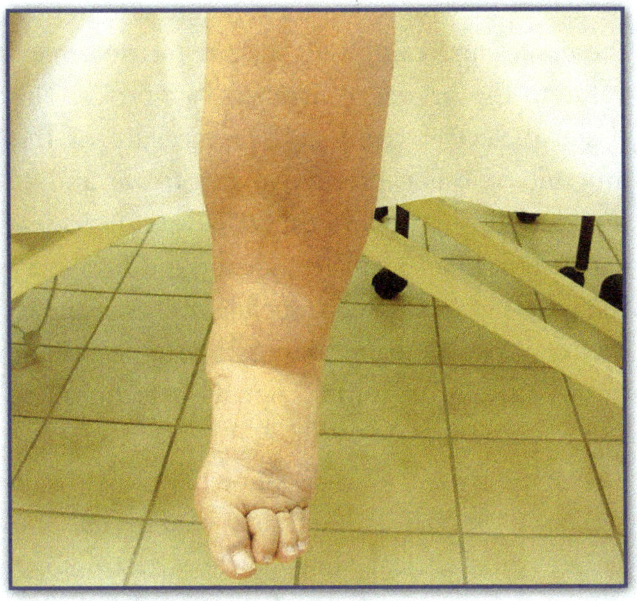

FIGURE 19. Benign lymphedema
Courtesy of Robyn Bjork, MPT, CWS, CLT-LANA, CLWT

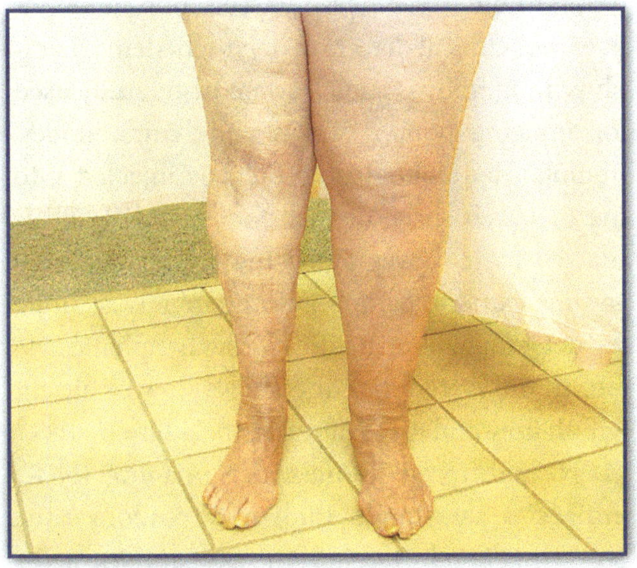

FIGURE 20. Malignant lymphedema
Courtesy of Robyn Bjork, MPT, CWS, CLT-LANA, CLWT

XII. Lipedema

Lipedema is a painful fat syndrome that can progress to lipolymphedema, a combination of lipedema and lymphedema. It can also present with concurrent CVI, in part due to poor connective tissue support for the vasculature and fragility of vascular walls. The combination of lipedema, CVI, and lymphedema is called lipophlebolymphedema (Figure 21). It is a chronic disease of unknown origin, although a genetic cause is suspected and family history likely, resulting in abnormal fat metabolism and accumulation of subcutaneous fatty tissue. The syndrome primarily affects females, with an onset usually during puberty, pregnancy, or menopause. Distinguishing characteristics are bilateral, symmetrical accumulation of fatty tissue from the waist to the ankle, resulting in large hips and thighs with disproportionately small trunk and arms. The feet are spared, and the Stemmer's sign is negative, unless there is concurrent lymphedema present. These patients have hypermobile joints, painful tissues, lipomas, and hypersensitivity to touch. The skin is less elastic and bruises easily because of the fragility of vascular walls. Thirty percent-90% of people with lipedema are also affected in their arms, with hanging fat lobes from the upper arms. Fatty cuffs, or inverted fatty "shelves," may be present at the wrist and ankles. Lipedema is not the same as simple obesity and persists despite diet and exercise. Related diseases are Dercum's disease, Madelung's disease or multiple symmetric lipomatosis, and familial multiple lipomatosis.[30]

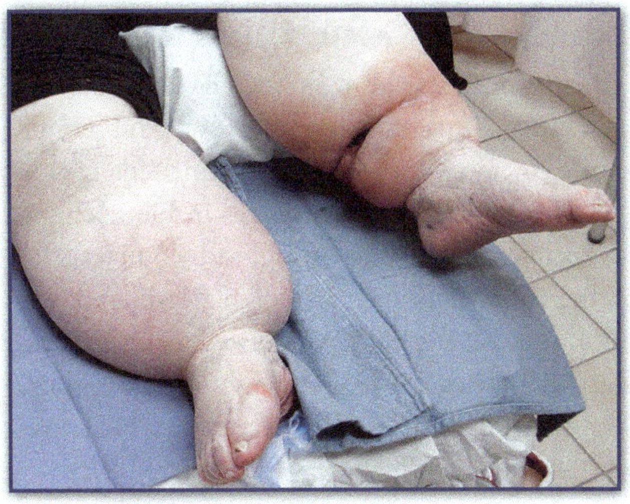

FIGURE 21. Lipophlebolymphedema with cellulitis and tunneling wound
Note relative sparing of the feet.
Courtesy of Robyn Bjork, MPT, CWS, CLT-LANA, CLWT

Relevance to case study

The patient presents with the characteristics of lipedema, including excess deposition of loose, lobular fatty tissue, with large hips and thighs, inverted fatty shelf at the ankle, and spared feet (Figure 1). Stemmer's sign is negative at the base of the second toe but does not exclude lymphedema, and a positive Stemmer's sign is evident in the tissue of the medial knees, confirming secondary lymphedema. The skin at the apex of the lymphedematous lobes of the medial knees is cobblestone in appearance, evident of papillomatosis, which is a unique characteristic of lymphedema. Hemosiderin staining of the gaiter area bilaterally is evidence of underlying, concurrent venous disease. The patient should receive routine testing that includes an ABI study, venous duplex ultrasound to rule out DVT, and a venous insufficiency study. She would not be a candidate at this time for corrective venous surgical procedures due to the Stage 3, uncontrolled lymphedema, high risk of secondary postsurgical infections and cellulitis, and high risk of exacerbation of lymphedema secondary to surgery.

XIII. Volumetric measurements and diagnostic tests

Diagnostic tests for lymphedema may include soft tissue imaging, lymph vessel and lymph node imaging, measures of volume, changes in electrical conductance, changes in biomechanical properties, genetic testing, and blood tests for other conditions that can look like lymphedema.[31] Limb volume can be calculated using circumferential measurements and a software program, water displacement, or perometry, which uses infrared light transmitters to detect the girth of a limb. Tissue texture can be quantified by estimating the percent of the limb that is hard and noncompressible, fibrotic, or soft and pliable. An indurometer or tonometer is a device that measures the amount of force required to indent the tissues and can give a specific measurement value to the degree of firmness or fibrosis. The tissue dielectric constant is a measure of the amount of water present in the tissue and is detected through a device that delivers an electrical current of a specific frequency and measures the reflected wave. Reproducible results of tissue dielectric constant and tonometry can be limited by technical difficulties, operator techniques, and environmental factors.[31]

MRI, CT, and US can show the presence of increased interstitial fluid but cannot tell the cause. Bioelectrical impedance spectroscopy (BIS) measures resistance (impedance) to small electrical currents. This is used to measure extracellular fluid differences between limbs and aids in earlier clinical detection of lymphedema. Lymphoscintigraphy is a nuclear medicine study used for imaging lymph vessels and lymph nodes. Radiolabeled colloid or protein is injected into the first web space of each foot or hand and is tracked as it moves along the lymphatics by a gamma camera. Lymphoscintigraphy is accurate for detecting abnormalities of the lymphatic system in the extremities and shows slow or absent lymph flow and areas of reflux (backflow).

Near-infrared fluorescence imaging (NIR) utilizes a substance known as indocyanine green that is injected into the skin and immediately imaged in real time using an infrared fluorescence camera. The dynamic function of the lymphatic vessels and dermal lymphatics can be visualized using this technique. For patients who have been diagnosed with primary lymphedema, genetic counseling and genetic testing may be appropriate.[31]

Relevance to case study

Although special diagnostic tests may be interesting, accessibility may be limited, and they are not needed to arrive at a definitive diagnosis of lymphedema. Further, special diagnostic tests will not change the treatment plan.

XIV. Role of surgery in lymphedema

Lymphedema is typically managed through complete decongestive therapy (CDT). CDT involves two phases: an initial reductive phase (Phase 1) followed by a maintenance phase (Phase 2). CDT is comprised of skin and nail care, manual lymph drainage (MLD), compression, therapeutic exercise, and patient education. CDT has been shown to be safe and effective, with numerous case studies demonstrating limb volume reductions of 50%–70% or more, improved appearance of the involved limb, reduced symptoms, fewer infections, and an improved quality of life.[(31)]

Surgery for lymphedema is not curative but may help manage severe cases. Surgical procedures to manage lymphedema have been around for over a century, with the Charles procedure being first reported in 1912[(32)] to manage scrotal lymphedema, which later became used on the lower extremities. This approach was named after Dr. Charles; however, he used the approach only for scrotal surgery. Subsequent physicians employed the techniques created by Dr. Charles (naming the procedure after him), which involved aggressive and extensive resection of all skin and soft tissue down to deep fascia to debulk the limb. This was followed by skin grafting, and typically resulted in significant disfigurement with limited success. Sistrunk in the 1920s and Thompson in the 1960s attempted to preserve lymphatic function through their surgical approaches; however, the results were often ineffective and disfiguring as well.[(33)]

Modern surgical approaches are much less invasive and involve microsurgical approaches to reduce lymphatic fluid or minimally invasive procedures to remove accumulated fatty and proteinaceous solids within the affected areas. It is important to note, however, that any surgical approach to treat lymphedema should be reserved for cases when traditional treatments have not been successful or when outcomes from CDT can no longer be maintained.[(34)] Further, even after surgery, patients should continue with compression and Phase 2 maintenance of CDT.[(31)] Current surgical options that are aimed to reduce fluid excess include vascularized lymph node transfer (VLNT), lymphaticovenous anastomosis (LVA), and lymphnodal-venous anastomosis (LNVA), or lymphaticolymphatic bypass. Suction-assisted protein lipectomy (SAPL) is a procedure to remove excess fatty and proteinaceous solids that have accumulated within the affected limb(s). A brief review of each procedure is outlined below.

A. VLNT

This procedure was first described in the literature in the early 1990s. VLNT is a microsurgical flap transfer of soft tissue containing lymphatic structures with its arteriovenous supply. Typically, the flap is taken from the lateral groin, chest wall, or neck and transferred to the affected limb, groin, or axilla.[(33)] Any obstructing scar tissue is released, and the vascular recirculation is reestablished in the transferred flap. Reduction in lymphatic swelling has been noted immediately after surgery in some instances. The main complication, although unlikely, is donor-site morbidity.

B. LVA and LNVA

Initially described in the 1970s, LVA involves the connection of multiple lymphatic vessels with small adjacent venules in an effort to decrease swelling.[(33)] This enables the excess lymph fluid to bypass areas of obstructed or low flow and drain directly into the venous system. LVA is considered a supermicrosurgical procedure as most lymphatic collectors range from 0.1 to 0.6 mm in diameter.[18] LNVA involves surgically attaching lymph nodes to veins to create a bypass from the lymphatic tissue to the venous tissue directly. The most likely reason that these techniques fail is that lymphatic pressure levels are lower than the venous pressure levels; therefore, the emptying capacity of the lymphatics is not strong enough to overcome the venous pressure.

C. Lymphaticolymphatic bypass

Baumeister et al.[35] first described this technique, which involves transferring healthy, functioning lymphatic vessels, usually from the inner thigh, and attaching the lymphatic vessels of the donor site directly to the lymphatic vessels of the affected extremity.[33] Improvements in volume reductions were noted to be more in the upper extremities compared to the lower extremities.

D. SAPL

This procedure is performed after a patient has received CDT to aspirate the fatty and proteinaceous solids using power-assisted liposuction cannulas that cannot be removed with traditional interventions. Suction-assisted protein lipectomy is a radically different form of liposuction and very different from techniques used in cosmetic surgery. It is imperative this technique is performed only by highly trained and experienced surgeons. When the procedure is properly performed, SAPL has been shown to be safe. Currently, there are no reported cases of patients whose lymphatics were further damaged after the procedure.[33] Although the procedure is effective at removing excess volume, it does not address the pathophysiology causing lymphedema. Therefore, the incorporation of individualized lymphedema therapy and compression use following SAPL surgery is critical in achieving and maintaining a good result. Granzow et al. have indicated that after SAPL surgery, there is an average volume reduction of 111% in the arms and 86% in the legs. Further, it has been reported that SAPL may reduce the risk of cellulitis by as much as 80%.[36] The procedure is recommended only for patients who are able to maintain long-term compression therapy after the procedure.

Although improvements in surgical procedures to treat lymphedema have been made, it is essential these procedures are performed only on carefully screened patients and that surgery does not replace complete decongestive therapy. Even after surgery, lymphedema precautions should be continued to reduce risk and ensure optimal outcomes.

XV. Interventions: complete decongestive therapy

Complete decongestive therapy (CDT) is considered the standard of care for lymphedema management. The focus of CDT is to achieve a reduction in limb volume and improve the quality and integrity of the skin. CDT is typically divided into two phases, an intensive phase and a maintenance phase. The intensive phase is best performed daily (or as frequently as possible) until maximal volume reduction is achieved. Once the lymphedematous limb has plateaued and is no longer achieving a reduction in volume, the patient is transitioned into the maintenance phase, which is continued for life. The components of CDT will be discussed in detail below.

Throughout both phases of CDT, patient education is paramount as self-care is critical for successful long-term outcomes.[37] Although there is no cure for lymphedema, it is a disease that can be successfully managed, improving function and quality of life.

CDT involves the following components which are guided by a trained lymphedema specialist during the intensive phase: 1) meticulous skin and nail care of the affected areas; 2) therapeutic exercises to promote lymphatic pumping; 3) approximately 60 minutes of manual lymph drainage (MLD), a gentle manual technique that helps redirect lymph flow; 4) multilayer, short-stretch compression bandaging; and 5) over-the-counter or custom compression garments once the limb has decongested. All aspects of CDT continue during the maintenance phase with a few modifications. The maintenance phase is also patient directed and is necessary for lifelong management of lymphedema.

During the maintenance phase, compression garments are worn during the day followed by short-stretch bandaging or the use of a proper compression system at night. Compression garments or systems can employ different closure mechanisms (such as Velcro), assisting the patient with donning and doffing and often improving adherence with use. During the maintenance phase, the utilization of intermittent pneumatic compression (IPC) may also be employed as an adjunctive device to help maintain fluid reduction. Of note, it is important to educate patients about the importance of diaphragmatic breathing which should become a regular part of the patient management regimen. Diaphragmatic breathing stimulates the thoracic duct (the largest lymph vessel in the body) as this structure pierces the diaphragm. This aids in a siphoning effect to promote fluid mobilization and edema reduction.

A. Skin and nail care

Educating patients about proper skin and nail care is essential, as patients with lymphedema are highly susceptible to infection. The protein-rich fluid is an ideal medium for bacteria and other pathogens to flourish. Skin changes associated with lymphedema often result in dry, scaly skin that can present with cracks and fissures. In some instances, the fluid burden is so high, the edema weeps through the skin, leading to denudement, fungal growth, and various forms of moisture-associated skin damage. Patients should learn and demonstrate proper cleansing and moisturizing techniques to reduce the incidence of infection and maintain skin integrity. Ointments, as well as soaps or other skin cleansers used in lymphedema management, should have good moisturizing qualities, contain no fragrances, be hypoallergenic, and be in either the neutral or acidic range of the pH scale (around pH 5).[38]

It is important to note that patients presenting with concomitant integumentary dysfunction require appropriate wound management interventions. Any comorbid conditions or diseases contributing to the development of the wound(s) should be addressed and medically managed. All aspects of CDT can be rendered, as long as the wound(s) and/or integumentary impairments are addressed according to standards of care. Typically, this can be a subset of the skin and nail care aspect of CDT. MLD can be performed around any lesions to help decongest and rid the wounds of lymph stasis, promoting closure. Appropriate dressing selection following the principles of wound bed preparation and moist wound healing should occur prior to the application of compression.

Relevance to case study

This patient requires diligent skin and wound care. The cellulitis should be managed with proper systemic and topical antibiotics. Her legs should be properly cleaned with a mild soap or cleanser, with special attention to carefully dry beneath the tissue folds. A skin fold management system could be employed to keep the folds clean and dry, and/or a fungal powder could be used if yeast or fungal infections are present in the folds. A neutral moisturizing agent should be applied to her skin prior to compression. The denuded skin areas would benefit from dressings that protect the areas, wick fluid away from the wounds, and function under compression. Nonstick foam dressing would be a good example. As she begins to reduce in volume through CDT, the wounds should spontaneously resolve, as should the hyperkeratosis.

B. Therapeutic exercise

Exercise is an important component of CDT. Exercise can stimulate the lymphatic system increasing the transport of lymph fluid and proteins. In addition, muscle activity and diaphragmatic breathing facilitate venous return, which positively affects fluid balance in the interstitial spaces. For patients with lymphedema, it is imperative that all exercise is performed while wearing compression to provide additional support to the lymphatic and venous systems. Compression facilitates lymphatic and venous return and provides a counterbalance to the development of additional lymphatic loads, which is a byproduct of exercise and increased circulation.

Although there is no consensus for a particular type of exercise regimen for patients with lymphedema, research does support a program of progressive exercises (i.e., starting with gentle exercises and increasing intensity moderately over time) tailored to each patient's needs and abilities.[39-40] An exercise regimen should involve a combination of stretching and flexibility, strength training, aerobic exercise, and diaphragmatic breathing (deep breathing or belly breathing). To maximize adherence, exercises and activities should be selected that the patient enjoys. An exercise regimen should be designed while being mindful of the patient's abilities as well as any concomitant health conditions or comorbidities.

Relevance to case study

Given the pain and functional limitations of this patient, a basic exercise regimen of toe curls, ankle pumps, and gentle heel slides would suffice to assist the calf muscle pump and stimulate lymphangiomotoricity without exacerbating her pain. Isometric contractions of her upper leg musculature and diaphragmatic breathing would also be beneficial. Ideally, the patient should perform these exercises five to ten times several times a day while wearing compression. Additional activities can be added depending upon her pain status and functional improvements. Simple, basic exercises are best to ensure adherence.

C. Manual lymphatic drainage therapy

The lymphatic system starts at the blood capillary level and parallels the venous system back to the heart. It is a slow-moving system, and lymph is propelled by rhythmic, smooth-muscle contractions of lymphangions, coupled with one-way valves. Flow progresses from the lymphatic capillaries in the dermis to precollectors residing in subcutaneous tissue to collectors running above the fascia, parallel to veins. Normally, lymph from the skin flows towards the nearest regional lymph nodes and, after being filtered through nodes, flows into lymphatic trunks that converge into ducts. The two largest ducts in the body, the thoracic duct and right lymphatic duct, dump the lymph back into the bloodstream at the venous angle in the neck where the internal jugular and the subclavian veins conjoin. From there, the lymph flows through the heart and is filtered through the kidneys, and excess fluid and waste is excreted from the body.

In the presence of lymphedema, normal flow patterns are compromised due to obstructions or congestion in the lymphatic system.

Manual lymphatic drainage therapy (MLDT) is an important component of CDT and is delivered by certified lymphedema therapists. The treatment begins with an assessment of the etiology of lymphedema and identification of congested pathways. Barriers to lymph flow are identified, and alternate pathways are mapped to help direct the overall treatment strategy. Specialized manual techniques are then aimed at specific lymphatic structures to facilitate flow and reroute lymph away from congested areas. A number of different manual techniques exist for MLDT. However, there is little evidence to demonstrate which is the most effective and for what clinical indications.[22]

Terminus

The superficial, epifascial lymph vascular system drains lymph from the dermis and hypodermis while the deep, subfascial lymph vascular system drains muscles, tendon sheaths, joints, and nerves.[21] Seventy percent of all lymph flow is generated from the superficial lymph vascular system.[19] MLDT starts at the end point of the lymphatic vasculature at the venous angles, also known as the "terminus." Hand techniques initially target the terminus and then progress to the lymphatic trunks, which propel lymph toward the venous angles.

Thoracic duct

The thoracic duct is the largest lymphatic trunk in the body and is 2–5 mm wide and 36–45 cm in length. It originates with the cisterna chyli, coursing proximally along the anterior spine, and perforates the diaphragm, along with the aorta at the aortic hiatus, en route to the left venous angle. The thoracic duct drains lymph from both legs, the lower quadrants of thorax, L head, neck and L upper extremity, equating to 75% of the body. Between 1.5 and 3 liters of lymph per day circulate through the thoracic duct; however, 40% of the liquid volume of lymph entering a lymph node is recirculated directly into the venous system through the node's veins, before it reaches the thoracic duct.[19] Thus, under normal physiologic conditions, up to 4.2 liters of lymph per day flows through pathways en route to the thoracic duct alone. Deep diaphragmatic breathing helps "milk" the thoracic duct, and increased negative pressure during inhalation pulls lymph from the thoracic duct into the bloodstream, facilitating a central vacuum effect in the lymphatic system.[21]

Lymph nodes

Lymph is filtered through at least two lymph nodes before it enters a lymphatic trunk. Lymph enters the node through multiple afferent vessels and exits via one to two efferent vessels, acting like a dam slowing down lymph for filtration. Macrophages in the node digest foreign material, and lymphocytes detect and fight bacteria by mounting a cell-mediated or humoral immune response. Thus, impairments in the flow of lymph toward regional lymph nodes can compromise the body's ability to recognize and respond to bacteria in the skin or a chronic wound. The major regional lymph node groups are located in the neck, axillae, abdomen, and inguinal areas. In MLDT, superficial and deep abdominal lymph nodes and regional lymph nodes are manually "pumped" to stimulate them and facilitate lymph drainage.

Collectors

Lymphatic collectors are transport vessels that "collect" lymph from the skin and hypodermis and propel it toward regional lymph nodes. Collectors are made up of bulbular, contractile units called lymphangions, meaning "little hearts," with 1-way bicuspid valves that prevent reflux of lymph. Because of the lymphangions, collectors look like a string of pearls. Lymph is propelled by rhythmic, peristaltic, smooth-muscle contractions of lymphangions. The lymphangion wall is smooth muscle, innervated by the sympathetic nervous system, that responds to stretch and lymph flow to increase its contraction rate. At rest, the contraction rate is five to eight times per minute.[19] When stimulated, such as through MLDT, the action of these tiny muscles can increase the flow through the lymphatic system by some 20–30 times.[19] Improved lymphatic contractile function after MLDT can be visualized using near-infrared fluorescence imaging.[41]

Lymphotomes, watersheds, and interterritorial anastomoses

Lymph from the skin naturally drains toward the nearest regional lymph nodes. Lymph draining from an area of skin, flowing in one general direction toward a group of regional lymph nodes, is called a "lymphotome" or "lymphatic territory." Watersheds are imaginary lines separating lymphotomes. In the watershed, lymph can flow in either direction because the collectors in this zone have valves on either side, which open in opposite directions.[42] Thus, MLDT can gently assist lymph across free-flowing capillary networks from 1 lymphotome to another, crossing the watersheds, in order to find alternate pathways through collectors to regional lymph nodes.

Within a lymphotome, there are very free anastomoses of collectors, called intraterritorial anastomoses, creating many drainage pathways from lymphotomes en route toward their corresponding nearest regional lymph nodes. In contrast, interterritorial anastomoses connect collectors between lymphotomes. Similar to a highway cloverleaf, congestion in regional lymph nodes causes back pressure in the system that opens valves in the interterritorial anastomoses and redirects lymph to a contralateral or ipsilateral, uncongested set of regional lymph nodes.

The most prominent interterritorial anastomoses used in MLDT are the anterior axillo-axillary (AAA) anastomosis, which creates a connection across the anterior chest between bilateral axillary regional lymph node groups; posterior axillo-axillary (PAA) anastomosis, which creates a connection across the back between bilateral axillary regional lymph node groups; right and left axillo-inguinal (AI) anastomoses, which create a connection between the axillary and inguinal lymph nodes of the right or left sides of the body; anterior inter-inguinal (AII) anastomosis, which crosses the pubic mound and creates a connection between bilateral inguinal regional lymph node groups; and the posterior inter-inguinal (PII) anastomosis, which crosses the sacrum and creates a connection between bilateral inguinal regional lymph node groups.

MLDT takes advantage of these alternate pathways by focusing on hand techniques to stimulate lymphatic structures in uncongested areas. This creates a siphoning effect that draws lymph away from the congested area, creating an alternate pathway for excess fluid in the interstitium to enter the lymphatic system. Draining a neighboring, unaffected area may increase the drainage of the affected area by 25%.[19]

Congestion zones

Congestion zones are not defined in previous literature. Congestion zones are defined as common areas of focal lymphatic congestion, often corresponding to the convergence of collectors, lymphatic bundles, or dependent areas of soft tissue where lymph tends to pool. Common congestion zones include the dorsum of the hands and feet, the medial aspect of the knees and elbows where collectors converge to cross the joints, the posterior-medial, fleshy aspect of the upper thighs and arms, and the posterior ankle on either side of the Achilles tendon. Other congestion zones include the anterior and posterior deltoid, the lateral hips in the areas of the greater trochanters, and the small of the low back. Targeting congestion zones as part of MLDT helps relieve congestion and soften fibrosis in these bottlenecked areas and is postulated to help speed up the treatment process.

Lymphatic capillaries and pre-collectors (initial lymphatics)

Within the superficial lymph vascular system, lymphatic capillaries form a dense, spider web–like network throughout the dermis, less than 3 mm from the surface of the skin. Lymphatic capillaries start at the arteriovenous capillary level as open-end, fingerlike projections. There are no valves in the dermal capillaries, which enables lymph to flow in any direction. There are three layers of lymphatic capillaries in the dermis that are interconnected to form a plexus. The superficial dermal plexus is at the border of the papillary and reticular dermis, the deep dermal plexus throughout the reticular dermis, and intermediate in between.[(42)] This dense network of lymphatic capillaries is also referred to as the initial lymphatics.

Pre-collector lymph vessels facilitate lymph flow from the lymphatic capillaries in the dermis to the superficial collectors, located below the hypodermis but above the fascia. They course through the subcutaneous fatty layer of the skin, or hypodermis, at an oblique angle. The pre-collectors have funnel-style valves that allow dermal backflow. Some pre-collectors have structural features like that of capillaries, and, because of the lymph absorption capabilities, some texts considered pre-collectors as part of the initial lymphatics. Some pre-collectors perforate the fascia and connect the superficial and deep lymphatic systems, acting as a release valve for edema of structures below the fascia.

Under normal conditions, lymph from the dermal capillary plexus tends to flow like a sink drain, perpendicular to the skin, into a pre-collector that drains an area 1.5 cm in diameter on the palms and soles of the feet and 3–4 cm elsewhere on the body.[(21)] However, in the presence of lymphedema, normal flow patterns are disrupted by back pressure in the system. Fortunately, the dense, valveless, and free-flowing capillary networks cover the entire body, allowing for virtually unlimited options for MLDT to move lymph in any direction. For example, lymph from the leg can be rerouted toward the axillary lymph nodes, after central decongestion has primed the system and helped create streaming through that alternate pathway.

The lymphatic capillary wall is a single layer of endothelial cells, with overlapping inner and outer flaps called "swinging tips." The openings between the cells can be as much as four to six times larger than in the arterial capillary wall, enabling large proteins and immune cells to enter the lymphatic capillary lumen, which is also larger.[(19)] Outer swinging tips anchor to elastic fibers of the skin via anchoring filaments; anchoring filaments also attach to the capillary wall. As edema increases in the tissues, the elastic fibers stretch and pull on the anchoring filaments, lifting the swinging tips and opening the lymph capillary lumen. At that moment, the lower fluid pressure in the opened lymphatic capillaries facilitates drainage of interstitial fluid into it.[(21)] As lymph fills the capillary, the inner flap closes to prevent reflux back into the interstitium.

MLDT techniques used to stimulate patent lymphatic capillaries are very light. The ideal hand pressure is 1–2 oz/cm^2 or 4–8 oz/in^2, or the weight of a nickel.[(19)] Superficial, directional stretches of the skin pull the anchoring filaments that, in turn, lift lymph capillary endothelial swinging tips and open the lymph capillary lumen. Dormant lymph capillaries and redundant pathways can be activated in patent areas using MLDT.

MLDT has been shown to have powerful pain-relieving effects in patients with breast cancer.[43] MLDT may help purge toxins from the body, boost the immune system, facilitate drainage of swelling secondary to injury or surgery, facilitate resolution of bruises, and help heal recalcitrant wounds. Some general contraindications include acute, untreated cellulitis, uncompensated congested heart failure (CHF), unstable kidney function, untreated cancer, acute DVT, and ascites.[18,22] Above all, using sound clinical judgment is most prudent.

MLDT results can often be felt during 1 treatment session. There is palpable softening of the tissues and "deflation" of the skin with appearance of wrinkles during the treatment. Figures 22 and 23 demonstrate dramatic soft-tissue changes after two days of CDT. Often, this visual effect can be seen in the extremities after central decongestion alone, even before the extremity itself is treated directly. Facilitated lymph flow can sometimes be felt as warmth. As flow is stimulated through the lymphatic system, and the protein load is circulated back into the bloodstream, increased filtration by the kidneys results in the patient's urgency to urinate by the end of the session, with increased output for several days thereafter. In combination with compression, significant reduction in limb volume is realized, but equally important, the texture of the skin and subcutaneous tissues gradually soften and become more pliable, and the chronic pathohistological state of chronic inflammation is normalized.

Relevance to case study

For this patient, one of the main focuses of MLDT should be to teach her how to perform a self-MLDT program on a regular basis, in conjunction with therapeutic exercises. During the very first session, the patient can be taught deep, diaphragmatic breathing to help empty the thoracic duct, which drains lymph from both legs through the inguinal regional lymph nodes. This should be monitored and corrective instruction provided throughout every subsequent treatment session. By the third treatment session, the patient should be taught self-MLDT that includes central decongestion of the trunk and facilitation of rerouting flow from the legs toward the regional lymph nodes in bilateral axillae. The certified lymphedema therapist (CLT) can provide both treatment and instruction at the same

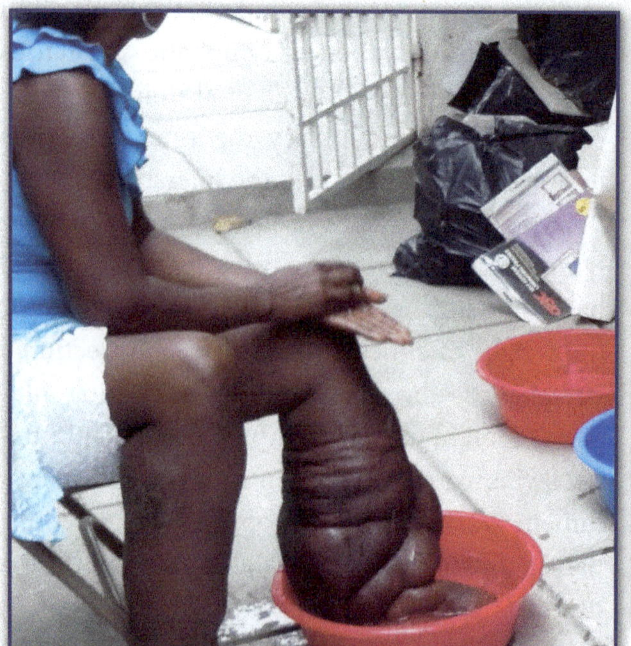

FIGURE 22. Before complete decongestive therapy
Courtesy of Robyn Bjork, MPT, CWS, CLT-LANA, CLWT

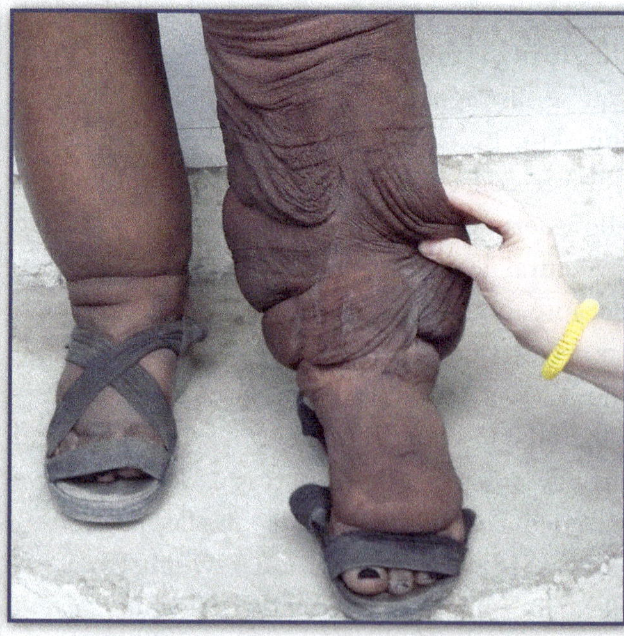

FIGURE 23. After two days of complete decongestive therapy
Courtesy of Robyn Bjork, MPT, CWS, CLT-LANA, CLWT

time. By quickly transitioning the patient to self-MLDT of the trunk, the CLT can focus on the most dysfunctional areas around the medial knees. MLDT will be utilized to soften the fibrotic changes through fibrosis techniques aimed at the hypodermis of this congestion zone. Lymph flow will also be rerouted, via the dermal lymphatics, from the medial knees to the lateral hips and then proximally, crossing watersheds along the lateral trunk, into collectors flowing toward the axillary regional lymph nodes. In order to be effective, MLDT must be combined with CDT, including multi-layered lymphedema bandaging.

D. Multilayered lymphedema bandaging (MLLB)

Multi-layered lymphedema bandaging (MLLB) is composed of multiple layers of short-stretch bandages, along with hygienic lining and padding materials, to create graduated compression with high containment (Figure 24). MLLB can be continually adjusted for limb volume reduction through frequent reapplication in the first few weeks of intensive CDT treatment. The bandages are worn 24 hours a day and are only removed for showering and hygienic care and then immediately reapplied. These bandaging systems are highly customized in the treatment of lymphedema, essential to CDT, and require specialized skills.

Before applying MLLB, peripheral blood flow should be assessed and an ABI conducted. Other factors to consider are the patient's protective sensation, skin tenderness, balance, footwear, cognition and judgment, incontinence, and patient adherence. Contraindications include acute, untreated conditions such as acute cellulitis, CHF, myocardial infarction (MI), DVT, cancer, and unstable kidney function. However, bandaging may be indicated to manage or reduce edema associated with these conditions after appropriate medical management has been initiated, and the physician clears the patient for compression therapy.

A common misconception is that compression therapy cannot be used in the presence of peripheral arterial disease (PAD). Compression is contraindicated in the presence of severe PAD with an ABI of less than 0.5 or an absolute ankle systolic pressure of less than 60 mmHg. However, Mosti et al. demonstrated that inelastic bandages are highly efficient in improving venous pumping function, increasing the reduced ejection fraction in venous disease by 72% under compression bandaging with pressures of 21 to 30 mmHg and by 103% with pressures of 31 to 40 mmHg. They found that in patients with venous ulceration and concurrent underlying arterial disease who had an ankle-brachial pressure index >0.5 and an absolute ankle pressure of >60 mm Hg, inelastic compression of up to 40 mm Hg does not impede arterial perfusion but may lead to a normalization of the highly reduced venous pumping function.[44]

Short-stretch bandages have an elongation of 30%–60% of the original length and, in MLLB, are typically applied with 50% tension and 50% overlap. Layering systems are created using bandages of increasing width as they are applied

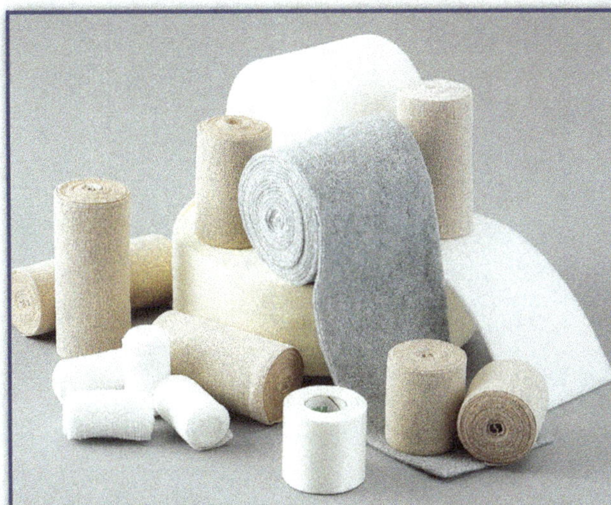

FIGURE 24. Bandaging supplies
Courtesy of Robyn Bjork, MPT, CWS, CLT-LANA, CLWT

distal to proximal on an extremity. Sub-bandage pressure can be altered using the principles of LaPlace's law. Increasing stretch/tension during application, applying more layers, and using bandages of smaller widths all increase the mmHg of applied pressure.

Short-stretch bandaging systems have high working pressure. The bandages resist muscle contraction and expansion, creating an inward force that pumps veins and lymphatics. Graduated short-stretch compression bandaging helps prevent regurgitation of fluid in the vessels and fluid displacement in the tissues, supports veins and lymphatic collectors, approximates weak, stretched-out valves, and improves calf muscle pump function.[45] Short-stretch bandages have low resting pressure, which is the bandage pressure exerted on a limb without muscle contractions. This makes short-stretch bandaging safer for patients with mild to moderate arterial disease.

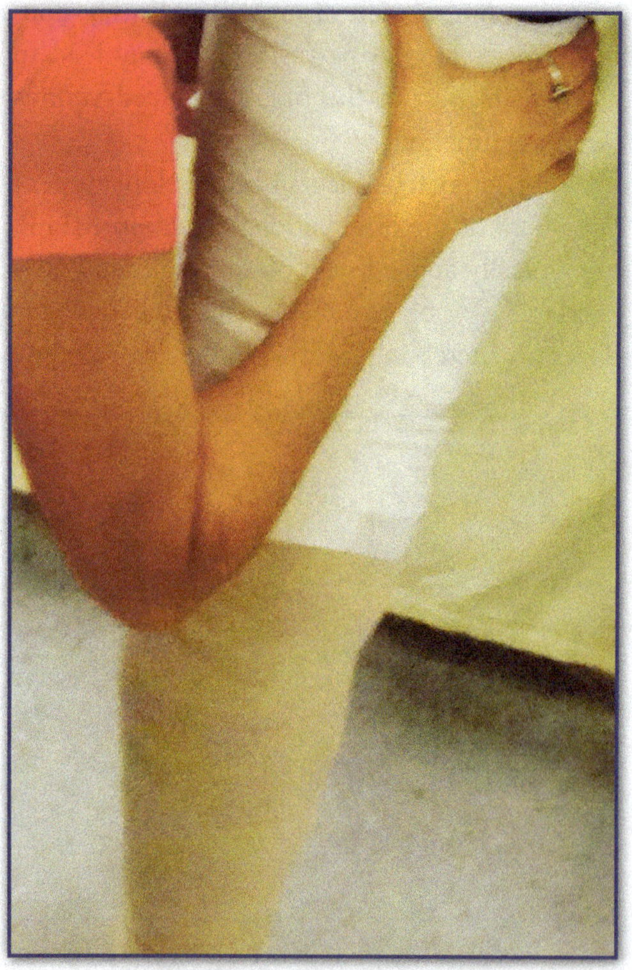

FIGURE 25. No-slip bandaging
Courtesy of Robyn Bjork, MPT, CWS, CLT-LANA, CLWT

Containment is the ability of compression to prevent expansion of edema. Recoil is the ability of the compression to accommodate or get smaller, as edema decreases. Short-stretch bandaging systems provide excellent containment. As lymphedema volume decreases with CDT, stretched-out skin lacks the elasticity needed to maintain the reduction; bandages provide an outside container to help maintain the reduction. The recoil of short-stretch bandages is limited by the two-way stretch within the weave of the cotton fibers. Unlike long-stretch bandages, they do not easily accommodate to large amounts of volume reduction. Consequently, the bandages must be frequently reapplied during the acute phase of treatment. Custom bags of foam with good rebound can be placed into the bandaging system to help soften fibrotic tissues as well as fill in spaces as the limb reduces to help keep the bandages in place. With a few adaptations, such as strategic placement of structural foam and grip layers, even thigh-high MLLB systems will securely stay in place. Pictured in Figure 25, a therapist is able to pull down firmly on the bandaging system with her body weight without slippage of the bandaging system.

Relevance to case study

One of the key problems with this patient was that compression was applied only below the knee. This contributed to the development of the lymphedematous lobes hanging from the medial aspects of her knees. Rather than Unna boots, MLLB can be used to treat the patient's lymphedema as well as heal her leg ulcers. At this point, applying MLLB will take a highly specialized skill set. Custom bags of foam pieces with exceptional rebound should be utilized to soften the fibrosis as well as help keep the system in place. The bandaging system will need to be separated into two sections, one from the toes to the knee, and a separate system to capture the knee, lobe, and thigh. Ten-meter-long, twelve-centimeter-wide bandages can be applied at an oblique angle to help lift the lobe and reposition it proximally, in order to redistribute weight and facilitate lymph drainage. A biker-short-style compression garment can be donned over the bandaging system to help hold it in place (Figure 26).

E. Compression garments

Although MLLB is essential in the early phase of lymphedema treatment, as the limb volume stabilizes, the patient needs to be transitioned into compression garments for lifelong management. Application of compression bandages on a long-term basis can be time consuming and exhausting for patients and caregivers. Lymphedema management requires compression therapy 24 hours per day. The development of a long-term compression therapy program and selection of appropriate compression garments is highly specialized and customized for each patient and requires close collaboration between the specialist, patient, and vendor.

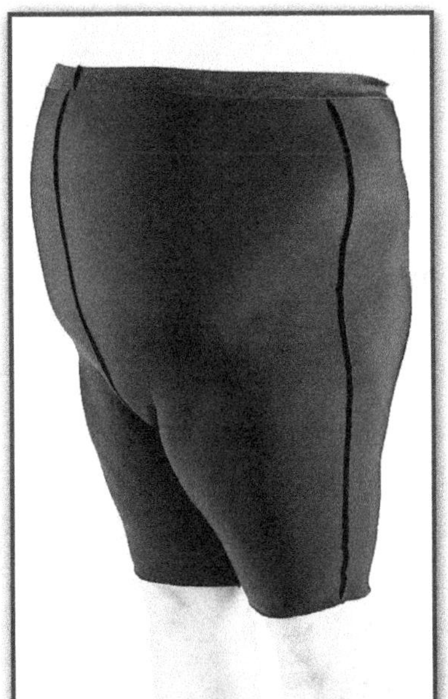

FIGURE 26. Biker short
Courtesy of Robyn Bjork, MPT, CWS, CLT-LANA, CLWT

A commitment to long-term compression should be discussed with the patient at the initial visit. Patient buy-in is necessary for successful outcomes. Poor adherence to appropriate compression can result in exacerbation of lymphedema and need for additional treatment. Recurrent cellulitis and hospitalizations may result from poorly managed lymphedema. CDT, including bandaging and compression garments, has been shown to reduce the average annual hospitalizations for cellulitis from 8.5 per year to 0.67 per year, a twelvefold reduction in hospitalization costs.[46] Unfortunately, many health-care plans still fail to provide adequate coverage for compression garments.

Considerations in choosing the appropriate long-term compression include assessment of the patient's cognition and judgment, range of motion, hand strength, adherence and commitment, potential assistance from family and friends, financial constraints, cosmetic preferences, incontinence issues, hygienic practices, climate, skin condition, level of containment needed, and location of lymphedema. Fortunately, there are many compression garment options that can meet various patient needs, with a wide variety of textile and color choices. Off-the-shelf standard sizes and custom-measured options are available. If needed, garments can be layered to achieve higher cumulative pressures. Compression garment options include knee-high, thigh-high, full or hemi pantyhose, biker shorts, capris, toe caps, gloves, gauntlets, arm sleeves, therapy bras, vests, and head and neck compression options. Pockets within garments can be utilized with inserts to manage focal lymphedema in the genitals, dorsum of the hand and foot, or breast and chest.

Garments used for lymphedema are less elastic than those used for watery forms of edema, due to the need for higher containment. They also tend to be thicker to provide the stiffness and ability to help shape the limb, hugging lobes and bridging gaps between lobes. Garments for lymphedema must have low fatigue, so as to maintain adequate compression throughout the course of the day and over the course of use. These properties are equally important to the actual mmHg of compression delivered by the garment.

Regarding the mmHg of compression delivered by a garment, classification systems vary. The U.S. classification system is Class 1: 20–30 mmHg, Class 2: 30–40 mmHg, Class 3: 40–50 mmHg, and Class 4: 50–60 mmHg designations. There are varying classification systems in Europe. The German RAL standard is Class 1: 18–21 mmHg, Class 2: 23–32 mmHg, Class 3: 34–46 mmHg, and Class 4: >49 mmHg.[22]

A circular-knit garment is knitted in a continuous circle to create a tube by a circular-knit machine. Circular-knit garments are seamless compression stockings, are lighter weight, are visually appealing, and come in a large variety of colors and textile options (Figure 27). They can be an excellent choice for day compression. However, it is important to consider the distribution of the compression pressures and the stiffness properties when choosing circular-knit garments for patients with lymphedema.

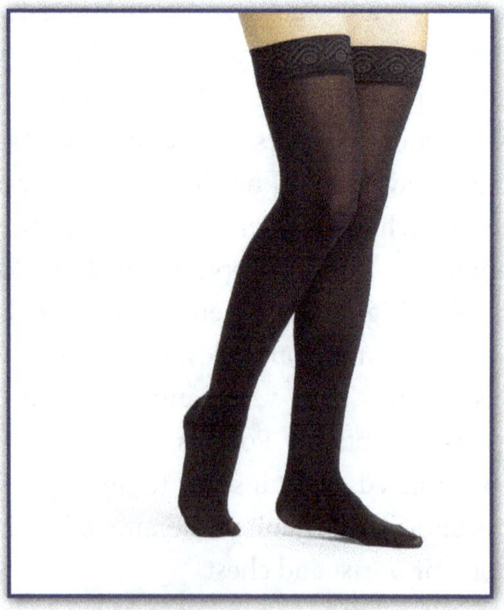

FIGURE 27. Circular knit
Courtesy of Robyn Bjork, MPT, CWS, CLT-LANA, CLWT

A flat-knit garment is knitted in a sheet by a flat-knit machine. It is knitted flat according to size, and then the edges are knitted together to create a seam. Seamless, 3-D knitting options are also available. Flat-knit garments are typically thicker, come in large variety of colors and textiles, provide excellent containment for day compression, and can be visually appealing (Figure 28 Flat Knit).

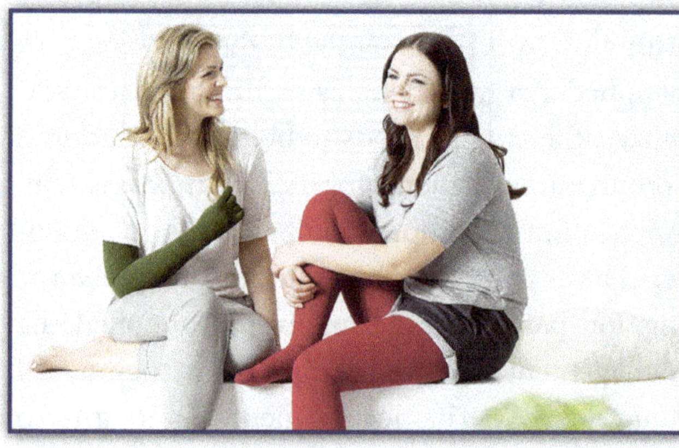

FIGURE 28. Flat knit
Courtesy of Circaid/Medi

Day compression, such as circular-knit or flat-knit garments, must be paired with a night garment to provide the 24-hour compression needed for the long-term management of lymphedema. Night garments are typically used for compression at night only, although they could also be worn during the day. Some night garments are constructed as foam-padded, pull-on sleeves that can be easily bandaged over using simple technique (Figure 29). Alternatively, a

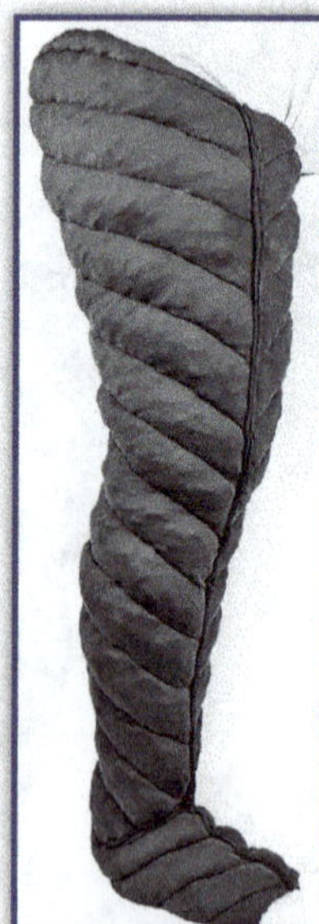

FIGURE 29. Pull-on leg sleeve
Courtesy of Robyn Bjork, MPT, CWS, CLT-LANA, CLWT

separate, thin elastic oversleeve can be donned over the night garment to add additional compression. Night garments may also be constructed as a padded garment, with hook and loop closures, that can be used in lieu of bandages (Figure 30).

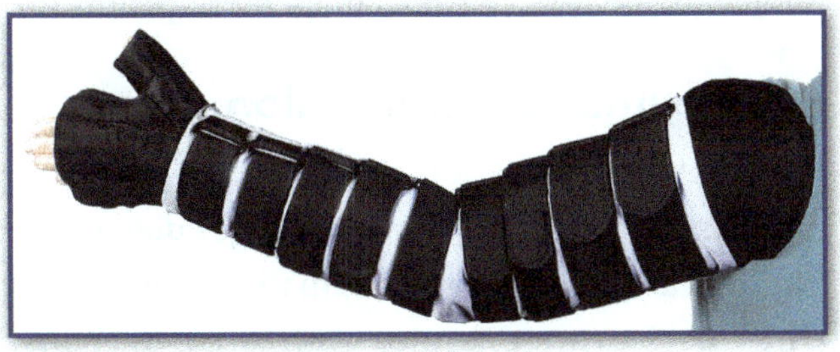

FIGURE 30. Arm sleeve with hook and loop closures
Courtesy of Robyn Bjork, MPT, CWS, CLT-LANA, CLWT

Inelastic, or short-stretch, wraps provide an alternate garment for compression that can be used both during the day and night (Figure 31). They are usually secured with hook and loop tabs and can be adjusted to accommodate for variations in lymphedema volume. Toe-caps and foot, leg, knee, and thigh wraps are available. They are easy to don and doff and provide high working pressure, with low resting pressure. Some wraps are constructed to allow for trimming or cutting to achieve a custom fit and resizing with lymphedema volume reductions. In some cases, inelastic wraps may be used in lieu of bandages for the acute phase of treatment.[47] (Figure 32 Circaid Reduction Kit)

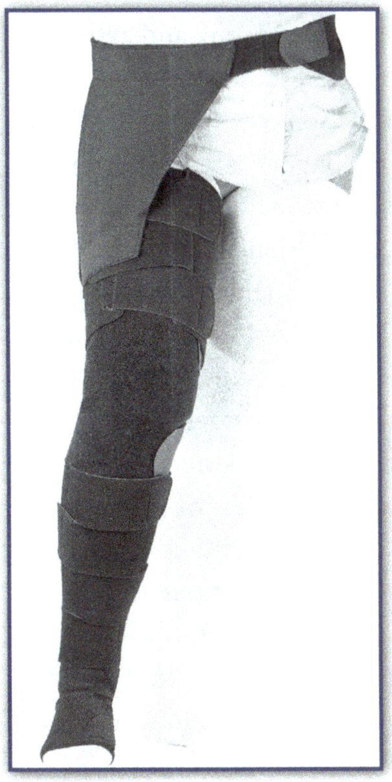

FIGURE 31. Alternate compression system
Courtesy of Robyn Bjork, MPT, CWS, CLT-LANA, CLWT

There are numerous aids that are indispensable in assisting patients and caregivers to don and doff garments. These include donning gloves, donning frames, gripper pads, fluid- or air-filled tubes, and aids made of parachute-type material. Patients should be thoroughly trained to don and doff their own compression garments. Validate this activity of daily living (ADL) skill through return demonstration, and monitor for effectiveness before discharging the patient. Day garments generally require replacement every six months, and using two sets, one to wash and one to wear, will extend wear time and improve adherence to a wearing schedule.

Relevance to case study

As soon as possible, the patient should be transitioned from multilayered lymphedema compression bandaging to compression garments. Because the patient has little swelling in her toes and feet, fairly uniform lower legs,

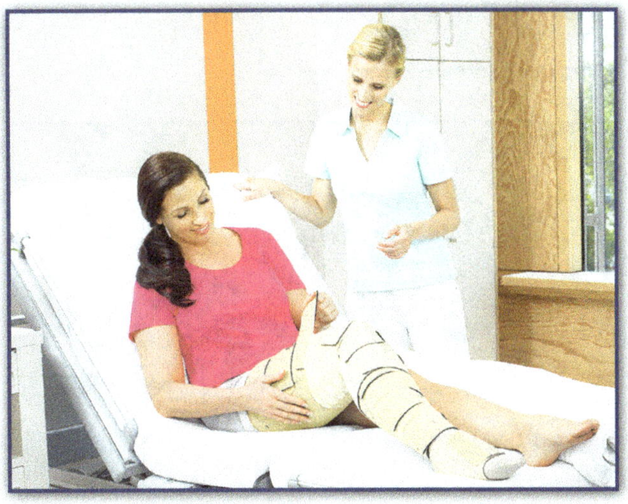

FIGURE 32. Circaid reduction kit
Courtesy of Circaid/Medi

inverted shelves at the ankles, limited mobility, and reduction of edema in the lower legs will plateau quickly, a short-stretch wrap would be a good choice for long-term management from the knee down (Figure 33). In contrast, the severe lymphedema at the knees will require custom bandaging for a longer period of time, perhaps two weeks of daily intensive treatment to achieve rapid volume reduction. However, as soon as it is feasible, the patient can transition into a custom compression garment with a lobule compression system (Figure 34). This will provide good containment, ease of use for the patient and spouse, and be able to accommodate to further volume reduction of the lobes; it should be used in conjunction with the lower leg wraps. By transitioning to compression wraps, more skilled clinic time can be utilized to focus on manually softening the fibrosis of the lobes, as well as the long-term management program.

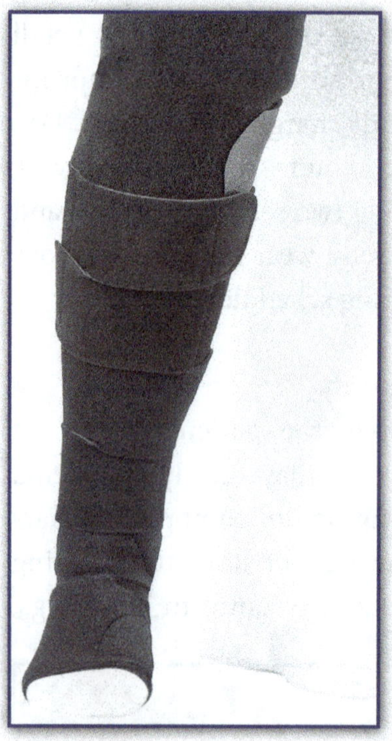

FIGURE 33. Lower leg compression
Courtesy of Robyn Bjork, MPT, CWS, CLT-LANA, CLWT

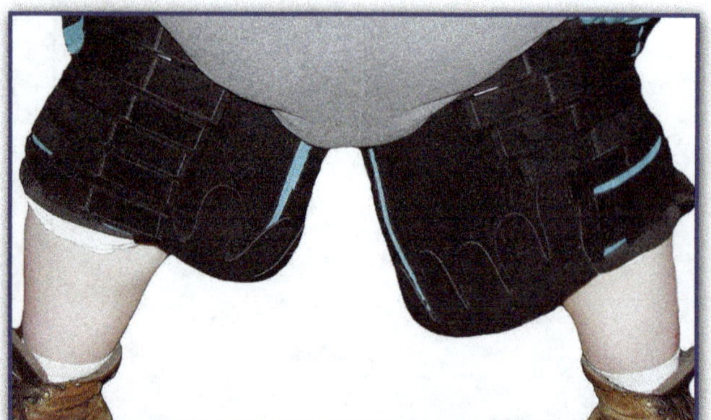

FIGURE 34. Lobule compression system
Courtesy of Robyn Bjork, MPT, CWS, CLT-LANA, CLWT

F. Pneumatic compression

Pneumatic compression devices have been utilized since the early 1950s to manage edema.[48-49] The initial intermittent pneumatic compression (IPC) devices were pumps with a single chamber pressure cuff that applied a uniform level of compression to the entire limb. In the 1970s, segmented compression devices were developed which evolved to allow pressure gradients, with the pressure in the distal chambers being higher than in the proximal chambers, enabling a sequential mechanism of pressure applied distal to proximal.[50] More recently, advanced pneumatic compression devices have evolved to allow for digital programming to mimic manual lymphatic drainage techniques and promote fluid clearance from the proximal trunk and extremity. Additionally, advanced IPC devices have appliances that can treat the torso as well as the limbs. These additional appliances are important as pumps that address only the fluid in an extremity can cause an increase in edema or fibrotic tissue (fibrosclerotic ring) above the pump's sleeve.[51]

Traditionally, IPC devices are not considered a component of the gold standard of CDT; however, IPC devices may be considered adjunctive to effectively manage lymphedema.[50] According to a recent systematic review of IPC devices, Feldman et al. reported that IPC is considered an effective and safe intervention particularly for patients with little access to medical care. Additionally, IPC devices can be used in the home and are well tolerated when used at the low to moderate pressure ranges.[50]

The decision to utilize an IPC device should be determined on a case-to-case basis. IPCs, when used properly on the right patient, may help maintain the benefits achieved during the intensive phase of CDT; however, many experts suggest IPC devices should not replace CDT as the only intervention. If utilized, they should be employed only after successful CDT to support the patient during the maintenance phase. Remember, the MLDT aspect of CDT helps to reroute and redirect lymph fluid by training the system to bypass the compromised areas. After the intensive phase of CDT and over time, the body's intelligence maintains these new routes of lymph flow. Although IPC can mobilize fluid from the affected body regions, it does not train the system to reroute itself. Instead, it tends to increase the fluid load on other areas, particularly the trunk and groin regions. Since it cannot remove protein, over time these areas tend to become more fibrotic and create a more treatment-resistant limb/body region. Further, pumps are time intensive and when not used properly, they can traumatize residual functioning lymph vessels.

According to Feldman et al., the IPC literature reports significant variability in IPC-related clinical outcomes, and no single best-practice guideline for IPC is preferred as no universal consensus on clinical recommendations is noted.[50]

Relevance to case study

For this patient, IPC is not a preferred intervention. Given the shapes of her lower extremities, it would be difficult to fit her properly with a sleeve that would encompass her legs and trunk. An improper fit would promote fluid redirection to other body regions (groin, trunk) and possibly lead to a fibrosclerotic ring at the top of the sleeve. For this patient, treatment should focus on CDT and wound and skin care, with an emphasis on patient education for lifelong management.

Summary

Proper identification and diagnosis is essential for patients with lymphedema. Recognizing the predisposing risk factors, signs, and symptoms of lymphedema will assist with differential diagnosis when faced with complex patient presentations. Many patients with lymphedema have concomitant comorbidities, which may complicate medical management. It is imperative to appreciate all contributing factors to individualize interventions and modify treatment approaches as applicable. Chronic wounds directly or indirectly related to lymphedema are not uncommon. Proper management involves addressing the underlying medical conditions or diseases that may be the likely cause of ulceration, while simultaneously addressing skin and nail care and providing proper complete decongestive therapy, modified according to the patient's specific needs, clinical presentation, and functional impairments. Referral to a certified lymphedema therapist and/or trained physician specialist is of utmost importance.

Review questions

1. ***True/False.*** Lymphedema is a vascular disorder that is either due to congenital malformations of the lymphatic system or related to an insult or injury to the lymphatic system.

2. **Although there is no cure for lymphedema, it can be successfully managed by:**
   a. complete decongestive therapy
   b. surgery
   c. pneumatic compression
   d. diuretics

3. ***True/False.*** Lymphedema results in a protein-rich edema that can lead to reactive fibrosis of the tissues.

4. **Patients with lymphedema are at high risk for which of the following conditions?**
   a. ingrown toenails
   b. cellulitis
   c. CHF
   d. ascites

5. ***True/False.*** Other distinguishing clinical features of lymphedema are papillomatosis and hyperkeratosis.

ANSWERS: 1) True
2) a
3) True
4) b
5) True

References

1. Stout N, Weiss R, Feldman, J, Stewart B, Amer J, Cormier J, Shi Y. A systematic review of care delivery models and economic analysis in lymphedema; health policy impact 2004-2011. Lymphology. 2013;46:27-41.
2. Sen CK, Gordillo GM, Roy S, et al. Human skin wounds: a major and snowballing threat to public health and the economy. Wound Repair Regen. 2009;17(6):763-71.
3. Kuhn BA, Coulter SJ. Balancing ulcer cost and quality equation. Nurs Econ. 1992;10(5):353-9.
4. Hess CT. Putting the squeeze on venous ulcers. Nursing. 2004;34(Suppl):8-13.
5. Driver VR, Fabbi M, Lavery LA, Gibbons G. The costs of diabetic foot: the economic case for the limb salvage team. J Am Podiatr Med Assoc. 2010;100(5):335-41.
6. Beebe-Dimmer J, Pfeifer J, Engle J, Schottenfeld D. The epidemiology of chronic venous insufficiency and varicose veins. Ann Epidemiol. 2005;15(3):175-84.
7. Bull R, Gane J, Evans J, Joseph A, Mortimer P. Abnormal lymph drainage in patients with chronic venous leg ulcers. J Am Acad Dermatol. 1993;28:585-90.
8. Collins P, Villavicencio J, Abreu S, Gomez E, Coffey J, Connaway C, et al. Abnormalities of lymphatic drainage in lower extremities: a lymphoscintigraphy study. J Vasc Surg. 1989;9:145-52.
9. Gloviczki P, Calcagno D, Schriger A, Pairolero P, Cherry K, Hallett J, et al. Noninvasive evaluation of the swollen extremity; experiences with 190 lymphoscintigraphic examinations. J Vasc Surg. 1989;9:683-9.
10. Cormier JN, Askew RL, Mungovan KS, et al. Lymphedema beyond breast cancer: a systematic review and meta-analysis of cancer-related secondary lymphedema. Cancer. 2010;116:5138-49.
11. Schook CC, Mulliken JB, Fishman SJ, Grant FD, Zurakowski D, Greene AK. Primary lymphedema: clinical features and management in 138 pediatric patients. Plast Reconstr Surg. 2011;127:2419-31.
12. Kim JH, Choi JH, Ki EY, et al. Incidence and risk factors of lower-extremity lymphedema after radical surgery with or without adjuvant radiotherapy in patients with FIGO stage I to stage IIA cervical cancer. Int J Gynecol Cancer. 2012;22:686-91.
13. Petrek JA, Senie RT, Peters M, Rosen PP. Lymphedema in a cohort of breast carcinoma survivors 20 years after diagnosis. Cancer. 2001;92:1368-77.
14. Wilke LG, McCall LM, Posther KE, et al. Surgical complications associated with sentinel lymph node biopsy: results from a prospective international cooperative group trial. Ann Surg Oncol. 2006;13:491-500.
15. Chang SB, Askew RL, Xing Y, et al. Prospective assessment of postoperative complications and associated costs following inguinal lymph node dissection (ILND) in melanoma patients. Ann Surg Oncol. 2010;17:2764-72.
16. Hunt KK, Askew R, Cormier JN. Measuring lymphedema in patients with breast cancer: go with the flow? Breast Cancer Res Treat. 2009;117:559-60.
17. Disipio T, Rye S, Newman B, Hayes S. Incidence of unilateral arm lymphedema after breast cancer: a systematic review and meta-analysis. Lancet Oncol. 2013;14:500-15.
18. Zuther JE, Norton S. Lymphedema management: the comprehensive guide for practitioners. 3rd ed. New York: Thieme; 2013.
19. Chikly B. Silent waves: theory and practice of lymph drainage therapy. 2nd ed. Scottsdale (AZ): I.H.H. Publishing; 2004.

20. Wikipedia: the free encyclopedia [Internet]. Wikimedia Foundation, Inc. 2001 - . Blood proteins; [cited 2016 Jun 25]. Available from: https://en.wikipedia.org/wiki/Blood_proteins.

21. Földi M. Textbook of lymphology. 3rd ed. Munich: Elsevier GmbH; 2013.

22. Framework L. Best practice for the management of lymphedema. International consensus. London: MEP Ltd.; 2006. p. 3-52.

23. Ortman JM, Velkoff VA, Hogan H. An aging nation: the older population in the United States. Washington (DC): U.S. Census Bureau; 2014 May 24. p. 25-1140.

24. International Society of Lymphology. The diagnosis and treatment of peripheral lymphedema: 2013 consensus document of the International Society of Lymphology. Lymphology. 2013;46(1):1-11.

25. WOCN. Ankle brachial index: quick reference guide for clinicians. J Wound Ostomy Continence Nurs. 2012;39(2 Suppl):S21-S29.

26. Nicolaï SP, Kruidenier LM, Rouwet EV, Wetzels-Gulpers L, Rozeman CA, Prins MH, Teijink JA. Pocket Doppler and vascular laboratory equipment yield comparable results for ankle brachial index measurement. BMC Cardiovasc Disord. 2008;8:26-30.

27. Rooke T, Hirsch A, Misra S, Sidawy A, Beckman J, Findeiss L, et al. 2011 ACCF/AHA focused update of the guideline for the management of patients with peripheral artery disease (updating the 2005 guideline): a report of the American College of Cardiology Foundation/American Heart Association Task Force on Practice Guidelines. J Am Coll Cardiol. 2011;58(19):2020-45.

28. Brenner E, Putz D, Moriggl B. Stemmer's (Kaposi-Stemmer-) sign – 30 years later. Phlebologie-Stuttgart. 2007;36(6):320.

29. Schultz-Ehrenburg U, Niederauer H, Tiedjen K. Stasis papillomatosis clinical features, etiopathogenesis and radiological findings. J Dermatol Surg Oncol. 1993;19(5):440-6.

30. Fat Disorders Research Society [Internet]. Fat Disorders Research Society. Lipedema; [cited 2016 Jun 25]. Available from: http://www.fatdisorders.org/.

31. National Lymphedema Network Medical Advisory Committee. NLN position statement: the diagnosis and treatment of lymphedema. NLN; 2011 Feb.

32. Charles H. Elephantiasis of the leg. In: Latham A, English TC, editors. A system of treatment. Vol. 3. London: Churchill; 1912.

33. Granzow J, Soderberg J, Kaji A, Dauphine C. Review of current surgical treatments for lymphedema. Ann Surg Oncol. 2014;21:1195-201.

34. Zuther J. Lymphedema: inform yourself and take control [blog on the Internet]. Joachim Zuther. Suction assisted protein lipectomy (SAPL) for the treatment of chronic lymphedema; 2016 May 6 [cited 2016 Jun 6]. Available from: http://www.lymphedemablog.com/2016/05/06/suction-assisted-protein-lipectomy-sapl-for-the-treatment-of-chronic-lymphedema/.

35. Baumeister RG, Siuda S, Bohmert H, Moser E. A microsurgical method for reconstruction of interrupted lymphatic pathways: autologous lymph-vessel transplantation for treatment of lymphedemas. Scand J Plast Reconstr Surg. 1986;20:141-6.

36. Granzow JW, Soderberg JM, Kaji AH, Dauphine C. An effective system of surgical treatment of lymphedema. Ann Surg Oncol. 2014;21(4):1189-94.

37. Lasinski B, Thrift, K, Squire D, Austin M, Smith K, Wanchai A, et al. A systematic review of the evidence for complete decongestive therapy in the treatment of lymphedema from 2004 to 2011. PM R. 2012;4:580-601.

38. Zuther J. Lymphedema: inform yourself and take control [blog on the Internet]. Joachim Zuther. Skin and nail care in lymphedema management [cited 2016 Jun 7]. Available from: http://www.lymphedemablog.com/wp-content/uploads/2011/04/Skin-and-Nail-Care-in-Lymphedema-Management.pdf.

39. Position statement of the National Lymphedema Network on exercises [Internet]. National Lymphedema Network [cited 2016 Jun 10]. Available from: http://lymphnet.org/pdfDocs/nlnexercise.pdf.

40. Zuther J. Lymphedema: inform yourself and take control [blog on the Internet]. Joachim Zuther. Why exercises should be part of your lymphedema treatment regimen [cited 2016 Jun 10]. Available from: http://www.lymphedemablog.com/2015/11/12/why-exercises-should-be-part-of-your-lymphedema-treatment-regimen/.

41. Tan IC, Maus EA, Rasmussen JC, Marshall MV, Adams KE, Fife CE, Smith LA, Chan W, Sevick-Muraca EM. Assessment of lymphatic contractile function after manual lymphatic drainage using near-infrared fluorescence imaging. Arch Phys Med Rehabil. 2011;92(5):756-64.

42. Forbes G. Lymphatics of the skin, with a note on lymphatic watershed areas. J Anat. 1938;72(Pt 3):399.

43. Hamner JB, Fleming MD. Lymphedema therapy reduces the volume of edema and pain in patients with breast cancer. Ann Surg Oncol. 2007;14(6):1904-8.

44. Mosti G, Iabichella ML, Partsch H. Compression therapy in mixed ulcers increases venous output and arterial perfusion. J Vasc Surg. 2012;55(1):122-8.

45. Moffatt C, Glover D. Compression therapy: a position document on compression bandaging. Lymphedema Pathw. 2012;Summer:5-8.

46. Arsenault K, Rielly L, Wise H. Effects of complete decongestive therapy on the incidence rate of hospitalization for the management of recurrent cellulitis in adults with lymphedema. Rehabil Oncol. 2011 Jan 1;29(3):14-20.

47. Linnitt N, Hunt K. Use of Juxta-Fit™ to reduce edema and promote self-management. J Lymphedema. 2011;6(2):94-100.

48. Brush, BE, TJ Heldt: A device for relief of lymphedema. J Am Med Assoc. 1955;158:34-5.

49. Brush BE, JH Wylie, J Beninson. The treatment of postmastectomy lymphedema. AMA Arch Surg. 1958;77:561-7.

50. Feldman J, Stout N, Wanchai A, Stewart B, Cormier J. Intermittent pneumatic compression therapy: a systematic review. Lymphology. 2012;45:13-25.

51. Boris M, Weindorf S, Lasinski B. The risk of genital edema after external pump compression for lower limb lymphedema. Lymphology. 1998;31(1):15-20.

Chapter 14
ARTERIAL ULCERS: EVALUATION AND TREATMENT

Boulos Toursarkissian, MD, RPVI, FACS
Mellick T. Sykes MD, FACS

KEY CONCEPTS

1. Arterial insufficiency ulcers represent a late manifestation of peripheral arterial disease (PAD).

2. Atherosclerosis is by far the most common etiology for PAD.

3. A word of caution is warranted in diabetic patients. A nonpalpable pulse may be merely a reflection of the noncompliant calcified yet patent vessel.

4. On another hand, there are many case reports of diabetic patients with palpable pedal pulses, yet with clear-cut angiographically documented high-grade stenosis or occlusions in the arterial tree.

5. A normal ABI in a diabetic patient is not helpful, since medial calcinosis of the tibial vessels will render them difficult to compress and may therefore artificially and erroneously elevate the ABI.

6. Transcutaneous oxygen measurements offer information regarding cutaneous arterial flow and are frequently used to guide amputation levels and wound healing failure.

7. The selection of open surgical versus endovascular approaches depends on a number of factors such as local expertise, renal function status, previous open or endovascular interventions, cardiac and medical risk factors, extent and location of disease, patient life expectancy, expected patency rates of intervention versus bypass in the individual case, and availability of conduit for bypass.

NOTE: The authors wish to acknowledge Ronald L. Blumoff, MD, MBA, FACS for his contribution to this chapter based on the content in Chapter 12: Arterial Insufficency Ulcers in Wound Care Practice.[15]

CONTENTS

Introduction

Arterial insufficiency ulcers represent a late manifestation of peripheral arterial disease (PAD), a spectrum of symptoms caused by progressive chronic stenosis of the arteries to the legs. Although atherosclerosis is by far the most common etiology, PAD may be caused by thromboangiitis obliterans (Buerger's disease), inflammatory arteritis, radiation arteritis, adventitial cystic disease, popliteal aneurysm, or popliteal entrapment syndrome. PAD is also known as chronic limb ischemia (CLI), lower-extremity occlusive disease (LEOD), lower-extremity arterial disease (LEAD), or peripheral vascular disease (PVD).

Ulceration of the feet may be caused by arterial insufficiency alone; however, coexisting PAD may exacerbate ulcers of other etiologies, such as venous insufficiency or neuropathy.

I. Case study

A 55-year-old patient presents to the emergency room with a necrotic fifth toe on the left foot. He attributes this event to the use of a poor fitting shoe three weeks earlier. What was initially a blister has progressed to gangrene with associated cellulitis on the dorsum of the foot. He has long-standing diabetes, hypertension, and hyperlipidemia. He has no history of claudication but has smoked for many years. He is on insulin and a beta blocker for his hypertension only. On exam, he has good femoral pulses, but the popliteal and pedal pulses are not palpable. He has a temperature of 101°F, a pulse of 110, and a blood pressure of 90 mmHg. His white cell count is 14,000, HbA1C 11%, and his creatinine is 1.8 mg/dL.

II. Epidemiology

Estimates suggest that 10 million individuals may be affected by PAD in the United States. For every person with symptomatic PAD, it is believed that there are six others who have asymptomatic disease,[1]

Depending on the age range and method of screening, prevalence ranges from 3% to 22%, increasing dramatically in the later decades. At 60 the prevalence is around 5%, rising to 20% for persons over 70.

Risk factors for development of symptomatic PAD include age, male sex, elevated homocysteine levels, smoking, hypercoagulable conditions and diabetes. In contrast to coronary artery disease, few patients develop PAD without identifiable risk factors.

III. Pathway

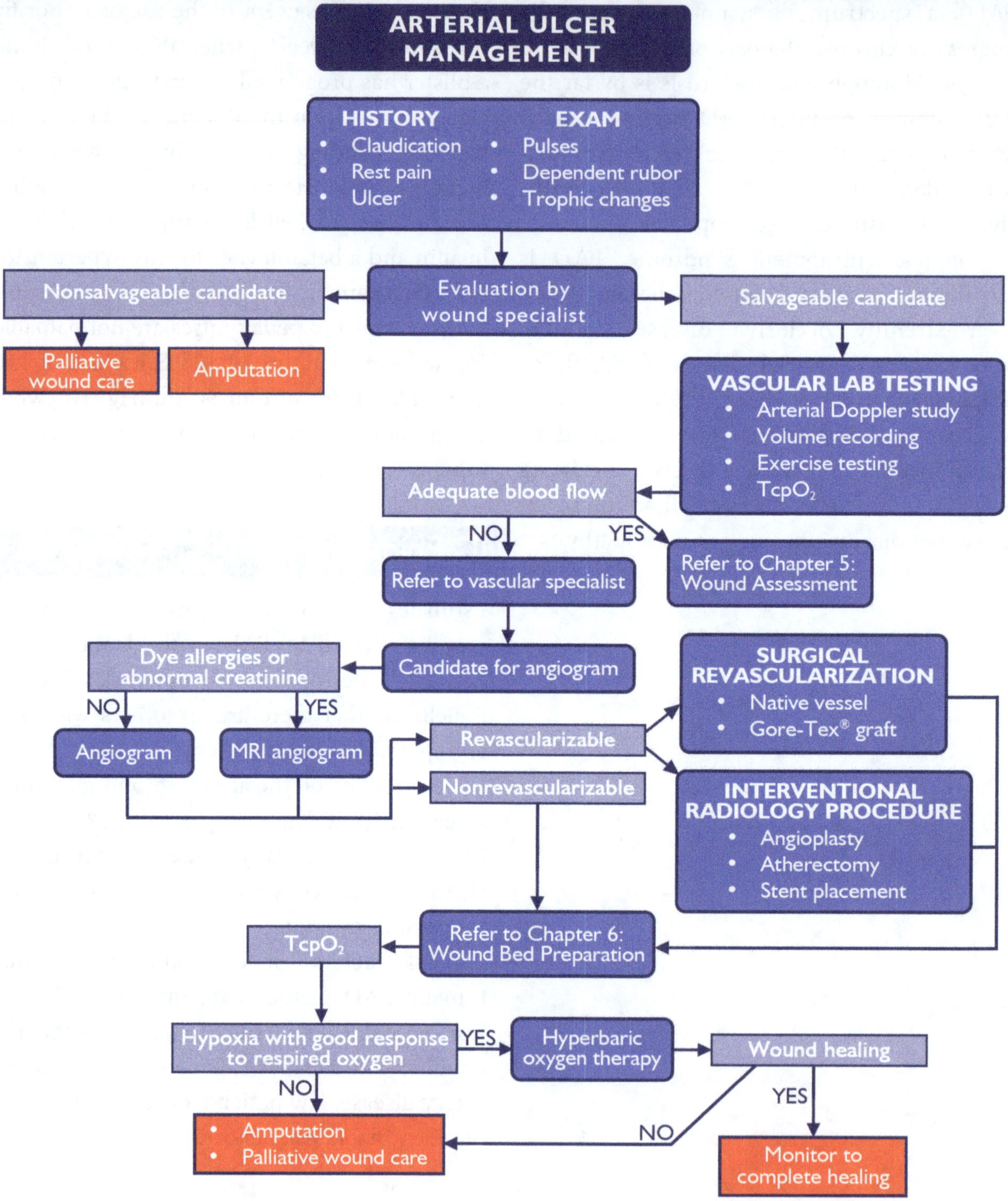
ARTERIAL ULCER MANAGEMENT
HISTORY
• Claudication
• Rest pain
• Ulcer
EXAM
• Pulses
• Dependent rubor
• Trophic changes
Evaluation by wound specialist
Nonsalvageable candidate
Palliative wound care
Amputation
Salvageable candidate
VASCULAR LAB TESTING
• Arterial Doppler study
• Volume recording
• Exercise testing
• $TcpO_2$
Adequate blood flow
NO
YES
Refer to Chapter 5: Wound Assessment
Refer to vascular specialist
Candidate for angiogram
Dye allergies or abnormal creatinine
NO
YES
Angiogram
MRI angiogram
Revascularizable
Nonrevascularizable
SURGICAL REVASCULARIZATION
• Native vessel
• Gore-Tex® graft
INTERVENTIONAL RADIOLOGY PROCEDURE
• Angioplasty
• Atherectomy
• Stent placement
Refer to Chapter 6: Wound Bed Preparation
$TcpO_2$
Hypoxia with good response to respired oxygen
YES
Hyperbaric oxygen therapy
Wound healing
NO
• Amputation
• Palliative wound care
NO
YES
Monitor to complete healing

IV. Pathophysiology

Poiseuille's equation describes blood flow in an ideal laminar tube. Flow within a vessel is proportional to the driving pressure gradient, the fourth power of the radius, and is inversely proportional to the length of the tube:

$$\text{Flow} = \pi P R^4 / 8 \eta L$$

Where

P = driving pressure; R = radius of the vessel;
η = viscosity; L = length of the vessel.

Thus, a stenosis that decreases the vessel radius by one-half causes a sixteen-fold decrease in maximum blood flow.

In a pulsatile arterial system, energy losses caused by turbulence within and distal to a stenosis also result in diminished flow.

A. Atherosclerosis and blood flow

Atherosclerosis (AS) reduces flow by several mechanisms: 1) AS plaque narrows the vessel radius, which diminishes distal flow exponentially; 2) irregular AS plaque produces turbulent flow, which further lessens the energy and flow to distal tissue; and 3) the intimal "cap" over the plaque may ulcerate or dissect, releasing atheroembolic plaque or thrombus to occlude distal vessels.

B. Absolute and relative ischemia

Ischemia occurs when local tissue demands exceed the supply of blood flow.

Ischemia = Demand > Supply

Ischemia may be caused by increased demand, decreased supply, or both. PAD causes a drop in the absolute blood flow to a limb (absolute ischemia), which may or may not cause clinical symptoms, depending on the tissue metabolic demands.

Exercise (such as walking), infection, and trauma are high-metabolic processes that greatly increase the demand for blood flow. If this is unavailable due to PAD, exercise ends prematurely in claudication, infection spreads, wounds fail to heal, and tissue dies. The concept of relative ischemia refers to a discrepancy between the amount of blood *available* and the amount of blood *needed* to carry on cellular function. Relative ischemia arises when supply becomes inadequate, demand increases, or both.

C. Trauma and ischemia

A severely ischemic foot has been likened to a dry forest, where a minor spark may start a fire. That spark might be an abrasion from a new ill-fitting shoe, a crack in dry skin, or minor trauma from nail trimming. This minor injury is often initially unrecognized. When the injury happens, the increased metabolic demands cannot be met because of inadequate circulation, leading to worsening necrosis or infection with a resultant vicious circle. This combination of poor arterial blood flow and tissue trauma creates the arterial insufficiency ulcer (Figure 1). The wound, ulcer, or infection is a secondary phenomenon. Breaking the vicious circle requires revascularization.

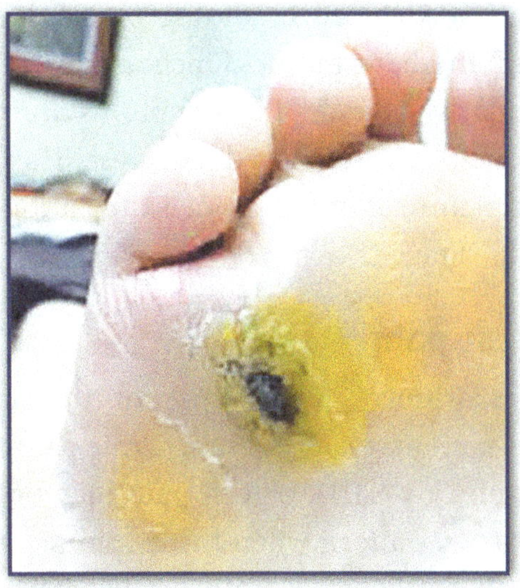

FIGURE 1. Ulcer of mixed arterial and neuropathic etiologies

V. Classification of PAD

Fontaine's simple description of the classic stages of chronic limb ischemia is useful in understanding the progression of PAD. Fontaine's classification starts from Stage 1 (asymptomatic) to Stage 2 (claudication), Stage 3 (rest pain), and Stage 4 (tissue loss).[17] The Rutherford classification is more recent and complex but follows the same principle in more detail.[16] Although these categories present gradually more severe symptoms, patients with PAD do not necessarily pass through all stages. Most Stage 2 claudicants never progress to critical limb ischemia, for example, and many diabetics present with Stage 4 gangrene as the first manifestation of arterial occlusive disease.

A. Asymptomatic

PAD progresses slowly and insidiously. The initial asymptomatic phase (Fontaine Stage I) involves gradual narrowing of the major limb vessels accompanied by a variable degree of collaterals development.[17] Inactive patients may never manifest intermittent claudication.

B. Intermittent claudication (IC)

As stenosis increase, most patients complain of exercise-induced cramping or tiredness of the calf, thigh, or buttock. Inclined surfaces are particularly difficult. The symptoms are highly reproducible, and relieved with rest. This is the classic picture of intermittent claudication (IC – Fontaine Stage II).[17]

C. Rest pain

With continued compromise of the arterial supply, patients experience ischemic pain at rest (Fontaine Stage III).[17] Rest pain may begin in a nocturnal pattern when the combined effects of leg elevation and central redistribution of cardiac output combine to further deprive the foot of circulation. Ischemic rest pain is typically located in the metatarsal and instep area. Patients may resort to sleeping in a chair or with the foot hanging off the bed. Edema may therefore develop. Caution is warranted in diabetic patients as sensory neuropathy may mask ischemic rest pain.

D. Tissue loss: ulceration and gangrene

With progression of PAD, minor trauma or infection produce ulcers or gangrene (Fontaine Stage IV).[17] In this category neuroischemic plantar ulcers which do not heal may be placed. A purely arterial ulcer (Figure 2) is usually located in the toes or metatarsals areas and tends to be very painful with irregular borders.

Critical limb ischemia (CLI) includes Fontaine's Stages III and IV, and Categories 4, 5, and 6 of Rutherford's scheme.[16-17] It is defined as a combination of desperate clinical presentation (rest pain, ulceration, or gangrene) plus objective evidence (see section below on Evaluation) that the pain or tissue lesion is caused predominantly by arterial insufficiency. CLI if untreated usually leads to limb loss.

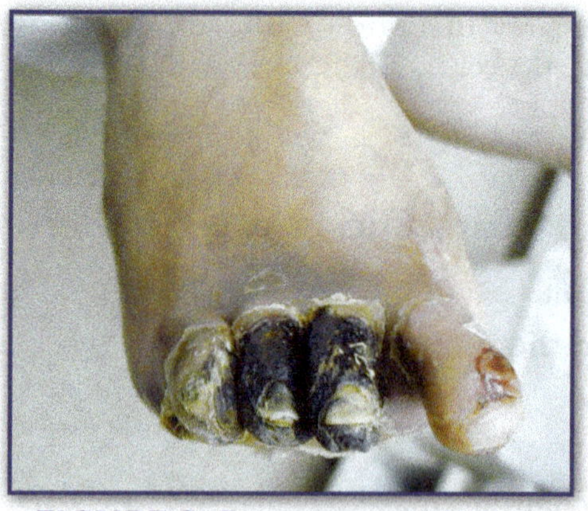

FIGURE 2. Dry gangrene of digits due to obstructive PAD

VI. Diagnosis of PAD

Assessment (see pathway on previous page) should begin with a careful palpation of the abdominal femoral popliteal dorsalis pedis and posterior tibial pulses, as well as auscultation for any associated bruits (Figures 3, 4, 5). A word of caution is warranted in diabetic patients: A nonpalpable pulse may be merely a reflection of the noncompliant calcified yet patent vessel. On another hand, there are many case reports of patients with palpable pedal pulses, yet with clear-cut angiographically documented high-grade stenosis or occlusions in the arterial tree. Pulses may also be difficult to palpate in obese individuals, muscular individuals, or in the presence of peripheral edema. An absent pulse at one level usually indicates the presence of arterial occlusive disease in the segment above it.

The leg and foot should be inspected for other signs of arterial insufficiency. Common findings include trophic changes from chronic tissue malperfusion; atrophy of skin and muscles, "baked potato toe" with loss of pulp space turgor, diminished lanugo hair, dependent rubor and elevation pallor, and nails that are hypertrophic from slow growth (Figure 6). The foot may be cool compared to the contralateral side. Signs of infection, such as cellulitis, plantar tenderness, or drainage should also be noted. Toes should be spread to find occult interdigital ulcers. The heel and plantar surface should be palpated for tenderness, suggesting deep infection.

A careful physical exam should be supplemented in most cases with a set of arterial noninvasive studies.[3] There is currently some confusion as to what exactly is included in arterial noninvasive studies. Any protocol should include a measurement of the ankle brachial index (ABI). An ankle brachial index is the ratio of the highest of either the dorsalis pedis or posterior tibial pressure as numerator to the higher of the two systolic brachial pressures as the denominator. A normal value is usually 0.9 to 1.2. A normal ABI in a nondiabetic patient has a good negative predictive value for the absence of PAD, whereas an abnormally low ABI in both

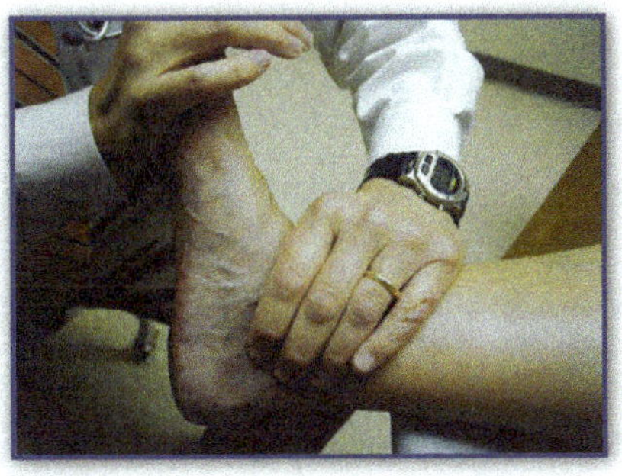

FIGURE 3. Posterior tibial pulse palpation aided by gentle dorsiflexion of foot

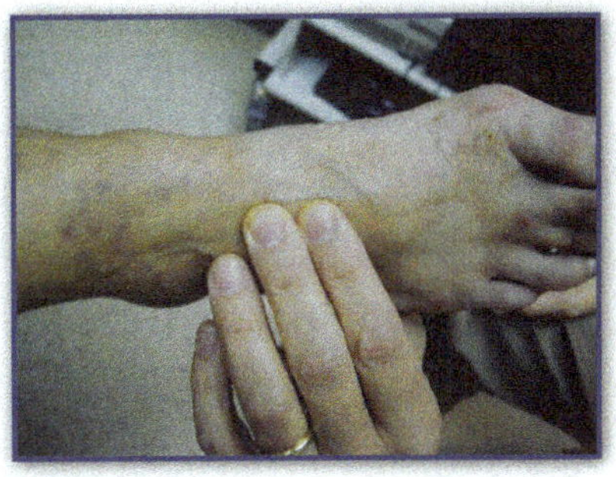

FIGURE 4. Dorsalis pedis pulse palpation

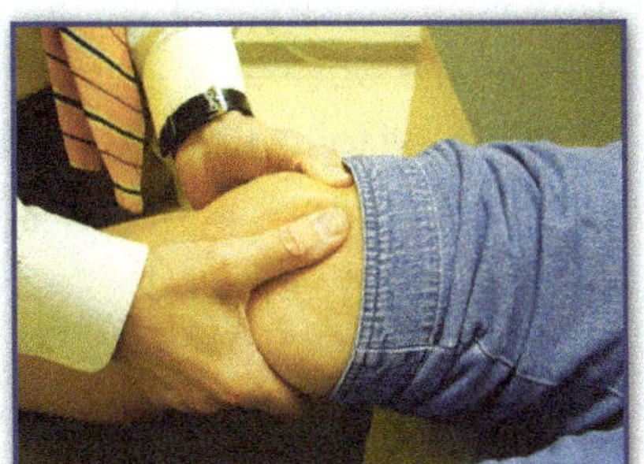

FIGURE 5. Popliteal artery pulse palpation

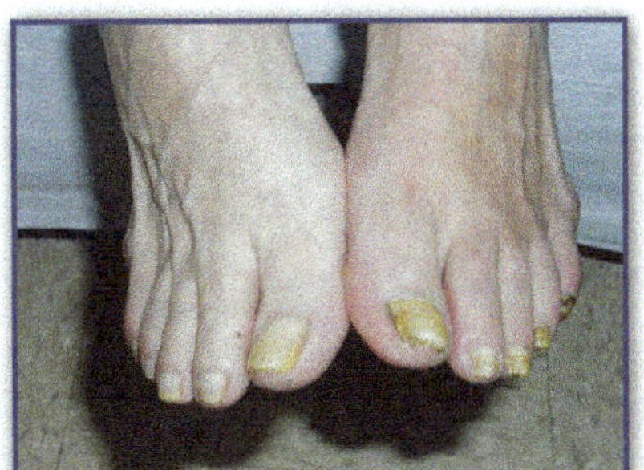

FIGURE 6. Dependent rubor left foot

TABLE 1. Differential Diagnosis of Foot and Ankle Ulcers

Type	Ischemic	Venous	Neuropathic
Location	Toes, interdigital, heel, lateral malleolus	Lower leg (gaiter), above medial malleolus	Plantar
Pain	Present, relieved with dependency	Mild, relieved with elevation	Absent
Appearance	Pale, irregular, dry, poor granulation	Beefy-red granulation	Deep tract, punched out
Pulses	Poor / absent	Present, may be hidden by induration	Normal
Skin	Trophic changes: thin, shiny, dry. Thick nails.	Stasis changes: thick, indurated, pigmented	Normal; callus
Bleeding	Poor	Venous	Brisk
Edema	None – muscular atrophy	Present	None
Risk Factors	For atherosclerosis, especially smoking, diabetes, age	Varicose veins, DVT	Diabetes, immobility
Key Treatment	Revascularization	Compression	Offloading
If treatment lags suspect:	Renal failure, infection, restenosis	Occult ischemia, inadequate compression	Occult ischemia, osteomyelitis

diabetic and nondiabetic patients has a good positive predictive value for the presence of PAD. A normal ABI in a diabetic patient is not helpful, since medial calcinosis of the tibial vessels will render them difficult to compress and may therefore artificially and erroneously elevate the ABI. Along the same lines, an elevated ABI greater than 1.2-1.3 is not helpful in terms of predicting the presence or absence of PAD. An ABI less than 0.5 indicates the presence of significant vascular disease.

The toe brachial index or TBI has been suggested as an alternative or supplement to the ABI. A normal TBI has a value of 0.7 or greater. A normal ABI in the presence of a low TBI may suggest forefoot arterial disease, or may be a finding in a diabetic patient with calcified stenotic tibial vessels. A TBI in diabetic patients may not be interpretable in up to a third of cases due to calcified pedal vessels or missing or infected digits.

Any pressure measurements should be accompanied by Doppler waveform (Figure 7) analysis of the femoral popliteal posterior tibial and dorsalis pedis levels. Doppler waveform interpretation is qualitative and not quantitative in nature. A normal waveform is triphasic with a major forward systolic flow, a small reversal at the onset of diastole, and a third smaller forward component due to elastic recoil of the vessel. With progression of disease, waveforms distal to the area affected will become biphasic, then monophasic, and eventually flat. Again, caution should be applied in diabetic patients

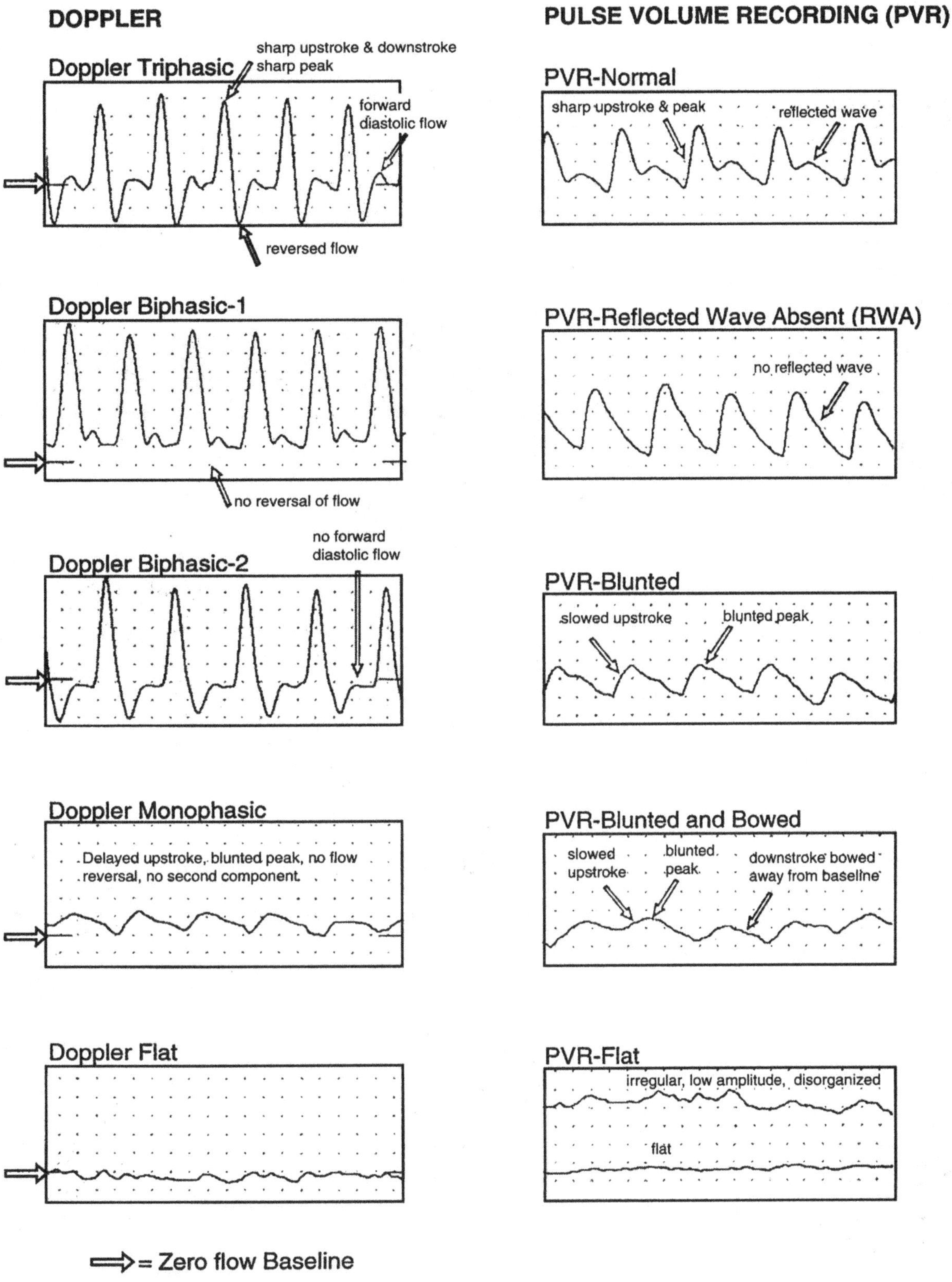

FIGURE 7. Arterial doppler and pulse volume recording

where stiff noncompliant vessels may show monophasic waveforms even in the absence of high-grade stenosis.

Another modality frequently used in noninvasive testing is pulse volume recording or PVR. The part of the extremity being studied is placed in a cuff, which is then inflated to a pressure sufficient to stop venous flow. Any arterial inflow into that part of the extremity leads to a compression of the fixed volume cuff with a resultant pressure tracing. A normal tracing has a sharp upstroke, a dicrotic notch in the early down slope, and a down slope that is curved toward the baseline. Early findings of disease will consist of a loss of the dicrotic notch, followed by a delayed upstroke, followed by outward bowing of the down slope, with ultimate flattening of the PVR tracing. Like Doppler, PVR interpretation is mainly qualitative and not quantitative. PVR in general has a tendency to underestimate the degree of arterial disease.

Duplex imaging of the arterial tree has been gaining increased acceptance more recently. Although it has many advantages in terms of visualizing the arterial tree, it lacks in perfusion pressure measurements that many vascular specialists rely upon to predict likelihood of wound healing or nonhealing. Therefore it ideally should be accompanied by ABI and TBI measurements. A complete duplex study should include visualization of the vessels from the aortoiliac level down to the foot with a grayscale imaging along with velocity measurements of blood flow peak systolic velocities at specific points in addition to velocity measurements at any suspicious points identified by grayscale scanning. An area where the peak systolic velocity doubles usually indicates a greater than 50% diameter stenosis, whereas a quadrupling of the velocity suggests a greater than 80% stenosis. The peak systolic velocity will usually be decreased distal to areas of significant stenosis once you are past the area of flow disturbance. A low distal velocity, especially if accompanied by a monophasic waveform, will usually indicate the presence of more proximal arterial occlusive disease. Velocities, however, can also be affected by other factors such as congestive heart failure or severe valvular disease. Duplex scanning will also be limited in the face of severe obesity or in the presence of severe calcification, which makes ultrasound penetration difficult.

VII. Assessment of healing potential

What constitutes adequate arterial perfusion to predict wound healing? It depends, of course, on the extent of the wound. It also depends on whether the patient is diabetic. A perfusion pressure above a certain threshold does not, of course, guarantee healing. A toe pressure greater than 40 mmHg in a nondiabetic and 60 mmHg in a diabetic is desirable (for a roughly 80% healing rate). An ankle pressure greater than 70 mmHg in a nondiabetic or 90 mmHg in a diabetic is also ideal. Very few wounds will heal with an ankle pressure less than 40 mmHg. There are no such values described for peak systolic velocities obtained by duplex, although velocities less than 20-30 cm/s are rarely associated with healing.

Transcutaneous oxygen measurements offer information regarding cutaneous arterial flow, and are frequently used to guide amputation levels and wound healing failure. They may be repeated after breathing 100% oxygen to determine possible benefit of hyperbaric oxygen therapy. Measurements are adversely affected by the presence of edema, open wounds, cellulitis, heart failure, and infection.

VIII. Imaging studies

Once a decision has been made that revascularization will be needed, imaging studies are required.

Duplex scan can be used, as discussed earlier. It has the limitations listed above. There have been occasional papers describing interventions and bypasses on the basis of duplex alone. Experience with that approach remains limited to very few places in the country that have extensive ultrasound experience.

Other imaging choices include conventional digital subtracted angiography, CT angiography, and magnetic resonance angiography. **Magnetic resonance angiography (MRA)** has the advantage of avoiding radiation exposure. Calcification, however, will lead to an over-estimation of the degree of disease. Prior areas of stenting would also appear as signal voids on the MRA. The use of gadolinium as a contrast agent is beneficial in enhancing details of imaging but has limited applicability in patients with any kind of renal insufficiency because of the risk of nephrogenic systemic fibrosis. Visualization of vessels below the knee will also require a dedicated acquisition sequence with gadolinium enhancement.

CT angiography offers the advantage of cross-sectional visualization of the vessels, leading to a better evaluation of potential emboligenic foci. However, it does require a significant contrast load, which can be a problem in patients with renal insufficiency. For vessels below the knee, the timing of the contrast bolus is critical for good visualization. This requires an experienced tech or a dedicated second bolus injection. Heavy calcification, especially below the knee, will still be a problem in terms of distinguishing the calcification from the contrast in the tiny vessels despite the use of calcium windows.

Conventional angiography (Figure 8) has the main disadvantage of being invasive, but it does afford the opportunity for endovascular intervention at the same setting if indicated. A judicious diagnostic study alone will use less contrast and a CT angiogram. Carbon dioxide can be used as a contrast agent for visualization of the aortoiliac and proximal femoral vessels. It is not helpful for vessels below the knee. It can, however, help limit the volume of contrast administered. Subtraction techniques coupled with contrast injection from a catheter parked in the popliteal artery can provide excellent images of the vessels in the foot. With the current increase in the use of endovascular techniques for revascularization, conventional angiography has become the most widely used modality.

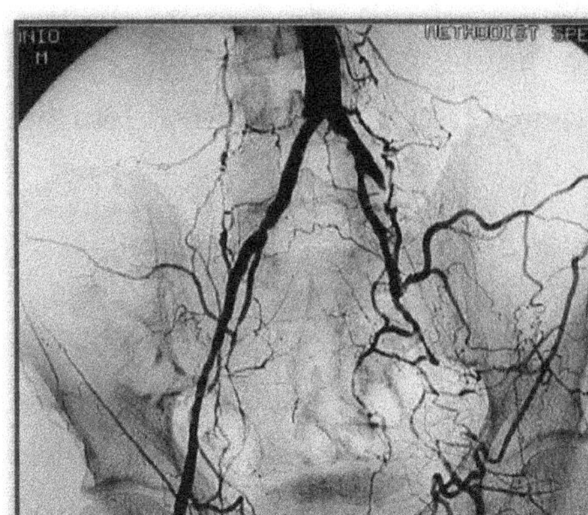

FIGURE 8. Left external iliac artery occlusion

IX. Treatment options

There are basically three treatment options: 1) conservative treatment, 2) revascularization, either open or endovascular, or 3) amputation. They are not mutually exclusive, and often all occur in the same patient. Treatment must be individualized not only to the patient but also to the local medical resources.[4-6]

A. Conservative treatment

Usually, a nonhealing ulcer is an absolute indication for expedient intervention. However, since revascularization, either endovascular or open, involves 1) some initial risk; and 2) a finite life-span, it is occasionally reasonable to defer revascularization in the presence of an ischemic ulcer if it appears small, and modifiable risk and wound factors may be improved.[7]

B. Control of risk factors

Although risk factors for atherosclerosis take years to produce arterial narrowing, acute modification of risk factors appears to have a surprisingly beneficial effect on the healing of arterial insufficiency ulcers.

Smoking should stop, blood glucose levels should be controlled to a Hgb A1C less than 7, blood pressure should be less than 130/90, and hyperlipidemia treatment should reach an LDL < 100 mg%. Suspected hypercoagulable factors (elevated homocysteine, fibrinogen, Hematocrit or platelet, etc.) should be identified and treated.

C. Wound care

A number of wound treatment regimens may be used, depending on the location and nature of the ulcer. These regimens are described elsewhere, but all follow the principles of regular debridement of devitalized tissue, control of infection, moist wound environment, protection from further trauma, and close follow-up. The particular characteristic of arterial insufficiency ulcers is that if ischemia is corrected, a number of wound care regimens may succeed; in the absence of revascularization, failure of healing is very common, although some studies have suggested that up to a third of superficial ulcers may heal with aggressive wound care measures. This is less likely the lower the presenting ABI.[7]

D. Amputation

A primary amputation should be considered in individuals who are neurologically impaired and/or nonambulatory on a long-term basis. It can also be considered in individuals who have failed many revascularization attempts and have limited other choices. Patients with overwhelming infections and extensive foot necrosis may also benefit from primary amputation. There are certain scenarios that have a high risk of limb loss even with successful revascularization. In some select cases, such as those, a primary amputation may be considered. A particular example is the dialysis patient with an extensive heel ulcer. If the patient is ambulatory, every effort should be made to preserve the knee joint, since it is easier to ambulate with a below-the- knee prosthesis than an above-the-knee prosthesis. For patients who are bedridden, an above-the-knee amputation is preferred because it has a much lower risk of wound complications than a below-the-knee amputation.

E. Revascularization

There are essentially three options for revascularization: Open surgery, endovascular interventions, and hybrid procedures incorporating elements of the first two.

Open surgical interventions include endarterectomy for focal lesions (such as a femoral endarterectomy) and bypass for longer or more extensive lesions or occlusions. Bypasses can be fashioned with autologous vein or prosthetic grafts. Prosthetic grafts do very well in the aortoiliac segment, whereas autogenous veins are definitely superior below the groin in terms of patency. Bypasses can be anatomic when they follow the normal vessel pathway or extra-anatomic when placed in a nonanatomic plane. An example of the latter is an axillofemoral bypass used to revascularize a leg in the setting of aortoiliac disease, when a direct aortoiliac approach is not possible. Infrainguinal bypasses constructed with autogenous vein can be in a reverse configuration when the vein is reversed to account for the valves, or it

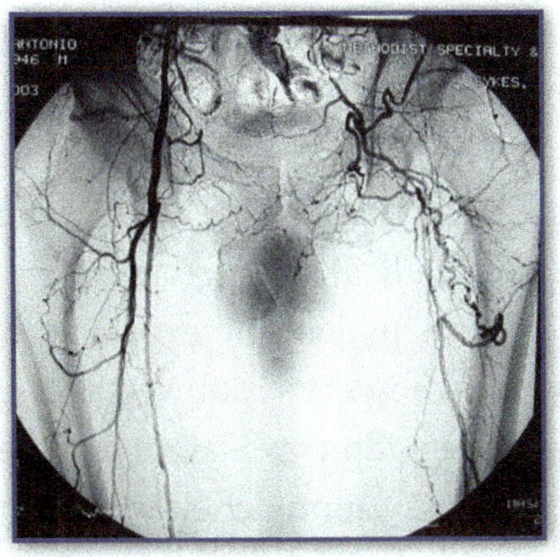

FIGURE 9. Superficial femoral artery occlusion on the left, most likely requiring fempop bypass

can be in situ when the vein is left in its bed undisturbed and the valves are lysed with one of several different types of valvulotomes. Patency rates are more or less equivalent for these approaches. For infrainguinal bypasses, in general, the more proximal the outflow site, the higher the patency rate. Therefore, a femoral-popliteal bypass (Figure 9) can be expected to have a superior five-year patency rate compared to a femoral to dorsalis pedis bypass (Figure 10), for instance. The principle of the good bypass relies on adequate inflow, adequate conduit, and adequate outflow. In other terms, a bypass should not have its inflow distal to an area of disease. Therefore, aortoiliac disease should be treated first before infrainguinal problems are addressed. In terms of conduits, the best patency rate is for one single segment of greater saphenous vein. Alternative conduits such as lesser saphenous vein or arm veins or spliced veins have inferior patency rates. In terms of outflow, a bypass should not be plugged into a vessel that has significant stenotic lesions farther distally down the leg. The mortality rate for lower-extremity bypasses still averages about 1-2%, mostly due to cardiac comorbidities. Wound complications are more frequent, however. Thirty-day failure rates vary in the literature but average around 5%. A femoropopliteal bypass with saphenous vein can be expected to have a 5-year primary patency of 85% versus 70% for a femoral-tibial graft.

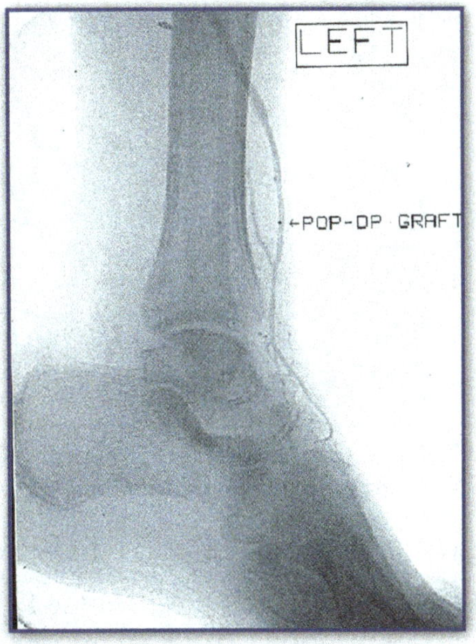

FIGURE 10. Femoral to dorsalis pedis bypass

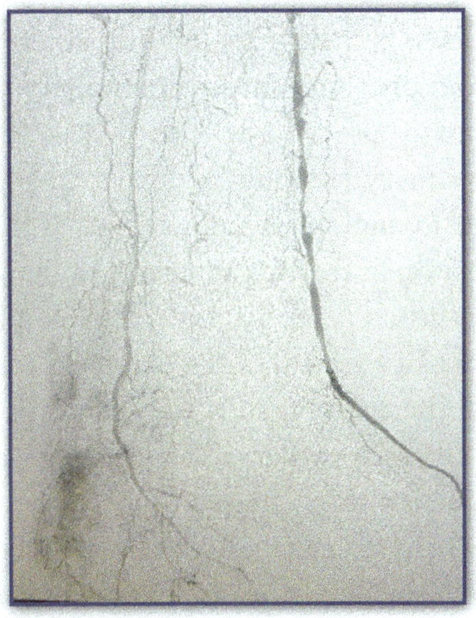

FIGURE 11. Severe tibial occlusive disease with multiple stenosis in the anterior tibial artery amenable to angioplasty

Endovascular approaches include angioplasty (Figure 11), stenting, atherectomy, and thrombolysis,[8] Angioplasty can be indicated for focal stenosis. There are currently drug-eluting balloons on the market that release paclitaxel when inflated. The paclitaxel inhibits smooth muscle proliferation, and these balloons have been shown to have lower rates of restenosis compared to conventional nondrug-eluting balloons. They are available for the treatment

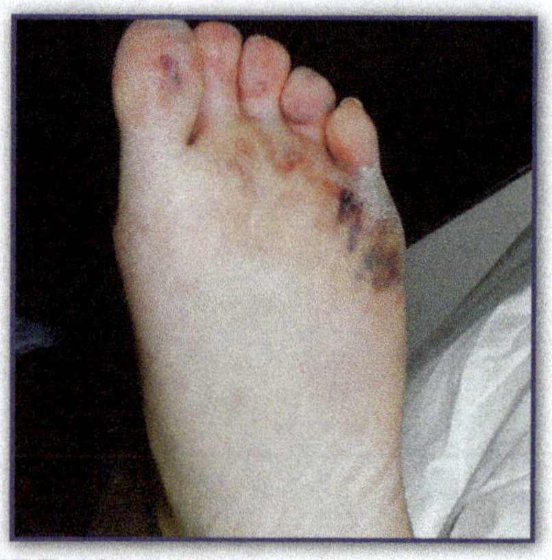

FIGURE 12. Atheroembolization to foot from a proximal source

of femoral lesions. Stenting is indicated for lesions that do not respond to angioplasty or develop complications from angioplasty such as acute recoil or flow-limiting dissection. In some cases, patients may develop atheroembolism from proximal source after angioplasty or atherectomy procedures (Figure 12). In some cases, primary stenting has been shown to be superior to angioplasty alone. Such is the case, for instance, in treating segments of iliac artery total occlusion. Atherectomy refers to physical removal of a segment of the plaque. It comes in various alternatives, such as directional excisional atherectomy or ablative using sanding techniques or using a laser. Some variants may be beneficial in calcified vessels. Atherectomy may offer a benefit in terms of improved patency rates in patients with diabetes compared to angioplasty alone. Thrombolysis refers to clot removal using chemical or aspirational techniques. It is infrequently indicated in patients with chronic disease where the problem is usually plaque and not clot. It is very helpful in cases of acute ischemia with a large clot burden. As far as endovascular interventions go, shorter lesions have better patencies, stenosis does better than occlusions, and a better runoff vessel enhances patency rates. Infrainguinal interventions will have about a 30% six-month recurrence rate on average.

The selection of open surgical versus endovascular approaches depends on a number of factors such as local expertise, renal function status, previous open or endovascular interventions, cardiac and medical risk factors, extent and location of disease, patient life expectancy, expected patency rates of intervention versus bypass in the individual case, and availability of conduit for bypass. The two approaches were compared in the British BASIL trial (balloon angioplasty versus surgery in limb ischemia), which compared a bypass first approach to an angioplasty first approach.[9] Limb-salvage rates were similar, but recurrence rates were higher in the endovascular group. The authors concluded that a surgical approach might be preferable if the patient has a reasonable midterm life expectancy. In general, the trend today is toward an endovascular-first approach. In some situations, such as iliac occlusive disease, the patency rates for stenting rival those of open surgery except possibly in the case of total aortic occlusion. To help physicians choose among the various options, various societies agreed upon a classification referred to as transatlantic inter-societal consensus (TASC) classification. It is based on the recommendation of a panel of experts reviewing the available literature. Lesions are classified as being A B, C, or D. In general, A lesions are best treated by endovascular means, whereas open surgery is preferred for D lesions. There is a TASC classification for aortoiliac disease, a separate one for superficial femoral-popliteal disease, and a third one for tibial occlusive disease. The last consensus recommendations date back to 2007. The problem with this approach is that endovascular techniques keep evolving and that aggressive interventional physicians keep pushing the envelope with more complex interventions.

F. Timing of revascularization

The question frequently arises as to the timing of revascularization. In cases of ulcerations that are noninfected or dry gangrene, revascularization should proceed before any podiatric procedures. This will allow for adequate demarcation of the nonviable tissue that will need to be resected. In cases of deep infection or wet gangrene, surgical debridement of the foot should be carried out first, followed by prompt revascularization, followed again by a formal podiatric closure of the foot wound.

When an endovascular intervention is done, the needed podiatric procedure should be done as expeditiously as possible. The reason for that is the high recurrence rates that are frequently seen with endovascular interventions. The goal, therefore, should be to achieve complete wound healing before any possible recurrence or stenosis. When a bypass is chosen as the revascularization option, the foot procedure can proceed on a more leisurely pace, although again the goal should be to achieve wound healing as soon as possible.

In general, wound healing after bypass surgery is achieved faster than after endovascular intervention (four months mean wound healing time versus seven months for endovascular interventions).[8]

X. Prognosis

Of all claudicants, almost 20% will require revascularization or amputation in their lifetime. More than 80% remain stable and do not require intervention.

Of patients with CLI, about 20% will die in the first year, and 33% after two years; a diagnosis of rest pain, foot ulcer, or gangrene, therefore, carries a worse overall prognosis for survival than many cancers!

XI. Follow-up

All revascularization procedures have the potential to fail with time, usually due to the build-up of intimal hyperplasia within the vessel – commonly at the site of anastomosis, angioplasty, stenting, valve, clamp site, or endarterectomy. This explains the life-long follow-up needed by these patients, with clinical and duplABI follow-up to detect and correct small problems before they cause graft or vessel thrombosis and amputation.

Summary

Arterial insufficiency ulcers are common, and arterial insufficiency is a common factor in poor healing ulcers even with another primary etiology. The combination of atherosclerosis-induced chronic limb ischemia and minor trauma produces ulceration, gangrene, infection, or rest pain—the classic manifestations of CLI that portend limb loss.

Evaluation involves assessing nature of the ulcer and its blood supply. Clinical history and physical exam can make a fairly secure qualitative exam. Objective verification of ischemia is important and may be obtained by the vascular lab.

Treatment by risk-factor modification and wound care may succeed in patients with simple small ulcerations. Most patients, however, require revascularization or amputation.

Case study recap

Control of infection should take first priority. The patient should be hydrated to improve blood pressure and started on broad-spectrum antibiotics. If necessary the offending toe should be amputated or debrided along with the foot and the wounds left open. No definitive closure should be done at this point. Simultaneously, the patient should undergo noninvasive arterial evaluation with ABIs and Doppler. He should be started on antiplatelet therapy as well as a statin. He needs better glycemic control as well. After stabilization, the patient should undergo angiography of the affected limb, assuming his creatinine has stabilized or improved. Endovascular management should be carried out if possible. If this is done, he can then be taken back for a definitive podiatric procedure soon after revascularization. Consideration should be given for adjunctive wound care measures as needed to treat any microcirculatory problems.

Review questions

1. **What is the major limitation of ABI measurement in diabetic patients?**

   a. artificial elevation due to calcified vessels

   b. inability to measure due to missing digits

   c. unreliability due to large limb size

   d. unnecessary unless the patient has nonpalpable pulses.

2. **The BASIL trial showed that**

   a. angioplasty is superior to surgery for limb salvage

   b. initial mortality is higher with angioplasty

   c. long-term results are better with angioplasty

   d. early results in terms of limb salvage were equivalent for angioplasty and surgery

3. **Atherectomy:**

   a. is the preferred endovascular modality in a majority of cases

   b. may have beneficial effects in diabetic patients in terms of improved patency

   c. should only be used below the knee

   d. has better results when the runoff vessels are occluded

4. **Major limb amputation:**

   a. should never be offered as a primary treatment

   b. should be below the knee in nonambulatory patients

   c. is more likely after angioplasty then bypass

   d. may be required despite successful revascularization in some cases, such as heel ulcers in dialysis patients

5. **Duplex imaging of the arterial tree:**

   a. is preferred to abi measurement in most cases

   b. can predict the likelihood of healing of digital amputation

   c. is not affected by vessel calcification or patient obesity

   d. provides anatomic information to supplement other forms of arterial evaluation.

ANSWERS: 1) a
2) d
3) b
4) d
5) d

References

1. Criqui MH, Peripheral arterial disease: epidemiological aspects. Vasc. Med. 2001;6(3):3-7.
2. Tendera M, Aboyans V, Bartelink ML et al. ESC guidelines on the diagnosis and treatment of peripheral artery diseases. European Heart Journal. 2011;32:2851-2906.
3. Sykes MT, Godsey JB. Vascular evaluation of the problem diabetic foot. Clinics in Podiatric Medicine and Surgery. 1998;15(1):49-83.
4. Norgen L, Hiatt WR, Dormandy JA et al. Inter-society consensus for the management of peripheral arterial disease (TASC II). Journal of Vascular Surgery. 2007;45(1):S5A-67A.
5. The TASC steering committee. An update on methods for revascularization and expansion of the TASC lesion classification to include below the knee arteries: a supplement to the inter-society consensus for the management of peripheral arterial disease. J. Endovasc. Ther. 2015;22:657-671.
6. Rooke TW, Hirsch AT, Misra S et al. 2011 ACCF/AHA focused update of the guidelines for the management of patients with peripheral artery disease (Updating the 2005 guideline): a report of the American College of Cardiology Foundation/American Heart Association task force on practice guidelines. J Am. Coll. Cardio. 2011;58(19):2020-2045.
7. Marston WA Davies SW, Armstrong B et al. Natural history of limbs with arterial insufficiency and chronic ulceration treated without revascularization. J. Vasc. Surg. 2006;44:108-114.
8. Obrien-Irr MS. Outcomes after endovascular intervention for chronic critical limb ischemia. J. Vasc. Surg. 2011;53:1575-1581.
9. Bradbury AW, Adam DJ, Forbes JF et al. Bypass vs. angioplasty in severe ischemia of the leg: analysis of amputation free and overall survival by treatment received. J. Vasc. Surg. 2010;51(5):18S-31S.
10. American Diabetes Association: http://www.diabetes.org/main [Internet].
11. American Association for Vascular Surgery: http://aavs.vascularweb.org/ [Internet].
12. Transatlantic Inter-Society Consensus (TASC) on the Treatment of Peripheral Vascular Disease. http://www.tasc-pad.org/ [Internet].
13. Society of Interventional Radiology: http://www.sirweb.org/ [Internet].
14. American Heart Association: http://www.americanheart.org/ [Internet].
15. Sheffield PJ, Fife CE, eds. Wound Care Practice. Flagstaff, AZ: Best Publishing Company; 2007.
16. Rutherford RB, Baker JD, Ernst C, Johnston KW, Porter, JM, Ahn S, et al. Recommended standards for reports dealing with lower extremity ischemia: revised version. J Vasc Surg. 1997;26:517-538.
17. Fontaine R, Kim M, Kieny R. Surgical treatment of peripheral circulation disorders. Helv Chir Acta. 1954;21:499-533.

SECTION 4

ATYPICAL WOUNDS AND BURNS

Editor - Jayesh B. Shah, MD, UHM(ABPM), CWSP, FAPWCA, FCCWS, FUHM, FACP, FACHM

Chapter 15
APPROACH TO COMMONLY MISDIAGNOSED ULCERS AND ATYPICAL ULCERS

Jayesh B. Shah, MD, UHM(ABPM), CWSP, FAPWCA, FCCWS, FUHM, FACP, FACHM

KEY CONCEPTS

1. Even with the technological innovations of the twenty-first century, history-taking remains the best and cheapest tool to make a good diagnosis.
2. All local and systemic factors need to be looked at when taking history of a patient with a wound.
3. Simple attention to the clinical clues is important before you even touch the wound.
4. When in doubt, consider a wound biopsy.
5. Underlying systemic conditions need to be treated before the wound can be healed.
6. A nonhealing wound that does not heal after 4 to 6 weeks of standard wound care should be referred to a specialty wound center for a comprehensive evaluation.

CONTENTS

Introduction

Some wounds demonstrate difficulty with healing despite seemingly appropriate management including good wound bed preparation principles.(1) In such situations, physicians should step back and look at the wound afresh. One should refocus at the complete history and physical, and consider performing a wound biopsy because often, failure to heal is a result of misdiagnosis.(2-4) Sometimes misdiagnosis occurs as a result of unusual presentation of a common condition and, in some instances, an unusual systemic condition presents as a wound.(2-7)

Most often, misdiagnosis results from overlooking simple clues. As the first step to healing a wound is to make an accurate diagnosis, the wound care physician, like a detective, should gather all the clues and try to put them together to make a correct diagnosis.(2)

I. Case study: unusual wound

See Figures 1-4. Mrs. SL is a pleasant 31-year-old black female with history of End Stage Renal Disease (ESRD) secondary to focal segmental glomerulosclerosis. The patient was on dialysis for two months before presenting to the hospital and she developed this wound two months before presentation. The patient says it started because of a fall. Initially it was red, and then it turned black. She started having lot of pain, so she was admitted to the hospital for further work-up where she was seen by multiple specialists including a rheumatologist, a nephrologist, and a wound care specialist. A wound biopsy was positive for vasculitis. She had a positive lupus anticoagulant, a negative anti-nuclear antibody (ANA), elevated complements and an elevated erythrocyte sedimentation rate (ESR) of 91. She was also found to have protein S deficiency. The patient was treated with steroids, debridement, negative pressure wound therapy, silver calcium alginate dressings and then collagen dressings.

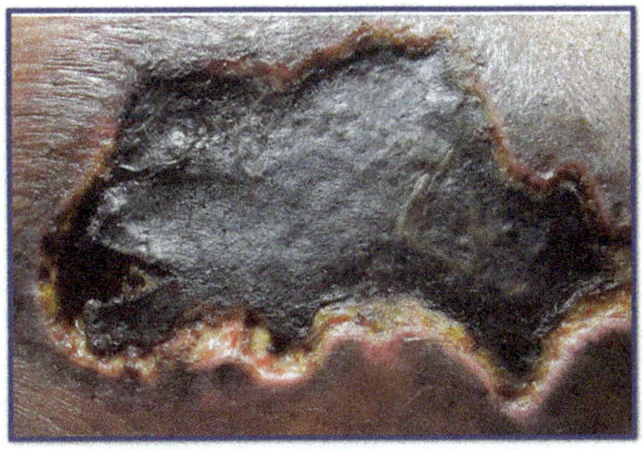

FIGURE 1. Patient with vasculitis and positive lupus anticoagulant on presentation

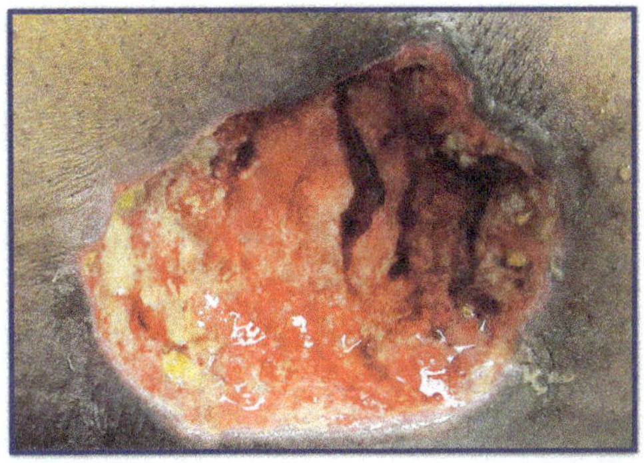

FIGURE 2. S/q to surgical debridement

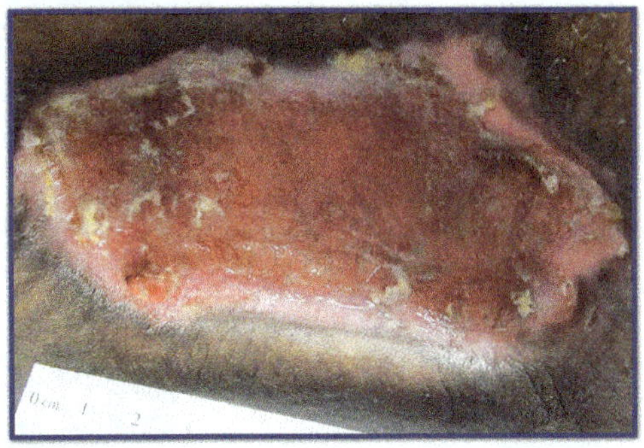

FIGURE 3. S/q to negative pressure therapy

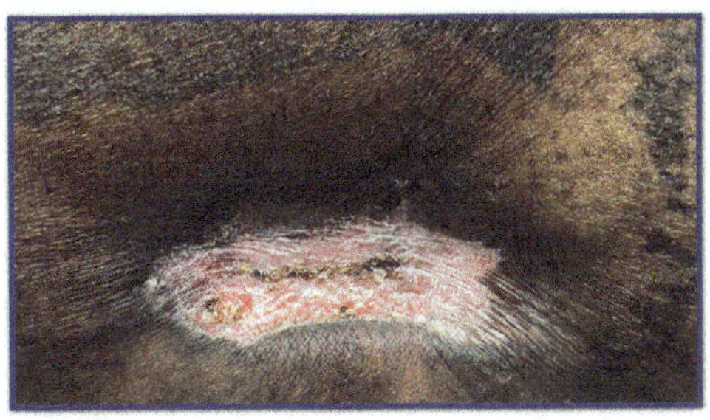

FIGURE 4. S/q to application silver alginate and then collagen dressing till complete epithelialization

II. Pathway for approach to commonly misdiagnosed wounds and unusual leg ulcers

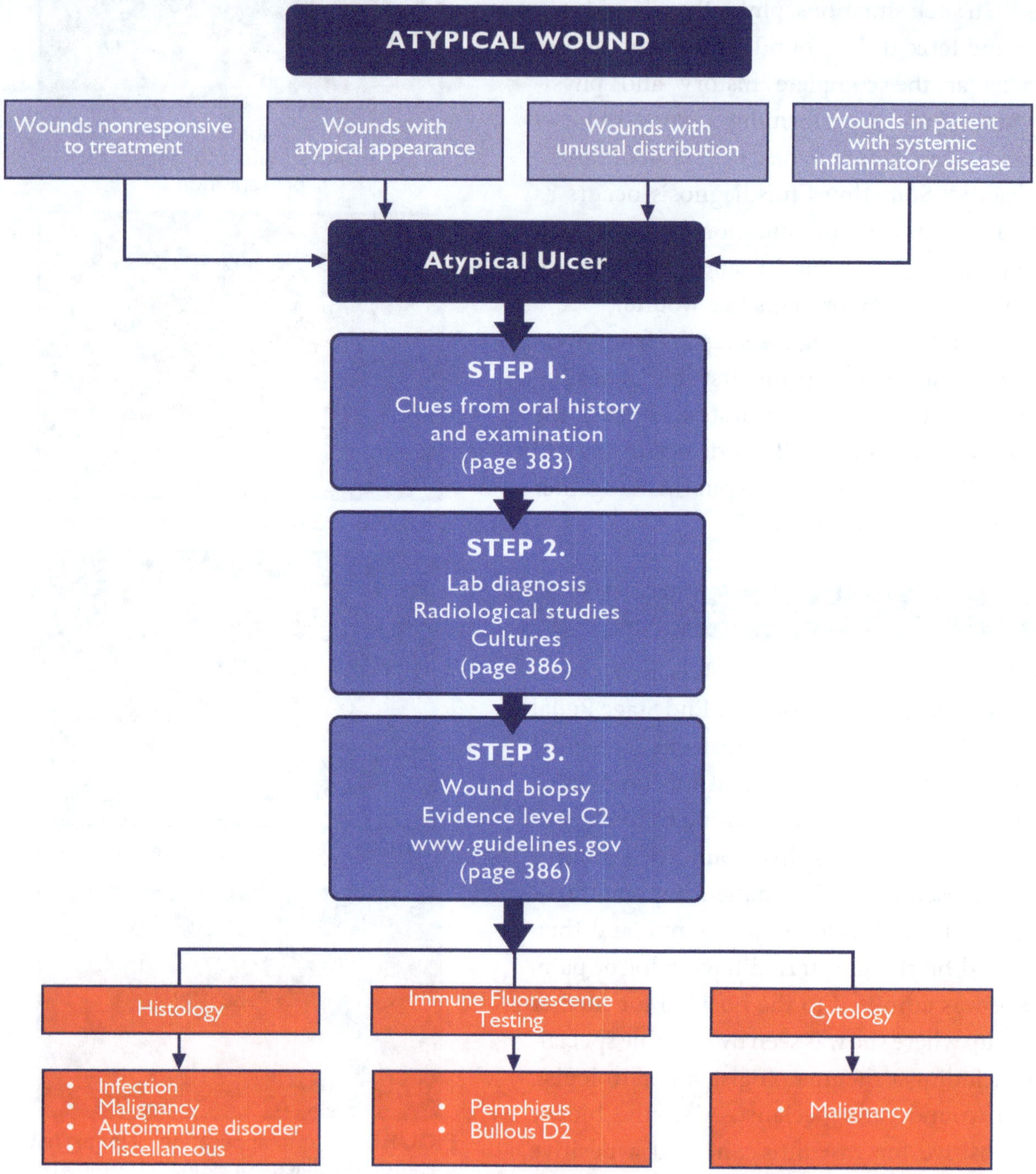

Step 1 from pathway

A. Clues from a good history [2,4,6]

Identify diagnosis by proper history and examination. Even with the technological innovations of the twenty-first century, history-taking remains the best and cheapest tool to make a good diagnosis. Recognizing clues from the patient's history can give important information about the patient's wound.

Inability to heal may be due to the following local or systemic factors.

a) Local factors

- Repeated external trauma because of inappropriate offloading
- Foot deformity causing abnormal pressure areas
- Uncontrolled edema
- Injury from use of toxic substances
- Inappropriate measures for exudate control
- Inappropriate infection control
- Tissue tension
- Hematoma formation
- Undebrided wound
- Poor blood supply
- Hypoxia

b) Systemic factors

- Arterial insufficiency
- Venous insufficiency
- Systemic conditions (collagen vascular disease, sickle cell disease, hemoglobinopathies, uremia, diabetes, jaundice)
- Immunosuppresive drugs (systemic corticosteroids, anticancer drugs, NSAIDS)
- Immunosuppressive diseases (HIV)
- Local or systemic malignancy
- Exposure to radiation
- Malnutrition
- Old age
- Systemic infection

All these local and systemic factors need to be looked at when taking history of a patient with a wound.

B. Clues from examination[2-6]

a) General appearance

- Cushingoid appearance – Corticosteroid use, disease with excessive release of corticosteroids
- Rheumatoid joints – Pyoderma gangrenosum, rheumatoid ulcer, vasculitis
- Cachexia – Malnutrition, AIDS, cancer, other infectious etiologies (tuberculosis)
- Scleroderma face (purse string mouth) – Calcinosis, Raynaud's syndrome
- Abnormal affect, posture, facial expression – Factitious disorder
- Facial palsy, weakness in 1 or more extremities – Cerebrovascular accident. If bed bound or wheelchair bound, more prone to pressure ulceration

b) Examination of skin and identifying skin disease morphology[3,5]

- Macule – A circumscribed, flat, nonpalpable lesion that is flush with the level of surrounding normal skin; smaller than 10 mm in diameter
- Patch – A flat, nonpalpable lesion that is flush with the level of surrounding normal skin; greater than 10 mm in diameter

TABLE 1. Significance of patient history[4]

Important clues found in the patient history	Significance to the patient's wound
General History	
Age and sex	Leg ulcers more common in older women; some rheumatic disease more common in women
Initial injury	Spontaneous or gradual appearance; trauma from accident, shoes, insect bite
Duration of wound	Acute—less than one week; subacute –one week to four weeks; chronic – more than three weeks
History of recurrence	Venous ulcers likely to be recurrent
History of previous DVT	Predisposing factor to venous disease
Previous vein surgery or pelvic trauma	Indicative of venous disease
Intermittent claudication	Indicative of arterial disease
Rest pain	Indicative of arterial disease
Systemic symptoms	Indicative of systemic disease leading to ulcers
Arthralgia	Associated with some ulcers associated with systemic disease
Social History	
Smoking	Predisposes to or worsens arterial disease
Alcohol	Vitamin deficiency
IV drug use	HIV or ulcers related to IV drug use
Past Medical History	
Diabetes	Wound could be related to neuropathy, foot deformity, or arterial disease associated with diabetes
Connective tissue disease	Wound could be related to vasculitis, pyoderma gangrenosum, cryoglobinemia, etc.
Sickle cell disease	Increased risk of small-vessel occlusion
Dietary History	Some vitamin deficiencies common in a vegetarian diet; poor nutrition and obesity influences healing
Drug History	Steroids delay healing; hydroxyurea interferes with healing
Travel History or geographic location of patient	For example, leprosy remains a common cause for nonhealing wounds in India; spider bites are only endemic in Southern, Western, and Midwestern areas of USA.
Allergies	Contact dressings, bandages, and ointment can add to existing skin damage

- Papule – A superficial, circumscribed, dome-shaped or-flat-topped palpable lesion elevated above the skin surface; less than 10 mm in diameter
- Plaque – A lesion that rises slightly above the surface of the skin; greater than 10 mm in diameter
- Nodule – A firm lesion that is thicker or deeper than the average plaque or papule; is palpable as differentiated tissue
- Vesicle – An elevated lesion that contains clear fluid; less that 10 mm in diameter
- Bulla – An elevated lesion that contains clear fluid; greater than 10 mm in diameter
- Pustule – An elevated lesion that contains pus
- Urticarial (hives) – An allergic reaction characterized by white fluid- filled blisters (termed wheals) surrounded by erythema (flares)
- Livedo reticularis pattern – A mottled, lace-like purplish discoloration of the skin caused by thrombotic occlusion of the capillaries that leads to swelling of the venules

c) **Appearance of the extremity/extremities**[2-4,6]

- Edema – Venous disease, deep vein thrombosis, lymphedema, congestive heart failure with dependent edema
- Foot deformities – Neuropathic wounds, diabetes with autonomic neuropathy, osteomyelitis, rheumatoid arthritis
- Cyanosis – Arterial disease, Raynaud's syndrome
- Dependent rubor – Arterial disease
- Erythema – Infection, contact dermatitis
- Livedo Reticularis – Cholesterol emboli, collagen vascular disease, cryoglobulinemia
- Sclerodactyly – Scleroderma, Raynaud's syndrome
- Lipodermatosclerosis/hemosiderin pigmentation – Venous disease
- Eczema – Irritation arising from previous treatments

d) **Appearance of the wound**[2-4,6]

- *Configuration/wound edge*
  - Undermining edge – Pressure, pyoderma gangrenosum
  - Irregular edge/intact fascia – Venous
  - Undulating/scalloped – Rheumatoid ulcer
  - Linear/geometric – Factitious
  - Fenestrated – Pyoderma gangrenosum
  - Eschar – Ischemia, pressure
  - Irregular, raised, discolored – Malignancy
- *Wound base*
  - Green – Pseudomonas infection
  - Pale – Pressure, ischemia
  - Black – Arterial insufficiency
  - Red – Good granulation/vascularity
  - Exposed tendon – Pressure, shear, tension, fistula
  - Exposed bone – Osteomyelitis, pressure

e) **Location of the wound**

- Weight-bearing surface – Neuropathic wound, pressure
- Digital ulcers – Ischemia

- Gaiter area – Venous disease
- Tibial area – Arterial disease, necrobiosis lipoidica diabeticorum
- Vaginal ulcers – Behcet's disease
- Underlying internal viscera – Fistula, abscess, Crohn's disease, radiation injury

f) Surrounding skin

- Edge necrosis – Pyoderma gangrenosum, vasculitis, ischemia
- Redness around the wound – Vasculitis, arterial disease, contact dermatitis
- Purpura – Vasculitis
- Purple discoloration – Pyoderma gangrenosum, vasculitis, cryoglobulinemia, cryofibrinogenemia,
- Micro livedo – Cryoglobulinemia, cryofibrinogenemia, antiphospholipid syndrome
- Red/yellow – Necrobiosis lipoidica diabeticorum

Step 2 from pathway

Identify diagnosis by proper lab diagnostics and radiological studies.[4-6,8-9]

- Complete blood cell count (CBC) to look for leukocytosis, anemia, or thrombocytopenia
- Basic metabolic panel to look for renal insufficiency and electrolyte abnormalities
- Serum protein, albumin, prealbumin, and transferrin level to evaluate patient's nutritional status
- Coagulation studies to evaluate for hypercoagulable disorders and bleeding tendencies
- Increase values of ESR and CRP indicates infectious or inflammatory process
- Increase values of ANA suggests possibility of lupus
- Increase values of RF, ESR suggests possibility of rheumatoid arthritis
- Increase values of SCL 70 suggests possibility of scleroderma

Radiological studies like plain X-ray, CT, and MRI may help in looking for underlying osseous abnormalities including (osteomyelitis) and to rule out foreign body.

Step 3 from pathway

A. Wound biopsy[2-7,10]

"When in doubt, consider wound biopsy."
—Jayesh Shah, MD

Identify diagnosis by proper wound biopsy. Wound biopsy is a simple bedside procedure performed to establish a definitive diagnosis in a chronic, nonhealing wound. The correct time to obtain a biopsy of a wound base and its margins remains controversial. Some clinicians advocate performing biopsies of wounds that have been present for longer than 3 months and wounds that have not responded to standard therapy. Some clinicians routinely biopsy all wounds. Considering the uncommon nature of malignant wounds, some authors suggest that only suspicious wounds undergo biopsy. The following indications can serve as general guidelines for performing a biopsy.

B. Indications

1. Indications for pathology diagnosis
   - Chronic wound refractory to healing by standard wound care

TABLE 2. Lab markers in diagnosing atypical wounds[8]

Hematologic tests	Chemistry tests	ımmunologic tests (autoimmune disorders, vasculitis)
Complete blood count with differential	Kidney (blood urea nitrogen, creatinine)	ESR (erythrocyte sedimenation rate)
C-reactive protein	Liver (liver enzymes, hepatitis panel)	C Reactive Protein
Protein S	Electrolytes	ASO(anti-streptolycin -o)
Factor V Leiden	Glucose	Rheumatoid factor (RF)
Prothrombin time/partial thromboplastin time	Fasting lipids	Serum and immune protein electrophoresis
	Iron	Antineutrophil cytoplasmic antibodies and protoplasmic-staining
	Folate	antineutrophil cytoplasmic antibodies
	Parathyroid hormone	Indirect immunogluorescence
	Phosphorus	Antiphospholipid antibodies (lupus anticoagulant, IgG, or IgM anticardiolipin antibodies)
	Magnesium	Scl 70 (scleroderma -70)
	Albumin	
	Prealbumin	
	Transferrin levels	
	Vitamins/minerals	

- Wound that have increased in size despite appropriate treatment
- Unusually painful wounds, or painless wounds in a patient who does not have neuropathy
- Wounds with excess granulation tissue that extends beyond the margins
- Wounds with irregular base or margin
- Wounds with excess bleeding or exophytic growth

2. Indications for biopsy for quantitative culture
   - Infected wounds
   - Maldorous wounds
   - Wounds that experience a change in drainage

C. Types of wound biopsy

1. Punch biopsy
   - Simple punch biopsy
   - Deep punch biopsy
   - Multiple punch biopsy
2. Wedge biopsy
   - Deep wedge biopsy
   - Deep incisional wedge biopsy
3. Shave biopsy
4. Excisional biopsy

D. Procedure for each type of biopsy

- Simple punch biopsy: biopsy in which the tissue is obtained by a punch (Figure 5); usually 0.4 mm or 0.5 mm punch is used.
- Deep punch biopsy: deeper tissues are taken for biopsy. Multiple punch biopsies are sometimes needed to make a diagnosis.
- Wedge biopsy: biopsy in which the tissue is removed by surgical cutting (Figure 6). Optimally, wound biopsy should include wound bed and the surrounding skin. Wedge biopsy is indicated if cancer is suspected. Biopsy should be extended well beyond the wound perimeter. Also, multiple wound biopsies from different areas of the wound should be performed. A biopsy should also be taken from the center of the wound bed (Figure 6). If biopsy results do not match the clinical findings then repeat biopsy should be performed.

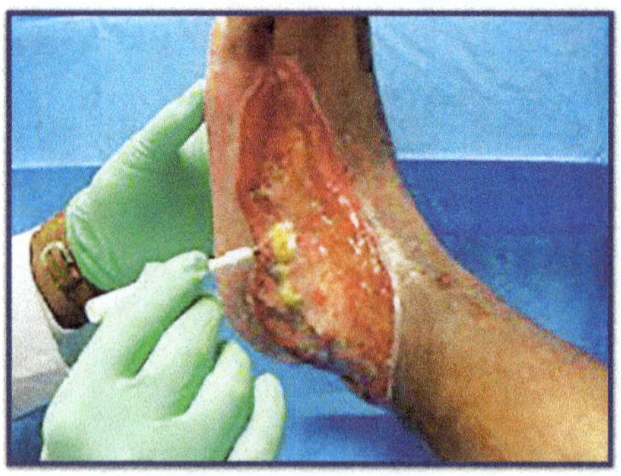

FIGURE 5. Punch biopsy

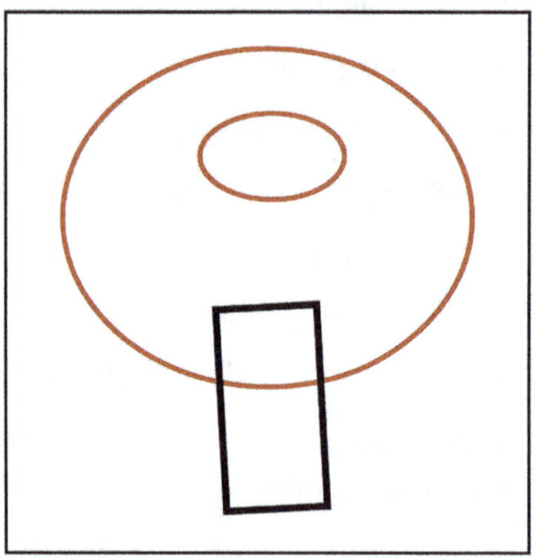

FIGURE 6. Sketch of wound sites for wedge biopsy

E. Complications

Biopsy sites in wounds usually heal and do not generally worsen the condition. Most common complication from biopsy can be bleeding from the biopsy site, which, in most cases, can be stopped with chemical cauterization.

F. Relative contraindications

- Blood dyscrasia
- Extremely vascular wounds or venous congestion
- Anticoagulation medications

III. Differential diagnosis of commonly misdiagnosed wounds and unusual leg ulcers

A. Common skin conditions seen by wound healing providers

1. *Contact dermatitis*

See Figures 7a-7c. Contact dermatitis is a very common skin condition. There are two types of contact dermatitis.

- Allergic
- Irritant

Pathophysiology

Allergic contact dermatitis is type IV delayed hypersensitivity reaction to a specific chemical, while irritant contact dermatitis is caused by a direct toxic effect on the epidermis from exposure to a chemical such as a cleaning agent, other caustic substances, or repeated wetting and drying and is not mediated by the immune system.[3,11-13]

Clinical presentation

Contact dermatitis is often mistaken as a wound infection. Usually patient with contact dermatitis has geometric, sharply bordered pattern of the rash in area of contact. Also, patient has lot of pruritus in that area, while patient with allergic contact dermatitis presents with geometric lines or splatters of red papules and vesicles especially on exposed areas. Patch testing may help to identify the causative allergens.[3,11-13]

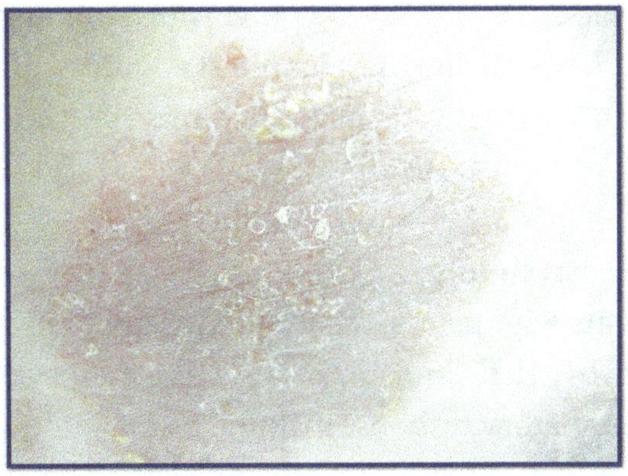

FIGURE 7a. Contact dermatitis on back after application of medication patch
Courtesy R. Singh

Common causes of contact dermatitis

- Plants: Poison ivy, poison oak, and poison sumac
- Nickel
- Neomycin and bacitracin[12]
- Transdermal medications such as clonidine, fentanyl[13]
- Soaps, moisturizers
- Certain wound dressings

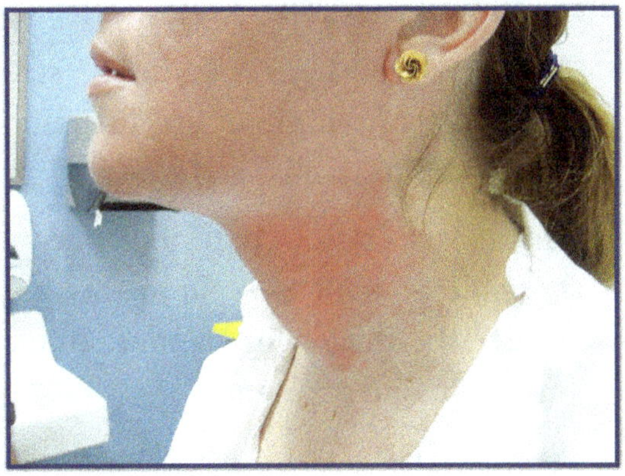

FIGURE 7b. Contact dermatitis on face after wearing jewelry Courtesy R. Singh

Differential diagnosis

- Wound infections
- Cellulitis
- Spider bite
- Atopic dermatitis
- Xerotic eczema
- Nummular dermatitis
- Stasis dermatitis

Treatment

It is curable by avoiding the causative material. Low-potency local steroid cream may be helpful. Systemic steroid might be necessary in some cases.

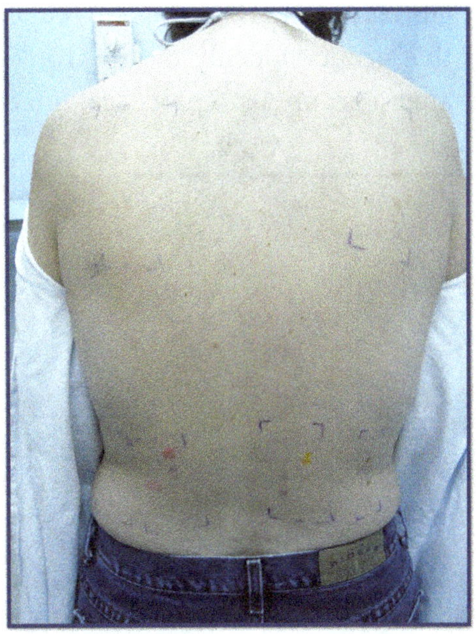

FIGURE 7c. Patch testing
Courtesy R. Singh

2. *Psoriasis*

See Figure 8. Psoriasis is a chronic inflammatory dermatosis that manifests with scaling, variably pruritic plaques that may be recalcitrant to topical therapy.[14]

Pathophysiology

Patients with psoriasis have increased inflammatory Th1, Th17, and Th22 cells. It is a multisystem inflammatory response including skin, joint, cardiovascular disease, and metabolic disorder.[14]

Clinical presentation

Multiple kinds of psoriasis[14]

- Psoriasis vulgaris: red, thick, scaling plaques concentrated on the elbows, knees, ankles, shins, and trunk
- Inverse psoriasis: red, thin plaques with variable amount of scale in the axillae, under the breasts or pannus, intergluteal cleft, and perineum
- Sebopsoriasis: red, thin plaques in the scalp, eyebrows, nasolabial folds, central chest, and pubic area
- Guttate psoriasis: 0.5 to 2 cm red plaques that erupt suddenly on the trunk often after a group A streptococcal infection

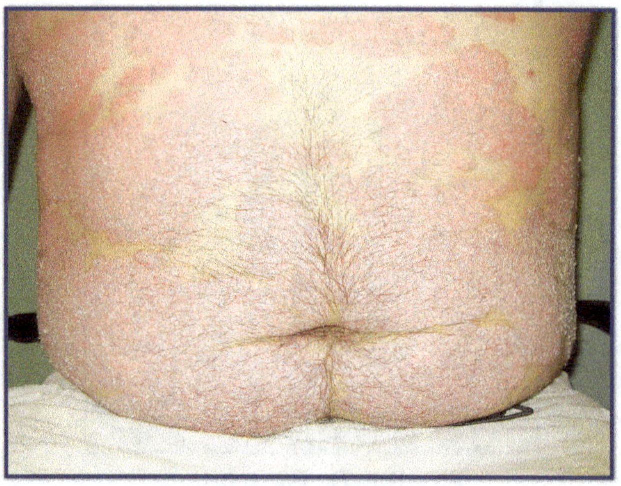

FIGURE 8. Psoriasis
Courtesy Dirk Elston, MD

- Nail psoriasis: indentations and "oil spot" often involving multiple nails

Treatment

Topical therapy[14]

- Intermittent pulses of medium- to high-potency topical glucocorticoids
- Topical vitamin D analogues
- Keratolytic agents

Systemic therapy[14]

Phototherapy

Traditional systemic agents or biologics should be considered for

- Severe (> 10% body surface area)
- ii. Psoriasis arthritis or
- iii. Psoriasis unresponsive to topical therapy

B. Common skin conditions with acneiform eruptions

1. *Acne*

See Figure 9. It is chronic inflammatory skin condition characterized by blackheads, whiteheads, papules, pustules, and nodules.[15-16]

Pathophysiology

Androgens stimulate increased sebum production. Acne lesions are formed because of proliferation and accumulation of keratinocytes that block the outflow of sebum.[15-16] The anaerobic bacterium *Propionibacterium acnes* proliferates in the comedones and causes inflammation and dermal leakage which leads to formation of papules, pustules, deep cysts, and nodules.[15-16]

Clinical manifestations

Shows coexisting open and closed comedones, papules, pustules, and nodular lesions primarily on face, neck, and upper trunk.[15-16]

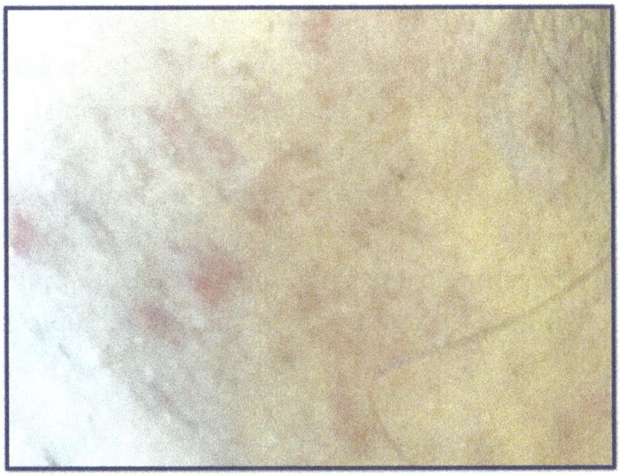

FIGURE 9. Acne

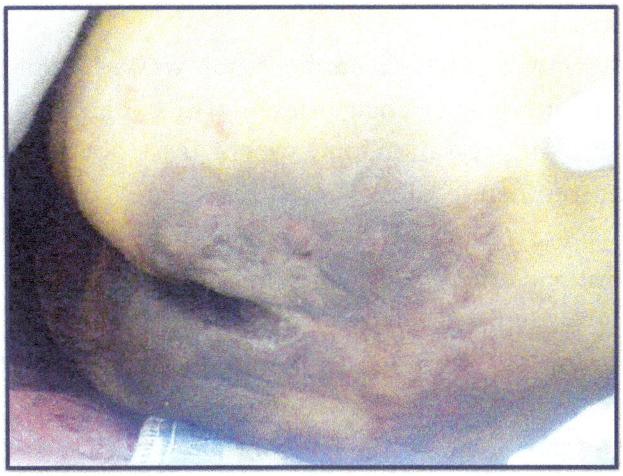

FIGURE 10. Hidradenitis suppurativa

Differential diagnosis

- Rosacea
- Medication-induced acneiform eruption
- Bacterial folliculitis

Treatment

In patients with mild to moderate acne could be treated with topical retinoids, salicylic acid, azelaic acid, benzoyl peroxide, and topical antibiotics (clindamycin, erythromycin).[15,16]

In patients with moderate acne could be treated with topical dapsone or oral doxycycline or minocycline and erythromycin.[15-16] Patient could also be treated with oral contraceptives or spironolactone.[15-16]

Patients with severe disease could be treated with oral isotretinoin.[15-16]

2. *Hidradenitis suppurativa (HS)*

See Figure 10. HS is also called 'acne inversa." It is a chronic inflammatory disease that predominantly affects the apocrine gland–bearing areas of the skin.[17]

Pathogenesis

HS begins with follicular occlusion but not infection or inflammation of apocrine glands; that is why it is called "acne inversa."[17] Following occlusion, there is buildup of secretions in follicular duct and results in rupture and subsequently develops inflammatory reaction resembling abscess.[17]

Clinical presentation

HS is commonly found in axilla, breast and inframammary creases, inguinal folds, and gluteal cleft.[17] It is usually characterized by comedones, inflammatory papules, nodules, cysts, and scarring.[17] Usually these lesions are painful and are characterized with foul-smelling drainage.[17]

Differential diagnosis

- Folliculitis
- Abscess
- Carbuncle
- Ruptured epidermal inclusion cyst
- Cutaneous manifestation of Crohn's disease
- Sexually transmitted disease like granuloma inguinale or lymphogranulom venereum

Treatment

For mild disease, antibacterial washes, topical antibiotics, analgestics, warm compresses, smoking cessation, and weight loss should be recommended.(17-18)

For moderate disease, oral antibiotics with antibacterial washes and/or topical antibiotics (1% clindamycin gel), analgesics, and wide local excision should be considered. In women, oral contraceptives and spironolactone should also be considered.(17-18)

For severe disease, referral to dermatologist for consideration of tumor necrosis factor alpha inhibitor or to surgeon for wide local excision should be considered.(17-18)

C. Ulcers associated with infections

1. *Folliculitis*

See Figure 11. Folliculitis is inflammation of hair follicles

Pathophysiology

Folliculitis can be noninfectious or infectious inflammation of hair follicles

Clinical presentation

It is characterized by erythematous papules and pustules that are centered around a follicle on the face, chest, back, or buttocks. It is most often caused by *Staphylococcus aureus*,(19-20) but it can occur secondary to gram-negative organisms (i.e., *Pseudomonas*), fungi such as *Malassezia* or *Candida* species, or from viruses, including herpes viruses.(19-20) Sometimes folliculitis could be noninfectious (i.e., acne vulgaris, eosinophilic folliculitis, or a reaction to shaving or topical medications).(15)

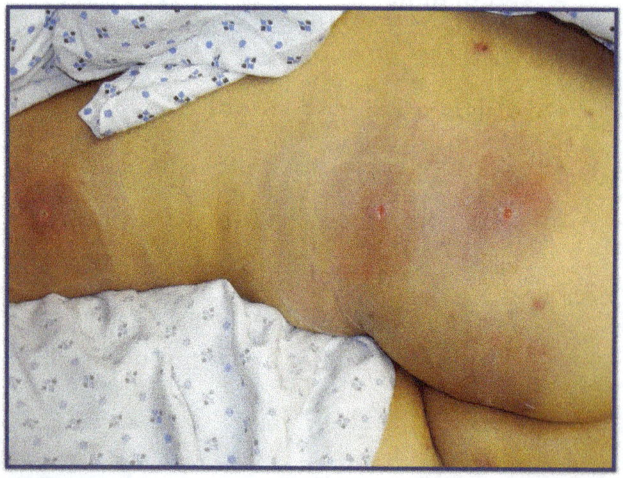

FIGURE 11. Multiple boils secondary to folliculitis

Differential diagnosis

- HS
- Acne

Treatment

Topical antibacterial agents such as chlorhexidine, topical antibiotics, or oral antistaphylococcal antibiotics.

2. *Abscesses, furuncles, and carbuncles*

Introduction and pathophysiology(19-20)

- **Abscess** (Figure 12a, Figure 12b) consists of collection of neutrophils and purulent material within the dermis or subcutaneous tissue
- **Furuncle** (Figure 13) is a small abscess because of infection which is centered on a hair follicle with pus extending into the dermis
- **Carbuncle** (Figure 14a, Figure 14b) is superficial inflammatory mass consisting of several inflamed hair follicles, and it has multiple sites of drainage

Clinical presentation

Usually presents with inflamed, tender, fluctuant dermal and subcutaneous nodule and associated warmth.(19-20) Erythema is present and can expand to represent surrounding cellulitis.(19-21) Purulent drainage may be expressed.

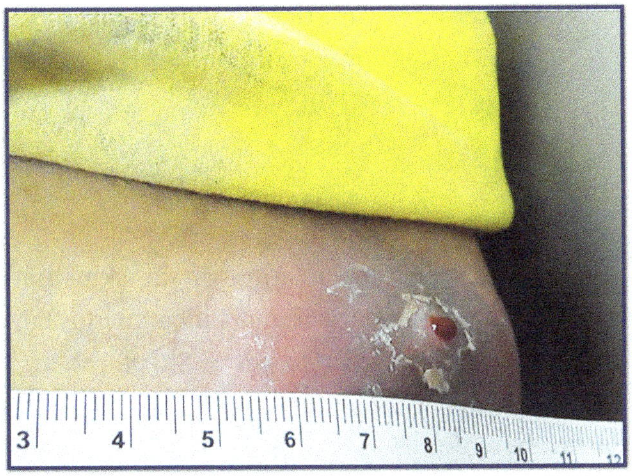

FIGURE 12a. Abscess of left hip

Differential diagnosis

- Inflamed epidermal inclusion cyst
- Sebaceous cyst

Treatment

- Incision and drainage with wound culture
- Warm compresses
- Local wound care with topical antibiotic cream
- Systemic antibiotics for associated cellulitis, systemic symptoms, a large abscess > 5cm, or multiple abscesses or in patient who is immunosuppressed.[19-21]
- Empiric antibiotics effective against MRSA (tetracycline, clindamycin, and trimethoprim-sulfamethoxazole) is usually first-line therapy.[19-21]

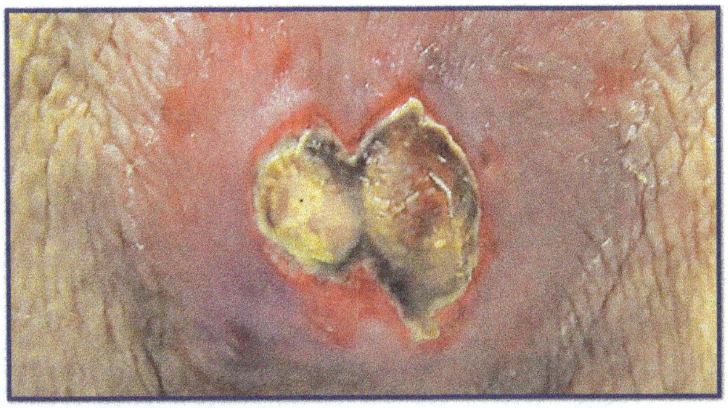

FIGURE 12b. Deep abscess right ischium

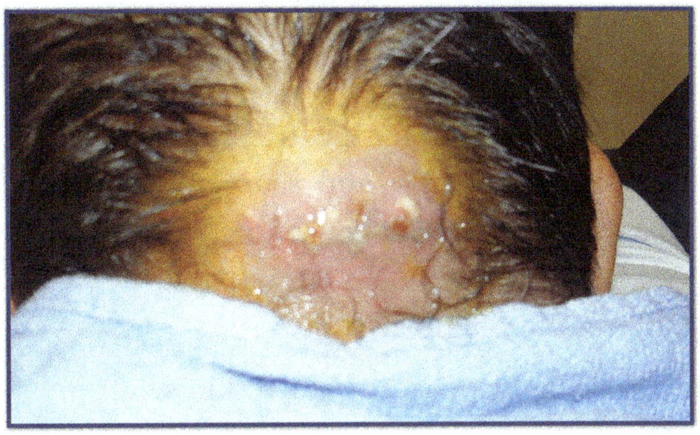

FIGURE 13. Furuncle

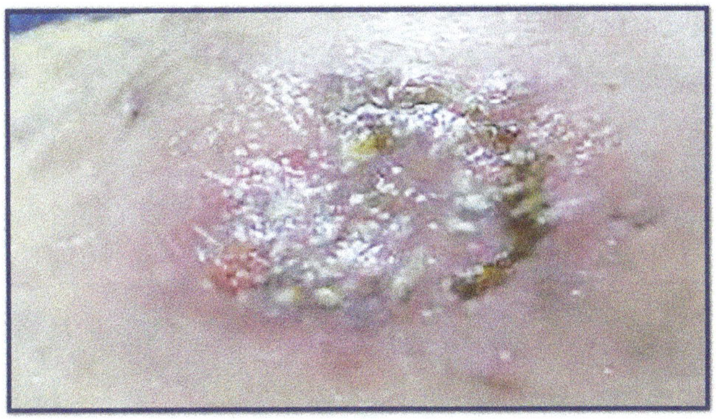

FIGURE 14a. Carbuncle before surgery

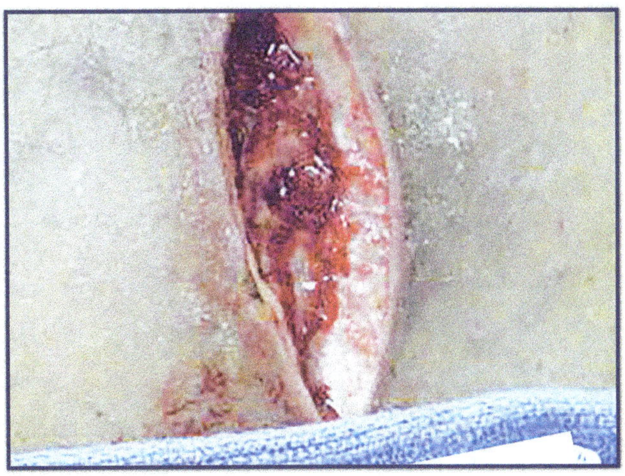

FIGURE 14b. Carbuncle after surgery

3. *Impetigo*

See Figure 15. Impetigo is an acute, highly contagious, and superficial skin infection caused by gram-positive organisms (*S. aureus* or *Streptococcus pyogenes*).[19-20]

Pathophysiology

Bullous impetigo is secondary to exfoliative toxin released by *S. aureus*.[19-20] Non-bullous impetigo is not toxin mediated.

Clinical presentation

Usually affects the face or extremities. It presents as vesicles, pustules, and sharply demarcated area with overlying honey-colored crust.[19-20]

Differential diagnosis

- Staphylococcal scalded skin syndrome
- Ecthyma gangrenosum

Treatment

- Topical mupirocin
- Washes with chlorhexidine
- Diluted bleach baths
- Systemic antibiotics (antistaphylococcal antibiotics) for more extensive infection[19-20]

4. *Cellulitis*

See Figure 16. Acute infection of the skin that involves the deeper dermis and subcutaneous fat, mainly caused by *Staphylococus* or *Streptococcus*.

Pathophysiology

Usually infection starts from superficial breaks, microscopic break, or trauma. Patients with diabetes mellitus, older age, lymphedema, and peripheral vascular disease have much higher risk for recurrent cellulitis.

Clinical presentation

Patient has four classical cardinal signs like erythema, pain, warmth, and swelling. Systemic symptoms may include fever, chills, and malaise. It is good idea to mark erythema with marker so progression of cellulitis can be monitored.

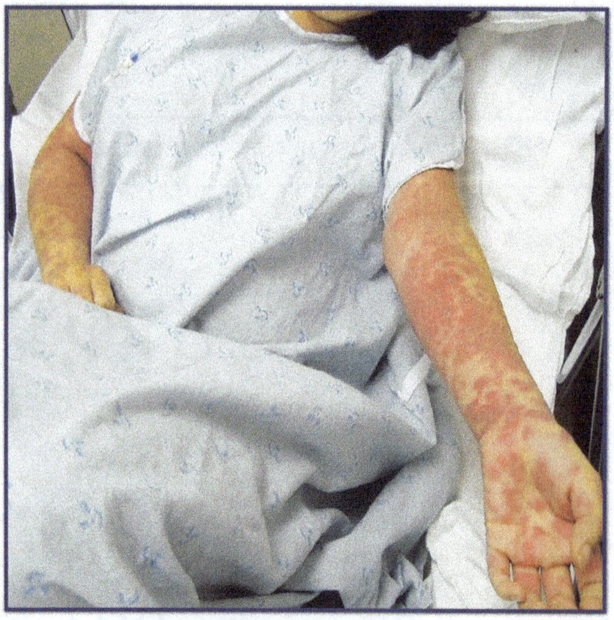

FIGURE 15. Impetigo
Courtesy of Rajinder Singh, MD

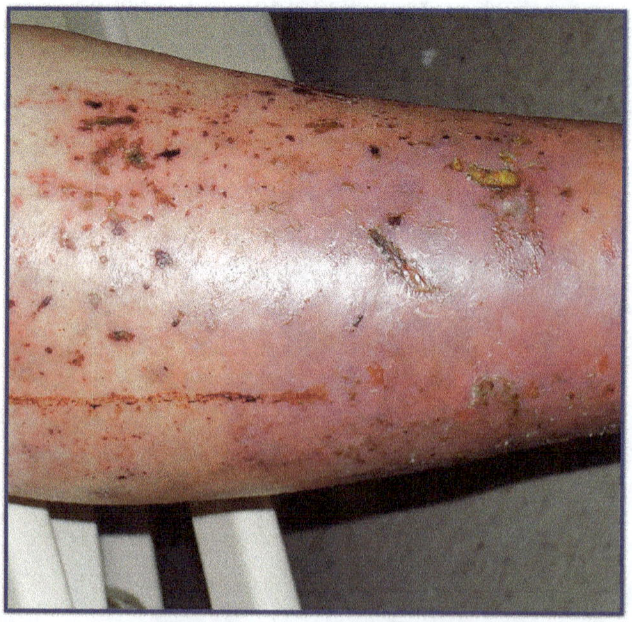

FIGURE 16. Cellulitis of leg

Differential diagnosis

- Acute stasis dermatitis
- Contact dermatitis
- Deep venous thrombosis
- Panniculitis
- Erysipelas

Treatment

Systemic antibiotics covering both *Streptococcus* and *Staphylococcus* with beta lactam antibiotics such as cephalexin or dicloxacillin, clindamycin, or a macrolide antibiotic can be used.[21]

5. *Actinomycosis*

Clinical types of actinomycosis are predominantly cervicofacial, abdominal, or thoracic. Actinomycosis of foot is rare but reported in the literature.[22-25]

Actinomycosis israelli is the most common cause of actinomycosis in humans.

Actinomyces organisms are gram-positive, non-spore-forming anaerobic bacilli (Figure 17c).

Pathophysiology

The infection is usually accompanied by the presence of some other bacteria that facilitates its invasion of tissue. Organisms also produce sulphur granules.[22-25]

Clinical presentation

Typical course of development is a painless swelling of the soft tissue that becomes indurated, followed by a period of apparent inactivity; then draining sinuses appear, followed by sinus tracts and osteomyelitis (Figures 17a-b).

Differential diagnosis

- Nocardiosis

Treatment

Recommended treatment is surgical excision of all necrotic tissue, sinus tracts, and infected bone, followed by a postoperative course of antibiotics for minimum of 6 months; ampicillin is the first drug of choice,[22-25] followed by doxycycline; sulfonamides and clindamycin may be used. Local wound management includes treating locally with topical antibiotics and antiseptic wound cleansers.

6. *Tuberculosis* (*Mycobacterium tuberculi*)

Tuberculosis is caused by bacteria belonging to the *Mycobacterium tuberculosis* complex. The disease usually affects the lungs, but in some instances it can cause cutaneous manifestations like abscesses, chronic ulcers (Figure 18), scrofuloderma, lupus vulguris, milliary lesions, and erythema nodosum.

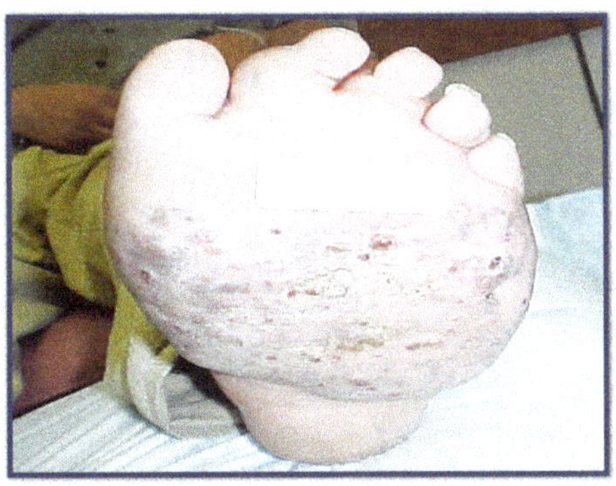

FIGURE 17a. 32-year-old Hispanic male presents with 3-year history of multiple sinuses of foot

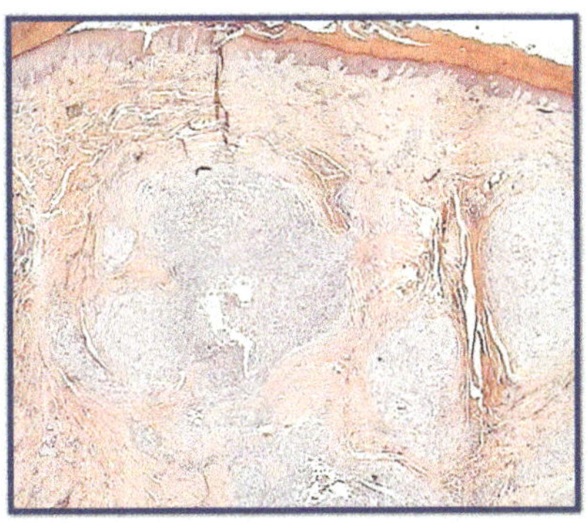

FIGURE 17b. Multiple abscesses on microscopic exam

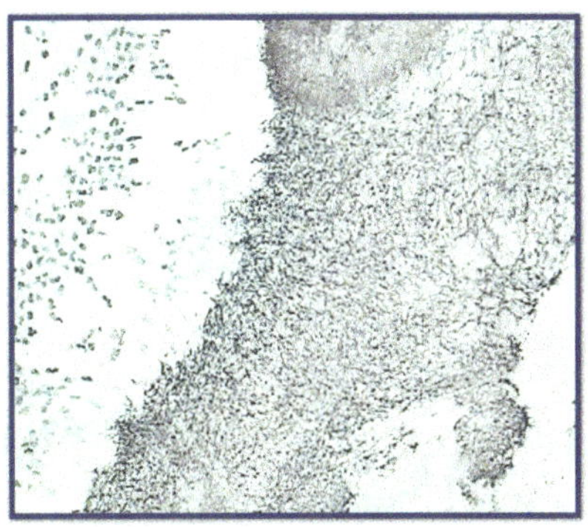

FIGURE 17c. Neutrophils and filamentous organisms (*Actinomycosis israeli*)

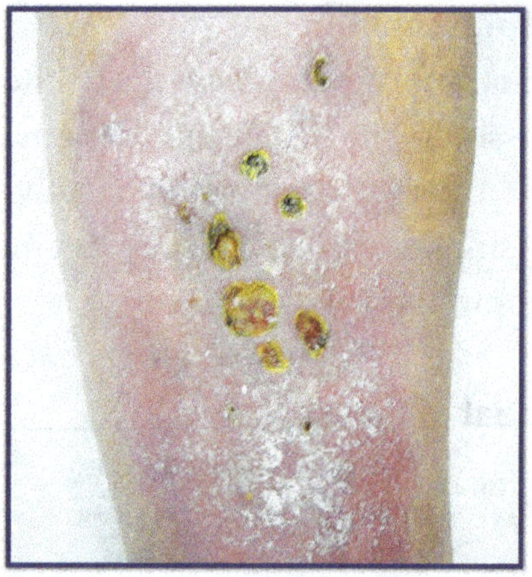

FIGURE 18. Mycobacterium tuberculosis ulcers
Courtesy of Bharat Shah, MD

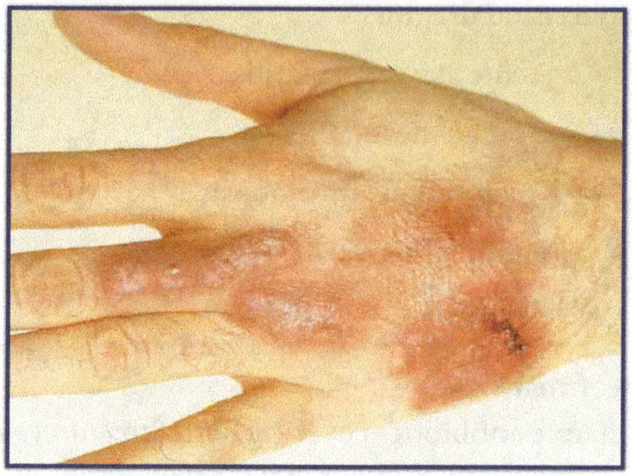

FIGURE 19. Mycobacterium marinum
Courtesy Dirk Elston, MD

Nontuberculous mycobacteria
Nontuberculous mycobacteria are ubiquitous environmental acid-fast bacilli belonging to species other than *Mycobacterium leprae* and Mycobacterium tuberculosis complex.

***Mycobacterium marinum* (swimming pool and fish tank granuloma)** - *Mycobacterium marinum* is slow-growing bacteria

Pathophysiology
Trauma-associated skin infection after exposure to fresh or salt water with contaminated tropical fish tanks, swimming pool, or saltwater fish for a period from one week up to two months.[26-27]

Clinical presentation
A small, violet papule, nodule, or pustule may appear at the site of minor trauma.[26-27] The lesion may evolve to form a crusted ulcer or small abscess (Figure 19). It is usually caused by *M. marinum*.

Treatment
Lesions often heal spontaneously; however, in case of persistence, lesions should be treated with rifampin in combination with ethambutol, trimethoprim/sulfamethoxazole, or minocycline for a period of at least three months.[26-27]

***Mycobacterium ulcerans* (Buruli ulcer)** -
In many tropical areas throughout the world but mainly found in Africa.[28]

Clinical presentation
M. ulcerans may cause an itching nodule on arms or legs, which then breaks down to form a shallow ulcer of variable size (Figure 20).[28]

Treatment
Usually consists of excision or treatment with rifampin, clofazimine, or trimethoprim sulfamethaxole.[29]

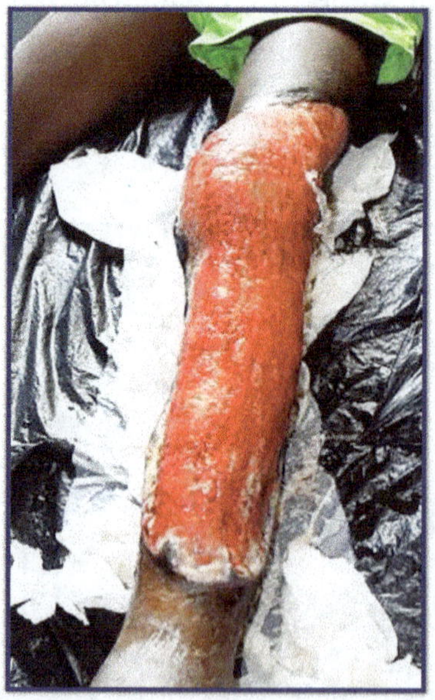

FIGURE 20. Buruli ulcer of leg
Courtesy of T. Treadwell

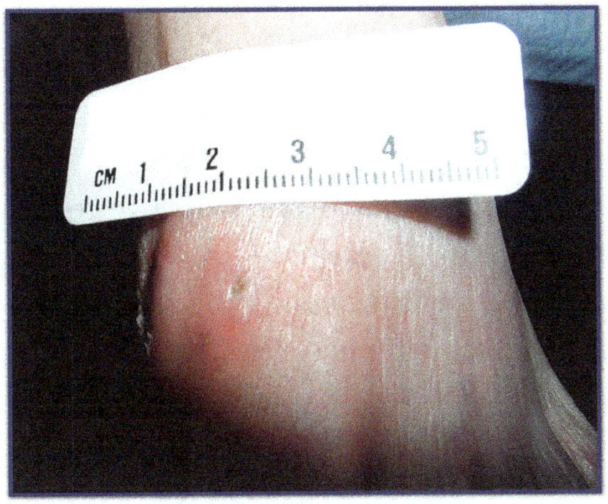

FIGURE 21. Mycobacterium fortuitum infection

Nodular skin lesions associated with *M. fortuitum* - It is skin infection found in patients who obtain pedicures at nail salons that use contaminated whirlpool footbaths.[30]

Pathophysiology

Occasionally, these kinds of mycobacteria are isolated from nodular skin lesions (Figure 21) of hospitalized patients, particularly those who are immunosuppressed and diabetics.[30] In some instances, there is associated lymphatic spread. They are rapidly growing mycobacteria, and punch biopsy usually reveals necrotizing granulomatous dermatitis.[30]

Clinical presentation

Usually found in distal lower extremity and appears initially as papule, and then it progresses to a boil before ulcerating (Figure 21).

Treatment

Usually all rapidly growing mycobacterial organisms are resistant to most antituberculous drugs.[30] Usually it is recommended to do susceptibility testing of amikacin, doxycycline, fluoroquinolones, tobramycin, sulfonamides, cefoxitin, clarithromycin, imipenem, and linezolid.[30] Recommendation is to give two to three drugs based on susceptibility for prolonged course.[30]

7. Leprosy

Leprosy remains as a common cause of non-healing wounds (Figure 22a) in developing countries like India, Brazil, Bangladesh, Indonesia, and Myanmar.[3,27]

Pathophysiology

Leprosy (Hansen's disease) is a chronic granulomatous disease, caused by *Mycobacterium leprae* that attacks superficial tissues, especially the skin and peripheral nerves.

Clinical presentation

Usually has neuropathy on both hands and feet. Patient also has foot deformity and ulcers with digital auto-amputations (Figure 22b).[3,27]

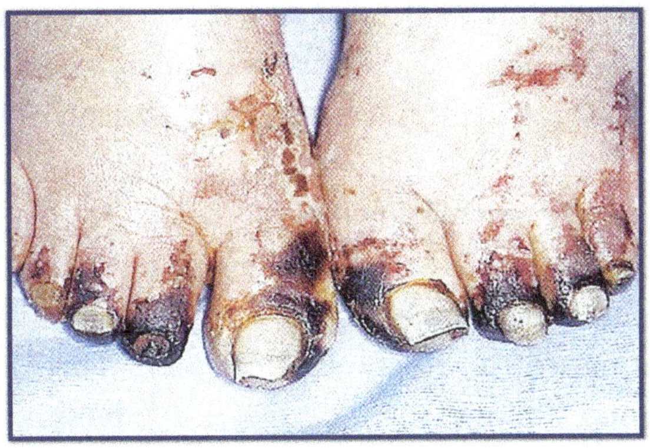

FIGURE 22a. Necrotic changes in multiple toes in leprosy patient

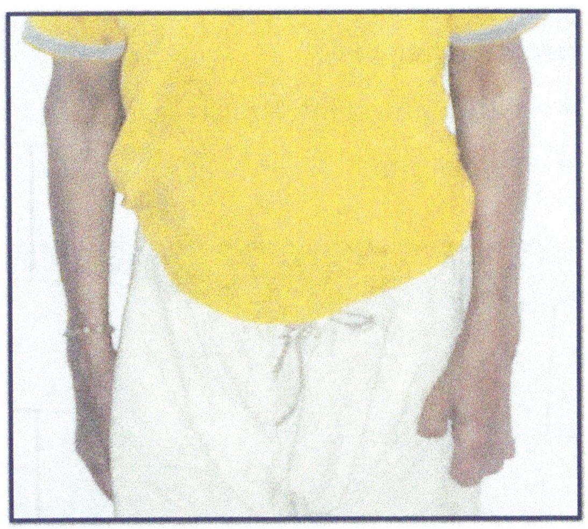

FIGURE 22b. Leprosy patient with auto-amputations of distal finger and toes

Treatment

- Paucibacillary disease – Dapsone at 100mg/d plus rifampin at 600mg/d for one year
- Multibacillary disease – Dapsone at 100mg/d plus rifampin at 600mg/d plus clofazimine at 50mg/d for two years

8. Sporotrichosis

Sporothrix schenckii is found in soil, moss, and other vegetation. Nursery workers, florists, and gardeners acquire this illness from roses, sphagnum moss, and other plants.(31)

Pathophysiology

Infection results from inoculation of *S. schenckii* (fungus) into subcutaneous tissue via minor trauma. Pulmonary and osteoarticular infections can happen in immunosuppressed patients.(31)

Clinical presentation

It usually presents as non-tender, red maculopapular granuloma confined to the site of inoculation which sometimes ulcerates (Figure 23). Similar lesions then occur along lymphatic channels proximal to the inoculation site. Diagnosis is established by culture.(31)

Differential diagnosis

- Other fungal infections
- Spider bite

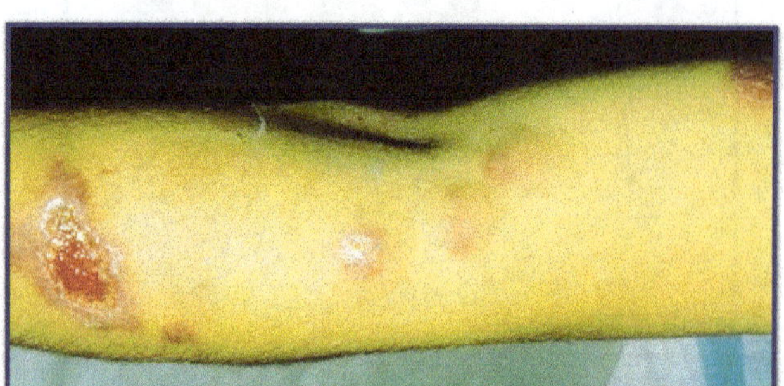

FIGURE 23. Sporotrichosis

Treatment

Oral itraconazole is the therapy of choice for cutaneous and osteoarticular sporotrichosis.(32-33) Other treatments that can be considered are saturated solution of potassium iodide, fluconazole, terbinafine, and amphothericin B.(31-32) Local wound treatment includes topical antifungal or application of saturated solution of potassium iodide or application of heat locally.(31-32)

9. Superficial fungal infections

Pathophysiology(33-35)

Tinea infections are specific fungal infections caused by dermatophytes that locate exclusively in keratin (i.e., stratum corneum, hair, nails). The most common tinea infections are caused by *Epidermophyton*, *Trichophyton*, or *Microsporum*. Tinea infections are categorized according to the area of the body that is involved. Histological features of tinea infections include neutrophils in the stratum corneum, often with parakeratosis and a variable inflammatory response in the dermis

Clinical presentation(33)

Usually presents as pruritic, annular erythematous patches with rim of scale and central clearing. Rarely lesions are pustular. Depending on the body part involved the affected area is named: Tinea capitis is infection of the hair follicles, typically of scalp but may involve eyebrows and eyelashes. Tinea barbae, tinea corporis (body) (Figure 24), tinea cruris (genital area), tinea pedis (feet) (Figure 25), and tinea unguium (Figure 26) or onychomycosis (nail) (Figure 27). Tinea nigra presents as hyperpigmented, scaly patch, often on the palmar aspect of the hands.

Diagnosis is made by visualizing organisms by periodic acid-Schiff (PAS) stain and potassium hydroxide (KOH) prep showing presence of branching hyphae.(33)

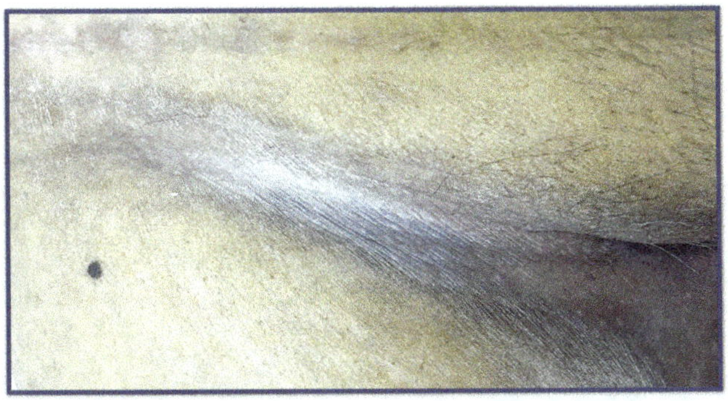

FIGURE 24. Tinea corporis infection in inguinal folds

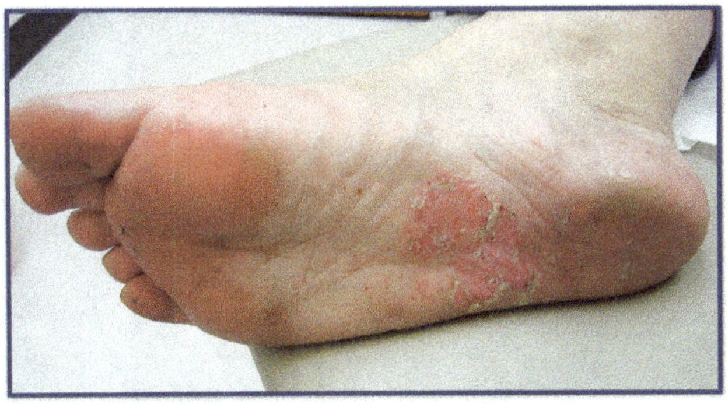

FIGURE 25. Tinea infections of foot

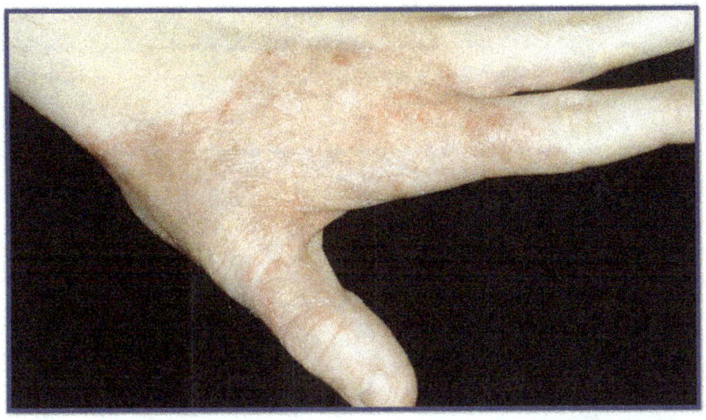

FIGURE 26. Tinea infection of hand
Courtesy of Dirk Elston, MD

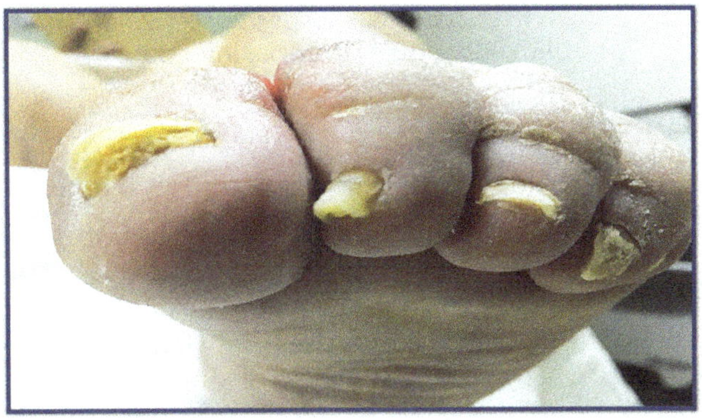

FIGURE 27. Tinea unguium-onychomycosis of nails

Treatment

Most superficial infections can be treated with topical antifungal agents such as miconazole, clotrimazole, ketoconazole, or terbinafine.[34] Nystatin is not found to be effective against dermatophytes. Combination of steroids and antifungal should be avoided because of risks of side effects and risks of treatment failure.[34] Oral antifungal agent with terbinafine or an azole may be necessary for severe infections, tinea capitis, and onychomycosis.[34]

10. *Herpes virus*

Pathophysiology

- Herpes simplex Type 1 – Oral or cold sores[36]
- Herpes simplex Type 2 – Genital Herpes[36]
- Herpes zoster – Varicella zoster or shingles[35]

Viruses usually are latent in the nerve dorsal root ganglia; they migrate to this area after initial infection where they can remain latent and cause subsequent reinfection and recurrence. Vesicles can involve the epidermis and dermis, with degenerative changes characterized by ballooning, multi-nucleated giant cells and eosinophilic intranuclear inclusions.

Clinical presentation

Classic presentation is a group of painful small vesicles on an erythematous base, transitioning to pustules and subsequent crusting of the lesions over time (Figure 28).[35-36] History and clinical presentation are often all that is necessary to establish the diagnosis of herpes; therefore, confirmatory tests such as the Tzanck smear, biopsy, or viral culture are rarely necessary.[35-36] In cases where herpes zoster involves first division of trigeminal nerve then urgent opthalmological consult is required.

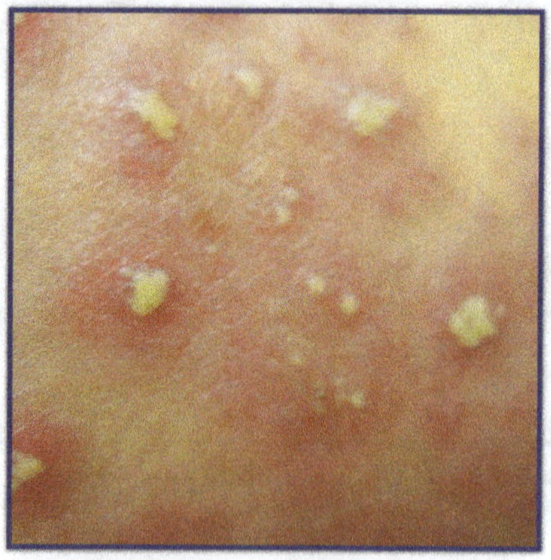

FIGURE 28. Herpes zoster with secondary bacterial infection

Differential diagnosis

- Other sexually transmitted disease (syphilis, chancroid, granuloma inguinale, lymphogranuloma venereum)
- Spinal nerve compression (pain)
- Poison ivy

Treatment

Oral antiviral agents are considered first-line therapies for herpes simplex infection and are most effective if instituted early on presentation.

Oral acyclovir, valacyclovir, or famciclovir, if initiated within 24–48 hrs of presentation, can shorten the course of herpes zoster and help prevent postherpetic neuralgia.

Herpes simplex can be treated with topical acyclovir.[36]

Locally thin hydrocolloid dressing also may be helpful to facilitate autolytic debridement.

11. *Necrotizing fascitis, Fournier's gangrene, myonecrosis (gas gangrene)*

Necrotizing fasciitis (NF)
(flesh-eating bacteria)

Necrotizing fasciitis is an acute, potentially fatal infection of the superficial and deep fascia of the skin and soft tissue, which progresses rapidly along the fascial planes with severe systemic toxicity.[37-42]

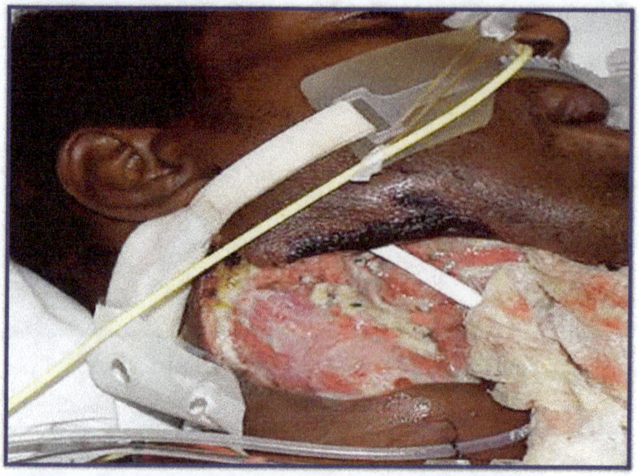

FIGURE 29a. Patient with gas gangrene on neck
Courtesy of Carolyn E. Fife, MD

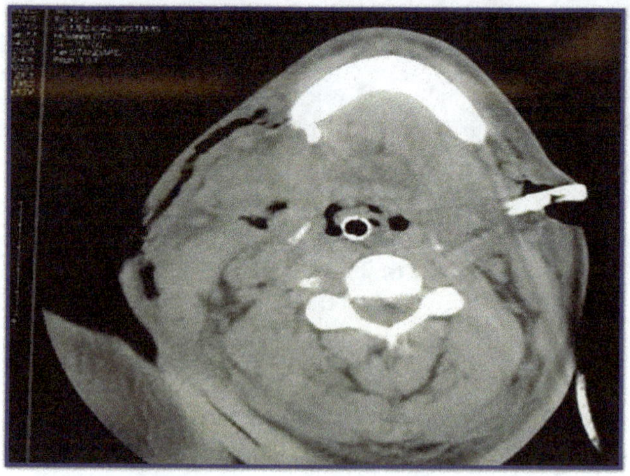

FIGURE 29b. CT Scan findings of gas
Courtesy of Caroline E. Fife, MD

Pathophysiology

Type 1 NF refers to polymicrobial infection comprising aerobic and anaerobic gram-positive and gram-negative organisms.[37,39]

Type II NF is a monomicrobial infection typically caused by *Streptococcus pyogenes* but it could also be caused by *S. aureus, Vibrio vulnificus*, or *Streptococcus agalactiae*.[37,39]

Type III NF (gas gangrene or clostridial myonecrosis) (Figure 29a, Figure 29b), primarily caused by *Clostridium perfringens*, usually develops after surgery or other significant trauma.[37,39]

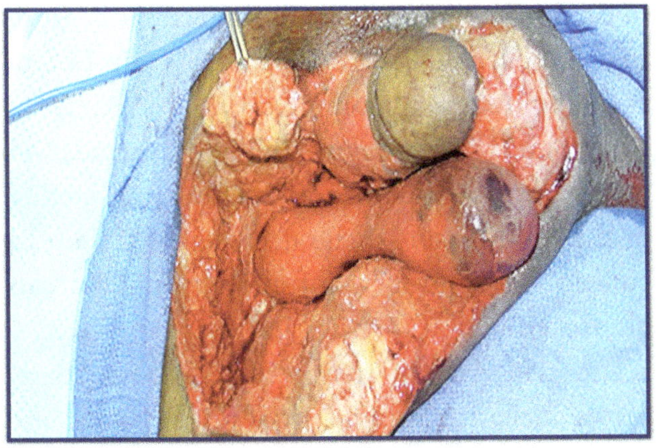

FIGURE 30. Fournier gangrene
Courtesy of Robert Michaelson, MD

Fournier's gangrene is an aggressive form of necrotizing infection of the perineum that may extend to the anterior abdominal wall, gluteal muscles, and in males, to the penis and scrotum (Figure 30). The causative organisms are a mixed collection of aerobic gram-negative bacteria, enterococci, and anaerobes, including *Bacteroides* and peptostreptococci.[40,42]

Usually arises after skin damage or trauma. It is more common in patients who have comorbidities, including diabetes mellitus, cancer, injection drug use, liver disease, and immunosuppression.[37-42]

Clinical manifestations

- Initially may resemble less complicated cellulitis.[37]
- Patient may have systemic toxicity with fever, chills, altered mental status, and hypotension.[37]
- Pain may be disproportionate to initial clinical findings.[37]
- Loss of sensation locally because of cutaneous nerve destruction.[37]
- Swelling with massive, "sausage-like" edema and "woody" induration and creptitus on palpation of the involved area.[37]
- Skin changes evolve rapidly and becomes ecchymotic, vesiculobullous, and gangrenous in appearance (Figure 31).[37]
- Labs suggestive of NF[38] are Creactive protein > 15 mg/dl, total leukocyte count > 15/micro liter, hemoglobin < 11 g/dL, sodium < 135 mEq/L, creatinine > 1.6 mg/dl, and glucose > 180 mg/dL.
- Plain X-ray may demonstrate subcutaneous gas (Figure 32), and MRI may help determine extent of infection.[37,39]

Differential diagnosis

- Cellulitis
- *Aeromonas hydrophila* cellulitis (recreational sports in freshwater lake)

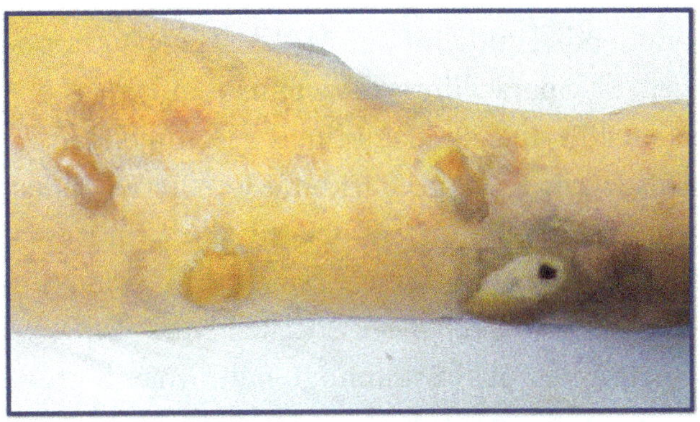

FIGURE 31. Necrotizing fasciitis

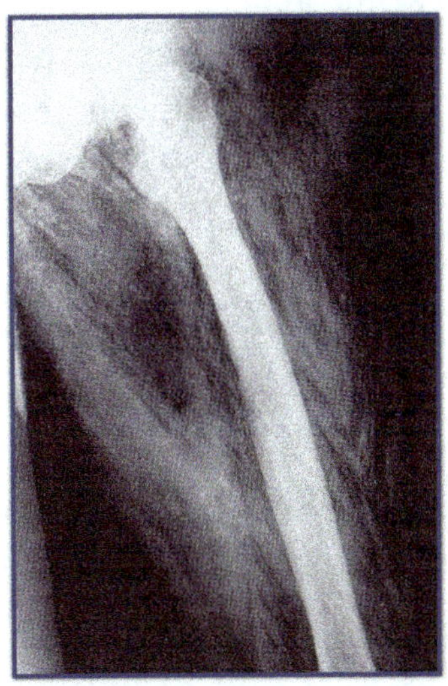

FIGURE 32. Gas gangrene – radiographic image of gas in thigh muscle
Courtesy of Caroline E. Fife, MD

- *Pasteurella multicida* (cat bite)
- *Capnocytophaga canmorsus* (dog bite)
- *Bacillus anthracis* (bioterrorism, contact with infected animal)
- *Francisella tularemia* (bite for infected animal i.e., cats or arthropod bites)
- *Mycobacterium marinum* (fish tank granuloma)
- *Mycobacterium fortuitum* (exposure to freshwater footbaths/pedicures at nail salon)
- *Vibrio vulnificus* (sea oysters)

Treatment

Early surgical exploration is the gold standard for diagnosis and treatment of necrotizing fasciitis.[37]

Empiric broad-spectrum antibiotics are recommended initially (anti-MRSA agent plus impenem or piperacillin-tazobactam.[37] In Type II NF penicillin and clindamycin is recommended.[37] Doxycycline plus ceftazidime is recommended for *Vibrio vulnificus*–associated NF,[37] and doycyline plus ciprofloxacin is recommended for *Aeromonas hydrophila*–associated NF.[37]

Intravenous immunoglobulin may be recommended in patients who have associated toxic shock syndrome.[37]

Adjunctive hyperbaric oxygen (HBO_2) therapy is recommended with the treatment protocol to be determined by the hyperbaric physician depending on many clinical variables. A typical regimen is at 2.0–2.5 ATA pressure for 90 minutes of oxygen given twice a day for mild to moderate cases[38] until there appears to be no further extension of necrosis in previously debrided area and infection is "controlled." In patients with gas gangrene, depending on the clinical situation, an even more aggressive regimen may be used with treatments given at 3 ATA for 90 minutes twice a day.[39] Afterwards patient can be switched to once-a-day treatment once the patient appears stabilized to be sure that the process does not flare up again before stopping treatment completely.

Wound management initially depends on amount of debridement, amount and quality of the residual soft-tissue necrosis, or if there is concern of continued infection.[6] Initially can be packed with 0.25% Dakin's solution or 0.25% acetic acid. Patient may require repeated surgeries including wound exploration. Once the wounds are more than 70% clean, negative-pressure wound therapy[40-41] can be used to help with wound bed preparation[6] before skin grafts or flaps. Patient may need admission to acute long-term care or rehabilitation unit.[42] Pain management and psychological care is also necessary in some cases.[42]

12. *Other infections*

Other rare infections to consider in patients with nonhealing wounds are coccidiomycosis, histoplasmosis, syphilis, viral infections such as herpes simplex or cytomegalovirus, and protozoal infections like leishmaniasis, to name a few.

D. Malignant wounds

Chronic nonhealing wounds of two to three months' duration, especially those which are refractory to healing, should be looked at with high index of suspicion for malignancy.[43] Malignancies and wounds can be related in two ways: there can be malignant transformation of chronic wound into cancer,[44] or malignancy can present as chronic wound.[45] Malignancy found within chronic wound, though rare, is well documented.[43-46]

The following clues should make a wound care physician suspicious of malignancy.[1-6]

- History of repeated trauma
- Wound with no obvious etiology
- Wound at unusual location

- Asymmetric wound
- Exuberant granulation tissue
- Rolled-out edges
- Fungating growth
- Purple-red color around the ulcer
- Ulcer in center of pigmented lesion (suspect melanoma)
- Wounds secondary to burns, trauma, radiotherapy, and diabetes are at a risk for malignant degeneration

Malignant wounds are more common in older patients with advanced cancer, although they can develop in patients with localized cancer and can be present for several years. In general, malignant wounds will not heal unless the malignancy is amenable to treatment with anticancer therapy. For basal or squamous cell cancer, complete excision or Mohs micrographic surgery is the treatment of choice.[47]

1. *Basal cell carcinoma (BCC)*

Pathophysiology

Basal cell carcinoma is a malignancy arising from epidermal basal cells usually as a result of prolonged exposure to ultraviolet light. In a study by Hansson et al., basal cell cancer was found to be the most common malignancy.[47-48]

Clinical presentation

Usually, basal cell cancer presents as a wound, outgrows its blood supply and erodes, and subsequently, ulcerates (Figures 33a-c). Often, this ulcer remains misdiagnosed for a long time, unless a wound biopsy is done early on.[49] Other characteristics include rolled edges, slightly raised, painless, and slow growing. BCC usually occurs on the head, neck, back, or chest where there has been sun exposure. They rarely metastasize; most have the ability to cause significant local tissue destruction if not removed. Multiple variants include superficial, infiltrative, and nodular basal cell carcinoma (with papules present).

Differential diagnosis

- Squamous cell cancer
- Vasculitis
- Venous stasis ulcer

Treatment

Mainly consists of surgery excision. Mohs micrographic surgery should be reserved for head and neck lesions. Superficial lesions may be treated topically. Sometimes after excision patient may require split-thickness skin graft (STSG).

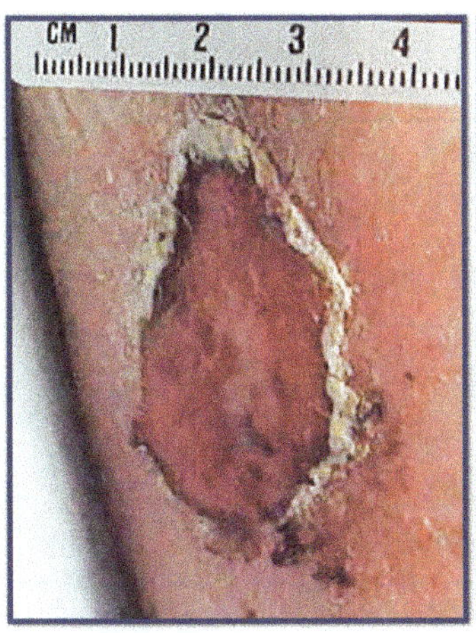

FIGURE 33a. Basal cell cancer on right leg

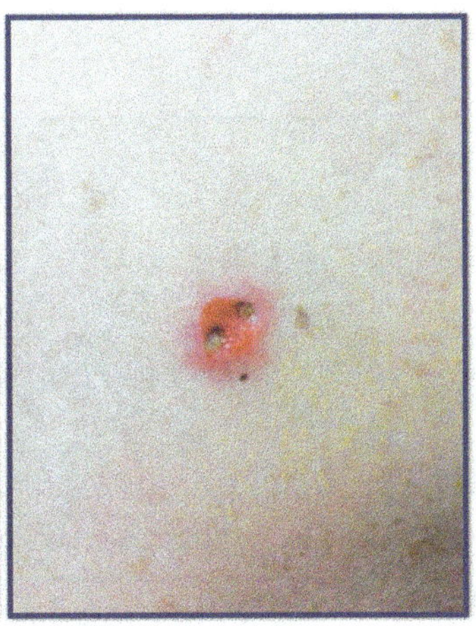

FIGURE 33b. Basal cell cancer on back

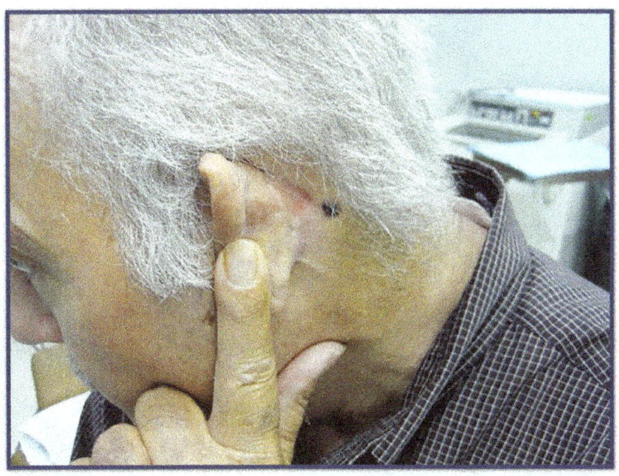

FIGURE 33c. Basal cell carcinoma on back of ear
Courtesy of Rajinder Singh, MD

2. *Squamous cell carcinoma (SCC)*

Pathophysiology

Primary cutaneous squamous cell carcinoma is a malignant neoplasm of keratinizing epidermal cells. It is the second most common form of skin cancer (Figure 34a).[44-51] Unlike basal cell carcinomas, which have a very low metastatic potential, squamous cell carcinoma can metastasize and grow very rapidly.[44,50-51] The development of squamous cell carcinoma has been reported in chronic wounds secondary to burns, trauma, hidradenitis suppurativa (Figure 34b), radiotherapy, diabetes, and draining sinus tract of chronic osteomyelitis.[44] It is the most common type of skin cancer seen in persons who are immunocompromised following solid-organ transplant.[51] Marjolin was the first to report that borders of a chronic wound underwent malignant changes.[50] If the SCC occurs in the area of a previous wound, for example, a burn, venous ulcer, or traumatic wound, years after the initial wounding, it is termed a Marjolin ulcer.[50] This type of SCC is usually very aggressive and requires excision beyond its margins and radiation therapy.[44,50-51]

Clinical presentation

SCC usually typically presents as red, scaly papules and nodules on sun-exposed skin. It is commonly hyperkeratotic or ulcerated and may metastasize and grow rapidly.

Differential diagnosis

- Basal cell cancer
- Vasculitis

Treatment

Localized SCC can be treated with Mohs micrographic surgery. Until recently, amputation had been the treatment of choice for squamous cell carcinomas that arose within chronic wounds associated with chronic osteomyelitis;[44] however, other reports have shown that other methods of ensuring complete local excision are also useful. If the SCC metastasizes, chemotherapy and radiation therapy are indicated, as well as excision of nodules and any regional lymph nodes that are involved.[44] Fine-needle aspiration can be used to diagnose any metastasis. Sometimes because of radiation therapy, patient may develop soft-tissue radiation necrosis and may require advance wound management including HBO_2 therapy, STSG (split thickness skin graft) and flap (Figures 35a-f).

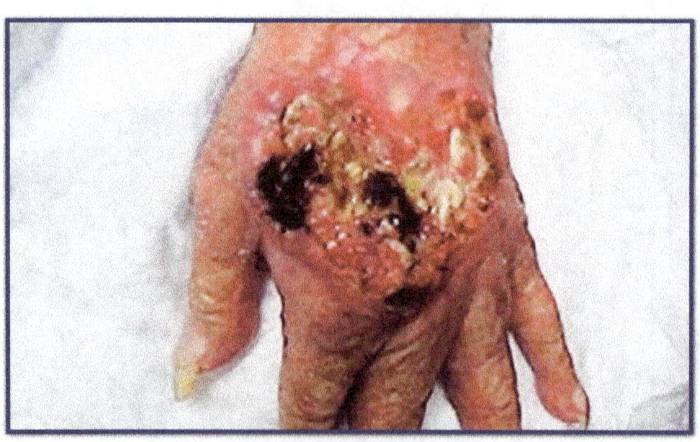

FIGURE 34a. Squamous cell cancer on left dorsal hand

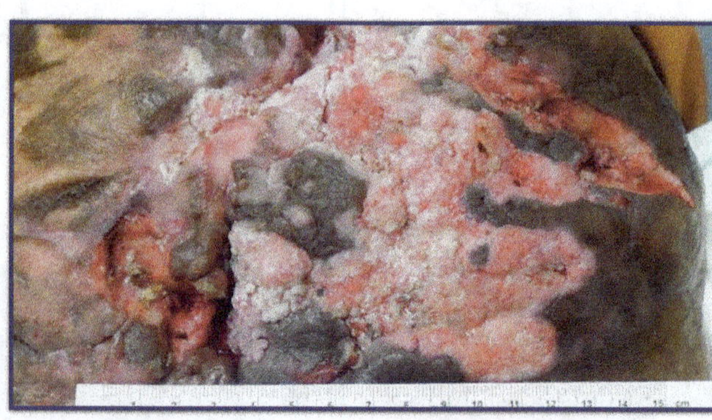

FIGURE 34b. Long-standing hidradenitis suppurativa patient who transforms to squamous cell cancer

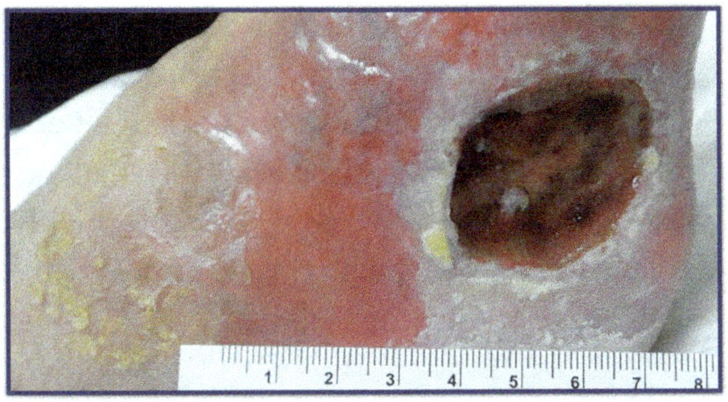

FIGURE 35a. 70-year-old male with history of squamous cell cancer s/q radiation therapy presents with complicated infected wound on right ankle

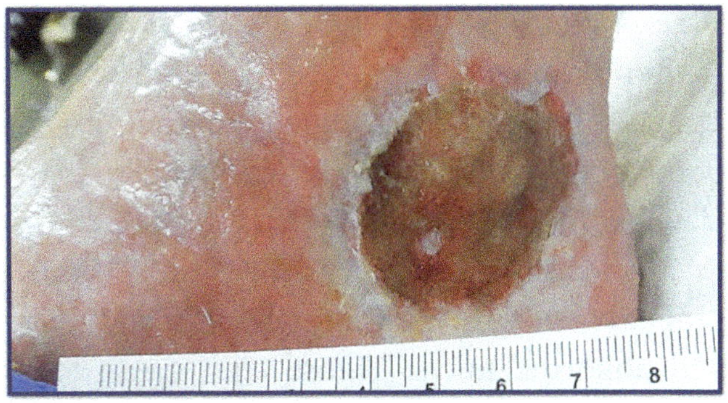

FIGURE 35b. S/q to debridement, antibiotics, silver and foam dressing, compression bandage and HBO_2

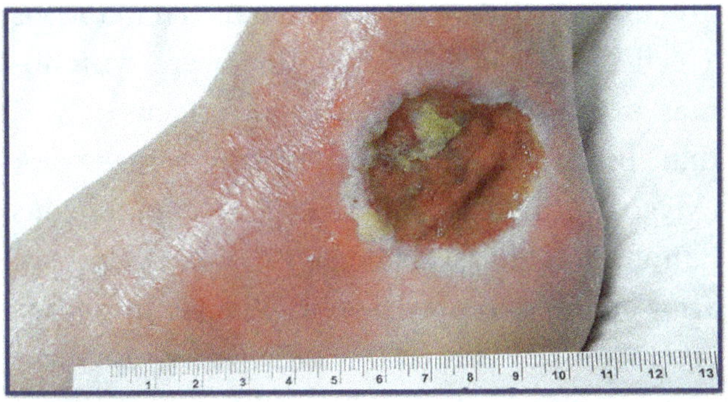

FIGURE 35c. Negative pressure therapy, silver dressing on the base, and HBO_2

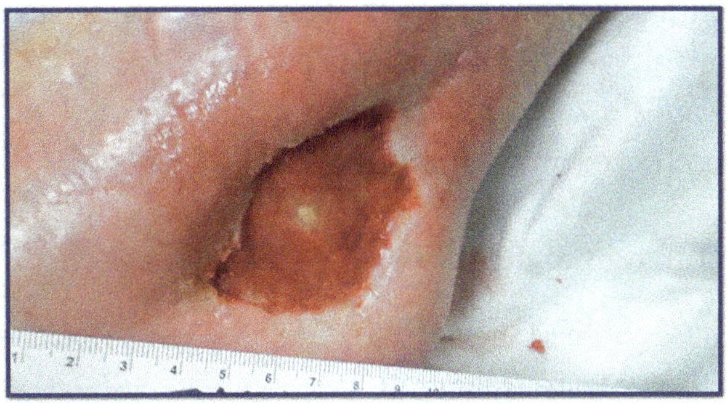

FIGURE 35d. S/q to bone resection, negative pressure therapy, and silver dressing

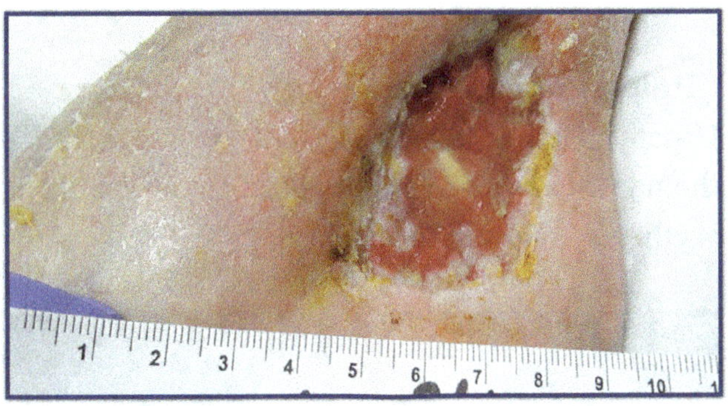

FIGURE 35e. S/q to epidermal grafting

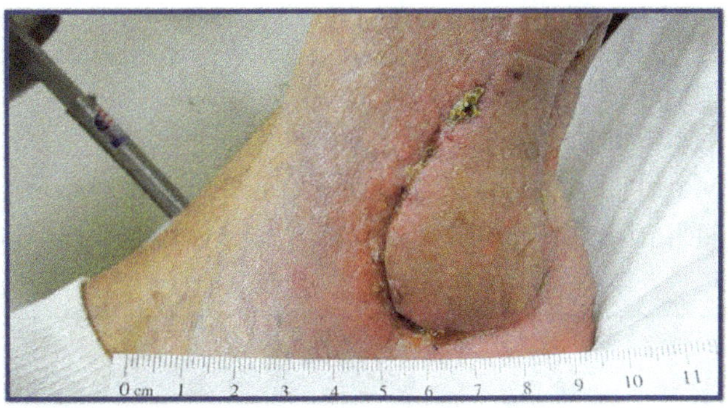

FIGURE 35f. Wound got better but tendon stayed exposed so required flap for complete closure

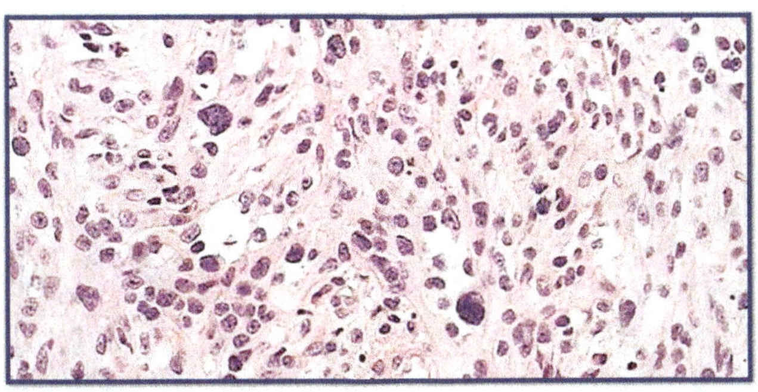

FIGURE 36. Microscopic exam of Kaposi sarcoma showing spindle cells and abnormal nuclei

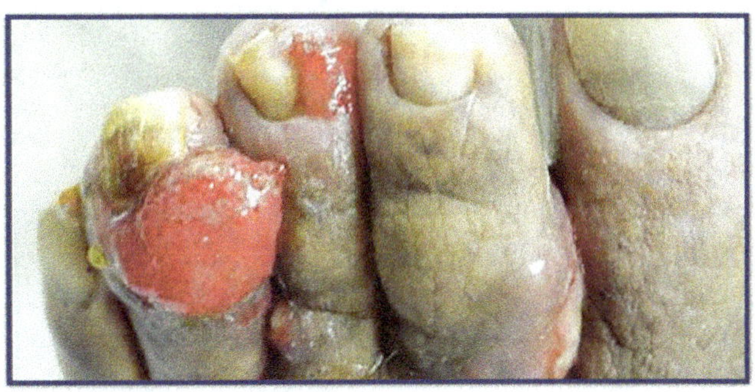

FIGURE 37. Kaposi sarcoma of right foot on initial presentation
Courtesy of Caroline E. Fife, MD

3. *Kaposi's sarcoma (KS)*

Pathophysiology

Kaposi's sarcoma is malignant tumor of the lymphocytic and endothelial cells highly associated with HIV and herpes simplex infection.[52] It is mainly associated with AIDS.[52] Microscopic exam will show spindle cells and cells with abnormal nuclei (Figure 36).

Clinical presentation

KS lesions are usually slightly raised, elongated with poorly demarcated edges. Lesions are usually purple-red maculae or patches (Figure 37). Kaposi's sarcoma, though rare, is reported to present as an ulcer associated with diabetes.

Differential diagnosis

- Diabetic wounds
- Venous wounds
- Pyogenic granuloma
- Squamous cell carcinoma
- Melanoma

Treatment

Mainly includes observation, surgical excision, radiation therapy, intralesion chemotherapy and systemic chemotherapy, using a combination of chemotherapy. Recently topical treatment with 9-cis-retinoic acid (alitretinoin gel) has been proven superior to vehicle gel.[52] In patients with KS associated with AIDS, HAART (highly active antiretroviral therapy) is recommended.

4. *Cutaneous lymphoma*

Pathophysiology

Cutaneous lymphoma may present as various types of skin lesions and rarely as an ulcer (Figure 38). The more common forms of cutaneous T-cell Non-Hodgkin's lymphoma are lymphomas expressing T-cell surface antigens (CD4) that infiltrate skin and initially cause rash (Mycosis fungoides).[52] Ulcerative cutaneous lymphomas are associated with poor prognosis. They are increasingly seen in severely immunocompromised patients.[53] Many of these lymphomas appear to be B-cell lymphomas, but occasionally, T-cell lymphoma can also be seen (Figure 39).

Clinical presentation

Usually begins with small area of pruritic erythema which progresses to raised plaques, diffuse erythema, and skin ulcers.[53]

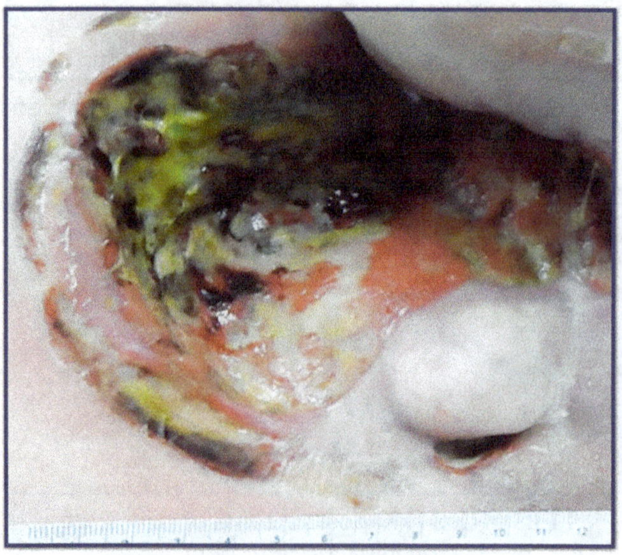

FIGURE 38. Non-Hodgkin's Lymphoma on left axilla s/q resection

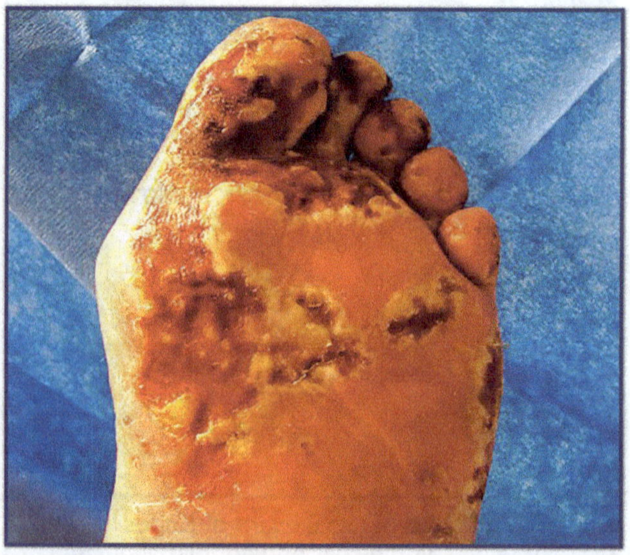

FIGURE 39. Cutaneous T-cell lymphoma

Differential diagnosis

- Fungal infection
- Kaposi's sarcoma
- Squamous cell cancer

Treatment

Early-stage cutaneous T-cell non-Hodgkin's lymphoma is treated with topical glucocorticoids, retinoids (when needed), psoralen, and ultraviolet light with interferon alfa.[53] Advance stated stage is treated with chemotherapy, purine analogues, histone deacetylase inhibitors, and monoclonal antibodies.[53] Allogeneic hematopoietic stem cell transplantation may be curative in young patients.[53]

5. *Melanoma*

Pathophysiology

Melanoma, the most lethal form of skin cancer, is a tumor of the melanocytes of the epidermis. Breslow depth scale is used as a prognostic indicator.[54] The scale indicates how deeply the tumor cells have invaded the epidermis/dermis/subcutaneous tissue in micrometers. The deeper the involvement worse is the prognosis.[54] It also predicts how likely a melanoma is going to spread. The cause of melanoma is exposure to ultraviolet light in the sun and from tanning beds.

Types of melanoma[54]

- Superficial spreading malignant melanoma
- Nodular melanoma
- Acral lentiginous melanoma
- Amelanotic melanoma
- Minimal deviation melanoma
- Desmoplastic melanoma

Clinical presentation

See Figures 40a-d. Melanomas are best described by the ABCDE presentation.

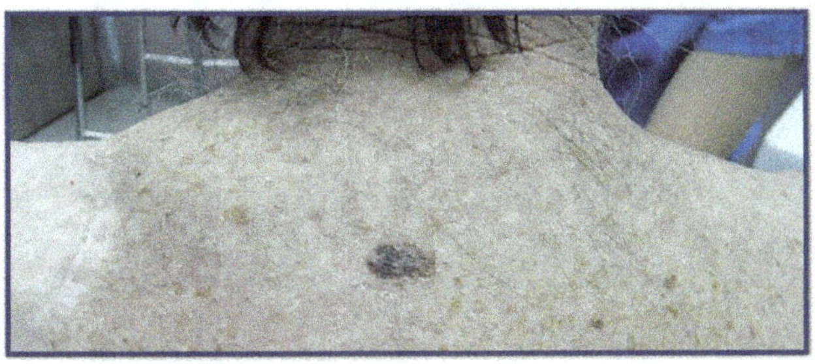

FIGURE 40a. Melanocytic nevus

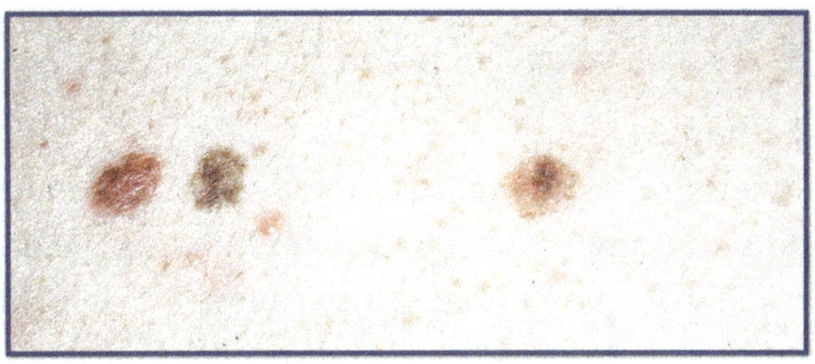

FIGURE 40b. Dysplastic nevi
Courtesy Rajinder Singh, MD

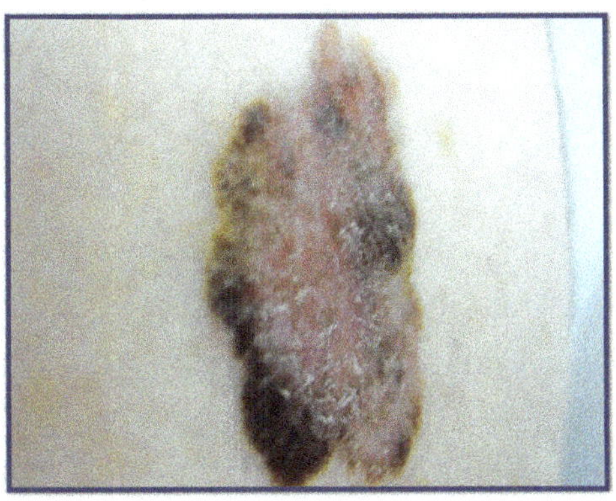

FIGURE 40c. Malignant melanoma
Courtesy Rajinder Singh, MD

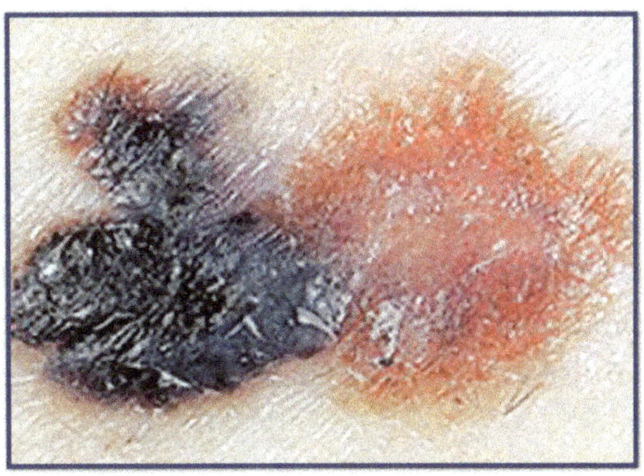

FIGURE 40d. Malignant melanoma
Courtesy of Rajinder Singh, MD

- Asymmetry of the discolored area
- Borders that are uneven and distinct
- Color that is dark brown or black
- Diameter more than 1 cm
- Evolution to larger, darker lesion

Treatment

Stage 1 and 2 melanomas are treated surgically, with the margin of excision dependent on the depth of invasion of the lesion.(55) Stage 3 melanoma is treated with wide local excision, lymph node dissection, and occasionally adjuvant interferon alfa.(55) Stage 4 melanoma is treated with chemotherapy or immunotherapy.(55)

E. Wounds associated with vasculitis and connective tissue disorders

This section will focus on inflammatory causes of leg ulcers with emphasis on connective tissue disorders, pyoderma gangrenosum, vasculitis, and microthrombotic disease.

1. *Pyoderma gangrenosum (PG)*

Pathophysiology

Pyoderma gangrenosum is a noninfectious autoimmune neutrophilic dermatosis that usually starts with sterile pustules,(56-58) which rapidly progresses to painful ulcers of variable depth and size with undermined violaceous borders. Pyoderma gangrenosum is most commonly associated with an underlying disease such as inflammatory bowel disease, rheumatologic disease, hematological disease, or malignancy.(56) Diagnosis of pyoderma gangrenosum is based upon any underlying disease, typical presentation, histopathology, and exclusion of other diseases that can lead to a similar appearance.(56-58)

Clinical presentation

The four different types of pyoderma gangrenosum include ulcerative, pustular, bullous, and vegetative.(56) In general, **ulcerative variant** is most common, has an association with inflammatory bowel disease and arthritis, and tends to evolve rapidly. Clinically, it is described as ulceration with a purulent base, undermined borders, and surrounding erythema (Figures 41a-b). **Pustular pyoderma gangrenosum** is most commonly associated with active inflammatory bowel disease. Clinically, the lesions consist of discrete pustules with an inflammatory border occurring on the normal skin. **Bullous pyoderma gangrenosum** is often noted in

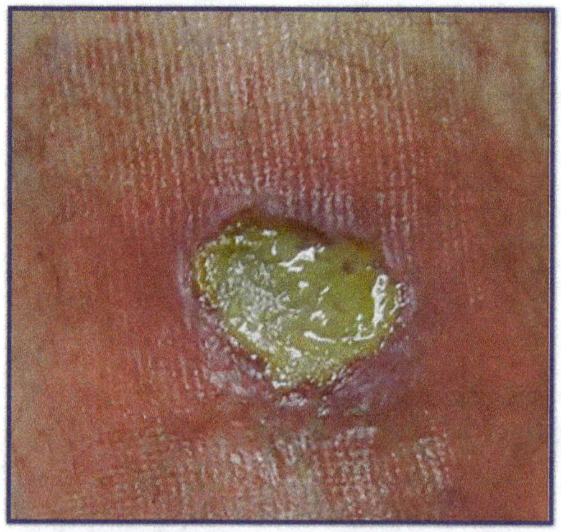

FIGURE 41a. Pyoderma gangrenosum before debridement

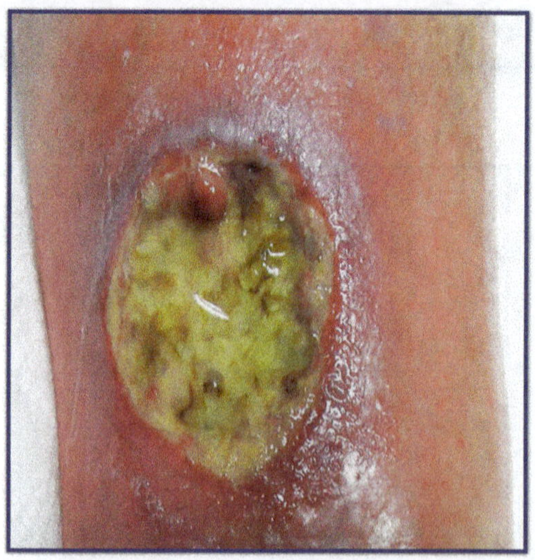

FIGURE 41b. Pyoderma gangrenousum after debridement

patients with leukemia and other myeloproliferative disorders. It is characterized by superficial and painful bullae with progression to erosion and ulceration. **Vegetative pyoderma gangrenosum** is the most indolent of the four clinical variants. Clinically, it is more superficial ulceration without any undermining border and purulent base as opposed to the more common ulcerative type. Diagnosing PG is challenging; all patients with suspected PG should be evaluated for potential underlying causes. Usually PG may be idiopathic, but it is associated with an underlying disease in 50% of patients.[56]

Diagnostic criteria[56]

Major

- History of rapidly progressing, painful ulcer with irregular, violaceous, undermined border
- Exclusion of other causes of ulceration (typically vasculitis, neoplasm, infection)

Minor

- Skin biopsy showing sterile neutrophilic inflammation
- Presence of pathergy (Figures 41a-b) or healing with cribriform scarring (Figure 41c)
- Presence of systemic disease associated with pyoderma gangrenosum (inflammatory bowel disease, IgA paraproteinemia, internal malignancy, systemic lupus erythematous, or other autoimmune disease)
- Response to systemic glucocorticoid therapy (1–2mg/kd/d, anticipate 50% decrease within four weeks)

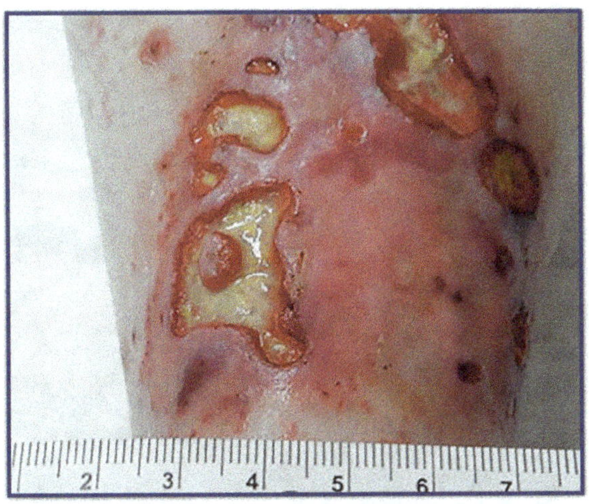

FIGURE 41c. Pyoderma gangrenosum healing with cribriform scarring

Differential diagnosis

- Vasculitis
- Venous stasis ulcer

Treatment

Treatment of pyoderma gangrenosum includes systemic corticosteroids 1–2 mg/kg/day;[57-58] combination of corticosteroids with cyclosporine and infliximab may also be effective;[57-58] combination of corticosteroids with sulfa drugs, such as dapsone, clofazimine, minocycline, and thalidomide.[57-58]

Alternative treatments may include local application of granulocyte-macrophage colony-stimulating factor, intravenous immunoglobulins, plasmapheresis, skin transplants, application of bioengineered skin, hyperbaric oxygen therapy.[57-58]

2. *Rheumatoid arthritis and ulceration*

Pathophysiology

Rheumatoid arthritis is a systemic autoimmune disorder of unknown etiology. The cutaneous manifestations include rheumatoid nodules over pressure points, vasculitic lesions (25%–30% of patients),[59] and leg ulceration (in approximately 8%–9% of patients).[60]

Clinical presentation

Typically, the ulcer in rheumatoid arthritis is smooth, undulating, with irregular "geographic" shape, and extremely painful (Figure 42).

Accompanying cutaneous findings include palpable purpura and livedo reticularis (Figure 43). Occasionally there is histological evidence of leukocytoclastic vasculitis.[59]

Some rheumatoid arthritis patients with several nodules have a constellation of symptoms collectively known as Felty's syndrome.[60] This syndrome is described as the combination of rheumatoid arthritis, splenomegaly, granulocytopenia, and leg ulcers.

Differential diagnosis

- Venous stasis ulcer
- Pyoderma gangrenosum

Treatment

Rheumatoid ulcers often require high-dose corticosteroids, cyclophosphamide, dapsone,alone or with colchicines, and certain disease-modifying drugs.[61] Wound treatment includes standard wound care plus growth factors or bioengineered skin.

3. *Systemic lupus erythematosus (SLE)*

Pathophysiology

"Lupus-specific" skin lesions are cutaneous signs of lupus that are characteristic of the disease and when biopsied show diagnostic histologic findings ("interface reaction" of lymphocytes at the dermal-epidermal junction causing damage to the base of the epidermis).[62]

Clinical presentation

The incidence of leg ulceration in SLE patients is between 2%–8%.[62] These ulcers can be extremely painful and are typically found over the pretibial surface and malleolar area. The ulcers may precede the diagnosis of SLE by many years. They are characterized by well-defined margins with a purulent bed and varying amount of granulation tissue (Figures 44a-d). Surrounding skin may be normal in appearance or erythematous with evidence of atrophie blanche. Livedo reticularis (Figure 43) is often observed in SLE and is associated with the antiphospholipid syndrome. Malar rash (Figure 45) consisting of bright erythematous patches over both cheeks and the nasal bridge is also a common clinical finding. Subacute cutaneous lupus erythematosus[63] is a drug-induced (examples of drugs includes hydrochlorothiazide, calcium channel blockers, ACE inhibitors, and

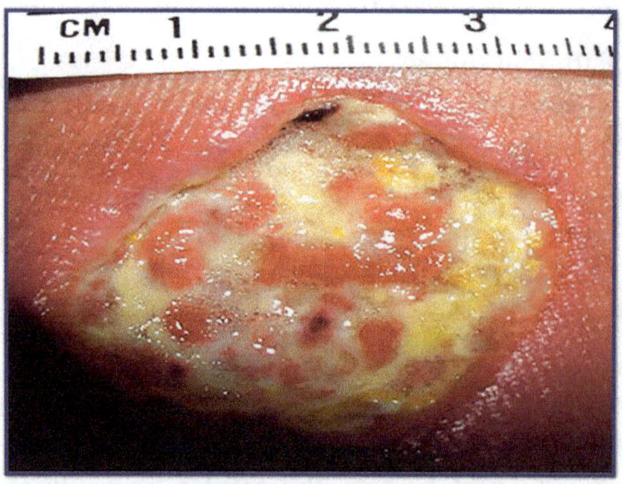

FIGURE 42. Rheumatoid arthritis with vasculitic ulcer

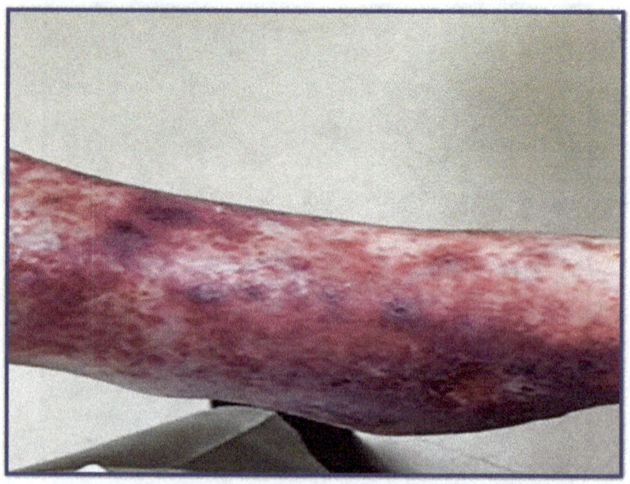

FIGURE 43. Palpable purpura and livedo reticularis pattern rash

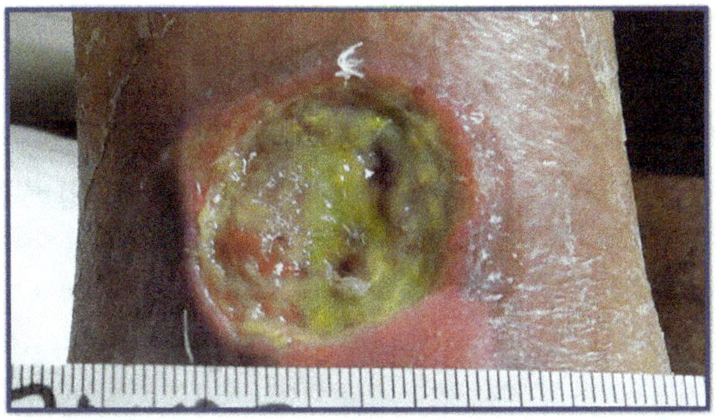

FIGURE 44a. 52-year-old female with history of lupus on immunosuppressants with vasculitic ulcer

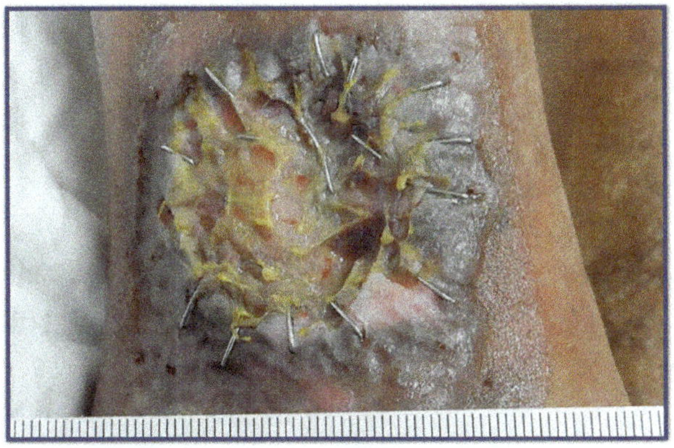

FIGURE 44b. Lupus vasculitis s/q debridement and STSG with nontake

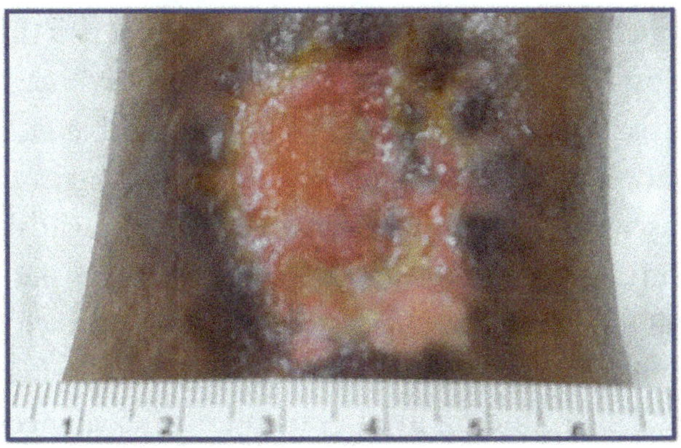

FIGURE 44c. Lupus vasculitis ulcer s/q application of theraskin

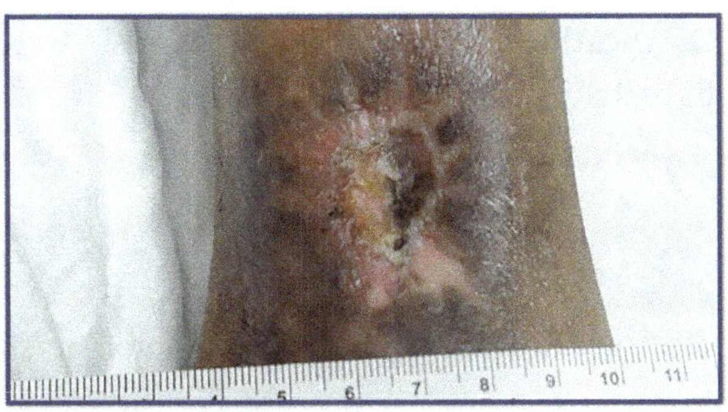

FIGURE 44d. Lupus vasculitis ulcer patient epithelialized after eight weeks of Theraskin application

terbinafine), photosensitive eruption of circular, scaly, erythematous patches over the forearms, chest, or upper back.

Treatment

Treatment is often challenging. Topical Vitamin A has been shown to improve granulation tissue in patients on systemic corticosteroids. Patients with antiphospholipid syndrome have shown promising results with stanozolol.[64] Intralesional triamcinolone acetonide (5 mg/ml) has also been used with success in some patients with lupus ulceration. Sun protection, topical glucocorticoids, and hydroxychloroquine are also used to treat cutaneous lupus erythematous.[62-63]

4. *Scleroderma*

Pathophysiology

Scleroderma is an autoimmune disorder of unknown etiology that usually affects women between the ages of 30 and 50.[65] It causes skin to become thick and hard (sclerotic) with a buildup of scar tissue. Skin involvement varies in both the extent of body surface involved and the severity of induration. Scleroderma patients usually have excessive collagen proteins.[5,65]

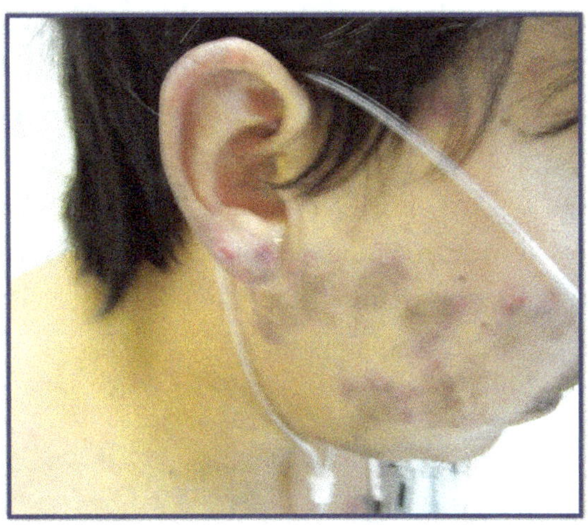

FIGURE 45. Lupus erythematous with rash on face. Courtesy of Rajinder Singh, MD

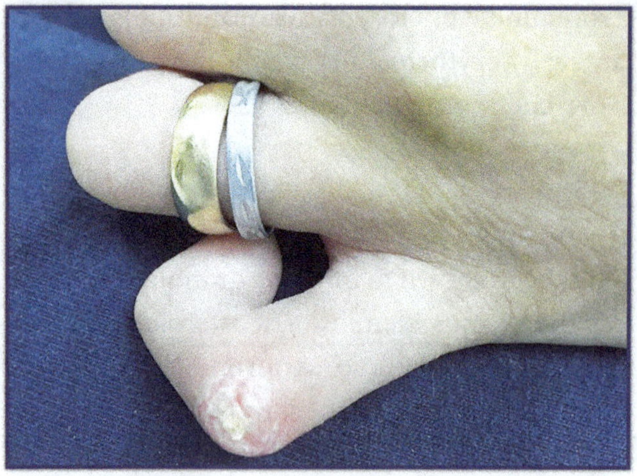

FIGURE 46. Scleroderma ulcer on right fifth finger knuckle

Often, patients will have a "purse-string mouth" and unusually smooth facial skin. Sclerodactyly is a hallmark, and ulcers usually develop over the digits and overlying bony prominences (Figure 46). Digital ulcers are difficult to re-epithelialize and are usually refractory to healing.[65] Thirty-five percent of scleroderma patients will develop skin ulcers.[65] Raynaud's syndrome (sequential white, blue, and red color changes in the digits precipitated by cold or stress) occurs in all almost all patients with scleroderma and may precede other disease manifestations including ulceration.[65] There are two types of scleroderma, localized and systemic. Localized scleroderma is further described as morphea (discolored patches on the skin) and linear (streaks or bands of thick, hard skin on arms and legs). Systemic scleroderma can be limited (affecting only the arms, hands, and face) or diffuse (rapidly progressing, affecting large area of skin and 1 more of the organs). CREST syndrome is associated with scleroderma in which patient has calcinosis, Raynaud's syndrome, esophageodactyly, sclerodactyly and telangiatiasis. [65]

Differential diagnosis

- Lupus vasculitis ulcer
- Rheumatoid arthritis vasculitis ulcer

Treatment

Occlusive dressings may provide pain relief and help with autolytic debridement.[1-2] Collagenase may be useful to help with enzymatic debridement.[1-2] Early inflammatory phase may respond to systemic glucocorticoids, weekly methotrexate, or other immunosuppressive therapies. Indurated, thickened phase of skin involvement responds poorly to therapy.[65] Patients with Raynaud's syndrome should be educated on wearing gloves and protecting the skin to prevent ulceration.[65]

5. *Vasculitis*

Pathophysiology

Vasculitis, or inflammation of blood vessels, can affect any size vessels. It plays a crucial role in a number of collagen vascular disorders.[66-67]

Clinical presentation

Vasculitis usually affects males and females equally and is most common in the elderly. The most common cutaneous vasculitis is small-vessel vasculitis, which presents as palpable purpura (nonblanching red papules). Medium-vessel vasculitis (such as polyarteritis or granulomatosis with polyangiitis) can lead to ulcers in the skin, but the lesions are often strikingly inflamed with an active erythematous-to-red border and often with surrounding livedo reticularis-like changes (Figures 47a-d).

Classification of vasculitis (adapted from Cupps TR, Fauci AS)[59]

- Polyarteritis nodosa group
  - Classic polyarteritis nodosa (classic PAN)
  - Allergic angiitis and granulomatosis
  - Systemic necrotizing vasculitis (overlap syndrome)

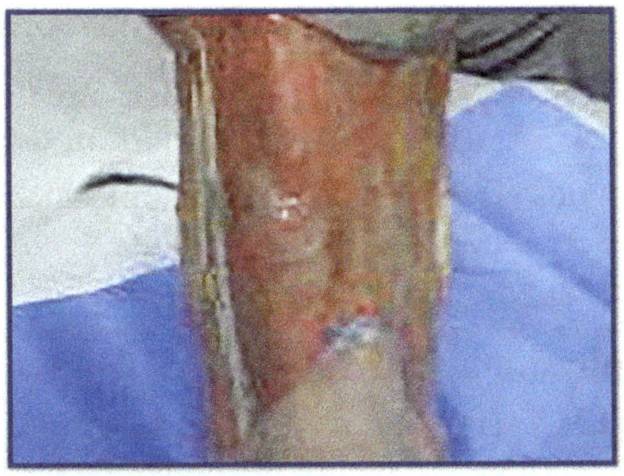

FIGURE 47a. Extensive lupus vasculitis ulcer on right leg

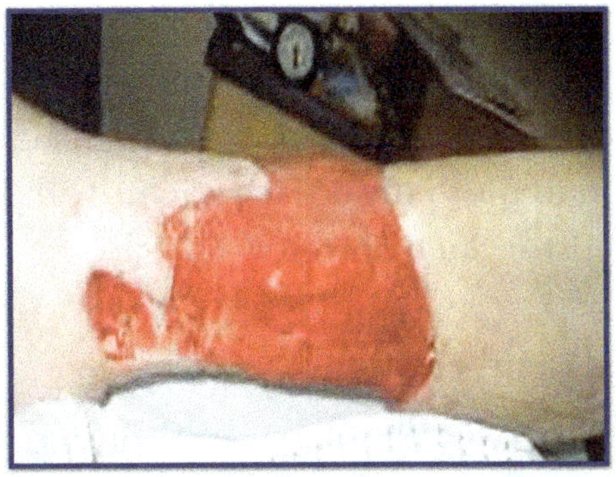

FIGURE 47b. S/q negative pressure therapy, silver dressing, and compression bandage

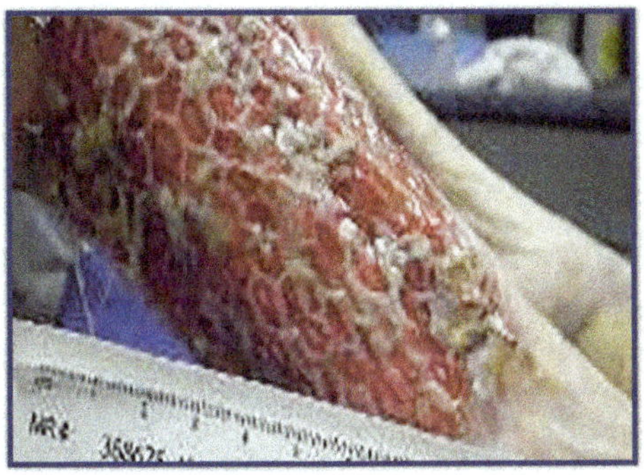

FIGURE 47c. S/q STSG

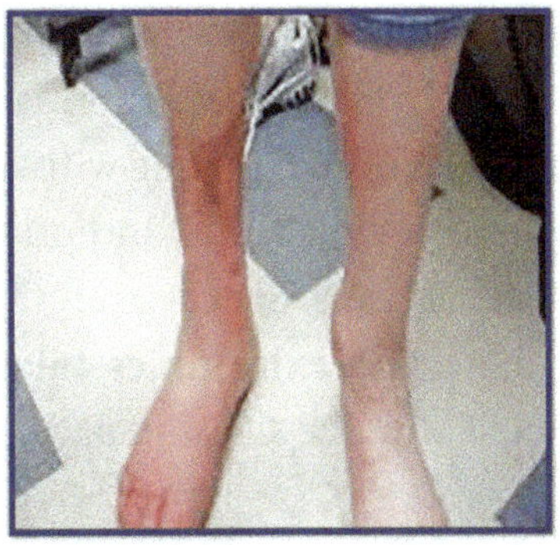

FIGURE 47d. Wound healed

- Hypersensitivity vasculitis
  - Vasculitis associated with
    - Infections
    - Chemical/drug exposure (Figure 48)
    - Connective tissue disease
  - Serum sickness
  - Henoch-Schonlein purpura
  - Erythema elevatum diutinum
  - Mixed essential cryoglobulinemia with vasculitis
  - Vasculitis associated with other primary disorders
- Wegener's granulomatosis
- Lymphomatoid granulomatosis
- Giant cell arteritis (temporal, Takayasu's)
- Other
  - Mucocutaneous lymph node syndrome
  - Thromboangiitis obliterans (Buerger's disease)
  - Central nervous system vasculitis

Treatment

Depends on accurate diagnosis of the underlying cause and is directed at eliminating the underlying cause, in addition to local and/or systemic anti-inflammatory and immunosuppressive agents.[67]

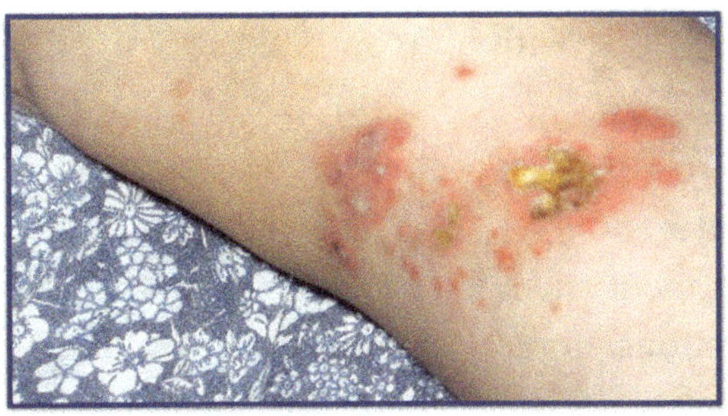

FIGURE 48. Lymphocytoclastic vasculitis secondary to sulfa drugs
Courtesy of Kirsten Smith, MD

6. *Necrobiosis lipoidica diabeticorum*

Pathophysiology

It is a disease of unknown etiology that is usually seen in morbidly obese patients with strong family history of diabetes.[68]

Clinical manifestations

Necrobiosis lipoidica diabeticorum (Figure 49) is a skin lesion or ulceration typically located on the shins and is usually found in diabetic patients and is often associated with retinal or kidney damage. The typical lesion is an irregular ovoid reddish brown plaque with a shiny yellow center and a violaceous, indurated border. Typically, the lesions occur over the anterior aspect of the lower extremities bilaterally but not symmetrically. The size and depth may vary.

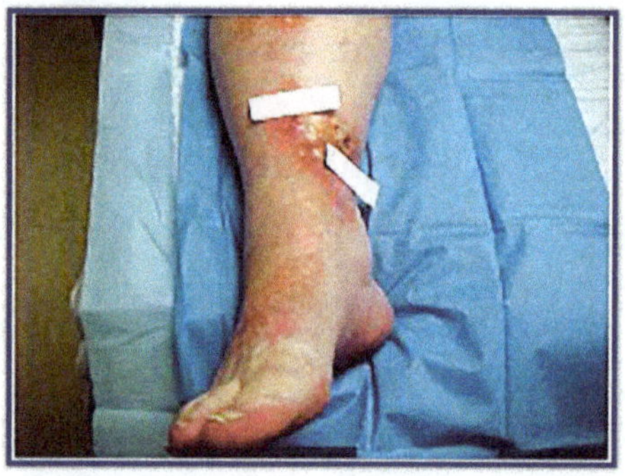

FIGURE 49. Necrobiosis lipoidica diabeticorum

Differential diagnosis

- Calciphylaxis
- Pyoderma gangrenosum
- Diabetes with peripheral vascular disease with necrosis
- Vasculitis

Treatment

Treatment includes intralesional corticosteroid injections, topical corticosteroids, and perilesional heparin.[68] There are some reports of using oral steroids, aspirin, and nicotinamide in refractory cases. There are reports of successful treatment of this condition with 0.1% topical tacrolimus.[69] Also topically applied bovine collagen has been found to be useful.[70] Photodynamic therapy has also been used with some success.[71]

7. *Pemphigus vulgaris*

Pathophysiology

Incidence varies by country and ethnicity and is estimated to be 0.5 to 3.2 cases per 100,000 persons per year. The autoimmune blistering disease is characterized by persistent pruritic to painful blisters with erosion and variable mucosal and ocular involvement and scarring.[72] Histopathology shows suprabasilar clefting in pemphigus vulgaris compared with subepidermal clefting seen in bullous pemphigoid.[72-73]

Clinical characteristics

Tender, fragile blisters and erosions seen in oral mucosa and skin, mucous membrane lesions much more common than in bullous pemphigoid (Figures 50a-b); Nikolsky sign (rubbing of the skin results in blister formation) is positive.

Differential diagnosis

- Bullous pemphigoid
- Porphyria cutanea tarda
- Dermatitis herpetiformis
- Paraneoplastic pemphigus

Treatment

For limited disease, potent topical glucocorticoids may be sufficient; in most patients, systemic therapy is required.[72-73] Oral prednisone is usually the first line of therapy. Additional immunosuppressive therapy (azathioprine, methotrexate, cyclophosphamide, mycophenolate mofetil) may be necessary to control the disease.[72-73] IV immunoglobulin and tetracycline antibiotics have also been used.[72-73]

8. *Bullous pemphigoid*

Pathophysiology

One of most common autoimmune blistering diseases. Histopathology shows subepidermal bullae without acantholysis and with prominent eosinophils. Direct immunoflourence shows linear IgG deposition at the basement membrane zone.[73]

Clinical manifestations

Tense blisters preceded by intense pruritus or urticarial lesions most commonly seen in the elderly on the trunk, limbs, and flexures; does not usually present with oral lesions (Figure 51).[73]

Differential diagnosis

- Bullus pemphigoid
- Porphyria cutanea tarda

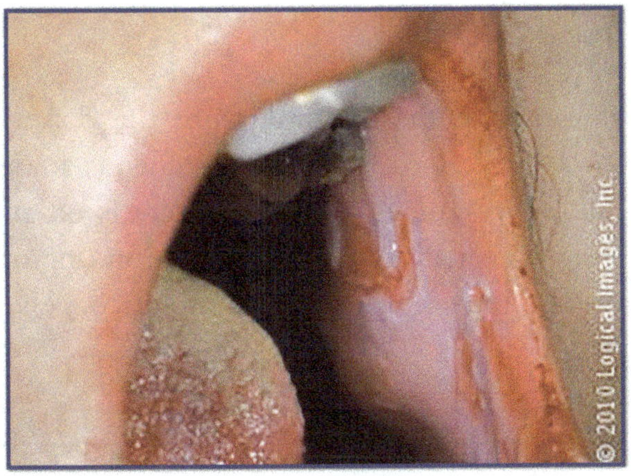

FIGURE 50a. Mucosal Lesion - *Pemphigus Vulgaris*

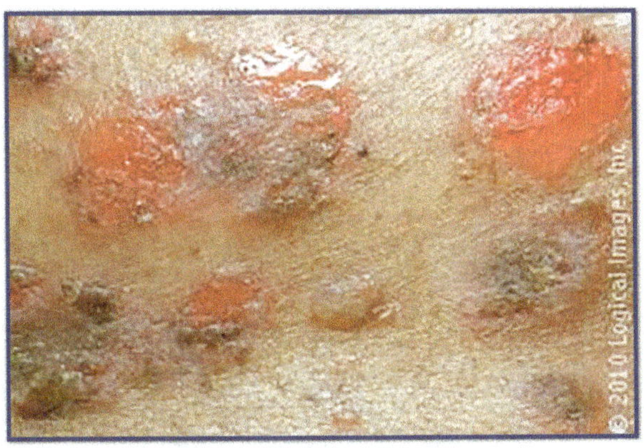

FIGURE 50b. Blistering skin lesion - *Pemphigus Vulgaris*

- Dermatiis herpetiformis
- Paraneoplastic pemphigus

Treatment

Same as pemphigus vulgaris (see above).

F. Ulcers due to microthrombotic disease

Disorders such as antiphospholipid syndrome, cryofibrinogenemia, cryoglobulinemia, cholesterol embolization, thrombocytosis, and warfarin necrosis can cause thrombi within the microvasculature, resulting in ulceration.

Usually patients with microthrombotic disease presents with i) livedo reticularis pattern. ii) purple discoloration of surrounding skin with cyanosis, and iii) intense pain out of proportion to the size of the wound.

1. *Antiphospholipid syndrome*

Pathophysiology

Antiphospholipid syndrome (Figure 52) is a disorder secondary to autoantibodies against phospholipids and phospholipid-binding proteins such as cardiolipin and Beta-2-glycol protein. It can be primary or secondary disorder associated with a multitude of disease states

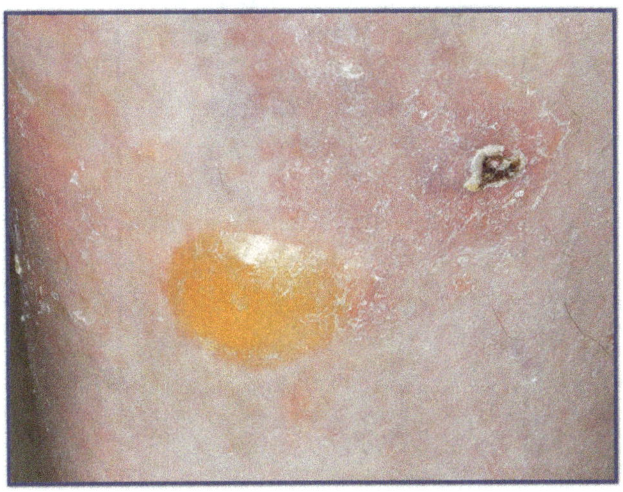

FIGURE 51. Bullous pemphigoid
Courtesy Dirk Elston, MD

including autoimmune disorder, malignancy, or drugs. Histopathologic specimens much demonstrate thrombosis in absence of inflammation of vessels.[74]

Clinical manifestations

In vitro, they can prolong clotting tests, but in vivo they increase risk of venous or arterial thrombosis. Patient may present with acute onset of gangrene (Figure 52). Patient usually gives history of (i) three or more unexplained, consecutive spontaneous abortions before tenth week of gestation, (ii) unexplained fetal death at or beyond the tenth week of gestation with normal fetal morphology, and (iii) one or more premature births of a morphologically normal neonate before the thirty-fourth week of gestation.[74]

Differential diagnosis

- Acute arterial insufficiency
- Cholesterol emboli
- Peripheral Vascular Disease (PVD)with gangrene

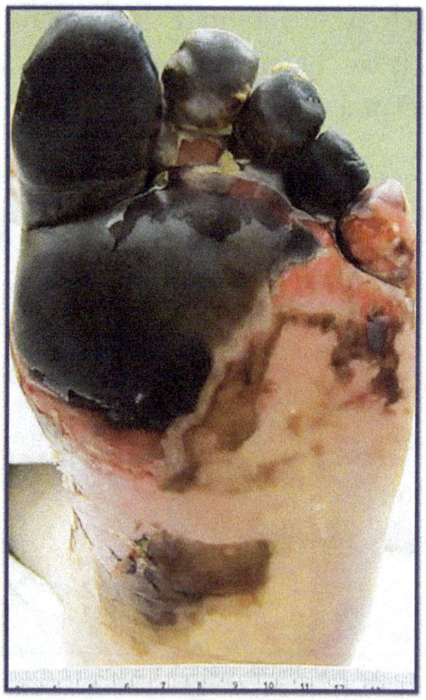

FIGURE 52. Antiphospholipid syndrome

Treatment

Long-term anticoagulation and treating the underlying disease is the mainstay of treatment. HBO_2 therapy may be useful in emergent basis to salvage the extremity.[74]

2. *Cryofibrinogenemia*

Cryofibrinogenemia is a disease associated with the presence of cryofibrinogen in plasma. It can be a primary process or secondary to a neoplastic, infectious, thrombotic, or connective tissue disorder.[75]

3. *Cryoglobulinemia*

Cryoglobulinemia (Figure 53) is a condition in which serum proteins precipitate at cold temperatures. It is often associated with hepatitis C, collagen vascular diseases, vasculitis, lymphomas, and myeloproliferative disorders.[75]

4. *Cholesterol emboli*

Cholesterol emboli results from the dissolution of cholesterol plaques. Cutaneous manifestations resemble vasculitis. There is often a history of recent surgical manipulation, angiography, or the commencement of anticoagulant therapy.[75]

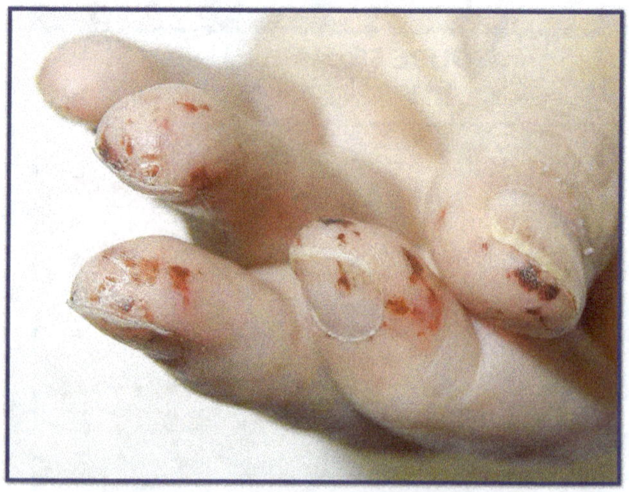

FIGURE 53. Cryoglobulinemia
Courtesy of Dirk Elston, MD

5. *Warfarin necrosis*

Warfarin necrosis (Figure 54) may occur with initiation of warfarin (Coumadin®) therapy (within the first week) of starting Coumadin.[76] It leads to skin necrosis. Although exact pathogenesis is unknown, it is understood that it could be secondary to protein C deficiency, protein S deficiency, and antithrombin III deficiency.[77] Sometimes there is reduced level of free proteins during antepartum and immediate postpartum period.[78]

Clinical presentation

The ulcerations and necrosis usually appear on the trunk. Other manifestations include ecchymoses, purpura, hemorrhagic necrosis, and purple toes.

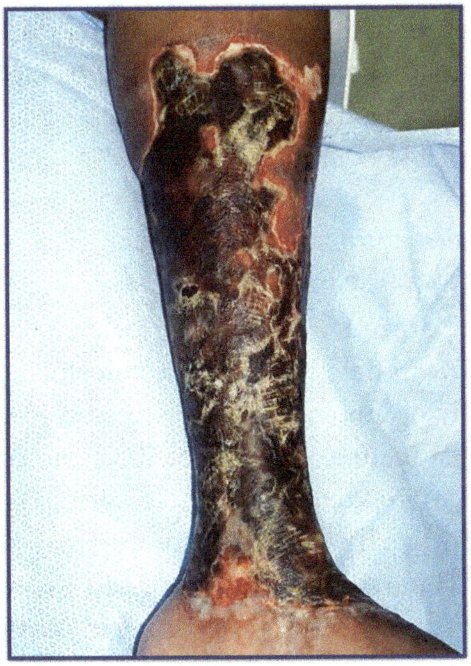

FIGURE 54. Coumadin-induced ulcerations
Courtesy of Mary Hirsch, MD

Differential diagnosis

- Antiphospholipid syndrome
- Calciphylaxis
- Vasculitis
- Pyoderma gangrenosum

Treatment

Most important treatment is discontinuation of Coumadin. Wound management includes debridement, infection control, moisture balance, and possible need for negative pressure therapy and skin graft.

G. Other unusual wound conditions

1. *Lipodermatosclerosis*

Lipodermatosclerosis (Figure 55) is manifested by indurated skin that usually occurs on the medial aspect of the lower leg in patients with venous disease. In the acute phase, the skin is intensely red with scaling and exquisitely painful. In the chronic phase, there is pronounced hyperpigmentation and painless induration.[79]

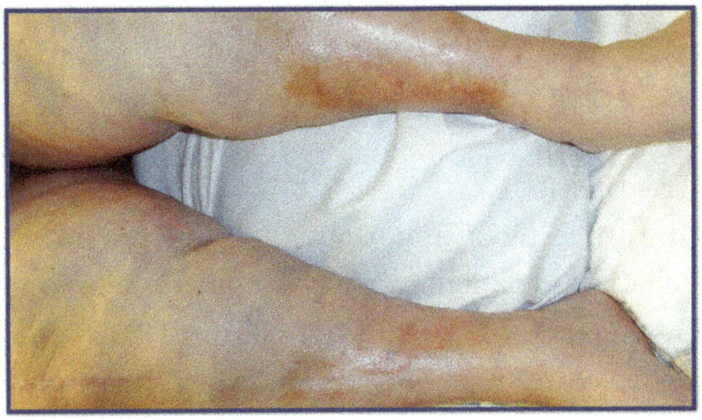

FIGURE 55. Lipodermatosclerosis

2. *Sickle cell ulcers*

Pathophysiology

Sickle cell disease is an inherited hemoglobinapathy wherein sickle-shaped red blood cells are formed that clog the capillaries and prevents normal flow to the tissues, which can lead to local hypoxia, thrombosis, and ischemia.[80] This disease affects about 0.6% of the African American population in the United States; approximately 50,000 cases are reported every year. The trait is present in approximately 40% of the general population in some areas of Africa and in descendents of Asiatic Indians, Italians, Greeks, or Mediterraneans. Although the exact cause of sickle cell ulcers is not clear, they have been associated with trauma, infection, severe anemia, warm temperatures, and venous insufficiency.[81]

Clinical manifestations

Sickle cell patients are prone to ulceration, and the ulceration can become chronic in nature. These ulcers are painful, debilitating, difficult to treat, and prone to recurrence and are usually found on the lower third of the leg, usually over the medial and lateral malleoli of the ankle (Figure 56). Sickle cell ulcers frequently become infected or heavily colonized with bacteria.

Differential diagnosis

- Pyoderma gangrenosum
- Venous stasis ulcers
- Hydroxyurea induced ulcers
- Vasculitis

Treatment

The three most important therapies for sickle cell disease patients are hematopoietic stem cell transplantation, prophylactic transfusions, and hydroxyurea therapy.[80-81] Transfusions should not be given unless they have symptomatic anemia or signs of end organ damage.

Oral zinc sulfate (200 mg 3 times a day) and a combination of L-Methylfolate with vitamin B6 and B12 (Metanx) may help in wound healing in patients with sickle cell ulcers by decreasing endothelial cell homocysteine and increasing nitric oxide levels.[81] It also helps to reduce pain associated with sickle cell ulcers and increase blood flow in microcirculation at the wound margin. Arginine therapy has also been found to help in patients with sickle cell ulcer by inducing nitric oxide production.[82]

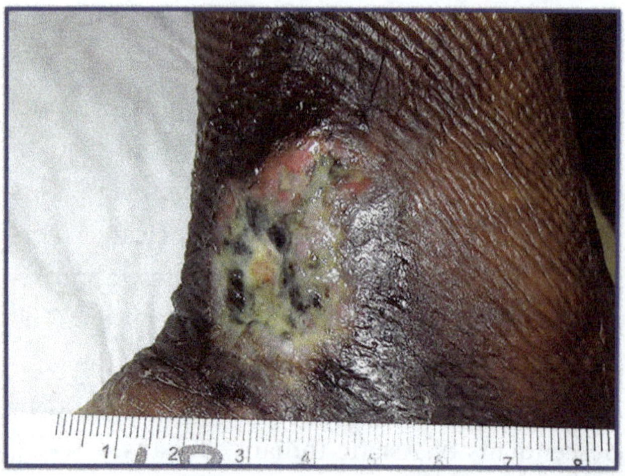

FIGURE 56. Sickle cell ulcers

Pentoxifylline (Trental) may also help to decrease viscosity and increase peripheral tissue perfusion.[81]

Wound management includes debridement, infection control including management of biofilm, edema control with compression therapy. Electrical stimulation and HBO_2 therapy have also been utilized in refractory wounds. Topical application of Molgramostim (GMCSF: granulocyte macrophage colony stimulating factor)[83] and bioengineered skin have been used successfully in sickle cell ulcer patients.[84]

3. *Calcific uraemic arteriopathy (calciphylaxis)*

Calcific uraemic arteriopathy (calciphylaxis) is a rare necrotizing cutaneous abnormality that typically occurs in patients with advanced kidney dysfunction and elevated calcium-phosphorus products usually associated with tertiary hyperparathyroidism.[85] Skin biopsy shows abnormal deposition of calcium within the lumen of arterial vasculature in dermis and subcutaneous tissue,[85] which then compromises flow and leads to increased thrombosis and downstream ischemia, resulting in subsequent painful tissue necrosis.

Clinical presentation

Calciphylaxis lesions are painful subcutaneous nodules or plaques with overlying red-brown discoloration and angulated purpuric patches,

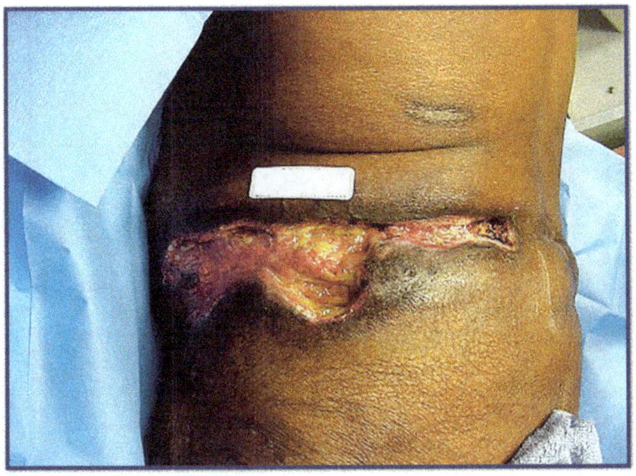

FIGURE 57. Calciphylaxis

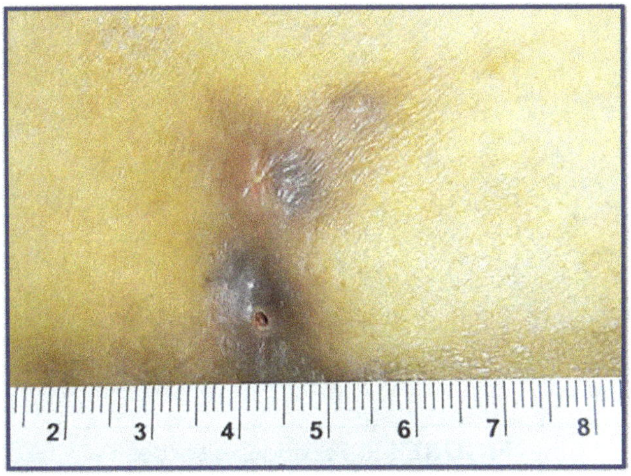

FIGURE 58. Cutaneous calcinosis cutis

often with central necrosis, and ulcerations. Ulcerations associated with calciphylaxis can be located on the trunk, heels, fingers, and toes and may manifest ischemic and gangrenous changes which are sudden in presentation (Figure 57). Ischemia and gangrenous necrotic changes may extend from skin to skeletal muscles.

Differential diagnosis

- Cutaneous cutis
- Pyoderma gangrenosum
- Necrotizing fasciitis
- Coumadin-induced skin necrosis

Treatment

Treatment is difficult and often unsuccessful with high mortality rate of 50%–100%.[85] Treatment includes standard wound care, parathyroidectomy, and hyperbaric oxygen therapy.[86-87] Low doses of warfarin or calcium channel blockers may be helpful.[85] Also, low-calcium hemodialysis is also found to be promising. Systemic antibiotics may be necessary for wound infections. Phosphate binders are indicated to decrease (calcium X phosphorus) product.[85] Sodium thiosulfate is used as a chelating agent for calcium deposits in the tissue.[85] Bisphosphonate therapy may be helpful in removing arterial calcification.[85] Cinacalcet may help to lower parathyroid levels and improve calcium-phosphorus homeostasis. Patient needs meticulous wound care including conservative debridement. For noninfected wounds, enzymatic or autolytic debridement is recommended. If wound is infected, then surgical debridement is necessary. There are some reports of successfully treating calciphylactic wounds by combination of surgical debridement, negative pressure therapy, HBO_2,[86-87] and bioengineered skin. Pain management and nutrition management are extremely important for patients with calciphylaxis.

4. *Calcinosis cutis*

Pathophysiology

Calcinosis cutis is a group of disorders in which calcium deposits form in the skin. It is of four types according to etiology: dystrophic, metastatic, iatrogenic, and idiopathic.[88] Dystrophic calcinosis is most common. In all cases of calcinosis cutis, insoluble compounds of calcium are deposited within the skin due to local and/or systemic factors.[88]

Clinical manifestations

Most lesions of calcinosis cutis develop gradually and are asymptomatic. In general, multiple, firm,

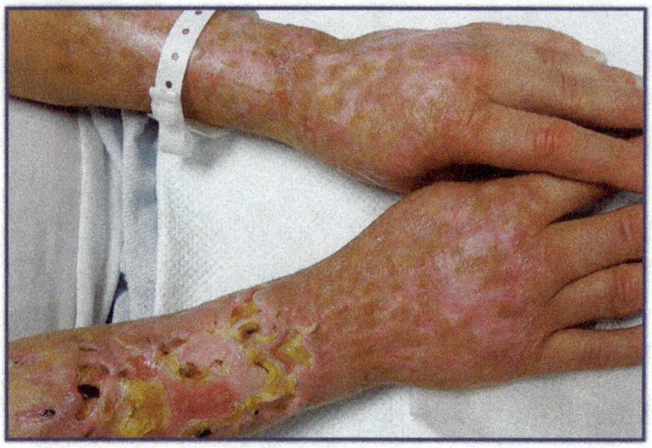

FIGURE 59. Factitious disorder

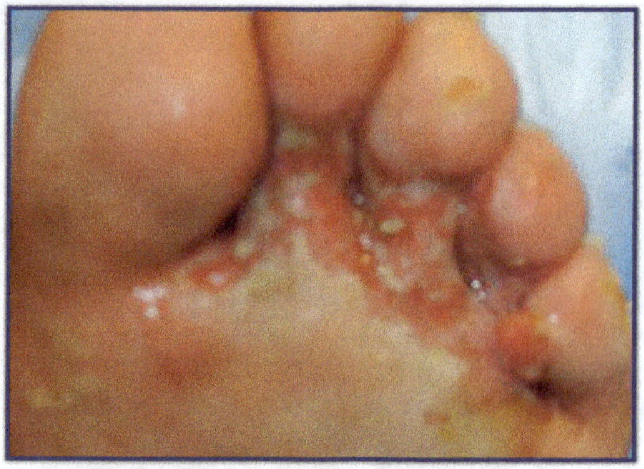

FIGURE 60. Pyogenic Granuloma

whitish dermal papules, plaques, nodules, or subcutaneous nodules are found. The lesions are usually studded with yellow-white gritty substance. The lesions spontaneously ulcerate, extruding a chalky white material (Figure 58). In some patients, severe vascular calcification can cause diminished pulses and cutaneous gangrene.

Differential diagnosis

- Xanthomas
- Calciphylaxis
- Osteoma cutis
- Gouty tophi

Treatment
Medical therapy is of limited benefit. When identified the underlying problem should be corrected. Intralesional corticosteroids may be beneficial.[88] Magnesium or aluminum antacids may be effective phosphate binders in patients with renal insufficiency. Sodium etidronate and diphosphonate may reduce bone turnover and inhibit growth of ectopic hydroxyapatite crystals.[88] Minocyline has been used in some cases of cutaneous calcinosis with success.[88] Surgical debridement is needed when there is pain, recurrent infection, or ulceration, but calcification might get worse as trauma may stimulate calcification.

5. *Factitious disorder*

This group of patients usually has unexplained urge to scratch and harm themselves. These patients have an associated psychiatric disorder.[89] Ulcers have geometric edges and good granulation tissue on the wound base (Figure 59). Diagnosis sometimes is made after excluding all other diagnoses.

6. *Pyogenic granuloma*

Pyogenic granuloma (Figure 60) is a relatively common skin growth and should not be confused with pyoderma gangrenosum. It is usually a small, red, oozing and bleeding bump that looks like raw hamburger meat. It is an acquired vascular lesion which may follow a laceration or skin puncture and grows rapidly over a period of a few weeks. The head, neck, upper trunk, and hands and feet are the most common sites. Treatment usually is by cauterization with silver nitrate, cautery, curettage, or laser removal.[90]

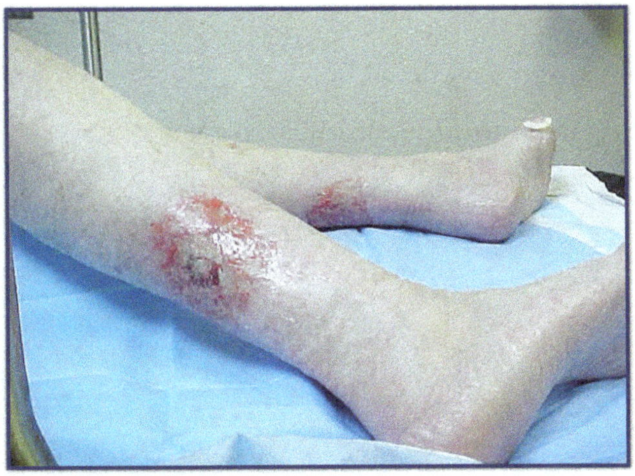

FIGURE 61. Hydroxyurea-induced ulcers

7. *Drug-induced ulcerations (i.e., hydroxyurea)*

Pathophysiology

Hydroxyurea is an antineoplastic agent commonly used to treat myeloproliferative disorders and other nonneoplastic conditions. Dermatologic side effects of hydroxyurea are fairly common and include hyperpigmentation, scaling, erythema and desquamation of the face and hands, and partial alopecia.[91] A less well-described and less well-characterized complication is leg ulcers.

Clinical manifestations

Usually ulcers are shallow but painful. Surrounding hyperpigmentation, scaling, and desquamation are present (Figure 61).

Differential diagnosis

- Venous stasis ulcer
- Vasculitis
- Pyoderma gangrenosum

Treatment

Discontinue hydroxyurea. Wound management includes debridement, edema control, and moist dressings.[91]

Summary

This chapter focuses on the importance of a complete history and physical for initiation of the wound healing process. It implies that if the wound does not heal in a reasonable amount of time, it should be reassessed for any misdiagnosis and for a possible need of wound biopsy. An attempt has been made to identify a variety of disorders that can be ongoing with a nonhealing wound. Underlying systemic condition needs to be treated before the wound can be healed.

A nonhealing wound that does not heal after four to six weeks of standard wound care should be referred to a specialty wound center for a comprehensive evaluation.

Review questions

1. All of the following are local factors contributing to nonhealing wounds except

a. hypoxia
b. edema
c. microvascular disease
d. malnutrition
e. necrosis

2. Malignancy should be suspected with

a. history of repeated trauma
b. exuberant granulation tissue
c. rolled-out edges
d. purple-red color around the ulcer
e. wounds secondary to burns
f. all of the above

3. Match the following

a. basal cell cancer	1. arises from keratinizing epidermal cells
b. Marjolin's ulcer	2. arises from epidermal basal cells
c. Kaposi's sarcoma	3. associated with hyperparathyroidism
d. pyoderma gangrenosum	4. associated with inflammatory bowel disease
e. calciphylaxis	5. associated with AIDS

4. Match the following

a. fish tank granuloma	1. *S. schenckii*
b. Buruli ulcer	2. gram-positive, non-spore-forming anaerobic bacteria
c. actinomycosis	3. *Mycobacteria leprae*
d. Hansen's disease	4. *Mycobacteria marinum*
e. sporotrichosis	5. *Mycobacteria ulcerans*

ANSWERS: 1) d
2) f
3) a -2, b-1, c-5,d -4, e-3
4) a-4, b-5, c-2, d-3, e-1

References

1. Schultz GS, Sibbald RG, Falanga V, et al. Wound bed preparation: a systemic approach to wound management. Wound Repair Regen. 2003:11(Suppl 1):S1-28.
2. Shah JB. Approach to commonly misdiagnosed wounds and unusual leg ulcers. In: Sheffield PJ, Fife CE, editors. Wound care practice. 2nd ed. Best Publishing; 2007. p. 579-602.
3. Shah JB. Dermatology review and unusual wounds. In: Shah JB, Fife CE, Sheffield PJ, editors. Wound care certification study guide. 2nd ed. Flagstaff (AZ): Best Publishing; 2016. p. 169-81.
4. Falanga V. *Cutaneous wound healing*. London: Martin Dunitz Ltd; 2001. p. 247-63.
5. Shah JB, Hamm R. Atypical wounds. In: Hamm's text and atlas of wound diagnosis and treatment. Mcgraw Hill Publications; 2015. p. 227-55.
6. Falanga V, Phillips T, Harding K, et al. *Text atlas of wound management*. London: Martin Dunitz Ltd; 2000. p. 189-227.
7. Weinstein D. Atypical wounds. In: Baronski S, Ayelo E 3rd, editors. Wound care essentials: practice principles. 2012. p. 491-511.
8. Hess CT. Checklist for laboratory tests to rule out atypical causes of leg ulcers. Adv Skin Wound Care. 2010;23:52.
9. Wheeless CR 3rd, editor. Wheeless' text book of orthopaedics [Internet]. Duke University Medical Center, Division of Orthopaedic Surgery. Available from: *http://www.wheelessonline.com. Joint publication with Data Trace Internet Publishing, LLC.*
10. Shah JB. Unusual wounds. WoundDoctor [application on Apple Store and Google Play].
11. Ashton RE. Teaching non-dermatologists to examine the skin: a review of literature and some recommendations. Br. J Dermatol. 1995 Feb;132(2):221-5.

12 Sasseville D. Neomycin. Dermatitis. 2010 Jan-Feb:21(1):3-7.

13. Corazza M, Mantovani L, Virgilli A, Strumia R. Allergic contact dermatitis from a clonidine transdermal delivery system. Contact Dermatitis. 1995 Apr;32(4):246.
14. Huerta C, Rivero E, Rodriguez LA. Incidence and risk factors for psoriasis in the general population. Arch Dermatol. 2007 Dec;143(12):1559-65.
15. Strauss JS, Krowchuk DP, Leyden JJ, et al., American Academy of Dermatology/ American Academy of Dermatology Association. Guidelines of care for acne vulgaris management. J Am Acad Dermatol. 2007 Apr;56(4):651-63.
16. Thiboutot D, Gollnick H, Bettoli V, et al. New insights into the management of acne: an update from the global alliance to improve outcomes in acne group. J Am Acad Dermatol. 2009 May;60(5 Suppl):s1-50.
17. Ailkhan A, Lynch PJ, Elsen DB. Hidradenitis suppurativa; a comprehensive review. J Am Acad Dermatol. 2009 Apr;60(4):539-61.
18. Rambhatla PV, Lim HW, Hamzavi I. A systemic review of treatments for hidradenitis suppurativa. Arch Dermatol. 2012 Apr;148(4):439-46.
19. Daum RS. Clinical practice. Skin and soft-tissue infections caused by methicillin-resistant Staphylococcus aureus. N Engl J Med. 2007 July 26;357(4):380-90.
20. Liu C, Bayer A, Cosgrove SE, et al. Clinical practice guidelines by the Infectious Diseases Society of America for the treatment of methicillin-resistant Staphylococcus aureus infections in adults and children. Clin Infect Dis. 2011;52:285-92.
21. Thomas KS, Crook AM, Nunn AJ, et al. Penicillin to prevent recurrent leg cellulitis. N Engl J Med. 2013 May 2;368(18):1695-703.
22. Bettesworth J, Gill K, Shah J. Primary actinomycosis of the foot: a case report and literature review. J Am Coll Clin Wound Spec. 2009;1(3):95-100.

23. Creighton R. Actinomycosis. A rare pedal infection. *J Am Podiatr Med Assoc.* 1993;83:637.

24. Mahgoub E, Yacoub A. Primary actinomycosis of the foot and leg: report of a case. *J Trop Med Hyg.* 1968;71:256.

25. Vogen K. A case report on actinomycosis of foot. *J Am Podiatr Med Assoc.* 1996; 86:238-240.

26. Wentworth AB, Drage LA, Wengenack NL, et al, Increased incidence of cutaneous nontuberculous mycobacterial infection, 1980 to 2009: a population-based study. Mayo Clin Proc. 2013 Jan;88(1):38-45.

27. Dodiuk-Gad R, Dyachenko P, Ziv M, et al. Nontuberculous mycobacterial infections of the skin: a retrospective study of 25 cases. J Am Acad Dermatol. 2007;57(3):413-20.

28. Kwyer TA, Ampadu E. Buruli ulcers: an emerging health problem in Ghana. Adv Skin Wound Care. 2006;19(9):479-86.

29. Nienhuis WA, Stienstra Y, et al. Antimicrobial treatment for early, limited mycobacterium ulcerans infection: a randomized controlled trial. Lancet. 2010;375(9715):664-72.

30. Winthrop KL, Abrams M, Yakrus M, et al. An outbreak of mycobacterial furunculosis associated with footbaths at a nail salon. N Engl J Med. 2002 May 2;346(18):1366-71.

31. Ramos-e-Silva M, Vasconcelos C, Carneriro S, et al. Sporotrichosis. Clin Dermatol. 2007;25(2):181-7.

32. Leroux S, Ulimann AJ. Management and diagnostic guidelines for fungal diseases in infectious disease and clinical microbiology: critical appraisal. Clin Microbiol Infect. 2013 Dec;19(12):1115-21.

33. Perfect JR. Fungal diagnosis: how do we do it and can we do it better? Curr Med Res Opin. 2013 Apr;29(Suppl 4):3-11.

34. Moriarty B, Hay R, Morris-Jones R. The diagnosis and management of tinea. BMH. 2012 Jul 10;345:e4380.

35. Cohen JI. Clinical practice: herpes zoster. N Engl J Med. 2013 Jul 18;369(3):255-63.

36. Karlsmark T, Goodman JJ, Drouault Y, Lufrano L, Pledger GW, Cold Sore Study Group. Randomized clinical study comparing Compeed cold sore patch to acyclovir cream 5% in the treatment of herpes simplex labialis. J Eur Acad Dermatol Venereol. 2008;22(10):1184-92.

37. Stevens DL, Bisno AL, Chambers HF, et al. Practice guidelines for the diagnosis and management of skin and soft tissue infections: 2014 update by the Infectious Diseases Society of America. Clin Infect Dis. 2014:59(2):147-59.

38. Wong CH, Khin LW, Heng KS, et al. The LRINEC (Laboratory Risk Indicator for Necrotizing Fasciitis) Score: a tool for distinguishing necrotizing fasciitis from other soft tissue infections. Crit Care Med. 2004 Jul;32(7):1535-41.

39. Jacoby I. Clostridial myositis, necrotizing fasciitis and zygomatic infections. In: Newman & Thom's physiology and medicine of hyperbaric oxygen therapy. Elsevier Publication; 2008. p. 397-419.

40. Ozturk E, Ozguc H, Yilmazlar T. The use of vacuum assisted closure in the management of Fournier's gangrene. Am J Surg. 2009;197(5):660-5.

41. Czymek R, Schmidt A, Eckman C, et al. Fournier's gangrene: vacuum-assisted closure versus conventional dressings. Am J Surg. 2009;197(2):168-76.

42. Balbierz JM, Ellis K. Streptococcal infection and necrotizing fasciitis – implications for rehabilitation: a report of 5 cases and review of the literature. Arch Phys Med Rehabil. 2004;85(7):1205-9.

43. Naylor W. Malignant wounds: aetiology and principles of management. *Nursing Standard.* 2002;16(52):45-54.

44. Kirsner R, Spencer J, Falanga V, et al. Squamous cell carcinoma arising in osteomyelitis and chronic wounds. Treatment with Mohs microsurgery versus amputation. *Dermatol Surg.* 1996;22:1015-28.

45. Trent J, Kirsner R. Wounds and malignancy. *Adv Skin Wound Care.* 2003;16:31-34.

46. Hansson C, Anderson E. Malignant skin lesions on the legs and feet at a dermatological leg ulcer clinic during five years. *Acta Derm Venereol.* 1998;78:147-8.

47. Rubin AI, Chen EH, Ratner D. Basal-cell carcinoma. N Engl J Med. 2005 Nov 24;353(21):2262-9

48. Goldman M. Nonhealing leg ulcers: a manifestation of basal cell carcinoma. *J Am Acad Dermatol.* 1992;26:791-2.

49. Franco R. Basal and squamous cell carcinoma associated with chronic venous leg ulcer. *Intern J Dermatol.* 2001;40:539-44.

50. Fleming M, Hunt J, Purdue G, Sandstad J. Marjolin's ulcer: a review and reevaluation of a difficult problem. *J Burn Care Rehabil.* 1990;11:460-9.

51. Alam M, Ratner D. Cutaneous squamous-cell carcinoma. N Engl J Med. 2001 Mar 29;344(13):975-83.

52. Gill K, Shah J. Kaposi sarcoma in patients with diabetes and wounds. *Adv Skin Wound Care.* 2006;19(4):196-201.

53. Taniguchi S, Kono T, Tanii T, et al. Secondary T-cell lymphoma presenting as a giant ulcer. Clin Exp Dermatol. 1992;17:379-81.

54. Balch CM, Gershernwald JE, et al. Final version of 2009 AJCC melanoma staging and classification. J Clin Oncol. 2009 Dec 20;27(36):6199-206.

55. Tsao H, Atkins MB, Sober AJ. Management of cutaneous melanoma. N Engl J Med. 2004 Sept 2;351(10):998-1012.

56. Powell F, Su W, Perry H. Pyoderma gangrenosum: classification and management. *J Am Acad Dermatol.* 1996;34:395-409.

57. Wollina U. Clinical management of pyoderma gangrenosum. *Am J Clin Dermatol.* 2002;3(3):149-58.

58. Miller J, Yentzer BA, Clark A, Jorizzo JL, Feldman SR. Pyoderma gangrenosum; a review and update on new therapies. J Am Acad Dermatol. 2010 Apr;62(4):646-54.

59. Cupps TR, Fauci AS. The vasculitides. *Major Probl Intern Med.* 1981;21:1-211.

60. Thurtle O, Cawley M. The frequency of leg ulceration in rheumatoid arthritis: a survey. *J Rheumatol.* 1983;10:507-9.

61. Hafner J, Schneider E, Burg G, Cassina PC, Gunter B, et al. Management of leg ulcers in patients with rheumatoid arthritis or systemic sclerosis: the importance of concomitant arterial and venous disease. J Vasc Surg. 2000;32(2):322-9.

62. Okon LG, Werth VP. Cutaneous lupus erythematosus: diagnosis and treatment. Best Pract Res Clin Rheumatol. 2013 Jun;27(3):391-404.

63. Lowe G, Henderson CL, Grau RH, et al. A systemic review of drug-induced subacute cutaneous lupus erythematosus. Br. J Dermatol. 2011 Mar;164(3):465-72.

64. Helfman T, Falanga V. Stanazolal as a novel therapeutic agent in dermatology. J Am Acad Dermatol. 1995;33:254-8.

65. Gelber AC, Manno RL, Shah AA, et al. Race and association with disease manifestations and mortality in scleroderma: a 20-year experience at the Johns Hopkins Scleroderma Center and review of the literature. Medicine (Baltmore). 2013 Jul;92(4):191-205.

66. Fauci A, Braunwald E, Isselbacher, et al. *Harrison's principles of internal medicine.* New York: McGraw Hill; 1998. p. 989-91, 1004-19.

67. Lawley T, Kubota Y. Vasculitis. *Dermatol Clin.* 1990;8:681-7.

68. Lowitt M, Dover J. Necrobiosis lipoidica. *J Am Acad Dermatol.* 1991;25:735-48.

69. Clayton TH, Harrison PV. Successful treatment of chronic ulcerated necrobiosis lipoidica with 0.1% topical tacrolimus ointment. Br J Dermatol. 2005;152(3):581-2.

70. Spenceri EA, Nahass GT. Topically applied bovine collagen in the treatment of ulcerative necrobiosis lipoidica diabeticorum. Arch Dermatol. 1997;133(7):817-8.

71. Heidenheim M, Jemec GB. Successful treatment of necrobiosis lipoidica diabeticorum with photodynamic therapy. Arch Dermatol. 2006;142(12):1548-50.

72. Schmidt E, Zillikens D. Modern diagnosis of autoimmune blistering skin diseases. Autoimmun Rev. 2010 Dec;10(2):84-9.

73. Di Zenzo G, Marazza G, Borradori L. Bullous pemphigoid physiopathology, clinical features and management. Adv Dermatol. 2007;23:257-88.

74. Alarcon-Segovia D, Deleze M, Oria C. Antiphospholipid antibodies and the antiphospholipid syndrome in systemic lupus erythematosus: a prospective analysis of 500 consecutive cases. *Medicine.* 1989;68:353-65.

75. Ramos-Casias M, Stone JH, Cid MC, Bosch X. The cryoglobulinaemias. Lancet. 2012 Jan 28;379(9813):348-60.

76. Thornsberry LA, LoSicco KI, English JC 3rd. The skin and hypercoagulable states. J Am Acad Dermatol. 2013 Sept;69(3):450-62.

77. Nazarian RM, Van Cott EM, Zembowicz A, et al. Warfarin–induced skin necrosis. J Am Acad Dermatol. 2009;61(2):325-32.

78. Cheng A, Scheinfeld NS, McDowell B, et al. Warfarin skin necrosis in postpartum woman with protein S deficiency. Obstet Gynecol. 1997;90:671-2.

79. Richmond NA, Maderal AD, Vivas AC. Evidence-based management of common lower extremity ulcers. Dermatol Ther. 2013 May-Jun;26(3):187-96.

80. Treadwell T. Sickle cell ulcers, chapter 17. In: Baranoski et al, editors. Wound care essentials. 3rd ed. Lippincott and Williams; 2012. p. 447-59.

81. Hamm RL, Weitz I, Rodrigues J. Pathophysiology and multidisciplinary management of leg wounds in sickle cell disease: a case discussion and literature review. Wounds. 2006;18(10):277-85.

82. Morris C, Kuypers FA, Larkin S, et al. Arginine therapy: a novel strategy to induce nitric oxide production in sickle cell disease. Br J Haematol. 2000 Nov;111(2):498-500.

83. Mery L, Girot R, Aractingi S. Topical effectiveness of molgramostim (GM-CSF) in sickle cell leg ulcers. Dermatology. 2004;208(2):135-7.

84. Gordon S, Bui A. Human skin equivalent in the treatment of chronic leg ulcers in sickle cell disease patients. J Am Podiatr Med Assoc. 2003;93(3):240-1.

85. Coates T, Kirkland G, Dymock R, et al. Cutaneous necrosis from calcific uremic arteriolopathy. *Am J Kidney Dis.* 1998;32(3):384-91.

86. Vassa N, Twardowski Z, Campbell J. Hyperbaric oxygen therapy in calciphylaxis-induced skin necrosis in a peritoneal dialysis patient. *Am J Kidney Dis.* 1994;23(6):878-81.

87. Podymow T, Wherrett C, Burns K. Hyperbaric oxygen in the treatment of calciphlaxis: a case series. *Nephrol Dial Transplant.* 2001;16:2176-80.

88. Nunley JR, Elston DM. Calcinosis cutis. Medscape [Internet]. Available from: emedicine.medscape.com/article/1103137-overview

89. Dimsdale JE, Creed F, Escobar J, et al. Somatic symptom disorder: an important change in DSM. J Psychosom Res. 2013 Sept;75(3):223-8.

90. Silverstein LH, Hanes PJ, Garnick JJ. Pyogenic granuloma. *J Fam Pract.* 1995 Aug;41(2):196.

91. Sirieix ME et al. Leg ulcers and hydroxyurea: forty-one cases. Arch Dermatol. 1999;135(7):818-20.

Chapter 16

ARTHROPOD-RELATED WOUNDS

Dirk Elston, MD

KEY CONCEPTS

1. Arthropod-related wounds may occur following insect bites and stings.
2. The wound manifestations may be the direct result of toxins within the venom, immune response to the venom, or ensuing infection.
3. A history of likely arthropod exposure as well as the color, morphology, and distribution of the lesions may be helpful in establishing a diagnosis.
4. A punch biopsy can be helpful to confirm a diagnosis of arthropod-related injury.
5. Brown recluse bites are over-diagnosed, and many suspected cases actually represent pyoderma gangrenosum and methicillin-resistant staphylococcus abscesses.

CONTENTS

Introduction

Arthropod-related wounds may occur following insect bites and stings. Some of the most serious arthropod-related wounds are caused by arachnids, including the brown recluse spider. The wound manifestations may be the direct result of toxins within the venom, immune response to the venom, or ensuing infection.

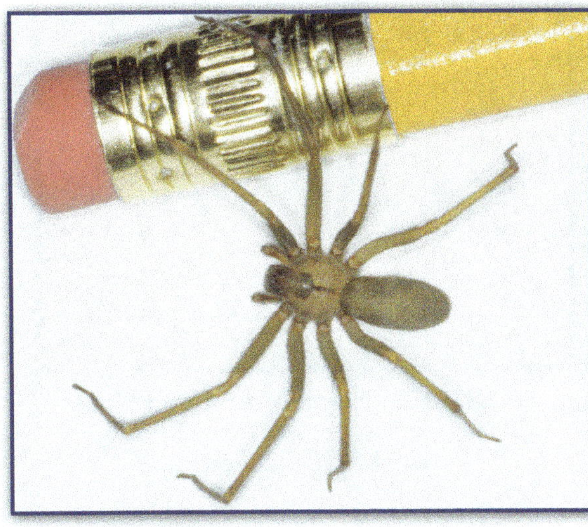

FIGURE 1. Brown recluse spider

I. Case history: arthropod-related wound

Mr. BR was cleaning his basement when he sustained a bite on his right lower leg. He brought the crushed spider into the office for identification. The spider was brown with three pairs of eyes and a fiddle pattern overlying the cephalothorax (Figure 1). The area surrounding the bite was edematous and dusky in color, with areas of ulceration and necrosis (Figure 2).

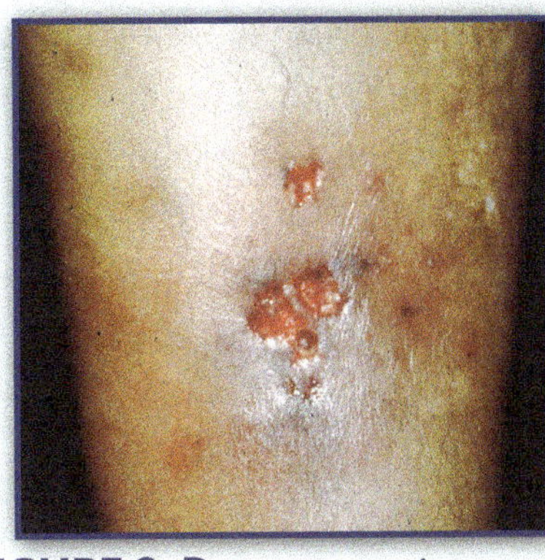

FIGURE 2. Dermonecrotic reaction secondary to a brown recluse spider bite

II. Approach to arthropod-related wounds

Step 1: Diagnosis is identified by proper history and examination.

1. Clinical clues toward diagnosis

A history of likely arthropod exposure as well as the color, morphology, and distribution of the lesions may be helpful in establishing a diagnosis. Cutaneous loxoscelism secondary to the bite of a brown recluse spider starts with a pruritic papule evolving to a wider zone of intense pain, accompanied by cyanosis, edema, and necrosis.

2. Clues from a good history

Spiders may be encountered year-round, while many other arthropod-related wounds are seasonal in nature. A history of outdoor activity or other likely exposure can be helpful. Pet-associated dermatoses from fleas or mites may persist year-round. Small arthropods, like biting midges, are rarely seen, whereas visual identification of a spider or tick is more likely and extremely important in guiding treatment and anticipating possible vector-borne illness.

3. Clues from examination

Spider bites are solitary, often with a dusky cyanotic hue, associated edema, and variable necrosis. Insect bite reactions may be grouped or disseminated erythematous urticarial papules. They are often excoriated because of the associated pruritus. Edematous plaques, nodules, and vesiculobullous reactions may be seen, and exaggerated bite reactions are common in patients with underlying chronic lymphocytic leukemia (Figure 3). Extreme hypersensitivity to mosquito

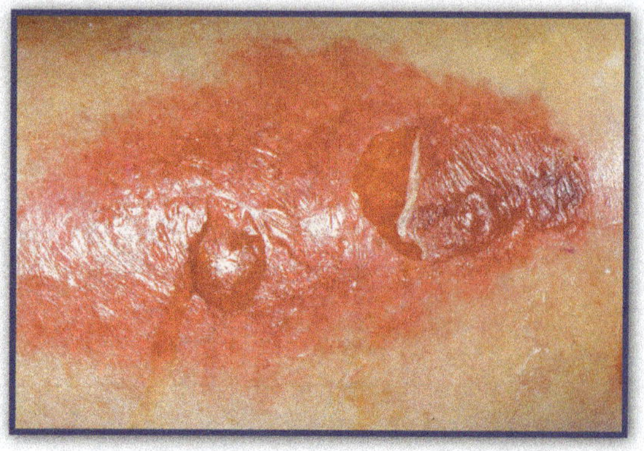

FIGURE 3. Exaggerated insect bite reaction in a patient with chronic lymphocytic leukemia

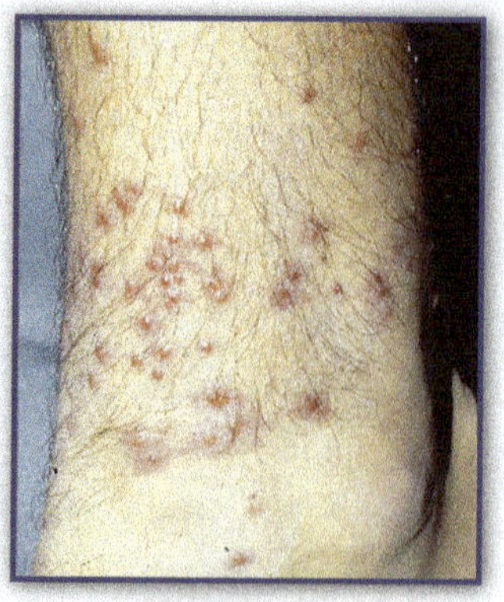

FIGURE 4. Chigger bites

bites with development of bullous or necrotic skin lesions has also been described in Asian and Hispanic children with chronic Epstein-Barr virus (EBV) infection and proliferation of EBV-carrying natural killer (NK) cells.[1] Screening for an underlying hematologic malignancy and latent EBV infection should be considered in patients with unusual and exaggerated arthropod bite reactions. Chigger bites are intensely pruritic and often grouped at the edge of tight clothing or elastic (Figure 4). Bedbug bites are often grouped and bites on the arms can resemble prurigo nodularis. Bee and vespid wasp stings typically produce immediate burning pain, followed by erythema and swelling. Atrial arrhythmias have been reported after bee stings, even in the absence of anaphylaxis. Killer bee and wasp attacks may produce myoglobinuria or hemoglobinuria and acute tubular necrosis.

Step 2: Diagnosis is identified by biopsy. A punch biopsy can be helpful to confirm a diagnosis of arthropod-related injury. Histologic features suggestive of an arthropod bite include a wedge-shaped perivascular lymphocytic infiltrate with eosinophils, endothelial prominence and overlying spongiosis, or focal epidermal necrosis.

Step 3: Diagnosis is identified by proper lab diagnostics. The diagnosis of a brown recluse spider bite can be confirmed by an enzyme immunoassay to detect Loxosceles venom in a skin biopsy, glycophorin A measurement, or passive hemagglutination inhibition test.

Step 4: This is a differential diagnosis. Brown recluse bites are over-diagnosed, and many suspected cases actually represent pyoderma gangrenosum and methicillin-resistant staphyloccoccus abscesses. Clues to the correct diagnosis of pyoderma gangrenosum include a history of pathergy (lesions occurring at sites of minor injury), a pustule which evolves into an ulcer with a violaceous, necrotic overhanging border, and necrotic pitting which resolves with cribriform scarring. Insect sting hypersensitivity with severe immediate reactions may also be an indication of underlying mastocytosis. Scabies can produce bullae with positive immunofluorescence studies mimicking bullous pemphigoid.

III. Pathogenesis

Immediate reactions are commonly related to histamine, serotonin, formic acid, or kinins contained within the venom, while delayed reactions are usually a manifestation of the host's immune response to proteinaceous allergens.

Sphingomyelinase D is the major toxin in brown recluse venom, and it interacts with serum amyloid protein. Hyaluronidase allows eschars to spread in a gravity-dependent fashion.

IV. Treatment

A. Brown recluse spider bites

Most brown recluse bites can be treated effectively with rest, ice, and elevation. Although intradermal injection of polyclonal anti-Loxosceles Fab antibody fragments has been shown to attenuate necrosis in an animal model up to four hours after envenomation, this treatment is often not necessary. Antivenin can reduce the ultimate size of the necrotic area even when administered up to 48 hours after envenomation.[2] Hyperbaric oxygen therapy may decrease the final size of ulceration, although results have varied. Studies with dapsone and colchicine have been inconsistent, and data suggest that with any significant delay in treatment there may be little to no benefit. Dapsone therapy is complicated by the potential for hemolysis, especially in individuals who have an inherited glucose-6-phosphatase dehydrogenase (G6PD) deficiency. Given the potential for harm and the lack of consistent data showing any benefit, it is not recommended to have routine therapy with any systemic agent except antivenin and prednisone (in the case of systemic reactions). On the basis of limited animal data, intralesional triamcinolone may be useful to reduce local necrosis.[3] The complement inhibitor eculizumab has demonstrated the ability to prevent venom-induced hemolysis in vitro, but in vivo data are needed before this agent is used for the treatment of bites in humans. Plasma exchange has been used in the setting of severe systemic reactions.[4-5] Early implementation of HBO_2 may be beneficial in patients with spider bite who have extensive progressive tissue necrosis.[14]

B. Funnel-web spiders

Tegenaria agrestis (the hobo spider) was imported to North America from Europe and is most commonly found in the northwestern states. It has been associated with dermonecrotic reactions similar to those of the brown recluse spider. Hadronyche and Atrax funnel-web spiders are endemic to eastern Australia. Their bites can result in bradycardia or tachycardia, hypertension, hypersalivation, muscle spasms, diaphoresis, and shock. Severe myocardial injury, including catecholamine-induced cardiomyopathy, has been reported.[6] Australian funnel-web spider venom contains small peptide neurotoxins including the δ-atracotoxins that slow tetrodotoxin-sensitive voltage-gated sodium channel inactivation resulting in catecholaminergic and cholinergic excess. Agatoxins from Agelenopsis apena, the native American funnel-web spider, target ion channels, suggesting the potential for antivenin therapy.[7]

C. Tarantulas

Tarantulas are large, hairy spiders common in the southwestern United States and Mexico. Although the bite of most tarantula species does not produce severe systemic toxicity, many species of tarantulas possess urticating hairs on the dorsal abdomen. Itching produced by these hairs may persist for weeks and corneal penetration can result in ophthalmia nodosa, a chronic granulomatous reaction that can lead to loss of vision.

D. General treatment of insect bites

Fluorinated topical corticosteroid creams can be applied to persistent bite reactions. Camphor and menthol lotion and gel formulations are useful in the control of pruritus. Topical anesthetic preparations containing pramoxine are readily available and present a low risk of contact dermatitis. When topical agents fail, intralesional injection of triamcinolone may be necessary.

Prevention of bites involves the use of protective clothing and repellents. DEET (N,N-diethyl-3-methylbenzamide, previously called N,N-diethyl-m-toluamide) and picaridin are the most widely used repellents. Newer agents for application to skin include IR3535, KBR 3023, and para-menthane-3,8-diol. Picaridin, IR3535, and p-menthane-3,8-diol perform reasonably well against a variety of mosquitoes and generally outperform soybean oil, citronella, neem oil, fennel oil, and geraniol.[8] For protection against the common mosquitoes Aedes aegypti and Culex quinquefasciatus, IR3535 appears comparable to DEET. The Mediterranean monk's pepper plant (Vitex agnus-castus) has demonstrated efficacy against Ixodes ricinus and Rhipicephalus sanguineus ticks as well as some mosquitoes, biting flies, and fleas.

Permethrin is largely used for fabric impregnation.[9] Impregnated clothing can protect against ticks and chiggers. Impregnated mosquito netting can help prevent malaria and leishmaniasis.[10]

Those allergic to bees and wasps should carry an epinephrine (adrenaline) auto-injector with them at all times. The EpiPen® autoinjector contains 0.3 ml of epinephrine 1:1000 (for individuals weighing >66 pounds [>30 kg]), while the EpiPen® Jr. contains 0.3 ml of epinephrine 1:2000 (for children weighing 33-66 pounds). Bee stingers should be removed as rapidly as possible. Venom immunotherapy has been shown to improve quality of life for patients allergic to stings.[11] Desensitization protocols vary and should be discussed with an allergist. Rush (accelerated) immunotherapy can be performed for those with severe reactions, and it has a reasonable safety profile.[12] Omalizumab has been used in conjunction with immunotherapy for patients refractory to standard regimens, and this may help to prevent immunotherapy-related anaphylaxis.[13]

Summary

Arthropod-related wounds resulting from toxins within the venom, immune response to the venom, or ensuing infection are common. The diagnosis should be based on a history of likely arthropod exposure as well as the color, morphology, and distribution of the lesions. When in doubt, a punch biopsy can be helpful to confirm a diagnosis of arthropod-related injury.

Review questions

1. **Brown recluse spider bites are most closely associated with which of the following?**

    a. hemolytic anemia

    b. hepatic necrosis

    c. cardiac necrosis

    d. renal tubular necrosis

    e. hypoglycemia

2. **Which of the following is most likely to mimic a brown recluse spider bite?**

    a. a scorpion sting

    b. a mosquito bite

    c. pyoderma gangrenosum

    d. urticarial vasculitis

    e. lupus profundus

ANSWERS: 1) a
2) c

References

1. Asada H. Hypersensitivity to mosquito bites: a unique pathogenic mechanism linking Epstein-Barr virus infection, allergy and oncogenesis. J Dermatol Sci. 2007;45:153–60.
2. Pauli I, Minozzo JC, da Silva PH, et al. Analysis of therapeutic benefits of antivenin at different time intervals after experimental envenomation in rabbits by venom of the brown spider (Loxosceles intermedia). Toxicon. 2009;53:660–71.
3. Elston DM, Miller SD, Young RJ, et al. Comparison of colchicine, dapsone, triamcinolone, and diphenhydramine therapy for the treatment of brown recluse spider envenomation. A double blind, controlled study in a rabbit model. Arch Dermatol. 2005;141:595–97.
4. Abraham M, Tilzer L, Hoehn KS, Thornton SL. Therapeutic plasma exchange for refractory hemolysis after brown recluse spider (Loxosceles reclusa) envenomation. J Med Toxicol. 2015 Sep;11(3):364-67.
5. Said A, Hmiel P, Goldsmith M, Dietzen D, Hartman ME. Successful use of plasma exchange for profound hemolysis in a child with loxoscelism. Pediatrics. 2014 Nov;134(5):e1464-67.
6. Isbister GK, Sellors KV, Beckmann U, Chiew AL, Downes MA, Berling I. Catecholamine-induced cardiomyopathy resulting from life-threatening funnel-web spider envenoming. Med J Aust. 2015 Oct 5;203(7):302-04.
7. Miller M, O'Leary MA, Isbister GK. Towards rationalisation of antivenom use in funnel-web spider envenoming: enzyme immunoassays for venom concentrations. Clin Toxicol (Phila). 2016 Mar;54(3):245-51.
8. Costantini C, Badolo A, Ilboudo-Sanogo E. Field evaluation of the efficacy and persistence of insect repellents DEET, IR3535, and KBR 3023 against Anopheles gambiae complex and other Afrotropical vector mosquitoes. Trans R Soc Trop Med Hyg. 2004;98:644–52.
9. Faulde MK, Pages F, Uedelhoven W. Bioactivity and laundering resistance of five commercially available, factory-treated permethrin-impregnated fabrics for the prevention of mosquito-borne diseases: the need for a standardized testing and licensing procedure. Parasitol Res. 2016 Apr;115(4):1573-82.
10. Rowland T, Davidson SA, Kobylinski K, Menses C, Rowton E. Efficacy of permethrin treated bed nets against Leishmania major infected sand flies. US Army Med Dep J. 2015 Jul-Sep:10-15.
11. Casale TB, Burks AW. Clinical practice. Hymenoptera-sting hypersensitivity. N Engl J Med. 2014 Apr 10;370(15):1432-39.
12. Nittner-Marszalska M, Cichocka-Jarosz E, Małaczyńska T, Kraluk B, Rosiek-Biegus M, Kosinska M, Pawłowicz R, Lis G. Safety of ultrarush venom immunotherapy: comparison between children and adults. J Investig Allergol Clin Immunol. 2016;26(1):40-47.
13. Palgan K, Bartuzi Z, Gotz-Zbikowska M. Treatment with a combination of omalizumab and specific immunotherapy for severe anaphylaxis after a wasp sting. Int J Immunopathol Pharmacol. 2014 Jan-Mar;27(1):109-12.
14. Hagood CO, Wilson JR. Necrotic wounds produced by spider bites. In: Sheffield PJ, Fife CE. Wound Care Practice 2nd Ed. Flagstaff, AZ: Best Publishing Company; 2007. p. 561-578.

Chapter 17

THE EFFECTS OF RADIATION ON WOUND HEALING

John J. Feldmeier, DO, FACRO, FUHM

KEY CONCEPTS

1. Usual treatments for carcinomas consist of doses of 5,000 to 7,000 cGy over five to eight weeks.
2. It is estimated that between 50% and 60% of patients diagnosed with malignancy will receive radiation as part of their cancer treatment.
3. Radiation effects on normal tissues can occur primarily in two different time frames. Acute reactions occur during or just after completion of radiation. Chronic radiation effects occur after a latent period of months to years, occurring most frequently from six months to two years after radiation.
4. Wounds can occur within radiation fields before radiation, just after radiation, or even many years after radiation.
5. Radiation impairs wound healing by reducing angiogenesis and by directly depleting both stem cells and certain mature cell lines (fibroblasts, vascular endothelial cells, and squamous cells) required for the healing process.
6. The induction of fibrosis, sometimes very marked, is also a major contributor to radiation damage.
7. Hypoxia perpetuates and enhances radiation-induced tissue damage and interferes with healing.
8. Significant vascular changes typically require a latent period of at least six months to become clinically manifest.
9. When surgery is to follow radiation, the vast majority of the time it will follow four to six weeks after completion of the radiation.

10. When preoperative radiation is planned before surgery, preferably at least three to four weeks and no more than six weeks should elapse between radiation and surgery.
11. If wound closure will require flap creation, ideally the vascular supply to that flap should originate from outside radiation portals.
12. When the treatment plan includes radiation after surgery, at least two weeks and no more than six weeks time should elapse before therapeutic radiation is begun.
13. Hyperbaric effects on radiated tissues include the induction of stem cells, the reduction of fibrosis, and the enhancement of angiogenesis.
14. The protocol for existing mandibular osteoradionecrosis is to deliver 30 presurgical treatments followed by 10 postoperative treatments. When hyperbaric oxygen is given to prevent ORN (osteoradionecrosis), the recommendation is for 20 pre-extraction treatments followed by 10 post-extraction treatments.
15. Marx has emphasized the importance of giving most of the hyperbaric treatments prior to surgical wounding to improve the vascularity and inherent quality of the tissues prior to surgical wounding.

CONTENTS

Introduction

The impact of radiation therapy on cancer care

Roentgen discovered X-rays in 1895, and within five years patients were receiving radiation therapy for malignancy. Initially a wide range of nonmalignant pathologies were also treated, but this is now uncommon. Coutard and other early clinicians discovered that cancer treatment was most successful and normal tissue reactions least severe when treatments were fractionated, or divided into many, usually daily treatments. Coutard established the standard radiation therapy regimen for external radiation that is used even to this day. It consists of one treatment per day, five days per week, at a daily dose of 180 to 200 cGy (centigray) per day or 900 to 1,000 cGy per week. Modern radiation occasionally deviates from this standard based on modern developments of targeted therapy and increased appreciation of radiation biology. Usual treatments for carcinomas consist of doses of 5,000 to 7,000 cGy over five to eight weeks. An exception to this fractionated dose delivery is radiosurgery where a small field is given a very targeted single dose typically delivering 1,000 to 2,000 cGy and has a much higher biologic effect than this dose divided over several treatments. The prescribed dose depends to a large extent on whether the radiation is the sole local modality or whether radiation is to be combined with surgery. For other more radiosensitive malignant tumors such as lymphomas or germ cell tumors, radiation doses are reduced to the range of 2,500 to 4,500 cGy. For sarcomas doses required are in the 6000 to 7000 cGy range. Because of normal tissue tolerance, total doses will rarely exceed 7,000 cGy except in brachytherapy or implant radiation therapy treatments. Palliative treatments are usually given to lower total doses but at a higher daily treatment fraction in order to complete the therapy in a shorter total time so as to maximize quality of life concerns.

It is estimated that between 50% and 60% of patients diagnosed with malignancy will receive radiation as part of their cancer treatment.[1] Typically, about one-half of these receive treatment as part of a treatment plan offered with curative intent. The other half will receive radiation with a high rate of successful quality-of-life-improving, palliative intent. Approximately 1.7 million new cases of invasive cancers (not including basal and squamous skin cancers) will occur this year. There are more than 15 million cancer survivors alive today in the United States.[2] More and more frequently, with current treatment regimens, radiation is combined with surgery, chemotherapy, or both as a component of a multimodality approach to treatment. Serious radiation complications are often delayed, and those who are long-term survivors of their treatment are at risk for developing complications even many years after treatment. Overall only about 5%–10% of those treated with radiation will develop serious complications.[3] However, traditional interventions for these complications are dissatisfying, often requiring complex and potentially complicated surgical interventions with removal of the injured part if possible.

Radiation doses employed with the intent of eradicating gross disease as the primary local treatment or residual microscopic tumor after surgical resection are well established and consistently employed at different centers across the world. These dose recommendations have been obtained empirically after many years of treatment experience although radiobiologic models have been developed to provide additional guidance. Often doses employed are very close to limits of tolerance for adjoining normal tissues in the average patient. Tolerance doses vary significantly in individual patients based on a wide range of individual idiosyncratic sensitivities to the effects of radiation. In some cases, this individual tolerance is exceeded during treatment and complications result. Certain genetic syndromes, most notably Ataxia Telangiectasia, significantly increase the likelihood of severe reactions and complications.[4] Total dose, dose per treatment, frequency of dose, and volume treated are the best-understood determinants of treatment complications.[5,6] We do not yet have dependable biochemical assays or imaging studies available to us, which will reliably predict complications (or tumor control for that matter) for a given individual patient though some show promise.

Radiation therapy is a local-regional therapy wherein sites of gross or suspected residual microscopic disease plus sites of potential nodal metastases are targeted for therapy. Complications affect only those organs or tissues receiving a significant dose. Radiation almost never causes complications outside of the radiation fields treated. The scope of treatment is contrasted with cytotoxic chemotherapy and other systemic therapies including immunotherapy where complications, and potentially therapeutic effects, are also systemic in nature. Modern radiation oncology uses modern three-dimensional imaging techniques such as CT, MRI, and PET to identify the treatment volume. It then delivers a targeted dose employing complex treatment plans typically composed of multiple intersecting shaped beams or the summation of multiple dynamic beamlets to deliver the intended dose to the desired tissues while avoiding normal critical organs and tissues. These targeted techniques include conformal therapy, intensity-modulated radiation therapy, and radiosurgery. However, even with sophisticated modern targeting techniques, normal tissues will necessarily receive some radiation dose. The final plan of dose delivery to shaped and modulated fields requires high-powered modern computers, complex planning algorithms, and iterative computer calculations until all the parameters of treatment are optimized. Computer-optimized plans are always reviewed by the physician before they are employed.

Radiation effects on normal tissues can occur primarily in two different time frames. Acute reactions occur during or just after completion of radiation. These occur mostly in tissues that, like cancers, are undergoing active

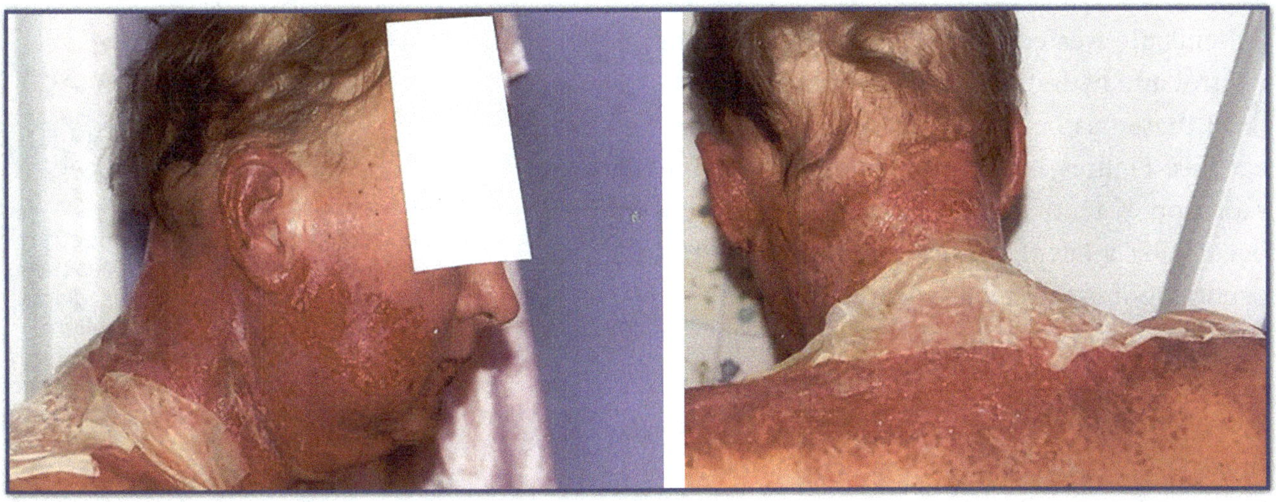

FIGURE 1. This patient suffered a severe acute radiation reaction and discontinued his treatment for his pharyngeal squamous cell cancer at 4,000 cGy of a planned dose of 7,000 cGy. The reaction did resolve over several weeks of supportive care. He had no further cancer treatment, and interestingly his cancer was controlled at this very low dose suggesting that both his normal tissues and his malignancy were exceptionally sensitive to radiation.

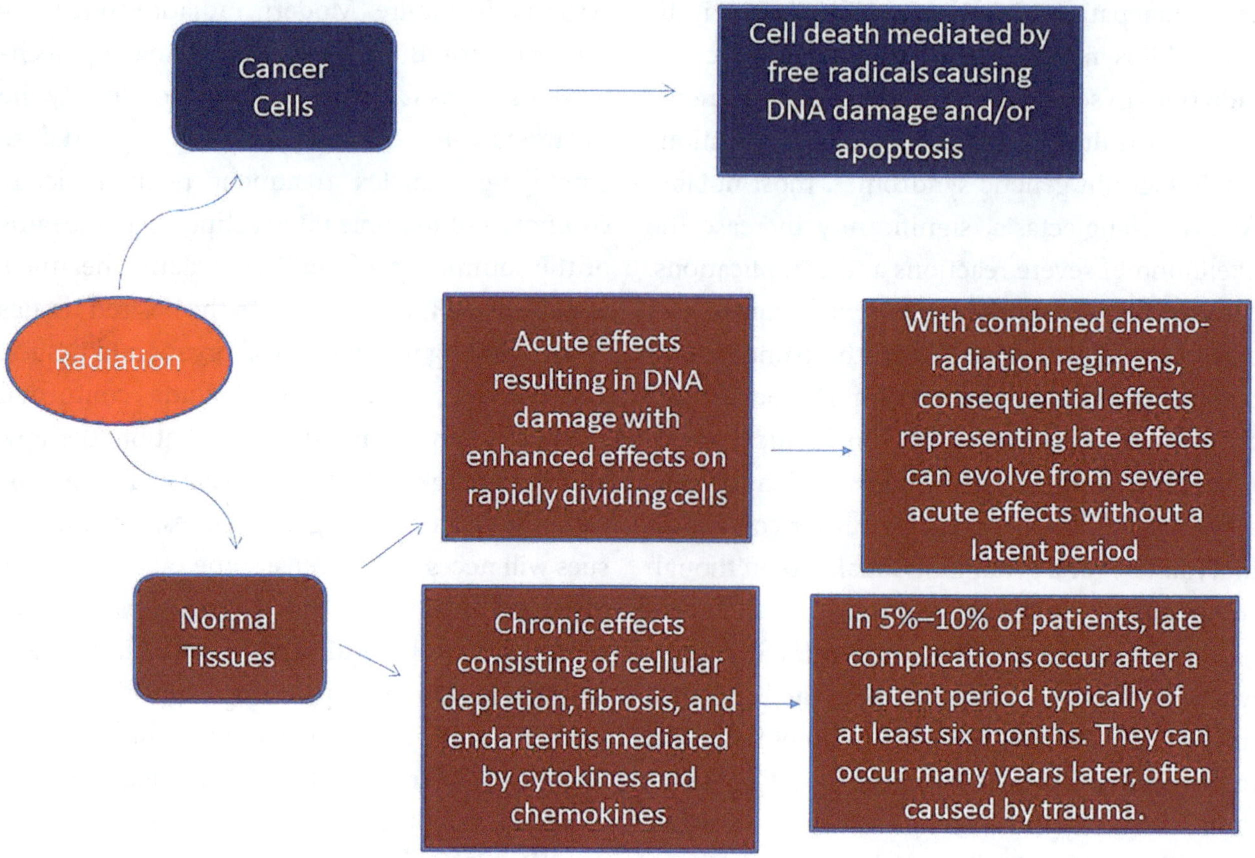

FIGURE 3. A schematic depiction of radiation effects

mitotic cellular division. Like cancer cells, these cells are damaged by direct effect on their DNA leading to chromosomal aberrations and cell death. For the most part, this damage is self-limited and typically resolves in a few weeks. Patients are treated with supportive care (pain control and hydration and nutritional support) until there has been a resolution of this damage. See Figures 1 and 2 for examples of acute radiation reactions. Chronic radiation effects occur after a latent period of months to years, occurring most frequently from six months to two years after radiation. These are the source of the most difficult and serious complications of radiation. They are often not self-limited. Sometimes with aggressive combined chemotherapy and radiation treatment regimens, patients will develop severe acute reactions, which evolve into serious chronic complications without the latent symptom-free period. See Figure 3 for a graphic depiction of acute and chronic radiation effects.

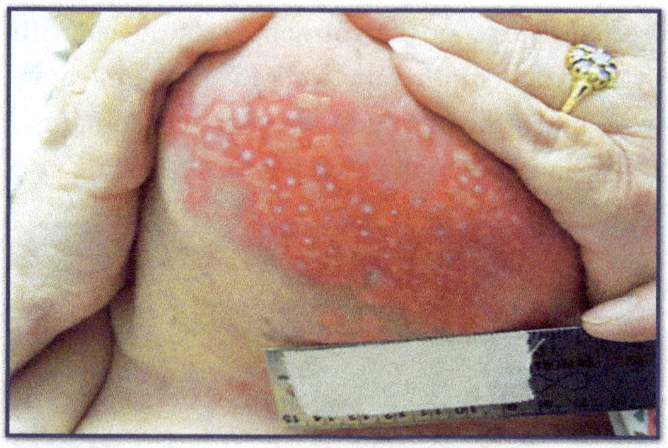

FIGURE 2. This patient received post-lumpectomy radiation and experienced a brisk acute reaction. The patient was given a break from radiation treatments. The photo shows that epithelium is rapidly spreading not only from the wound edges but also from islands of residual epithelium in the center of the wound not recognized until the wound began to show rapid epithelialization.

Brachytherapy or implant radiation has been reported in at least some publications to cause higher rates of treatment-related complications.[7] Brachytherapy consists of placing radioactive sources inside the body within tumor masses interstitially or next to the tumor if a body cavity is adjoining. A time-tested application for brachytherapy is gynecologic tumors where encapsulated radioactive isotopes are placed into applicators through the vagina and often into the uterus to treat cervical, endometrial, or vaginal cancers. These gynecologic implants are almost always temporary where the isotope is removed once the prescribed dose has been delivered. Traditionally, this dose is delivered to the patient as part of patient hospital admission for two to three days. The patient is kept in an isolated hospital room to prevent exposure to other patients, visitors, and staff. An alternative and frequent method employed now is to combine several sessions of outpatient treatment utilizing a remote-controlled machine that introduces a single highly radioactive source (usually the isotope Iridium-192) that moves through the implanted applicator with precise computer control. This technique is called HDR (high-dose-rate) brachytherapy. The dose is typically given in just a few minutes and is repeated several times.

A common treatment for prostate cancer is the implantation of permanent radioactive Iodine-125 seeds. These seeds slowly deliver the prescribed dose over 12 months. Sometimes over 100 seeds will be placed with real-time ultrasound guidance. In brachytherapy treatments, doses may exceed 16,000 cGy or about twice the operational dose limit for a course of external beam radiation. However, these brachytherapy doses are delivered to a very small volume. With permanent implants as in the prostate, the dose is delivered at a slow, steady rate, which is predicted by radiation biology principles to be the most protective of radiation dosing schemes for normal tissues. Brachytherapy is usually a cooperative procedure involving the radiation oncologist, surgeon, and radiation physicist and requires a high skill level in the team accomplishing the procedure. The outcome is very dependent on the placement of the isotopes. They must be placed precisely to avoid failure to dose the entire tumor or hot spots of dose in critical normal tissues, which are likely to cause complications.

I. Case study

Figure 4 is an example of a difficult chronic irradiated wound in the groin treated with pre-graft hyperbaric oxygen followed by skin grafting with the final photo in the series showing a nearly healed, healthy-appearing wound.

II. A brief review of the wound healing timeline

Wounds can occur within radiation fields before radiation, just after radiation, or even many years after radiation. Special considerations in combining surgical wounding and radiation must include a discussion of the evolution of radiation effects dependent upon the timing of surgery and radiation relative to each other. Obviously, when surgery and radiation are planned as part of the original treatment plan, these considerations can be taken into account to help minimize the toxicity of combined treatment by optimizing the relative timing of both and the dose of radiation to maximize both anti-cancer effect and successful wound healing.

The complex mechanisms and involved biochemical reactions necessary to support wound healing are discussed in detail elsewhere in this text and in many comprehensive publications elsewhere.[8-9] However, in order to discuss the impact of radiation on wound healing we must discuss very briefly the phases of wound healing. The effects of radiation do differ at different stages

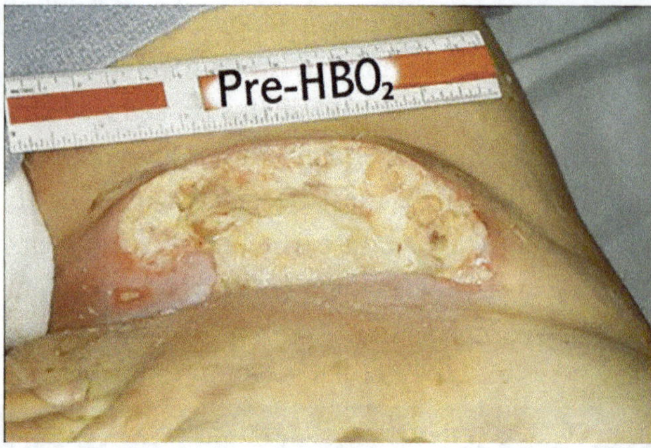

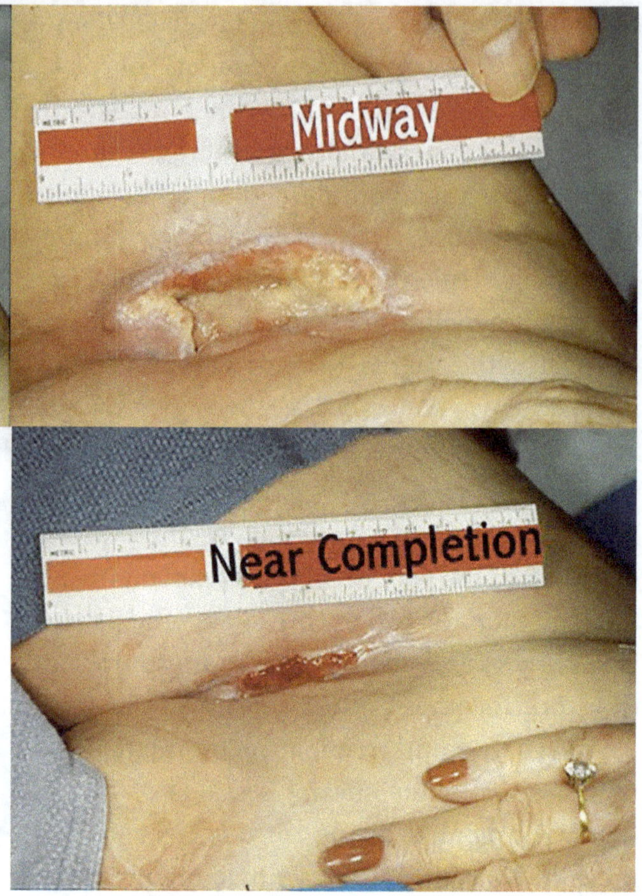

FIGURE 4. This patient underwent vulvectomy and groin dissection followed by radiation. She had a chronic nonhealing wound which responded well to hyperbaric oxygen. The last photograph shows considerable contraction and excellent granulation tissue.

of the process. For the most part our knowledge of healing of all wounds comes from experience with approximated surgical wounds. Three stages of wound healing have been described in an approximated surgical wound.(10) In chronic wounds, including those involving radiated tissues, these stages are not as well defined as in the approximated surgical wound. These wounds may ultimately heal by secondary intention or require flaps or grafts to achieve closure. Phases of wound healing in a chronic wound may be prolonged or even repeated several times during the healing process. Though this model may not exactly fit the process of healing a radiated wound, especially a chronic one, the model does highlight essential elements of the wound healing process and establish a timeline that is often useful in developing strategies to heal the irradiated wound by identifying and addressing the barriers to healing.

The following three stages of healing have been described:

A. The inflammatory phase
B. The proliferative phase
C. The maturation or remodeling phase

A. The inflammatory phase

During the first three or four days after wounding, the dominant physiologic response is an inflammatory response. Hemostasis has been achieved. A wound matrix has been formed which will attract fibroblasts and monocytes to it. The fibrin clot is responsible for giving the wound what integrity it has at this point. At this time the wound typically has only 5% of the tensile strength of a fully healed wound.(10) For surgical wounds, this time period has been reported to be the most susceptible to inhibition by radiation or chemotherapy because these cytotoxic interventions are likely to decrease the various inflammatory cells involved at this stage of the healing process. The actions of platelets, macrophages, and granulocytes are very prominent in the healing process during this phase. Many cytokines released from these cells and from other sources are active in the healing process at this time. Platelet-derived growth factor (PDGF), transforming growth factor-beta (TGF-beta), and basic fibroblast growth factor (bFGF) are produced and are active in inducing mitogenesis and angiogenesis.[8-9] Vascular dilation is observed, and this dilation permits cellular and growth factor migration.[10-12] Fibroblasts proliferate, and epithelialization begins with basal cell migration over the dermis.[13] During the inflammatory phase macrophages provide enzymes, which shape the extracellular matrix and prepare the wound for continued remodeling.[14]

B. The proliferative phase

The proliferative phase is the second identifiable stage in wound healing. It dominates for the next three weeks after the inflammatory phase. This phase is characterized by the production of collagen, which is enhanced by the presence of PDGF (platelet-derived growth factor) and TGF-beta.[15] Fibroblasts move to the wound and proliferate under the influence of several cytokines. Much of the process is controlled by macrophage-released bFGF [15-16] and further influenced by TGF-beta, which increases the release of tissue inhibitors of metalloproteinases (TIMP). These dissolve and permit the remodeling of the wound matrix.[17-18] Oxygen is a required substrate for healing during the proliferative phase since it is needed for hydroxylation of proline and lysine and release of collagen from proliferating fibroblasts. Myofibroblasts appear at this time. They function to provide wound contraction. By reducing the size of the void into which proliferating cells must move, they facilitate the formation of the collagen matrix of a healed wound. Basal keratinocytes move from the wound edges to provide epithelial coverage of the wound.

Collagen production reaches a maximum at about Day 7 after wounding but then continues at an accelerated rate for about four weeks after wounding. Many growth factors including VEGF (vascular endothelial growth factor) are released from activated macrophages and these serve to stimulate angiogenesis.[8] Tissue hypoxia at this time is a major stimulant for angiogenesis directly and indirectly through the production of lactic acid. At the end of the proliferative phase of wound healing, the wound now has about 30% of normal tissue strength.[10]

C. The maturation or remodeling phase

The final phase of wound healing, the maturation or remodeling phase, lasts for approximately two years following the proliferative phase. Collagen matures, and more cross-linkage occurs providing enhanced tensile strength to the wound. As the maturation phase progresses, there is a decrease in fibroblast and macrophage presence in the wound. Collagen content has progressively increased, as has the bursting strength of the wound.[8] By the completion of the maturation phase, the wound has achieved a tensile strength of about 80% of the strength of surrounding normal tissues.[10]

III. Radiation and surgical wounds: the importance of timing

Some wounds in radiated tissues are due to spontaneous breakdown. A more common concern is surgical wounding and the deleterious effects of radiation on surgical wound healing. Wounding of tissues in a radiated field occurs under a number of different circumstances. Radiation may be delivered in a planned preoperative fashion as part of the initial approach to treatment. The usual intent here is to enhance the successful resection of the tumor. Patients may require radiation following surgery as an adjunct or for gross residual tumor, and the incompletely healed surgical wound may receive significant radiation. This circumstance is seen frequently after an abdominal-perineal resection (APR) for rectal cancer where healing is often prolonged and adjuvant radiation may sometimes have to be initiated before complete wound healing has been achieved. Some patients require salvage or palliative surgery within the radiation field if a local recurrence or persistence of tumor occurs. Sometime after radiation, even many years later, the patient may require surgery within the irradiated field for either a benign or oncologic indication which may or may not be related to his or her original cancer. Each of these circumstances may present a somewhat different challenge. In all cases, though, wound healing is slowed and complication rates are higher due to the prior radiation exposure. The root cause of complications originates in insults to and defects of both vascular and constitutive elements of the radiated tissues.

IV. Radiation's broad effects on wound healing

There is general agreement that radiation impairs wound healing by reducing angiogenesis and by directly depleting both stem cells and certain mature cell lines (fibroblasts, vascular endothelial cells, and squamous cells) required for the healing process.(6) The induction of fibrosis, sometimes very marked, is also a major contributor to radiation damage. As noted above, the impairment of local immune response is especially deleterious during the first phase of healing. Researchers have recently demonstrated prolonged effects of radiation on fibroblast density and function and the resultant impact of these effects in impairing wound healing in radiated tissues.(15) Radiation does impact the progression of wound healing by specific effects peculiar to that phase of healing in which the wound finds itself at the time radiation is delivered. In addition to considering the phases of wound healing, it should be noted that the impact of radiation on wound healing is likely permanent and probably progressive impairment over time. Surgical wounding of irradiated tissues sometime after the completion of that irradiation for benign pathologies such as cholecystitis or diverticulitis or for salvage of recurrent tumor presents a special problem. In this setting the vascular damage caused by endarteritis and the impairment of angiogenesis, which progresses to a plateau within the first six to twelve months after irradiation, is usually well established. The resultant hypoxia presents significant difficulties in regard to wound closure. Some within the radiation oncology community believe that tissue quality will improve with the passage of time and that wound healing should have less impairment with this improvement. In the author's experience, improvement and less complicated wound healing is not readily evident with the passage of time. After the first one to two years after radiation, these changes progress at a much slower rate than do the initial changes. Further deterioration in the health of these tissues with time explains the occasional occurrence of spontaneous tissue necrosis occurring many years after radiation. Often, but not always, expressed radiation injury is related to traumatic events such as surgery or accidental tissue injury. Certainly, as patients age, there are progressive senescent changes in the vasculature in part due to arteriosclerotic changes from hyperlipidemias.

Anscher and coauthors [15] in a review article have given us a nice summary and further elucidated the chain of events, which result from therapeutic radiation contributing to difficulties in wound healing. This group explains that reactive oxygen species (ROS) resulting from radiation exposure initially cause biologic damage in both benign and malignant tissues and organs. The initial damaging events are triggered by the release of pro-inflammatory cytokines, chemokines, and profibrotic cytokines. Their model for delayed radiation tissue injury predicts that following the initial DNA damage carried out by ROS, increased cellular permeability results causing edema and an accumulation of fibrin in the extracellular matrix. An inflammatory response follows resulting in an accumulation and activation of macrophages. These macrophages release a wide variety of cytokines. Tissue hypoxia results in part from the increased metabolic demand of these macrophages enhanced by vascular damage caused by radiation-induced endarteritis and reactive fibrosis. This hypoxia leads to additional ROS production with more tissue damage and more fibrosis. The cytokine, TGF-beta, has a major role in causing tissue fibrosis and in turn stimulates VEGF. Endothelial cells, damaged by the radiation, do not respond normally to the VEGF released, and many die due to a combination of prior damage combined with the stress of new stimuli for proliferation from VEGF. Hypoxia therefore perpetuates and enhances radiation-induced tissue damage and interferes with healing. ROS continue to be generated along with tissue-damaging cytokines.

It is hoped that the evolving understanding of these mechanisms will permit strategies for interrupting this chain of events at some discrete point or points along their continuum. Additionally, future research may help to explain the mechanisms whereby hyperbaric oxygen has utility in the treatment of these injuries. These mechanisms are likely to include the reactive production of free radical scavengers and the production and release of growth factors that can lead to the repair of radiation-damaged tissues.

V. Preclinical models of irradiated wound healing

As previously discussed, the first three days after wounding are dominated by an inflammatory response. When radiation occurs before or during this time, a depletion of this inflammatory reaction and the associated inflammatory cells, especially neutrophils and macrophages, occurs, and wound healing is delayed due in part to the loss of the growth factors released by these cells.

In a clinical setting, external radiation is avoided fastidiously during this time because radiation oncologists are well aware of the deleterious effects radiation delivered too soon after surgery would have on wound healing. Experimental animal study data does verify the predicted impact that radiation has if given at this time. However, there are instances in which brachytherapy or implant radiation sources are placed at the time of a surgical procedure. Initiation of the brachytherapy treatment immediately following surgery has been reported by some authors to be associated with a higher incidence of wound complications.[7] This observation will be discussed in more detail below.

Gu and coauthors[21] have reported the results of an animal model designed to investigate the effects of radiation during the inflammatory phase of wound healing. Using rats, they caused consistent wounds of identical depth, width, and length in the dorsal skin of these study animals. One half of the animals were followed as unirradiated controls. Animals in the study group were then immediately irradiated after wounding to a single dose of 15 Gy to a field, which included the wound plus a 0.5-cm margin. The authors assessed wound healing using several different measures. These included gross and microscopic morphometry, immunohistochemical assay of type III collagen, in situ hybridization assay of type I collagen, and WBC and platelet assays.

These authors found that white blood cell counts and platelets were decreased in the circulation of irradiated animals initially but recovered to normal by 12 days postirradiation. They observed reduced levels of both type I and III collagen in the wounds of study animals on Day 7. Interestingly, by Day 14, both types of collagen increased in the irradiated animals to levels higher than those of non-irradiated controls.

In this study, at Day 7, infection was also detected in 8 of 12 irradiated wounds, and no sign of infection was seen in the unirradiated controls. When compared at three days postradiation, microscopic morphometry of wounds demonstrated decreased infiltration by neutrophils and macrophages and decreased granulation tissue in irradiated wounds compared to control wounds. Examination on Day 7 showed much less and thinner granulation tissue in the study group. When examined on Day 7 and again on Day 14, the wounds of irradiated animals contained so called "radiation" fibroblasts and fibrocytes, which fail to exhibit the activity and collagen production of normal fibroblasts.

In another study by Wang and associates[22] also employing a rat skin model, both light and electron microscopy were applied to determine the impact of radiation on the healing process. Electron beam irradiation (which biologically mimics X-rays but physically has less penetration) consisting of a single dose of 9.6 Gy had been delivered to the animals' dorsal skin seven days prior to wounding. Wounds were designed to be identical, full thickness, and incisional. Animals were euthanized at various times following wounding (1, 3, 7, and 14 days). Examination showed depressed levels of inflammatory cells and tissue exudates in irradiated specimens compared to unirradiated controls. The authors also observed a slowing of epithelial migration and decreased numbers of fibroblasts in the irradiated specimens. Granulation tissue was decreased up to the 7th day in the radiated animals but was found to have recovered by Day 14. These investigators conclude that the process of healing was slowed but not prevented in their model.

Bernstein and coworkers,[23] employing guinea pigs, have completed a study to investigate the effects of radiation on wound healing. Animals were irradiated with 18 Gy orthovoltage (low energy X-rays) radiation to a skin flap, which was isolated and then threaded through a slit in a lead shielding box. The intent was to limit the dose by this shielding and therefore limit the effect on surrounding tissues. In this model wounds were circular in shape of identical size cut into the dorsal skin of study animals with a 6-mm skin biopsy punch two days after irradiation. Each animal received six such wounds. Half of these wounds were created within the radiation field. The other one-half were created in the contralateral unirradiated skin. These matched wounds were examined at 5, 7, 10, and 14 days after wounding. At days 10 and 14 the wounds on the irradiated side were larger, and these differences were statistically significant.

Impairment of wound contraction as the result of irradiation was demonstrated by Yanase and coworkers[24] in a cell culture model. This study focused on the effects of radiation on both fibroblast proliferation and function including those of myofibroblasts. It therefore showed impact primarily on the proliferative phase of wound healing during which fibroblasts increase in great numbers. In this model, human oral mucosal fibroblasts were harvested, grown in cell culture, and then irradiated with escalated single doses of radiation. This dose escalation began at 2 Gy and continued to 10 Gy. Unirradiated controls were also cultured in a similar fashion for comparison. After trypsinization, separated cells were then placed in a 3-dimensional collagen gel media. The dimensions of this collagen gel media were measured repetitively over 10 days for both irradiated and non-irradiated cells. No evidence in initial contraction of the gels was detected by their average measured diameters. However, two weeks after irradiation the contraction of the irradiated gels showed significantly less contraction in a dose-dependent fashion compared to controls. Gel diameters for unirradiated cells had decreased to about 50% of those irradiated to doses of 6 Gy or greater. At eight weeks after irradiation there was some recovery, and the diameter of irradiated gels was only about 20% larger than controls.

These investigators also examined fibroblasts morphologically after staining for actin filaments. As before there was no significant difference between irradiated and unirradiated control cells initially. However, by two weeks after radiation, the irradiated cells exhibited an obvious decrease in the number of actin filaments, also in a dose-related fashion. Those cells irradiated to 6 Gy or more had very few identifiable actin filaments. There was recovery in irradiated cells by eight weeks after irradiation with considerable increase in actin filaments visible at that time.

These authors conclude that their model is consistent in demonstrating only a temporary but noteworthy inhibition of myofibroblasts in the irradiated cells, which in vivo would likely reduce wound contraction. The level of inhibition was found to be radiation dose dependent.

In yet another rat model, Aricini and coauthors[25] have studied the effects of radiation on vascular microanastomoses. The study employed four groups of animals: group one served as the control and had no radiation; group two received radiation two weeks before surgery; group three had radiation immediately followed by surgery. In the fourth and final group, animals had surgery followed by radiation two weeks later. Study animals were irradiated to a dose of 20 Gy to groin fields including the femoral artery. Surgery was identical in all four groups. This consisted of transection followed by microsurgical reanastomosis of the femoral artery. After one month, all animals were grossly examined under anesthesia. The femoral artery including the anastomosis was removed for light and electron microscopy. The patency of the anastomosis did not differ in any meaningful way when all groups were compared. From clinical experience, we know that significant vascular changes typically require a latent period of at least six months to become clinically manifest.

It is possible that this model failed to show any damage on group comparison because an inadequate time had elapsed to allow clinically manifest radiation changes to develop before the animals were sacrificed and examined.

Doyle and coworkers[26] studied the impact of radiation on wound angiogenesis in a rat model employing polytetrafluoroethylene (PTFE) sheet implants. The study animals had either two or three fractions of irradiation at daily intervals. Daily radiation doses consisted of 3 Gy. Those animals who received only two radiation exposures had no decrease in angiogenesis in the PTFE sheets compared to unirradiated controls. However, in those animals who received three radiation exposures (9 Gy) the authors observed a statistically significant decrease in neoangiogenesis compared to control.

In the preclinical studies discussed so far, researchers concentrated on the effects of radiation on the healing of skin and subcutaneous tissues. Radiation does impact on the healing of other tissues and organs. In most cases a deleterious impact on the healing of deep tissues is likely to have more impact on patient survival and even quality of life than is just the skin. The impact of radiation on colonic anastomoses in irradiated animals has also been studied and is discussed below.

In 1998, Kuzu and co-investigators[27] reported the results of a rat study comparing unirradiated controls to animals receiving 22 Gy in four fractions of 5.5 Gy to their whole pelvis. Animals had left-colon resection with primary reanastomosis. The surgery followed the radiation by four days. Animals were assessed at three and seven days after surgery at autopsy. The authors did not demonstrate differences between irradiated and control groups in adhesions or anastomotic failure. Bursting strength determinations were used to assess any relative weakness of the anastomoses. At both three and seven days, burst strength was reduced in irradiated animals in a statistically significant way. The same group replicated this study in 1999,[28] but this time they studied radiation and 5-fluorouracil together instead of radiation alone as potential causes of delayed healing and weakness in the anastomoses. The study with combined chemotherapy and radiation also showed statistically significant detrimental effects on healing in the left-colonic anastomosis as demonstrated by measurements of bursting strength. However, even when chemotherapy and radiation were combined, there were no increased failures of the physical integrity of the anastomosis prior to euthanasia nor was there a delay in healing of the skin incision. This study also potentially fails to relate to the common clinical dilemma since it does not allow enough time after the radiation to transpire to permit the full clinical expression of delayed radiation damage.

Ceelen and coworkers accomplished another animal study of the impact of radiation on colonic anastomoses.[29] This was also a rat study. In this study only one limb of the colonic anastomosis was irradiated, and the other was shielded. Radiation was delivered in standard daily doses of 2 Gy with accelerating total doses of 40, 60, or 80 Gy. A control group of unirradiated animals was also available for comparison. One day following completion of irradiation, the anastomosis was completed. Animals were euthanized 10 days after radiation. This group found no intergroup difference in peritonitis, anastomotic leaks, burst strength, or hydroxyproline content among animal groups. The irradiated animals were found to have lower weights than control animals. These authors conclude that, when one limb of the anastomosis is shielded, radiation has no effect on anastomotic healing and integrity.

If we consider the preclinical animal studies on the whole, we find that they do help to increase our understanding of the scope and mechanisms of the problem. When radiation is delivered early after wounding, the animal experience consistently shows diminishment of the typical initial inflammatory response and a consistent delay in wound healing. The studies do have limitations in their design, which makes it harder to relate them to our clinical challenges. Most animal studies look at radiation just before or just after surgical wounding. The studies do not mimic a clinical course where surgery is routinely delayed for at least two and usually four weeks after radiation. The radiation dosing schemes are not usually standard typically using only one or a few high doses per treatment fractions. They are also not adequate models for surgery occurring before irradiation when there are still open wounds. Finally, they do not investigate surgery in an irradiated field many months or even years after completion of irradiation.

VI. Clinical experience in irradiated wounds

In 1968 Rubin and Casarett[4] published the classic work in radiation pathology that continues to be a major source of our understanding of radiation injury to and tolerance of normal tissues for radiation damage. In 1998, Emami and his coauthors[5] updated our understanding of the risks for radiation injury to normal tissues based on several factors. Important determinants include total radiation dose, dose per individual radiation fraction, number of treatments per week (assuming daily treatment), and volume of tissue or in some cases the relative volume of an individual organ included in the high-dose region. It is accepted that patients are distributed in a normal distribution for their individual sensitivities to radiation injury. Some patients are unusually resistant to radiation injury while some are unusually sensitive. Various tissues and organ systems display lower tolerances to radiation compared to others. Comorbid disorders such as diabetes or collagen vascular disease have been shown to lower the threshold for serious radiation complications.[30] For example, in the past, a diagnosis of lupus erythematosis had been considered by some to present an absolute contraindication for definitive radiation following conservative surgery in early breast cancers.[31] A case report of a radiation-induced death in a patient receiving pelvic radiation for cervical cancer due to extreme sensitivity and resultant injury in a patient with lupus has been published.[32]

This author has himself cared for a patient with a nonspecific collagen vascular disorder who was also irradiated for cervical cancer and rendered cancer free by this treatment. Unfortunately, this patient also rapidly succumbed to severe radiation complications including radiation enteritis, cystitis, and proctitis.

Porock and her colleagues[33] reviewed the factors associated with severe acute skin injury in patients receiving radiation for breast cancer. These authors reported that injury is more likely to be severe for patients who smoke, patients with large breasts, patients who experience a lymphocele postoperatively, patients taking Tamoxifen, and patients with a past history of skin cancer.

Often a cancer treatment strategy is developed which will include both surgical resection and radiation. When developing such a treatment plan, the optimal sequencing of the two modalities must be determined. There are several putative advantages for the radiation to precede the surgery. Preoperative radiation may decrease the shedding of viable malignant cells released from the tumor at the time of resection. Cells in the periphery of the tumor are more likely to be released by surgical manipulation. When postoperative surgical scarring has not disrupted the circulation to the tumor, these peripheral tumor cells are characteristically well oxygenated and more sensitive to successful cell kill by the radiation dose since oxygen status is a large determinant of radiosensitivity. If these cells are killed by the radiation, they will not be able to produce metastases. Another major reason to consider preoperative radiation is that tumors, which are marginally resectable, have a major improvement in successful resection if they are reduced in size by preoperative irradiation.[34]

There is published clinical experience demonstrating the success in enhancing surgical resectability with preoperative radiation. These publications report this strategy in sarcomas, early-stage but bulky cervical cancers, head and neck cancers, especially those fixed to major vessels, and rectal cancers, especially those fixed in the pelvis. Pre-resection radiation has become the standard treatment for rectal cancers, especially low-lying tumors where up-front surgical resection would require an APR (abdomino-perineal resection)and permanent colostomy. When preoperative radiation precedes surgical resection, the radiation dose is typically reduced to 5,000 cGy or less.[34] When there is not likely to be a clear-cut advantage for preoperative radiation in terms of tumor control or resectability, the more common practice in the United States is to complete the surgery before the radiation. This practice would apply to most head and neck cancers that are planned for surgical resection. (More and more now, head and neck cancers and tumors at other sites are being treated with chemotherapy-sensitizing radiation, saving surgery for salvage). Most American surgeons prefer to complete resection of the tumor prior to radiation because of their concerns about wound healing complications and sequence treatment so that adjunctive radiation follows after two weeks or more allowing for adequate initiation of healing.[35]

Brachytherapy (implant radiation) represents a special consideration in conjunction with surgical resections of tumors, including soft-tissue sarcomas, and has been briefly mentioned above. In many centers, it is standard therapy to insert brachytherapy catheters into the resection bed at the time of tumor resection. These catheters are fixed into the tumor bed with sutures, and one end of the catheter is externalized for access after loading radioactive sources. Shortly after the surgery, radiation treatment is initiated either by manually loading radioactive isotopes in strands or ribbons into the catheters or by using a remote high-dose-rate after loading the device. This high-dose-rate unit contains a single very intense radioactive source attached to an insertion cable and computer controlled to move through the catheters to deliver the prescribed radiation dose. Usually, the isotope for either the manual insertion or the remotely controlled insertion is Iridium 192. The manually inserted sources deliver their intended dose slowly, classically over several days of inpatient status, and the patient is kept in an isolated shielded room to prevent exposure to other patients or health-care workers. We call this procedure low-dose-rate brachytherapy. An increasingly popular alternative treatment is to accomplish the catheter placement in the same fashion, and then bring the patient to the radiation department and connect his or her catheters to a high-dose-rate brachytherapy unit in a suite with appropriate shielding. With high-dose-rate brachytherapy, the equivalent of one day's treatment with low-dose-rate brachytherapy is accomplished in less than one hour. When the patient treated with high-dose-rate brachytherapy has multiple interstitial catheters, the patient must still be an inpatient, but can receive visitors and does not present a radiation exposure risk to nursing staff, other health-care personnel, and visitors. In many cases, the high-dose-rate patient may be treated as an outpatient. As previously noted, this described brachytherapy treatment is essentially the only time during which radiation is delivered during the initial phases of wound healing. Several publications have reported that any increase in wound complications associated with this technique can be significantly reduced by not loading the appliance until five days or more after the surgical resection and wound closure.

In general, acute radiation complications including wound healing delays occur during and just after the radiation dose has been administered. These acute changes are generally self-limited, and no care other than analgesic, nutritional, and other supportive care is needed. Characteristic of delayed radiation injuries which are usually more serious than acute injuries and often dose limiting and not self-limited is that they occur after a latent period of six months or more. Animal models and microscopic examination of clinical specimens have shown that the endarteritis, fibrosis, and cellular depletion (apoptosis) associated with delayed radiation injuries are not fully expressed for at least several months after the completion of radiation. Open wounds can occur in these tissues sometimes spontaneously, though trauma including surgical procedures may impose a metabolic demand on the irradiated tissues. These tissues may not have the reserve in terms of stem cells and vascularity to meet the added demand of wound healing. These wounds may become chronic and fail to heal and even progress to extend into critical structures such as major blood vessels. This progression can lead to impaired quality of life and function and occasionally become a fatal injury in spite of medical intervention.

As the patient is seen in follow-up, recurrent tumors may be detected within the radiation field. Of course this recurrence may occur at any time following radiation although for many tumors the recurrence is usually seen within two years. Surgery may follow radiation not only when recurrence is detected but often after radiation given as part of a planned treatment plan. We have already discussed some of these issues above. When surgery is to follow radiation, the vast majority of the time it will follow four to six weeks after completion of the radiation. This planned interval is designed to allow for maximum shrinkage of the tumor, resolution of the acute effects of radiation, but also the avoidance of excessive delay, which might permit tumor progression or maturation of delayed radiation changes which will increase the likelihood of wound healing complications. As already observed above, surgery may be needed within the radiation field many months or years later, either for oncologic reasons or for addressing benign disorders such as cholecystitis.

VII. Strategies to prevent and treat problem irradiated wounds

Prevention is always preferable to dealing with established complications. The following general guidelines discussed below offer strategies designed to decrease the likelihood of wound complications secondary to radiation.

When preoperative radiation is planned before surgery, preferably at least three to four weeks and no more than six weeks should elapse between radiation and surgery. When given in this fashion, radiation should not depress the initial inflammatory response which is so necessary to initiate the healing process.[35] This choice of timing for postradiation surgery between three to six weeks after radiation is considered a "window of opportunity" during which there should be no significant increases in wound healing complications.

If wound closure will require flap creation, ideally the vascular supply to that flap should originate from outside radiation portals. The intention of this design is to provide the flap with a vascular supply undamaged by prior radiation. For similar reasons, if surgery will require bowel resection, complications can be reduced when one limb of the anastomosis has not been irradiated.

When the treatment plan includes radiation after surgery, at least two weeks and no more than six weeks should elapse before therapeutic radiation is begun.[35-36] The selection of this time interval is based on balancing the dual concerns of treating any residual cancer while the tumor burden is its lowest and at the same time minimizing the negative impact of radiation on wound healing. Intuitively, in terms of tumor control, radiation should begin as soon after surgery as possible because any residual malignant cells will have the opportunity to go on dividing without additional treatment. In point of fact, clinical experience has not shown a worsening of tumor control or patient survival when postoperative adjuvant radiation is given within six weeks of surgery.[37] Occasionally, the surgical wound is still open at six weeks and beyond. A published review of head and neck cancer patients treated at the University of Florida has shown that even when radiation is initiated before wound healing, most of these wounds (67%) healed without additional surgical intervention, and another 15% were successfully closed with additional surgery. The remaining 18% of patients either died or were lost to follow-up before the wounds had healed.[36]

Early intervention is indicated when problem wounds develop within radiated fields as the result of surgery many months or years after completion of the irradiation. Progression of these wound complications can lead to wound enlargement and even extensive necrosis. This progression can become life threatening if the wound is located near major vasculature. Many of these issues have been discussed above. After the latent period during which acute radiation problems have resolved and chronic deleterious tissue changes have matured, depletion of stem cells, damage to vasculature, and induction of fibrosis create a milieu wherein the complex events related to healing are seriously inhibited.

Surgery may be indicated in heavily irradiated tissues for one of several reasons. Surgical salvage may be offered to the patient for locally recurrent tumors, for intervention designed to deal with radiation-induced injury, or for a medical indication unrelated to the original malignancy. For example, a patient may experience a local recurrence of a larynx tumor after full-dose radiation with or without chemotherapy. In the face of no metastatic disease, a salvage laryngectomy may be curative, but postoperative complications have been reported to be as high as 67.5%.[38] As an example of surgery in a radiated field for the second circumstance, we would include resection of radiation-damaged small bowel some time after successful treatment of a rectal cancer. The final situation would include a patient who developed bladder cancer after primary and successful radiation of a prostate cancer and who requires cystectomy for a second malignancy.

For all of these circumstances, surgical approaches have been recommended to avoid or minimize postoperative wound complications. Fascia and underlying muscle should not be dissected from skin and subcutaneous tissues whenever possible. No potential dead space should be left unfilled. Wounds closure should be without tension and appropriately drained. Any resultant seroma or hematoma should be evacuated. Skin sutures should be left for a longer period of time than usual (some recommend up to one month). For patients with lower-extremity wounds, bed rest should be maintained for several additional days.[10] In her review, Tibbs has recommended that complications occurring within two weeks are an indication to return the patient promptly to the OR for debridement or flap design and closure or both.[10] She also observes that if healing is progressing normally during the first three to four weeks, the patient will most likely have continued successful healing without subsequent difficulties.

In their review from 1998, Frank and colleagues[12] extensively discuss the issue of wound-dressing materials for the radiation-associated wound. Of course their discussion is outdated given the rapid development of wound care products and dressing materials that have been developed in the intervening years. A comprehensive discussion of dressing materials is beyond the scope of this chapter, and wound care products are discussed elsewhere in this text. Frank does list several qualities that are desirable for dressings in an irradiated wound. The authors recommend that wound materials 1) optimize perfusion and oxygenation, 2) optimize wound environment including pH and eradication of infection, 3) retain serum to stimulate migration and adhesion of cellular constituents involved in healing, and 4) protect the wound mechanically and reduce inflammation.

In a review article from 2012, Iyer and Balasubramanian[39] have published a fairly comprehensive article discussing irradiated wounds. This article begins with a discussion of the pathophysiology of radiated wounds. It discusses radiation fibrosis of the skin, nonhealing ulcers due to radiation-induced necrosis, chondro- and osteoradionecrosis, radiation-induced neural plexopathies, and radiation-induced lymphedema. The actual management portion of the article advocates flaps including rotational flaps and especially free flaps in the closure of radiated wounds.

VIII. The role of hyperbaric oxygen

Since the 1970s, hyperbaric oxygen has been investigated and applied to treat or prevent radiation injuries, including problem wounds. Hyperbaric oxygen offers some specific therapeutic advantages to irradiated tissues. Recall that our understanding of the pathophysiology of delayed radiation injury includes the depletion of stem cells, the induction of fibrosis, and the diminishment of circulation to the radiated tissues. Figure 5 gives a very-much-simplified depiction of hyperbaric effects on radiated tissues, namely the induction of stem cells,[40] the

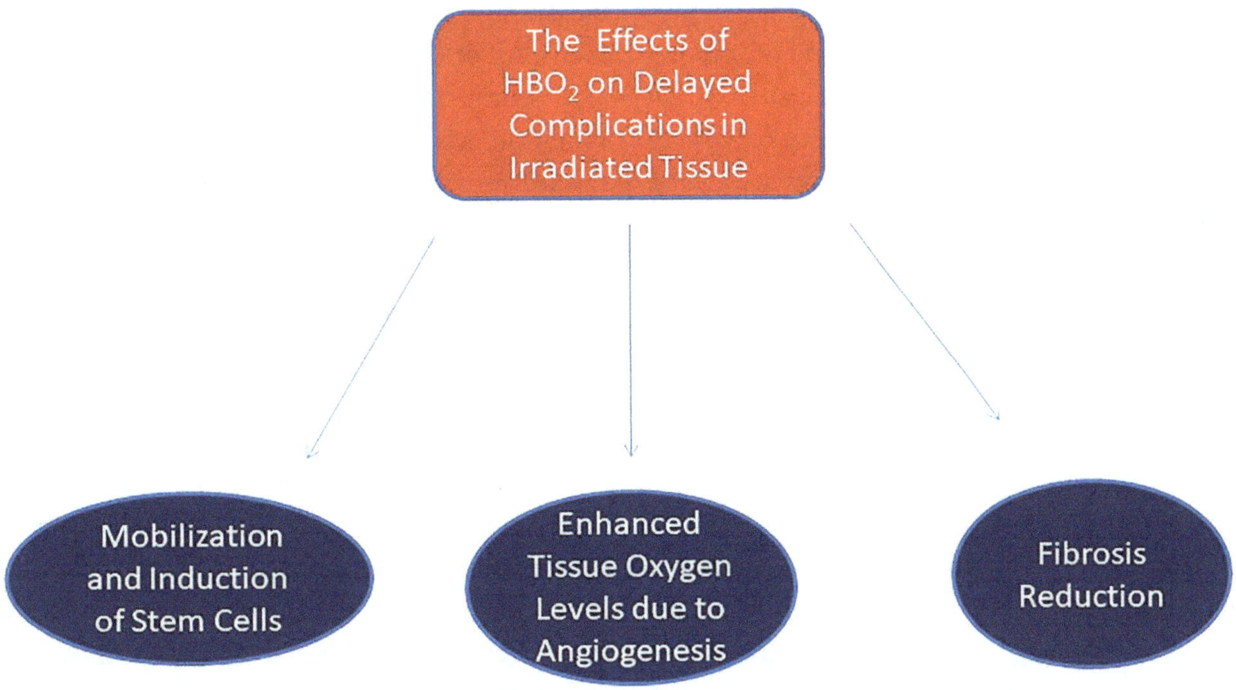

FIGURE 5. A very simplified depiction of the effects of hyperbaric oxygen on chronically damaged radiated tissues

reduction of fibrosis,[41] and the enhancement of angiogenesis.[42]

Robert Marx,[43] who pioneered the rational application of hyperbaric oxygen to the treatment and prevention of mandibular osteoradionecrosis (ORN), was the first to advocate that the majority of treatments in a planned course of hyperbaric oxygen for radiation injury should come before surgery. The sequencing of these therapies is designed to improve the quality of these radiated tissues, especially their vascular status, before surgical wounding. The protocol for existing mandibular osteoradionecrosis is to deliver 30 presurgical treatments followed by 10 postoperative treatments. When hyperbaric oxygen is given to prevent ORN, the recommendation is for 20 pre-extraction treatments followed by 10 post-extraction treatments. Marx is a strong advocate of treatment at 2.4 atmospheres absolute pressure in part based on a dose escalation study he did with colleagues in a rabbit model.[42] These patients are treated for 90 minutes of 100% oxygen at pressure.

In the randomized controlled study, Marx[44] investigated the role for prophylactic hyperbaric oxygen in preventing ORN and promoting healing of the tooth socket resulting after dental extractions. He reported an incidence of 5.4% of necrosis in the hyperbaric group versus a 29.9% incidence in the nonhyperbaric group who did receive penicillin. In the rabbit model, previously mentioned, Marx reviewed the effects of increasing pressure on vascular density in an animal model of high-dose mandibular radiation. In this model, Marx demonstrated a dose-dependent enhancement of vascular density after hyperbaric oxygen.[41] In a clinical series, Marx[45] also demonstrated an improvement in the subsequent oxygen status of head and neck cancer patients previously irradiated. Serial transcutaneous oxygen measurements in these patients showed significant continuous improvement during hyperbaric oxygen ultimately achieving levels many times higher than original levels but not quite reaching the levels at a control site outside the radiation portals.

Grandstrom,[46] a prominent oral maxillofacial surgeon from Sweden, and Marx[47] independently have reported a major benefit for hyperbaric oxygen in supporting dental implants inserted into radiated jaws. Their studies have shown a significantly higher success rate for osteointegration of these implants and a lower risk for ORN. Many clinicians feel that prior high-dose radiation to the jaws is a strong contraindication to attempting these implants because of the high risk for failure and the possibility of precipitating osteoradionecrosis. These treatment protocols also emphasize the importance of presurgical hyperbaric oxygen.

Feldmeier and colleagues[48] have reported a similar successful application of hyperbaric oxygen in enhancing the healing of wounds in a radiated group at high risk for complications. This group of 32 patients received hyperbaric oxygen as soon after surgery as they were stable enough to come to the chamber for treatment. All of these patients had recurrent cancer after initial treatment that included full-dose radiation. Many of these salvage surgeries were radical resections within the field of high-dose radiation. These patients underwent a short course (10 to 15 treatments at 2.4 ATA) of hyperbaric oxygen. This early intervention led to prompt healing in 87.5% of patients without serious wound complications in any patient. These results compare very favorably to published complication rates of 60% in patients undergoing salvage therapy in previously heavily radiated head and neck fields who do not receive hyperbaric oxygen. Historically, death due to carotid artery blowout is not unheard of in this group of high-risk patients.[49]

The same principles applied to preventing wounds discussed above apply to the management of established wounds in radiated tissues. Surgical articles emphasize the importance of debriding necrotic tissues. Marx[50] in his description of the comprehensive management of mandibular osteoradionecrosis directs that all necrotic bone must be surgically debrided. Subsequently, Feldmeier et al.[51] in their case series reviewing the management of chest wall radiation necrosis observed that here, too, when bone is involved, all necrotic bone must be surgically removed to ensure success. Figure 6 is a clinical example where a patient suffering from a combination of osseous and soft-tissue necrosis had a sustained response to hyperbaric oxygen combined with debridement of necrotic bone and skin grafting. Rudolph[52] has previously reported a 100% failure rate when simple skin grafts were applied to radionecrotic wounds. In the same paper, he also reported a 43% occurrence of complications in myocutaneous flaps applied to the closure of radiation-induced skin ulcers. Since this paper was published, many improvements have been made in flap design. When flaps are needed to close the defect, either an axial flap based on a sizeable (usually named) artery or a free flap is recommended. Ideally, all pedicle flaps should have their blood supply originate outside the radiation field. Arnold and colleagues[53] have reported a fairly extensive experience in employing myocutaneous flaps in the reconstruction of 100 radiation-related wounds. In this series about one-half of the flaps had had their blood supply irradiated. The other one-half of the flaps were supported by unirradiated blood supply. When the vasculature had been irradiated, the complication rate was 32%, and complete loss of muscle was experienced in 14%. In those flaps with blood supply originating outside the radiation field, complications were 19%, and none of these flaps were completely lost. Free flaps have also been used to close defects in irradiated wounds with good success reported. Teknos and coworkers[54] have reported a complication rate of 20% in 10 patients where radial forearm free flaps were employed in the reconstruction of defects of the hypopharynx after surgical salvage for recurrence after full-course radiation. The combination of hyperbaric oxygen and the best surgical techniques is the most appropriate intervention for chronic wounds complicated by radiation.

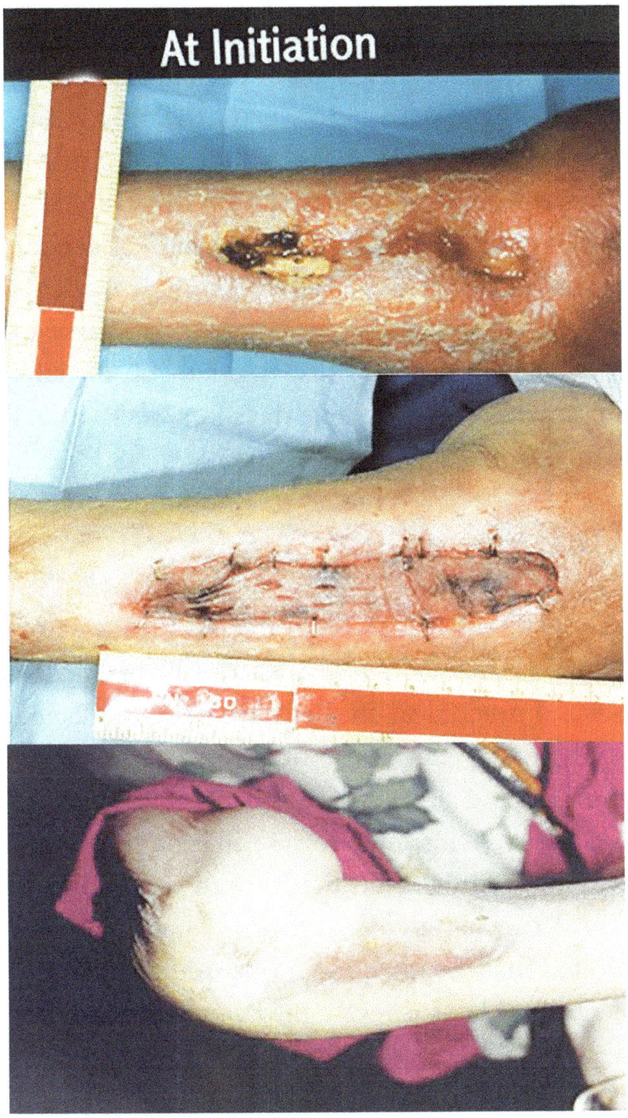

FIGURE 6. This patient had resection and post-operative radiation for a sarcoma of the forearm. She developed bone necrosis and a nonhealing wound. She underwent presurgical HBO_2 for about six weeks predebridement including necrotic bone with skin grafting and additional HBO_2. Final photo is a 10-year follow-up showing sustained healing and good function.

There are a number of publications supporting the use of hyperbaric oxygen in the treatment of radiation-wounded tissues. Some of these relate to visceral damage such as radiation-induced cystitis and proctitis and do not exhibit skin wounds. However, most of the studies including injuries to the head and neck and other sites include a skin wound. In 2002, Feldmeier and Hampson[55] published a review of 74 reports addressing this issue from an evidence-based approach. The review includes discussions of wounds in the head and neck, chest wall, extremities, and abdomen and pelvis. Results from many different centers are consistently positive with successful resolution typically in the 65% to 85% range. One of the most impressive reports is that of Marx[56] wherein he discusses the application of hyperbaric oxygen combining pre- and postoperative hyperbaric oxygen in a protocol identical to that already discussed above for the treatment of mandibular necrosis. In this publication, Marx reports the results in 160 patients in whom surgery was planned for repair of radiation necrosis or resection of recurrent tumor. This study was controlled but not randomized. Marx reports the incidence of complications in the hyperbaric group versus the control group in the following fashion: 1) wound infection 6% versus 24%, 2) wound dehiscence 11% versus 48%, and 3) delayed wound healing 11% versus 55%.

Neovius and associates, though with limited numbers, published a very positive publication for hyperbaric oxygen.[57] The authors report the results in applying hyperbaric oxygen to 15 patients with soft-tissue wounds after preoperative radiation with doses of 64 Gy, which preceded surgical resection for laryngeal or pharyngeal cancers. Postoperatively, these patients had nonhealing wounds and began hyperbaric oxygen. Typically, they were treated at pressures of 2.5 ATA once daily. Treatments ranged in number from 10 to 40 although most received 30 or more treatments. Twelve of 15 of this group healed completely and two improved. Only one did not respond to hyperbaric oxygen. The authors compared their results in this group with a carefully matched historic control group. Only seven of these 15 patients ultimately healed without additional surgery. Two patients sustained severe postoperative hemorrhage, and one of these died as a result of the hemorrhage.

Hampson and associates[58] in 2012 reported their extensive single-institutional experience in applying hyperbaric oxygen to delayed radiation injuries. Their series included 411 patients treated between 2002 to 2010. In this series, there were 58 evaluable patients with cutaneous wounds. Eighty-two percent of these patients had a strong positive response to a course of hyperbaric oxygen with a median of 40 daily treatments (typically five days per week) at 2.4 atmospheres absolute pressure.

IX. Possible future strategies to prevent or treat irradiated wounds

Several preclinical studies have been published applying topical exogenous growth factors or unirradiated fibroblasts to wounds. This strategy has shown some promise in models of irradiated wounds. Gorodetsky and colleagues[59] and Kruegler and coauthors[60] have demonstrated that the injection of unirradiated syngeneic fibroblasts directly into wounds enhances healing in study animals.

The topical application of both TGF-beta and PDGF has promoted healing in irradiated wounds in other animal models.[13,17,61] In a publication previously cited, Anscher and his colleagues[20] have discussed several pharmacologic therapeutic strategies including free-radical scavengers, anticytokine antibodies, antichemokine antibodies, and antiapoptotic agents.

Werier and colleagues[62] have developed a rat model of deep incisional wounds after radiation and shown that porcine small bowel can be applied to radiated wounds with some success in enhancing wound healing.

Delanian and Lefaix[63] have advocated the use of pentoxyfifylline for the treatment or prevention of soft-tissue or bony radiation necrosis.

A more recent review by Haubner and associates[64] addresses the application of special wound dressings, the injection of multipotential cells, and the topical administration of various active substances and growth factors. These substances include hydrogel membranes, silver membranes, injections of autologous fibroblasts, and stem cells. Also included are brief discussions of several topical agents and growth factors including TGF-beta, platelet-derived growth factor, and granulocyte macrophage-colony stimulating factor. Nearly all of the experience with these strategies has been in animal models of irradiated wounds, and many do show promise. Reasonably sized and designed clinical trials will have to be completed before these become standard care.

Stanirkowsi and coworkers[65] from Poland have reported a review in treating difficult gynecologic wounds including irradiated wounds with growth factors, silver dressings, and wound vacs in various combinations. They state that their review suggests that these wound care strategies may improve clinical outcomes. They point out that these promising results are very preliminary and must be subjected to clinical trials. Clinical trials have been launched to investigate the blockage of the renin-angiotensin by ACE (angiotensin converting enzyme) inhibitors. Preclinical models have shown promise with this approach.[66]

In a rat model, Huang and coworkers[67] from Taiwan have reported that radiated ulcers demonstrate improved angiogenesis and more rapid healing after injection with adipose-derived stem cells compared to those not treated.

Summary

Radiation presents significant changes in the quality of tissues requiring special considerations when dealing with associated wounds. Our increasing understanding of the complex biochemical reactions associated with wound healing and an enhanced appreciation for the multistep process needed to achieve a closed wound permits us to combine all cancer treatment modalities in an optimum fashion for both cancer control and minimization of untoward effects. Preclinical studies and clinical experience have demonstrated the importance of applying this knowledge to avoid increased complications both in incidence and severity. Preclinical work suggests that the addition of growth factors or stem cells or untreated fibroblasts can reverse some difficulties identified during the early phases of wound healing, namely delayed angiogenesis and wound contraction. Well-established surgical principles emphasize the use of flaps especially those whose vascular supply originates outside the radiation portals. Hyperbaric oxygen has proven to be very effective as an adjunct when approaching wounds in heavily irradiated tissues. Marx has emphasized the importance of giving most of the hyperbaric treatments prior to surgical wounding to improve the vascularity and inherent quality of the tissues prior to surgical wounding. Both animal studies and clinical reports show an improvement in vascularity and a reduction of fibrosis as a result of hyperbaric oxygen. A fertile area for future studies is the combination of growth factors and hyperbaric oxygen for the treatment and prevention of radiation-associated wounds.

Review questions

1. **Which of the following statements is most correct regarding the impact of radiation therapy on wound healing?**

    a. Radiation has no impact on surgical wound healing, and no special considerations are necessary when combining radiation and surgery.

    b. It is common to initiate radiation after surgery as soon as the patient can be safely transported.

    c. Radiation therapy should always follow surgery by at least two months to prevent serious wound healing problems.

    d. Whether given before or after surgery, radiation therapy can significantly impact wound healing, and careful consideration should be given to the timing of the various therapies and care of the resulting wound.

2. **With regard to the optimal timing of radiation relative to surgery, which of the following statements is most correct?**

    a. Radiation is usually given right up to the day of surgery to have the best impact on cancer control with the least effects on wound healing.

    b. Radiation should be given as soon as the patient can be transported after surgery (preferably the same day) to have the best impact on tumor control.

    c. Typically, radiation follows only after surgical healing is well underway, and usually this means at least two weeks after surgery.

    d. It is mandatory that at least two months separate surgery and radiation, otherwise postoperative radiation will cause wound breakdown in a majority of patients.

3. **Which of the following is most correct in regard to the impact of radiation on wound healing?**

    a. Radiation potentially has the biggest impairment of wound healing during the maturation phase of wound healing.

    b. Radiation has minor impact on wound healing during the inflammatory phase of wound healing because neutrophils and macrophages involved in the inflammatory process are known to be exceptionally radioresistant.

    c. Timing presents no issues for postoperative radiation but for preoperative radiation it is crucial that surgery is done within a few days.

    d. Postoperative radiation can impact on wound healing during any phase of wound healing but practically speaking often follows surgery by two to four weeks without causing an increase in wound breakdown.

4. **Which of the following is <u>not</u> correct in regard to the wound healing problems caused by radiation therapy?**

   a. Careful surgical technique including the design of flaps with their blood supply outside the radiation field can prevent wound problems.

   b. Experimental studies have shown that the topical application of certain growth factors is likely to enhance wound healing in radiated wounds.

   c. Hyperbaric oxygen has been shown to have a role in preventing wound healing difficulties and should be considered when surgery needs to be accomplished within the radiation field.

   d. When radiated wounds begin to break down in the immediate postoperative time period, the surgeon should not intervene because these complications always occur and most are self-limited.

5. **Which of the following is most correct in regard to radiation and wound healing?**

   a. Even doses of radiation received in common diagnostic procedures can impair wound healing.

   b. Radiated wounds are frequently treated in the clinic with topical growth factors and cytokines with established positive clinical results.

   c. Hyperbaric oxygen has been shown in several clinical reports to enhance healing in radiated wounds.

   d. Hyperbaric oxygen is so effective in healing radiated wounds that no consideration should be given to surgical flaps or grafts, as they will not be necessary.

ANSWERS: 1) d
2) c
3) d
4) d
5) d

References

1. NIH National Cancer Institute. U.S. Department of Health and Human Services. Radiation therapy for cancer [Internet]. Accessed 2010, June 30. Available from: www.cancer.gov/about-cancer/treatmet/types/radiation-therapy/radiation-fact-sheet.
2. American Cancer Society. Cancer facts & figures 2016. Atlanta: American Cancer Society; 2016.
3. Rieger KE, Hong WJ, Tusher VG, et al. Toxicity from radiation therapy associated with abnormal transcriptional responses to DNA damage. Proc Natl Acad Sci. 2004;101(17):6635-40.
4. Rubin P, Cassarett GW, editors. Clinical radiation pathology. Philadelphia: WB Saunders; 1968.
5. Emami B, Lyman J, Brown A, Coia L, Goitein M, Munzenrider JE, Shank B, Solin LJ, Wesson M. Tolerance of normal tissue to therapeutic radiation. Int J Radiat Oncol Biol Phys. 1998;2 (1):109-22.
6. Stone HB, Coleman CN, Anscher MS, McBride WH. Effects of radiation on normal tissue: consequences and mechanisms. Lancet Oncol. 2003 Sep;4(9):529-36.
7. Emory CL, Montgomery CO, Potter BK, Keisch ME, Conway SA. Early complications of high-dose-rate brachytherapy in soft tissue sarcoma: a comparison with traditional external-beam radiotherapy. Clin Orthop Relat Res. 2012;470(3):751-58.
8. Hunt TK, Hopf H, Hussain Z. Physiology of wound healing. Adv Skin Wound Care. 2000;13(2 Suppl):6-11.
9. Witte MB, Barbul A. General principles of wound healing. Surg Clin North Am. 1997;77:509-28.
10. Tibbs MK. Wound healing following radiation therapy: a review. Radiother Oncol. 1997;42(2):99-106.
11. Drake DB, Oishi SN. Wound healing considerations in chemotherapy and radiation therapy. Clin Plast Surg. 1995;22(1):31-37.
12. Frank J, Barker JH, Marzi I, Mutschler W. Modern theraoy of chronic wounds with respect to radiation. Strahlentherapie und Onkologie. 1998;174(Suppl 3):69-73.
13. Mustoe TA, Purdy J, Gramates P, Deuel TF, Thomason A, Pierce GF. Reversal of impaired wound healing by platelet-derived growth factor-BB. Am J Surg. 1989;158:345-50.
14. Tokarek R, Bernstein EF, Sullivan F, Utto J, Mitchell JB. Effect of therapeutic radiation on wound healing. Clin Dermatol. 1994;12:57-70.
15. Anscher MS, Chen L, Rabbani Z, et al. Recent progress in defining mechanisms and potential targets for prevention of normal tissue injury after radiation therapy. Int J Radiat Oncol Biol Phys. 2005;62(1):255-59.
16. Pierce GF, Tarpley JE, Yangihara D, Mustoe TA, Fox GM, Thomason A. Platelet-derived growth factor (BB homodimer), transforming growth factor-beta 1 and basic fibroblast growth factor in dermal wound healing. Neovessel and matrix formation and cessation of repair. Am J Pathol. 1992;140:1375-88.
17. Bernstein EF, Harisiadis L, Salomon G, Norton J, Sollberg S, Uitto J, Glatstein E, Glass J, Talbot T, Russo A, Mitchell JB. Transforming growth factor-beta improves healing of radiation-impaired wounds. J Invest Dermatol. 1991;97:430-434.
18. Wahl SM, Wong H, McCartney-Francis N. Role of growth factors in inflammation and repair. J Cell Biochem. 1989;40:193-199.
19. Armstrong FG, Jude EB. The role of matrix metalloproteinases in wound healing. J Am Podiatr Med Assoc. 2002;92:12-18.
20. Anscher MS, Chen L, Rabbani Z, et al. Recent progress in defining mechanisms and potential targets for prevention of normal tissue injury after radiation therapy. Int J Radiat Oncol Biol Phys. 2005;62(1):255-59.

21. Gu Q, Wang D, Cui C, Gao Y, Xia G, Cui X. Effects of radiation on wound healing. J Environ Pathol Toxicol Oncol. 1998;17(2):117-23.
22. Wang Q, Dickson GR, Abram WP, Karr KE. Electron irradiation slows down wound repair in rat skin: a morphologic investigation. Br J Dermatol. 1994;130:551-60.
23. Bernstein EF, Harisiadis L, Salomon GD, Harrington F, Mitchell JB, Uitto J, Glatstein E, Russo A. Healing impairment of open wounds by skin irradiation. J Dermatol Surg Oncol. 1994;20:757-60.
24. Yanase A, Ueda M, Kaneda T, Torii S, Matsuyama M. Irradiation effects on wound contraction using a connective tissue model. Ann Plast Surg. 1993;30:435-440.
25. Arcini A, Topalan M, Aydin I, Solakoglu S, Olgac V, Merla R, Erer M. Effects of early pre- and postoperative radiation on the healing of microvascular anastomoses. J Reconstr Microsurg. 2000;16(7):573-76.
26. Doyle JW, Li YQ, Salloum A, Fitzgerald TJ, Walton RL. The effects of radiation on neovascularization in a rat model. Plast Reconstr Surg. 1998;98:129-35.
27. Kuzu MA, Koksoy C, Akyol FH, Uzal D, Kale T, Demirpence E. Effects of preoperative irradiation on left colonic anastomoses in the rat. Dis Colon Rectum. 1998;41:370-76.
28. Kuzu MA, Kuzu J, Koksoy C, Akyol FH, Uzal D, Kale IT, Orhan D, Terzi C. Histological evaluation of colonic anastomotic healing in the rat following preoperative 5-fluorouracil, fractionated radiation, and combined treatment. Int J Colorectal Dis. 1998;13(5-6):235-240.
29. Ceelen W, El Malt M, Cardon A, Berrevoet F, De Neve W, Pattyn P. Influence of preoperative high-dose radiotherapy on postoperative outcome of colonic anastomotic healing: experimental study in the rat. Dis Colon Rectum. 2001;44(5):717-21.
30. Linengood CH, Soper JT, Clarke-Pearsson DL, Addison WA. Necrotizing fasciitis in irradiated tissue from diabetic women: a report of two cases. J Reprod Med. 1991;36:455-458.
31. Fleck R, McNeese MD, Ellerbroek NA, Hunter TA, Holmes FA. Consequences of breast irradiation in patients with pre-existing collagen vascular diseases. Int J Radiation Oncology Biol Phys. 1989;17:829-33.
32. Olivotto IA, Fairey RN, Gillies JH, Stein H. Fatal outcome of pelvic radiotherapy for carcinoma of the cervix in a patient with systemic lupus erythematosis. Clin Radiol. 1989;40:83-84.
33. Porock D, Kristjanson l, Nikoletti S, Cameron F, Pedler P. Predicting the severity of radiation skin reactions in women with breast cancer. Oncol Nurs Forum. 1998;25(6):1019-1029.
34. Tobin RL, Mohiuddin M, Marks G. Preoperative irradiation for cancer of the rectum with extrarectal fixation. Int J Radiat Oncol Biol Phys. 1991;21(5):1127-32.
35. Sause WT. Principles of combining radiation therapy and surgery. In: Cox J, editor. Moss' radiation oncology: rationale, technique, results. St. Louis (MO): Mosby; 1994.
36. Isaacs JH, Siles WA, Cassisi NJ, Million RR, Parsons JT. Postoperative radiation of open head and neck wounds—updated. Head Neck. 1997;19:194-99.
37. Vikram B, Shaw EW, Shah J, et al. Failure in the neck following multimodality treatment for advanced head and neck cancer. Head Neck Surg. 1984;6:724-29.
38. Hasan Z, Dwivedi RC, Gunaratne DA, Virk SA, Palme CE, Riffat F. Systematic review and meta-analysis of the complications of salvage total laryngectomy. Eur J Surg Oncol. 2016.
39. Iyer S, Balasubramanian D. Management of radiation wounds. Indian J Plast Surg. 2012;45(2):325-31.

40. Thom SR, Bhopale VM, Velazquez OC, Goldstein LJ, Thom LH, Buerk DG. Stem cell mobilization by hyperbaric oxygen. Am J Physiol Heart Circ Physiol. 2006;290:378-86.

41. Feldmeier JJ, Davolt DA, Court WS, Onoda JM, Alecu R. Histologic morphometry confirms a prophylactic effect for hyperbaric oxygen in the prevention of delayed radiation enteropathy. Undersea Hyperb Med. 1998;25(2):93-97.

42. Marx RE, Ehler WJ, Tayapongsak P, Pierce LW. Relationship of oxygen dose to angiogenesis induction in irradiated tissue. Am J Surg. 1990;160:519-524.

43. Marx RE. A new concept in the treatment of osteoradionecrosis. J Oral Maxillofac Surg. 1983;41(6):351-57.

44. Marx RE, Johnson RP, Kline SN. Prevention of osteoradionecrosis: a randomized prospective clinical trial of hyperbaric oxygen versus penicillin. J Am Dent Assoc. 1985;11:49-54.

45. Marx RE. Radiation injury to tissue. In: Kindwall EP, editor. Hyperbaric medicine practice. 2nd ed. Flagstaff (AZ): Best Publishing; 1999, p. 668-73.

46. Granstrom G, Jacobsson M, Tjellstrom A. Titanium implants in irradiated tissue: benefits from hyperbaric oxygen. Int J Oral Maxillofac Implant. 1992;7(1):15-25.

47. Marx RE. Radiation injury to tissue. In: Kindwall EP, editor. Hyperbaric medicine practice. 2nd ed. Flagstaff (AZ): Best Publishing; 1999, p. 693-97.

48. Feldmeier JJ, Newman R, Davolt DA, Heimbach RD, Newman NK, Hernandez LC. Prophylactic hyperbaric oxygen for patients undergoing salvage for recurrent head and neck cancers following full course irradiation [abstract]. Undersea Hyper Med. 1998;25(Suppl):10.

49. McDonald MW, Moore MG, Johnstone PA. Risk of carotid blowout after reirradiation of the head and neck; systematic review. Int J Radiat Oncol Biol Phys. 2012 Mar 1;82(3):1083-1089.

50. Marx RE. Radiation injury to tissue. In: Kindwall EP, editor. Hyperbaric medicine practice. 2nd ed. Flagstaff (AZ): Best Publishing; 1999. p. 703-15.

51. Feldmeier JJ, Heimbach RD, Davolt DA, Court WS, Stegmann BJ, Sheffield PJ. Hyperbaric oxygen as an adjunctive treatment for delayed radiation injury of the chest wall: a retrospective review of 23 cases. Undersea Hyperb Med. 1995;22:383-393.

52. Rudolph R. Complications of surgery for radiotherapy skin damage. Plast Reconstr Surg. 1982;70(2):179-85.

53. Arnold PG, Lovich SF, Pairolero PC. Muscle flaps in irradiated wounds: an account of 100 consecutive cases. Plast Reconstr Surg. 1994;93:324-326.

54. Teknos TN, Myers LL, Bradford CR, Chepeha DB. Free tissue reconstruction of the hypopharynx after organ preservation therapy: analysis of wound complications. Laryngoscope. 2001;111:1192-1196.

55. Feldmeier JJ, Hampson NB. A systematic review of the literature reporting the application of hyperbaric oxygen prevention and treatment of delayed radiation injuries: an evidence based approach. Undersea Hyperb Med. 2002;29:10-30.

56. Marx RE. Radiation injury to tissue. In: Kindwall EP, editor. Hyperbaric medicine practice. 2nd ed. Flagstaff (AZ): Best Publishing; 1999. p. 682-89.

57. Neovius EB, Lind MG, Lind FG. Hyperbaric oxygen therapy for wound complications after surgery in the irradiated head and neck: a review of the literature and a report of 15 consecutive patients. Head Neck 1997;19:315-322.

58. Hampson NB, Holm JR, Wreford-Brown CE, Feldmeier J. Prospective assessment of outcomes in 411 patients treated with hyperbaric oxygen for chronic radiation tissue injury. Cancer. 2012;118:3860-3868.

59. Gorodetsky R, Mc Bride WH, Withers HR, Miller GG. Effect of fibroblast implants on wound healing of irradiated skin: assay of wound strength and quantitative immunohistology of collagen. Radiat Res. 1991;125:181-86.

60. Kruegler WWO, Goepfert H, Romsdahl M, Herson J, Withers RH, Jesse RH. Fibroblast implantation enhances wound healing as indicated by breaking strength determinations. Otolaryngology 1978;86:804-11.

61. Cromack DT, Porras-Reyes B, Purdy J, Pierce GF, Mustoe TA. Acceleration of tissue repair by transforming growth factor beta 1: identification of an in vivo mechanism of action with radiotherapy-induced specific healing deficits. Surgery 1993;113:36-42.

62. Werier J, Ferguson P, Bell R, Hill R, Wunder J, O'Sullivan B, Kandel R. Model of radiation-impaired healing of a deep excisional wound. Wound Rep Reg. 2006;14:498-505.

63. Delanian S, Lefaix JL. Current management for late normal tissue injury: radiation induced fibrosis and necrosis. Semin Radiat Oncol. 2007;17(2):99-107.

64. Haubner F, Ohmann E, Pohl F, Strutz J, Gassner HG. Wound healing after radiation therapy: review of the literature. Radiat Oncol. 2012;7:162.

65. Stanirokowski PJ, Wnuk A, Cendowski K, Sawicki W. Growth factors, silver dressings and negative pressure wound therapy in the management of hard-to-heal postoperative wounds in obstetrics and gynecology: a review. Arch Gynecol Obstet. 2015:292(4):757-775.

66. Ward WF, Molteni A, Ts'ao C, Hinz JM. The effect of captopril on benign and malignant reactions in irradiated rat skin. Br J Radiol. 1990;63(749):349-54.

67. Huang SP, Huang CH, Shyu JF, Lee HS, Chen SG, Chan JY, Huang SM. Promotion of wound healing using adipose-derived stem cells in radiation ulcer of a rat model. J Biomed Sci. 2013;20(1):51.

Chapter 18

PRACTICAL APPROACH TO BURNS

Julie A. Rizzo, MD
Matthew P. Rowan, PhD
Kevin K. Chung, MD

KEY CONCEPTS

1. The size and depth of the burn and the patient's age are important predictors of morbidity and mortality in burn injury.
2. Tools such as the Wallace Rule of Nines and the Lund-Browder Diagram should be used to help determine the total burn size.
3. The distinction between irst- and second- or third-degree burns is the most clinically signi icant decision in the outpatient and emergency room setting.
4. Early referral to a specialized burn center should be considered for burn injuries that meet speci ic criteria.

CONTENTS

Introduction

Burn wounds present a unique challenge to clinicians due to a number of factors, including varied presentation, unique clinical requirements for wound diagnosis and treatment, and systemic complications from large burns requiring resuscitation. The goal of this chapter will be to present a brief introduction of the epidemiology and pathophysiology of burns, as well as some clinical considerations for the diagnosis and treatment of burn wounds.

I. Case history

Mr. JM is a 42-year-old male who was pouring gasoline on a brush fire when he sustained burns to his face and upper and lower extremities. He was transported to a community hospital emergency department where he was found to have 12% total body surface area partial- and deep partial-thickness burns to his hands, arms, and legs and superficial, first-degree burns to his face. He was transferred to an American Burn Association–verified burn center where he was evaluated by a burn surgeon and admitted to the burn center, placed in silver nylon dressings, and given maintenance intravenous fluids. His burns were re-evaluated three days later and determined to be healing with nonoperative management. He was transitioned to topical bacitracin and discharged home. He was evaluated in the clinic one week later where he demonstrated further evidence of healing and was transitioned to lotion over his burned areas.

II. Pathway

This simple pathway may be utilized by clinicians to appropriately triage burn patients to the right level of care while providing guidance on the management of relatively simple burns.

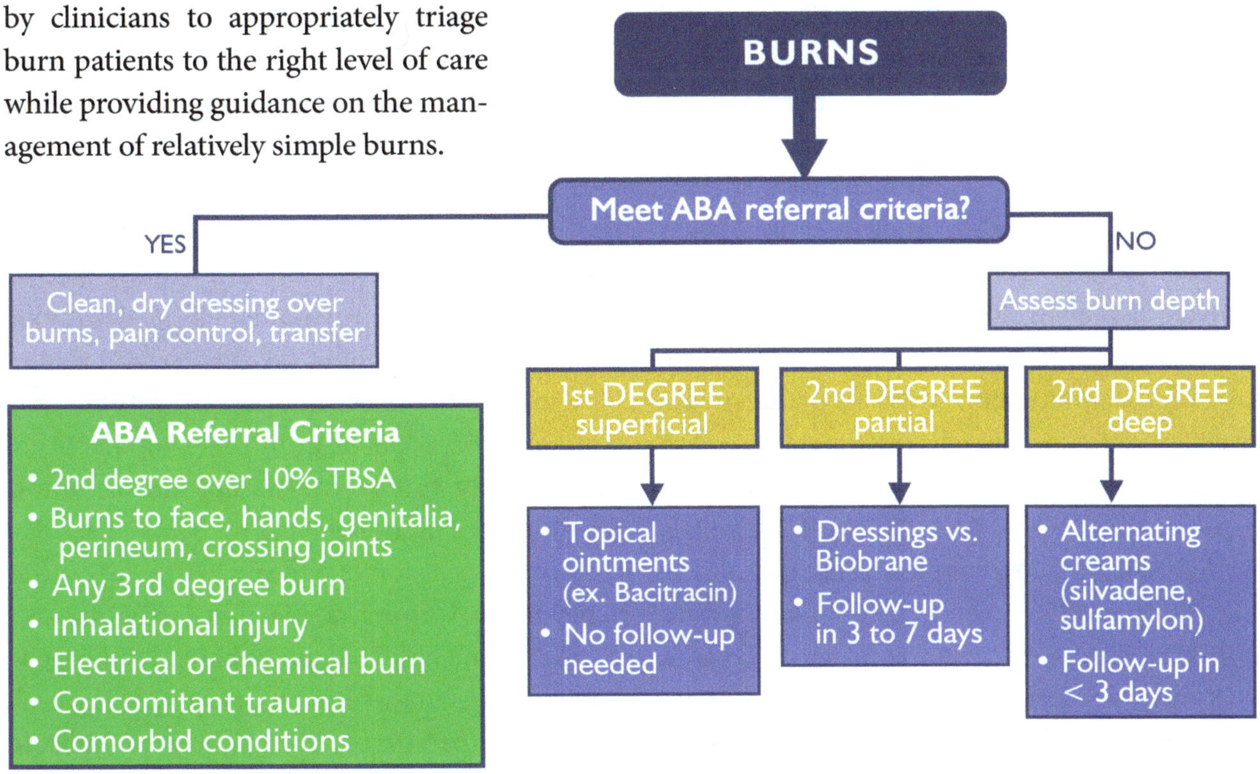

Printed with permission by Kevin Chung, MD, Julie A. Rizzo, MD, and Matthew P. Rowan, PhD

III. Epidemiology of burns

Nearly half a million burns receive medical treatment every year in an emergency room, urgent care facility, clinic, or physician's office. While the vast majority of these burns are minor and do not require hospitalization or specialized treatment, approximately 25,000 burns are treated annually at specialized burn centers that contribute data to the National Burn Repository (NBR) of the American Burn Association (ABA).[1] The 2015 NBR Annual Report compiled and analyzed data from 27,737 burn injuries treated at ABA-verified burn centers in 2014 and 203,422 total from 2005-2014. Information contained in the NBR provides valuable insight into patient demographics and injury characteristics that can be used to impact patient care, both for burns requiring specialized care and for minor burns treated in an outpatient setting.

Improvements in patient care, including improved antibiotics, early excision and grafting, improved methods of ventilation, and increased attention to patient nutrition, have resulted in steady reductions in burn patient mortality since the 1940s.[2] However, the incidence rate of burns has not decreased; in fact, burn centers have seen an increase in cases over the past decade, from under 15,000 in 2005 to over 27,000 in 2014.[1] Of the burns with known etiology treated at burn centers over the past decade, the majority (86%) of burns are received through contact with fire, flame, hot liquids, or other objects at home (73%), and as the result of an accident (72%). Most burns (81%) are small, covering less than 20% of the total body surface area (TBSA), and require a hospital stay of just over eight days. Overall mortality in <20% TBSA burns is under 1%, but mortality is directly related to burn size, as burns covering 20–40% TBSA are accompanied by an 11% mortality rate, and burns covering >40% TBSA are associated with a 39% mortality rate. Mortality from burns is affected by many factors, including age and the incidence of complications such as pneumonia, cellulitis, urinary tract infection, wound infection, and septicemia. Since the majority of burns treated each year are small, accidental burns received in the home as a result of contact with fire/flame/liquids, and infectious complications, among others, increase mortality risk. Understanding of the pathophysiology of burn wounds and keys to proper diagnosis and treatment will improve patient outcomes and functional recovery.

IV. Pathophysiology of burn wounds

Burn wounds present a unique challenge to clinicians because in addition to local injury at the site of burn, severe thermal injury over a large area of the body results in acute systemic responses that affect treatment requirements.[3] Damage from burn injuries may be limited to only the epidermis (first degree), or may extend down to the superficial dermis (second degree, "superficial partial thickness"), deeper dermis (second degree, "deep partial thickness"), or all of the dermis (third degree, "full thickness"). The important clinical distinction of the degree of burn damage is used to distinguish which wounds will heal without intervention, commonly first-degree and superficial partial-thickness injuries, from those that will require an operation in order to effectively heal, namely the deeper partial-thickness and full-thickness injuries.

The progression of a burn wound during the acute phase starting at the time of injury and lasting for the first 48 hours is based on the well-known model of three zones of injury.[4] The central zone of necrosis or coagulation is nonviable tissue with no possibility of revitalization. A zone of stasis or ischemia surrounds this, which is marginally viable tissue that possesses the ability to live if perfusion is maintained but can easily progress to necrosis without support. It is thought that this zone of stasis is the area responsible for the worsening of burns initially evaluated to be partial thickness but upon re-evaluation 24-48 hours later, found to be a deeper injury. The outermost zone of hyperemia is clearly viable tissue that appears erythematous, as it possesses the greatest number of inflammatory mediators.

The three phases of wound healing are well described and apply to recovery from burn injury as well.[5] Specific to burn injury, the inflammatory phase is characterized by increased fluid extravasation into the surrounding tissue causing profound edema. The proliferative phase is focused on fibroblast activation and keratinocyte migration, which is responsible for the appearance that the burn heals inward from the wound edges.[6] The final phase of wound healing is the remodeling phase which determines the final appearance of the healed burn wound, which can take up to 12 months to complete. This is longer than most remodeling phases, likely secondary to the prolonged hypermetabolic state of burn injury.[7]

V. Diagnosis

A. Burn size

Thermal and chemical burns are classified based on their size (% TBSA) and depth. Several

TABLE 1. Lund-Browder Chart ©American Burn Association

Lund and Browder Chart

Estimate of % Total Body Surface Area (TBSA) Burn

AREA	BIRTH - 1 YEAR	1 - 4 YEARS	5 - 9 YEARS	10 - 14 YEARS	15 YEARS	ADULT	TOTAL
Head	***19***	***17***	***13***	***11***	***9***	***7***	
Neck	2	2	2	2	2	2	
Anterior trunk	13	13	13	13	13	13	
Posterior trunk	13	13	13	13	13	13	
Right buttock	2.5	2.5	2.5	2.5	2.5	2.5	
Left buttock	2.5	2.5	2.5	2.5	2.5	2.5	
Genitalia	1	1	1	1	1	1	
Right upper arm	4	4	4	4	4	4	
Left upper arm	4	4	4	4	4	4	
Right lower arm	3	3	3	3	3	3	
Left lower arm	3	3	3	3	3	3	
Right hand	2.5	2.5	2.5	2.5	2.5	2.5	
Left hand	2.5	2.5	2.5	2.5	2.5	2.5	
Right thigh	***5.5***	***6.5***	***8***	***8.5***	***9***	***9.5***	
Left thigh	***5.5***	***6.5***	***8***	***8.5***	***9***	***9.5***	
Right lower leg	***5***	***5***	***5.5***	***6***	***6.5***	***7***	
Left lower leg	***5***	***5***	***5.5***	***6***	***6.5***	***7***	
Right foot	3.5	3.5	3.5	3.5	3.5	3.5	
Left foot	3.5	3.5	3.5	3.5	3.5	3.5	
Total							

*Rows in **bold italics** indicate areas of difference between adult and pediatric patients. All other areas are the same for adults and children.*

methods are commonly used for estimating burn size, but the most common are the Lund-Browder chart[8] and the Wallace Rule of Nines[9] (Table 1 and Figure 1 respectively). The Rule of Nines estimates the burn TBSA by assigning approximate percentages to regions of the body: the head, chest, abdomen, and each arm are 9%; the back and each leg are 18%; and the groin is 1% for a total of 100%. The Lund-Browder chart provides adjustments to the body region percentages for adults and children and provides a more detailed breakdown of subregions, including upper and lower extremities, hands, feet, and others. An easy unit of measurement that can be used at the bedside and is particularly useful for small, scattered areas of burn is to use the patient's hand size as 1% TBSA.

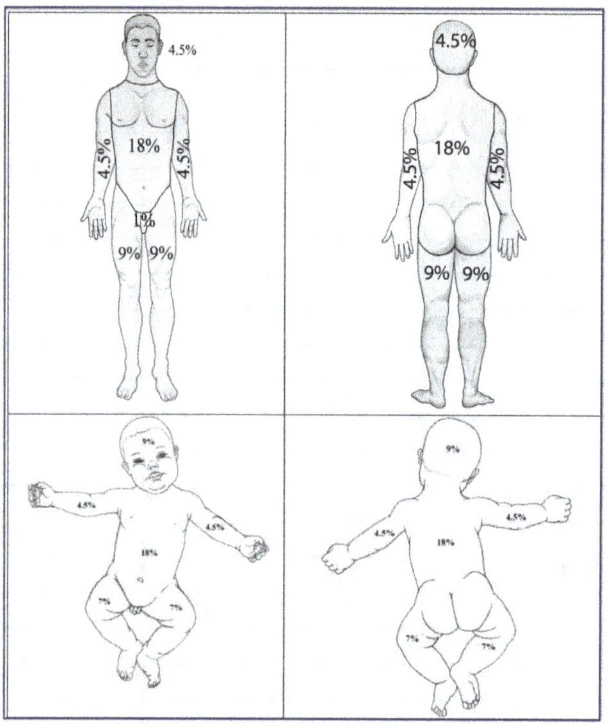

FIGURE 1. Wallace Rule of Nines
©American Burn Association
Used with permission.

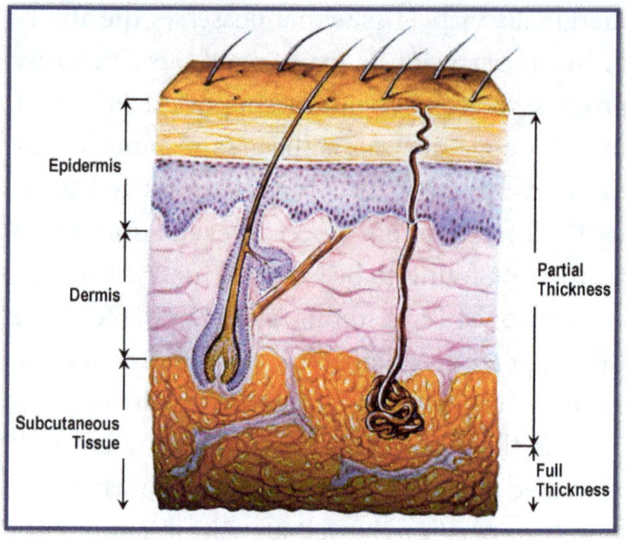

FIGURE 2. Burn depth
Courtesy of Julie A. Rizzo, MD
US Army Institute of Surgical Research

B. Burn depth

Along with the age of the patient and TBSA involved, the depth of the burn is an important prognostic indicator of mortality. Accurate assessment of the burn wound remains an important clinical goal, and several methods have met with variable success when used individually. However, when used together, the accuracy of measurements of depth and prognosis is significantly increased. Clinically, the ability to distinguish between wounds that will spontaneously heal by re-epithelialization within two to three weeks and not require surgical intervention from those that are deep enough to require surgery is critically important. The most common method used in the evaluation of burn depth is clinical evaluation[10-11] to identify features such as blanching, pain, tenderness, and blistering that might suggest a partial-thickness burn that should heal without surgical intervention. Insensate wounds without normal capillary refill are more likely to be deeper wounds that will require intervention in order to heal. Clinical evaluation can be performed quickly without the need for instrumentation by trained providers and can be repeated as needed throughout the patient's stay.

Clinical evaluation of burns also carries many limitations. No single clinical feature or combination of features will provide for a perfect assessment of burn depth every time. In fact, burn depth is commonly overestimated.[12] The timing of assessment and the effects of resuscitation on the burn wound present a potential issue regarding inaccuracy, as hypoperfusion can lead to conversion of a partial-thickness wound to a full-thickness wound.[4] The accuracy of burn depth estimations is correlated with provider experience in diagnosing burn injuries, with inexperienced and experienced providers achieving 50% and 64–75% accuracy rates, respectively.[13-14]

Tissue biopsy and subsequent histologic analysis have long been considered the gold standard to which other modalities of burn depth determination have been compared.[10] Denatured collagen and thrombosed vessels on hematoxylin, as well as eosin staining, are indicators of full-thickness injury.[11] The utilization of other staining techniques has increased the accuracy of burn depth determination.[15-16] However, the routine use of biopsies to assess burn depth is not commonly practiced. Biopsies are invasive, result in additional scarring, and carry the possibility of sampling error if the biopsy taken is not representative of the burn wound as a whole.[11] The experience of the pathologist, much like the burn surgeon performing a clinical evaluation of burn depth, also contributes to the accuracy of measurements.[17] The most common current use of burn wound biopsy is to determine colonization versus invasive infection of fungal elements, which has direct implications on mortality.[18]

Measurement of tissue perfusion with dyes has been explored as a method to gauge burn depth. Indocyanine green is the most accurate dye currently available,[19] and along with the addition of videography, has allowed dynamic changes in tissue perfusion within the burn wound to be observed.[20] The limitations of dyes include the need for intravenous injections, expensive imaging equipment, and specialized personnel.[21] Furthermore, dressings and topical ointments can affect imaging results, so these should be removed prior to scanning.[22]

Laser Doppler Imaging (LDI) is the most widely studied imaging technology in the assessment of burn depth and currently the only modality approved by the FDA for the assessment of burns. After imaging a burned area, a color-coded perfusion map is generated that correlates to varying burn depths. In non-infected wounds, accuracy of up to 99% has been reported.[23] Optimal conditions for scanning are difficult to achieve, as image accuracy is affected by ambient and skin temperatures, the presence of tissue edema, and the angle of scanning over curved surfaces.[24] Despite limitations, LDI is the most advanced technology currently available for imaging-based assessment of burn depth.

While certainly not all-inclusive, several methods of determining burn depth have been presented here that each have advantages and limitations. A combination of clinical evaluation by an experienced burn-care provider and another modality, such as LDI, holds the most promise in providing an accurate diagnosis of burn depth.

C. Burn wound infection

All burn wounds are colonized with bacteria, most commonly skin flora, which does not constitute an infection. All burn wounds, both before and after intervention, require constant surveillance for the development of infection, which may present as cellulitis or more severely as an invasive infection. Burn wound cellulitis most often presents three to five days after initial injury and is more common in males, in lower extremity burns, and in scald injuries. Erythema around the burn wound, increased pain, warmth, and induration are clinical features consistent with cellulitis. Treatment is typically intravenous antibiotics that are targeted against gram-positive organisms as these are the most likely causative organisms.[25]

More invasive infections can present with a wide constellation of symptoms, to include eschar separation or discoloration to black, violet, or dark brown. This diagnosis is confirmed by either histopathological examination of the wound identifying an infectious organism invading into viable tissue or a bacteremia with no other identifiable source. A histological classification system[26] is in place to characterize the severity of the burn wound infection (Table 2). These severe infections require immediate surgical excision and intravenous antimicrobial therapy.[27]

VI. Treatment

A. Pre-hospital care

Pre-hospital care of minor burns (under 10% TBSA) should focus on stopping the burning process and removing all items in contact with the skin that could continue to conduct heat, such as clothing and jewelry. Dissipating the heat from the site of the burn injury is beneficial in limiting edema formation and aids in pain control. There are several ways to locally cool the wound, including over-the-counter burn gels and cooling pads and running cool tap water or saline over the burn. Using ice and other colder substances should be avoided due to the potential for increased tissue damage.[28]

B. Care in an outpatient setting

Minor burns can be treated in the outpatient setting. Providing adequate pain control and appropriate local wound care are the main objectives in the emergency department or outpatient clinic. Narcotics are used as first-line treatment, especially while performing local wound care. Nonsteroidal anti-inflammatory drugs (NSAIDs) can be used as an adjunct if bleeding risk and kidney injury is considered. Topical pain agents (sprays or lotions) or subcutaneously injected pain medications are currently not recommended in the treatment of pain related to burn injury.

Local wound care should focus on removing clearly devitalized tissue and providing a clean wound environment. There is no consensus on

TABLE 2. Histologic classification of burn wound infection

Class 1A – Superficial colonization	Organism present on wound surface
Class 1B – Penetration	Organism penetrating eschar
Class 1C – Proliferation	Organism multiplication in the subeschar space
Class 2A – Microinvasion	Organism in viable tissue adjacent to subeschar space
Class 2B – Generalized invasion	Multifocal/widespread presence of organism in viable tissue
Class 2C – Microvascular invasion	Involvement of small vessels and lymphatics

the treatment of blisters associated with partial-thickness burn injuries, as some advocate to remove the blistered skin[29] while others propose that leaving the blister intact provides coverage for the underlying open wound.[30] If a blister is left intact, it should begin to resolve spontaneously within 7 to 10 days. If this does not occur, consideration should be given to transfer to a specialized burn center, as the burn is considered deeper than originally gauged.

C. Care at a specialized burn center

The American Burn Association has published criteria on burn injuries that should be referred to a specialized burn center: any partial-thickness injury greater than 10% TBSA; burns involving the face, hands, feet, genitalia, or perineum or crossing major joints; any third-degree or full-thickness injury; electrical and chemical burns; the presence of or concern for inhalational injury; concomitant trauma; or patients with pre-existing medical conditions that could affect management or recovery or impact mortality should be transferred.[31] If a patient is determined to go to a burn center, burn wounds should be covered with clean, dry dressings to facilitate evaluation immediately upon arrival.

D. Treatment strategies

For partial-thickness injuries that are expected to heal via re-epithelialization, dressings are chosen based on their ability to promote healing, minimize the risk for infection, and encourage maximal function during the healing process. Many burn dressings are silver-impregnated secondary to silver's antimicrobial properties. Several studies have examined different silver-impregnated dressings, such as Acticoat[32] (Smith & Nephew, London, UK) and Silverlon[33] (Argentum, Geneva, IL), both of which are commonly used at the U.S. Army Burn Center, and found that healing outcomes, such as number of people healed and time to complete wound healing, were improved with the use of silver-impregnated dressings.[34] The addition of a silicone interface to a silver dressing, such as those found in Mepilex Ag[35] (Gothenburg, Sweden), have demonstrated the same increased healing rates due to the presence of silver but without the epidermal damage and delayed re-epithelialization that has been suggested to be a problem with silver dressings.[36]

Synthetic and biosynthetic dressing options are popular options in the treatment of partial-thickness injuries. A commonly used dressing is Biobrane (Dow-Hickham, Sugarland, TX), which is composed of a dual-layer membrane with an inner layer of mesh that allows ingrowth of healing tissue and an outer layer of silicone that provides a barrier against moisture and bacteria. Careful wound selection and frequent monitoring are essential as this dressing must be applied to fresh, noninfected partial-thickness burns without eschar which must be kept clean and dry. Due to the occlusive outer layer, frequent monitoring for entrapment of moisture of infected fluid is necessary but is facilitated by the transparent nature of the dressing.[37]

Topical agents have a long tradition of being used in the emergency department setting as well as by burn providers for the treatment of smaller burns. The most popular agent is 1% silver sulfadiazine, also known as Silvadene (Pfizer, New York, NY), that is indicated for smaller burns with eschar overlying the burn injury. Silver sulfadiazine is often used on partial-thickness wounds without eschar, despite growing literature that demonstrates that wound healing is in fact impaired by delayed re-epithelization.[37-38] The most common observed side effect of silver sulfadiazine is a transient leukopenia that usually resolves without intervention.[39] Silvadene should not be used in patients with a sulfa allergy.

Mafenide acetate, also known as Sulfamylon (Mylan International, Rockford, IL), has been used as a topical burn treatment for decades and is available as a high-concentration (11.1%) cream or more dilute (5%) solution. Application of either form is painful, which limits use. With excellent eschar penetration and antimicrobial activity against many gram-negative species, it continues to have a role in early, nonoperative management of burns. Systemic toxicity presents in the form of metabolic acidosis and is secondary to the inhibition of carbonic anhydrase.[40] Developed at the U.S. Army Burn Center is a regimen that alternates mafenide acetate cream in the mornings with silver sulfadiazine in the evenings for deeper burns with overlying eschar.[3]

Sodium hypochlorite (NaOCl), commonly known as Dakin's solution (Century Pharmaceuticals, Indianapolis, IN), is a broad-spectrum bactericidal and antifungal agent that is used to control colonization of the burn wound and burn wound infection.[41] The bactericidal activity of sodium hypochlorite is dependent on the concentration of the solution and the time of exposure.[42] The solutions are available in various concentrations and can be used alone or in conjunction with a longer-acting antibacterial agent, such as mafenide acetate, to decontaminate the skin but leave viable epidermal cells for healing.

Early excision and grafting is the standard for deep partial-thickness and full-thickness burn injuries in order to reduce the risk of infection, decrease scar formation, shorten hospital stay, and reduce cost.[43] Split-thickness skin grafting, utilizing skin from an unburned donor site, is the most effective way to cover excised burns. The donor site, which is now considered an additional open wound, contributes significantly to pain, insensible fluid losses, and the overall wound healing burden.

Care of the donor site is quite variable, and the ideal donor site dressing is still much debated. Donor site dressings are broadly categorized into moist and nonmoist. Common moist dressings include Opsite (Smith & Nephew, London, UK) and Tegaderm (3M, St. Paul, MN) and examples of commonly used nonmoist dressings include Xeroform (DeRoyal Industries, Powell, TN) and Scarlet Red (no longer available). Studies that have examined different donor site dressings focused on outcomes such as pain, infection rate, and healing rate. Moist dressings were found to be associated with less pain and trended toward association with a lower rate of infection and faster healing.[44] Silver dressings have also been examined but due to their impairment of re-epithelialization and cytoxic effects on fibroblasts and keratinocytes, silver dressings are not recommended as a coverage option for donor sites.[45]

For patients with a large TBSA who do not have enough donor skin to cover all burned areas, the patient is surgically addressed in stages, utilizing temporary coverage with allograft (most commonly deceased donor skin), xenograft (most commonly porcine), skin substitutes, or dermal analogs. Allograft prepares the wound bed by promoting dermal regeneration and is not typically rejected by the body for approximately two to three weeks.[46] This time period of coverage with allograft allows for healing of unburned donor skin used in earlier surgical stages so that it may be harvested again for autograft coverage. Coverage with xenograft has been shown to reduce the systemic inflammatory response, which may play an important role in reducing the incidence of sepsis.[47] Several skin substitutes and dermal analogs exist, which can provide only epidermal replacement or a dermal regenerative scaffold. Epidermal substitutes are a few cell layers thick and require meticulous handling during placement and wound care in order to survive.[48] Integra (Plainsboro, NJ) is a dermal substitute that contains an external layer of silicone and an internal layer of bovine collagen/chondroitin sulfate matrix, which promotes fibroblast proliferation of the wound bed and can be used with success over exposed tendons, bone, and joints to build a wound bed favorable for autografting.[(49)]

Summary

The accurate diagnosis and effective treatment of burn injuries often requires highly specialized training, so patients receiving burn injuries are often transferred or otherwise referred to specialized burn centers, many of which are ABA-verified. However, it is estimated that over 500,000 burn injuries are received each year, and only 25,000 of these are treated at burn centers. Despite the large number of injuries that are likely to be treated in the home without any additional medical intervention, the vast majority of burns each year receive treatment in nonspecialized centers (emergency room, urgent care facility, clinic, or physician's office). Therefore, it is crucial that all clinicians are aware of the fundamental pathophysiology of burn injuries, as well as proper methods for diagnosis and treatment.

Review questions

1. **The best way to diagnose a burn wound infection is:**
    a. culture swab of the wound
    b. biopsy of the wound
    c. blood cultures
    d. physical examination

2. **A common complication of Sulfamylon for burns is:**
    a. neutropenia
    b. acidosis
    c. hyponatremia
    d. hyperkalemia

3. **A common complication of Silvadene for burns is:**
    a. neutropenia
    b. acidosis
    c. hyponatremia
    d. hyperkalemia

4. **What is the best outpatient management of a partial thickness burn?**
    a. silvadene
    b. excision and grafting
    c. sulfamylon solution
    d. watchful waiting

5. **All of the following patients require referral to a burn center EXCEPT:**
    a. a 15% TBSA third-degree burn to the chest of a 30-year-old man
    b. a 5% TBSA third-degree burn to the face of a 40-year-old man
    c. a 3% TBSA third-degree burn to the hand of a 25-year-old woman
    d. a 9% TBSA second-degree burn to the back of a 50-year-old man

ANSWERS: 1) b
2) b
3) a
4) a
5) d

References

1. National Burn Repository 2015 report of data from 2005-2014 [Internet]. Chicago: American Burn Association; 2015. Available from: http://www.ameriburn.org/2015NBRAnnualReport.pdf.
2. Mann R, Heimbach D. Prognosis and treatment of burns. West J Med. 1996;165(4):215-20.
3. Rowan MP, Cancio LC, Elster EA, Burmeister DM, Rose LF, Natesan S, Chan RK, Christy RJ, Chung KK. Burn wound healing and treatment: review and advancements. Crit Care. 2015;19:243.
4. Jackson DM. The diagnosis of the depth of burning. Br J Surg. 1953;40(164):588-96.
5. Gurtner GC, Werner S, Barrandon Y, Longaker MT. Wound repair and regeneration. Nature. 2008;453(7193):314-21.
6. Pastar I, Stojadinovic O, Yin NC, Ramirez H, Nusbaum AG, Sawaya A, Patel SB, Khalid L, Isseroff RR, Tomic-Canic M. Epithelialization in wound healing: a comprehensive review. Adv Wound Care (New Rochelle). 2014;3(7):445-64.
7. Atiyeh BS, Gunn SW, Dibo SA. Metabolic implications of severe burn injuries and their management: a systematic review of the literature. World J Surg. 2008;32(8):1857-69.
8. Lund CC, Browder NC. The estimation of areas of burns. Surg Gynecol Obstet. 1944;79:352-58.
9. American Burn Association. Advanced burn life support course, provider manual. Chicago: American Burn Association; 2007.
10. Heimbach D, Engrav L, Grube B, Marvin J. Burn depth: a review. World J Surg. 1992;16(1):10-15.
11. Watts AM, Tyler MP, Perry ME, Roberts AH, McGrouther DA. Burn depth and its histological measurement. Burns. 2001;27(2):154-60.
12. Niazi ZB, Essex TJ, Papini R, Scott D, McLean NR, Black MJ. New laser Doppler scanner, a valuable adjunct in burn depth assessment. Burns. 1993;19(6):485-89.
13. Heimbach DM, Afromowitz MA, Engrav LH, Marvin JA, Perry B. Burn depth estimation--man or machine. J Trauma. 1984;24(5):373-78.
14. Hlava P, Moserova J, Konigova R. Validity of clinical assessment of the depth of a thermal injury. Acta Chir Plast. 1983;25(4):202-08.
15. Chvapil M, Speer DP, Owen JA, Chvapil TA. Identification of the depth of burn injury by collagen stainability. Plast Reconstr Surg. 1984;73(3):438-41.
16. Nanney LB, Wenczak BA, Lynch JB. Progressive burn injury documented with vimentin immunostaining. J Burn Care Rehabil. 1996;17(3):191-98.
17. Jaskille AD, Shupp JW, Jordan MH, Jeng JC. Critical review of burn depth assessment techniques: part I. Historical review. J Burn Care Res. 2009;30(6):937-47.
18. Horvath EE, Murray CK, Vaughan GM, Chung KK, Hospenthal DR, Wade CE, Holcomb JB, Wolf SE, Mason AD Jr, Cancio LC. Fungal wound infection (not colonization) is independently associated with mortality in burn patients. Ann Surg. 2007;245(6):978-85.
19. Jerath MR, Schomacker KT, Sheridan RL, Nishioka NS. Burn wound assessment in porcine skin using indocyanine green fluorescence. J Trauma. 1999;46(6):1085-88.
20. Kamolz LP, Andel H, Haslik W, Donner A, Winter W, Meissl G, Frey M. Indocyanine green video angiographies help to identify burns requiring operation. Burns. 2003;29(8):785-91.
21. Devgan L, Bhat S, Aylward S, Spence RJ. Modalities for the assessment of burn wound depth. J Burns Wounds. 2006;5:e2.

22. Haslik W, Kamolz LP, Andel H, Winter W, Meissl G, Frey M. The influence of dressings and ointments on the qualitative and quantitative evaluation of burn wounds by ICG video-angiography: an experimental setup. Burns. 2004;30(3):232-35.

23. Jeng JC, Bridgeman A, Shivnan L, Thornton PM, Alam H, Clarke TJ, Jablonski KA, Jordan MH. Laser Doppler imaging determines need for excision and grafting in advance of clinical judgment: a prospective blinded trial. Burns. 2003;29(7):665-70.

24. Jaskille AD, Ramella-Roman JC, Shupp JW, Jordan MH, Jeng JC. Critical review of burn depth assessment techniques: part II. Review of laser Doppler technology. J Burn Care Res. 2010;31(1):151-57.

25. Heard JP, McDonald KM, Xing Y, Kluesner KM, Liao J, Wibbenmeyer LA. Regional and national review of factors associated with burn wound cellulitis. J Burn Care Res. 2015;36(1):23-32.

26. Pruitt BA Jr, McManus AT, Kim SH, Goodwin CW. Burn wound infections: current status. World J Surg. 1998;22(2):135-45.

27. Gibran NS, Wiechman S, Meyer W, Edelman L, Fauerbach J, Gibbons L, Holavanahalli R, Hunt C, Keller K, Kirk E, et al. Summary of the 2012 ABA Burn Quality Consensus conference. J Burn Care Res. 2013;34(4):361-85.

28. Jandera V, Hudson DA, de Wet PM, Innes PM, Rode H. Cooling the burn wound: evaluation of different modalites. Burns. 2000;26(3):265-70.

29. Rockwell WB, Ehrlich HP. Should burn blister fluid be evacuated? J Burn Care Rehabil. 1990;11(1):93-95.

30. Swain AH, Azadian BS, Wakeley CJ, Shakespeare PG. Management of blisters in minor burns. Br Med J (Clin Res Ed). 1987;295(6591):181.

31. Mackersie RC. Field triage, and the fragile supply of "optimal resources" for the care of the injured patient. Prehosp Emerg Care. 2006;10(3):347-50.

32. Muangman P, Chuntrasakul C, Silthram S, Suvanchote S, Benjathanung R, Kittidacha S, Rueksomtawin S. Comparison of efficacy of 1% silver sulfadiazine and Acticoat for treatment of partial-thickness burn wounds. J Med Assoc Thai. 2006;89(7):953-58.

33. Heggers J, Goodheart RE, Washington J, McCoy L, Carino E, Dang T, Edgar P, Maness C, Chinkes D. Therapeutic efficacy of three silver dressings in an infected animal model. J Burn Care Rehabil. 2005;26(1):53-56.

34. Wasiak J, Cleland H, Campbell F, Spinks A. Dressings for superficial and partial thickness burns. Cochrane Database Syst Rev. 2013;3:CD002106.

35. Gee Kee EL, Kimble RM, Cuttle L, Khan A, Stockton KA. Randomized controlled trial of three burns dressings for partial thickness burns in children. Burns. 2015;41(5):946-55.

36. Aziz Z, Abu SF, Chong NJ. A systematic review of silver-containing dressings and topical silver agents (used with dressings) for burn wounds. Burns. 2012;38(3):307-18.

37. Barret JP, Dziewulski P, Ramzy PI, Wolf SE, Desai MH, Herndon DN. Biobrane versus 1% silver sulfadiazine in second-degree pediatric burns. Plast Reconstr Surg. 2000;105(1):62-65.

38. Hansbrough JF, Achauer B, Dawson J, Himel H, Luterman A, Slater H, Levenson S, Salzberg CA, Hansbrough WB, Dore C. Wound healing in partial-thickness burn wounds treated with collagenase ointment versus silver sulfadiazine cream. J Burn Care Rehabil. 1995;16(3 Pt 1):241-47.

39. Choban PS, Marshall WJ. Leukopenia secondary to silver sulfadiazine: frequency, characteristics and clinical consequences. Am Surg. 1987;53(9):515-17.

40. Asch MJ, White MG, Pruitt BA Jr. Acid base changes associated with topical Sulfamylon therapy: retrospective study of 100 burn patients. Ann Surg. 1970;172(6):946-50.

41. Heggers JP, Sazy JA, Stenberg BD, Strock LL, McCauley RL, Herndon DN, Robson MC. Bactericidal and wound-healing properties of sodium hypochlorite solutions: the 1991 Lindberg Award. J Burn Care Rehabil. 1991;12(5):420-24.

42. Coetzee E, Whitelaw A, Kahn D, Rode H. The use of topical, un-buffered sodium hypochlorite in the management of burn wound infection. Burns. 2012;38(4):529-33.

43. Still JM Jr, Law EJ, Belcher K, Thiruvaiyarv D. Decreasing length of hospital stay by early excision and grafting of burns. South Med J. 1996;89(6):578-82.

44. Voineskos SH, Ayeni OA, McKnight L, Thoma A. Systematic review of skin graft donor-site dressings. Plast Reconstr Surg. 2009;124(1):298-306.

45. Nikkhah D, Gilbert P, Booth S, Dheansa B. Should we be using silver based compounds for donor site dressing in thermal burns? Burns. 2013;39(6):1324-25.

46. Lineen E, Namias N. Biologic dressing in burns. J Craniofac Surg. 2008;19(4):923-28.

47. Feng X, Shen R, Tan J, Chen X, Pan Y, Ruan S, Zhang F, Lin Z, Zeng Y, Wang X, Lin Y, Wu Q. The study of inhibiting systematic inflammatory response syndrome by applying xenogenic (porcine) acellular dermal matrix on second-degree burns. Burns. 2007;33(4):477-79.

48. Atiyeh BS, Costagliola M. Cultured epithelial autograft (CEA) in burn treatment: three decades later. Burns. 2007;33(4):405-13.

49. Ryan CM, Schoenfeld DA, Malloy M, Schulz JT 3rd, Sheridan RL, Tompkins RG. Use of Integra artificial skin is associated with decreased length of stay for severely injured adult burn survivors. J Burn Care Rehabil. 2002;23(5):311-17.

Section 5

WOUND CARE IN SPECIAL POPULATIONS

Editor - Dianne Rudolph, DNP, GNP-BC, CWOCN

Chapter 19

WOUND CARE IN PEDIATRIC PATIENTS

Margie Rodriguez, RN, MSN, WCC

KEY CONCEPTS

1. Little research has been conducted to determine prevalence, incidence, and risk factors associated with pressure ulcers in infants and children.
2. Children with special needs constitute a large portion of acute and chronic wounds/pressure injuries.
3. Evidence presented by Pallija et al. depicts 20%–43% pressure ulcer incidence rates among patients with spina bifida.
4. In pediatric cases, aggressive debridement should not be the first line of treatment.
5. When at bedside during wound dressing changes in children, it is extremely important to have the discipline of child life/music therapy for pain management.
6. The wound care clinician must work closely with the medical team of the children with special needs

CONTENTS

Introduction

The estimated cost of treating a single full-thickness pressure ulcer is as high as $70,000, with the annual total costs for treating pressure ulcers in the United States at $11 billion.[1] In the United States, chronic wounds affect around 6.5 million patients. It is claimed that an excess of $25 billion is spent annually on treatment of chronic wounds.[2] These numbers may or may not reflect and/or distinguish the pediatric population. Little research has been conducted to determine prevalence, incidence, and risk factors associated with pressure ulcers in infants and children.[3] Nevertheless, the pediatric population also experiences wounds such as pressure injuries (ulcers), chronic wounds, acute wounds, and/or acute wounds that escalate into chronic wounds. These chronic wounds can sometimes last up to a year or more to heal due to the multifactorial medical complexities associated with the pediatric population. It is essential to look at any illness the child presents as a confounding factor to the healing process and watch that these conditions remain stable during the healing process. Children with special needs constitute a large portion of acute and chronic wounds/pressure injuries. Evidence presented by Pallija et al. depicts 20%–43% pressure ulcer incidence rates among patients with spina bifida as one example of special needs population.[3] Of the 53.9 million school-aged children (aged 5 to 17) in the U.S. civilian noninstitutionalized population, about 2.8 million (5.2%) were reported to have a disability in 2010.[4] From 2005 through 2011, the neonatal mortality rate (deaths under age 28 days per 1,000 live births) declined 11%, and the post-neonatal mortality rate (deaths at ages 28 days to under one year per 1,000 live births) declined 14%.[5] Because of technological advances, some of the special needs pediatric population is able to thrive for long periods of time when illness, congenital anomaly, or neurological impairment occurs. It is then fair to say this population remains underrepresented when it comes to wound care literature and/or research. The literature reveals limited information on pediatric skin care issues in comparison to the adult population.[6]

This chapter examines wound care issues in the pediatric population. It includes discussion of the difference between adult and pediatric skin, the most common wounds (acute and chronic) in the pediatric population, wounds over scar tissue (as in recurrent breakdown), debridement methods, biofilm and its role in pediatric wound care, prevention of pressure injuries in children, and dressings useful for the pediatric population.

I. Cases

Six-month-old female admitted to a pediatric nursing skilled facility for wound care s/p IV extravasation. (Figure 1) She was treated with 0.9% saline gel to wound bed, moisture barrier film to wound edges, pink foam dressing with surfactant properties to keep it clean as primary dressing, and Tegaderm™ as secondary dressing. These were changed once a day. This dressing allowed for autolytic debridement of the eschar and slough. When scar tissue formed, it was

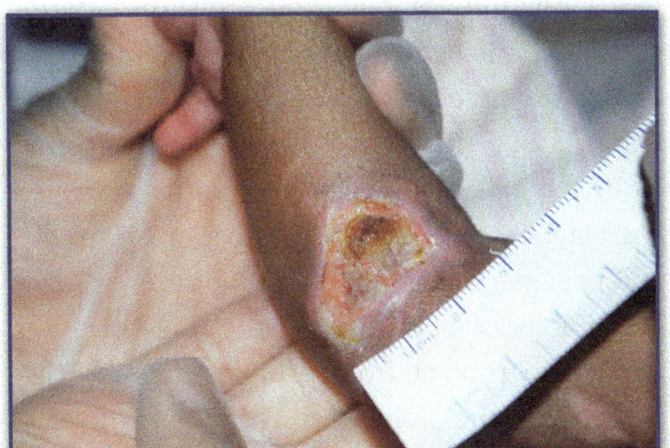

FIGURE 1. Extravasation

light but did not avoid contracture to the joint. Moisturization to scar tissue was ongoing with silicone based ointment.

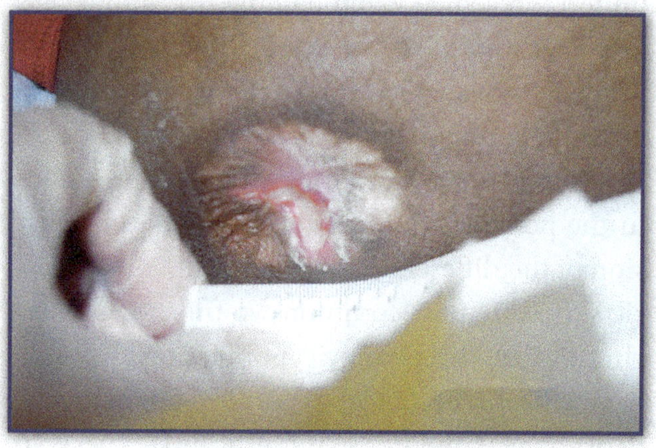

FIGURE 2. Scar tissue wound

Nine-year-old male – a medically complex child – with skin breakdown to right trochanter due to friction and shear over previous scar tissue s/p Stage 4 pressure injuries sustained when he was seven years old related to his wheelchair. (Figure 2) He outgrew his chair and no one noticed the skin breakdown while living at home. At the time, he was hospitalized for four to six months in acute care setting for B/L trochanter Stage 4 pressure injuries with complications of infection both bacterial and fungal. When stable, he was transferred to long-term care facility. Two years post admission, a full-thickness wound occurred due to friction and shear over scar tissue. It was a small abrasion that with time, biofilm, and moisture deteriorated the scar tissue, widening the wound base. Nonviable tissue was present on wound base. Upon taking the child for opinion at a wound clinic for stalled wound, osteomyelitis was ruled out via CT scan with contrast (negative result), and collagen matrix with bacteriostatic primary dressing was applied. Silicone dressing was applied to protect from primary dressing dislodgement and epidermal stripping. The surrounding skin (scar tissue) was moisturized lightly with silicone-base ointment. The wound healed and took one year controlling its biofilm growth with silver dressing. Dressing treatment was alternated/changed every two to three weeks; various forms of silver and collagen dressings were used. It was extremely important to continue to change treatment whenever there was no progress. Offloading was achieved by keeping the child in a supine position over an air mattress.

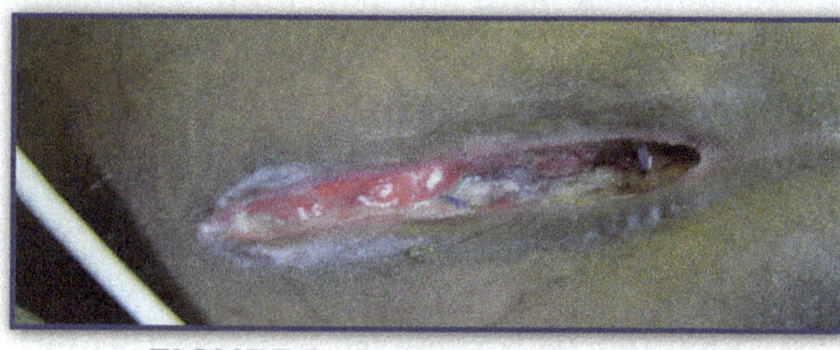

FIGURE 3. Abdominal dehiscence

10-year-old male with abdominal dehiscence post exploratory abdominal surgery. (Figure 3) Very active, special needs, nonambulatory, nonverbal, alert and interactive, moves all extremities freely. Patient was healed in three weeks with daily dressing changes that consisted of 0.9% saline gel to wound bed (provided autolytic debridement and environment for healing) and moisture barrier film to wound edges to prevent maceration of edges. Packed with collagen matrix for empty space (lightly), as primary dressing and pink foam dressing as secondary with Tegaderm to hold in place and not allow child to touch or remove.

Six-year-old female, ambulatory, nonverbal, gastrostomy tube, alert, interactive, very fearful of dressings placed on her. (Figure 4) Surrounding this open skin from tracheotomy tube (hard plastic), there is hypertrophic scar tissue. It is difficult to treat this area so close to tracheostomy and in a child who refuses to have anything placed. She received treatment for her scar tissue with silicone-based tape dressing developed by a company for scar tissue. The silicone scar tape was placed over site once a day after bath. Child healed in 10 days posttreatment, scar tissue decreased, erythema resolved, no edema, and the opening closed with minimal to no scar formation. The dressing changes were painless as the silicone dressing was removed with ease and was nontraumatic since it did not cause adhesive stripping. There was diminishing fear of dressing changes for the child.

Pain is managed in the pediatric population by using medications prior to dressing changes, music therapy, and ancillary staff playing with child. Children become apprehensive when hearing your voice and anticipate the dressing change; fluctuation in vital signs with higher heart rates and decrease in oxygenation is also observed.

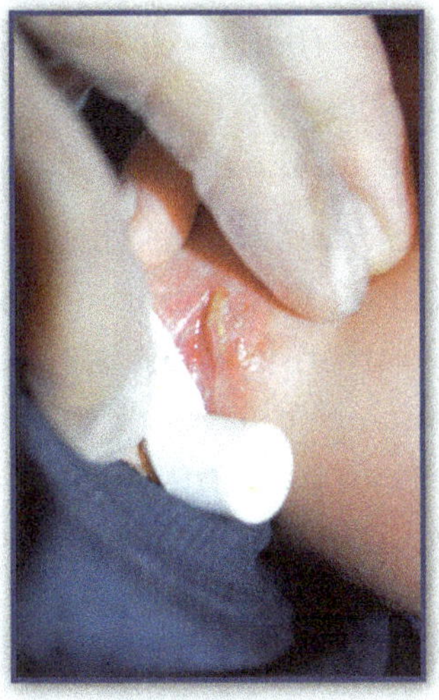

FIGURE 4.
Tracheostomy wound

Two-year-old male with arthrogryposis of B/L lower extremities s/p B/L amputation below the knees and grafting of sites. (Figures 5-7) Grafts did not take, and surgeon was planning to regraft. Prior to surgery, it was requested to do wound care and watch to remove dead tissue (graft) and redo. Child treated with 20% saline gel to sites for 10 days, using pink foam dressing as primary dressing and gauze dressing as secondary and a tube-like cotton sock to go over it and hold all in place. Child was verbal, alert, and interactive, eating by mouth and playful. Prior to dressing changes, child received pain medications as well as ancillary therapies for pain management, i.e., music therapy. After 10 days, continued with autolytic debridement with 0.9% saline gel, pink foam dressing, and gauze wrap as well as the cotton tube-like dressing for another 14 days. At that time, all viable dermal tissue was

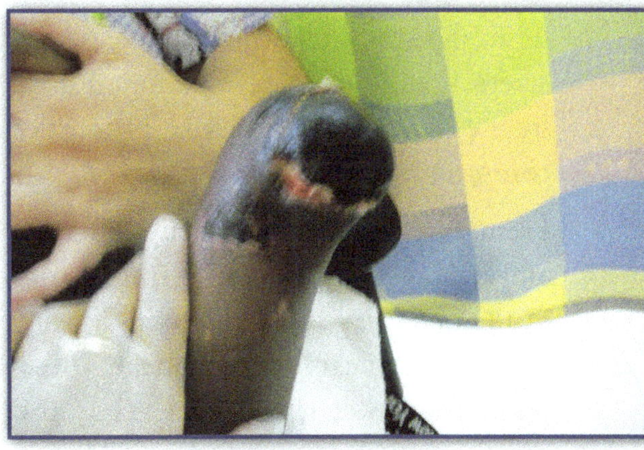

FIGURE 5. Graft #1

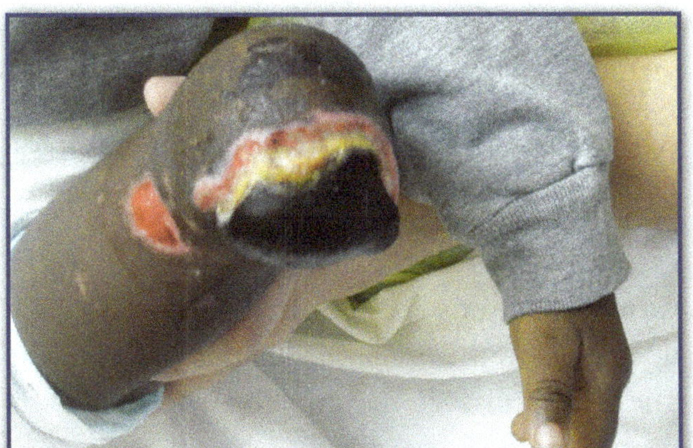

FIGURE 6. Graft #2

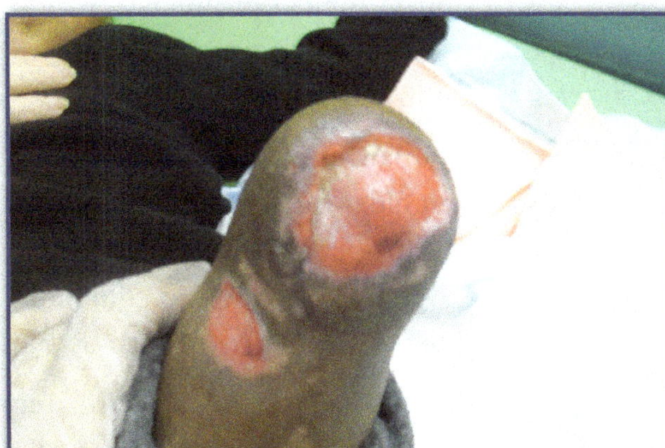

FIGURE 7. Graft #3

present, and when the child followed up with surgeon, there was no need for further surgical intervention. He was sent back to the skilled nursing facility for complete healing of stumps. Upon four weeks' treatment, stumps were healed, and rehab therapy took over to try and begin the process of prosthetic fitting and therapy.

II. Difference between adult and pediatric skin

Functions of the skin remain essentially the same in all phases of life, including barrier, photo protection, thermoregulation, immune surveillance, hormonal synthesis, insensible fluid loss prevention, and sensory perception.[7] Differences in pediatric skin that affect healing include the following:[8]

- Premature neonate skin appears translucent due to underdeveloped epithelium; the stratum corneum has few cell layers; and the epidermal junction is fragile, leaving skin barrier properties compromised.
- Premature junction between epidermis and dermis fragility due to immaturity of the anchorage structures that results in high permeability, significant transepidermal water loss (TEWL), and increased risk for infection. Higher absorption of topical products through the skin can place the newborn at risk for systemic toxicity.
- Newborn infants have less subcutaneous tissue than older infants and young children, and this plays a role in the inadequate skin function of thermoregulation, leaving the newborn to lose heat.
- Infant skin has a larger ratio of skin area to body weight.
- Infant skin is thinner than older children due to immature epidermis which matures around 30 to 32 weeks of life, post birth.[8] The dermal layer remains thinner than adults.
- Dermal thickness increases slowly after one year of age and doubles between the ages of three years through seven years.
- Sebaceous glands are functional at birth, but sebum production remains low until ages eight years through 10 years, providing less protection against evaporation and drying.
- Infants and small children are at higher risk for superficial bacterial infections associated with systemic symptoms, allergenic reactions, and inflammatory processes that form blisters/furuncles/carbuncles as the epidermis separates easily from the dermis.

Given these differences in pediatric skin versus adult skin, it is important to keep them in mind when treating wounds, especially when choosing dressings to lay over their skin. Adhesive stripping can cause further skin breakdown and scarring in the pediatric population.

III. Definition of wounds

Disruption to the integrity of tissue(s) whether surgical or due to trauma. Types of wounds include:

Acute wounds present with a sudden onset; for example, while a child is playing with a toy he/she acquires a laceration (cut).

Chronic wounds are nonhealing wounds. They do not follow the predefined patterns of growth. These wounds are common in children with special needs.

Palliative wounds are wounds whose goal is not healing; however, 50% achieve healing.[9] In the author's experience, children at the end of life or in hospice experience palliative wounds just as in the adult population. All three types of wounds exist in the pediatric community.

The phases of wound healing are as follows:

- Phase 1: hemostasis
- Phase 2: inflammation
- Phase 3: proliferation
- Phase 4: remodeling[10]

In phases 3 and 4, contraction of the wound occurs. Contraction, movement of wound edges that facilitates closure of a wound defect, essentially begins concurrently with collagen synthesis. The maximal rate of contracture is 0.75 mm/day and depends on the degree of tissue laxity and shape of the wound. Loose tissues contract more than tissues with poor laxity, and square wounds tend to contract more than circular wounds.[11] The above concept becomes extremely important for wound healing over scar tissue, as this scar tissue is poor in laxity.

Maturation of a healed wound can last up to two years and returns to approximately 80% of its prewound tensile state, leaving the area with a predisposition of recurrence, thus the importance of preventive measures to be implemented for patients with history of pressure injuries/wounds in order to minimize a potential of recurrence.

To know in what phase the wound is stalled allows us to choose the right dressing for it and guides us toward what product will be needed for wound bed preparation. In the pediatric special needs population, this becomes crucial as these children often receive multiple surgical interventions throughout their life spans. Avoiding invasive interventions like sharp debridement is recommended. The author has had many successes in healing wounds in the pediatric population without sharp debridement by using some of these products and understanding the basics of wound healing.

Wound healing is the body's normal response to injury and the attempt to restore the injured tissue to a relatively normal state. It happens in one of three ways.

Primary intention – as in surgical incision – wound edges approximate; no tissue loss; no local infection, minimal scar formation.

Secondary intention – healing from the bottom up, healing through granulation of cavity, takes longer than primary intention, scar formation is excessive.

Tertiary intention – this type of wound healing is also known as "delayed" or "secondary closure." It is indicated where there is a reason to delay suturing or closing a wound to some other day, for example, when there is poor circulation to the injured area. These wounds are closed later.[12]

IV. Guidelines in healing pediatric wounds within the three major intentions of healing

Guidelines created and used by author for wound healing in the pediatric population follow.

A. Wounds healing by primary intention

Goal

Maintain free from infection, maintain free from friction and shear, and maintain free from water submersion.

First 72 hours' postsurgical intervention maintains sterile technique when performing care/dressing change if needed (inflammation phase of wound healing). During the proliferation phase (14–21 days), maintain skin cleanliness, control moisture to incision line/avoid maceration, and assess for signs of dehiscence. If signs of dehiscence occur, it would then heal by secondary intention.

Guidelines on healing wounds by primary intention

Post 72 hours – Dressing remains intact. If dressing needs changing before this time due to soiling and/or saturation, it will be a sterile technique dressing change. If after 72 hours of first dressing, cleanse with sterile water or normal saline top to bottom, side to side each time changing the gauze, using aseptic techniques. Wipe surrounding skin down (2–5 cm) lateral to wound bed. End with wiping the suture line again, apply topical bacterial ointment, and reapply dressing. The dressing should stay intact and in place ~three to five days before exposing again to evaluate if suture line is healed. The exception would be that the dressing has been soiled or is 75% saturated, in which case it would need to be changed. Once sutures are removed, and no further dressing is necessary, moisturize lightly the scar tissue. This will help to avoid gross scar tissue formation of skin as well as promote laxity to the scar tissue.

B. Wounds healing by secondary intention

Goals

Maintain free from infection, control bioburden and/or debridement, apply moist wound healing technique, and document progress towards healing seven days (weekly). Documentation should include measurements of height x width x depth, tissue descriptions (epithelium, dermis, slough, necrosis), and appearance of the surrounding skin. When documenting the affected places of these tissues on the wound bed, use of the clock is recommended (e.g., at six o'clock the wound bed presents with 2% of slough). Wound healing timeline varies, especially in the pediatric special needs population, as many factors play into the premise of optimal healing, some of which include multiple medical complexities, where the child lives (home versus facility), and risk factors that may prolong the healing process. Change dressing daily. Avoid friction and shear at the affected site in order to minimize tissue disruption during the healing phases.

Guidelines on healing wounds by secondary intention (bottom up)

Using aseptic technique, cleanse wound bed and surrounding skin by using wet gauze with sterile water or normal saline. Using a gauze allows patting of the wound bed but also removing manually any nonviable tissue that may be loose, using one gauze at a time and discarding each time. End with cleansing wound bed again, and assess for signs and symptoms of infection (friable granulation tissue, hypergranulation tissue, edema, odor, amount of exudate, escalating pain, vital signs). Protect wound edges from maceration when performing care and choosing dressings, using the premise of moist wound healing as it shortens days of healing. It is gentle to tissues promoting cellular growth. For protection of wound bed edges, use of a moisture barrier film (wound prep) is very helpful prior to preparing wound bed. Debride nonviable tissue as well as excessive biofilm on the wound bed to jump-start the healing phases of the wound. For any wound cavities (tunneling, sinus tract), fill the empty space. Apply primary nonadhesive dressing to the wound bed – it allows no tissue disruption upon removal from the wound bed. Adhesive dressing may be applied as a secondary dressing. Change dressing daily if dressing maintains its integrity and is not saturated 75% with exudate or soiled.

C. Wounds healing by tertiary intention

Goal

The goal is to heal. Follow the goals and premise of primary intention for the first 72 hours post-surgical intervention. Follow the goals and premise of secondary intention for remainder of the healing on all those complex wounds needing further treatment and surgery more than once.

D. Palliative care

Goal

A wound is considered in "palliative care" when healing is not the goal of treatment. However, because the wound is receiving palliative care, it should not be assumed that the patient is receiving palliative or end-of-life care. It is true that healing is seldom the goal of patients who are receiving end-of-life care. Many patients at the end of life actually heal their wounds, and this is particularly true of pediatric patients. A wound may be considered for palliative care if one or more of the contributory factors that impair healing cannot be controlled (e.g. nutritional deficits, contracture).

Healing is not the goal; however, even under palliative wound care, 50% of wounds achieve healing. Prevent and relieve suffering by means of early detection, assessment, and treatment of pain. Also address physical, psychosocial, and spiritual health during palliative wound care treatment. When patients are actively dying, wound care might cause undue discomfort. In those cases, the need to measure wounds at least weekly can be suspended. The National Pressure Ulcer Advisory Panel's white paper titled "Pressure Ulcers in Individuals Receiving Palliative Care" states,states that healing is usually not the goal for patients receiving hospice or palliative care. There is no need to measure the wound size or deterioration because intervention is not planned.[13]

How do we as clinicians determine when to call a wound palliative? Ask these questions: Is the patient/resident at the end of life, and does the wound care impede quality of life with undue discomfort? Is the family and/or patient/resident requesting relief of undue discomfort due to wound care? Would the patient's quality of life improve significantly if the wound heals? If the answer is no to these questions, palliative wound care should be considered.

Guidelines for palliative wound care

Use aseptic technique when cleansing—follow the goal of controlling odor and exudate and preserving patient's/resident's self-esteem. Apply dressing that will produce less pain upon removal when it is time to change, and change only when necessary—soiled, saturated, or deteriorated. No need for continual follow-up or to perform measurements. Assess deterioration of wound, and avoid infection if possible. In extreme end-of-life cases, pressure ulcers are unavoidable. Though palliative care is defined as comfort care, hospice care is end-of-life care. Although no formal survey on pediatric service has been performed since 2007, data from the National Hospice Palliative Care Organization's 2013 National Summary on hospice care shows that 14.1% of participating agencies have formal pediatric palliative care services with specialized staff. The most common primary diagnosis for these services is the following: 41% genetic/congenital, 39% neuromuscular, 19.8% malignancy, with median time from consult to death 107 days.[14] Children are also part of the population of palliative and hospice care.

Factors that affect wound healing in the pediatric population include the following: 1) neurological deficits, 2) metabolic instability, 3) genetic anomalies, 4) ischemia, 5) infection versus. bioburden, 6) nutritional deficiency (e.g., esophageal atresia, gastrostomy, jejunostomy, prolonged periods of total parenteral nutrition [TPN]), 7) edema, 8) arterial insufficiency, 9) neuropathy, 10) mechanical injury, 11) venous insufficiency, 12) contractures, 13) cytotoxic topical agents, 14) insensate regions in the body, 15) medical conditions causing immune suppression, 16) spasticity, 17) behavioral issues (e.g., self-stimulating behavioral children with special needs would not tolerate dressings on skin), and 18) multiple medical/surgical interventions that could impact the wound healing process.

E. Wounds over scar tissue

In the world of the pediatric special needs population, clinicians understand that scars are a huge factor that affects wound healing. Scar tissue develops as a consequence of the disruption in the skin/tissue integrity and the healing process. Collagen, the "glue" of the body, helps with the regeneration of skin. An overactive healing process causes hypertrophic scars and keloids. This produces an excessive amount of collagen at the wound site.[15] These scars may in fact have a recurrence of tissue interruption which causes a unique challenge to clinicians for management/treatment of open scar tissue. Contracture scars are caused by the loss of a large section of skin due to burns or other injury. The scar contracts or tightens around the wound. This contracted scar could impact a person's mobility. If the scar deepens, it could affect muscles and nerves.[15] Contracted scar tissue in the special needs pediatric population poses great challenges. For example, when IV infiltration happens in a newborn or infant, it might result in development of contracted scar formation that may lead to limited limb mobility, impacting range of motion.

Guidelines for wounds over scar tissue

When a new scar forms, moisturize the scar for up to six to eight weeks post healing, especially if there is formation of hypertrophic or keloid tissue. When treating an area that has reopened, wound moisture must be monitored closely. Excessive moisture to this scar tissue (minimally vascularized over a bony prominence with minimal adipose tissue) will decompensate under those conditions, and the wound will deteriorate. On the other hand, no moisture will dry the wound bed, and it becomes deeper with minimal to no remodeling phase occurring. What to do? Control the moisture in the wound bed by applying petrolatum-based impregnated gauze as primary dressing, applying a small piece only in the wound bed. On the surrounding scar tissue, use a silicone-based ointment, and apply lightly to protect from secondary dressing that will cover the wound. It will allow for laxity of the skin and promote healing. This laxity of the skin will optimize wound healing, and in scar tissue this is minimal to none. Assess for any biofilm, and apply secondary dressing that will contain silver to keep this biofilm under control.

These wounds may take more time to heal than first-time tissue-interrupted wounds in well vascularized, non-medically compromised children. Once healed, protection of the scar tissue and prevention is key. Instruction should be given to avoid friction and shear for up to two years. Even after two years, the wounded area never gets 100% of tensile strength, and the wounded area will remain vulnerable to breakdown.

V. Treatment of wounds in the pediatric population

What the wound needs and the products available determine the treatment options for wounds in both adult and pediatric populations. There is widespread consensus in both Europe and the United States regarding the healing benefits of moist wound healing environments as the preferred method of treatment.

A moist environment accelerates the rate of wound repair as compared to letting the wound dry out and allowing a scab to form. In addition, as a result of moist wound healing, there is a reduction in the risk of scarring. Principles of modern-day wound management began with George Winter, PhD, University of London, who questioned if allowing a wound to dry out was the best method of healing. In 1962, he conducted a study by creating multiple small partial-thickness wounds on the backs of pigs. Some of the wounds were allowed to dry out and form scabs. Others were covered with polymer film. Wounds that had been covered by polymer film epithelialized twice as quickly as the wounds exposed to air. Dr. Winter demonstrated that moist healing can heal wounds in half the time.[16-17] As a guideline for treating pediatric wounds, moist wound healing is used by the author all the time. Moist wound healing mimics the function of the epidermis in limiting transepidermal water loss. It provides a natural environment for cells, allowing for an environment where they can thrive. A dry cell is a dead cell. Hydration and cell proliferation cannot thrive in a dry environment.

Benefits of moist wound healing include, but are not limited to increased angiogenesis, enhanced autolytic debridement, cell life enhancement, proteolytic enzymes carried to the wound bed, increased re-epithelialization, painless debridement, and decreased overall pain at wound site. Using moist wound healing insulates the wound and protects nerve endings, thereby reducing overall pain.

In pediatric cases, aggressive debridement should not be the first line of treatment. Methods of debridement in general include sharp, enzymatic, autolytic, biological (maggots), and mechanical. In the author's experience, two of these five methods for debridement work well in the pediatric population: autolytic and enzymatic. Healing many pediatric wounds, these two methods assist with minimal pain and discomfort to the child. They also achieve debridement of nonviable tissue in the wound bed preparation process.

Other advantages of enzymatic and autolytic methods of debridement are 1) they can be used in children of all ages and 2) they can effectively be used on both superficial and deep wounds. Enzymatic ointments work, but slowly. It has been the author's observation in the pediatric special needs population that enzymatic ointment sometimes acts as an occlusive agent and stalls wound healing in the debridement process.

The author recommends autolytic debridement with use of gels as the preferred method for children. The advantages are 1) gels have increased water base, and they debride and heal in half the time in the author's experience, and 2) dressing changes are done with minimal discomfort and/or no pain. The author recommends a customized and individualized approach of wound healing treatment in children. The concept of wound bed preparation is similar to the adult population and is described well in Chapter 5: Wound Assessment.[18]

VI. Dressings

Dressings are classified primarily into primary and secondary. Primary are those which touch the wound bed. Secondary are those which serve as a protective function to secure the primary dressing. In pediatrics, we often use both; one to treat the wound bed, and the other to secure it in place for the child, allowing for an improved quality of life while undergoing wound care. An ideal dressing protects the wound, is biocompatible, and provides ideal hydration. The cardinal rule is to keep the tissues moist and the surrounding skin intact, dry, and protected from adhesive stripping, especially in the pediatric population. Silicone-based dressing works really well in the pediatric population because of its soft and conforming properties. For superficial lesion, nonexudating wounds, low-profile hydrocolloid dressing works well. For light to moderate exudating wounds, polymer foam dressing with cleansing properties has worked with such speed in healing, it is of great benefit. It is oftentimes used by the author for Stage 2 pressure injuries that heal in three to five days. A Stage 3 pressure injury in a special needs child due to BIPAP dependence healed completely in five days. For heavily exudating wounds, an alginate with silver is used and works quickly in wicking away excessive moisture from the wound bed. The rule of thumb is to leave the dressing in place at minimum for 24 hours or more. The product and whether the dressing is saturated, deteriorated, or is soiled will determine the length of time it may be left in place.

Change three times a week as a rule of thumb or once a week using the above description to determine the time frame and progress of the wound healing. Techniques for changing dressings should include the following:

- lay out all of your material before you begin new dressing
- clean barrier
- obtain garbage bag where you will place old dressing
- maintain aseptic technique, cleanse wound bed and include the surrounding skin
- cleanse the wound bed, measure, and then apply new dressing
- initial the dressing and include date and time (doing this will provide a time frame between dressing changes and a clear idea as to its progress of healing or deterioration. In the pediatric population, the most difficult challenge is to obtain the correct size of products for dressings.)

VII. Prevention

To be proactive in education of the pediatric population is the first step in prevention. Prevention begins with the history of the child obtained with meticulous intention, accurate assessment of at-risk children for skin breakdown (daily activities, medical equipment evaluations, medical complexities, nutrition, medications, shear, friction, and/or pressure). Once the child is identified as "at risk," implement measures accordingly (weight redistribution surfaces, products to relieve disruption of tissues [foam/soft], education, etc.). Identifying and being well informed of the products that are effective in healing (e.g., collagen, gels, enzymatic debridement, silicone dressing, silicone tapes, silver dressings, scar control products, etc.) is key. It is important to organize a medical team including parents/guardians/patient (if verbal) for history-taking and management. This is a huge asset in prevention. Constant communication and documentation – telling the story of each child as he or she progresses or deteriorates – is equally important. This will allow the medical team to implement interventions that will prevent escalation.

Summary

Wounds in the pediatric population are sometimes very challenging, requiring consultation with a specialist. They present difficulties with medical complexities and are a population that is underrepresented and understudied. They are treated by clinicians who specialize in wound care and work with most impossible circumstances within their unique population. When at the bedside during wound dressing changes in children, it is extremely important to have the discipline of child life/music therapy for pain management. When children are traumatized due to medical interventions, it stays with them for a very long time. It is through the help of the other disciplines like child life, music therapy, and art therapy that the child can work through these invasive procedures and cope. These are some of the things in which pediatric wound care differs, and in light of these things, to educate your team/parents/guardians is to have a foot in the right direction towards healing, as well as to have an informed caregiver to oversee their status.

First: Intake of history is the first step of healing a wound in a pediatric patient. Gathering information of what the life of that child consists of and asking for an example of a typical day for the child will elicit information as to risk factors that can stall or impair wound healing both in the well and in the special needs pediatric population.

Patience is the first virtue to practice when healing children's wounds. Moist wound healing is the rule of thumb as well as using products that will keep control of biofilms and/or the use of autolytic debridement for wound bed preparation and healing.

Second: The wound care clinician must work closely with the medical teams of children with special needs. These children are often medically complex and have multifaceted confounding factors that may inhibit wound healing. Once they are stable or controlled, the wounds heal. For example, spasticity, a common diagnosis in neurological deficits in children with special needs, is a confounding factor for healing. Spasticity increases the energy expenditure (consumption of oxygen) as well as predisposes the child for increased friction and shear to the skin. These movements may increase with time. The wound care clinician can then work with the rehabilitation team and medical team on a plan. The wound care clinician should work closely with the health-care team of the child in managing risks, wound care, and the wound healing process. This population of children with special needs with wounds/pressure injuries is underrepresented in the literature and research.

Review questions

1. ***True/False.*** In treating pediatric patients with wounds, heightened attention is given to the special needs population because this population is considered to be a high-risk population for acquiring wounds that may be difficult to treat.

2. **Newborn infants are at risk of toxicity with topical products due to all of these except:**

    a. premature junction between epidermis and dermis

    b. topical products are absorbed through the skin

    c. epidermis and dermis fragility

    d. there is no difference in adult versus newborn skin

    e. immaturity of the anchorage structures between epidermis and dermis

3. ***True/False.*** Infant/small child is at higher risk for superficial bacterial infections associated with systemic symptoms, allergenic reactions, inflammatory processes that form blisters/furnuncles/carbuncles as the epidermis separates easily from the dermis.

4. ***True/False.*** The pediatric population does not present with multiple medical complexities, and therefore wounds heal faster.

5. **The optimal wound healing processes for the pediatric special needs population will depend on the clinician's knowledge of:**

    a. pediatric disease processes and individual presentation(s)

    b. assessment of biological impact of the patient's physical status as in nutrition, disease processes, and medications

    c. knowledge of wound healing products and their adaptability to the pediatric patient

    d. obtaining history of child's activities of daily living in order to identify risk factors that will impact wound healing and/or cause potential skin breakdown, especially in the pediatric special needs population.

    e. all of the above

ANSWERS: 1) True
2) c
3) True
4) False
5) e

References

1. Schindler CA, Mikhailov TA, Kuhn EM, et al. Protecting fragile skin: nursing interventions to decrease development of pressure ulcers in pediatric intensive care. Am J Crit Care. 2011;20(1):26-34.

2. Sen CK, Gordillo GM, Roy S, Kirsner R, Lambert L, Hunt T K, et al. Human skin wounds: a major and snowballing threat to public health and the economy. Wound Repair Regen. 2009 Nov-Dec;17(6):763–71.

3. Pallija G, Mondozzi M, Webb AA. Skin care of the pediatric patient. J Pediatr Nurs. 1999;14:80-7. Cited in: Baharestani MM, Ratcliff C. Pressure ulcers in neonates and children: an NPUAP white paper. Adv Skin Wound Care. 2007 Apr; 20(4):208-20. Available from: http://www.npuap.org/wp-content/uploads/2012/01/peds_white_paper.pdf.

4. Brault MW. School-aged children with disabilities in U.S. metropolitan statistical areas: 2010. American community survey briefs [Internet]. U.S. Department of Commerce, U.S. Census Bureau. 2011 Nov. Available from: https://www.census.gov/prod/2011pubs/acsbr10-12.pdf.

5. MacDorman MF, Hoyart DL, Mathews TJ. Recent declines in infant mortality in the U.S., 2005-2011. National Center for Health Statistics data brief. No. 120 [Internet]. U.S. Department of Health and Human Services, Centers for Disease Control and Prevention, National Center for Health Statistics; 2013 Apr. Available from: www.cdc.gov/nchs/products/databriefs/db120.htm.pdf.

6. Butler CT. Pediatric care: guidelines for assessment, prevention and treatment. Pediatr Nurs. 2006 Sep/Oct: 443-50. Available from: http://search.proquest.com/openview/3751da32500f7e32bded37aff100d8ba/1?pq-origsite=gscholar.

7. Fluhr JW, Darlenski R, Taieb A, et al. Functional skin adaptation in infancy – almost complete but not fully competent. Exp Dermatology. 2010;19(6):483-92. Cited In: Lio P. How does infant skin differ from adult skin? Medscape [Internet]. 2011 Jun 20. Available from: http://www.medscape.org/viewarticle/743529.

8. Skin and wound resource manual. Lake Geneva (WI): Wound Care Education Institute; 2006. Section 8: Pediatric skin care; p. 115-22.

9. Herbert G. Palliative wound care: part 1: although wound healing may no longer take priority, palliative wound care is far from a do-nothing approach. Wound care advisor [Internet]. 2015 Jan/Feb;4(1). Available from: http://woundcareadvisor.com/wp-content/uploads/2015/02/PALLIATIVE_J-F15.pdf.

10. Chin G et al. Chapter 2: Biochemistry of wound healing in wound care practice. In: Sheffield and Fife's Wound Care Practice. 2nd ed. 2007; p. 51-78.

11. Simon PE, Romo T, Moutran HA. Skin wound healing. Medscape [Internet]. 2016 Jan 20. Available from: http://emedicine.medscape.com/article/884594-overview.

12. RN Central [Internet]. Olin J. Wound healing – a process almost all RNs encounter; Jun 5. Available from: http://www.rncentral.com/blog/2012/wound-healing-a-process-almost-all-rns-encounter/.

13. Langemo DK, Black J, NPUAP. Pressure ulcers in individuals receiving palliative care: a National Pressure Ulcer Advisory Panel white paper. Adv Skin Wound Care. 2010 Feb 23;23(2):59-72. Available from: http://www.npuap.org/wp-content/uploads/2012/01/Pressure_Ulcers_in_individuals_Receiving.7.pdf.

14. Freibert S, Williams C. NHPCO's facts and figures pediatric palliative and hospice care in America [Internet]. National Hospice and Palliative Care Organization; 2015. p.1-8. Available from: http://www.nhpco.org/sites/default/files/public/quality/PediatricFacts-Figures.pdf.
15. Swain L. Gale Encyclopedia of Medicine. 3rd ed. 2006. Scars. Available from: http://www.encyclopedia.com/doc/1G2-3451601445.html.
16. Winter GD. Formation of the scab and the rate of epithelization of superficial wounds in the skin of the young domestic pig. Nature. 1962 Jan 20;193:293-94.
17. Junker J, Kamel RA, Caterson EJ, Eriksson E. Clinical impact upon wound healing and inflammation in moist, wet, and dry environments. Adv Wound Care (New Rochelle). 2013 Sep;2(7):348-56.
18. Wound care centers [Internet]. eDoctors. Infected wounds. Available from: http://www.woundcarecenters.org/article/wound-types/infected-wounds.

Chapter 20

SKIN CARE ISSUES IN THE OLDER ADULT

Dianne Rudolph, DNP, GNP-BC, CWOCN

KEY CONCEPTS

1. Between 2000 and 2010, the population 65 and older grew 15.1%, while the total U.S. population grew 9.7%.
2. There are three hallmark features of intrinsic skin aging: atrophy of the dermis as a result of collagen loss, degeneration of the elastic fiber network, and loss of hydration.
3. Extrinsic aging is often referred to as photoaging.
4. Collagen disruption that occurs with aging lends itself to poor tensile strength, which can lead to skin tears and wound dehiscence.
5. Moisture-associated skin damage should NOT be documented as a Stage 1 or 2 pressure ulcer.
6. Wounds at the end are a significant problem for the nearly 1million hospice patients and millions of other frail, elderly persons living with chronic disease.
7. The Kennedy Terminal Ulcer presents as an unavoidable ulcer occurring during the dying process, often within the last 24 hours of life.

CONTENTS

Introduction

Diseases of the older adult are becoming increasingly important as life expectancy gradually increases worldwide. According to the 2010 Census, there were 40.3 million people 65 and older on April 1, 2010, increasing by 5.3 million since the 2000 Census when this population numbered 35 million. The percentage of the population 65 and older also increased during the previous decade. In 2010, the older population represented 13% of the total population, an increase from 12.4% in 2000. [1]

Between 2000 and 2010, the population 65 and older grew 15.1%, while the total U.S. population grew 9.7%. The opposite happened between 1990 and 2000, when the growth of the older population was slower than the growth of the total population, with growth rates of 12% and 13.2%, respectively.[1]

In order to promote healthy aging, it is important to care for diseases that affect older adults. Because a complete review is beyond our intended scope, the focus of this chapter is on special considerations for some of the more common skin issues. This includes presentation, contributing factors, and management.

I. Senescent changes in the skin

It is readily apparent from physical examination of the skin that major changes in its mechanical properties occur with aging. Cutaneous aging occurs through both intrinsic and extrinsic aging. Intrinsic aging is a process that occurs naturally and results from a slow degradation of the epidermis and dermis. There are three hallmark features: atrophy of the dermis as a result of collagen loss, degeneration of the elastic fiber network, and loss of hydration. As skin ages, it becomes wrinkled, lax, and easier to tear. Histologically, the rete pegs (also known as rete ridges) become flattened or retracted. Cellular turnover slows, and there is a progressive loss of cells within the dermis and epidermis. This subsequently leads to a loss of the extracellular matrix. The epidermis thins, and reduces stratum corneum biosynthesis impairs barrier function and permeability. There is a decrease in cutaneous blood flow, diminished numbers of sweat glands, and loss of subcutaneous fat.[2]

In contrast to intrinsic aging, extrinsic aging is due to environmental factors; ultraviolet (UV) exposure is the main cause of extrinsic aging. Extrinsic aging is often referred to as photoaging. A microscopic characteristic of photoaging is massive accumulations of abnormal elastotic material in the upper and middle dermis. UV radiation has been shown to activate signaling pathways that induce matrix metalloproteases, which degrade the ECM. Chronic UV exposure also contributes to progressive loss of cutaneous vasculature.

Hormone therapy with estrogens appears to ameliorate aging of the skin. Estrogen restores skin thickness by increasing collagen synthesis while limiting excessive collagen degradation. Wrinkling is improved following estrogen treatment, since estrogen enhances the morphology and synthesis of elastic fibers, collagen type III, and hyaluronic acids. Dryness is also alleviated through increased water-holding capacity, increased sebum production, and improved barrier function of the skin. Furthermore, estrogen modulates local inflammation, granulation, re-epithelialization, and possibly wound contraction, which collectively accelerates wound healing at the expense of forming lower-quality scars.[3-4]

Despite its promises, long-term estrogen replacement therapy (ERT) has been associated with harmful systemic effects, which include increased risk of coronary artery disease, stroke, breast cancer, and thromboembolic events such as venous thrombus and pulmonary emboli.[2,4]

Skin loses its elasticity at an early age but appears to maintain its extensibility up to the seventh decade of life. With aging, the synthesis of collagen gradually declines; however, the stiffness of the dermal collagen increases. Collagen content in extrinsically (photo) aged skin is up to 56% less than collagen content in intrinsically aged skin. Collagen disruption that occurs with aging lends itself to poor tensile strength, which can lead to skin tears and wound dehiscence. Long-term solar irradiation also leads to a decrease in skin extensibility and elastic recovery, although elderly skin is also easier to reapproximate than younger skin. This may be because the rigidity of the aged dermis, due to changes in collagen, decreases the skin's ability to resist shearing forces.[3-5]

II. Case study: skin tears

Case Study, Mrs. Z.

Mrs. Z. is an 84-year-old female who resides in an assisted-living facility. Her medical history is significant for atrial fibrillation on warfarin therapy, hypertensive heart disease, congestive heart failure, mild cognitive impairment, macular degeneration, and osteoarthritis. She has a BMI of 18. She ambulates with a walker and tripped over her cat and fell in her bedroom, striking her left arm against her bureau. She sustained a laceration to her left arm and forearm. Focal exam revealed a full thickness, irregular injury of her left upper arm with moderate serosanguinous exudates. Area was moderately tender to palpation. There were no obvious deformities, and her range of motion (ROM) was intact.

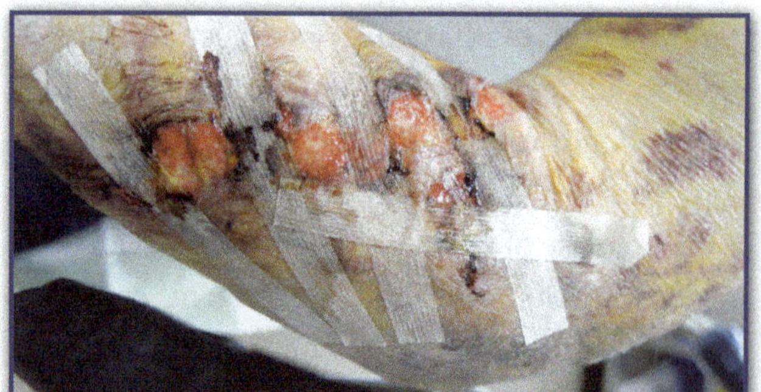

FIGURE 1. Patient presenting 24 hours after fall. Nurses at the facility attempted to reapproximate the edges with Steri-Strips; however, there was significant flap loss at the time of presentation.

Mrs. Z. clearly had a number of risk factors that placed her at risk for the development of a skin tear. She was of advanced age with many of the characteristics of aging skin: she was on warfarin therapy, had a history of cardiovascular problems, had low vision and cognitive impairment, and used a walker. She sustained a Type 2 skin tear. Given her history of warfarin use, which elevates the International normalized ratio (INR), she experienced a significant amount of oozing from her wound.

Discussion

The appropriate management of patients with skin tears remains an ongoing challenge for health-care clinicians. These traumatic wounds are acute in nature, painful, and mostly preventable. It is critical for clinicians to identify persons at risk for skin tears and implement preventive strategies to mitigate risk. Approximately 1.5 million skin tears occur each year in institutionalized adults in the United States. The prevalence of skin tears, particularly in the long-term care setting, closely resembles that of pressure ulcers, yet frequently these wounds are not afforded the attention they require and are often not distinguished as unique wounds.[5,6]

Despite some data that suggests that skin tears may be more prevalent than pressure ulcers in the aging population, there has been a paucity of literature until recently on the prevention and management of this common skin issue in the older adult.

According to the International Skin Tear Advisory Panel (ISTAP), a skin tear is a wound resulting in separation of skin layers, either partial-thickness (separation of the epidermis from the dermis) or full-thickness (separation of both the epidermis and dermis).[7]

There are currently several classification systems for skin tears. The Payne-Martin Classification System was developed in 1993 and was the only known method for classifying skin tears. The authors maintained that the system demonstrated internal and external validity, but it was not widely used in clinical practice. Carville et al. developed the STAR system in 2006, but it was used mostly in Australia. The need for a universally accepted definition as well as comprehensive treatment strategy led to the establishment of a consensus panel of wound care experts in 2011 and subsequent development of the International Skin Tear Advisory Panel (ISTAP) with subsequent recommendations to include a toolkit and clinical pathway.[7-9]

According to the International Consensus on Skin Tears (2011), the following are some risk factors for skin tears:

- Very young (neonate) and very old (>75 years old)
- Sex (female)
- Race (Caucasian)
- Impaired mobility (chair- or bed-bound)
- Undernutrition
- Long-term corticosteroid use (oral and topical)
- History of previous skin tears
- Altered sensory status
- Cognitive impairment
- Limb stiffness (joint stiffness/contractures) and spasticity
- Presence of Neuropathy
- Having blood drawn/phlebotomy procedures
- Polypharmacy
- Presence of ecchymosis
- Dependence on other for activities of daily living (ADLS)
- Using assistive devices (walkers, canes, etc.)
- Applying and removing stockings
- Removing tape or dressings
- Vascular, pulmonary, or cardiac problems
- Visual impairment/low vision
- Need for transfers assistance
- History of falls
- Prosthetic devices (splints, braces, use of prosthetic limb)
- History of incontinence
- Improper use of skin cleansers and skin sealants

(International Consensus on Skin Tears, 2011)

ISTAP developed a skin tear risk assessment pathway in 2013. The pathway incorporates an assessment of the patient's general health factors such as chronic diseases, polypharmacy, and sensory impairments, mobility, and history of previous skin impairments. If there are no risk factors, periodic assessment is advised. If risk factors are identified, then implementation of a skin tear risk reduction program is recommended.[7]

III. Classification of skin tears

According to ISTAP, skin tears are classified as Type 1, in which there is no skin loss; Type 2, indicating partial flap loss; and Type 3, which involves total flap loss.[7] Treatment of skin tears is aimed at treating the cause of the injury (i.e, general health, mobility, skin condition), providing local wound care, and addressing patient-centered concerns such as ADL needs, pain control, and education.

IV. Best practices for care and prevention

Initial treatment for a skin tear with an intact flap is to irrigate the wound with saline and use moistened sterile-tipped applicators in an attempt to reapproximate the wound edges. If the edges can be approximated, then the clinician can secure them with either Steri-Strips or a cyanacrylate adhesive (i.e, Dermabond) and cover with a nonadherent dressing such as a silicone dressing, oil emulsion gauze, or bismuth gallium impregnated gauze dressing. If there is a moderate amount of exudate formation, an absorbent product such as a calcium alginate, foam, or hydrofiber dressing can be used. Avoid the use of adhesives if possible and consider applying roll gauze to secure the dressing followed by the use of elastic netting. In Mrs. Z.'s case, the use of a calcium alginate with silver was used to absorb the exudates. Her dressing was changed every three days until it re-epithelialized approximately 21 days later.

In regard to prevention, it is important to consider that Individuals frequently acquire skin tears during routine activities such as dressing, bathing, positioning, and transferring. Those who are dependent on others but are independent in ambulation report high numbers of skin tears, which tend to occur more frequently on the lower extremities. Other common causes of skin tears include equipment injury, patient transfers, falls, activities of daily living (ADLs), treatment, and dressing removal.[7-9]

Clinicians must educate caregivers on gentle handling of older adults with fragile skin. Any unintended friction or shear force can create a skin tear. Patients and families should understand the importance of proper positioning, turning, lifting, and transferring. Use lift sheets to move patients up in bed. Provide padding for side rails, wheelchair arm and leg

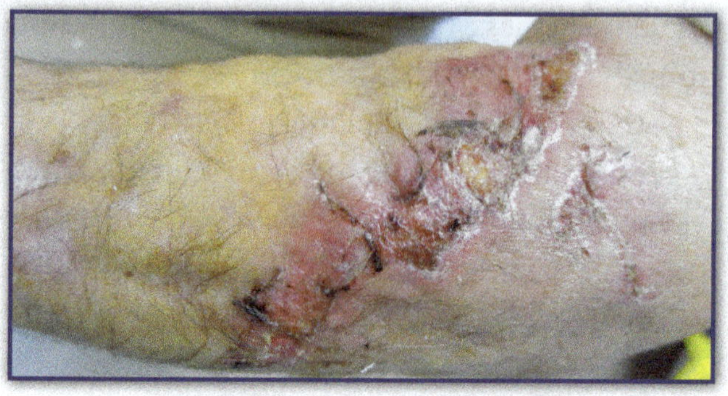

FIGURE 2. Skin tear at 16 days with epithelialization occurring

supports, and other equipment. Patients at risk are encouraged to wear long sleeves and trousers/pants for added protection. Specialized sleeves, called "Geri sleeves," are composed of a soft fabric with an elastic cuff that extends from the back of the hand to just above the elbow and can be very effective at mitigating trauma.

Patients and caregivers should keep their fingernails short; use no-rinse, pH-balanced soap for bathing, and moisturize the skin with creams or emollients rather than lotions. Lotions tend to have a higher percentage of water and are less effective at retaining moisture within the epidermal layers. Creams or emollients tend to have a higher percentage of oils or petrolatums, which tend to have better moisture-retentive properties.

Falls pose a serious risk of skin tears for older adults. Preventing falls in older adults requires several different approaches to mitigate factors that may predispose them to this type of

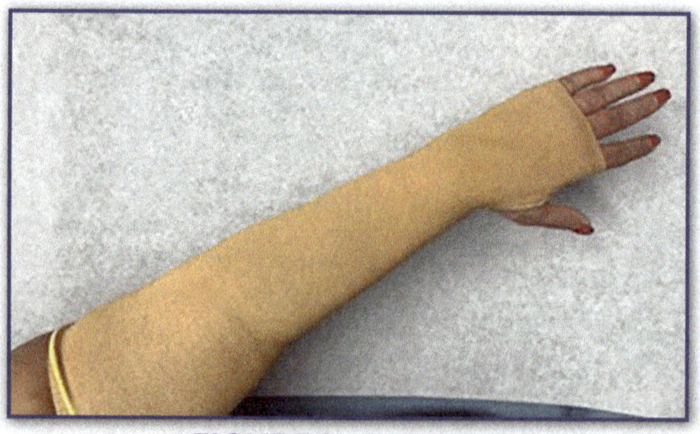

FIGURE 3. Geri sleeve

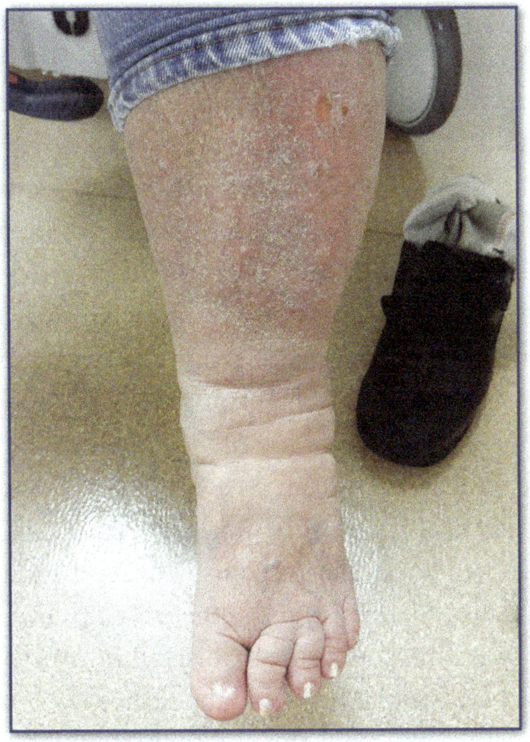

FIGURE 4. 74-year-old male with lymphedema and cutis xerosis

injury. According to the World Health Organization (WHO), a fall is defined as a sudden, unintentional change in position, which results in an individual's hitting either the ground or another object below his or her starting point. The American Medical Directors Association (AMDA) reports that falls are a significant cause of injury and death in older adults living in long-term care facilities. Falls are also the leading cause of fatal and nonfatal injuries among Americans 65 or older, resulting in more than two million emergency department visits. Predisposing factors for falls include unsteady gait and balance, weak muscles, poor vision, medications, and dementia. Other factors that may contribute to falls include poor lighting, loose rugs, poorly fitting shoes, floor clutter, urinary urgency, and beds or toilets without handrails. Medical conditions that may lead to falls in older adults include orthostatic hypotension, stroke, Parkinson disease, arthritis, poorly controlled diabetes, thyroid disorders, poorly controlled epilepsy, and other neurocognitive disorders. An important step in reducing skin tear risk is the introduction of a falls-prevention program supported[7,10] by the individual at risk, care provider, and health-care setting. Implementing a best-practice fall-prevention program has proven to be successful in reducing falls in older adults; however, best-practice guidelines can be successfully implemented only with adequate planning, resources, organization, and administrative support.

V. Moisture-associated skin damage

Case study, Mr. P.

Mr. P. is a 72-year-old male with a history of urge incontinence with frequent accidents, severe osteoarthritis, obesity, and diabetes. He presented to his primary care provider's office with reports of a rash to his groin and inguinal areas, which he described as burning, stinging, and moderately pruritic. He wears adult incontinence briefs when leaving his home. He had not used any treatments on the rash. Focal exam indicated the presence of excessive moisture in his inguinal area and perineum with moist desquamation and a macular, erythematous rash with satellite lesions.

Moisture-associated skin damage (MASD) occurs when excessive moisture in urine, stools, and wound exudate leads to inflammation of the skin, with or without erosion or secondary cutaneous infection.[11] Perineal dermatitis, diaper rash, incontinence-associated dermatitis, or moisture-associated skin damage are all names used to describe damage to skin caused by moisture. Regardless of what the condition is called, this damage is painful and costly. Moisture can come from many sources, including perspiration or wound drainage, but fecal and/or urinary incontinence are the most common causes.

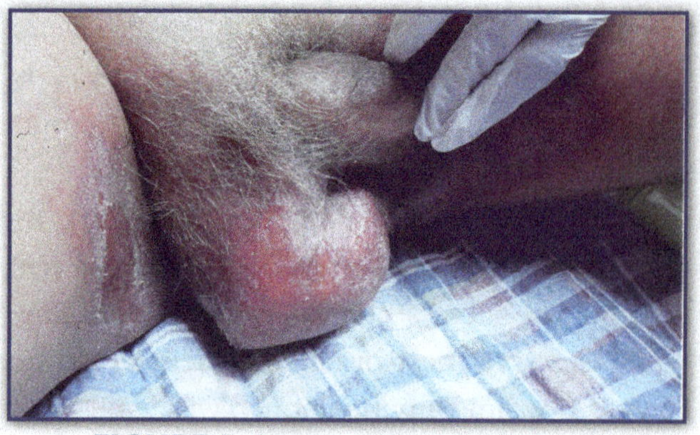

FIGURE 5. Patient with erythema and denudement of intertriginous areas

Lesions caused by the moisture are characterized by an erosion of the epidermis and a macerated appearance of the skin. A secondary cutaneous infection may also occur. Occasionally this type of skin damage is incorrectly attributed to pressure ulcer formation. It is essential for the clinician to be able to accurately identify the cause of skin damage and determine the appropriate treatment pathway.[11-12] See Table 1.

The etiology of moisture-associated skin damage is complex. Moisture from any source increases the skin's permeability and decreases its barrier function. The stratum corneum layer of the epidermis is slightly acidic and, when intact, protects the body from pathogens. When the skin is compromised by moisture alone or moisture with friction, a break in the surface may occur, allowing pathogens to enter. The most common pathogens are *Candida albicans* and *Staphylococcus aureus*. In addition, the alkaline nature of urine increases the skin's pH, changing it from acidic to alkaline. Alkaline urine may promote the enzymatic activity of proteinases and lipases when fecal incontinence is present and further erode the skin's surface. Cleaning the skin frequently, especially with soap and water, also decreases the acid mantle and promotes a chemical and physical irritation of the area with associated epidermal damage. When the skin is moist, the effects of friction are more damaging. Sliding across bed linens during transfer or repositioning may cause friction injury to the wet skin. Even in persons with containment briefs, the microclimate between the brief and the skin is warm and moist; this may make the skin more susceptible to moisture-related damage and friction.[11-13]

It is sometimes difficult even for an expert to distinguish between moisture-associated skin damage and a Stage I or II pressure ulcer as both conditions may occur over the buttocks in some Stage l patients. Consequently, it is necessary to correctly identify the causative issue or issues to provide appropriate treatment. Moisture-associated skin damage should NOT be documented as a Stage I or II pressure ulcer.[11,13]

TABLE 1. Characteristics of moisture-associated skin damage versus pressure ulcers

Characteristics	MASD	Pressure ulcer
Etiology	Moisture from any cause	Pressure, friction, shear
Location	Skin folds, periwound areas, peristomal areas, perineum	Bony prominences or under medical devices
Presence of necrosis	none	May be present with deeper ulcers
Depth	Shallow, partial thickness	Variable, partial to full thickness
Edges	Irregular, indistinct	Well defined
Pain	Burning, itching, soreness	May or may not be present depending upon depth and patient level of sensation

Treatment starts with identification of the moisture source. The clinician should consider testing as indicated to determine the type of urinary incontinence[14] or if there are underlying causes of fecal incontinence such as *Clostridium difficile* or tube feeding–related diarrhea. Note the time of day the incontinence occurs and monitor that for patterns. Foods such as caffeine, carbonated beverages, spicy foods, or acidic foods such as citrus products and fruit juices may trigger bladder spasms that lead to incontinence. Some incontinence cases can be treated surgically or with medication.[14-15] See Table 2.

Treatment of UI is directed at mitigating or eliminating the problems that are causing the UI. This may include medications, surgical interventions, behavioral techniques, biofeedback, and dietary changes.

In some cases, medications may cause constipation, which can worsen or contribute to fecal incontinence due to straining at stool or because the rectal vault is full of hard stool that is pressing on the bladder. The incidence of fecal incontinence is increased if stool is liquid. Fiber added to food may help, or active yogurt cultures, such as *lactobacillus* GG or *Saccharomyces boullardi*, may be given. If the diarrhea is related to tube feeding, the dietitian should be consulted to adjust the rate or type of formula. The skin needs to be protected from exposure to further irritants.

TABLE 2. Types of urinary incontinence (UI)

Type of UI	Symptoms	Etiology
Stress	Loss of urine with sneezing, coughing or laughing; any increase in intra-abdominal pressure may be a cause	The scaffolding that helps support the bladder including pelvic floor muscles, vagina and ligaments weaken, and the bladder moves downward. This prevents muscles that force the urethra shut from squeezing as tightly, and as a result, urine leaks into the urethra. In men this may occur following prostatectomy surgery.
Urge	Suddenly feeling the urge to urinate; may be due to inappropriate bladder contractions. The bladder contracts without its owner's permission	May be due to inappropriate bladder contractions; some fluids or medications, such as diuretics, or anxiety may worsen this condition.
Overflow	Bladder does not empty properly and "spills" over; may be accompanied by dribbling or incomplete sense of emptying	May be from nerve damage, weak bladder muscles, a tumor, or a partially blocked urethra (prostatic hypertrophy)
Functional	Unable to get to the bathroom due to functional limitations	Dementia, arthritis, chairbound, any factor that impairs mobility

Skin should be cleansed gently using a no-rinse skin cleanser with a pH similar to normal skin. These types of cleansers are as effective as soap and water in removing both Gram-negative and Gram-positive bacteria from the skin and are preferred over towel drying. Cleansing should occur as soon as possible following an episode of incontinence to limit contact with urine and stool. After cleansing, a barrier ointment or a no-sting barrier film should be applied to protect the skin from the constant moisture. Products should be applied according to the manufacturer's directions or after each incontinent episode and cleaning. Keeping the patient clean and dry, changing underpads or briefs after soiling, and using barrier creams or ointments to replace intercellular lipids and promote moisture barrier function of the skin are usually all that is required for moisture-associated dermatitis to resolve. It is helpful to keep the individual off the affected area to promote dryness and reduce potential friction.[15]

Referral to a continence specialist should be considered for assessment and treatment of the underlying incontinence.

In some cases, diversion devices, such as Foley or condom catheters, or fecal containment devices are used to keep the skin dry. However, use of these devices also has risks, including bladder infection, ulceration of the penis, or anal mucosal erosion. Be sure to monitor for such complications.

If a secondary infection is present, appropriate treatment should be implemented. Types of secondary infection include fungal or yeast infections and bacterial infections. These infections are a result of invasion of opportunistic pathogens into compromised skin. *Candida albicans* easily penetrates the compromised epidermis and appears as a maculopapular rash with satellite lesions. The skin is usually very erythematous and pruritic and may be tender and very itchy. Lesions may take on a macular appearance from friction, and the rash may extend from the groin into the buttocks and thighs. Treatment usually consists of a liberal and consistent application of a topical antifungal product such as nystatin, miconazole, or clotrimazole two to three times daily until clear. In some cases, it may be necessary to treat for two to four weeks. Especially severe cases may also require an oral agent such as fluconazole to eradicate the infection.[11-12,16]

Bacterial infections are typically caused by bacteria that reside normally on the skin but may cause infection when the acid mantle of the skin is disrupted. Manifestations of bacterial infection causing a cellulitis include redness, tenderness, induration, and localized edema. Treatment may include the application of topical antimicrobials but usually requires an oral antibiotic for seven to 14 days to clear the infection.[11,16]

Case study, Mr. Z.

Mr. Z. was evaluated and had a urine culture, which indicated a urinary infection that was increasing his episodes of bladder irritability and incontinence. He was treated with a 10-day course of antibiotics with significant improvement in his symptoms. He was also given a prescription for a topical antifungal twice a day. He was instructed to keep his skin as clean and dry as possible and to use an over-the-counter pH-balanced soap for routine bathing. A consult was placed for him to see a urologist for further evaluation of his symptoms. A two-week follow-up indicated complete resolution of his rash.

VI. Peristomal skin damage

In some cases, MASD can occur around peristomal areas or wounds. In the case of peristomal skin damage, the cause is usually a leaking appliance or an allergic dermatitis caused by exposure to adhesive, paste, or the skin barrier/

wafer itself. The main ingredient in most skin barriers is hydrocolloids. Hydrocolloids absorb moisture from the skin as well as stoma effluent. If the amount of moisture in contact with the skin barrier is significant, the barrier absorbs the moisture, eroding the barrier, eliminating its protective function, and allowing stool or urine to come into contact with the peristomal skin. Erosion of the solid skin barrier depends on the amount, moisture content, and composition (e.g. enzymes, bacteria) of the stoma effluent, skin moisture levels (e.g. perspiration, humidity), and the type of skin barrier (regular or extended wear). Failure of the skin barrier can allow the stoma effluent to contact the skin around the stoma and cause peristomal moisture-associated dermatitis.[17]

The majority of peristomal irritant dermatitis occurs from leakage of the stoma effluent under the seal. Prevention is aimed toward maintaining the peristomal skin by using the most appropriate pouching system. Selecting an optimal pouching system in the patient with peristomal moisture–associated dermatitis focuses on the skin barrier. High liquid output (urostomy, ileostomy) is best managed with the use of an extended-wear barrier, which erodes more slowly in the presence of liquid output. Low-volume, low-moisture effluent such as found in a person with a left-sided colostomy would best be managed with a standard- wear skin barrier. The opening in the skin barrier must be cut to match the size and shape of the stoma. As a newly created stoma changes shape and size for at least six weeks following creation, repeated measuring is advised to ensure that the barrier aperture conforms to both the size and shape of the stoma. Moldable solid skin barriers can also be fit to conform to the stoma shape. The use of a convex barrier should be considered when the stoma lumen is not above skin level or has creases or folds around the stoma in the sitting or standing position. In some cases, accessory products can be considered to enhance the seal: skin barrier paste, skin barrier strips or rings, skin barrier powder, liquid skin protectants, and belts. Custom-made convex barriers are also an option for difficult cases.

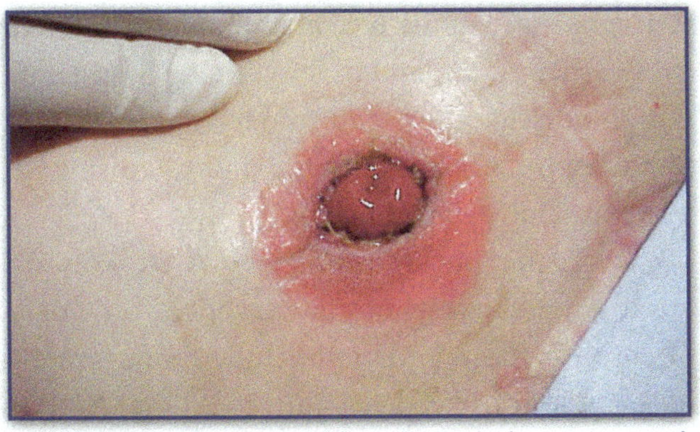

FIGURE 6. 69-year-old female with ileostomy and MASD of the peristomal area due to cutting the opening in the ostomy wafer too large and allowing effluent in contact with the skin

If peristomal MASD develops, close surveillance is needed to gauge the effectiveness of the interventions and to monitor for complications. Treatment initially focuses on altering the pouching system in order to prevent further exposure to irritants. Achieving success is challenging because patients often fail to recognize effluent leakage that harms the skin. It is recommended that the patient establish a pouch change schedule, to continually monitor the skin barrier seal for undermining or erosion, and to seek treatment if the skin becomes irritated. Healing irritated skin can be done using several techniques, but topical therapies are limited to products that will allow the adhesive seal to be secured. Skin barrier powder can be dusted over the moist skin (skin barrier powder contains hydrocolloids that can absorb the moisture) and facilitate a seal of the solid skin barrier to the skin. Some experts suggest the use of a polymer acrylate liquid skin protectant over the powder as a sealant. An astringent may be applied prior to pouch placement to dry the peristomal skin.

In cases of severe irritation, a steroid spray may be used to diminish the inflammatory process. Peristomal candidiasis, which results from a proliferation of a *Candida* organism, is associated with excessive moisture on the peristomal skin. Peristomal candidiasis appears as a pustule and is generally encountered under the adhesive seal of the pouching system; erythema, maceration, itching, and burning may also be present.

Treatment involves identifying and correcting the moisture source, then applying a topical antifungal (generally a powder) that will not interfere with adhesion of the solid skin barrier. Depending upon the severity of the candidiasis and the response to topical therapy, oral antifungal therapy may be indicated.[16-17]

VII. Skin and wound care issues at the end of life

Wounds at the end are a significant problem for more than 1.3 million hospice patients and millions of other frail, elderly persons living with chronic disease.[18] End-of-life patient care includes a variety of wound care challenges. Much of current evidence-based wound care practice focuses on the outcome of healing, which may not be an expected or desired outcome at the end of life. Patients under palliative care or hospice care deserve to have symptoms of all types managed, and this should include wound management. This section describes evidence-based assessment and current management of wounds in palliative care.

Current philosophies in evidence-based wound care are similar to palliative wound care defined by Emmons and Lachman in 2010. Palliative wound care is approach that is holistic and integrated to include i) managing patient's symptoms, ii) improving psychosocial well-being, iii) using a multidisciplinary team approach, and iv) patient/family driven goals.[19]

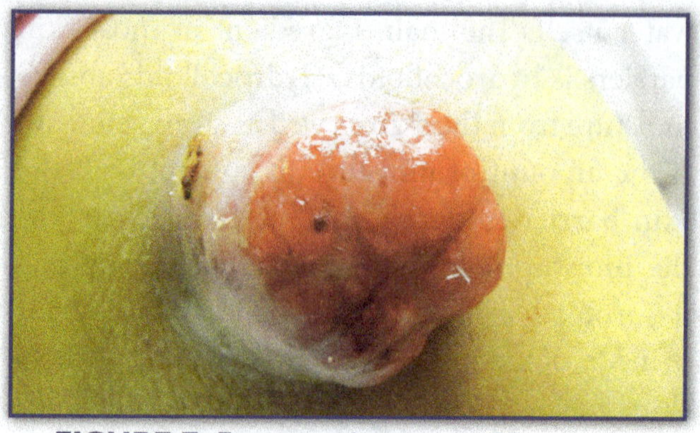

FIGURE 7. Fungating lesion in a 75-year-old female with lung cancer

According to Farris et al., a palliative wound care is a holistic approach, helping to relieve suffering and improving quality of life for patients suffering from chronic wounds.[20]

It can often be a difficult issue for patients and family members to accept that some chronic wounds may not heal due to factors beyond the control of the patient and clinician. In these instances, severe comorbidities, nutritional deficits, and immobility impact the ability of the wound to heal. There may also be some ethical considerations that emerge if there is conflict between patient and family regarding the goals of treatment.[21]

Common types of wounds seen in palliative and hospice patients include pressure ulcers, malignant or fungating wounds, skin tears, arterial ulcers, venous ulcers, and diabetic ulcers, and malignant or fungating wounds. A fungating wound is a malignant lesion that infiltrates the skin and its supporting blood and lymph vessels. They tend to develop in the last few months of a patient's life and often impair psychosocial well-being.[22]

While the specific etiologies of these wounds are discussed elsewhere in this book, the goals of care for these patients include management of pain, odor, exudate, and bleeding. At the same time, there is strong focus on maintaining self-image, dignity, and quality of life.

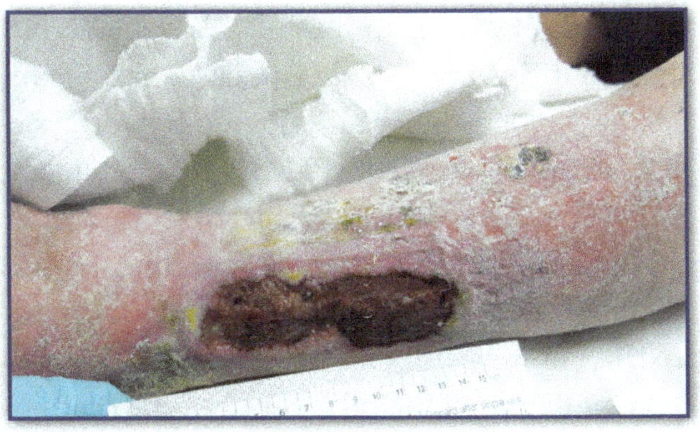

FIGURE 8.

Case study, Mr. E.

Mr. E. is an 89-year-old with a history of multiple medical problems that include congestive heart failure, dementia, peripheral vascular disease, hypertension, coronary artery disease, and venous hypertension. He is on hospice for end-stage cardiovascular disease. He has a history of a nonhealing ulcer on his left lower leg for more than two years that has been refractory to treatment. He has significant pain in his wound and has been unable to tolerate most topical therapies.

A. Pain

Pain control is central in the effective management of patients receiving palliative wound care. It is the clinician's responsibility to comprehensively assess the pain experience, including location, duration, intensity, quality, onset, and impact on daily living so the type of pain can be identified. Pain can be categorized into three types: cyclic, noncyclic, and chronic. Cyclic pain occurs with intermittent treatment or movement. Removal of a dressing or a position change can cause cyclic pain. Noncyclic occurs as a result of a single incident such as wound debridement. Chronic pain is more persistent but can be exacerbated. Recognizing the different types of pain and understanding that patients can have acute and chronic pain at the same time, can assist the clinician in developing interventions to address specific causes.[23]

Dressing changes are a frequent cause of cyclic pain. Selecting nonadherent dressings that are atraumatic on removal can significantly reduce the pain experience.[24] Choose dressings that can remain in place and require less frequent dressing changes.

If the best dressing option you have, such as for optimal exudate absorption, does not provide an atraumatic layer, an additional option is to place a nonadherent contact layer down first. Other methods of reducing cyclic pain include positioning off for the painful site/pressure redistribution, topical medications, skin barriers to protect from chemical irritation, and systemic pain medications. In general, less frequent dressing changes are better for the wound as they reduce the cyclic pain experience.[24-25] Noncyclic pain is often associated with wound debridement. Debridement may be necessary to reduce malodorous necrosis caused by bacteria. To reduce noncyclic pain, premedicating either systemically or topically is essential. All procedures should have a mechanism in place for "time-outs" to allow the patient to take a break if increased and prolonged pain is experienced. Reducing bacteria with antimicrobials can also be effective in reducing pain, as infection or increased bacteria can contribute to pain.[26] Chronic pain can be managed with a combination of the above techniques, as well as with systemic and local pain medications. The World Health Organization (WHO) Clinical Ladder for systemic pain medication remains the standard for treating chronic pain, especially for those with wounds.[26] This stepwise approach starts with nonsteroidal anti-inflammatories and works up to strong opiates. The use of adjunctive pain medications recommended by WHO, such as tricyclic antidepressants or anticonvulsants, can be beneficial for neuropathic pain.[26-28] When systemic medications do not reduce pain to an acceptable level, clinicians should consider the use of topical pain medications.[29]

Management of pain requires a holistic, interdisciplinary approach to care.[30] In addition to a pain regimen that includes both a sustained or long-acting medication as well as a short-acting agent for breakthrough pain, there are some other specific interventions that target the patient with severe wound pain. There is some data suggesting that morphine, for example, has a local effect on the receptors of peripheral nerves. Opioids have actions on nociceptors or free nerve endings in superficial layer of skin, therefore have a local action. All classes of opioid receptors have action on peripheral nerve terminals similar to the way opioids work in the CNS. One off-label option for severe wound pain includes the use of Morphine SO_4 injection 10 mg mixed with 8-10 gms of amorphous hydrogel (1% mixture). This agent can be applied directly to the wound and covered with an occlusive dressing and left for 24 hours.[30-31] Other non-opiate options for wound care include EMLA 3-150 gms or Lidocaine 2-5%, viscous or ointment. These agents can be applied from 45 to 60 minutes prior to wound care or gentle debridement.[21] The use of ibuprofen topically has been shown to convey some benefit as well. A foam-based product impregnated with ibuprofen is available in non-U.S. markets and has been shown to be effective in reducing pain in elderly patients with venous leg ulcers. Anecdotal evidence suggests that a compounded formulation of ibuprofen and hydrogel (400 mg/10 ml) has been effective in mitigating pain in patients with chronic wound pain and can last up to 24 hours. The mechanism of action appears to be related to a suppression of thromboxane release. Thromboxane is a substance made by platelets that causes blood clotting and constriction of blood vessels. It also encourages platelet aggregation. There are two thromboxanes. Thromboxane A2 (TXA2) is active but is very unstable and has a half-life of only 30 seconds before it undergoes hydrolysis to form thromboxane B2 (TXB2), which is inactive. The thromboxanes are derived from arachidonic acid and are related to prostaglandins. There are no known allergic reactions or local toxicity; however, topical anesthetics may cause tissue inflammation and local wound irritation and may potentially decrease wound healing as result of suppression of substance P, a neuropeptide involved in regulating the inflammatory response in wound healing. Clearly more research is required, as most reports have been limited to case studies and anecdotal reports. Further investigation about side effects and systemic uptake is needed. Conversely, the use of topical agents may prove to be a helpful adjunctive therapy for patients with severe wound pain, especially at the end of life.[29,32]

B. Odor

Wound odor can be extremely distressing for patient and can make them uncomfortable and cause intense physical and psychological suffering, feelings of rejection, disgust, and social isolation. Some patients feel that they are expected to have to live with the odor. The goal of palliative wound care or care at the end of life is to reduce odor, pain, and infection. Cure is usually not a goal, but palliation of symptoms should be a priority. Wound odor usually occurs from the bacteria within the wound, especially on necrotic tissue. With fungating tumors, necrotic tissue can occur when the tumor outgrows the blood supply. A fungating wound is a malignant lesion that infiltrates the skin and its supporting blood and lymph vessels. They tend to develop in the last few months of a patient's life. Fungating wounds have a tendency to expand rapidly, and they show a propensity to become locally invasive or form shallow craters. Initially, they present as multiple non-tender nodules that are skin-toned, pink, violet-blue, or black-brown in color, but they go on to develop into papillary lesions (resembling a cauliflower stalk) that may be complicated by an ulcer, sinus tract, or fistula. Bacterial growth, release of volatile fatty acids, and liquefaction of non-viable tissue will cause an increase in both exudate and odor.[20-22,33]

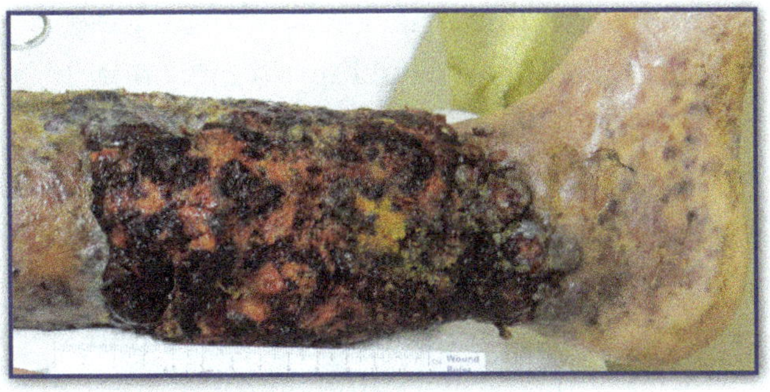

FIGURE 9. Fungating angiosarcoma of the left lower leg

Case study, Mr. J.

Mr. J. was a 100-year-old male with a one-year history of a lump on his leg. He was referred to the wound clinic by his primary care physician. Upon initial presentation, the wound was fungating in appearance with irregular surface, large amounts of exudates, and a strong odor.

Treatment for odor encompasses multiple aspects of wound care. Elimination of odor can be accomplished through a combination of cleansing, debriding, and decreasing bacterial load.

Wound cleaning can occur with each dressing change or even in the shower by gently allowing the water to wash over the lesion, particularly in malignant wounds. In some cases, topical antiseptics such as the use of Dakin's solution or acetic acid can be used to cleanse a wound and also for light packing to quickly reduce bacterial loads and associated symptoms. Low-strength Dakin's solution has good bacterial coverage and can quickly reduce the amount of bacteria and associated symptoms without harming the patient or wound. Unfortunately, the dressing changes for Dakin's solution are usually at least daily to get the maximum effect. After the Dakin's solution has significantly reduced the bacteria and odor, it is recommended to switch to a dressing that can be left in place for several days in order to minimize discomfort with dressing changes.[33,34]

The use of antiseptics should be limited to a short period of time until the desired effect is reached. Gentle debridement through the body's ability to autolytically debride the wound is accomplished by using moisture-retentive dressings, and it is the preferred method. In highly colonized wounds or in infected wounds, systemic antibiotics may be appropriate if there is evidence of clinical infection. However, excessive use of antimicrobial agents should be avoided because it can lead to overgrowth of resistant organisms such as methicillin-resistant *Staphylococcus aureus* and vancomycin-resistant *enterococcus,* and some antibiotics increase the risk of nausea and vomiting. In some cases, a wound care specialist may be called to remove loosely adherent necrosis without causing pain to the patient to quickly reduce the amount of dead tissue that promotes bacterial growth. Reducing bacterial loads can be successfully accomplished by using topical antimicrobials.[16,30,32]

Silver dressings are a good choice because they typically release silver over several days, negating the need for frequent dressing changes. They are also impregnated into most dressing categories, so it is possible to have the benefit of a foam, alginate, or hydrogel with the added antimicrobial benefits of the silver. Silver dressings cannot be mixed with Dakin's solution or oil-based dressings as it deactivates the silver. Iodine cadexomer dressings are also available in several preparations and can be left in the wound for several days at a time. They are effective for infected and malodorous wounds, but they too have contraindications for anyone who cannot be exposed to iodine.[30]

Metronidazole has been widely used as a topical agent for reducing wound odor. It is readily available in most settings and is relatively inexpensive. It is a synthetic antimicrobial drug, which works against anaerobic bacteria and protozoa; however, it may take several days before odor is reduced. The wound should be cleansed with normal saline and the metronidazole applied liberally and covered with a secondary dressing. For heavily exudative wounds, consider the use of crushed metronidazole tablets sprinkled over the wound surface and covered with a petroleum-jelly-coated dressing. For dry wounds, the gel form of metronidazole is more appropriate. Metronidazole should not be used in conjunction with any other topical creams, gels, or ointments because its effectiveness and antimicrobial activity could be potentially diluted. Although it has been shown to be effective in many odorous wounds, it is ineffective in wounds that are too moist or dry.[22-23]

Honey has been used as a dressing since ancient times, and due to the emergence of antibiotic-resistant strains of microorganisms, there is an increased interest in its wound healing properties. Medical-grade honey derived from the Leptospermum species, found in the manuka flower of Australia and New Zealand, inhibits bacterial growth in several ways. It has an acidic pH, which prevents biofilm formation. It results in the slow release of hydrogen peroxide, which is toxic to microbes, and in addition has a high osmolality, which inhibits bacterial growth. Honey also acts as a debriding agent with several mechanisms of action. It encourages autolytic debridement due to its strong osmotic action of pulling fluid from the wound and washing the base to remove debris and slough. The production of hydrogen peroxide contributes to debridement by activating proteases to break down unwanted tissue. Odor control is attributed to inhibition of bacterial growth and removal of necrotic tissue from the wound base. However, topical honey may be difficult to apply and requires the use of an absorbent secondary dressing. Therefore, it may not be an option for wounds that are too moist. Advances in technology have provided several forms of honey-impregnated dressings, including alginates and hydrocolloids that may be more effective in the management of fungating wounds.

Charcoal dressings also may be used to alleviate odor. Because the molecules that are responsible for the malodor are attracted to the carbon surface, the activated charcoal dressing acts as a filter to absorb these molecules, preventing them from being released into the air. In order to be effective, a charcoal dressing must be fitted as a sealed unit directly on the wound. There are limitations for application of charcoal dressings in fungating wounds as these types of dressings are only effective in wounds that produce minimal amounts of exudates.[20,22]

Nonpharmacologic management of wound odor, based primarily on anecdotal evidence, includes the use of peppermint oil or lavender oil, aromatherapy products, dryer sheets, and cat litter or baking soda under the bed These methods only cover up the odor and do not stop the production of odor-causing bacteria, so they are best used in conjunction with appropriate topical therapies.[35]

C. Exudate

Exudate is part of the normal inflammatory process, but an increase in the amount and type is impacted by several factors, including edema and bacterial load. The general concepts of appropriate dressing selection to manage exudate include products that absorb exudate without drying the wound bed, provide an effective bacterial barrier, and are atraumatic upon removal, leaving no dressing debris when possible. Typical dressings to manage exudate include foams, alginates, hydrofibers, and cellulose polyacrylate fiber dressings. Using combinations of these dressings increases the amount of exudate held within the dressings and increases dressing wear time, thereby reducing the other symptoms associated with frequent dressing changes. The polyacrylate dressings appear to be the most absorbent option for exudate control but may be cost-prohibitive in some settings. In extreme cases, pouching a wound with a wound manager or ostomy pouching system may be the best option. For wounds on the lower extremity related to venous insufficiency, reducing the edema by elevation and light compression will help to significantly reduce the amount of exudate.[20-22]

D. Bleeding

The best management of bleeding in a wound is prevention. Ensuring that dressings do not stick to the wound bed will help reduce the incidence of traumatic bleeding. These dressings include dressings with nonadhesive layers, silicone, and most dressings that remain moist and do not dry to the wound bed. Friable wounds bleed easily because they are heavily colonized with bacteria or are infected. Reducing the bacterial load will reduce the occurrence of bleeding. Malignant wounds are known to bleed frequently because of their vascularization. Bleeding occurs in 4-6% of malignant wounds. Usually this involves small vessels or capillaries but can be arterial in nature as well. For some patients, this causes a sensation of potentially "bleeding to death" and can be a continual reminder of disease and impending death. Bleeding can also be exacerbated by coagulopathies and/or anticoagulation.[25-26,36]

Medications such as topically applied epinephrine, aminocaproic acid, and sucralfate paste are effective at stopping widespread oozing. For pinpoint bleeding, silver nitrate can be applied to cauterize the area. Hemostatic agents used in surgery, such as gelling hemostatic agents and hemostatic gauze, can also be used at the bedside if available. Silver calcium alginate can be applied to successfully stop bleeding as well. This dressing should be left in place until it falls off on its own to avoid bleeding upon removal. Moh's paste has also been used with success in cases of bleeding due to advanced cancers. Moh's paste is made of a mixture of zinc chloride (50 g), distilled water (25 mL), zinc starch (19 g), and glycerol (15 mL). Zinc chloride in Moh's paste changes into zinc ions by ulcerative exudate, and then the zinc ions precipitate wound proteins. Tissues, vessels, and cell membranes of bacteria are fixed chemically. This generally works with the initial application and has been effective in bleeding breast tumors and genital bleeding from cervical cancer.[36-38]

If modifiable, systemic factors should be addressed, such as the concurrent use of anticoagulants. In cases of more severe bleeding, the use of systemic therapy may be required. Fibrinolytic Inhibitors such as aminocaproic acid or tranexamic acid competitively inhibit the activation of plasminogen to plasmin by binding to specific sites of plasminogen and plasmin, a molecule responsible for the degradation of fibrin.[30,35-37]

Nonpharmacologic management of bleeding in cases where it cannot be stopped at the end of life (terminal hemorrhage) aims at providing a calm, comfortable environment that minimizes the impact of bleeding, such as using dark sheets and towels (purple, navy blue, or brown) to contain large blood loss.[39]

E. Skin changes at life's end

The continued decline of the patient results in skin changes that occur at the end of life as patients enter the dying process. End-of-life patient care includes a variety of wound care challenges. Much of current evidence-based wound care practice focuses on the outcome of healing, which may not be an expected or desired outcome at the end of life. Patients under hospice care deserve to have symptoms of all types managed, and this should include wound management.[40]

Skin changes that occur at the end of life are sometimes confused with pressure ulcers. Pressure ulcers and skin failure are not the same. A pressure ulcer is a localized injury to the skin and/or underlying tissue, usually over a boney prominence, as a result of pressure or pressure in combination with shear.[41] Skin failure occurs without the presence of pressure and/or shear. A pressure ulcer and skin failure can and frequently do occur together, as an area of skin failure exposed to pressure and/or shear would be much more vulnerable to breakdown. This would not be uncommon in a patient with hemodynamic instability or whose position cannot be changed or can only be changed infrequently or minimally.[42] Understanding of skin failure versus pressures ulcers has continued to evolve. In 1989, the Kennedy Terminal Ulcer was first described. This type of ulcer presents as an unavoidable ulcer occurring during the dying process, often within the last 24 hours of life. This type of ulcer presents as a red, yellow, or purple irregular lesion on the coccyx or sacrum[43] In 2006 Langemo and Brown described skin failure as "an event in which the skin and underlying tissue die due to hypoperfusion that occurs concurrent with severe dysfunction or failure f other organ systems."[44] In 2009 an interdisciplinary panel of 18 experts convened to develop a consensus on skin changes at the end of life.[45]

A consensus statement on Skin Changes At Life's End (SCALE) was published in 2009 to explore the issues surrounding skin conditions associated with dying patients. The SCALE Final Consensus Statement reflects the current evidence and best practices surrounding Skin Changes At Life's End. The 10 statements represent the expert opinions of thought leaders from around the world. There is clear agreement that more research needs to be undertaken to enhance our understanding of the multiple and complex skin change phenomena that occur during the dying process. In the meantime, the 10 consensus statements give practical and focused suggestions for clinical management. [45-46]

In addition to summarizing best practices for clinicians providing end of life care, the SCALE consensus statements underscore the importance of recognizing that under some conditions, patients will develop skin breakdown despite optimal care.[45]

Palliative or end-of-life care concentrates on managing the symptoms of disease, including the wound characteristics, rather than trying to cure or reverse the progression of the disease process. In this situation, the goal of care is to prevent or mitigate suffering and to improve the quality of life for patients with serious or advanced illness. Managing pain, odor, exudates, bleeding, and other distressing symptoms is an important goal of palliative wound care. Evidence-based wound care should be an integral component in providing wound care at life's end. Current literature and clinical practice suggest that wound care in palliative settings is a common issue with negative effects on both the patient and family. Unfortunately, there is a paucity of research that specifically focuses on the assessment and management of palliative wounds. Clearly there is a need for more research in this area.[47-49]

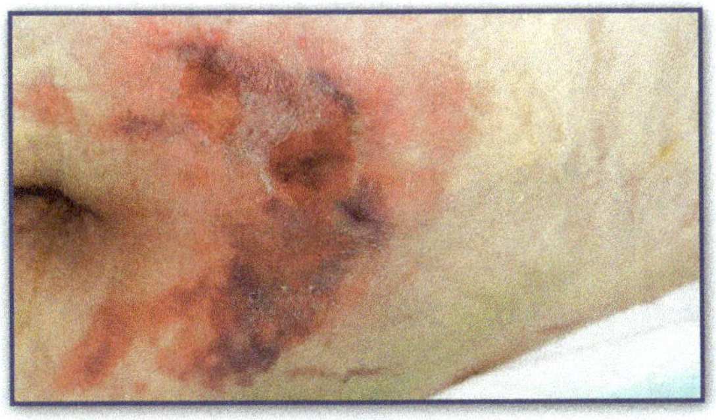

FIGURE 10.

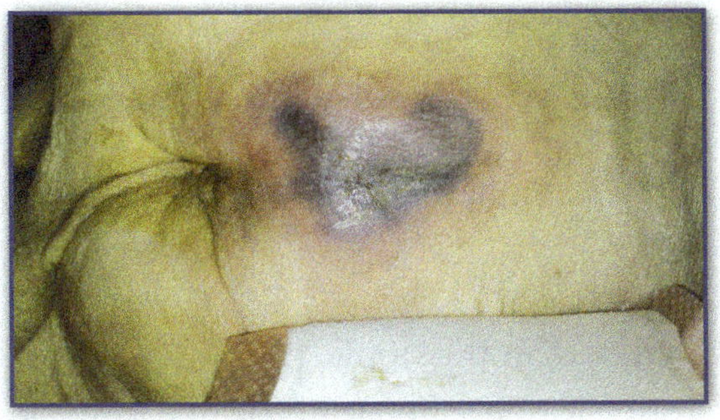

FIGURE 11.

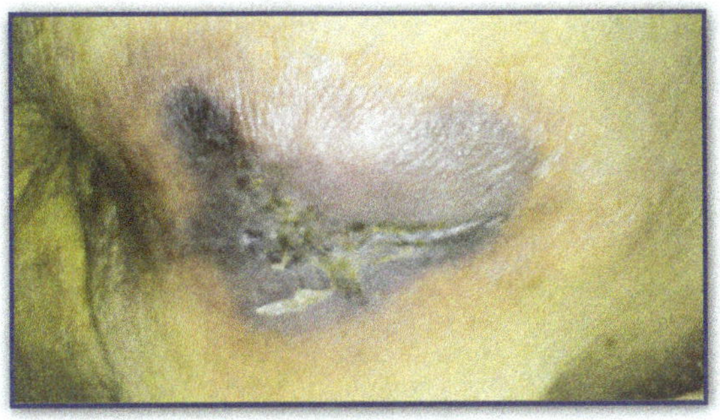

FIGURE 12.

FIGURES 10-12. Images of Kennedy ulcers - appearance of terminal, ischemic wounds in patients with impending death. These wounds typically appear hours to days before death and are usually unavoidable.

Summary

Elderly patients have a number of skin issues that present a challenge for most wound care clinicians. The combination of multiple comorbid medical conditions, impairments in functional status and mobility, as well as the physiologic impact of aging, can make it difficult to accurately identify the issue(s), goals of care, and appropriate treatment plan. Use of clinical pathways, when available, is strongly recommended. Clinical pathways are standardized, evidence-based, multidisciplinary management plans, which identify an appropriate sequence of clinical interventions, timeframes, milestones, and expected outcomes for a homogenous patient group. Implementation of best practices, an interdisciplinary approach, and use of clinical pathways can help guide the care of this challenging population of patients.

Review questions

1. **Which of the following are considered to be risk factors for skin tears?**

   a. poor mobility or history of falls

   b. advanced age

   c. multiple chronic illnesses

   d. previous skin trauma

   d. all of the above

2. **Strategies to reduce the risk of skin breakdown around a stoma include:**

   a. scrubbing the area around the stoma with soap and water

   b. cutting the opening in the wafer just slightly larger than the stoma

   c. properly using skin protectants and pastes

   d. both b and c

   e. all of the above

3. **Wound odor in a chronic wound can be treated with:**

   a. metronidazole

   b. hydrogel

   c. collagen particles

   d. topical lidocaine

4. ***True/False.*** Skin changes at the end of life are a result of physiologic changes in the dying process and are unavoidable.

5. ***True/False.*** Moisture-associated skin damage (MASD) is due to moisture from any cause and more common in patients with incontinence.

ANSWERS: 1) d
2) d
3) a
4) True
5) True

References

1. 2010 census shows 65 and older population growing faster than total U.S. population [Internet]. U.S. Census Bureau. 2011 Nov 30 [cited 2016 May 1]. Available from: https://www.census.gov/newsroom/releases/archives/2010_census/cb11-cn192.html.
2. Na CR, Wang S, Kirsner RS, Federman DG. Elderly adults and skin disorders: common problems for nondermatologists. Southern Medical Journal. 2012 Nov;105(11):600-606.
3. Shu Y, Maibach HL. Estrogen and skin: therapeutic options. Am J Clin Dermatol 2011;12 (5):297-311.
4. Gurll NJ, McCord DE. Anatomical and physiological basis for corneotrophic care of the skin. Adv Skin Wound Care. 2009;22(9):402-411.
5. Helfrich YR, Sachs DL, Voorhees JJ. Overview of skin aging and photoaging. Derm Nurs. 2008 June;20(3):177-183.
6. Hussain SH, Limthongkui B, Humphreys TR. The biomechanical properties of the skin. Dermatol Surg 2013;39:193–203.
7. LeBlanc K, Baronoski S. skin tears: state of the science: consensus statements for the prevention, prediction, assessment, and treatment of skin tears. Adv Skin Wound Care. 2011:24(9):2-15.
8. Lichterfeld A, Hauss A, Surber C, Peters T, Blume-Peytavi U, Kottner J. Evidence-based skin care: a systematic literature review and the development of a basic skin care algorithm JWOCN 2015 Oct;42(5):501–524.
9. LeBlanc K, Baronoski S, Christenson D, Langemo D, Sammon MA, Edwards K, Holloway, S, Gloeckner M, Williams A, Sibbald RG, Regan M. International Skin Tear Advisory Panel: A tool kit to aid in the prevention, assessment, and treatment of skin tears using a simplified classification system. Adv Skin Wound Care. 2013 Apr;26(10):459-476.
10. World Health Organization: Falls fact sheet [Internet] [updated 2017 Aug; cited 2017 May 7]. Available from: http://www.who.int/mediacentre/factsheets/fs344/en/.
11. Gray M, et al. Moisture-associated skin damage: overview and pathophysiology. Journal of Wound, Ostomy and Continence Nursing.2011;38(3):233-241.
12. Voegeli D. Moisture associated skin damage: an overview for community nurses. British Journal of Community Nursing. 2013;18(1): 6-12.
13. Doughty D. Differential assessment of trunk wounds: pressure ulceration versus incontinence-associated dermatitis versus intertriginous dermatitis. Ostomy and Wound Management. [Internet] 2012 Apr. Available from: http://www.o-wm.com/files/owm/pdfs/OWM_April2012_Doughty.pdf.
14. Vasavada SP Urinary Incontinence. Medscape. [Internet] 2016 Nov.Available from: http://emedicine.medscape.com/article/452289-overview.
15. Neki S. Urinary incontinence in the elderly. JKIMSU. 2016 Jan-Mar; 5(1[Internet]. Available from: http://citeseerx.ist.psu.edu/viewdoc/download?doi=10.1.1.735.4271&rep=rep1&type=pdf.
16. Erfurt-Berge C, Renner R. Recent developments in topical wound therapy: impact of antimicrobiological changes and rebalancing the wound milieu. BioMed Research International. 2014 (2014), Article ID 819525[Internet]. Available from: https://www.hindawi.com/journals/bmri/2014/819525/.
17. Shelton S, Zukowski K, Ayello EA. Practice Implications for peristomal skin assessment and care from the 2014 World Council of Enterostomal Therapists International Ostomy Guideline. Advances in Skin and Wound Care. 2015. [Internet]. Available from: https://goo.gl/3Dg2d1

18. Hospice Care. Centers for Disease Control and Prevention. 2016. [Internet]. Centers for Disease Control and Prevention. [cited 2016 May 1]. Available from: https://www.cdc.gov/nchs/fastats/hospice-care.htm.

19. Emmons KR, Lachman VD. Palliative wound care: a concept analysis. J Wound Ostomy Continence Nurs. 2010;37(6):639-644.

20. Ferris F, Khateib A, Fromantin I, et al. Palliative wound care: managing chronic wounds across life's continuum: a consensus statement from the International Palliative Wound Care Initiative. J Palliat Med. 2007;10(1):37-38.

21. Shah P, Aung TA, Ferguson R, Ortega G, Shah J. Ethical considerations in wound treatment of the elderly patient. J Am Coll of Clin Wound Spec. 2016;(6):46–52.

22. Bergstrom KJ. Assessment and management of fungating wounds. J Wound Ostomy Continence Nurs. 2011;38(1):31-37.

23. Hampton S. Chronic pain in wounds; a report on 11 case studies. Nurs Times. 2007;103(15):48-50.

24. Meaume S, Téot L, Lazareth I, Martini J, Bohbot S. The importance of pain reduction through dressing selection in routine wound management: the MAPP study. Journal of Wound Care. 2004 Nov;13(10).

25. Rippon M, Davies P, White R. Taking the trauma out of wound care: the importance of undisturbed healing. Journal of Wound Care. 21(8):359–360, 364–368.

26. Price P, Fogh K, Glynn C, Krasner DL, Osterbrink J, Sibbald RG. Managing painful chronic wounds: the wound pain management model. International Wound Journal. 4(Suppl. 1):4–15.

27. World Health Organization. WHO's Pain Relief Ladder. [Internet}. World Health Organization. [cited 2016 May]. Available from: http://www.who.int/cancer/palliative/painladder/en/.

28. Roden A, Sturman E. Assessment & management of patients with wound-related pain. Nursing Standard. 23(45):53-62.

29. Gallagher R. The management of wound-related procedural pain (volitional incident pain) in advanced illness. Curr Opin Support Palliat Care. 2013 Mar;7(1):80-85. doi: 10.1097/SPC.0b013e32835ac704.

30. Emmons KR, Dale B, Crouch C. Palliative wound care, part 2: application of principles. Home Health Care Nur. 2013 Apr;32(4):210-222.

31. Ribeiro MD, Joel SP, Zeppetella G. The bioavailability of morphine applied topically to cutaneous ulcers. Journal of Pain and Symptom Management 2004; 27(5): 434–439.

32. Gallagher R. Management of painful wounds in advanced disease. Can Fam Physician. 2010 Sep;56(9):883–885.

33. Seaman S. Management of malignant fungating wounds in advanced cancer. Seminars in Oncology Nursing. 2006;22(3):185–193.

34. Suzuki K. Current insights on treating gangrenous, odorous and painful wounds. [Internet]. Podiatry Today. 2013;26 (11). Available from: http://www.podiatrytoday.com/current-insights-treating-gangrenous-odorous-and-painful-wounds-0.

35. Hebert GR. Palliative wound care, part 2, Wound care Advisor. [Internet]. 2015;4(2). Available from: https://woundcareadvisor.com/palliative-wound-care-part-2/.

36. Recka K, Montagnini M, Vitale CA. Management of bleeding associated with malignant wounds. Journal of Palliative Medicine. 2012;15(8):952–954.

37. Shintaro Y, Douzono H, Yanazume Y, Lio K, Douchi T. New hemostatic method using Moh's paste for fatal genital bleeding in advanced cervical cancer. Gyn Onc Case Reports. 2013;4: 47-49.

38. Graves ML, Sun V. Providing quality wound care at the end of life. JHPN. 2013 Apr;15(2): 66-71.

39. Bogagu U, Harris DG. Guideline for the management of terminal haemorrhage in palliative care patients with advanced cancer discharged home for end-of-life care. [Internet]. 2012;2(4). Available from: http://dx.doi.org/10.1136/bmjspcare-2012-000253.

40. Langemo DK. When the goal is palliative care. Adv Skin Wound Care. 2006;19(3):148-154.

41. National Pressure Ulcer Advistory Panel (NPUAP) Pressure Ulcer Guidelines. [Internet]. Available from: http://www.npuap.org/resources/educational-and-clinical-resources/npuap-pressure-injury-stages/.

42. White-Chu EF, Langemo D. Skin failure: identifying and managing an under recognized condition. [Internet]. Annals of LTC. 2012 July 20(7). Available from: http://www.annalsoflongtermcare.com/article/skin-failure-identifying-and-managing-underrecognized-condition.

43. Kennedy-Evans, KL. Understanding the Kennedy Terminal Ulcer. [Internet]. Available from: http://www.kennedyterminalulcer.com/.

44. Langemo DK, Brown G. Skin fails too: acute, chronic and end stage skin failure. Adv Skin Wound Care. 2006;19(4):206-211.

45. Sibbald RG, Krasner DL, Lutz JB, et al. The SCALE expert panel: skin changes at life's end. Final Consensus Document. 2009 Oct 1.

46. Langemo DK. General principles and approaches to wound prevention and care at end of life: an overview. Ostomy Wound Manag. 2012;58(5):24-344.

47. Tippett A. Wounds at the end of life. Wounds. 2005;17(4):91-98.

48. Alvarez OM, Kalinski C, Nusbaum P, et al. Incorporating wound healing strategies to improve palliative (symptom management) in patients with chronic wounds. J Palliat Med. 2007;10 (5):1161-1189.

49. Maida V, Ennis M, Corban J. Wound outcomes in patients with advanced illness. Int Wound J. 2012;10(1111):1742-1748.

Chapter 21

MANAGEMENT OF ENTEROCUTANEOUS FISTULA

Dianne Rudolph, DNP, GNP-BC, CWOCN

KEY CONCEPTS

1. A fistula is an abnormal communication between two epithelialized surfaces.
2. ECFs (enterocutaneous fistulas) are fairly common presentations in surgical units, and despite advances in the management of them, they are still responsible for a significant mortality (5-20%), due to associated sepsis, nutritional abnormalities, and electrolyte imbalances.
3. The etiology of ECFs can thus be characterized as postoperative, traumatic, or spontaneous.
4. Protection of the skin and containment of exudates is a critical component in the effective care and management of the patient with an ECF.
5. Psychological support is sometimes overlooked but is of great importance in management of ECF.

CONTENTS

Introduction

An enterocutaneous fistula (ECF) is an abnormal connection that develops between the intestinal tract or stomach and the skin. As a result, contents of the stomach or intestines leak through to the skin. Most ECFs occur after bowel surgery. Enterocutaneous fistulas may result from a wide variety of conditions and circumstances. Care of these patients can be quite challenging, frustrating, and, ultimately, rewarding. The patient with an enterocutaneous fistula presents the health-care provider with a variety of challenges, and a command of related anatomy and physiology is necessary to successfully meet these challenges. With an understanding of management principles, it is possible to care for these medically complex individuals.

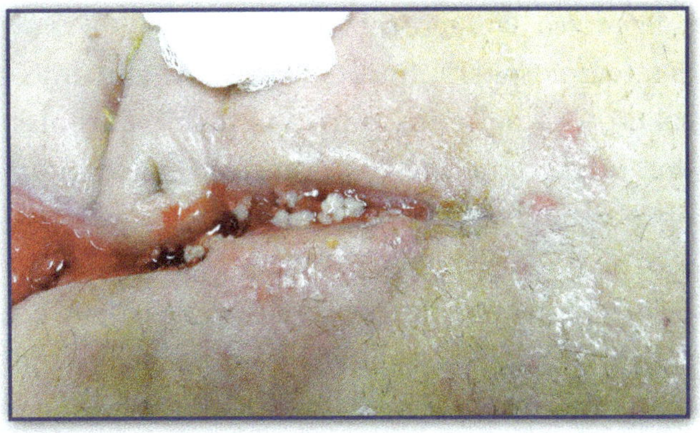

FIGURE 1. Patient with open wound with ileostomy (covered with gauze), mucous fistula and entercutaneous fistula draining mucopurulent exudates into proximal aspect of wound

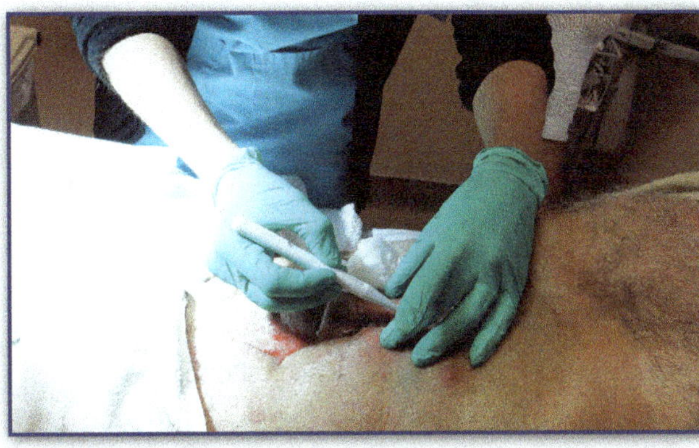

FIGURE 2. Wound being gently curetted/cleansed

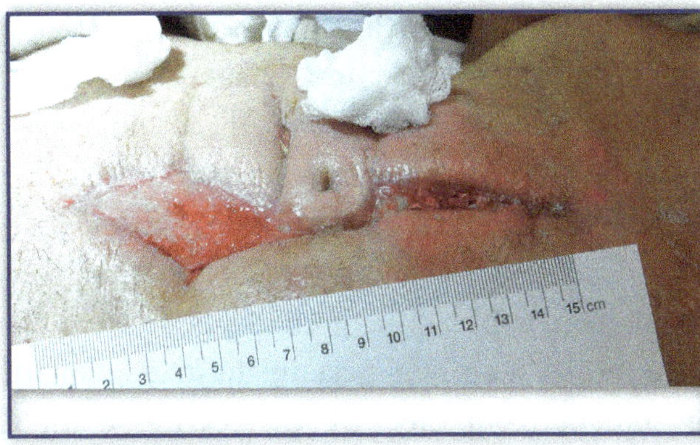

FIGURE 3. Post-debridement/cleansing

I. Case study

Mr. S. is a 66-year-old male with a past medical history of chronic abdominal pain and recurrent small bowel obstructions. His medical history includes diabetes, anemia, hypertension, hypothyroidism, osteoporosis, and renal insufficiency.

Surgical history includes numerous abdominal surgeries, including multiple laparotomies and lysis of adhesions, as well as sigmoidectomy with loop colostomy and subsequent colostomy takedown, open cholecystectomy, and small bowel resection. With the last small bowel obstruction, he underwent exploratory laparotomy and four-hour lysis of adhesions. He experienced complications, including a deep vein thrombosis and postoperative wound infection with methacillin-resistant Staphylococcu aureus, and wound dehiscence with an enterocutaneous fistula. He was being treated with dry gauze dressings that were being changed three to four times a day.

II. Definition

A fistula is an abnormal communication between two epithelialized surfaces; an enterocutaneous fistula (ECF), as the name indicates, is an abnormal communication between the small or large bowel and the skin. Fistula means "flute or pipe" in Latin. An ECF can arise from the duodenum, jejunum, ileum, colon, or rectum. The ileum is the most common site. Enteric fistulas are categorized as enterocutaneous fistulas (ECFs) or enteroatmospheric fistulas (EAFs). Enteroatmospheric is a newer term used to describe fistulas that originate in the bowel and terminate in an open wound. In many cases, EAFs are still categorized as ECFs.[1] ECFs may occur in specific disease processes or iatrogenically. Patients who suffer with this condition manifest signs and symptoms of fluid and electrolyte imbalance, malnutrition, and pain. Despite improvements in management and treatment modalities, mortality and morbidity rates remain high. ECFs are devastating complications of bowel disease, abdominal surgery, and/or open abdomen. Enteric fistulas are associated with a mortality rate varying from 1% to 33%; the main cause of death is sepsis. Coordinated and skillful efforts of an interdisciplinary professional team are required in customizing successful treatment regimens appropriate to each patient's unique clinical scenario.[2]

Multiple factors influence healing of postoperative abdominal wounds. Factors that may hinder proper wound healing include poor circulation, edema, infection, diabetes mellitus, immobilization, anemia, use of steroids, age, smoking, obesity, coagulopathy, and vasculitis. Development of an ECF is also associated with delayed healing and often requires surgical management. A major challenge in treating a wound with an ECF pertains to management of effluent from the ECF that carries a high potential for moisture-associated skin damage if allowed to come into contact with the periwound skin. Drainage of the effluent and protection of the periwound skin are applied to ensure both wound healing and closure of the ECF. However, systemic factors such as malnutrition and/or a compromised immune system that can impede wound healing must be addressed prior to administration of any treatment program.

It is estimated that about 95% of ECFs are postoperative, and the ileum is the most common site. Approximately 49% of fistulas are considered high-output (> 500 ml per 24 hours), and 51% are considered low-output (< 200 ml per 24 hours). Fistulas are commonly described according to the anatomic locations involved.

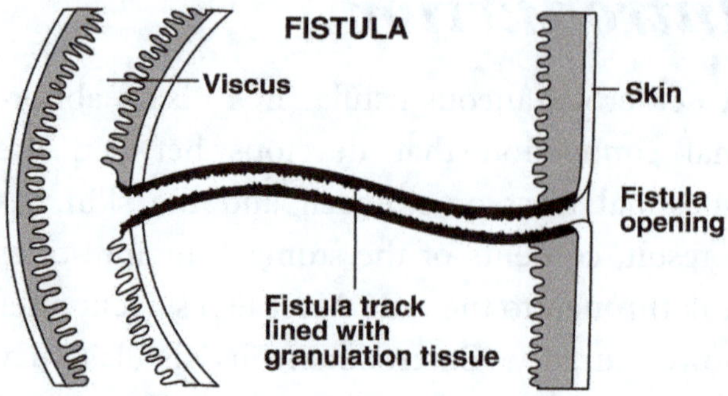

FIGURE 4. An ECF, classified as an external fistula (as opposed to an internal fistula, which is an abnormal communication between two hollow viscera), is a complication that is usually seen after surgery on the small or large bowel.

TABLE 1. Fistula Terminology[3]

FROM	TO	NAME	TYPE
Bladder	Skin	Vesicocutaneous	External
Bladder	Vagina	Vesicovaginal	Internal
Colon	Skin	Colocutaneous	External
Colon	Bladder	Colovesical	Internal
Intestine	Colon	Enterocolonic	Internal
Intestine	Skin	Enterocutaneous	External
Intestine	Bladder	Enterovesical	Internal
Intestine	Vagina	Enterovaginal	Internal
Rectum	Vagina	Rectovaginal	Internal

The type of ECF, as based on the output of the enteric contents, can have a significant impact on the patient's health status. ECFs are usually classified into three categories:[4]

- Low-output fistula (<200 mL/day)
- Moderate-output fistula (200-500 mL/day)
- High-output fistula (>500 mL/day)

ECFs are fairly common presentations in surgical units, and despite advances in the management of them, they are still responsible for a significant mortality (5-20%), due to associated sepsis, nutritional abnormalities, and electrolyte imbalances.

Understanding the pathophysiology of, as well as the risk factors for, ECFs should help to reduce their occurrence. Moreover, the well-established treatment guidelines for these fistulas, along with some newer treatment options, should help clinicians to achieve a better outcome in patients with an ECF.[4-5]

An ECF can occur as a complication following any type of surgery on the GI tract. Indeed, more than 75% of all ECFs arise as a postoperative complication, whereas about 15-25% result from abdominal trauma or occur spontaneously in relation to cancer, irradiation, inflammatory bowel disease (IBD), or ischemic or infective conditions. The etiology of ECFs can thus be characterized as postoperative, traumatic, or spontaneous.

III. Postoperative ECF

Postoperative causes of ECFs include disruption of an existing anastomosis, inadvertent enterotomy, or inadvertent small bowel injury. Disruption of anastomosis can result from inadequate blood flow due to an improper vascular supply, especially when extensive mesenteric vessels have to be ligated. Tension on anastomotic lines following colonic resection, restoration of continuity without adequate mobilization, or a minimal leak or infection can lead to perianastomotic abscess formation, resulting in disruption. This is sometimes seen in patients with anterior resection for rectal carcinoma. If anastomosis is performed in an unhealthy bowel, such as a diseased or ischemic bowel, it can lead to disruption and cause an ECF.

Inadvertent picking up of the bowel during abdominal closure can result in a small-bowel fistula; this especially can occur with the use of open inlay mesh or intraperitoneal mesh repair by the laparoscopic method, when the viscera comes in contact with the mesh, leading to adhesions and sometimes to disruption.

Gastroduodenal fistulas are seen most often after surgery for perforated peptic ulcer, especially in developing countries, where perforated peptic ulcer is more common. In patients with a perforated duodenal ulcer, when the perforation is large, extensive contamination is present. When the duration between the perforation and the surgery is long, there is a high possibility of a leak following surgery, leading to a lateral duodenal fistula. This problem is difficult to treat, and the mortality rate is high. Other causes of gastroduodenal leak include surgery for cancers of the stomach and the biliary tract.

A colocutaneous fistula can develop after colonic surgery, especially when the blood supply to a low colorectal/anal anastomosis is compromised or when there is tension at the anastomotic suture line. This type of fistula can also result from diseases of the colon, such as inflammatory bowel disease (IBD) or malignancy leading to perforation, pericolic abscess formation, and ECF. Surgery for appendicitis, appendicular perforation at the base, or drainage of an appendicular abscess can also lead to a colocutaneous fistula. Radiation therapy is also another major cause of colonic fistula. In rare cases, migration of a polypropylene or composite mesh from a hernia repair can lead to ECF formation.

IV. Spontaneous ECF

Spontaneous causes of ECF, which are seen in about 15-25% of cases, include malignancy, radiation enteritis with friable bowel that perforates, intra-abdominal sepsis and inflammatory bowel disease. Crohn's disease is a more common etiology for ECF than ulcerative colitis (UC). Ulcerative colitis can also lead to spontaneous ECF, but most cases of ECF associated with this IBD occur as a postoperative complication.

V. Surgical management

ECFs are treated via a surgical or nonsurgical approach. Although many enterocutaneous fistulas close spontaneously, if the ECF remains open after two months, surgical intervention is likely to be needed as spontaneous closure is unlikely after this interval. The timing of corrective surgery in relation to the initial operation(s) is important, as it affects the incidence of further complications. Major abdominal surgery stimulates the formation of dense adhesions, especially when complicated by intra-abdominal sepsis. This reaction is most severe between three weeks and three months after operation, and further surgery during this time is more likely to be complicated by fistula recurrence. Delayed surgery also allows time for metabolic and nutritional deficiencies to be corrected.[6-7]

The initial stage of EC fistula management consists of its identification, followed by general supportive care with fluid and electrolyte replacement, control of sepsis, nutritional support, and control of fistula drainage by pharmacologic means as well as through skin protection. Once a postsurgical or spontaneous EC fistula is identified, obtaining anatomic information is of the utmost importance to predict the site of intestinal opening and assess the need for surgery. Favorable external fistulas include esophageal, duodenal stump, pancreaticobiliary, and jejunal fistulas with small enteric defects (< 1 cm) and long tracts (> 2 cm). In contrast, gastric, lateral duodenal, ligament of Treitz, and ileal fistulas are less likely to close spontaneously. Additionally, nonhealing ECFs are associated with a number of factors that can be described using the mnemonic FRIEND: **F**oreign body, **R**adiation, **I**nflammation, **I**nfection, **I**nflammatory bowel disease, **E**pithelization of the fistula tract, **N**eoplasms, and **D**istal obstructions. The presence of any FRIEND component in ECF is generally an indication for surgical intervention; however, surgery should be performed only after sufficient time has been afforded to restore overall patient condition and allow lysis of the intra-abdominal fibrous adhesions from previous operations.

Determining the optimal time for surgical intervention has not been well defined in the literature. However, surgery should be delayed until the intra-abdominal and systemic conditions of the patient are conducive to major surgery. The timing of definitive surgery should be individualized according to patient characteristics. In some cases, surgery is performed within several weeks to several months after initial surgery.[8]

The aims of surgery for EC fistulas are: 1) refunctionalization of the entire bowel; 2) resection of the fistula with end-to-end anastomosis of the bowel; and 3) secure abdominal wall closure. Once surgery is planned, care should be taken not to injure the adjacent bowels while opening the abdomen. The fistula tract is detected by staining with methylene blue or guided probes. After identifying the fistula opening in the bowel, resection of the diseased bowel and end-to-end anastomosis is the preferred method compared to over-sewing the fistula opening of the bowel, as recurrent fistula is more likely after over-sewing (36%) than resection (16%). To facilitate early feeding and decompression of the proximal bowel, selected cases require gastrostomy, diverting ileostomy, or jejunostomy.

Abdominal closure is challenging when fistula closure is attempted. Skin defects and the increased probability of wound contamination make secure skin closure difficult. Wound complications can result in new or recurring EC fistulas. To promote normal healing of the abdominal wound after surgery, optimal parenteral or enteral nutrition with a supplement comprised of trace minerals and vitamins is essential.[4,8]

VI. Nonsurgical management

Conservative treatment should usually be administered for a period ranging from a few weeks to a few months. The principles of nonsurgical therapy for ECFs include rehydration, administration of antibiotics, correction of anemia, electrolyte repletion, drainage of obvious abscess, control of fistula drainage, skin protection, and nutritional support.[1,9]

VII. Nutritional requirements of ECF patients

Patients with ECFs have high calorie and nutritional requirements. Clinical dietitians play an instrumental role in determining these requirements as well as the best options for delivering adequate nutrition. Each patient requires an individualized calculation of the requirement depending on his condition, route of feeding, and feeding tolerance. Patients who were given 1,500–2,000 kcal/day had a mortality rate of 16%, and those who were given less than 1,000 kcal/day had a mortality rate of 58%. Moreover, they reported that 89% of fistula closure achieved among ECF patients with optimal nutrition support (1,500–2,000), and only 37% of those who were underfed (1,000 kcal/day).[1,7,10]

A. Routes of feeding in ECF patients

Several factors influence the selection of route of feeding, including origin of fistula, length of healthy bowel available for absorption, and fistula output. If there is sufficient functioning bowel for adequate nutrients absorption and no intra-abdominal sepsis and manageable fistula output, the enteral feeding would be the optimal choice. If the nutritional requirement could not have been achieved enterally or the fistula output is high, then total parenteral nutrition (TPN) feeding should be used.

Total parenteral nutrition (TPN) is administered intravenously by a central line. It is indicated for patients with high output who cannot tolerate other forms of feeding and is recommended for use for limited periods of time. Tight control of blood glucose level is necessary to avoid hyperglycemia. Carbohydrate, fat, and protein calories ratio in TPN are modified according to patient's medical history, (i.e. presence of comorbidities such as diabetes mellitus). Pulmonary disease may require increased fat and decreased dextrose percentages in order to reduce the carbon dioxide production by dextrose oxidation. The electrolytes requirements (sodium, potassium, chloride, calcium, phosphorus, manganese) were provided in crystalloid nutrient form, and all trace elements and vitamins (fat, water soluble) were included in the TPN bag. Adjustment of the acetate, bicarbonate, phosphate, and chloride was essential to maintain the acid-base balance.

Enteral feeding in clinical practice is recommended unless it is contraindicated, due to its relatively lower cost, greater availability, and fewer complications. Early enteral nutrition in ECF has been associated with earlier fistula closure, lower rates of pneumonia, and lower rates of fistula recurrence. Enteral feedings also help to protect the mucosal integrity and maintain immune and hormone function. Highly absorbable formulas with low-residue nutrients should be administered. Contraindications of enteral feeding include intestinal discontinuity, ileus, short bowel length (75 cm of small bowel is required for successful enteral feeding), inability to obtain enteral access, and inability to tolerate enteral feedings. An increase in fistula output, or a high-output fistula, can also preclude the use of enteral feedings and can potentially compound metabolic and management issues.

In enteral feeding, the volume and the concentration of tube feeding are usually low at the beginning of feeding, and then increase gradually to achieve the full strength as tolerated. In some cases, it may take several days to achieve the total requirement.

B. Oral feeding

Oral feeding starts when the patient can tolerate fluids and solid food. The recommendation is that patients be educated as to how to select a high-calorie, high-salt, low-fiber, and low-residual diet. In some cases, despite the patient's having normal gut absorption, oral feeding might increase the fistula output, especially if the food is solid. Again, this would require the close observation and management by the clinical dietitian and other members of the interdisciplinary team.

Fistuloclysis has been defined as a technique of using fistula as the primary enteral portal for access and infusion of food stuff, formula, or gastrointestinal secretion.[11] It has been considered an efficient and successful method of feeding in ECF patients. Fistuloclysis has not been a popular practice in fistula management due to technical and anesthetic issues. It has been indicated when the fistula location was in the small bowel and not distal enough to allow adequate enteral absorption, or when TPN was not available or contraindicated. Fistuloclysis may be a suitable choice if there is enough unobstructed bowel distal to the fistula to enable adequate nutrient absorption. In some cases, fistuloclysis can replace TPN for patients using polymeric formula. It appears to be a viable option to be considered in order to increase the tolerance of tube feeding and maintain fluid and electrolyte homeostasis. The technique of fistuloclysis needs specialized and experienced enterostomal care to stabilize the feeding tube in the fistula; otherwise the effluents would be leaked and lead to skin corrosion, and the tube could be pulled into the bowel by the peristalsis movement of the bowel.[11-12]

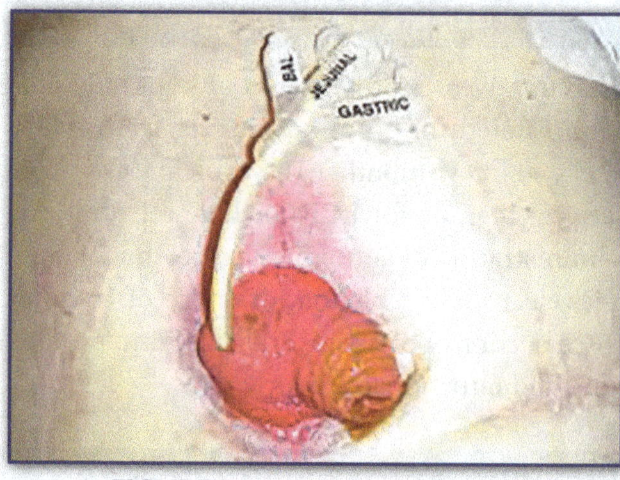

FIGURE 5. Insertion of feeding tube into proximal limb of small bowel fistula

VIII. Options for management of fistulas

Protection of the skin and containment of exudates are critical components in the effective care and management of the patient with an ECF. There are a variety of techniques available for the clinician to use, including nonpouching options, pouching options, and the use of negative pressure wound therapy (NPWT).

A. Nonpouching options for containment of fistula effluent

Nonpouching options are indicated when ECF output is less than 100 cc in 24 hours, there are no odor issues or if the contours of the skin prevent pouching. Options for management include the use of barrier products for skin protection and absorbant dressings. Petrolatum, zinc, or dimethicone barrier ointments can be used for skin protection with low volume, odorless fistula that does not require pouching. Absorbent wound dressings are indicated if the dressing change is require several times a day or more.[4-5]

1. Dressings

Typical dressings to manage exudate include foams, alginates, hydrofibers, and cellulose polyacrylate fiber dressings. Using combinations of these dressings increases the amount of exudate held within the dressings and increases dressing wear time, thereby reducing the other symptoms associated with frequent dressing changes.[4,7]

Hydrofiber or calcium alginate dressings

Alginate dressings are biodegradable, absorb up to 20 times their weight in wound fluid, and serve as hemostatic agents. The polyacrylate dressings appear to be the most absorbent option for exudate control but may be cost prohibitive in some settings.[4,7]

Case study: Mr. S.

Mr. S., as depicted previously, had a low volume fistula with <100 cc output per hour. In his case, management of his fistula was successfully achieved with the use of a petrolatum barrier product and a cyanoacrylate dressing (Sorbion Sachet, Alliqua Biomedical, Inc) that was changed daily and as needed. He spontaneously closed in several weeks and was able to return home with home health care.

2. Closed suction system

In acute-care settings, a closed suction system can be employed for management of higher volumes of drainage that cannot be managed with absorbent dressings. This may be an effective option for patients with high-output ECF who are of limited mobility and essentially bedbound. This method of management has been in use for several decades and was published by Chariker, Jeter et al.[13] In this method, a suction catheter hooked to continuous or intermittent suction is placed in the distal portion of the wound bed to the fistula to drain effluent. The suction catheter is used in conjunction with normal saline dressings and a film dressing.

In this technique, the perifistular skin is cleansed and protected with a liquid polymer or skin film. Solid barrier rings, strips or paste are applied to line the edges of the fistula. A layer of nonadherent dressing (xerform, oil emulsion gauze) is applied to the wound/fistula base to protect the tissue. A layer of gauze is placed over the nonadherent dressing, a drain is placed over the gauze and the entire area is covered with a transparent dressing. The system is then attached to low wall suction (60 to 80 mmHg) to create an airtight seal. Apply a border dressing or seal connections with waterproof tape. It is important that the catheter not be placed in the fistula tract, as it will be recognized as a foreign body and potentially delay closure. The continuous suction helps reduce dressing changes by diverting drainage to the suction system. Only soft, flexible suction catheters should be used. The advantages of this technique, is that it allows for ongoing collection and measurement of effluent volume, decreases the frequency of dressing changes and protects the skin. Disadvantages of this technique include the fact that its use is limited to the inpatient setting. The

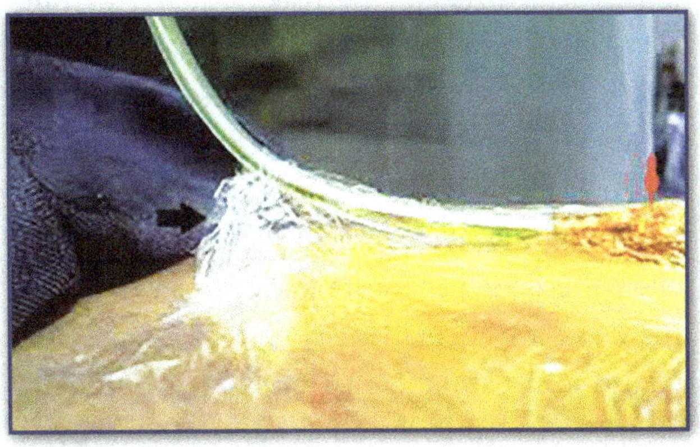

FIGURE 6. Use of closed suction technique for ECF

tubing is attached to wall suction and can significantly limit a patient's mobility, thus it may be most useful for acutely ill patients for brief periods of time.

B. Pouching options for containment of fistula effluent

For ECFs that have larger volumes of exudate, i.e, >100 cc per day, wound drainage collectors, fistula pouches or ostomy appliances can be very useful.

Wound drainage collectors/fistula pouches are special pouches that are disposable and are designed to collect and contain wound drainage. They are especially useful for fistulas and wounds with large volumes of exudate and replace dressings allowing accurate measurement of fluid. They typically have skin barriers attached to protect periwound skin from moisture and trauma. Some systems have windows that allow for wound care between changes of the wound managers. These systems are also available with adaptors that allow them to be attached to gravity or a continuous low-suction drainage system to prevent the device from overfilling.

A one-piece or two-piece urostomy or drainable ostomy appliance with a hydrocolloid skin barrier may also be suitable for a fistula with an output greater than 100 cc/24 hours. These can also be used for patients with low-volume output for convenience. Fecal, urinary, adult-size or pediatric-size may be used. There are some customized pouching solutions that are well described in the literature. These include the trough technique, bridging technique, and the saddle bag technique.

Troughing is a pouching technique used when the fistula is located within a wound. In this case, a wall or dam is created around the wound and fistula. Strips of solid skin barrier are applied around the outer edges of the wound and fistula, then covered with a transparent film dressing. A small opening is then made in the transparent film dressing, and a drainable ostomy pouch is applied over this opening.

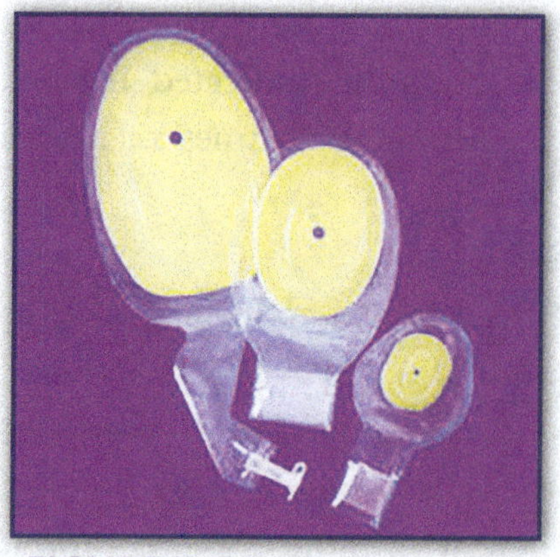

FIGURE 7. Eakin fistula pouches

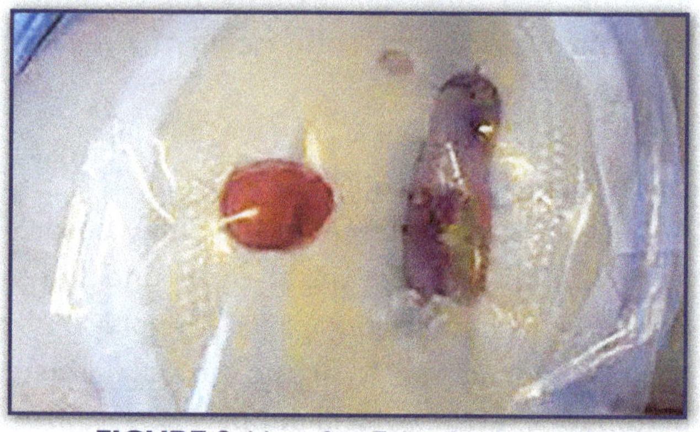

FIGURE 8. Use of an Eakin fistula pouch to contain ileostomy and ECF

EXAMPLES:

Hollister Wound Drainage Collectors
—access caps for the management of wounds with copious drainage. Available with and without skin barriers, sterile and nonsterile. *Small:* for wounds up to 3". *Medium:* for wounds up to 3(3/4)". *Large:* for wounds up to 4"x8". www.hollister.com

Wound Manager
—sterile drainage pouch utilizes a one-piece pouch design with a large-surface, flexible Durahesive body-side skin barrier for protection against wound drainage. 3"x3", 3"x7", 4"x9" www.convatec.com

Eakin Fistula and Wound Pouch
—www.convatec.com d. Special fistula pouches for use with unusual shape or size fistulas or wounds. www.nu-hope.com

POUCHING TIPS FOR SUCCESS(14)

A. Shave the hair in the area around the wound or fistula to increase adhesion of the appliance or dressing.

B. Set up all equipment before starting procedure. Fistula function is unpredictable and may occur before adhesives are set up.

C. Follow universal precautions with clean technique during procedures. Sterile products are an unnecessary expense and are not shown to control infection.

1. Clean technique. Clean means free of dirt, marks, or stains.
2. Clean technique involves strategies used in patient care to reduce the overall number of microorganisms or to prevent or reduce the risk of transmission of microorganisms from one person to another or from one place to another.
3. Clean technique involves meticulous handwashing, maintaining a clean environment by preparing a clean field, using clean gloves and sterile instruments, and preventing direct contamination of materials and supplies. No "sterile to sterile" rules apply. This technique may also be referred to as non-sterile.

D. Hold nonsterile gauze against the fistula opening while preparing for appliance placement to wick away the drainage and prevent leakage on the skin. Another option is to hold suction catheter close to the orifice of the fistula to remove the effluent. This prevents spillage onto the perifistular skin prior to appliance placement. Do NOT insert the suction catheter into the fistula or bowel.

E. Empty the appliance frequently, especially before the patient ambulates.

1. Attach the appliance to a bedside drainage system to prevent the weight of the effluent from disrupting the appliance seal and to increase the appliance wear time.
2. Minimize pooling of effluent over skin barrier by angling tail of pouch off to reclining patient's side.
3. Accurate measurement of effluent is critical to success of fluid and electrolyte resuscitation.

F. Change the appliance at least every seven days.

1. Increase the frequency of the appliance change if extensive corrosion on the inner edge of the appliance is noted when removing the old appliance.
2. Plan the time of the appliance change to avoid times when the fistula is active, such as after meals.
3. Do not attempt to "patch up" a leaking appliance, as this is rarely effective.
4. Appliance changes can take time to complete. Although possibly labor-intensive, a well applied system remains leakproof and thus ensures patient comfort.

G. Apply paste to any irregular indentations or creases in the periwound area to create a smooth surface.

H. Instruct the patient to rest in bed for at least 30 minutes after an appliance change to prevent leakage.

I. Implement odor-control measures.

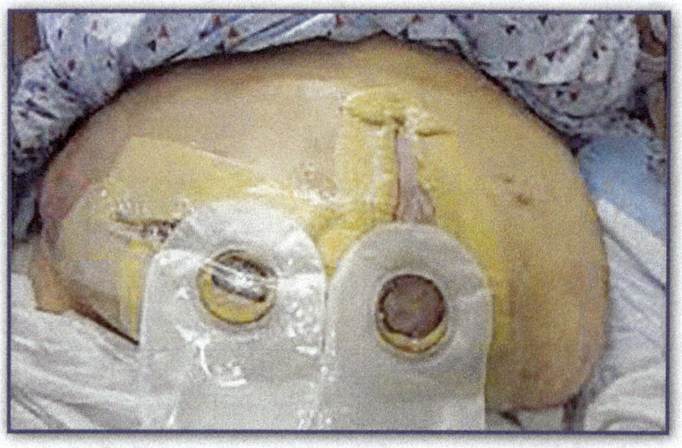

FIGURE 9. Trough technique used for ECFs

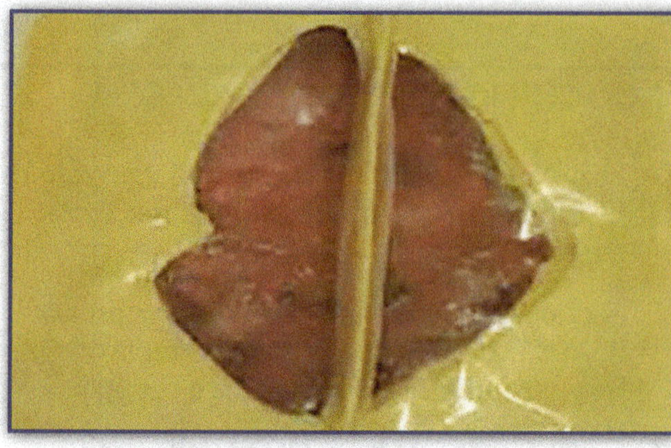

FIGURE 10. Saddle bag technique using two separate Eakin pouches

Trough technique does not prevent fistula output from contaminating the wound site.

Bridging is a pouching technique used when fistula is located within a wound to prevent fistula output from contaminating the wound. In this case the wound is separated from the fistula. Solid skin barrier is cut into small pieces to fill the wound at the selected bridge location and layered into place. A pouching system is then applied over the bridge that now exists in the wound. This helps to prevent the fistula output from getting into wound. This technique also works well with negative pressure wound therapy (NPWT) and will be discussed later in this chapter.

Saddle bagging is a technique employed to pouch over a large wound surface by attaching two open-end drainable pouches along the adhesive surface in order to create a large adhesive surface. In this case a large solid skin barrier is then attached to the combined adhesive surface. This allows the fistula to drain into both pouches. Adaptations can be made to ostomy pouches to accommodate the effluent.

Implementation of pouching techniques can be of great advantage in managing patients with higher-output ECFs. Basic principles of management and a trial-and-error approach are necessary to create a temporary solution for patients with ECFs.

C. Negative pressure wound therapy

Negative pressure wound therapy (NPWT) using a vacuum-assisted closure device (VAC Therapy; Acelity USA, Inc., San Antonio, Texas) and reticulated open cell foam (ROCF) has been shown to benefit for abdominal wounds complicated by ECF by removing effluent from the fistula and preventing moisture-associated skin damage (MASD) of the periwound skin. The use of NPWT helps to facilitate wound healing by providing a closed, moist wound environment, promoting granulation tissue formation through cell migration and proliferation, reducing edema, removing infectious material, and drawing the wound edges together.

There are a number of novel approaches to using NPWT in the literature.[15-16] These novel techniques combine critical thinking with application of topical techniques to manage wounds with ECF.

In terms of candidate selection, treatment of ECF with NPWT requires a determination of the goals of therapy and whether the ECF being treated is acute, acute complex, or chronic in nature as this will inform the technique used for the application of NPWT. An acute, complex ECF can be treated with NPWT to promote direct closure. In this case the goal of therapy is to close the wound by collapsing or holding together the ECF so that it self-seals. An acute ECF is one that is of recent onset, as its name implies, and has no evidence of epithelial cells. The opening must be easily visualized and accessible. In this case the patient should be nothing by mouth (NPO) or on TPN, and the effluent should be minimal to moderate in volume and slightly viscous in nature.[16-17] In order to accomplish this, the wound is cleansed and irrigated with sterile saline. The mouth or opening of the fistula is covered with petrolatum gauze, and any exposed bowel is also covered with gauze. White foam is then applied, followed by GranuFoam [reticulated open-cell, foam (ROCF)] and drape. Patient is placed on continuous pressure of 150-175 mmHg with dressing changes two or three times per week.[17-18]

With chronic ECF, the goal of therapy is to segregate the fistula from the wound bed. This diverts the effluent from the wound bed and allows the use of NPWT to be used to for wound healing. Chronic ECF patients include those who are not surgical candidates, have chronic formation/evidence of stomatization of the fistula, and are NPO or on TPN. There are a variety of techniques that can be used to accomplish this. In this case, NPWT is applied at 125 mmHg with dressing changes two or three times a week and as needed.[18]

Case study: Mr. R.

Mr. R. was a 58-year-old male with a history of a small bowel obstruction who underwent exploratory laparotomy and resection. His postoperative course was complicated by sepsis, acute respiratory failure requiring mechanical ventilation, and acute kidney injury. He developed a large wound dehiscence complicated by the development of several ECFs within his abdominal wound. He was maintained on TPN. He was producing a large amount of effluent requiring dressing changes five or six times daily.

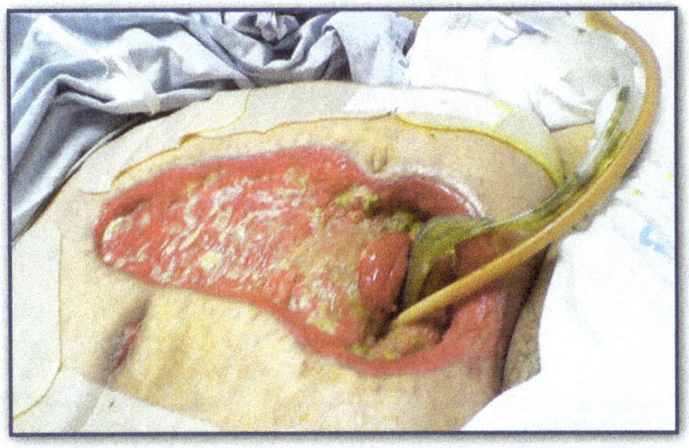

FIGURE 11. Patient with chronic stomatized ECF There is an ostomy take-down site in the right upper quadrant.

D. Fistula solutions

Recently Acelity has developed several accessories that are designed to be used in conjunction with NPWT to help improve the management of patients with enteric fistulas and other wounds. These products are referred to as the wound crown, fistula funnel, and isolator strip. These devices have been used effectively with the separation technique on fistulas and stomas that drain into open abdominal wounds with moderate- to high-output levels to extend dressing change intervals and accelerate wound healing.

The wound crown is designed to isolate small intestinal fistulas and ileostomies. The fistula funnel was created to isolate small fistulas, sidewall fistulas, and deep crevice wound bed areas. The isolator strip is used to isolate large fistulas, groups of fistulas, and large or uniquely shaped wound bed areas. While the same principles of NPWT apply, these accessories were designed to make the use of NPWT in ECFs more user friendly.[22] Heineman et al. have used the product with very positive outcomes.[23] Since these products are very new at the time of publication, it is not yet clear what the widespread experience of clinicians has been with them. As with any novel product, time will tell.

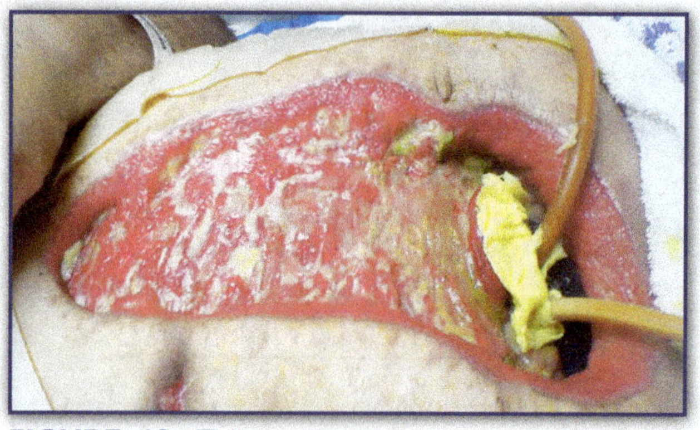

FIGURE 12. Tubing placed at mouth of ECF and covered at base with Xeroform gauze. Hydrocolloid was applied to the periwound areas for protection.

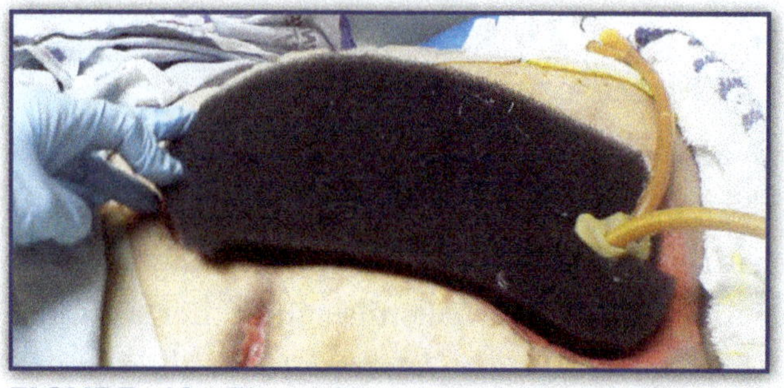

FIGURE 13. The ECF was segregated from the remainder of the wound bed using Eakin cohesive seals and stomahesive paste. A large piece of GranuFoam was cut to fit within the exposed wound bed.

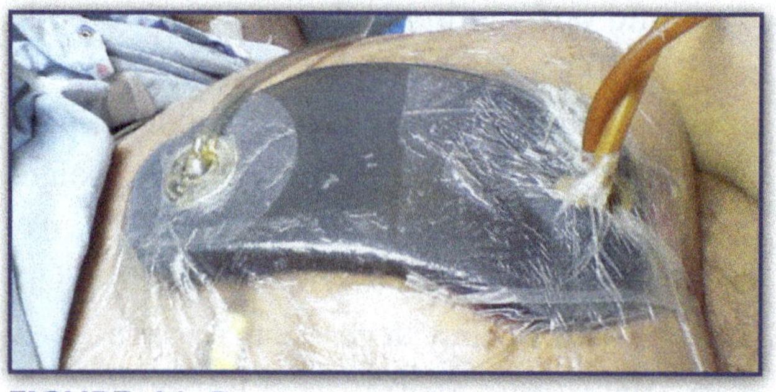

FIGURE 14. Drape was applied over the foam and around the dressing. A previous ostomy take-down site in the right upper quadrant was filled with Eakin barrier to level out the periwound surface.

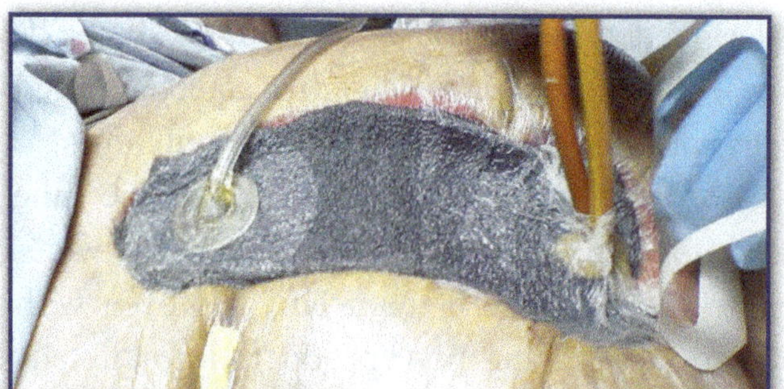

FIGURE 15. NPWT applied at 125 mmHg with good seal obtained.

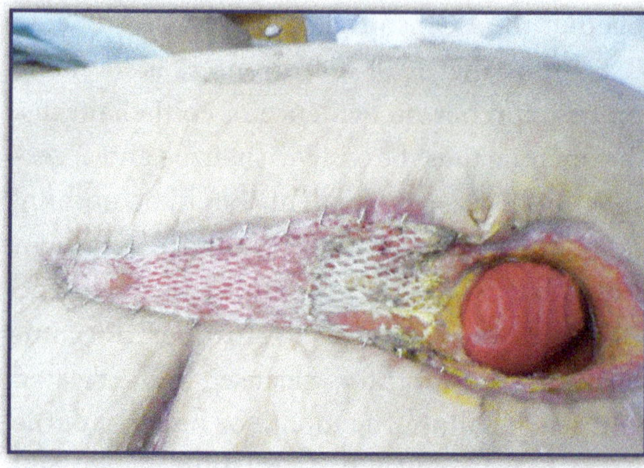

FIGURE 16. Patient was treated with NPWT for 60 days with significant reduction in wound size. He underwent a STSG to close the wound. He continued with a stomatized ECF that was managed with a wound manager.

IX. Prognosis

ECF is unfortunately a common condition in surgical units. Mortality has fallen significantly since the late 1980s, from as high as 40-65% to as low as 5-20%, largely as a result of advances in intensive care, nutritional support, antimicrobial therapy, wound care, and operative techniques. Even so, the mortality is still high, in the range of 30-35%, in patients with high-output ECFs. Once a patient develops an ECF, the morbidity associated with the surgical procedure or the primary disease increases, affecting the patient's quality of life, lengthening the hospital stay, and raising the overall treatment cost. Malnutrition, sepsis, and fluid electrolyte imbalance are the primary causes of mortality in patients with an ECF. If sepsis is not controlled, progressive deterioration occurs and patients succumb to septicemia. Other sepsis-related complications include intra-abdominal abscess, soft-tissue infection, and generalized peritonitis. However, patients with an ECF with favorable factors for spontaneous closure have a good prognosis and a lower mortality.[17-20]

A. Favorable factors for spontaneous closure

Spontaneous closure of an ECF is determined by certain anatomic factors. ECF that have a good chance of healing include the following:

- End fistulas (i.e., those arising from leakage through a duodenal stump after Pólya gastrectomy)
- Jejunal fistulas
- Colonic fistulas
- Continuity-maintained fistulas - these allow the patient to pass stool
- Small-defect fistulas
- Long-tract fistulas

In addition, a fistulous tract of more than 2 cm has a higher possibility of spontaneous closure. Spontaneous closure is also possible if the bowel-wall disruption is partial and other factors are favorable. If the disruption is complete, surgical intervention is necessary to restore intestinal continuity.[21]

B. Unfavorable factors for spontaneous closure

When an ECF is associated with adverse factors, spontaneous closure does not commonly occur and surgical intervention, despite its associated risks, is frequently required. In these patients, the outcome is less likely to be good.[21]

Factors preventing the spontaneous closure of an ECF can be remembered by using the acronym FRIEND, which represents the following:

- Foreign body
- Radiation
- Inflammation/infection/IBD
- Epithelialization of the fistula tract
- Neoplasm
- Distal obstruction – A distal obstruction prevents the spontaneous closure of an ECF, even in the presence of other favorable factors; if present, surgical intervention is needed to relieve the obstruction.[4,21]

X. Psychosocial aspects

Psychological support is sometimes overlooked but is of great importance. Patients with ECFs have usually undergone major surgery and suffered significant complications. They also face the prospect of a prolonged hospital stay. In addition, the combination of an open wound and the production of fistula effluent is likely to have a detrimental effect on body image. This, in turn, can have a detrimental impact on the patient's interpersonal relationships. Prolonged illness associated with ECF can lead to disability, loss of employment, and financial stress as well. All of these factors lead to psychological distress that must be addressed. Ascertaining that the patient has adequate social support, counseling, and resources is an important responsibility of the interdisciplinary team. Consultation with social services, psychology, and psychiatry can be helpful in ensuring that the patient's quality of life is maintained to the greatest extent possible. [6,17]

Summary

The management of ECFs can be a challenge for wound care providers and involves an understanding of the pathophysiology of the fistula as well as incorporation of key management principles. Goals of care include maintenance of quality of life, management of psychosocial concerns, addressing fluid and electrolyte as well as nutritional issues, and protecting the intact skin from damage. Small-output fistulas can be addressed with nonpouching options, while high-output fistulas will likely require a pouching or containment device or the use of NPWT. Understanding the goals of care and involving surgical expertise in a timely manner are crucial. An interdisciplinary approach is critical in providing a holistic approach to care with optimal outcomes.

Review questions

1. **Which of the following factors are associated with nonhealing ECFs?**

    a. radiation

    b neoplasm

    c. epithelialized fistula tract

    d. inflammatory bowel disease

    e. all of the above

2. **Fistuloclysis is an appropriate method of providing nutrition in which of the following?**

    a. fistula located in the distal end of the small bowel

    b unable to use parenteral nutrition

    c. obstructed bowel distal to the fistula

    d. palliative or terminal conditions

    e. both a and b

3. **Negative pressure wound therapy (NPWT)**

    a. can be used to treat acute and chronic fistulas

    b. should be used at a pressure no greater than 75 mmHg

    c. is contraindicated in patients with recent radiation

    d. all of the above

4. ***True/False.*** Goals of fistula management include skin protection, containment of effluent, maintenance of dignity, and in some cases, odor control.

5. ***True/False.*** Nonpouching options are contraindicated when ECF output is less than 100 cc in 24 hours, there are no odor issues, or if the contours of the skin prevent pouching.

ANSWERS: 1) e
2) b
3) a
4) True
5) False

References

1. Willcutts K. The art of fistuloclysis: nutritional management of enterocutaneous fistulas. Practical Gastroenterology. [Internet] 2010. Available from: https://med.virginia.edu/ginutrition/wp-content/uploads/sites/199/2014/06/WillcuttsArticle.pdf.
2. Willcutts K, Mercer D, Ziegler J. Fistuloclysis: an interprofessional approach to nourishing the fistula patient. J Wound Ostomy Continence Nurs. 2014;42(5):549-553.
3. Colwell JC, Goldberg MT, Carmel JE. Fecal and urinary diversions: management principles. Philadelphia, PA: Mosby; 2004.
4. Vikram K. Enterocutanous fistula. Medscape. [Internet] 2016. Available from: http://emedicine.medscape.com/article/1372132-overview.
5. Stein SL. Overview of enterocutaneous fistula. [Internet]. UpToDate. 2016. Available from: http://www.uptodate.com/contents/overview-of-enteric-fistulas.
6. Lloyd DAJ, Gabe SM, Windsor CJ. Nutrition and management of enterocutaneous fistula British Journal of Surgery. 2006;93:1045–1055.
7. Schecter WP. Management of enterocutaneous fistulas. Surg Clin North Am. 2011 Jun; 91(3):481-491.
8. Lee S. Surgical management of enterocutaneous fistula. [Internet] Korean J Radiol. 2012 Jan-Feb;13(suppl 1):S1-S17. Available from: http://www.ncbi.nlm.nih.gov/pmc/articles/PMC3341456/.
9. Joyce MR, Dietz DW. Management of complex gastrointestinal fistula. Curr Prob Surg. 2009 May;46(5):384-430.
10. Badrasawi M, Shahar S, Sagap I. Nutritional management in enterocutaneous fistula: what is the evidence? Malays J Med Sci. 2015 Jul-Aug;22(4):6-16.
11. Tong CY, Lim LL, Brody RA. High output enterocutaneous fistula: a literature review and a case study. Asia Pac J Clin Nutr. 2012;21(3):464-469.
12. Cawich S, McFarlane M, Mitchell D. Fistuloclysis: a novel approach to the management of enterocutaneous fistulae. The Internet Journal of Surgery. 2006;9(2). Available from: http://ispub.com/IJS/9/2/12591.
13. Chariker ME, Jeter KF, Tintle TE, Bottsford JE. Effective management of incisional and cutaneous fistula with closed suction wound drainage. Contemp Surg. 1989;34:59-63.
14. McNaughton V. Canadian Association for Enterostomal Therapy ECF Best Practice Recommendations Panel, Brown J, Hoeflok J, Martins L, McNaughton V, Nielsen EM, Thompson G, Westendorp C. Summary of best practice recommendations for management of enterocutaneous fistulae from the Canadian Association for Enterostomal Therapy ECF Best Practice Recommendations Panel. J Wound Ostomy Continence Nurs. 2010 Mar-Apr;37(2):173-184.
15. Reed T, Economan D, Wiersema-Bryant L. Colocutaneous fistula management in a dehisced wound: a case study. Ostomy Wound Manage. 2006;52(4):60-66.
16. DeLeon JM. Pressure wound therapy for the management of enterocutaneous fistula in the long term care setting. J Wound Ostomy Continence Nurs. 2013;40(5):481-488.
17. Bryant RA, Rolstad BS. Management of draining wounds and fistulas. In: Bryant RA, Nix DP, editors. Acute And Chronic Wounds: Current Management Concepts; 2012; p. 517- 533.

18. Galarza L. Enterocutaneous fistula. [Internet]. Available from: http://www.kci1.com/cs/Satellite?blobcol=urldata&blobheadername1=Content-type&blobheadername2=Content-disposition&blobheadername3=MDT-Type&blobheadervalue1=application%2Fpdf&blobheadervalue2=inline%3B+filename%3D965%252F431%252F12-054ProfEd%252BFistul%252B82113%252B6pm.pdf&blobheadervalue3=abinary%3B+charset%3DUTF-8&blobkey=id&blobtable=MungoBlobs&blobwhere=1226705658697&ssbinary=true.

19. Skovgaard R, Keiding HA. Cost-effectiveness analysis of fistula treatment in the abdominal region using a new integrated fistula and wound management system. JWOCN. 2008;35(6):592-595.

20. Hahler B, Schassberger D, Novakovic R, Lang S. Managing complex, high output enterocutaneous fistulas: a case study. Ostomy Wound Manage. [Internet]. 2009;55(10). Available from: http://www.o-wm.com/content/managing-complex-high-output-enterocutaneous-fistulas-a-case-study.

21. Dionigia G, Dionigia R, Roveraa F, Bonia L, Padalinoa P, MinojabG, Cuffarib S, Carrafiello G. Treatment of high output entero-cutaneous fistulae associated with large abdominal wall defects: single center experience. International Journal of Surgery. 2008;(6) 51–56.

22. Acelity Fistula Solutin devices. [Internet]. Available from: http://www.acelity.com/products/fistula-solution-devices.

23. Heineman JT, Garcia LJ, Obst MA, Chong HS, Langin JG, Humpal R, Pezella PA, Dries D. Collapsible enteroatmospheric fistula isolation device: a novel, simple solution to a complex problem. J American Coll Surg. 2015 Aug; 221(2): e7–e14.

Additional resources

1. Baranoski S, Ayello EA, editors. Wound care essentials practice principle, Third Edition. Lippincott Williams & Wilkins; Ambler, PA, 2012.
2. Canadian Association for Enterostomal Therapy ECF Best Practice Recommendations Panel. Best practice recommendations for management of enterocutaneous fistulae. 2009.
3. Clarke L. Caring for fungating tumors. J Wound Care. 1992;88:66-70.
4. FDA Safety Communication: Update on serious complications associated with negative pressure wound therapy systems. 2011 Feb 24.
5. Franklin C. The suction pouch for management of simple or complex enterocutaneous fistulae. JWOCN. 2010:37(4):387-392.
6. Gibbs K. Absorptive dressings: alginates and hydrofibers. In: Advances in wound care: Volume 1, 2010; p. 142-147.
7. Krasner D, editor. WoundSource 2012: The Kestrel wound product sourcebook, Fifteenth Edition. Kestrel Health Information Publishers.
8. Metcalf C. (1999). Enterocutaneous fistulae. Journal of Wound Care. 8(3):141-142.
9. Owen R, Love TP, Perez SD, Srinivasan JK, Sharma J, Pollock JD, Haack, CI, Sweeneny JR, Galloway JR. Definitive surgical treatment of enterocutaneous fistula outcomes of a 23-year experience. JAMA Surg. 2013;148(2):118-126.
10. Rolstad S, Boarini J. Principles and techniques in the use of convexity. Ostomy/Wound Management. 1996; 42(1):24-32.
11. Rowley S, Clare S, Macqueen S, Molyneux R. ANTT v2: An updated practice framework for aseptic technique. Br J Nurs. 2010;19:S5-S11.
12. Stevens P, Burden S, Delicata R, Carlson G, Lal S. Somatostatin analogues for treatment of enterocutaneous fistula. Cochrane Library. 2013 Apr. Available from: http://onlinelibrary.wiley.com/doi/10.1002/14651858.CD010489/full.
13. Willcutts K, Scarano K, Eddins CW. Ostomies and fistulas: a collaborative approach. Practical Gastroenterology. 2005 Nov:63-79.
14. Tuncel U, Turan A, Bayraktar A, Erkormaz U. Clinical experience with the use of gauze based negative pressure wound therapy. WOUNDS. 2012;24(8):227-233.
15. Wound, Ostomy and Continence Nurses Society (WOCN) Wound Committee; Association for Professionals in Infection Control and Epidemiology, Inc. (APIC) 2000 Guidelines Committee. Clean vs. sterile dressing techniques for management of chronic wounds: a fact sheet. J Wound Ostomy Continence Nurs. 2012 Mar-Apr;39(2 Suppl):S30-34.

Section 6

WOUND CARE IN DIFFERENT SETTINGS

Editor - Helen B. Gelly, MD, FUHM, FCCWS

Chapter 22

WOUND CARE IN HOSPITAL-BASED OUTPATIENT WOUND CLINICS

Michael White, MD, MMM

KEY CONCEPTS

1. Location of care can impact patient outcomes with respect to chronic wounds.
2. Dedicated comprehensive wound care centers have been shown to have a greater healing rate compared to those patients who received "fractionated care" in the community setting.
3. Given the number of diabetic patients and its impact on patient outcomes and mortality, hyperbaric oxygen therapy can have a very positive impact on patient care but rarely is what keeps an outpatient wound center "a loat" inancially in a critical access or community hospital.
4. Tertiary care centers are in a much better position to offer 24/7 hyperbaric oxygen therapy, as the mechanism to receive transfer patients is usually in place, and the required surgical services are generally established.

CONTENTS

Introduction

It is estimated that 2% of the general population of the United States suffers from a chronic wound.[1] This represents over six million people with a chronic wound, using the 2016 U.S. population data. There are multiple reasons as to why we are seeing this explosion in chronic wound sufferers, including increasing rates of obesity and diabetes and an aging population.[2] These patients are treated in a variety of clinical locations, including physician offices, long-term care settings, acute care hospitals, at-home via home-health agencies, and in specialized wound care centers. The location of care and the attitudes of the care providers towards the wounded patient can influence outcomes. In this chapter, we will examine how the above factors can be leveraged to positively to affect wound healing and will discuss the components of a comprehensive wound healing center.

Obesity and type 2 diabetes have a direct correlation. In 2014, it was estimated that 422 million persons worldwide have diabetes and that the number is expected to rise to 642 million by the year 2040.[3] It is not unexpected that the rates of obesity worldwide are also on the rise. Since 1975, obesity rates have risen 167% worldwide from 3.2% to 10.8%.[4] Many health-care providers benignly neglect or are unaware of the effects that diabetes and its complications can have on the morbidity and mortality of their patients. The diabetic patient that presents with a nonhealing ulcer has a five-year mortality rate comparable to many cancers.[5] There must be a paradigm shift in the approach to this patient, from a chronic disease to a potentially fatal complication. Cardiovascular disease is the major causal factor, and the diabetic foot ulcer should be viewed as a harbinger of increased morbidity and mortality. Additionally, it has been estimated that 30%–40% of patients with diabetic foot ulcers are not being treated according to standard evidence-based guidelines, and up to 20%–30% of patients with diabetic foot ulcers are mistreated.[6]

TABLE 1. Five-year mortality rates of various disease processes[5]

Disease Process	Five-Year Mortality Rate (percentage)
Prostate cancer	8
Breast cancer	18
Acute myocardial infarction (MI)	30
Neuropathic ulcer (DFU)	45
Neuropathic ulcer with amputation	47
Colon cancer	48
Ischemic ulcer	55
Peripheral arterial disease	64
Pancreatic cancer	97

Diabetes is only one of many contributory factors in complicated and delayed healing of chronic wounds. As our population ages, venous insufficiency, pressure injury, and the direct effect of aging also impact wound healing. Given the stark realities of the disease burden of the wounded patient and the lack of adequate care, now, more than ever, comprehensive wound care centers stand to make a direct impact not only on mortality but also on patients' quality of life.

Location of care can impact patient outcomes with respect to chronic wounds. Dedicated comprehensive wound care centers have been shown to have a greater healing rate compared to those patients who received fractionated care in the community setting.[7] Lack of clinician education can also affect wound care outcomes. It is estimated that physicians receive less than nine hours of training in wound care over their four-year medical school training.[7] Therefore, multidisciplinary teams have been shown to improve outcome in wound care and limb salvage.[1,7]

There are many important components to a successful wound center. Proper planning from wound center inception can increase the chance of the wound center succeeding in its mission. The scopes of practice of wound centers are as varied as the hospitals that start them. However, there are some common elements in planning, execution, and ongoing management of the wound center that can be applied to all hospitals. These elements include the facilities, personal finances, and, most importantly, clinical outcomes. If the hospital is diligent in planning and oversight of the wound center, then not only will the center be financially successful but also will more importantly have a positive outcome on the lives of the patients it serves.

Hospitals start outpatient wound care centers for a variety of reasons. However, proper planning, implementation, and oversight can be the difference between a center that is successful and one that becomes "something we tried in the past." Hospital margins tend to run very thin, so the decision to start a wound center should be taken with some trepidation. There are obviously financial factors involved. No hospital wants to start a program to become a loss leader. Community impact should also be taken into account. Hospitals should examine the patient population they serve and consider if a wound center would be of benefit to those patients. There are a number of questions that should be asked prior to starting a wound center. In addition to the "Five Ws," (Who, What, When Where, Why), the hospital should also ask the question of How to open a wound center.

I. Why

There are very few hospitals that do not have a ready-made population of diabetic patients. There may also be other patient populations that may be served by the wound center. There may be a hospital-owned or community long-term care center that may have a population of patients with pressure injuries. Hospitals with cancer centers may have a group of patients who are at risk for the late effects of radiation. It may also be that the hospital administration desires to get into the outpatient wound care business because administrators see it as a potentially lucrative revenue stream. The decision to start a wound center must have the support of both the administration and the medical staff, and those two groups may have very different expectations of the wound center. It is also good to have a "physician champion" who can tout the benefits of a wound center, which may help garner support on the medical staff.

A. Pre-planning steps

- Decision made by hospital to start an outpatient wound center
- Market analysis/pro forma (catchment area analysis should be positive financially)
- Physician champion/medical staff buy-in

II. Who

Various hospital stakeholders should have input into the planning phase of the wound center. Encouraging stakeholder participation builds consensus to have a smooth opening to the wound center.

Adequate staffing and management is essential for smooth, successful operation of the wound center. Staffing is generally divided into clinical and nonclinical staff. Nonclinical staff may include front office staff and program

TABLE 2. Hospital stakeholders and their role in planning the wound center

Stakeholder	Role in planning the wound center
Physician	Need physician engagement/support for the idea of the wound center; determine physician interest in staffing
CEO	Must be willing to support the idea of a wound center and be able to "sell" it to the hospital board or governing authority; must decide on reporting structure
CFO	Must allocate adequate monies towards wound center opening and operations
Patient Financial Services Director	Perform charge master changes/additions; set billing process changes and mechanism for charge capture; wound care/hyperbaric coding education
IT	Decision to use dedicated wound care electronic medical records (EMR) or use hospital legacy EMR; addition of phone/data lines; possible interfaces with wound-care-specific EMR
Marketing	Develop both internal and external marketing plans
Materials Management	Begin process of determining start-up supplies/equipment and ongoing supply needs; work with wound-care/hyperbaric-specific vendors to have materials in place for opening
Nursing	Assess needs for nursing staff; add wound-center-specific policies
Human Resources	Hiring of staff; job descriptions
Facilities Planning	Construction/remodeling of space
Environmental Maintenance	Cleaning/linen needs

manager, although the program manager may also be a clinical staff member. Clinical staff members include nurses, patient care technologists, physician staff members, medical director, safety director, and hyperbaric chamber operators. In many centers, individuals may fill one or more of the roles. As the patient volume increases, the staffing requirements will also increase in a stepwise fashion.

III. What

The scope of practice of the wound center must be defined. Hospital capabilities, physician pool, and the decision to have hyperbaric oxygen therapy must be considered. Critical access hospitals (no more than 25 beds and paid on a cost report basis) or community-based hospitals may not see enough cases to feel comfortable treating diagnoses like necrotizing fasciitis, burns, or decompression illness. Additionally, there may be services that the hospital does not offer, such as vascular surgery, orthopedic surgery, or plastic surgery. The decision to offer hyperbaric oxygen therapy should be made both clinically and financially. The decisions revolve around the types of patients seen and the hours of operation. "Outpatient only" is usually the easiest type of schedule. This helps keep personnel costs under relative control and is by and large the most common scenario. Seeing both outpatients and inpatients adds another level of complexity to the center and may require more personnel and/or a call schedule. Additionally, outpatient-only departments typically work eight to nine hours a day on weekdays, whereas 24/7 operations are just that and can carry more cost but expand what can be treated clinically.

Hyperbaric oxygen therapy is expensive with new monoplace chambers costing over $100,000. Multiplace chambers can be well over $500,000; however, there are many outlets for obtaining used equipment as well. There are also additional costs for oxygen piping and sprinklers, and a separate liquid oxygen farm may be needed. Many CEOs and CFOs look at the potential revenue to be made from hyperbarics as the main driver to offer hyperbaric medicine; however, the clinical impact should take main priority. Hyperbarics can add significant, if irregular, revenue to a hospital, but its impact on the wound healing process and amputation prevention is most important. Given the number of diabetic patients and its impact on patient outcomes and mortality, hyperbaric oxygen therapy can have a very positive impact on patient care but rarely is what keeps an outpatient wound center "afloat" financially in a critical access or community hospital. Tertiary care centers are in a much better position to offer 24/7 hyperbaric oxygen therapy, as the mechanism to receive transfer patients is usually in place, and the required surgical services are generally established.

IV. Where

The location of the wound center is driven by the scope of service, types of patients seen, hours of operation, and cost to operate. From a strictly real estate standpoint, centers located in off- or on-campus medical office buildings are cheaper to operate on a per-square-foot basis than those in the physical plant of the hospital. Centers that treat only outpatients can do well in a medical office building. Those that operate 24/7 with hyperbarics or treat inpatients should consider location in the physical plant of the hospital. Other considerations include room size, hallway size, and access to Americans with Disabilities Act (ADA)–compliant bathrooms. Many patients come in wheelchairs of varying size or on stretchers. When planning the layout of the wound center, these factors must be taken into account.

Recent changes in Federal regulations governing the development of new outpatient centers is addressed in Chapter 23: Reimbursement and Compliance Issues with Hospital Outpatient Department (HOPD)—Hospital-Based Wound Healing Centers.

V. When

The planning and implementation process can take as little as four months or up to one year. What is important is that the process must not be rushed, or the chances of success will diminish. Proper planning and a diligent implementation phase will increase the chance of operating a financially viable, clinically competent wound care center.

VI. How

The question of "how" is the most complex question to answer. Hospitals must decide if they want to open a wound center on their own, use a management company, or use an independent consultant.

All personnel should have an introductory course in wound care and/or hyperbaric medicine. These courses are offered in various forms, but hospitals are urged to make sure they are sponsored by national accrediting agencies such as the Undersea and Hyperbaric Medical Society (UHMS). It is worthwhile to send the nonclinical personnel to these courses to gain

TABLE 3. Decision Factors

Questions	Hospital Alone	Hospital and Wound Care Management Company	Hospital and Consultant
Pre-planning	Must have the resources and talent in-house for success	Generally a templated model with copious external consultants	Adds to in-house talent for the hospital; usually cheaper than a full-blown management company, but support may not be as robust
Financial	Hospital keeps (or loses) all monies; responsible for billing and coding	Fees of varying amounts with multiyear contracts that ensure the management company is paid	May be expensive in the short term but usually time limited (3–12 months)
Marketing	Hospital responsible for marketing	Contract may include some marketing materials and budget	Hospital responsible for marketing, but consultant may aid in development
Personnel	Hospital responsible for all staffing; physician staffing models vary	Some or all nonphysician personnel covered by the contract; physicians may be as well	Hospital responsible for all staffing; physician staffing models vary
Equipment	Responsible for equipment lease and/or purchases	May have some or all equipment (including equipment maintenance and repair [EMR]) provided, but it is then owned by the management company	Responsible for equipment lease and/or purchases, but consultant can aid in choosing cost-effective equipment and documentation systems

an understanding of the language and scope of wound care. There is also a need for ongoing updates and continuing education offered by a number of agencies such as the following:

- National Fire Protection Agency (NFPA)
- Undersea and Hyperbaric Medical Society (UHMS)
- American College of Hyperbaric Medicine (ACHM)
- Baromedical Nurses Association (BNA)
- National Board of Diving and Hyperbaric Medical Technology (NBDHMT)
- Wound Healing Society (WHS)
- Association for the Advancement of Wound Care (AAWC)
- National Pressure Ulcer Advisory Panel (NPUAP)

For start-up and ongoing management, there are four components to a successful wound care program: patient volume, operational efficiency, revenue cycle management, and regulatory compliance.[8] Patient volume should continue to climb each quarter and year the wound center is in operation. However, patient volume is limited by staffing models. Additionally, clinical outcomes are an important driver of volume as word of mouth and satisfied patients are the best marketing tools. Clinical outcomes cannot be stressed enough; the goal should be to obtain a 50% reduction in wound area every four weeks. If this is not happening, then those cases should be brought to an "outlier" meeting where they can be discussed. There are numerous reasons why a patient's wound is slow to heal, and trying to make sure that everything that needs to be done for the patient has been done is of paramount importance. These meetings can be an opportunity to educate the physicians and nurses and fine-tune patient care.

Operational efficiency is important for streamlining the patient evaluation and care process but also to gain financially. Once a patient is admitted to the wound care center, necessary records should be immediately available, testing and labs easily ordered, and supplies readily available to care for the patients. All wound care supplies and equipment should be evaluated for clinical efficacy and cost. It is sometimes desirable to use a more expensive product or piece of equipment if the clinical results are going to be better or the wound healed faster.

There is an old saying in medicine: "No margin, no mission." It is imperative that hospitals engage in a robust revenue cycle management program from the inception of the wound center. There must be a process to account for each bill sent out and revenue received. Denials from insurance companies must be vigorously fought with clinician engagement. Given the relatively thin margins in health care, hospitals must try to collect each dollar they are reasonably due. Coders may need specialized training in the nuances of wound care and hyperbaric medicine. Many wound-care-specific electronic health records (EHR) systems have features that can aid in revenue cycle management and coding.

Lastly, regulatory compliance must not be ignored. There are numerous organizations that publish policies that must be adhered to. Some of these organizations include the following:

- Centers for Medicare and Medicaid Services (CMS)
- Medicare Administrative Contractors (MAC)
- National Fire Protection Agency (NFPA)
- Occupational Health and Safety Agency (OSHA)
- The Joint Commission (TJC)
- State health-care authorities
- Det Norske Veritas (DNV)
- Medical societies

Attention to these factors will greatly increase the chances of implementing and running a successful wound care center. Patients will thank you for it.

Summary

In summary, wound care is a beneficial service line for many hospitals. Not only can wound care be financially viable, but also, more importantly, it can improve patients' clinical outcomes, heal chronic wounds, and prevent unnecessary amputations. The difference between having a successful wound center and a failed project is by paying careful attention to the planning and execution phases and consistently reviewing both clinical and financial metrics.

Review questions

1. **What percent of the U.S. general population suffers from a chronic wound?**

    a. 5%

    b. 10%

    c. 2%

    d. 0.5%

2. **What is the five-year mortality rate for a neuropathic ulcer?**

    a. 10%

    b. 50%

    c. 3%

    d. 45%

3. **Organizations that publish policies that directly affect outpatient wound care centers include which of the following?**

    a. Centers for Medicare and Medicaid Services (CMS)

    b. Det Norske Veritas (DNV)

    c. National Fire Protection Agency (NFPA)

    d. Medicare Administrative Contractors (MAC)

    e. all of the above

4. **It is estimated that physicians receive less than __ hours of training in wound care over their four-year medical school training.**

    a. 5

    b. 20

    c. 37

    d. 9

5. **Achieving a decrease in wound volume by 50% every __ weeks is one benchmark of adequate, effective wound healing.**

    a. 2

    b. 4

    c. 10

    d. 16

ANSWERS: 1) c
2) d
3) e
4) d
5) b

References

1. Kim P, Evans K, Steinberg J, Pollard M, Attinger C. Critical elements to building an effective wound care center. J Vasc Surg. 2013;57(6):1704-09.
2. Pruneda R, Sheffield P. Development of comprehensive wound care center. In: Sheffield P, Fife C, editors. Wound care practice. 2nd ed. Flagstaff (AZ): Best Publishing Co.; 2007. p.1107-32.
3. Shaw J, Sicree R, Zimmet P. Global estimates of the prevalence of diabetes for 2010 and 2030. Diabetes Res Clin Pract. 2010;87(1):4-14.
4. NCD Risk Factor Collaboration (NCD-RisC). Lancet. 2016;387(10026):1377-96.
5. Armstrong D, Wrobel J, Robbins J. Guest editorial: are diabetes-related wounds and amputations worse than cancer? Int Wound J. 2007;4(4):286-87.
6. Snyder R, Kirsner R, Warriner R, Lavery L, Hanft J, Sheehan P. Consensus recommendations on advancing the standard of care for treating neuropathic foot ulcers in patients with diabetes. Ostomy Wound Manage. 2010;56(Suppl 4):S1-24.
7. Ennis W, Fibeger E, Messner K, Meneses P. Wound healing outcomes: the impact of site of care and patient stratification. Wounds. 2007;19(11):286-93.
8. Fife C. Health & wellness plan for managing YOUR wound clinic. Today's Wound Clinic. 2015;9(7):10-13.

Additional resources

1. Attinger CE, Hoang H, Steinberg J, Couch K, Hubley K, Winger L, Kugler M. How to make a hospital-based wound center financially viable: the Georgetown University Hospital Model. Gynecol Oncol. 2008;111(2 Suppl):S92-97.
2. Fife C. Measuring quality in wound care. Today's Wound Clinic. 2011;5(11).
3. Fife C. Reassessing your outpatient wound clinic: building tomorrow's wound care facility today. Today's Wound Clinic. 2014;8(7):12-16.
4. Flattau A, Thompson M, Meara A. Developing and integrating a practice model of health finance reform into wound healing programs: an examination of the triple aim approach. Ostomy Wound Manage. 2013;59(10):42-51.
5. Wiersema-Bryant L et al. The outpatient wound clinic. In: Chronic wound care: the essentials: a clinical source book for healthcare professionals. HMP Communications LLC; 2014. p. 331-40.

Chapter 23

REIMBURSEMENT AND COMPLIANCE ISSUES WITH HOPD (HOSPITAL OUTPATIENT DEPARTMENT) – HOSPITAL-BASED WOUND HEALING CENTERS

Caroline E. Fife, MD

KEY CONCEPTS

1. Provider-based departments (PBDs) were created by Centers for Medicare & Medicaid Services (CMS) to manage patients who are too complicated to be cared for by their primary care physicians but not sick enough for hospitalization.

2. The cost of seeing a patient in the PBD or hospital outpatient department (service 19 or 22) is typically higher (often over 50% higher) in a physician's office because Medicare pays a hospital component as well as a physician component. PBDs are under intense scrutiny as payers question whether the added expense delivers additional value.

3. Wound centers operated as PBDs are not intended to be just simple dressing change clinics.

4. The reimbursement implications of the site of service designation are huge. It is absolutely vital that physicians use the correct place of service on claims submitted to Medicare because otherwise they can inadvertently receive overpayments and jeopardize the hospital facility fees.

5. Just like physicians, hospital outpatient departments must bill their services DAILY.

CONTENTS

Introduction

The way we deliver wound care changed in 2000 when the hospital outpatient department (HOPD) was created.[1] The Office of the Inspector General (OIG)[2] and the Medicare Evidence Development & Coverage Advisory Committee (MEDCAC)[3] have both questioned the value of the provider-based setting. As a result, reimbursement for new off-campus HOPDs has been reduced dramatically, and it is possible that the reimbursement for on-campus HOPDs will be reduced in the future. This could change the economic model for the provision of wound care services. It is important for wound care clinicians to clearly understand the federal regulations that are applicable to the site of service in which they provide services. The OIG continues its scrutiny of the HOPD[4] because compliance with the applicable regulations has been generally poor. Provider-based departments (PBDs) were created by Centers for Medicare & Medicaid Services (CMS) to manage patients who are too complicated to be cared for by their primary care physicians but not sick enough for hospitalization. What we call wound centers are actually just a small percentage of HOPDs paid under the Medicare Outpatient Prospective Payment System (OPPS). The other PBDs (e.g. emergency departments, dialysis departments, and infusion departments) care for relatively complex patients, and wound centers should care for patients with similar acuity levels. The concept is that if a patient can reasonably receive his or her chronic wound care in a physician's office, he/she simply does not need to be seen in a provider-based department.

Originally, the definition of a Medicare provider as set forth in Regulation 42 C.F.R. §413.65 included hospitals, skilled nursing facilities, and several other types of facilities. However, it was amended in 2002 to limit the provider setting to hospitals. There are very specific requirements that a hospital-based outpatient department (HOPD) must meet in order to bill as a provider-based setting. These requirements pertain to practice licensure, the integration of clinical services, financial operations, and medical records. Hospitals should verify, via an attestation, that their Medicare Administrative Contractor (MAC) agrees that their wound care HOPD meets the OPPS requirements. Hospitals are not required to submit an attestation to their MAC, but they can decide to voluntarily submit an attestation documenting that an HOPD facility meets the OPPS requirements. If their MAC agrees with the attestation, the hospital receives a letter from the MAC attesting that the hospital has permission to bill Medicare under the PBD rules. If a hospital decides to simply open a wound care department and does not go through the attestation process, the CMS may recoup overpayments if the MAC later audits the program and determines it does not meet the requirements of a PBD. The overpayment amount is the difference between the OPPS allowable rate and the Medicare Physician Fee Schedule (MPFS) allowable rate in a physician's office. According to an OIG report[2], more than three quarters of 50 hospitals reviewed had not voluntarily attested for their PBDs: these facilities may be billing Medicare improperly and may be receiving overpayments.

I. Provider-based requirements

1. **Licensure:** the HOPD and the main provider (hospital) must be operated under the same license, unless state laws prohibit this or require separate licenses.

2. **Clinical services integration:** The HOPD and the main hospital provider must have integrated clinical services evidenced by the

physician staff having clinical privileges at the main hospital. The hospital maintains the same monitoring and oversight of the HOPD as it does for any other hospital department; the medical director of the HOPD maintains the same reporting relationship with the hospital's chief medical officer as the other medical directors; medical staff committees at the hospital are responsible for medical activities in the HOPD (e.g. quality assurance, utilization review, etc.); the hospital and the HOPD have a unified retrieval system for medical records; and inpatient and outpatient services of the HOPD and the hospital are integrated, and patients have full access to all services of the hospital.

3. **Financial integration:** The hospital and the HOPD must have fully integrated financial operations.

4. **Public awareness:** The HOPD is held out to the public and other payers as part of the hospital with a shared name, websites, and other examples to show that the facility is part of the main provider.

5. **Compliance with hospital rules:** The HOPD must comply with applicable hospital health and safety rules and must also meet Medicare payment rules.

This OPPS payment is typically higher (often over 50% higher) than Medicare payment in a physician's office. When patients with chronic wounds are evaluated and managed by physicians and other qualified health-care professionals (QHPs) in PBDs, the patient and the payer receive two bills: 1) from the PBD for the component of the service related to the facility's operating costs, and 2) from the physician/QHP for the professional component of the same service. Because Medicare beneficiaries are responsible to pay 20% of all Medicare Part B allowable rates, their co-insurance payments are typically 50% or more higher when they receive wound care in PBDs than when they receive care in their physicians' offices.

II. Direct supervision

Wound centers are not intended to be dressing-change clinics. Physicians' offices can easily perform dressing changes for patients who cannot be taught to change their dressings and/or do not have caregivers who can change their dressings at home. HOPDs are expected to conduct thorough evaluations of the factors contributing to higher acuity chronic wounds and to develop and implement appropriate treatment plans, which may include procedures such as surgical debridement, total contact casting, multilayer high-compression bandage systems, negative pressure wound therapy (both disposable and durable medical equipment), cellular and/or tissue-based products for skin wounds (CTPs), hyperbaric oxygen therapy, etc.

Since the OPPS was initiated by CMS in 2000, several OPPS final rules have reiterated that direct supervision is required for all services performed in PBDs[(5)]. Direct supervision means that the MD, DPM, DO, NP, PA, or CNS must be immediately available to the PBD during all patient encounters. For wound care there are only a few services that can be provided by a nurse without the physician being directly involved in the visit: 1) application of Unna boot; 2) application of multilayer high-compression bandage system; 3) behavioral change smoking cessation 3-10 minutes; and 4) behavioral change smoking cessation >10 minutes. To provide these services, the advanced practitioner must be physically in the clinic but does not have to physically see the patient on that encounter. Remember that patients with chronic wounds are referred to wound care physicians who work in hospital-based wound care centers for excellence, that are designated as PBDs, when their wound management is beyond the expertise of their current physicians. The referring physicians and their patients expect these wound care physicians to diagnose why the patients' wounds are not healing, develop and implement appropriate care plans, and manage the patients' wounds until the patients are ready to return to their referring physicians. The hospital supplies the space, the office staff to handle scheduling/insurance benefit verification/coding/billing, the clinical staff to assist the wound care physician, the equipment and supplies, etc. Therefore, the regulations require direct supervision of PBDs by the wound care physician. The issue is not that the staff (e.g. WOCN) are not competent to manage wounds. The issue is that, from a regulatory standpoint, the patient is making a visit specifically to be seen by the wound care physician or advanced practitioner. Without the wound care professional, a patient cannot be seen in a PBD, regardless of how skilled the nurse is, or regardless of the fact that the nurse is a certified wound nurse.

III. Site of service

The OIG, the CMS, and the Medicare Payment Advisory Commission (MedPAC) continue to question the value of the higher costs in PBDs. The OIG conducted an audit of PBDs that revealed widespread disregard for the PBD billing rules. In their June 2016 report pertaining to this audit, the OIG recommended that CMS eliminate the "provider-based department" designation. The MedPAC, a nonpartisan legislative branch agency that provides Congress with analysis and policy advice on the Medicare program, also made the same recommendation. So far, the CMS has chosen not to implement the OIG and MedPAC recommendations, but reimbursement for new off-campus PBDs was reduced significantly in 2017. For the time being, it appears that wound centers will continue to exist, but there is a trend for more wound care to be provided in the private physician's office.

The reimbursement impact of site of service designation is huge. It is absolutely vital that physicians use the correct place of service on claims submitted to Medicare. On January 1, 2016, CMS began requiring physicians to use different place of service codes to distinguish between services performed at on-campus (service 22) and off-campus (service 19) hospital outpatient clinics. Off-campus outpatient departments are defined as those more than 250 yards but less than or equal to 35 miles from the main buildings of the main hospital. The on-campus versus off-campus designation is not something that can be determined by the providers. This designation must be confirmed by CMS through a letter of attestation. When physicians provide patient care in their private offices, they would bill site of service 11. If a physician providing services in the outpatient wound center (site of service 19/22) puts site of service 11 on a claim, he or she is telling Medicare that the hospital is actually a private office. Because the hospital provides the wound care PBD space, the nurses, the supplies, and all the overhead, CMS pays wound care physicians less for most of the services and procedures provided in a PBD (service 19 or 22) than in their offices (service 11). If the wound care physicians perform wound care in their own offices, they personally incur the additional expense associated with providing space, staff, supplies, and overhead. Therefore, if the wound care physician working in place of service 19 or 22 reports place of service 11 on his or her claim, two problems result:

1. The wound care physician is overpaid by Medicare, and that constitutes Medicare fraud due to improper billing – even if the provider did it unknowingly.

2. The wound care physician jeopardizes the hospital's payment because place of service 11 on the professional claim form tells the payer that the work was performed in a private office – not in a wound care PBD as was reported by the hospital. One of the requirements for the hospital to bill under OPPS is that the hospital MUST ensure that all the wound care physicians report place of service 19 or 22 on their claims. Hospital wound care PBD program directors must ensure that the physicians' claims report the correct place of service (19 or 22). In fact, that is part of the attestation process allowing the hospital to bill under the OPPS.

IV. Daily billing versus monthly billing

Hospitals often have little or no understanding of the way outpatient billing works. Because hospitals primarily bill for inpatient services, they assume that outpatient billing works the same way and that they can bill for services monthly.[6] This is not the way that physicians bill for services, and it is not the way that outpatient clinics bill for services. Hospital outpatients must bill their services DAILY, per encounter. Remember that PBD status indicators and National Correct Coding Initiative (NCCI) edits are typically enforced per claim.[7] Therefore, if two or more procedures were performed at different encounters but submitted on the same claim, the status indicators or NCCI edits may cause payment for some of the procedures to be denied. If the PBD had submitted separate claims, each of the procedures would probably have been paid. Imagine only being reimbursed for one procedure per month, no matter how many procedures were reported on the claim. That is what happens to hospital-based outpatient departments that bill hyperbaric oxygen therapy using serial (monthly) billing. One hyperbaric treatment per month is paid.

The regulations that govern the hospital-based outpatient department are complicated, and the billing rules are arcane. The stakes are high. Mistakes in billing and coding can cost millions of dollars, and the legal ramifications go far beyond monetary concerns. However, the need for advanced wound care services has never been greater. Wound care is effectively provided in long-term care facilities, nursing homes, and other sites of care. It is likely that the financial pressures of healthcare reform will induce changes in the delivery of wound care services as payment shifts away from volume toward a system based on value.

Summary

Since 2000 when CMS created HOPDs, the majority of wound care services have been delivered in hospital-based outpatient departments, which are either on-campus (250 yards or less from the main campus) or off-campus. In these settings, care is provided incident to the supervision of an advanced practitioner (e.g. MD, NP), and the advanced practitioner must be present in the department for services to be rendered. Medicare pays both a facility fee and a physician's fee for patient care, but there is considerable debate whether the additional cost incurred in the HOPD provides additional value to Medicare beneficiaries. The specific site of service (e.g. on-campus, off-campus, doctor's office) must be designated on claim forms using the proper numeric code because reimbursement for both the hospital and the practitioner may vary by site of service.

Cost pressures have led to a dramatic reduction in facility reimbursement for off-campus departments. Hospitals are not required to but are encouraged to request a letter of attestation from CMS verifying that they are able to bill as an on-campus provider-based department to ensure that in case of an audit, their facility fees will not be jeopardized. Hospitals should verify that practitioners have the correct site of service on their claim forms. Practitioners providing care in the HOPD but listing site of service 11 (doctor's office) on their claim forms are jeopardizing the hospital facility fees.

HOPDs exist to care for patients who are too ill to be seen in a doctor's office. Poor documentation practices that fail to represent all the comorbid conditions to justify care in the HOPD, failure to have the advanced practitioner in attendance or to provide documentation of such, and failure to meet all the other requirements of provider-based billing have brought the scrutiny of the OIG on wound centers. A transition of wound care to the doctor's office or other freestanding departments is possible in the future.

Review questions

1. **For a hospital wound center to charge a facility fee, which of the following are required?**

    a. The advanced practitioner who is responsible for the patient's care must have hospital privileges at the main hospital.

    b. The clinic has to be 250 yards or less from the main campus.

    c. The wound center's medical records have to co-exist with the hospital's medical records.

    d. There has to be a sign in the clinic stating that it is a hospital entity.

    e. all of the above

2. **If the advanced practitioner working in the on-campus hospital-based outpatient department (site of service 22) lists site of service 11 (doctor's office) on his or her claim forms, what may be the result?**

    a. The practitioner is likely being systematically overpaid for debridements, since those are paid at a higher rate in site of service 11.

    b. Per the False Claims Act (FCA), which makes keeping overpayments a crime, the practitioner will likely need to self-report all the overpayments and pay them all back.

    c. The practitioner is jeopardizing the hospital facility fees because he or she is telling CMS that the hospital clinic is actually his or her private office.

    d. all of the above

3. **Hospital-based outpatient wound centers provide services under the *direct supervision* of an advanced practitioner (e.g. MD, DPM, DO, NP, PA, or CNS). Which of the following scenarios is <u>NOT acceptable</u>?**

    a. An RN changes an Unna boot on an established patient as ordered by the MD who is in the department but does not go into the room to see the patient.

    b. A certified wound and ostomy continence nurse (CWOCN) sees an established wound center patient for a NPWT dressing change when the doctor is home with the flu.

    c. An NP performs an initial visit on a new patient with a pressure ulcer.

    d. The MD trained in HBO_2 therapy evaluates a hyperbaric patient prior to starting HBO_2 therapy and then is down the hall (but in the department) seeing wound care follow-ups while HBO_2 therapy is being administered.

4. ***True/False.*** A letter of attestation as an on-campus provider-based department is required in order to bill a facility fee.

5. ***True/False.*** Unlike inpatient billing, hospital *outpatient* charges must be billed daily, just like physician billing, if hospitals wish to be able to collect on the expensive advanced therapeutics they provide.

ANSWERS: 1) e
2) d
3) b
4) False
5) True

References

1. Medicare prospective payment system for hospital outpatient departments [Internet]. Washington (DC): Federal Register; 2000 [cited 2017 July 16]. 18450-18451. Available from: https://www.gpo.gov/fdsys/pkg/FR-2000-04-07/pdf/00-8215.pdf.
2. CMS is taking steps to improve oversight of provider-based facilities, but vulnerabilities remain [Internet]. Washington (DC): Department of Health and Human Services (US), Office of Inspector General. Available from: https://oig.hhs.gov/oei/reports/oei-04-12-00380.pdf.
3. 2014 MedPAC Report to Congress [Internet]. [cited 2017 July 16]. Available from: http://www.medpac.gov/docs/default-source/reports/mar14_entirereport.pdf.
4. 2017 OIG Work Plan [Internet]. Washington (DC): Department of Health and Human Services (US), Office of Inspector General [cited 2017 July 16]. Available from: https://oig.hhs.gov/reports-and-publications/archives/workplan/2017/hhs%20oig%20work%20plan%202017.pdf.
5. 2017 Federal Register OPPS [Internet]. [Washington (DC). Available from: https://www.federalregister.gov/documents/2016/11/14/2016-26515/medicare-program-hospital-outpatient-prospective-payment-and-ambulatory-surgical-center-payment?linkId=31128855.
6. Turner T. Work that happens before the patient is seen: the chargemaster and the billing cycle. Today's Wound Clinic. 2011;5(2). Available from: http://www.todayswoundclinic.com/work-happens-patient-seen-chargemaster-and-billing-cycle.
7. National correct coding initiative edits [Internet]. Baltimore: U.S. Centers for Medicare & Medicaid Services [cited 2017 July 16]. Available from: https://www.cms.gov/Medicare/Coding/NationalCorrectCodInitEd/index.html?redirect=/NationalCorrectCodinitEd/.

Chapter 24

WOUND CARE AND HYPERBARIC OXYGEN THERAPY IN THE PHYSICIAN'S OFFICE

Helen B. Gelly, MD, FUHM, FCCWS

KEY CONCEPTS

1. Almost 89% of hyperbaric treatments were delivered in an outpatient hospital setting in 2014 (Medicare claims data).
2. Almost 6% of hyperbaric treatments were delivered in a physician office setting in 2014 (Medicare claims data).
3. The provision of wound care in the physician office is hampered by the lack of CPT codes that reflect the inherently higher cost of providing service to the wound care patient.
4. Safety concerns are pre-eminent in the establishment of any hyperbaric facility, and this does not change in the office-based hyperbaric center.
5. An experienced hyperbaric physician with an extensive familiarity with safety guidelines is also a necessary component of a safe and well-run program.

CONTENTS

Introduction

Provision of outpatient wound care services in the office setting was *de rigueur* prior to the advent of payment for outpatient hospital-based services in 2000. In that year, the Centers for Medicare & Medicaid Services (CMS) published new regulatory guidelines for outpatient hospital-based services, the Medicare Outpatient Prospective Payment System (OPPS). The impetus behind this change was to provide a platform for the provision of complex services as an outpatient, thereby reducing inpatient hospitalizations. In order to facilitate this, a facility charge was created to reflect the cost of providing these services in the hospital outpatient department (HOPD) setting, with a commensurate reduction in the reimbursement to physicians. Since the physician was not providing the bricks and mortar, or the staff and supplies, reimbursement is based on their "work."

This change in the formula for reimbursement resulted in an explosion of outpatient service lines, including wound care and hyperbaric oxygen therapy. The establishment of a "facility charge" for the services that were historically provided by physicians' offices has resulted in an increased cost to the patient. The original intent was to use this setting to provide care to patients who were too sick to be seen in the private doctor's office, but whose acuity did not warrant admission. It is fair to say that the acuity level of most patients treated in outpatient wound centers do not meet this definition. As a result, procedures that were historically provided in the physicians' setting for a global fee are now being delivered in an HOPD, many times at a much higher cost to the patient as well as to Medicare.

I. Medicare Part B utilization data for 99183

Analysis of Medicare Part B claims in 2014 for 99183 (supervision of hyperbaric oxygen therapy by a physician or other qualified health-care provider) reveals that almost 89% of hyperbaric treatments were delivered in an outpatient hospital setting. This reflected almost 598,000 treatments. Claims from the office setting were about 6% (representing about 40,000 treatments), which had remained essentially unchanged for the previous few years.

The Medicare Evidence Development & Coverage Advisory Committee (MEDCAC) has been advocating for "site neutrality" for a number of years, and the Medicare Access and CHIP Reauthorization Act (MACRA) of 2015 has taken the first step toward changing the payment formula, by making it more difficult for hospitals to open new HOPD that are not on the main hospital campus.

II. Regulatory landscape

Full MACRA implementation will reduce the number of HOPD that are opening in the future. In 2015, CMS made 99183 (supervision of hyperbaric oxygen therapy by a physician or other qualified health-care provider) equivalent in payment regardless of the site of service. In order to compensate for the removal of the practice component, CMS deleted the OPPS charge of C1300 (facility charge for 30-minute segments of hyperbaric oxygen therapy) and replaced it with G0277, a code that may be billed across all lines of service, including the physician's office . The relative reimbursement for G0277 is considerably less in the office setting (about 60% of the OPPS rate). This raises concern about the potential for a reduction in reimbursement across the board, especially in hospital departments that are physically remote from the main campus, which do not treat inpatients, the critically ill, or who do not take calls 24/7. The factors that differentiate outpatient hospital or provider-based reimbursement are being scrutinized by CMS as a cost-saving measure that will have impact on the provision of wound care and hyperbaric services.

The provision of wound care in the physician office is hampered by the lack of CPT codes that reflect the inherently higher cost of providing service to the wound care patient. More of our patients are elderly, more have significant disabilities that make the provision of care more challenging, and the level of nursing care (WOCN) makes the cost per encounter higher than in a primary care office. Additionally, the cost of "standard" wound dressings is not well accounted for in the global cost, as more expensive specialty dressings have become "standard." One wonders if the long-held belief that wet-to-dry dressings are the best for all wound types [(1)] is based on monetary considerations when the surgical procedure is covered by a 90-day global period, and all dressing changes in the surgeon's office are "free"?

III. Clinical requirements for an effective wound care center: site of service neutral

The elements that are required to optimize the care of complex wound care patients do not change when the site of service changes. Elements that have been outlined with respect to outpatient hospital wound care departments[(2)] such as a multidisciplinary team including podiatrists, vascular surgeons, nutritionists, diabetic educators amongst many others, specialized nursing care, and advanced wound care modalities are also available in the office setting. There are additional needs that must be addressed when the convenience of a hospital-based outpatient department is not available; however, these are not much different than the challenges faced by physically remote HOPDs.

Vascular screening needs to be available on a same-day basis, as well as laboratory services and access to advanced modalities. It is essential for the organizational structure that these relationships be developed so that patient care is not hampered by delays in access. Anticipatory discussions with varied providers establish the necessary protocols for structured and time-sensitive access to needed modalities.

Additional care must be taken to design an office space that can accommodate the stretcher patient and the wheelchair patient, as well as the obese patient with mobility issues. Podiatric chairs and their bariatric counterparts must be accommodated as well as lifts that allow for ease of transfer for these patients. Universal precautions must be available in each examination room, and the disposal of contaminated dressings should be appropriately addressed. If it is impossible to accommodate these patients with special needs, then the range and scope of care will need to be narrowed and will result in the loss of patient referrals.

IV. The hyperbaric patient in the office setting

The treatment of patients with hyperbaric therapy in the office setting is not a new concept, as such practices have been in existence since at least 1993. However, there is a perception in the hyperbaric medical community that such practices are somehow less than an equivalent HOPD. The establishment of an office-based hyperbaric therapy practice must be conceived as the equivalent of the HOPD.

The majority of hospital-based hyperbaric facilities that have been initiated in the past decade not only occupy the same building as private physician offices, but are virtually indistinguishable from a doctor's office, both in physical appearance and in hours of operation. In many cases, the difference between the HOPD hyperbaric facility and the private office hyperbaric facility may be only that of classification.

Safety concerns are preeminent in the establishment of any hyperbaric facility, and this does not change in the office-based hyperbaric center. The center must comply with all NFPA guidelines at the time of construction and maintain the equipment on an annual basis with trained and certified technicians. It is imperative that no "short-cuts" are taken when safety is the overriding objective.

In the United States, the most recent and tragic clinical hyperbaric fire occurred in Florida in 2009. When the causative factors were analyzed, they highlighted the importance of regular and appropriate maintenance of all equipment, attention to line-of-sight observation by qualified hyperbaric technicians/nurses, and the necessity of a culture of safety to prevent such occurrences. The UHMS has established an accreditation program that includes nonhospital hyperbaric programs and a number of such programs have established and maintained accreditation for decades.[3] This process is important in the establishment and maintenance of high quality hyperbaric oxygen therapy programs that are not hospital affiliated. In fact, UHMS accreditation has been made a prerequisite for Medicaid payment, regardless of location, for at least one state.[4] This accreditation process, with its focus on equipment maintenance and upkeep, continued safety drills and training, and appropriate and continued education for all provider levels, is an excellent mechanism for ensuring the best care of the hyperbaric patient regardless of venue.

V. Managing the wound care/ hyperbaric patient in the office setting

The management of the patient in the office setting is much like the management of a similar patient in the HOPD setting. However, the provision of service may have some subtle differences due to the cost structure. When CMS decided to bundle cellular and or tissue-based products (CTP) into a high-cost and low-cost reimbursement, they excluded the physician fee schedule from this bundle. Likewise, there is no concomitant facility fee for the visit, and the average 28% increase in physician reimbursement for many CPT codes may not reflect the cost of providing the service. It is imperative that the physician who is contemplating an office-based wound care practice be cognizant of the regulatory and reimbursement environment at the time of decision making and be aware of changes as they occur. This entails an ongoing familiarity with changing governmental guidelines and is best achieved by subscribing to various trade journals and attending national educational meetings and seminars.

Electronic health records that are specifically designed for the hyperbaric and wound care space are readily available, and the importance of their use cannot be over emphasized. Reviews and requests for medical records by insurers are becoming more common, and an appropriate and easily understood medical record is extremely helpful in the review process. Additionally, the ability to participate in quality measure reporting is becoming more integral in the payment process of both governmental and commercial plans, and this is facilitated by participation in a certified registry for reporting.

The mix of commercial, private pay, and governmental plans that the office chooses to participate with will impact the financial feasibility of the practice. Many commercial plans do not reimburse a facility fee; however, other CPT codes can be negotiated to reflect the cost of care for these patients. The rule of thumb is that the payer mix should be approximately 50/50 between commercial plans and Medicare/ Medicaid to make the practice viable.

VI. Licensing requirements

Although licensing requirements are different in each state, and some states require clinics be licensed[5] to provide hyperbaric and wound care services, these are the exception. Most states do not require special permission to open a hyperbaric and wound care center, although the cost of the equipment and buildout may trigger the requirement for a certificate of need in some jurisdictions. However, the requirement of doing chamber side blood glucose monitoring necessitates the request for a Clinical Laboratory Improvement Amendments (CLIA)[6] certificate of waiver.[7] This will allow performing finger stick blood sugars in compliance with federal statute.

VII. Cost to the patient

Due to the provider-based status of HOPD, the patient and Medicare typically pays two bills, one for the physician and one for the facility charge. Although the physician reimbursement is approximately 28% less than if the same service was provided in an office setting, the facility fee typically exceeds the nonfacility physician fee, making the entire encounter more costly. The patient is faced with two copayments, rather than one. The dramatic increase in hospital acquisition of physician practices, and their subsequent conversion to outpatient departments has resulted in the passage of the Bipartisan Budget Act of 2015[8] that includes Section 603 which addresses the question of site neutrality for some noncampus-based outpatient departments.

The issue becomes more relevant to patients with commercial insurance, as many plans do not cover the outpatient hospital facility fee, and the patient remains responsible for the charges. Rice et al.[9] examined the charges generated by patients with diabetic foot ulcers (DFU) in the year prior to and then after the development of the ulcer. Examining all-cause medical costs, the Medicare DFU patients averaged $28,031 vs. $26,881 in commercial DFU patients. However, the outpatient/physician charges differed significantly, $8,418 (Medicare) vs. $4,888 (commercial). As the numbers of patients "shopping" for best pricing for their care increases, freestanding offices may provide more cost-effective care.

The implementation of the Merit Based Incentive Program (MIPS) has introduced another dimension of complexity to the payment formula. Quality reporting will be publically available and a metric that patients may turn to when choosing providers. Advanced practitioners in private practice have been more engaged in the quality reporting required MIPS, perhaps because they are entirely dependent on Medicare Part B payments for economic survival and because they control the data in their electronic health records. Hyperbaric and wound care relevant quality measures (available through the US Wound Registry) are allowing practitioners in the private setting to demonstrate and publicly report their commitment to high quality, evidence-based care while many hospital-based practitioners are struggling to do so. The financial implications could be profound for practitioners that practice in a system that does not facilitate specialty specific quality data.

Summary

The provision of hyperbaric and wound care services in the nonhospital affiliated or office setting is financially viable and possible with meticulous attention and financial oversight. A market analysis will provide much needed information about the payer mix and the viability of the services rendered. An aggressive marketing campaign to acquaint referring physicians of the scope of services available and the presence of a physician champion in the office are invaluable to the success of an office-based practice. An experienced hyperbaric physician with an extensive familiarity with safety guidelines is also a necessary component of a safe and well-run program. Although it requires more hands-on work and commitment, the practice of hyperbaric medicine and wound care in the private setting can be rewarding both professionally and financially.

Review questions

1. **Hospital-based outpatient services were initially established to provide:**

    a. complex services that would allow for earlier inpatient discharges

    b. an easy way for hospitals to make additional revenue

    c. the same level of care as a physician office based practice

    d. all of the above

2. **The components of the physician payment system include:**

    a. work RVUs

    b. practice expense RVU

    c. malpractice expense RVU

    d. all of the above

3. **The explosion of HOPDs and rising costs have captured the attention of CMS. One of the remedies to this increase in utilization is:**

    a. make it easier to open a HOPD

    b. make it harder to open HOPD that are not on the hospital campus

    c. make payments for similar service site neutral

    d. both c and d

4. ***True/False.*** In office based hyperbaric oxygen centers, NFPA-99 hyperbaric facilities guidelines do not apply.

5. ***True/False.*** UHMS accreditation is limited to hospital-based programs and there are NO non-hospital or freestanding centers accredited.

ANSWERS: 1) a
2) d
3) d
4) False
5) False

References

1. Armstrong MH et al. Wet to dry gauze dressings: fact and fiction. Wounds. 2004;16(2).
2. Kim PJ et al. J Vasc Surg. 2013;57:1703-09.
3. Undersea & Hyperbaric Medical Society [Internet]. North Palm Beach (FL): Undersea & Hyperbaric Medical Society. Accredited facilities. Available from: https://www.uhms.org/accredited-facilities.html.
4. Workman WT. Clinical hyperbaric facility accreditation – is the juice worth the squeeze? Today's Wound Clinic. 2008 Fall;2(4).
5. Florida Agency for Health Care Administration [Internet]. Florida Agency for Health Care Administration. Health care clinics. Available from: http://www.fdhc.state.fl.us/mchq/health_facility_regulation/healthcareclinic/index.shtml.
6. CMS.gov: Centers for Medicare & Medicaid Services [Internet]. U.S. Department of Health & Human Services, Centers for Medicare & Medicaid Services. Clinical Laboratory Improvement Amendments (CLIA). Available from: https://www.cms.gov/Regulations-and-Guidance/Legislation/CLIA/index.html?redirect=/clia/.
7. CMS.gov: Centers for Medicare & Medicaid Services [Internet]. U.S. Department of Health & Human Services, Centers for Medicare & Medicaid Services. Certificate of Waiver Laboratory Project. Available from: https://www.cms.gov/regulations-and-guidance/legislation/clia/certificate_of_-waiver_laboratory_project.html.
8. CONGRESS.GOV [Internet]. U.S. Library of Congress. H.R. 1314 – Bipartisan Budget Act of 2015. Available from: https://www.congress.gov/bill/114th-congress/house-bill/1314/text.
9. Rice JB, Desai U, Cummings AKG, Birnbaum HG, Skornicki M, Parsons N. Burden of diabetic foot ulcers for medicare and private insurers. Diabetes Care. 2014;37:651-58.

Chapter 25

WOUND CARE IN THE ACUTE LONG-TERM CARE HOSPITAL

David A. Johnson, MD, FAAFP, CWSP
Jaime Wise, MD, CWSP
Pedram Zendehrouh, MD, PhD, FACS

KEY CONCEPTS

1. The long-term acute-care hospital (LTCH) has evolved as an important care setting for medically complex patients after acute hospital stay with ongoing nursing needs, patients in need of extensive rehab, or patients in need of medical therapies that cannot be delivered in the outpatient setting.

2. Certain patients with acute or chronic wounds benefit from long-term acute care due to the potential threat to life and limb requiring this higher level of continued medical management.

CONTENTS

Introduction

Chronic wounds are often the manifestation of uncontrolled, unmanaged, comorbid medical conditions. The successful evaluation and management of such wounds depend on the ability of the wound care practitioner to diagnose and treat these comorbid conditions. Many wound patients suffer from acute and chronic illnesses and complex wounds that cannot be adequately treated in the outpatient setting and require hospitalization. Examples include wounds with overwhelming infection, osteomyelitis, and severe protein and calorie malnutrition. Complicated or infected surgical wounds may also require a higher level of care.

Acutely ill and worsening patients are frequently admitted to the local, acute-care hospital for their initial evaluation and management. Due to the nature and severity of some wounds, and their associated comorbidities, acute hospital-level care may still be necessary after discharge from the short-term, acute-care setting. To respond to this need for ongoing higher acuity, intensive-level care, there has been a great deal of growth in the availability of long-term acute-care hospitals (LTCHs). Between 1993 and December 2005, the number of LTCHs grew from 108 to 383.[1]

The long-term acute-care hospital is certified as any other acute-care hospital with one notable difference. LTCHs are unique in that the definition of their patient population is based on length of stay rather than diagnosis or intensity of care. Patients admitted to an LTCH stay, on average, more than 25 days. The types of patients treated in the LTCH are usually medically complex with ongoing nursing needs, patients in need of extensive rehab, or patients in need of medical therapies that cannot be delivered in the outpatient setting.[1] The LTCH serves a distinct role in the continuum of care of the patient compared to the skilled nursing facility (SNF). Patients that are discharged to a SNF have lower acuity needs compared to the LTCH but still require skilled level of care for comorbidities, skilled nursing observation and evaluation of wounds, prescription management, and consideration for psychosocial circumstances before outpatient settings are appropriate.

I. The wound patient in the LTCH

Wound management is a complex process that requires a collaborative multidisciplinary approach to diagnosis and treatment to promote timely wound healing and minimize complications. Certain patients with acute or chronic wounds benefit from long-term acute care due to the potential threat to life and limb requiring this higher level of continued medical management.

II. Case study

A 72-year-old female has a history of uncontrolled diabetes peripheral vascular disease and amputation of her right second toe due to osteomyelitis. In May 2015, she had an ingrown toenail removed from her right great toe. The wound became gangrenous and she underwent amputation of the proximal and distal phalanx of the right great toe in June 2015. The patient was discharged home with negative pressure wound therapy and home health three times per week to manage the negative pressure dressing. The wound failed to close during six weeks of outpatient treatment and she presented to the emergency room with cellulitis of the right foot with an abscess of the plantar fascia.

Past medical history: Uncontrolled diabetes with HbA1c of 10.5, coronary artery disease with a history of myocardial infarction in March

2015, angioplasty with stent placement in the left anterior descending and circumflex arteries, healed pelvic fracture from a previous fall, and lack of follow-up with her primary care provider to manage her chronic medical conditions.

Social history: She lives with her husband in their private residence. She is ambulatory with assist only. Her husband prepares the meals but serves only high-carbohydrate/low-protein, nutritionally poor food. She eats one to two meals per day. She denies alcohol or tobacco use.

She was admitted to the acute-care hospital (ACH), where the wound care team was consulted. Her acute-care hospital admission revealed the following diagnoses:

1. Cellulitis of the right foot and abscess involving the deep plantar support structures of the foot
2. Critical limb ischemia with complete occlusion of the anterior tibial artery, hemodynamically significant stenosis of the popliteal and peroneal arteries
3. Uncontrolled diabetes with Hemoglobin A1c of 11.1
4. Protein calorie malnutrition
5. Poor insight into her chronic medical conditions and a low global assessment of function

In her acute hospitalization, infectious disease was consulted and the patient was started on a six-week course of antibiotic therapy. She underwent angioplasty of the right popliteal and peroneal arteries. She then underwent debridement of the abscess and necrotic tissue of the plantar surface of the right foot.

She was then admitted to the local long-term acute-care hospital (LTCH) under the criteria of necrotic wound with an ongoing infectious disease process requiring prolonged treatment. She initially received ongoing antibiotic therapy with negative pressure wound therapy, nutrition consultation and support, aggressive blood sugar management with diabetic teaching, and serial debridements of necrotic tissue.

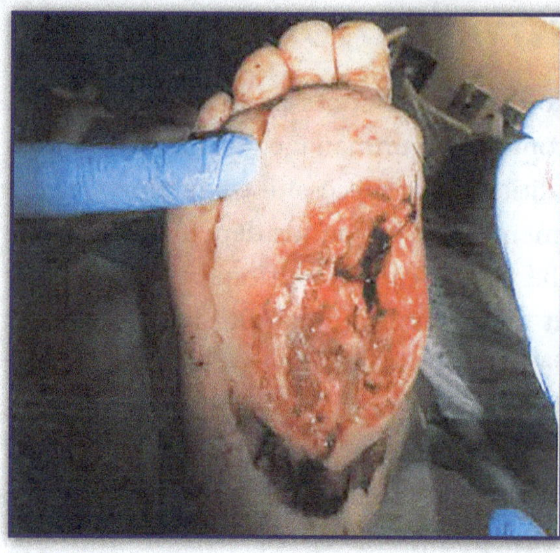

FIGURE 1. She was admitted to a long-term acute-care hospital (LTCH) under criteria of necrotic wound with ongoing infectious disease process requiring prolonged treatment.
Courtesy of David A. Johnson, MD

Despite three additional weeks of negative pressure wound therapy of the wound and treatment of her comorbidities, she suffered further necrosis of the wound base and margins

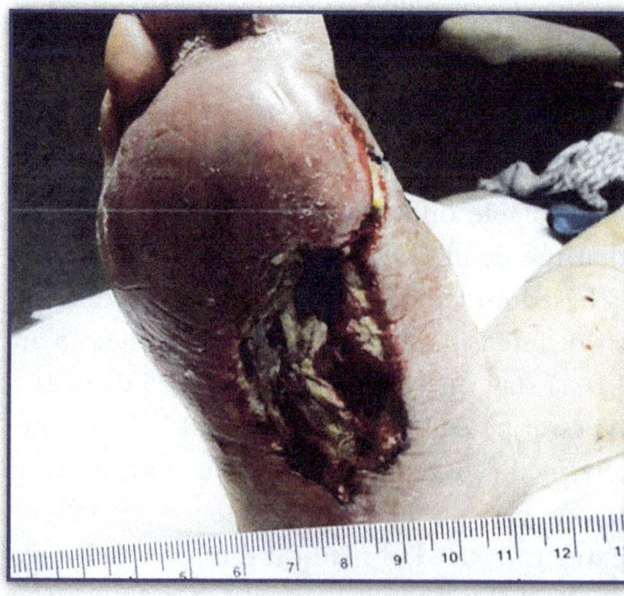

FIGURE 2. Inpatient HBO_2 therapy was initiated.
Courtesy of David A. Johnson, MD

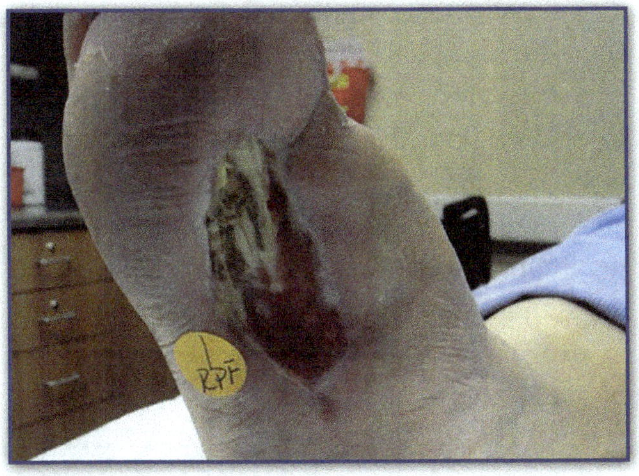

FIGURE 3. Wound shows significant improvement after five weeks in long-term acute-care hospital.
Courtesy of David A. Johnson, MD

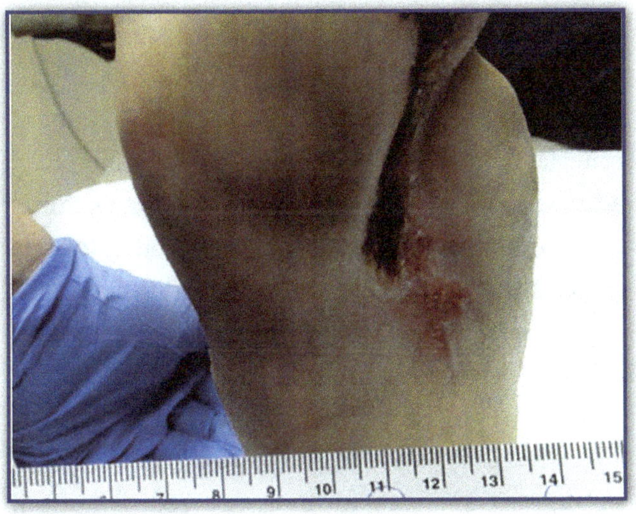

FIGURE 4. She was able to transition home
Courtesy of David A. Johnson, MD

requiring further debridement, and an amputation was considered.

Transcutaneous oxygen measurement of the foot demonstrated that the oxygenation of the foot was suboptimal to achieve wound healing but responsive to oxygen challenge. Inpatient hyperbaric oxygen therapy (HBO_2 therapy) was initiated, and an in-chamber $TcPO_2$ was 425 mmHg, which indicated a moderate to good response to HBO_2 therapy. This represents adequate oxygenation during treatment, an indication supporting potential healing.[2]

Her wound showed signs of significant improvement after five weeks in the long-term acute-care hospital. With the help of nutritional support, social services, and diabetes education, she was able to transition to her own home with ongoing management of her wound. She continued negative pressure wound therapy, HBO_2 therapy, and antibiotic therapy in the outpatient wound care center.

III. LTCH as a resource

Many wound care patients suffer from a complex interplay of competing medical conditions, any one of which is sufficient to impede wound healing. Some of these factors are unmodifiable chronic medical conditions such as end-stage renal disease or microvascular disease. Certain conditions, if addressed adequately, can mean the difference between healing a wound versus limb loss or death. These modifiable chronic conditions can be complicated by a patient's psychological, social, financial, or familial circumstances. For example, a paraplegic patient with a Stage 4 pressure ulcer who lives independently and is unable to offload effectively through the course of his activities of daily living may require LTCH level care. Access to an LTCH can be an important tool for the treatment of the most complicated wound care patients.

It is important, however, to make a distinction between the patient who would benefit from services in the LTCH as opposed to the patient who is appropriate for acute hospital care or outpatient care. In order to take advantage of this resource, it is important for the wound care specialist to be familiar with the admission and treatment criteria of the LTCH.

IV. LTCH criteria

There are some intensive treatment plans and modalities, which are easily managed out of the hospital through the outpatient, advanced wound care center. However, some patients would be better served by receiving these therapies and other treatments in an acute hospital setting. These patients are identified by criteria, which take into account the severity of illness as well as the intensity of service. InterQual Level of Care Criteria[3] and the National Association of Long Term Hospitals (NALTH) admission criteria are generally accepted standards for determining which patients are appropriate for the level of service and length of stay that can be provided in the long-term acute-care hospital.

Medicare defines long-term care hospitals as certified acute-care hospitals that treat patients hospitalized on average more than 25 days.[1] The typical patient is admitted following a stay at an acute-care hospital.[4] Specific admission criteria have not yet been established by CMS. Beyond that basic definition, there is much variation of services provided by individual LTCHs. Criteria for admission and treatment are determined by Quality Improvement Organizations (QIOs), which are authorized to define whether or not the care in an LTCH is appropriate or could be provided in a more cost-effective way.[1] Although QIOs are not directed to use any particular standardized criteria, Medicare and most private industry-sponsored QIOs utilize InterQual admission and treatment criteria.[1] Recommended guidelines, currently used by multiple private insurers, define LTCH admissions for wound care patients under certain clinical indications and treatment criteria. Clinically, a patient with an infected ulcer, a diabetic ulcer, osteomyelitis or complex ostomy care would be considered for admission as long as he or she was suffering with one additional medical condition requiring ongoing care. Admission criteria for wound care treatment include higher complexity wound care with advanced modalities, advanced dressings and specialty equipment such as support surfaces for pressure redistribution. Additionally, a wound care specialist would manage and direct the treatment care plan and perform procedures as indicated. The coexisting medical condition(s) require ongoing assessments,

TABLE 1. General wound categories for admission

Infected wounds requiring prolonged treatment
Complex ostomy or fistula patients
Dehisced surgical wounds
Demarcating vascular wounds
Diabetic ulcers
Full thickness wounds
Infected wounds
Morbid obesity with wounds requiring special equipment
Necrotic wounds
Open abdominal wounds
Open traumatic or amputation wounds
Postoperative grafts or flaps
Stage III or IV pressure ulcers
Third-degree burns
Wounds with underlying vasculitis
Autoimmune wounds
Oncologic wounds

TABLE 2. Treatment criteria

One concurrent medical condition requiring active intervention
Complex wound care requiring at least two interventions
Wound care clinician directing care and regular assessment
Acuity requiring acute level care: • Frequent laboratory monitoring • IV medication administration • Cardiac monitoring

monitoring, and interventions in addition to the wound care treatment.[5]

To summarize, LTCH patients are suffering with complex wounds requiring multiple specialty directed interventions in addition to comorbid conditions, which need continued higher acuity level care.

The case study presented met the wound care LTCH admission criteria. Clinically, she was suffering from a diabetic wound with active infection requiring prolonged treatment. She had protein calorie malnutrition, and her diabetes was uncontrolled. Treatment criteria for this patient were met due to her wound requiring complex wound care. She required a specialty wound dressing by means of a vacuum-assisted wound closure device and regular debridement and assessment by the wound care clinician. Additional treatment interventions with long-term IV antibiotics, regular laboratory monitoring, and multidisciplinary care were all considered as qualifying this patient as an appropriate LTCH admission.

Summary

As medically complex and critically ill patients continue to become a growing segment of the hospitalized population, the LTCH has evolved as an important care setting for this patient population after their index acute-care hospital (ACH) stay. Analyses of the degree of LTCH specialization in certain diagnosis-related groups (DRGs) indicate that wound-related conditions account for substantial proportion within a facility, ranging from 10% to 41.5%.[1]

The goal of the short-term ACH stay is to stabilize and control the comorbid condition that may be associated with the wounds, such as respiratory failure, sepsis, and multi-system organ failure. Furthermore, the ACH stay may involve complex surgical management such as surgical dehiscence cases, multisystem trauma with damage-control surgery, abdominal compartment syndrome from trauma or burn resuscitation requiring decompression laparotomy and acute limb salvage requiring revascularization procedures, surgical management of abscess, necrosis, and gangrene with concurrent control of infection. The intent of the LTCH is to limit the ACH stay and provide hospital-level care for the ongoing convalescence such as weaning from mechanical ventilator support, rehabilitation after ICU stay, IV antibiotic therapy, and management of complex surgical wounds such as the open abdomen or enterocutaneous fistula and ongoing advanced wound care required for limb salvage as described in the case presentation.

The wound care specialist is essential for management of the latter conditions as a member of the integrated, multidisciplinary team. Hospital-level, complex wound care is performed at the LTCH, using advanced healing modalities including aseptic technique, wound packing, serial debridements, and negative pressure therapy, as well as frequent assessments for wound complications such as infection or ischemia/vascular compromise. The wound care specialist can ensure the adherence to essential steps required for wound healing. Ongoing nutritional support, intensive blood glucose control, infection control, and education are provided in the LTCH to ensure optimized outcomes. Additional advanced wound healing tools such as HBO_2 therapy may be available on a center-by-center basis.

The LTCH functions to improve health, provide cost-effective care, and improve patient experience to beneficiaries that require hospital-level care for relatively extended periods. In order to achieve these outcomes, CMS and private insurers in the industry, InterQual and the National Association of Long Term Hospitals (NALTH) have developed the guidelines discussed for admission and treatment goals. This ensures that patients with compromised functional status, which would impede recovery and require a prolonged hospital level of care, can receive appropriate, high-quality, cost-effective care in a setting that is consistent with their clinical condition and needs. Claims data review indicates stable or declining unadjusted rates of readmission, death in the LTCH, and death within 30 days of discharge for the top 25 Medicare severity long-term care diagnosis-related group in 2012, including wound and wound-related conditions with major complications or comorbidity.[(6)] This data reflects the successful interventions that are available for wound care patients. LTCH care should be considered for the appropriate patient, as this level of care can significantly impact clinical outcomes.

Review questions

1. ***True/False.*** The wound care specialist is not essential in the management and care of some LTCH patients.

2. ***True/False.*** LTCH level of care does not include nutrition monitoring and intervention.

3. **General wound categories for admission to an LTCH include all of the following except:**

    a. Stage 3 or 4 pressure ulcers
    b. third-degree burns
    c. wounds with underlying vasculitis
    d. autoimmune wounds
    e. Stage 1 or 2 pressure ulcers

4. **Medicare defines long-term care hospitals as certified acute-care hospitals that treat patients hospitalized on average more than:**

    a. 10 days
    b. 30 days
    c. 25 days
    d. 14 days

5. **LTCH treatment criteria include all of the following except:**

    a. one concurrent medical condition requiring active intervention
    b. acuity requiring basic level care
    c. complex wound care requiring at least two interventions
    d. wound care clinician directing care and regular assessment

ANSWERS: 1) False
2) False
3) e
4) c
5) b

References

1. Gage B, Pilkauskas N, Dalton K, Constantine R, Leung M, Hoover, S et al. Long-term care hospital (LTCH) payment system monitoring and evaluation [Internet]. Baltimore (MD): Center for Medicare and Medicaid Services; 2007. Available from: https://www.cms.gov/medicare/medicare-fee-for-service-payment/longtermcarehospitalpps/downloads/rti_ltchpps_final_rpt.pdf.

2. Smith BM, Desvigne LD, Slade JB, Dooley JW, Warren DC. Transcutaneous oxygen measurements predict healing of leg wounds with hyperbaric therapy. Wound Repair Regen. 1996;4(2):224-229.

3. InterQual level of care criteria 2013. Long-term acute care adult. Newton (MA): McKesson Corporation; 2013.

4. Liu K, Baseggio C, Wissoker D, Maxwell S, Haley J, Long S. Long-term care hospitals under Medicare: facility-level characteristics. Health Care Financing Review [Internet]. 2001;23(2):1-18. Available from: https://www.cms.gov/Medicare/Medicare-Fee-for-Service-Payment/LongTermCareHospitalPPS/downloads/ltchurban.pdf.

5. National Association of Long Term Hospitals. Admission criteria worksheet; 2005.

6. MedPAC [Internet]. Washington (DC): Medicare payment policy: long-term care hospital services. 2014. Available from: http://www.medpac.gov/documents/reports/mar14_entirereport.pdf?sfvrsn=0.

Chapter 26

WOUND CARE IN THE NURSING HOME SETTING

Christina Ramsey, RN, MSN, GNP-BC, LNCC, CWS

KEY CONCEPTS

1. Managing a comprehensive wound care program in the nursing home setting requires a systematic methodology for preventing pressure ulcers.

2. Nursing homes are utilizing wound care-based physician groups to enhance wound care assessment and treatment while diminishing disruption of the resident's daily activity, decreasing pain from transportation back and forth to wound care centers, and decreasing cost of transportation.

3. Two of the quality measures relating to pressure ulcers include calculations of 1) percentage of high-risk residents with pressure ulcers for long-stay residents and 2) percentage of short-stay residents with pressure ulcers that are new or worsened. These quality measures are available on the Nursing Home Compare website.

4. Nursing homes commonly have wound care protocols for wound care treatments based on wound stage and characteristics.

CONTENTS

Introduction

Managing a comprehensive wound care program in the nursing home setting requires a systematic methodology for preventing pressure ulcers, identifying residents at risk for skin deterioration, immediate identification and reporting of alterations in skin integrity, prompt implementation of treatment plans, and ongoing evaluation for wound healing. This requires a multidisciplinary team collaboration between the facility's certified nursing assistants (CNAs), charge nurses, treatment nurses, minimum data set (MDS) coordinator, director of nurses, and physicians. It is imperative that the facility engages in a daily dialogue between the multidisciplinary team members to create an environment of wound healing and reduced facility-acquired pressure ulcers.

Nursing homes have become more skilled providers of wound care and are engaging in advanced wound care concepts, products, and participation in advanced wound healing devices. Nursing staff have become more educated in prevention and treatment of a variety of wound care conditions with the ongoing development of published guidelines regarding pressure ulcers in the long-term care setting and the increased availability of these resources through the Internet.[1] Nursing homes are utilizing wound care-based physician groups to enhance wound care assessment and treatment while diminishing disruption of the resident's daily activity, decreasing pain from transportation back and forth to wound care centers, and decreasing cost of transportation.

I. Evolution of wound care in long-term care

Several factors have contributed to the improvement and development of more advanced wound care in long-term care:

- Nursing homes are regulated by the Centers for Medicare and Medicaid Services and have extensive written regulations regarding appropriate practices in *The Centers for Medicare and Medicaid Services - State Operations Manual*, Appendix PP – "Guidance to Surveyors for Long-Term Care Facilities, §483.25(c) Pressure Sores. This guidance provides detailed recommendations regarding assessment, interventions, monitoring, and treatment of pressure sores.[2] Nursing homes have utilized this very valuable resource to provide staff education, develop wound care programs, and implement quality assurance and improvement programs to meet regulatory requirements.
  - Regulatory requirements related to the identification, prevention, and care of pressure ulcers are interwoven throughout the federal regulations in the state operations manuals. These federal regulations are commonly referred to as "F-Tags" and facilities can be cited with F-Tag deficiencies by state or federal surveyors. These deficiencies can range from F157 - failure to notify the physician of a change in condition, (e.g., identified pressure ulcer) to F501 – failure of the medical director to review and update policies and procedures to reflect current standards of practice for resident care (e.g., pressure ulcer prevention and treatment).[2]
  - Intent of F-Tag rule related to wound care is to:
    (a) Promote prevention,
    (b) Prevent additional pressure ulcers.
    (c) Promote healing.
    (d) Prevent Infection.
  - Facilities must adhere to these strict regulation guidelines or risk being cited

with F-Tag deficiencies that can occur at anytime during a on-site facility survey and currently include F157, F222, F272, F274, F309, F314, F317, F315, F323, F328, F403, and F501. While these F-Tags specially include the wording "pressure ulcer(s)", facilities can still be cited with other deficiencies indirectly related to pressure ulcer prevention, identification, and care, such as, F498 – Proficiency of Nurse Aides if they fail to "demonstrate skills and techniques necessary to the care of the resident's needs . . ."[2]

- Facility is assigned deficiencies based on
  a. Scope
     1. *Isolated* – less than 3 resident's affected.
     2. *Pattern* – more than 3 residents but less than 75% of the nursing home population.
     3. *Widespread* – affects more than 75% of nursing home population.

  b. Severity

     Level 1 - Letters A, B, and C – Deficiencies in this range are not serious

     Level 2 - Letters D, E, and F – Deficiencies in this range causes not actual harm but results in minimal discomfort to the resident

     Level 3 - Letters G, H, and I – Deficiencies in this range are cited if there is actual harm to the patient (i.e avoidable pressure ulcer or a skin tear)

     Level 4 - Letters J, K, and L – These deficiencies are classified under Immediate Jeopardy Territory (IJ) which is usually associated with a nice big fine.

- The Centers for Medicare and Medicaid Services adopted nursing home quality measures developed in the 1990s and implemented in 2004 to provide information to the public about the quality of care in nursing homes, give nursing homes measurements of high-risk care areas, to provide facilities data to facilitate quality improvement efforts, and to give data to the State Survey Agency for inspection. Two of the quality measures relating to pressure ulcers include calculations of 1) percentage of high-risk residents with pressure ulcers for long-stay residents and 2) percentage of short-stay residents with pressure ulcers that are new or worsened. These quality measures are available on the Nursing Home Compare website.
- Increased availability of physician-based wound care groups providing wound care in the long-term care facilities.
- The increased number of wound care product manufacturers have created a competitive market resulting in lower cost for low-air-loss beds; negative pressure wound therapy devices, and a variety of wound care products, which were previously cost-prohibitive.[3]

II. Components of a comprehensive wound care program

Nursing homes should have a comprehensive wound care program to provide optimal wound care through prevention, assessment, treatment, and evaluation.

A. Prevention – assessment

A key component to preventing the development of pressure ulcers in long-term care is through identification of those residents at risk for developing pressure ulcers by identifying risk factors for developing impaired skin integrity and utilizing standardized assessments, such as the Braden Scale for Predicting Pressure Sores or the Norton score.

1. Identify etiologic factors contributing to pressure ulcer occurrence.

a. Pressure
b. Shear
c. Friction
d. Moisture

2. Identify risk factors for pressure ulcer development.

a. Inability to perceive pressure/pain
b. Incontinence/moisture
c. Decreased activity level
d. Inability to reposition self
e. Poor nutritional intake
f. Friction and shearing from transfers/bed mobility

3. Recognize the presence of factors affecting tissue tolerance.

a. Age
b. Vascular competency
c. Glycemic control in diabetes mellitus
d. Body weight/malnutrition
e. Medications

4. Conduct pressure ulcer risk assessments using a valid and reliable tool.

a. Select a risk assessment method or tool appropriate to the population. Facilities often utilize the Braden Scale as their methodology for identifying residents at risk for skin breakdown due to the tested reliability and validity as well as the user-friendly format.[4]

b. Perform risk assessment
   (i) Admission
   (ii) Weekly for the first four weeks after admission
   (iii) With each facility readmission
   (iv) Calculate an individual's risk assessment score using the Braden Scale

c. Interpret the significance of the score

d. Reassess as significant changes occur in a patient, such as but not limited to:
   (i) Significant weight loss
   (ii) Decreased physical functioning
   (iii) Incontinence

5. Conduct ongoing assessments to identify residents at risk for pressure ulcer development.

Stop and Watch
Early Warning Tool

INTERACT
Version 4.0 Tool

If you have identified a change while caring for or observing a resident, please **circle** the change and notify a nurse. Either give the nurse a copy of this tool or review it with her/him as soon as you can.

S Seems different than usual
T Talks or communicates less
O Overall needs more help
P Pain – new or worsening; Participated less in activities

a Ate less
n No bowel movement in 3 days; or diarrhea
d Drank less

W Weight change
A Agitated or nervous more than usual
T Tired, weak, confused, or drowsy
C Change in skin color or condition
H Help with walking, transferring, toileting more than usual

☐ Check here if no change noted while monitoring high risk patient

Patient / Resident

Your Name

Reported to *Date and Time (am/pm)*

Nurse Response *Date and Time (am/pm)*

Nurse's Name

Facilities must have a systematic approach to maintaining an ongoing assessment and identification process for identifying residents at risk for pressure ulcer development. This can be achieved by many varied processes from conducting weekly skin assessments of residents by a licensed nurse to skin assessments during bathing by the certified nursing assistants.

A new approach adopted by many facilities includes implementation of a key component of the INTERACT Quality Improvement Program Tool, referred to as the Stop and Watch Early Warning Tool.[5] This simple tool is utilized by certified nursing assistants to communicate generalized changes in facility residents to their charge nurse for further assessment.

6. Conduct a thorough skin assessment, taking into account the individual's uniqueness.

a. Assess skin on admission and routinely.
b. Document findings and incorporate into plan of care.
c. Assess bony prominences and other areas of exposure to etiologic factors.
d. Observe indications of tissue ischemia (defined by stages) in accordance with the National Pressure Ulcer Advisory Panel (NPUAP):
   (i) Stage 1
   (ii) Stage 2
   (iii) Stage 3
   (iv) Stage 4
   (v) Deep-tissue injury (DTI)

**Stages define level of tissue injury and NOT progression of ulcer development.

B. Prevention – interventions

Nursing homes are required, at a minimum, to provide basic interventions to prevent impairment of skin integrity. These include but are not limited to:

1. Use of pressure relief devices for all residents at high risk
2. Prevention of shearing, friction, and prolonged pressure to bony prominences
3. Providing incontinence care and skin protectants
4. Completing nutritional assessment for all residents at risk for skin impairment, monitoring nutritional intake and providing supplements as needed
5. Maintaining adequate hydration
6. Weekly skin assessment by licensed nurses
7. Frequent repositioning of residents
8. Residents identified to be at risk for impaired skin integrity should have a comprehensive nutritional assessment completed by the facility dietitian and/or dietary consultant to implement necessary interventions to address nutritional deficits.[6]
9. Individualized care plans are implemented based on risk factors and resident-specific physical/medical characteristics.

Prevention measures have been well established and are identified in multiple publications.[7] Resources frequently utilized by nursing homes include:

- National Pressure Ulcer Advisory Panel (NPUAP), www.npuap.org
- The Centers for Medicare and Medicaid Services (CMS), *State Operations*

Manual, Appendix PP - Guidance to Surveyors for Long-Term Care Facilities, §483.25(c) Pressure Sores, www.cms.gov/Regulations-and-Guidance/Guidance/Manuals/downloads/som107ap_pp_guidelines_ltcf.pdf

- The Wound, Ostomy, and Continence Nurses Society (WOCN), www.wocn.org
- American Medical Directors Association (AMDA), www.amda.com
- The Quality Improvement Organizations, Medicare Quality Improvement Community Initiatives, www.medqic.org

C. Treatment

Lab monitoring

a. *Wound cultures:*

Cultures of pressure ulcers are ordered by the physician and are not routinely performed on all residents with pressure ulcers. Ulcers should be periodically assessed to determine whether a culture is necessary based on the appearance as defined below.

- Colonized versus infected wound

  "Colonized" refers to the presence of bacteria on the surface or in the tissue of a wound without the signs and symptoms of an infection.

  "Infected" refers to the presence of micro-organisms in sufficient quantity to overwhelm the defenses of viable tissues and produce the signs and symptoms of infection.

- Chronic wounds not responding to treatment or showing signs of healing may be cultured.
- Wound cultures can be obtained by:
  — Deep-tissue or punch biopsy
  — Needle aspiration
  — Swab culture - most commonly used technique because it is practical, noninvasive, and cost effective. Most commonly used is the Levine technique - twirling the end of cotton-tipped applicator on a 1 cm square area of the wound bed with enough pressure to cause minimal bleeding.[8]

b. *Pre-albumin, albumin, cholesterol, hemoglobin, and hematocrit (H&H)*

Laboratory values are assessed to determine nutritional status and/or impaired ability for wound healing. The lab tests are ordered by the physician and are not routinely performed on all residents with pressure ulcers.

i) Pre-albumin is done to evaluate nutritional status, more specifically visceral protein status, which is assessed by measuring concentrations of prealbumin in the plasma. Although other transport proteins, such as albumin or transferrin, can also be used, pre-albumin is a more reliable choice because of its shorter half life.

Normal levels are 15-29, with abnormal levels indicating malnutrition:

— Level 12-15 equals **mild** malnutrition

— Level 8-10 equals **moderate** malnutrition

— Levels < 8 equal **severe** malnutrition

ii) Albumin is done to determine low albumin levels, which can be an indicator of chronic malnutrition. Generally albumin levels of less than 3.0 will impede wound healing.

iii) Cholesterol is done to evaluate nutritional status because prolonged low cholesterol levels can indicate malnutrition.

iv) Hemoglobin and hematocrit is done to detect for anemia. Please refer to Chapter 4: Nutritional Assessment and Management and Chapter 11: Pressure Ulcers for further information.

Nutritional assessment and supplements

Part of the treatment plan includes a comprehensive nutritional assessment to include:

- Estimated nutritional requirements individualized to resident age, weight, height, and comorbidities to include caloric, protein, and fluid needs
- Comparison of current nutritional intake to estimated requirements
- Laboratory tests
- Factors that interfere with the resident's ability to maintain good nutrition/hydration
- Recommendations for nutrition interventions
- Development of care plan to address nutritional needs and monitoring of interventions for effectiveness

Research in nutrition and wound healing is limited, making evidence-based recommendations difficult. It is necessary to apply clinical judgment in each case. There are basic nutrition guidelines for wound healing as follows:[6]

- 30-35 calories/kilogram (kg) body weight
- Encourage extra hydration if not contraindicated to the resident's condition. At least 1 milliliter (mL) of fluid/kilocalorie (kcal) consumed/day.
  — 1.25-1.5 grams (g) protein/kg body weight/day – adjust based on renal function
- Provide adequate vitamins and minerals:
  — Multivitamin, one daily

  — Multivitamin liquid 5-10cc daily for swallowing difficulty or residents receiving tube feeding

  — Vitamin C 500 mg twice a day

  — Zinc sulfate 220 mg daily – usually for two to three weeks to prevent zinc overload

There are a variety of protein/calorie supplements that can be provided to meet the resident's nutritional needs.

a. Protein supplements such as fortified shakes, broth, pudding, meal enhancements, etc. provided by the dietary department to residents during meal times. The facility would need to implement a method of evaluating and documenting the supplement intake.

b. A two-calorie liquid formula or equivalent that includes two calories per cc can be administered in 60-90 cc doses two to four times a day during medication administration times by the nursing staff. This allows for better evaluation and documentation of the protein supplement intake.

c. Specialized supplement formulas for residents with renal insufficiency/failure or diabetes to meet their nutritional needs.

d. Liquid protein supplements offer 10gms of protein/oz up to three times/day in fluid of choice/mixed with the resident's food to meet their protein supplement needs. Better monitoring of actual intake is achieved when administered by the nursing department during medication administration times.

f. Arginaid supplement

g. Protein-enriched tube-feeding formula to meet increased protein needs. Conversion of calories will need to be calculated, since the protein-enriched formula may have more calories/ml.

Pressure relief and devices

The use of pressure-relief devices is a basic wound prevention and treatment intervention. With the advancement in pressure relief devices and competitive market, nursing homes have access to a variety of economical pressure-relief devices.

a. A pressure-relief (reduction of interface pressure below 32 mmHg capillary closure pressure) replacement/overlay bed mattress should be in use for any resident who is at risk for pressure ulcer development or impaired skin integrity. Care should be taken with a pressure-relief overlay mattress due to the increased height of the bed and potential for falls.

b. An automatic pressure-relief low-air-loss mattress usually provides more pressure relief than the replacement/overlay mattress and should be used for those residents with pressure ulcers on the trunk and/or heels.

c. An overlay air mattress can be used but is not preferred because the air pressure must be manually checked by the staff daily to ensure that the air pressure is maintained at an acceptable level so that it is neither over-inflated, which would cause increased pressure nor under-inflated. which would not provide pressure relief.

d. Pressure relief foam heel protectors/padded boots should be used on residents who are assessed to be at risk or who have developed any stage pressure ulcers on their heels. The manufacturer's specifications should be checked to ensure that the device offers pressure relief and not merely comfort.

e. Bridging of the heels by elevating the lower extremity to a level whereby the heels do not touch the bed is an acceptable intervention for pressure relief and is referred to as offloading. The resident must be assessed frequently for foot drop, which can be a complication of this intervention.

f. A pressure-relief cushion should be used in the resident's chair, wheelchair, or Geri-chair for residents identified as at risk or residents who have developed any stage pressure ulcer, which could be foam, gel foam, or gel pad.

g. Residents with any stage pressure ulcer should be kept off the identified pressure area and turned to alternate sides.

h. Residents with trunk ulcers should have physician's orders indicating whether sitting up in a chair is permitted and, if so, applicable time limits.

i. Compression therapy

Wound care

Nursing homes commonly have wound care protocols for wound care treatments based on wound stage and characteristics. These protocols are usually approved by the facility's medical director for use in the facility. Protocols should coincide with treatment standards from NPUAP.

Wound care-based physician groups provide weekly in-house wound care assessments and orders with sharp debridement as needed.

Wound care centers offer wound care treatment orders, as well as advanced wound care procedures such as HBO_2 (hyperbaric oxygen therapy), mist therapy-ultrasonic wound healing, and debridement.

NPWT (negative pressure wound therapy) manufacturers offer economical choices.

D. Evaluation

There are many documentation monitoring flow sheets or tools to evaluate healing of wounds. Most nursing homes utilize standard weekly skin assessment forms, which include stage, size, depth, drainage, odor, and pain. The assessments are documented weekly and reviewed during the weekly quality assurance and improvement program meetings to evaluate wound healing and identify whether additional interventions are needed.

Another evaluation tool is the Pressure Ulcer Scale for Healing (PUSH) tool developed by the National Pressure Ulcer Advisory Panel (http://www.npuap.org/wp-content/uploads/2012/02/push3.pdf). This is a quick and reliable tool for monitoring change in pressure ulcer status over time.[9]

Treatment(s) should be monitored and evaluated weekly for effectiveness and progress. Allow at least two weeks prior to determining effectiveness unless there is a decline in the condition of pressure ulcer(s), at which time the physician should be contacted and the treatment changed.

Documentation guidelines

1. Weekly skin assessment and documentation should be done on all residents with wounds to include stage, size, depth, color, odor, and drainage.

2. Tunneling should be documented, using the clock method. The resident's head is utilized as a reference point with the head indicating 12 o'clock, the foot indicating 6 o'clock, the right side indicating 3 o'clock, and the left side indicating 9 o'clock. A cotton swab should be used to measure the tunneling and measured at various different points of the pressure ulcer and recorded using the clock method.

3. Additional assessment and documentation should be completed for any unusual changes in the wounds with physician notification.

E. Quality assurance and improvement program (QAIP)

Review statistical data of facility wounds monthly for:

a. Pressure Ulcer Quality Measures from CMS Database[10]
b. Facility resident census and condition report regarding pressure ulcers
c. Percentage of total residents with pressure ulcers
d. Percentage of residents admitted with ulcers
e. Percentage of nursing home-induced pressure ulcers

Summary

Long-term care facilities need to continue to expand their wound care programs by increasing knowledge and training regarding the complexity of wound healing, implementing new interventions in pressure ulcer prevention, and incorporation of wound care-based physician groups both onsite and offsite of the facility. Developing a comprehensive wound care program will benefit the facility with increased quality of care, increased patient satisfaction, improved patient outcomes, increased reimbursement, and increased facility census.

Review questions

1. **What factors have contributed to the improvement of wound care in long-term care?**

   a. deficiencies during survey, decreased wound care costs, increased patients with wounds
   b. expanded regulation guidelines by CMS, quality measures, increased availability of physician-based wound care groups coming into long-term care facilities
   c. increased competitive market for wound care products, lawsuits, patient demand
   d. increased reimbursement, decreased wound care costs, lawsuits

2. **A comprehensive wound care program in long-term care should include which of the following?**

   a. treatment
   b. assessment
   c. prevention
   d. evaluation
   e. all of the above

3. ***True/False.*** Wound cultures are routinely performed on all residents with draining pressure ulcers.

4. **Completing a Pressure Ulcer Risk Assessment Tool is part of the __________ component of the comprehensive wound care program.**

   a. evaluation
   b. treatment
   c. assessment
   d. none of the above

5. **A comprehensive wound care program in long-term care is:**

   a. a multidisciplinary team collaboration
   b. responsibility of the director of nursing and the physicians
   c. is a set of regulations developed by the Centers for Medicare and Medicaid
   d. based on physician availability

ANSWERS: 1) b
2) e
3) False
4) c
5) a

References

1. Pressure ulcers in the long-term care setting. American Medical Directors Association [Internet]. 2008 [cited 2016 May 20]; Available from: https://www.guideline/gov.
2. State Operations Manual. Appendix PP – Guidance to surveyors for long term care facilities [Internet]. Centers for Medicare. 2016 [cited 2016 May 25]. Available from: http://www.cms.gov/regulations-and-guidance/legislation.
3. Wound care: advanced tools and talented care teams lead to solid wound management. McKnight's. 2009;30(3).
4. Prevention Plus [Internet]. Bradenscale.com. 2016 [cited 2016 June 2]. Available from: http://www.bradenscale.com.
5. Ouslander JG, Perloe M. INTERACT – Interventions to reduce acute care transfers [Internet]. Interact2.net. 2016 [cited 2016 May 19]. Available from: https://interact2.net.
6. Nutrition guidelines: skin and wound care for long-term care residents. Nutrition411 [Internet]. Nutrition411.com. 2015 [cited 2016 May 30]. Available from: http://www.nutrition411.com/wounds-center-your-patients/articles/nutrition-guidelines-skin-and-wound-care-long-term-care/page/0/1.
7. Maguire J. Wound care management. Geriatric Medicine. 2014;7(2):14.
8. Spear M. Best technique for obtaining wound cultures. Plast Surg Nurs. 2012:32(1):34-36.
9. PUSH Tool. The National Pressure Ulcer Advisory Panel – NPUAP [Internet]. Npuap.org. 1998 [cited 2016 May 28]. Available from: http://www.npuap.org/resources/educational-and-clinical-resources/push-tool/.
10. Quality Measures – Centers for Medicare & Medicaid Services [Internet]. Cms.gov. 2016 [cited 2016 May 29]. Available from: https://cms.gov/Medicare/Quality-Initiatives-Patient-Assessment-Instruments/NursingHomeQualityInits/NHQIQualityMeasures.html.

Section 7

CHALLENGES AND OPPORTUNITIES IN WOUND CARE PRACTICE IN THE NEW ERA

Editor - Caroline E. Fife, MD, FAAFP, CWS, FUHM

Chapter 27

INCORPORATING RESEARCH INTO WOUND CARE AND HYPERBARIC MEDICINE PRACTICE

Thomas E. Serena, MD, FACS, FACHM, MAPWCA

KEY CONCEPTS

1. A research program can greatly enhance the impact on a community by offering access to much-needed novel therapies.
2. Beyond the initial planning and preparation, one of the most important elements of a sustainable research program is a research culture.
3. Before becoming involved in wound care research, a thorough understanding of the regulatory environment is essential.
4. A multidisciplinary team of clinicians and coordinators, as well as regulatory and administrative staff, is vital for the overall success of the research program.

CONTENTS

Introduction

Recently, there has been a resurgence of interest in the field of wound care and hyperbaric medicine. Although hyperbaric oxygen (HBO_2) therapy has been employed for almost 45 years, the precise effects of HBO_2 on individual cells and tissues are just beginning to be revealed in both animal and human studies. The physiological benefits of oxygen include cell proliferation, angiogenesis, activation of immune cells, changes in cytokine production, and modulation of inflammatory mediators. One of the most important applications of HBO_2 is in the treatment of chronic nonhealing wounds. As an adjunct to standard of care (SOC), HBO_2 can improve healing, particularly for diabetic foot ulcers (DFUs), and can result in a significant reduction in amputations.

Despite a growing need for clinical research in wound care and hyperbaric medicine, many hospitals remain on the sidelines. A research program can greatly enhance the impact on a community by offering access to much-needed novel therapies. An efficiently managed program also can create sustainable revenue for the hospital. This chapter discusses the essential requirements for a research program in wound care and hyperbaric medicine. In addition, current research trends and significant findings from preclinical and clinical studies on HBO_2 are presented along with implications for future research.

I. Incorporating research in wound care: research culture

The value of embracing high-quality wound care research has long been recognized; however, hospitals and wound care practices often lack awareness of the resources, infrastructure, and commitment needed to establish a sustainable research program. Establishing a research program requires considerable effort and support in planning, fiscal oversight, and retention of a qualified research team.

Beyond the initial planning and preparation, one of the most important elements of a sustainable research program is a research culture. To establish a research culture, the program needs leadership and engagement from principal investigators (PIs) dedicated to clinical research. Experienced PIs, clinical research coordinators (CRCs), nurses, and other administrative staff can build a collaborative ecosystem where best practices can be shared and promoted.

It is critical to garner leadership support from executive staff and key stakeholders who can promote the research program and increase awareness of it. One of the challenges that the research staff must overcome is building a research capacity across the full continuum of care; this requires effective collaboration among departments that often work in silos.

The shift to a research culture occurs gradually as trust and rapport are built and lines of communication are open across the institution. Effective management of relationships is essential in ensuring that research continues to be valued and prioritized. Additionally, dissemination of research findings to hospital leadership, administrators, and key stakeholders is necessary to increase awareness of the impact research is having on patients.

II. Research facility

A. Needs assessment

A systematic approach should be used in the initial planning to assess the ability of the organization to conduct research. Often organizations have limited administrative infrastructure and their leaders may not see research as a priority. At a busy wound care practice, it can be challenging to find time for clinical trials even for clinicians committed to research. Thus, an assessment of the current state of the organization is critical. An extensive needs assessment, including internal departmental interviews, can help determine available resources, infrastructure, interest in the planned study, knowledge and operational experience of the staff, availability of target patient population, recruitment potential, and retention capability.

Appointing a steering committee is an important step in ensuring oversight for the overall direction and strategy of the clinical research program. The steering committee should include key members of the clinical staff, institutional review board (IRB), and contract and legal team. The most important function of the steering committee is to act as the ultimate decision maker in handling organizational, political, cost, and management issues related to the clinical research program. To help your organization navigate the complex and changing regulatory landscape, it may be helpful to engage a consultant for the initial groundwork. Having the right support and expertise from the get-go will ensure the long-term success of a clinical research program.

B. Organization and structure

Generally the most effective approach is to build upon the existing administrative infrastructure of an organization to gain widespread acceptance from existing legal, administrative, and regulatory departments. Aligning priorities across various departments, hospital management, and governing boards can help move toward consolidation and consensus of policies and procedures. Effective collaboration and consolidation of function across the departments also can shorten times for contract negotiations and IRB approvals while allowing investigator and clinical staff to manage research studies more effectively. Regulatory agencies and funding sources (e.g. NIH) strongly recommend the use of a central IRB for multicenter trials. In addition, pending legislation would mandate the use of a central IRB for trials involving more than one site.

1. Affiliation with a cooperative group

Hospitals and wound care practices can apply for affiliation with a cooperative group to participate in a clinical study. Cooperative groups or research consulting groups, such as those sponsored by the National Cancer Institute, have successfully promoted and supported clinical trials in most fields of medicine. Working with a cooperative group or research consulting groups helps to meet the growing need for wound centers with the capacity to conduct clinical research. They also help to bridge the gap for potential organizations interested in research by offering support in study management and regulatory compliance.

2. General requirement

A dedicated research area within the facility where participants will be seen and research activities will take place should be well organized. Exam rooms should comply with applicable local, state, and Occupational Safety and Health Administration (OSHA) requirements. Additionally, there should be dedicated space for storage of study-specific regulatory files or binders and other study-related documentation. Depending on the study, the facility also may need a refrigerator, freezer, and shelving to store products and supplies. If a facility has its own laboratory, documentation of a College of American Pathologists (CAP) laboratory accreditation or Clinical Laboratory Improvement Amendments (CLIA) Certificate or a certificate of waiver will be required. Workspace for administrative aspects of the study for research staff and for the monitor for on-site visits also is needed. Ability to incorporate web-based electronic data capture (EDC) applications into the practice usually is required in addition to internet access, telephone, and a fax machine. During a qualifying visit, the sponsors of a research study will assess the facility to ensure it meets the basic requirements.

3. Regulatory environment

Before wound care research begins, a thorough understanding of the regulatory environment is essential. The PI must be familiar with good clinical practices (GCP) and Code of Federal Regulations (CFR) Title 21, as this person ultimately is responsible for the conduct of the study. Compliance with GCP ensures protection of the rights, well-being, and confidentiality of study participants. Additionally, it ensures the collection of reliable data for submission to the regulatory agency. For device studies, investigators will need to complete an Investigator Agreement. It is important to note that Regulations 21 CFR 50, 54, and 56 still apply in additional to 21 CRF 803, 812, and 814. Investigator obligations can be found in 21 CFR 812.

4. Developing a research team

A multidisciplinary team of clinicians and coordinators, as well as regulatory and administrative staff, is vital for the overall success of the research program. The research staff plays an important role in ensuring smooth day-to-day study operations. It is important to underscore that although a PI may delegate duties to the research staff, he or she remains responsible legally and ethically. Thus, it is critical to train the research staff and maintain close oversight.

As research grows in scope and complexity, the demand for a well-trained CRC continues to rise. An experienced CRC is highly desired as he/she can play an essential role in ensuring the quality of the research program. A CRC is responsible for accurate maintenance of the records for the trial as well as many other important aspects of the study, including patient interactions during the informed consent process, study visits, and safety reporting. It is ideal to have a CRC who is cross-trained in multiple disciplines. A CRC who is clinically competent and can assess vital signs and draw blood will be less dependent on the investigator and the nursing staff. Moreover, cross-trained CRCs can help with other tasks such as budget preparation, negotiation, and IRB submission.

The research team needs standardized training in research as well as specialized training specific to the protocol. Investigators and all study personnel are required to obtain training in Good Clinical Practices (GCP). Several online resources are available, such as NIH (https://phrp.nihtraining.com/users/login.php) and CITI. (https://about.citiprogram.org/en/series/good-clinical-practice-gcp/).

Responsibilities related to the Health Insurance Portability and Accountability Act (HIPAA), ethical considerations and human subject protections, clinical requirements, regulations, compliance, and GCP should be highlighted as major training topics. All research staff must complete and achieve competency before beginning any substantive involvement in a research study.

5. Protocol assessment/study feasibility

Protocol assessment or study feasibility is often overlooked in the excitement to start a trial. The importance of a thorough and thoughtful review of a protocol cannot be overemphasized. It is important to take a more rigorous approach to evaluating study design, goals and objectives, and criteria for patient population, along with ethical and regulatory considerations.

Investigators should take on studies that fit their patient populations. This requires a careful consideration of the types of patients coming to the wound practice and the common types of ulcers being seen. It is essential to take a close look at the eligibility criteria to verify that they are not too restrictive and do not exclude patients coming to your practice. The study should be appropriate for the largest proportion of your patients.

While assessing your organization's suitability for a study, you should consider the demands being placed on the site and determine whether you have all the resources to meet the requirements of the protocol. You should determine whether additional training is required to administer specific procedures and tests required for the study. The treatment visits and schedule of activities also should be assessed carefully to determine whether compliance with the protocol would be difficult. If you are taking on multiple studies, you need to critically evaluate whether enrollment will compete with other studies.

6. *Study budget considerations*

Identifying cost at your facility will be helpful in determining the actual cost of the study. Having a survey of standard charges in your area may help in negotiating additional funds. Study budget line items may vary depending on the nature of the study and the location where subjects will be seen. Subject-related costs associated with study-specific procedures, physician exam, vitals, tests, and lab services should be considered along with up-front IRB fees and incident reporting fees for potential adverse events (AE) and serious adverse events (SAE). Some of the common mistakes in preparation of study budgets include underestimation of the time commitment by the research site, failure to include overhead, and unforeseen protocol revision, which may change the demands on the research staff. The study budget should be critically reviewed by the PI and research staff to ensure that the budget is fair and covers all study-related costs and overhead.

7. *Participant requirement and retention*

The study staff often mistakenly believes that once the site is up and the study is activated, patients will flock to the site; however, successful recruitment requires an active enrollment plan. The first place to look for patients is in your electronic health records (EHRs). Eligible patients can be found using the ICD-10 diagnosis code. It is a good practice to prescreen patients to determine who might be eligible for participation in the study.

Taking subject referrals from other wound care practitioners in the community is another approach to recruiting volunteers. A template letter describing the study, intervention, and benefit to the patient is generally helpful when requesting referrals from physicians. Additionally, investigators can reach out to advocacy groups, such as the Association for the Advancement of Wound Care (AAWC), Amputee Coalition of America (ACA), and Patient Access Network (PAN).

Advertising also can be effective in recruiting participants. Note that since FDA considers direct advertising to be a part of the informed consent process, ads need to be reviewed and approved by the IRB. A sponsor of a study also can assist in developing advertising materials for the site; all advertising must have written IRB approval.

To increase subject retention during a trial, it is essential for the research staff to stay in close communication with the participants. Lack of contact can lead to decreased compliance and withdrawal. Participants' concerns or questions around a trial should be addressed as part of the informed-consent process. If the population of the trial is older, make sure that any special needs are addressed. Putting the patient's needs first and maintaining a strong relationship with him/her will go a long way toward establishing a successful clinical trial.

III. Current trends in research

A. Preclinical studies

The positive and anti-inflammatory effects of HBO_2 have been shown in preclinical studies. HBO_2 promotes angiogenesis, improves fibroblast activity, enhances leukocyte function, and assists in bacterial clearance.[1] HBO_2 affects the release of a number of cytokines and growth factors important in wound healing. Studies have shown that it is important in up-regulation of fibroblast growth factors (FGF) and collagen synthesis.[2-5] HBO_2 also has been shown to inhibit inflammatory reactions, preventing leukocyte aggregation, and decreasing the secretion of tumor necrosis factor alpha (TNF-α), interleukin 1 (IL-1) and interleukin 6 (IL-6).[6-7] Furthermore, a more recent study using a validated ischemic wound model, Sprague-Dawley rats, showed that HBO_2 significantly decreased MMP1, MMP2, and MMP8 in ischemic wound tissue while increasing tissue inhibitor of metalloproteinase 2 (TIMP2).[8]

Improved survival of skin flaps and grafts has been established with HBO_2. Renner et al. found that HBO_2 improved auricular composite graft survival in rabbits treated with HBO_2.[9] This adds to the data from previous studies, showing enhanced flap survival, angiogenesis, and an increase in microvasculature.[10-11] A more recent study on streptozotocin (STZ)-diabetic rats demonstrated that HBO_2 improved oxygen saturation and the quantity of hemoglobin in micro blood vessels. It also improved the tissue breaking strength, but this did not reach statistical significance ($p=0.1$).[12]

B. Challenges and limitations

One of the challenges presented with current animal models is that it is difficult to represent the clinical features of chronic wounds. Chronic wounds are uncommon in small animals and additional measures are required to reproduce authentic wounds. Some models that have been extensively used include rabbit ear ulcer models, STZ-diabetic rats, and rodents and pig flap models.

Small mammals, however, have several anatomical and physiological differences. They have a relatively thin epidermal layer and the sub-epithelial layer is rich with skeletal muscle fibers.[13] In animals with subcutaneous panniculus carnosus muscle, the wound repair may be aided by contraction.[14-15] Porcine skin may be a better model as it is structurally similar to human skin and has similar patterns of hair follicles and blood vessels. Pigs contain dermal collagen and elastin content, which is similar to human. Furthermore, they have similar physical and molecular responses to various growth factors. However, the drawback is that they are not as cost-effective as smaller animal models. Although porcine studies are suitable for investigating the effectiveness of therapeutic interventions, rodents can be optimal models for understanding fundamental genetic, cellular, and molecular mechanisms.

C. Clinical studies

A number of randomized controlled trials (RCTs) using HBO_2 adjunctively with standard of care (SOC) have shown improved healing by six weeks.[16-25] Although a recent review of pooled data did not confirm the effect on major amputation, there are indications that hyperbaric oxygen may decrease major amputation in patients with DFUs.[26] Previously, pooled data from three studies examining wound healing and amputation revealed that a major amputation (95% confidence interval [CI], 0.13–0.71) could be prevented for every four patients treated (95% CI, 3–11).[27]

Over the past two decades, about a dozen pivotal RCTs have been published that compare the effect of HBO_2 on chronic wound healing. An overwhelming majority of these trials have centered on DFUs, with the sample size ranging from 18 participants to 100 participants. The treatment schedule also has varied between these trials from 3.0 ATA for 45 minutes to 2.2 and 2.5 ATA for between 60 and 120 minutes. Only five trials, enrolling a total of 205 participants, have reported proportion of ulcers healed at six weeks. The pooled results of these DFU trials show an increase in the rate of healing with HBO_2 (95% CI 1.19 to 4.62; p= 0.01).[26]

A limited number of studies have been completed on venous leg ulcers (VLUs) and other types of ulcers. In a more recent study by Kaur et al., which included both nonhealing DFUs and VLUs, there was a significant benefit of HBO_2 in reduction of ulcer area (95% CI 41.91 to 81.85, $p < 0.00001$).[28] In this study, a total of 30 HBO_2 sessions were delivered at 2.5ATA for 90 minutes, 6 days a week. An earlier study by Hammarlund also showed a significant reduction in wound area (95% CI 19 to 47) at week 6.[29] A treatment session of 2.4 ATA for 90 minutes was employed for a total of 30 sessions in patients with VLUs.

D. Implications for future research

It is important to note that data from current trials are limited by a small number of participants, varying wound characteristics and size, and different methodological approaches used for reporting of the trial. Moreover, the treatments and schedules used have varied among trials. Whereas some studies employed a control, others have not. Future studies should use appropriate control. Further, the effects of HBO_2 on chronic wounds caused by venous disease, arterial disease, and pressure damage need to be investigated. With the rapidly evolving movement toward quality and cost-effectiveness, there continues to be a need for future studies to undertake an economic evaluation.

Summary

The value of embracing high-quality wound care research has long been recognized. A systematic approach should be used in the initial planning to assess the ability of the organization to conduct research. An extensive needs assessment, including internal departmental interviews, can help determine available resources, infrastructure, the interest in the planned study, the knowledge and operational experience of the staff, availability of target patient population, and the recruitment potential and retention capability.

The research team needs standardized training in research as well as specialized training specific to the protocol. Responsibilities related to HIPAA, ethical considerations and human subject protections, clinical requirements, regulations, compliance, and GCP should be highlighted as major training topics. A multidisciplinary team of clinicians and coordinators, as well as regulatory and administrative staff, is vital for the overall success of the research program.

While assessing your organization's suitability for a study, you should consider the demands being placed on the site and determine whether you have all the resources to meet the requirements of the protocol. A research program can greatly enhance the impact on a community by offering access to much-needed novel therapies.

Review questions

1. **What is the most important consideration for wound care practices interested in participating in a clinical study?**

    a. Start with a study that would benefit at least 25% of your patient population.

    b. Take on studies that provide a steady stream of income.

    c. When determining clinical trial offering at your practice, it is essential to select studies that fit your practice and maximizes the benefit to your patients and your community.

    d. A wound care practice should consider the time and duration of the study.

2. **Responsibilities of a principal investigator include all of the following EXCEPT:**

    a. implementing informed consent

    b. performing data collection

    c. participating in quality assurance process

    d. maintaining an adequate rate of patient accrual

3. **The most effective way to determine a suitable study for your practice include:**

    a. Evaluate the demands being placed on the site and determine whether you have all the resources to meet the requirements of the protocol.

    b. Evaluate whether enrollment will compete with other studies.

    c. Consider whether eligibility is too restrictive and whether it will exclude patients coming to your practice.

    d. all of the above

4. **The challenges presented with current animal models include:**

    a. It is difficult to represent the clinical features of chronic wounds.

    b. Chronic wounds are uncommon in small animals.

    c. Wound repair may be aided by contraction.

    d. all of the above

5. **Although a number of pivotal RCTs that compare the effect of HBO_2 on chronic wound healing have been conducted over the past two decades, they have been limited by a number of factors including:**
    a. The treatment schedule has varied among these trials from 3.0 ATA for 45 minutes to 2.2 and 2.5 ATA for between 60 and 120 minutes.
    b. varying wound characteristics and size
    c. a small number of participants
    d. all of the above

ANSWERS: 1) c
2) b
3) d
4) d
5) d

References

1. Mader JT, Guckian JC, Glass DL, Reinarz JA. Therapy with hyperbaric oxygen for experimental osteomyelitis due to Staphylococcus aureus in rabbits. Infect Dis. 1978; 138:312-318.
2. Ishii Y, Myanaga Y, Shimojo H, Ushida T, Tateishi T. Effects of hyperbaric oxygen on procollagen messenger RNA levels and collagen synthesis in healing of rat tendon laceration. Tissue Eng. 1999;5:279-286.
3. Bonomo SR, Davidson JD, Yu Y, Xia Y, et al. Hyperbaric oxygen as a signal transducer: upregulation of platelet derived growth factor-beta receptor in the presence of HBO_2 and PDGF. Undersea Hyperbaric Med. 1998;24(4):211-216.
4. Bayati S, Russell RC, Roth AC. Stimulation of angiogenesis to improve the viability of prefabricated flaps. Plast Reconstr Surg. 1998;101(5):1290-1295.
5. Wu L, Pierce GF, Ladin DA, Zhao LL, et al. Effects of oxygen on wound responses to growth factors: Kaposi's FGF, but not basic FGF stimulates repair in ischemic wounds. Growth Factors. 1995;12(1):29-35.
6. Wilson HD, Wilson JR, Fuchs PN. Hyperbaric oxygen treatment decreases inflammation and mechanical hypersensitivity in an animal model of inflammatory pain. Brain Res. 2006;1098:12612-12618.
7. Zelinski LM, Ohgami Y, Chung E, Shirachi DY, Quock RM. A prolonged nitric oxide-dependent, opioid-mediated antinociceptive effect of hyperbaric oxygen in mice. J Pain. 2009;10:167-172.
8. Zhang, Qixu et al. Hyperbaric oxygen reduces matrix metalloproteinases in ischemic wounds through a redox-dependent mechanism. Journal of Investigative Dermatology. 2013;134(1):237–246.
9. Renner G, McClane SD, Early E, Bell P, Shaw B. Enhancement of auricular composite graft survival with hyperbaric oxygen therapy. Arch Facial Plast Surg. 2002;4:102-104.
10. Marx RE, Ames JR. The use of hyperbaric oxygen therapy in bone reconstruction of the irradiated and tissue deficient patient. J Oral Maxillofac Surg. 1982;52:412-420.
11. Nemiroff PM, Lungu AL. The influence of hyperbaric oxygen and irradiation on vascularity in skin flaps: a controlled study. Surg Forum. 1987;38:567-7.
12. Tuk B, Tong M, Fijneman EMG, van Neck JW. Hyperbaric oxygen therapy to treat diabetes impaired wound healing in rats. 2014. PLoS ONE. 9(10):e108533.
13. Perez R, Davis SC. Relevance of animal models for wound healing. Wounds. 2008; 20(1):3–8.
14. Wong VW, Sorkin M, Glotzbach JP, Longaker MT, Gurtner GC. Surgical approaches to creating murine models of human wound healing. J Biomed Biotechnol.2011.
15. Dorsett-Martin WA. Rat models of skin wound healing: a review. Wound Repair Regen.2004; 12(6):591–599. doi:WRR12601 [pii] 10.1111/j.1067-1927.2004.12601.x.
16. Abidia A, Laden G, Kuhan G, Johnson BF, Wilkinson AR, Renwick PM, et al. The role of hyperbaric oxygen therapy in ischemic diabetic lower extremity ulcers: a double-blind randomised-controlled trial. European Journal of Vascular and Endovascular Surgery. 2003;25:513–518.
17. Duzgun AP, Satir HZ, Ozozan O, Saylam B, et al. Effect of hyperbaric oxygen therapy on healing of diabetic foot ulcers. Journal of Foot and Ankle Surgery. 2008;47(6):515-9.
18. Kessler L, Bilbault P, Ortega F, Grasso C, et al. Hyperbaric oxygen accelerates the healing rate of nonischemic chronic diabetic foot ulcers. Diabetes Care. 2003;26:2378-2382.

19. Doctor N, Pandya S, Supe A. Hyperbaric oxygen therapy in diabetic foot. Journal of Postgraduate Medicine. 1992;38(3):112–114.

20. Faglia E, Favales F, Aldeghi A, Calia P, et al. Adjunctive systemic hyperbaric oxygen therapy in treatment of severe prevalently ischemic diabetic foot ulcer. A randomized study. Diabetes Care. 1996;19(12):1338-1343.

21. Lin TF, Chen SB, Niu KC. The vascular effects of hyperbaric oxygen therapy in treatment of early diabetic foot. Undersea and Hyperbaric Medicine. 2001;28:67.

22. Londahl M, Landin-Olsson M, Katzman P. Hyperbaric oxygen therapy as adjunctive treatment of chronic diabetic foot ulcers. 2010;33(5):998-1003.

23. Ma L, Li P, Shi Z, Hou T, et al. A prospective, randomized, controlled study of hyperbaric oxygen therapy: effects on healing and oxidative stress of ulcer tissue in patients with a diabetic foot ulcer. Ostomy Wound Manage. 2013;59:18-24.

24. Khandelwal S, Chaudhary P, Poddar DD, Saxena N, et al. Comparative study of different treatment options of grade iii and iv diabetic foot ulcers to reduce the incidence of amputations. Clin Pract. 2013;3:e9.

25. Wang CJ, Wu RW, yang YJ. Treatment of diabetic foot ulcers: a comparative study of extracorporeal shockwave therapy and hyperbaric oxygen therapy. Diabetes Research and Clinical Practice. 2011;92(2):287-293.

26. Kranke P, Bennett M, Martyn JM, Schnabel A, Debus SE, Weibel S. Hyperbaric oxygen therapy for chronic wounds (Cochrane Review). In: The Cochrane Library, Issue 6, 2015. Chichester, UK: John Wiley & Sons, Ltd.

27. Kranke P, Bennett M, Roeckl-Wiedmann I, Debus S. Hyperbaric oxygen therapy for chronic wounds (Cochrane Review). In: The Cochrane Library, Issue 2, 2004. Chichester, UK: John Wiley & Sons, Ltd.

28. Kaur S, Pawar M, Banerjee N, Garg R. Evaluation of the efficacy of hyperbaric oxygen therapy in the management of chronic nonhealing ulcer and role of periwound transcutaneous oximetry as a predictor of wound healing response: A randomized prospective controlled trial. J Anaesthesiol Clin Pharmacol.2012;28:70–75.

29. Hammarlund C, Sundberg T. Hyperbaric oxygen reduced size of chronic leg ulcers: a randomized double-blind study. Plastic and Reconstructive Surgery.1994;93(4):829–833.

Chapter 28

TELEMEDICINE

Stephen D. Guthrie, MD, PhD†
Barbara R. Guthrie, MD

KEY CONCEPTS

1. Telemedicine (TM), if used correctly, allows provider amplification without the hazard of potentially diluting the quality of the care provided.
2. On every continent, and in both urban and rural settings, TM has been shown to improve the management of chronic conditions.
3. Adding a TM component to an existing hospital-based outpatient wound center or hyperbaric medicine department or medical practice can help a practitioner fulfill the requirements of the Merit Based Incentive Payment System (MIPS).
4. The practice of TM is regulated differently in each U.S. state. The American Telemedicine Association (ATA) website provides a state-by-state summary of the status of relevant legislation pertaining to telemedicine as well as interactive forums so that up-to-the-minute information can be accessed.
5. Patients with chronic wounds often transition through multiple sites of care (e.g. inpatient hospital, outpatient wound center, home nursing, home health care, or nursing home), making continuity of care extremely challenging. TM can provide the needed continuity of care for complex wound management, limb salvage, and hyperbaric medicine patients.

CONTENTS

Introduction

One basic reality in the clinical arena of complex wound management is generally accepted: The population requiring these specialized services is growing rapidly while the provider pool is not.[1-2] Traditionally, an increase in the need for specialized medical services has been met by increasing the number of physician extenders (NPs, ANPs, and PAs).[3] While that tactic closes this gap, it does so with significant infrastructure costs and inefficiencies. Another solution, with demonstrable efficacy and utility, is explored in this chapter. At the risk of introducing yet another title to an already crowded cast of characters, the concept embraced here is that telemedicine (TM) allows provider amplification without the hazard of potentially diluting the quality of the care provided.[4]

"If the presence of electricity can be made visible in any part of the circuit, I see no reason why intelligence may not be transmitted instantaneously by electricity." Samuel Morse, 1848.

While Samuel Morse's most remembered saying is his first telegraph message sent in 1844, *"What hath God wrought,"* the precept captured in the quote above lies at the heart of why the virtual exchange of patient information supplies that desired "amplification" of the highly experienced practitioner.

The origin, the moment, and the nature of human language are vigorously debated, with expert opinions ranging from 500,000 to 30,000 years ago.[5] Regardless of which date is chosen, inchoate human communication was verbal and face-to-face. The printing press, while it removed the exchange from what we recognize as conversation,[6] enormously increased the breadth of information transfer. Digital communication provided another quantum expansion of individual-to-individual information exchange. At present most of our communications are no longer face to face, but rather interface to interface. Despite whatever impersonalization digital communication imposed, it has mitigated the tyranny of distance and the poverty of limited expertise.

I. Objectives

Upon completing this chapter, the reader should understand, and be able to comfortably communicate, basic ideas concerning the history of TM, the use of this modality to remotely transact diagnostic and therapeutic tasks on complex wound patients, and the technical infrastructure necessary to initiate a new TM program. The following text, photographs, and diagrams delineate these aims.

II. History

The earliest recognized use of distant communication for medical purposes was probably the practice of African villagers using smoke signals to warn neighboring communities of the presence of diseases at their locality.[7] In the early 1900s, people living in remote areas of Australia used two-way radios, powered with a dynamo driven by a set of bicycle pedals, to communicate with the Royal Flying Doctor Service.[8] In 1961, the National Institutes of Health (NIH) funded a two-way closed-circuit TV link between two psychiatric hospitals in Nebraska.

Since face-to-face physician encounters were often obviated by the circumstances, the National Aeronautics and Space Administration (NASA) was an early adopter of this technology. By the mid-1970s NASA and the U.S. military had 15 separate telemedicine programs in place. The military also recognized the application of this technology for wound management[9] and this utility quickly found a place in civilian medicine.[10-13] The meta-analysis of controlled studies (Cochrane

Database of Systematic Reviews)[14] in a variety of clinical settings, has documented telemedicine efficacy and economy with the only hazard noted, in one study, that being a slightly higher morality in the remotely managed cohort.[15] This is conceivably a risk with all telemedicine.[16]

Establishing that electronically transmitted patient data allowed practitioners to perform at their established standard was demonstrated more than 40 years ago.[17] In 1974, NASA examined the minimal television system requirements for accurate telediagnosis. A high-quality videotape was made of an actual medical exam conducted by a nurse but supervised by a physician watching on closed-circuit television. These videotapes were systematically electronically degraded to less than broadcast quality. The original and degraded videos were then shown to randomly selected groups of physicians who attempted to reach a correct diagnosis. The results included: 1) Diagnostic decisions were not impaired until the resolution was reduced below 200 lines or until the frame rate was below 10 frames a second; 2) There was no significant difference in the overall diagnostic results as the pictorial information was altered; 3) There was no significant difference in remote treatment designations of TV system type that would cause detriment to patients; and 4) The supplementary study of transmissions of 25 cases using televised radiographic film showed no diagnostic differences between the televised evaluations and direct assessments.

III. Available resources and applications

A. Professional organizations

The American Telemedicine Association (ATA) (http://www.americantelemed.org) was founded in 1993 and currently has 10,000 members. The ATA is the linchpin national organization and the most immediate source for information regarding accreditation, risks and benefits, federal and state mandates for payers, practice guidelines, and educational resources. The ATA also offers the most reliable advice on private administration companies for institutions or individuals interested in entering this discipline.

B. Institutional organizations

The regional implementation of TM capability has been uneven but is expanding rapidly. There are regions where several institutions are linked through a state framework such as in Maine where in 1995 four hospital systems joined to create and manage a single, state-administered TM system (maine.gov/Maine IS Technology). Similarly, the Upper Midwest Telehealth Resource Center (http://www.umtrc.org) has sites in Indiana, Ohio, and Iowa. And there are several organized and experienced TM systems based at individual teaching hospitals – University of Vermont, University of Virginia, University of Michigan, University of Mississippi, and the Cleveland Clinic, to name just a few.

C. Private sector

There are several commercial entities with established experience in this field, ranging from individual consultants to providers of infrastructure and network construction. And there are entities that serve as clearinghouses for such information (i.e., http://itelemedicine.com/telemedicine-organizations-and-associations/, or http://www.telehealthresourcecenter.org/toolbox-module/organization-telemedicine-services).

IV. Current utilization

A. Internationally

In the World Health Organization's 2010 survey, 60% of all nations had some form of TM. Thirty-eight percent of all nations had programs in teledermatology, a hint at what utilization of this modality for wound care could achieve. Ajami and Lamoochi reviewed the worldwide application of this modality in 2014, emphasizing its crucial role in large disasters and in accessing remote locations.[18] There are no summary statistics on the number of TM encounters for wound management worldwide, but there is a monitoring entity – European Wound Management Association(EWMA) that will soon do such an accounting globally.

On every continent, and in both urban and rural settings, TM has been shown to improve the management of chronic conditions[19-20] to improve decision making in acute situations[21] to compensate for local scarcity of health-care resources[22-23] and to provide access to scarce expertise.[24-25]

Innovative programs, some very aggressive and far-reaching, continue to be implemented. The Paris Ile de France Regional Health Agency has authority over health-care policy in that city, where a population of 12 million is served by 419 hospitals and 2,000 long-term and social-care institutions. In 2015 this governing body inaugurated eight TM studies (two randomized trials and six before-and-after studies) examining: 1) clinical effectiveness, 2) cost effectiveness, 3) security of the application, 4) patient satisfaction and quality of life, and 5) provider perception. As of this date, only the study design and initial implementation results have been published.[23] The initial 2,500 patients will be doubled or tripled. Populations were selected on the basis of need for specialized medical care and provider availability obstacles. Three of the eight studies are directed specifically at patient populations where access to care is recognized as a weakness in the current health system. Those inclusion criteria and the size of the study should produce valuable information over the five-year course of this project.

B. Nationally

In 1996 the NIH, through the Library of Medicine's Telemedicine Initiative, awarded 19 multi-year grants to evaluate the cost, the efficacy, and the improved access afforded by telemedicine. Now, 20 years later, TM is a significant and rapidly growing component of health care in the United States. There are currently about 200 TM networks, with 3,500 service sites in the U.S. In 2014 the Veterans Health Administration delivered more than 300,000 remote consultations using telemedicine.[26] More than half of all U.S. hospitals now use some form of telemedicine. Some larger health-care systems have begun telemedicine consultation for dermatological conditions, both simple and complex, in populations historically subject to limited specialty access. The Health Plan of San Joaquin (HPSJ) is a MediCal-managed plan with 380,000 enrollees. HPSJ dramatically increased the access to this specialty service with 75% of all new enrollees now engaging with their dermatologists via TM.[27]

V. General features and benefits of telemedicine in a wound care clinic

There are two primary modes of telemedicine: 1) synchronous and 2) asynchronous. Synchronous programs are those occurring in "real time" during which there is a two-way, live-time interaction, usually between a patient and a provider, although a primary care provider may also interact with a specialist. Asynchronous TM involves accessing electronic data at a later time. Currently, reimbursement in the U.S. for TM is limited to synchronous TM, but asynchronous TM may play a valuable role in the provision of wound care services for provider training and patient diagnosis.[51] In wound care, electronically transmitted patient information can assist in the management of individual patients and in managing data from multiple sites, including facilitating the management of clinical trials as described by Serena and colleagues.[52] More than a decade ago, the use of TM began by facilitating the improved management of a patient (as depicted), but the literature is now replete with reports covering a broad spectrum of clinical scenarios.[1-2,10,15,28] Once individual facilities have the core TM elements in place, the ability to link multiple sites for data exchange and collation will allow the analyses necessary to make fundamental practice pattern decisions. The exemplar of this capability is already a reality with the U.S. Wound Registry, and in the Future section below, other intriguing possibilities are presented.

A. Telemedicine as an instrument for program development

TM may be integrated horizontally within an institution and vertically among other institutions or providers. For example, a reconstructive surgeon, while performing a complex repair in the operating room, might easily benefit from reviewing the fluorescence vascular angiogram (FVA) of that patient's wound as it was being treated in the outpatient wound center. This could then be compared to the intra-operative FVA.

TM can broaden the reach of the wound care practitioner or service line. From the most basic provider-patient interaction (a home visit) to the most complex exchange (a real-time peer-to-peer consultation), the ability to communicate directly and to simultaneously view wounds and diagnostic data will: 1) improve patient care and outcomes; 2) contain costs by obviating unnecessary outpatient visits or actual admissions; 3) strengthen and expand referral bases; 4) serve as a powerful educational platform.

An example of its use as an educational platform is remote Medical Quality Management (MQM) of wound care physician services through asynchronous telemedicine. The project with the U.S. Wound Registry (USWR) is still ongoing, but results after three years were reported for six physicians in five U.S. wound centers managed by Precision Health Care. Physician learners undergo scheduled audits on a rotating basis. Over a three-year period, an average of 16% of the total 5,950 initial patient visits were reviewed, including wound and patient photographs. In 18% of reviewed cases, the primary diagnosis was questioned (e.g., likely arterial ulcer classified as venous ulcer) and in approximately 27% of cases reviewed, some deficiency was noted (e.g., failure to follow clinical practice guidelines, error in diagnosis coding, and/or incomplete charting). In some cases, photographs revealed a possible atypical ulcer or condition (e.g., inflammatory ulcer, cancer, and/or lymphedema). Over the monitoring episodes, all physicians improved their performance. This pilot project suggests that remote medical quality monitoring can enhance quality of care for wound care patients and improve physician practice.

Infrastructure cost per patient encounter

Institutions routinely calculate their costs for specific provider-patient encounters. If administrators compared the cost for managing an increase of 20% in volume by increasing employees, floor space, and mechanical infrastructure versus handling those additional encounters with a TM system, the virtual alternative would prevail for obvious reasons. A synchronous TM encounter would not necessarily require the following:

- Additional employees and all their attendant expenses
- Additional treatment rooms, with all their attendant costs, as the providers' offices already exist

- Any costs during periods of nonuse – unlike material and staff that have costs when not engaged, the TM utility is costless when not in use.

There are, of course, costs incurred when establishing a synchronous TM capability, but the expensive elements (seasoned practitioners, computers, and Internet access) are already in hand. The cost savings, both the mechanical and the personnel expenses, realized by managing complex wounds in a virtual manner have been amply documented.[12,26,29]

B. Telemedicine as an instrument for meeting the Merit Based Incentive Payment System (MIPS)

There is available excellent written guidance for institutions and practitioners regarding the increasingly complex world of professional compliance.[30-32] When a new TM unit is being established, the practitioners involved will typically be called upon to draft the institutional requisites as well as the professional best practices and privileges guidelines. This is a unique opportunity, allowing those practitioners to both shape the operational profile of the facility and to use their TM unit activities to discharge many of their professional obligations.

Simply establishing a TM arm in an existing hospital-based outpatient department (HOPD) providing wound care and hyperbaric oxygen therapy (HBO_2) fulfills many of the mandates for Quality Reporting under the Affordable Care Act (ACA) (https://www.cms.gov/Medicare/Quality-Initiatives-Patient-Assessment-Instruments/PQRS/2015_Physician_Quality_Reporting_System.html). However, Medicare Part B payments to physicians are now determined by the specifications of the Medicare Access and CHIP Reauthorization Act of 2015 (MACRA). The majority of practitioners are subject to the Merit Based Incentive Payment System (MIPS), which requires quality reporting, the meaningful use of electronic health records (now called "advancing care information"), and participation in clinical practice improvement activities. These activities may provide opportunities for the development of telemedicine services. The initial founding of the telemedicine unit, its ongoing evolution, and the educational services using this platform also serve the practicing physicians well. These can be used to fulfill their Focused Professional Practice Evaluation and Ongoing Professional Practice Evaluation credentialing requirements and their Continuing Medical Education licensing obligations.

C. Patient acceptance

Despite numerous patient attestations embracing synchronous TM technology in their care, it is surprising that implementation of TM has been slow.[25] This general approval by patients, and its clinical efficacy, are seen across the spectrum of medical care[23,33-34] and specifically in the problem wound population.[35] In one study, designed to examine the efficacy of TM remote management of ICU patients, a fascinating ancillary finding was the profound reluctance of the involved physicians to accept this technology.[36] This was despite the study findings that remotely managed patients had the same mortality, morbidity, and length of stay, as did patients managed on site. Given the consistent finding that patients readily accept and consider TM as another laudable action by their physician, it may be that provider hesitancy is one of the biggest hindrances to implementation of this technology.

VI. Clinical examples

In 2000, a cooperative effort was launched between a metropolitan New York City Hospital (Nassau County Medical Center, NCMC) and the Visiting Nurse Services of New York City (VNSNY) to monitor topical wound care for patients who had completed their HBO_2 therapy at NCMC. The primary outcomes measured were: 1) reducing the number of hospital follow-up visits required, 2) achieving outcomes consistent with patients who did have their follow-up at the hospital, and 3) interdicting healing problems before any limb-threatening circumstances developed. All three of these outcomes were achieved.

One patient in this study was a 54-year-old female with insulin-dependent diabetes who underwent an open TMA for limb salvage, followed by 40 hyperbaric oxygen treatments until all bony elements were covered and the skin envelope was healing secondarily. However, at the conclusion of her course of HBO_2, she still required active wound management. At that time, metropolitan New York City had only three wound and hyperbaric centers, and the patient's travel time from the Bronx to NCMC was almost two hours. VNSNY provided the necessary home care with remote monitoring, thus avoiding any further in person visits to NCMC. Figure 1 was taken upon discharge from the hospital-based wound center. A follow-up photo of the same patient (Figure 2) was taken in the home setting and electronically transmitted to NCMC. It shows the wound to be contracting nicely with continuing re-epithelialization. Uneventful secondary closure was achieved. In 2000, this project was accomplished long before the era of smart phones, using equipment capable only of asynchronous (store-and-forward functionality), but which allowed transmission from residencies without Internet service.

From 2011 to 2014, at another metro NYC hospital (Hudson Valley Hospital Centers in Peekskill, New York), a telemedicine link was established with a regional rehabilitation/long-term care facility (North Westchester Restorative-Rehabilitation Center in Mohegan Lake, New York; NWRT). In addition to involving the same providers who managed the complex wounds during their inpatient stay and preempting readmissions, this system had real-time-interaction capability for assisting with complicated negative-pressure-wound-therapy (NPWT). Figures 3 and 4 depict a complex, undermined diabetic foot wound that required accurate assessment of the tunneling and a nonstandard, layered packing

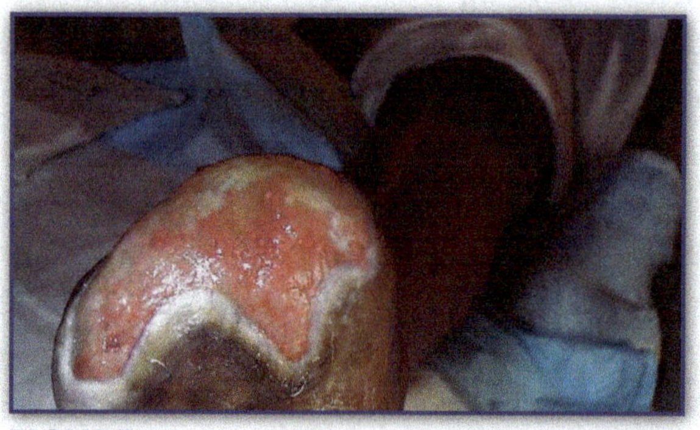

FIGURE 1. In 2000, a cooperative effort between Nassau County Medical Center and the Visiting Nurse Services of New York City allowed for asynchronous transmission of wound photographs. The first photo was taken on the day of discharge. The patient is a 54-year-old female with insulin-dependent diabetes, status post transmetatarsal amputation (TMA) for limb salvage and 40 HBO_2 therapy.

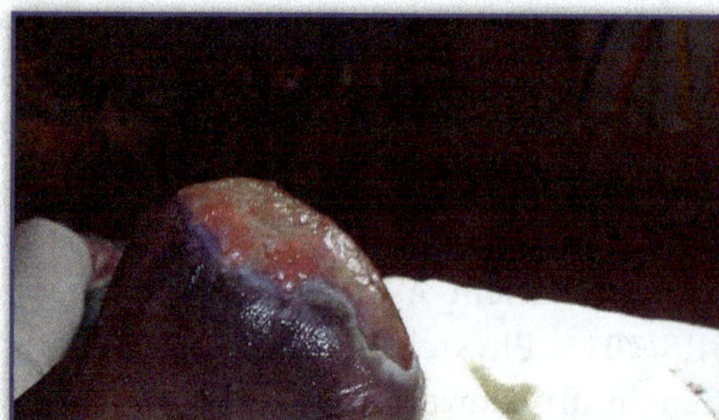

FIGURE 2. A follow-up of the same patient taken from home and transmitted to NCMC asynchronously in order to avoid a long commute for the patient into the city.

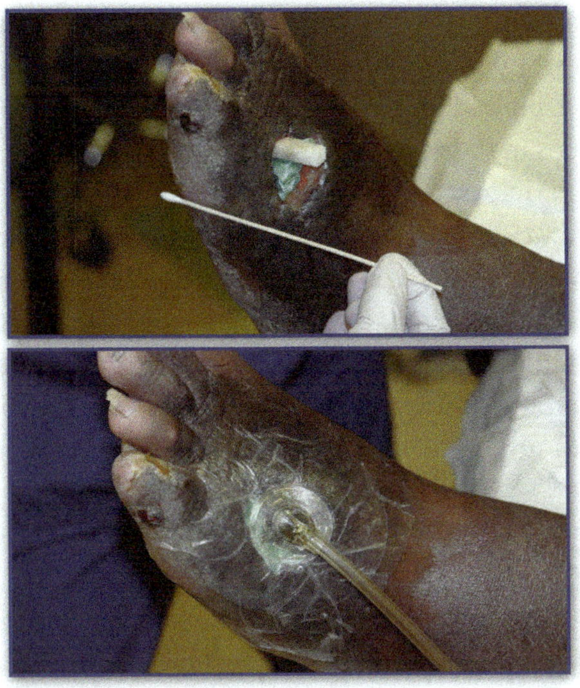

FIGURES 3 and 4. From 2011 to 2014, Hudson Valley Hospital Centers in Peekskill, New York, established a telemedicine link with North Westchester Restorative-Rehabilitation Center in Mohegan Lake, New York, a regional rehabilitation/long-term care facility. Photos depict a complex diabetic foot ulcer requiring accurate assessment of the tunneling and a nonstandard, layered packing arrangement for NPWT. Although photographs are reproduced here, the NPWT dressing change could be observed as a real-time interaction without having to transport the patient to the hospital's wound center.

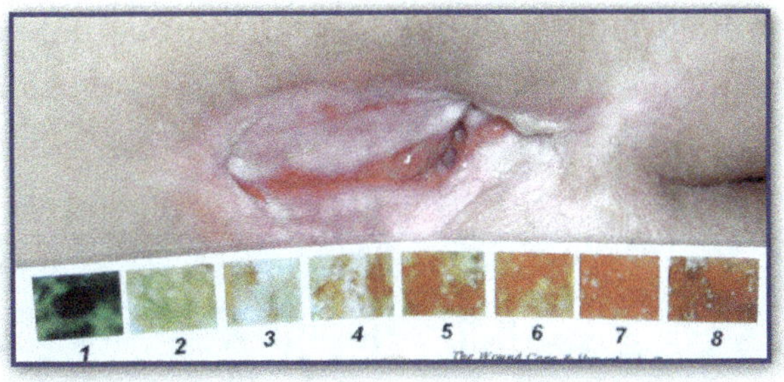

FIGURE 5. A patient with a Stage 4 sacral pressure ulcer cared for as an inpatient at HVHC. Photo taken at discharge showing the use of the low-tech granulometer.

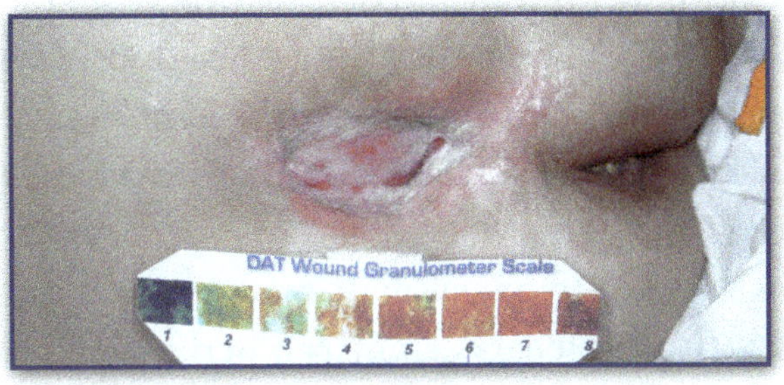

FIGURE 6. Two weeks post-discharge, a real-time virtual encounter provided the wound's dimensions, demonstrated the absence of further undermining, and an improvement in the "granulometer" score. The need for a clinic visit was avoided, and all further follow-up care was conducted by skilled home health care.

arrangement for NPWT. Although photographs are reproduced here, the NPWT dressing change could be observed as a real-time interaction via the link, without having to transport the patient to the hospital's wound center. Any practitioner who has had to manage the complications of an improperly applied NPWT dressing or struggled to educate a home health-care provider regarding the intricacies of a specific patient's NPWT application can appreciate the advantages provided by a real-time interaction.

Due to the visual nature of wound care, there is currently considerable focus on technology to automate wound measurement and/or to quantify various aspects of wound healing. Sophisticated cameras and photo analytic tools are proliferating as is the use of artificial intelligence (AI). However, not all solutions must be highly sophisticated. A relatively accurate assessment of bioburden and granulation density can be done with a simple, low-tech colorimetric grading scale, the granulometer.[37] This calibration of granulation percentage has been used since 1998 to empirically evaluate a wound base regarding its ability to accept an autologous skin graft. Until the advent of fluorescence vascular angiography, there has not been method beyond the observer's subjective opinion to get an immediate appraisal of a wound bed's reparability.[38-39] There are several other measures of a wound's "capacity for unaided secondary healing" (CUSH) such as quantitative cultures, growth factors, inflammatory markers, and MMPs, but none with the immediacy of visualization. Figures 5 and 6 demonstrate the use of this low-tech tool to help a viewer quantify granulation tissue over time if more sophisticated tools are not available, or if the wound is being viewed in real time.

VII. Establishing a telemedicine facility

A. General concerns

The fundamentals essential to developing a TM facility have been analyzed in the United States[15] as well as in a broad spectrum of health-care systems in developed and developing countries.[40-41] One of the more detailed expositions involves the MAST analysis (Model for Assessment of Telemedicine; http://www.mast-model.info) begun in 2010 at a plenary seminar in Berlin with representatives from six European countries. Video and PowerPoint presentations ranging from TM system implementation through practice paradigms, efficacy, and acceptance reports, to comprehensive legal considerations are available at the MAST website. The RAFT telemedicine network (*Réseau en Afrique Francophone pour la Télémédecine;* http://www.who.int/workforcealliance), originating and managed through Geneva University Hospitals, now services 10 African countries and provides a similar array of developmental tools for new TM programs.[41]

Common in all these reports is the conclusion that the institutional intent and the technological infrastructure are rarely serious impediments to building an effective TM program. Rather, the typical reluctance of the uninitiated practitioner, as discussed above,[35-36,42-43,46] and the construction of the interfacility network are the most common hurdles. Five challenges were frequently encountered: 1)capacity building; 2) network development and deployment of equipment; 3) implementation of clinical telemedicine; 4) implementation of activities related to continuing medical education, delivered from within the country and from abroad; and 5) establishment and use of the electronic virtual library.[40] Certainly both the host institution and the practitioners must work accordantly at all steps in the development of a TM system.

Malpractice coverage for the practitioner and risk management by the institution are valid considerations and are not addressed collectively. Fortunately, experience in both these realms is extensive, and the requisite experts are legion.[45-47] The following section details specific TM practice obligations and offers direction.

B. Current licensing and regulatory requisites

The morass of licensing demands, regulatory obligations, and clinical guidelines that bear upon a TM practice is real and cannot be ignored. However, it is not the complexity but the rapid evolution of these requirements that is actually most forbidding. The ATA maintains an almost continually updated compendium of the state legislative and regulatory enactments on these matters.[50] The ATA website provides such summary statements regarding the laws moving through each state's legislature and also provides interactive forums covering individual states so that up-to-the-minute information can be accessed. Up-to-date information by state is crucial because many states are in the process of removing the requirement for an initial face-to-face encounter in order to bill subsequent synchronous TM visits.

The issues monitored by the ATA relate to 1) payment parity; 2) practice guidelines; 3) rehabilitative/physical therapy practices; 4) state regulatory board actions; and 5) network adequacy requirements. Although in many states the licensing and regulatory decisions were initially quite restrictive, increased awareness and the universally positive impact of TM have moved mainstream medicine toward enthusiastic embrace of this discipline. The regulations for rehabilitation practices usually do not have direct applicability to a wound and hyperbaric medicine practice, but in the other four areas, examples are provided below to illustrate how effectively TM is being facilitated.

1. Payment parity

The ATA website provides a map of reimbursement parity, which shows that Rhode Island has no payment parity regulations and 18 other states have parity only with Medicaid patients. The remaining states have regulations enforcing reimbursement parity from both CMS and private payers. In 2015 a bipartisan bill was introduced in Congress (H.R.2948 - Medicare Telehealth Parity Act of 2015) that would codify this at the federal level. Concurrently, many states are in the process of enacting their own parity requirements. For example in Iowa, Medicaid parity was enacted in 2015 (SB 20) and there is pending legislation on parity for all state employees (HSB 502). The important message is that clinicians need to pay close attention to the regulations of their states.

2. Practice guidelines

At the ATA website the "Resources" tab accesses practice guidance documents ranging from the very general (Core Operational Guidelines for Telehealth Services Involving Provider-Patient Interactions) to the very specific (Guidelines for TeleICU Operations). Several medical specialties have their individual TM best practices directives available through the ATA. TM guidelines documents are also available from specific specialties. The most experienced organization with the largest number of documents relevant to TM is The American College of Radiology (http://www.acr.org/~/media/AF1480B0F95842E7B163F09F1CE00977.pdf).

3. State board regulatory actions

The ATA website also allows detailed scrutiny of TM practice regulations by issue and by state (http://www.americantelemed.org/policy/state-policy-resource-center/state-telemedicine-regulatory-tracker#.VzpCXGOcmkY).

For example, an issue that might be overlooked is that of defining an "on call" policy for the TM practitioner, a topic that was addressed by the Texas State Board in 2016 and which can be accessed on the ATM website.

4. Network adequacy requirements

Many health plans are required to meet network adequacy standards set by applicable regulatory and accrediting bodies. Generally speaking, these regulatory standards now focus simply on whether "enough" providers and facilities are included in the network based on prevalent norms. On December 2, 2015, CMS released its Patient Protection and Affordable Care Act; CMS Notice of Benefit and Payment Parameters for 2017 proposed rule. CMS issues a similar notice each year to amend federal rules governing the health insurance market under the Affordable Care Act. In establishing a TM system, while it may not be the responsibility of the institution or the practitioners to create the payer network in compliance with network adequacy directives, those health-care deliverers should expect their payers to provide assurance they are confirming to those standards.

VIII. The future

The immediate expectation for TM is for increased implementation of what has already proven to be effective and efficient. This will be in response not only to the logic of the issue but also in acknowledgement of rapidly changing health-care policies. If there is any doubt as to the importance and immediacy of this transformation of wound care, limb salvage, and hyperbaric medicine practices, a cursory review of the programs now operational at the University of Pittsburgh (http://www.upmc.com/healthcare-professionals/physicians/telemedicine/services/Pages/wound-care.aspx) and the entire Cleveland Clinic system (http://my.clevelandclinic.org/online-services/express-care-online) will quickly erase those disbeliefs.

Beyond that simple view of what the future holds, there are more ingenious applications of the TM technology once it is in place. Some of these have been alluded to above but deserve to be listed here.

1. Within the host hospital, the integration and immediate access to the hyperbaric center's data was illustrated above, but other circumstances reinforce this point. We often call upon our radiology colleagues to examine, and treat, arterial inflow obstructions. During such events in the radiology suite, having immediate access to the very distal microvascular images from FVA procedures done in the hyperbaric center provides information on actual tissue-level perfusion otherwise not seen.

2. The ability for a TM system to recruit new patients from established or previously untapped sources (visiting nurse services, LTAC/Rehabilitation Centers, and other hospitals) has been demonstrated.[38-39]

3. Establishing the host hospital as the regional nexus for physician TM consultations and patient educational information will enhance that institution's territorial presence.

4. The experts at the TM center can also serve as professional mentors for practitioners seeking to acquire new skills as their wound and hyperbaric centers evolve. This practice has been exemplified by the remote training of radiologists in MRI imaging advances.[48] Two such innovations in the wound care field are: 1) fluorescence vascular angiography (FVA)[38-39] and 2) bioelectric impedance analysis (BIA).[49] The potential for such data to be collected, collated, and analyzed at a national or regional center would be of immense value to the practitioners of wound care, limb salvage, and hyperbaric medicine.

5. The Learning Healthcare System (LHS) is the integration of clinical care, patient participation, quality improvement (QI), and comparative effectiveness research (CER), which has long been the ultimate goal of the electronic health-care revolution. In an LHS, knowledge is obtained continuously through electronic clinical documentation at the point of care, and turned into guidance through clinical decision support (CDS), with a resulting vast repository of data on treatment effectiveness to enhance RCTs and evidence-based medicine. Although few such systems have actually been realized, a recent publication describes a network-based learning health-care system by a consortium of wound care clinics that integrates wound care management, quality improvement, and comparative effectiveness research by harnessing structured real-world data within a purpose-built electronic health record at the point of care. Centers participating in the consortium submit their clinical data and quality measures to a qualified clinical data registry for wound care (the USWR), enabling benchmarking of their data across this national network. This consortium can transform wound care clinical research and raise the standards of care, while helping physicians achieve success with MIPS. Remote monitoring of

quality and identification of patients eligible for clinical trials is made possible via store-forward telemedicine.

Summary

The discrete specialty of complex wound management, limb salvage, and hyperbaric medicine is generally a referral practice. Depending on the applicable state law, an initial face-to-face encounter may not be required. The preponderance of available literature on TM, including two meta-analyses by the Cochrane Review[14] and the American College of Physicians,[46] are decidedly positive. The central question is not ***whether*** this technology will affect our discipline but ***how*** its use will shape the field, particularly with the advent of bundled payments. Given the visual nature of wound care, the frailty of our patients affecting their mobility, the number of different sites of care through which they matriculate, and the relatively low availability of wound care services in some geographic areas, TM would seem a logical solution to the dilemma of achieving continuity of care for these complex patients. TM may also help us meet the challenge of training enough wound care experts for an epidemic of wounds, in the absence of a recognized medical specialty.

Review questions

1. **Arguments for creating a telemedicine program in conjunction with a wound care program include:**

   a. TM can provide much needed continuity of care as patients transition through many different sites of care.

   b. TMs can help bridge gaps that may exist in availability of experienced wound care practitioners.

   c. TM can help contain the cost of care.

   d. broadening the reach of the wound care service line

   e. all of the above

2. **Which of the following statements about telemedicine is FALSE?**

   a. Synchronous TM involves accessing electronic data at a later time.

   b. Both synchronous and asynchronous TM may play a valuable role in the provision of wound care services.

   c. Currently only synchronous TM is reimbursed directly by payers.

   d. In wound care, electronically transmitted patient information can assist in the management of individual patients and in managing data from multiple sites.

3. **Realistic concerns when starting a TM program include all of the following EXCEPT:**

   a. malpractice coverage and risk management for the practitioner and/or institution

   b. a general unwillingness of the public to accept the concept of TM

   c. reimbursement parity which may differ by state

   d. state board regulatory actions and policies

   e. network adequacy requirements

4. ***True/False.*** The implementation of TM is expected to increase since it has already proven to be effective and efficient.

5. ***True/False.*** The visual nature of wound care makes it particularly amenable to the use of TM to solve a number of challenging health-care delivery issues.

ANSWERS: 1) e
2) a
3) b
4) True
5) True

References

1. Hellingman AA, Smeets HJ. Efficacy and efficiency of a streamlined multidisciplinary foot ulcer service. J Wound Care. 2008 Dec;17(12):541-544.

2. Barshes NR, Sigireddi M, Wrobel JS, Mahankali A, Robbins JM, Kougias P, Armstrong DG. The system of care for the diabetic foot: objectives, outcomes, and opportunities. Diabet Foot Ankle. 2013;4:10.

3. Cooper RA. New directions for nurse practitioners and physician assistants in the era of physician shortages. Acad Med. 2007 Sept; 82(9):827-828.

4. Guthrie SD, Guthrie BR, Arja MA. The evolvement of telemedicine in complex wound management & prospects for effectiveness in the wound clinic. Today's Wound Clinic. 2016 March;10(3).

5. Tallerman M, Gibson, KR. The Oxford handbook of language evolution. New York: Oxford University Press; 2012.

6. Warren, M. Features of Naturalness in Conversation. John Benjamins Publishing; 2006.

7. Nakajima I, Sastrokusumo U, Mishra SK, Komiya, R, Malik AZ, Tanuma, T. The Asia Pacific telecommunity's telemedicine activities 2006; 280-282. Available from: http://ieeexplore.ieee.org/Xplore/home.jsp?reload=true DOI: 10. 1109/HEALTH.2006.246471.

8. Strehle EM, Shabde N. One hundred years of telemedicine: does this new technology have a place in paediatrics? Arch. Dis. Child. 2006 Dec;91(12):956–959.

9. Kirkpatrick AW, Tien H, LaPorta AT, Lavell K, Keillor J, Wright Beatty HE, McKee JL, Brien S, Roberts DJ, Wong J, Ball CG, Beckett A. The marriage of surgical simulation and telementoring for damage-control surgical training of operational first responders: a pilot study. J Trauma Acute Care Surg. 2015 Nov;79(5):741–747.

10. Ablaza VJ, Fisher J. Telemedicine and wound care management. Home Care Provider. 1998 Aug; 3(4)206-211.

11. Jones SM, Banwell PE, Shakespeare PG. Telemedicine in wound healing. International Wound Journal. 2004 Dec 1(4): 225-230(6).

12. Dobke M, Renkielska A, De Neve J, Chao J, Bhavsar D. Telemedicine for problematic wound management: enhancing communication between long-term care, skilled nursing, and home caregivers and a surgical wound specialist. Wounds. 2006 Sept; 18(9): 256-261.

13. Lowery JC, Hamill JB, Wilkins EG, Clements E. Technical overview of a web-based telemedicine system for wound assessment. Advances in Skin & Wound Care.2002 July/August;15(4):165-169.

14. Flodgren G, Rachas A, Farmer AJ, Inzitari M, Shepperd S. Interactive telemedicine: effects on professional practice and health care outcomes. Cochrane Database Syst Rev. 2015 Sept 7; 9:CD002098.

15. Rasmussen BS, Jensen LK, Froekjaer J, Kidholm K, Kensing F, Yderstraede KB. A qualitative study of the key factors in implementing telemedical monitoring of diabetic foot ulcer patients. Int J Med Inform. 2015 Oct;84(10):799-807.

16. Wilcox ME, Adhikari NKJ. The effect of telemedicine in critically ill patients: systematic review and meta-analysis. Critical Care.201216:R127. DOI: 10.1186/cc11429.

17. Davis, JG. Video requirements for remote medical diagnosis. NASA Technical Reports Server (NTRS). Document ID# 19740024412; 1974 June 1.

18. Ajami S, Lamoochi P. Use of telemedicine in disaster and remote places. J Educ Health Promot. 2011; 4(3): 26.

19. Oliveira TC, Branquinho MJ, Gonçalves L. State of the art in telemedicine – concepts, management, monitoring and evaluation of the telemedicine programme; Alentejo (Portugal) Stud Health Technol Inform. 2012;179:29–37.

20. Chanussot-Deprez C, Contreras-Ruiz J. Telemedicine in wound care. International Wound Journal. 2008 Dec; 5(5):651–654.

21. Demaerschalk BM, Raman R, Ernstrom K, Meyer BC. Efficacy of telemedicine for stroke: pooled analysis of the stroke team remote evaluation using a digital observation camera (Stroke DOC) and Stroke DOC Arizona telestroke trials. Telemed J E Health. 2012;18:230–237.

22. Maddry JK, Sessions D, Heard K, Lappan C, McManus J, Bebarta VS. Wartime toxicology: evaluation of a military medical toxicology telemedicine consults service to assist physicians serving overseas and in combat (2005–2012). J Med Toxicol. 2014;10:261–265.

23. Charrier N, Zarca K, Durand-Zaleski I, Calinaud C. Efficacy and cost effectiveness of telemedicine for improving access to care in the Paris region: study protocols for eight trials. BMC Health Serv Res. 2015;16:45.

24. Drop SLS, Mure P-Y, Wood D, El-Ghoneimi A, Faisal Ahmed S. E-consultation for DSD: a global platform for access to expert advice. J Pediatr Urol. 2012;8:629-632.

25. Ong CA. Telemedicine and wound care. Stud Health Technol Inform. 2008;131:211-225.

26. Russo JE, McCool RR, Davies L. VA telemedicine: an analysis of cost and time savings. Telemed J E Health. 2016 Mar; 22(3):209-215.

27. Uscher-Pines L, Malsberger R, Burgette L, Mulcahy A, Mehrotra A. Effect of teledermatology on access to dermatology care among Medicaid enrollees. JAMA Dermatol. Published online 2016 May 4.

28. Ratliff CR, Forch W. Telehealth for wound management in long-term care. Ostomy Wound Manage. 2005;51(9):40-45.

29. Brainard JS, Ford JA, Steel N, Jones AP. A systematic review of health service interventions to reduce use of unplanned health care in rural areas. J Eval Clin Pract. 2016 Apr;22(2):145-155.

30. Fife CE, Walker D, Thomson B. Electronic health records, registries, and quality measures: what? why? how? Adv Wound Care (New Rochelle). 2013 Dec; 2(10):598–604.

31. Fife CE. The wound care clinician's quality reporting survival guide. Today's Wound Clinic. 2015 Mar;9(2).

32. Fife CE. Update on quality reporting & data registries for 2015. Today's Wound Clinic. 2015 Jan/Feb;9(1).

33. Komet, H. An analysis of the home health marketplace: how telehealth technology may assist home health agencies with changes in home care delivery under the prospective payment system. Home Health Care Management & Practice. 2001;13(2):142-148.

34. Wiseman JT, Fernandes-Taylor S, Barnes ML, Tomsejova A, Saunders RS, Kent KC. Conceptualizing smartphone use in outpatient wound assessment: patients' and caregivers' willingness to use technology. J Surg Res. 2015 Sept;198(1):245-251.

35. Hofmann-Wellenhof, R, Salmhofer, W, Binder, B, Okcu, A, Kerl, H, Soyer, HP. Feasibility and acceptance of telemedicine for wound care in patients with chronic leg ulcers. Journal of telemedicine and telecare. 2006;12(S1):15-17.

36. Thomas EJ, Lucke JF, Wueste L, Weavind L,Patel B. Association of telemedicine for remote monitoring of intensive care patients with mortality, complications, and length of stay. JAMA. 2009 Dec23/30; 302(24).

37. Cohen M, Giladi M, Mayo A, Shafir R. The granulometer – a pocket scale for the assessment of wound healing. Ann Plast Surg. 1998 June;40(6): 641-645.

38. Guthrie, SD, Guthrie, BR. Utilizing indocyanine green wound imaging in the management of hyperbaric therapy. Today's Wound Clinic 2014;.8 (8):19-22.

39. Guthrie, SD, Guthrie, BR. Detecting sbnormal sngiogenesis in on healing wounds with ICG micro-angiography. Today's Wound Clinic 2014. 2015 Nov/Dec; 9(9).
40. Latifi R, Dasho E, Merrell RC, Lopes M, Azevedo V, Bekteshi F, Osmani KL, Qesteri O, Kucani J, Lecaj I. Cabo Verde telemedicine program: initial results of nationwide implementation. Telemed J E Health. 2014 Nov;20(11):1027-1034.
41. Bediang G, Perrin C, Ruiz de Castañeda R, Kamga Y, Sawadogo A, Cheick Oumar Bagayoko CO, Geissbuhler A. The RAFT telemedicine network: lessons learnt and perspectives from a decade of educational and clinical services inlLow- and middle-incomes countries. Front Public Health. 2014;2:180.
42. Rosenthal MB. Beyond pay for performance — emerging models of provider-payment reform. N Engl J Med 2008;359:1197-1200.
43. Grol R. Successes and failures in the implementation of evidence-based guidelines for clinical practice. Med Care. 2001;39(8 Suppl 2):1146–1154.
44. Cabana, MD, Rand CS, Powe NR, Albert W. Wu AW, Wilson MH, Abboud PC, Rubin HR. Why don't physicians follow clinical practice guidelines? JAMA. 1999;282(15):1458-1465.
45. Stanberry B. Legal and ethical aspects of telemedicine. J Telemed Telecare. 2006;12(4):166-175.
46. Daniel H, Sulmasy LS. Health and Public Policy Committee of the American College of Physicians. Policy recommendations to guide the use of telemedicine in primary care settings: an American College of Physicians position paper. Ann Intern Med. 2015 Nov 17;163(10):787-789.
47. Kahn EN, La Marca F, Mazzola CA. Neurosurgery and telemedicine in the United States: assessment of the risks and opportunities. World Neurosurgery; 2016 May 89: 133–138.
48. Hata N, Tokuda J, Hurwitz, S, Morikawa S. MRI-compatible manipulator with remote-center-of-motion control. J Magn Reson Imaging. 2008 May; 27(5):1130.
49. Lukaski HC, Moore M. Bioelectrical impedance assessment of wound healing. J Diabetes Sci Technol 2012;6(1):209-212.
50. 2017 ATA state policies pertaining to telemedicine [Internet]. American Telemedicine Association [cited 2017 March 16]. Available from: https://higherlogicdownload.s3.amazonaws.com/AMERICANTELEMED/3c09839a-fffd-46f7-916c-692c11d78933/UploadedImages/Policy/State%20Policy%20Resource%20Center/State%20Legislation%20Matrix_2017.pdf.
51. Fife CE, Carey D, Spong K, Strba B, Wall V. Remote medical quality management: improving physician practice standards in wound care via Ttelemedicine. J of Wound Technology, 2013 April;(20): 46-50.
52. Serena TE, Fife CE, Eckert KA, Yaakov RA, Carter MJ. A new approach to clinical research: integrating clinical care, quality reporting, and research using a wound care network-based learning healthcare system. WWR. 2017 *in press*.

Chapter 29

ELECTRONIC HEALTH RECORDS IN WOUND CARE

Challenges and Opportunities

Caroline E. Fife, MD, FAAFP, CWS, FUHM

KEY CONCEPTS

1. Electronic medical records are not simply paper records viewable in electronic form; they also store information in a form that can be *processed and shared.*
2. EHRs are changing expectations regarding the timing of charting for all clinicians.
3. Point-of-care (POC) documentation reduces inefficiencies, decreases the probability of documentation errors, promotes information transfer, and makes clinical decision support possible.
4. Point-of-care charting might improve use of evidence-based care because clinicians will receive point-of-care reminders while they are in the room with the patient.
5. The hospital-based outpatient wound center is a provider-based setting making the physician responsible, medically and legally, for the care provided by all clinicians, regardless of whether the physician employs those caregivers, and making the physician ultimately responsible for the entirety of the clinical record.
6. The American Health Information Management Association (AHIMA) states that organizations should develop policies and procedures related to copying and pasting within the EHR, and that these actions should be considered "not OK until proven otherwise."
7. Pilot studies have already shown that clinical decision support can improve clinical practice standards with regard to offloading, compression, and vascular screening.

CONTENTS

Introduction

The medical record is the systematic documentation of a patient's medical history and care. Electronic medical records are not simply paper records viewable in electronic form; they also store information in a form that can be *processed and shared.* We no longer merely want access to the information in just one patient's chart; we want access to the information in all the charts. Processing all this information is what allows functions such as benchmarking, quality reporting, and information sharing, all of which are vital components of the modern health system.

Although quality documentation has been shown to be linked to quality of care, as a nation, the data suggest we do not do a particularly good job of either one. Americans receive appropriate, evidence-based care only 55% of the time, regardless of where they live, how much money they have, their race, their education, or their health insurance.[1-2] A major impetus for the adoption of electronic health records was that a decade ago, only 15% of physicians could generate a "registry list" from their patient data (e.g., a list of patients with a specific type of disease), 33% had to repeat tests because the results were unavailable, and few physicians had data on patient outcomes.[3] In an attempt to reduce costs and improve care through the use of health information technology (HIT), on February 17, 2009, the Health Information Technology for Economic and Clinical Health (HITECH) Act was signed into law.[4] It was hoped that the nationwide adoption of electronic health records (EHRs) would save as much as $81 billion annually due to fewer redundant tests, fewer treatment errors, and better evidence-based care.[5] The HITECH Act mandated standards that would allow the nationwide electronic exchange of health information. To foster the EHR adoption process, HITECH included up to $44,000 per physician in stimulus money, paid in installments, as practitioners achieved various stages of the meaningful use (MU) of their EHR. In addition to adopting an EHR certified to newly established (and progressively higher) standards, clinicians had to demonstrate its interoperability by activities like exchanging data with a registry and participating in quality reporting. These requirements also underpin the evolving redesign of physician payment under the Merit-based Incentive Payment System (MIPS).[6]

I. Structured data, the key to interoperability

It is fair to say that payer skepticism regarding a costly advanced therapeutic like hyperbaric oxygen therapy (HBO_2) is, at least in part, due to the lack of reliable cost-effectiveness data. Health-care organizations need actionable data to decide how to spend their resources in an era when technology is advancing, but health-care dollars are shrinking. Well-designed EHRs can provide that data. Unfortunately, EHRs are spoken of as if they are all identical when, even among products with the same level of certification as recognized by the Office of the National Coordinator for Health IT (ONC), they differ widely in functionality, usability, and value. Products that appear to have similar "front ends" may have dramatically different programming platforms, which affect reliability, customizability, data security, efficiency, and usefulness for clinical research.

The Affordable Care Act[7] is pushing health-care organizations towards value-based reimbursement models determined by measurable outcomes. The methods required to demonstrate improved outcomes and decreased cost rely on the use of discrete, highly controlled vocabularies or structured data. Structured data is information that is organized in a predefined manner, making it computer processable and identifiable for data mining and analytic purposes. Most clinicians are already familiar with two controlled vocabularies: ICD-10 (International Statistical Classification of Diseases – version 10), which is used to describe diagnoses, and CPT (Common Procedural Terminology) codes, which are used to describe clinical encounters and procedures. Other examples of structured language include LOINC (Logical Observation Identifiers Names and Codes), SNOMED CT (Systematized Nomenclature of Medicine – Clinical Terms), and RxNorm. Structured data is often captured within an EHR by the use of drop-down lists, radio buttons, and check boxes. Information that is entered as free text (typing) is not structured and therefore not processable or analyzable. Given current standards for interoperability, selecting an EHR because it is compatible with voice recognition software (which turns voice into unstructured free text) is like looking for the best carriage whip to use with your new car.

Unfortunately, many hospital EHRs provide only large vanilla "boxes" where clinicians can free-text their observations regarding a wound, its measurements, or its treatments. If the hospital EHR fails to provide any structure around wound care documentation, the data are not analyzable, and thus it is not possible to track trends in wound surface area or volume changes, transmit standardized data from one EHR to another, or document what products or therapies are used. Without data structure, it is not possible to understand outcome in relation to treatment. Structured data is particularly important because all certified EHRs must be able to create and display Continuity of Care Documents (CCDs) summarizing the key elements of medications, past history, diagnoses, labs, and studies.[8] The CCD is derived from preprogrammed vocabularies. Most EHRs use HL7 (Health Level 7) as the standard for HIT interoperability, to format the flow of data between systems. CCDs are based on the HL7 Version 3 standard Clinical Document Architecture (CDA). The CDA specifies that the content of a document consists of a mandatory, "human-readable" textual part, which ensures human interpretation of the document, and structured parts for software processing. The possible value of CCDs for wound care research will be discussed at the end of this chapter.

II. Point-of-care charting and workflow management

Many clinicians have become accustomed to dictating a note out of the hearing of the patient, perhaps even days after the encounter. EHRs are changing expectations regarding the timing of charting. Features such as clinical decision support (CDS), which include, for example, warnings about drug-drug interactions when a new drug is prescribed, are of no value if the clinician receives them hours after the patient is seen. Point-of-care (POC) documentation reduces inefficiencies, decreases the probability of documentation errors, promotes information transfer, and makes clinical decision support possible.[9] Even though the benefits have been exhaustively described and scientifically validated, the transition to POC charting has been difficult. Initially, physicians raised concerns that patients would not accept them using a computer during the patient encounter. Many studies have been performed to assess patient perception of clinician EHR use, and, almost without exception, they show that patient acceptance of POC documentation with EHRs is high. Clinicians tend to spend slightly more time in the exam room when using an EHR, and time in the room is directly linked to patient satisfaction. It can be helpful to begin encounters by explaining to patients that you will be using the computer to accurately record all the information they are going to provide and that you are listening to them even during those times you may not be looking directly at them. Most patients find this explanation acceptable and often remark that they feel the clinician is listening to them simply because they do their documentation in the room. With a properly designed EHR that maximizes structured language using features such as menus, the need for typing is dramatically reduced. Adoption of POC EHR charting may create a fundamental shift in the workflow within the wound center, but this can reduce wasted time by the staff. With point-of-care documentation, all the documents needed for the patient encounter (history and physical, home nursing orders, outpatient testing, and medical device orders) can be generated by the conclusion of the patient visit. Patients can exit the clinic with copies of their home nursing orders or letters to referring physicians or with instructions on how to access these and other documents via the EHR's patient portal. Electronically prescribed medications can be transmitted directly to the pharmacy. POC documentation can save countless phone calls for the physician and the staff. The only way that all the advantages of the EHR can be fully realized is if charting is done at the point of care.

There is another reason for point-of-care charting. The concept of the "Learning Healthcare System" put forth by the Institute of Medicine envisions an environment in which clinicians will improve their use of evidence-based care because they will receive point-of-care reminders while they are in the room with the patient. Additionally, the observations they make and document in the EHR will contribute to a vast repository of information, which can inform future decisions. It is now possible for predictive models to be incorporated within EHRs in such a way that clinicians can interact with the EHR to help make decisions about the best treatment options for a patient. We can already predict which wounds are not likely to heal with conservative care and even perhaps which patients are most likely to benefit from HBO_2. Whether patients or payers will support the use of models for this purpose is not clear, but it may be a better way to allocate increasingly scarce resources than the methods we are currently using.[10]

III. e-Prescribing

Electronic prescribing (eRx) represents one of the most advanced aspects of clinical decision support.[11] As a result of the highly structured vocabularies used for drugs and allergies, eRx systems automatically check new prescriptions against known allergy lists, look for drug-drug interactions with the patient's current medication list, and send the prescription directly to the patient's local pharmacy, checking coverage policy (and copay) with the patient's payer while the patient is still in the exam room. In many cases, e-Prescribing is a program, which is "bolted on" to the clinical EHR. Electronic prescribing vendors maintain compliance with the way in which prescribing rules differ from state to state, as well as rules pertaining to advanced care practitioners, narcotic prescriptions, and many other complex requirements.

IV. EHRs and billing

Data structure affects the ability of the EHR to perform internal auditing functions for activities like billing. According to the Healthcare Information Management Systems Society (HIMSS), with a properly programmed EHR, a clinician should perform no additional tasks in order for the billed level of service to be determined after the visit is documented.[12] If the clinician has to make any type of selection at the conclusion of the visit (e.g., use a checklist to calculate the visit level), then the calculations are not internal to the software.[13-14] Billing using a checklist is a compliance nightmare since human auditors are still necessary to ensure that proper documentation is actually present in the chart. Because internal auditing functions are characteristics of programming and thus not obvious to the user, it can be difficult for the clinician to tell the difference between systems that have internal logic and those that do not. However, most people are familiar with the way in which personal tax preparation software performs internal calculations to provide the user with the answer to the question, "How much do I owe in taxes?" To answer this question, data are entered into a software program, and the user understands that the purpose of the software is to apply a complex rule set (e.g., the tax code) to many different fields in order to produce an answer. Likewise, some EHRs are able to apply the complex physician or facility billing rules to determine the appropriate billed level of service based on the actual documentation within the chart. The difference between an internal audit function with programmed logic versus a checklist (which is a simple calculator) should be apparent. Failure to understand the difference between EHRs that perform internal, automated chart audits and those that do not can make the difference between a financially secure wound center and one which is open to Medicare recoupment.

V. HIPAA and EHRs

Ever since Congress enacted the Health Insurance Portability and Accountability Act (HIPPA) in 1996, it has controlled the way we manage patient information.[15] Originally, the act was passed to facilitate the stability of health-care benefits as individuals changed jobs. Health insurance companies and health-care providers asked Congress to find a simple way to transfer records in a standardized manner as patients moved their coverage (that is the portability part). However, protecting the privacy of the medical records was a substantial obstacle in transferring these data, so many of the HIPAA provisions have to do with privacy. The HITECH Act expanded many of the provisions of HIPAA because it addresses the privacy and security concerns associated with the electronic transmission of health information. The HITECH Act substantially increased penalties for breaching privacy regulations and extended the complete Privacy and Security Provisions of HIPAA to business associates of covered entities. That means if you work with a management company for wound care or hyperbaric medicine services, their contract must include the updated language.

To make information more portable, HIPAA requires that the provider identify the designated record set (DRS) for a patient. The DRS is a superset of information that includes the EHR as well as data housed in many other systems including billing, quality, research, and operational databases. This means that the health-care system must define all the documents, which together are going to consist of the medical record for a patient, regardless of whether those documents are maintained on paper or electronically. A common oversight in the discussion of the EHR is exactly what will be the DRS for the wound or hyperbaric center. Will it be what is in the electronic files, will it be paper documents printed from the EHR, or will it be some combination of both?

In defining the DRS, one must determine where all the parts of the record are to be found. This is a challenge for any wound and hyperbaric programs which are not managed together, because the medical justification for a hyperbaric treatment series may be contained within the wound center records. If the records of the hyperbaric center are brought up for audit, would all of the pertinent documents be available there, or would the reviewer need to go somewhere else to find these records? This is a particular consideration for EHRs provided as part of hyperbaric chamber services. How will that documentation be integrated into the rest of the chart? The custodian of medical records should be able to delineate where all the various parts of a wound and hyperbaric patient's chart are to be found, including all the photographs. If he or she is not able to do that, then this likely represents a HIPAA violation.

When one enters data into the EHR, one does so in order to create documents such as a history and physical, a progress note, a nurse's note, or a procedure note. The data entered into the EHR may be formatted a number of different ways. Hospitals often forget to ask the incredibly important question, "What will those documents LOOK like?" In the past, no clinic would have dreamed of implementing new documents without taking them through the hospital forms committee, yet many hospital EHR systems are selected without anyone ever seeing the actual documents generated by the data fields. In some cases, although the screens seemed very well organized, once the actual documents are created, it is not possible to tell which measurements refer to which wounds. This is a common problem among hospital inpatient EHRs.

VI. Photographs and protected health information

Photographs are now required by some Medicare Administrative Contractors (MACs) in order to document procedures such as debridement. The decision regarding whether or not to photograph, how, and by whom should be made by the individual facility or clinician, and institutions must understand the rules, which apply to their electronic storage. In response to HIPAA, in December of 2000, Congress authorized the U.S. Department of Health and Human Services (DHHS) to write standards to protect the privacy of individually identifiable health information, so-called protected health information (PHI). These standards are found in the U.S. Code of Federal Regulations and collectively are called the Standards for Privacy of Individually Identifiable Health Information, known as the Privacy Rule.[(16)] The Privacy Rule is intended to prevent covered health-care providers from using or disclosing health information without patients' authorization. Protected health information (PHI) is defined as any information gathered by a health-care provider that contains data that may be used directly or indirectly to identify the patient. Most clinicians are aware that the usual identifiers are PHI (e.g., name, Social Security number, and date of birth) but forget that date of service is considered an identifier, as are patient initials and the patient's medical record number (MRN). With regard to photographs, while the face is obviously PHI, so are unique birth marks or tattoos. In addition, photographs of relatives, employers, or household members can be considered PHI, according to Section 164.514(b)(2).

Most experts agree that if a wound is photographed, and there is no identifying feature in the photograph, then the photograph alone does not contain PHI as long as no written information containing PHI is in the photograph. However, the common practice of placing a ruler with either date, patient initials, medical record number, or any other link to the patient turns what would otherwise have been a de-identified photograph (falling outside of the PHI regulations) into a photograph with protected heath information. Once you have done this, all the regulations of the HITECH Act and HIPAA now apply. This has important implications regarding how photographs are stored and secured.

VII. Photographs and the designated record set

A hospital wound ostomy continence nurse (WOCN) reported that, after years of encouraging patient photographs, the hospital attorney told her to stop taking wound photographs. The decision was made, not out of medicolegal concerns, but because the hospital was adopting an electronic health record (EHR) provided by a major vendor. The hospital had chosen not to purchase photographic data storage for the EHR. In compliance with HIPAA, the hospital had determined that the designated record set would be only what was inside the hospital EHR. Thus, if the WOCN took photographs, where would these photos live from the standpoint of the record set? The nurse had been carrying around a camera in her pocket, using it to photograph various patients' wounds. To ensure that she did not place a photograph in the wrong chart, she put a ruler with the date and patient initials in each photograph. At the end of the day, she went to her office and printed out the photographs, taped the printed photos into the patient's paper chart, and stored the digital files in her office computer. This meant that a nurse was walking around the hospital with a camera in her pocket full of patient photos, which contained PHI (initials or MRN and date). If the camera was stolen or lost, there would be a breach of patient confidentiality. In addition, the computer in her office also contained photos with PHI. The only HIPAA-compliant answer, given the facility's unfortunate decision about photo management in their EHR, was to stop taking photographs on patients in the hospital. If your DRS is paper, the best option is likely to print out the digital photos and incorporate them into the paper chart and then delete the digital images from all computers and cameras. If your DRS is electronic, then the digital images would ideally be stored as part of that electronic medical record.

In response to the HITECH Act, the DHHS has exhaustively detailed the requirements for electronic data security, and these same requirements for security apply to electronic photographic data. To ensure confidentiality, storage systems must deploy strong encryption in both the actual storage and the data pathways leading in and out. The HITECH Act itself does not mandate that electronic data be encrypted. However, under the HITECH act, there are substantial penalties for breaches, which are specifically avoided if the data are strongly encrypted both "at rest" and "in motion." This means clinicians are ill-advised to leave photographs containing PHI at rest, unencrypted, in a camera. Although clinicians are accustomed to carefully securing the rest of a patient's chart, whether paper or electronic, they often handle patient photos in a cavalier fashion. The HITECH Act establishes penalties for breaching PHI, which is not encrypted "at rest." Since a camera cannot provide encryption, photos cannot stay in a camera but must instead be placed inside some sort of encrypted electronic file, preferably the EHR.

VIII. Understanding metadata

Metadata is a word that means data about data. It provides information about an item's content. For example, a text document's metadata may contain information about who the author is or when the document was written. The GPS location information on a smartphone picture is an example of metadata. Most users of EHRs do not realize that the EHR is creating metadata whenever it is being utilized. Using metadata, it is possible to determine when and who viewed an EHR and when documentation was added. More than one malpractice case has been won or lost using metadata. Your vendor will be able to tell you what type of metadata is collected within your EHR.

IX. Storage and backup

The storage system for records must be capable of providing long-term retention guarantees. Since it is conceivable that the failure of storage servers, as well as obsolescence of technology and formats, will require migration of records, the storage system must provide trustworthy and verifiable migration mechanisms. There must exist strong backup and restore operations. The backup copies should be located in a separate off-site location to ensure survival in case of fire or natural disasters. Organizations outsourcing some of their record management tasks, including the storage of photographs, must ensure that the third parties also comply with HIPAA.

X. Security and sign-off

Clinicians sign charts so frequently they may give little thought to the meaning of a signature. However, CMS states individuals who sign the chart are responsible for the authenticity of the information. This is true even when using an electronic signature.[17] When a clinician signs the chart, he or she is indicating that he or she has accepted the accuracy of the chart as his or her own. At the present time, there are no universal standards regarding electronic signatures for EHRs. Even if your EHR requires you to submit data periodically as you complete forms, unless you are actually entering a password or some other security device, you are not actually authenticating the document. Remember that the hospital-based outpatient wound and hyperbaric department provides patient care incident to a physician service. That means that the physician is responsible medically and legally for the care provided by all the other clinicians, even though those caregivers are not employed by the physician. In that setting, when the physician signs the chart, he or she is acknowledging the documentation of all the individuals in the chart and is attesting (1) that he or she has read the chart and is familiar with its contents, and (2) that he or she knows what treatments were performed and is responsible for the care provided by all the staff members in the wound and hyperbaric center. For this reason, no physician should ask for or use a "sign all unsigned charts" feature. According to the American Health Information Management Association (AHIMA), auto-authentication, defined as signing multiple documents at one time without opening the documents, falls short of federal and state authentication requirements and could place the organization at legal risk.[18] The EHR should not allow more than one chart to be signed at a time.

XI. Copying and pasting

For many years, clinicians dictated notes, which were transcribed into the clinical chart. As a new generation of clinicians emerged who were capable of typing, they began to enter notes directly into the EHR but quickly realized that since many procedures and observations were repetitive, they could avoid typing the same notes over and over by copying and pasting notes from one chart to another. Unfortunately, this process has introduced many possible errors into the medical record. A quality improvement project was carried out at the

Veteran's Administration Health Care System in Puget Sound, Washington, to evaluate the impact of copying and pasting in the electronic health record.[19] A sample of 1,479 patients were selected in which there were 167,076 notes written between 1990 and 2002. Within these notes, there were 90,762 copy events. After filtering frequent, trivial duplications, approximately 5% of charts were assessed as having misleading information resulting from copy/paste activities, incurring either some or a major health-care risk. After each chart was read by an advanced health-care professional, it was determined that there were 338 specific instances where patients might have been put at risk as a result of copy/paste activities, affecting about 5% of the total patients. In addition to the risk and liability, copy/paste documentation may result in an unwarranted increase in payment by making it appear that the provider did more work than he or she actually did, generating charges which are not likely to withstand an audit. The American Health Information Management Association (AHIMA) states that organizations should develop policies and procedures related to copying and pasting within the EHR, and that these actions should be considered not OK until proven otherwise.

XII. What's next

Wound care clinicians often express tremendous frustration that, although large hospital EHR vendors represent that they have a documentation solution for the outpatient wound center, in reality, the clinicians are expected to build the wound care documentation modules themselves. The process is time-consuming, and developing it is often low on the list of priorities after hospital-wide EHR implementation. The hospital EHR is not designed to perform the internal calculations, which can inform wound care physician or facility billing. Even documenting debridements or cellular products involves arcane rules which require the wound care practitioner to combine the skills of a billing and coding expert with that of a software engineer in a process that moves at a glacial pace. Contributing to data registries and quality reporting, which primarily benefit the clinician and are of less benefit to the facility, are luxuries not likely to be addressed. Clinicians provide the EHR vendors with their time and expertise, usually without receiving compensation. This process is repeated at hospitals all over the country, developing documentation modules that cannot share data because they each collect data differently. No mechanism exists by which the best ideas can be utilized by others.

In contrast, when the smartphone first arrived on the market, the decision was made to expose some parts of the source code so developers could build tools for use with the phone. The code that is exposed is called an application programming interface (API), a set of routines and protocols for building software applications commonly referred to as apps. The collective creativity of the marketplace has developed more apps than the originators of the smartphone could have ever imagined. Similarly, the next evolutionary step for EHR vendors is Open API. Large hospital EHR vendors will create a platform that can accept apps that visualize clinical data, offer decision support capabilities, and integrate data with outside sources like population health tools and registries. The Open API initiative will facilitate the installation of wound care quality measures and standardized wound care documentation modules throughout the United States. This will change the future of wound care clinical research.

XIII. Capitalizing on the opportunities

With near-universal hospital EHR adoption and growing physician acceptance (or at least, resignation) to their uses, the time is right for the opportunities inherent in EHRs to be realized, particularly in the field of wound care. The potential value of an EHR that can utilize logic is enormous for wound care because internal logic can, for example, help select dressings on the basis of wound descriptors, identify wounds that might benefit from cellular products or advanced therapeutics, and trigger clinical decision support based on a particular type of wound. Pilot studies have already shown that CDS can improve clinician adherence to off-loading, compression, and vascular screening.

Despite the fact that the prevalence of chronic wounds in the United States is roughly the same as that of heart failure and may cost the taxpayer considerably more in Medicare expenditures, wound healing has had nowhere near the commitment of research funding as cardiovascular disease. There is a desperate need for analyzable, real-world data, and the EHR revolution may make this possible. As a result of the HITECH Act, all certified EHRs are currently capable of automatically transmitting a CCD summary document using a standard format, which contains (at a minimum) the patient's medications, allergies, diagnoses, labs, procedures, studies, and treatments. This vast repository of data would once have required hours of labor to enter into a research database or registry, but now, once it exists as part of the medical record, it can be automatically transmitted to specialty registry without the need for any special computer interfaces or secondary data entry. Furthermore, the requirements of meaningful use mandate that clinicians participate in such registries or risk losing a percentage of their Part B Medicare payments. The U.S. Wound Registry[20] sponsors a number of meaningful use registries including the Hyperbaric Oxygen Therapy Registry, the Negative Pressure Wound Therapy Registry, the Cellular and Tissue-based Product Registry, the Podiatry Registry, and the Venous Leg Ulcer Registry, all of which are listed on the National Institute of Health (NIH) Clinical Trials website. These various registries receive data via CCD, transmitted directly from certified EHRs. The mechanism by which they can be used for clinical research will be discussed further in Chapter 30: Moving from Volume to Value in Wound Care. Structured data automatically transmitted from EHRs participating in the Hyperbaric Oxygen Therapy Registry (HBOTR) was provided to the American Medical Association's Relative Value Committee when it evaluated the work component of hyperbaric oxygen therapy chamber supervision.[21] Because the data were transmitted using structured language, rapid analysis was possible (within hours of the request). EHR data from more than 100 hospital-based outpatient hyperbaric centers demonstrated that the average hyperbaric patient has 10 major comorbid conditions and takes an average of 12 medications. This rapid analysis was able to preserve reimbursement for the work that hyperbaric physicians perform when they supervise hyperbaric oxygen therapy treatments due to the complexity of the patients involved. It would be nice to think that the frustrations experienced by clinicians to adopt EHRs could tangibly benefit the field of wound care and hyperbaric medicine if we can successfully harness the HIT revolution.

XIV. Core principles for EHR adoption in the wound and hyperbaric center

These principles below form the basis for an understanding of the way in which the EHR should be used within a hospital-based outpatient wound center and should be reflected in specific policies and procedures developed for the implementation of an EHR.

1. Recognition of provider-based departmental status: A wound and hyperbaric facility operating as a hospital-based outpatient department is a provider-based service. While the nurses and other staff members may be employed by the hospital, they provide patient care incident to the advanced practitioner. Therefore, the advanced practitioner has the legal responsibility for all of the patient care and thus all of the documentation made by all the staff members.

2. The legal chart is a file-based representation of an actual event (e.g., a progress note). It should be represented as a document, which is generated at a point in time and preserved without alteration after the clinician signs off.

3. The provider-based status of the wound and hyperbaric center services make the physician or other advanced practitioner ultimately responsible for the correct establishment of the diagnoses for which the patient is treated. The EHR should not allow other individuals to alter diagnosis codes once the physician has signed and locked the chart (e.g., hospital coders should not be able to change diagnoses in the chart) without the knowledge of the advanced practitioner.

4. The time period during which locked charts can be unlocked for changes should be defined and limited: for some period of time (e.g., 24–48 hours), it is acceptable for a locked chart to be able to be unlocked by the advanced practitioner in order to finalize or complete missing documentation. However, after some reasonable time period, and certainly after any charges have been dropped, no further changes can be made to the chart without clearly designating these changes as amendments to the original.

5. The designated record set (DRS) for the department will be clearly defined: the DRS will include all of the documents which might be necessary to justify charges should an audit occur. In other words, if the hyperbaric department is audited, and the wound center program is operated independently, the DRS is understood to contain the wound center records as well. The custodian of medical records can identify the location of all elements of the DRS, including data, which may reside, for example, in a hyperbaric chamber vendor database.

Summary

Electronic health records are the systematic collection of patient information in a form that can be *processed and shared.* Data sharing is contingent on the use of controlled vocabularies and facilitates functions such as internal auditing of charges and quality reporting. Wound and hyperbaric centers must define the designated record set and ensure that if photographs are taken, they are properly incorporated into the DRS and secured. The structure of an EHR has significant implications for the manner in which it functions within the clinic and how data and documents are created and secured. The new Quality Payment Program (QPP)[22] necessitates reporting to CMS a set of clinical quality measures, participating in clinical practice improvement activities, and transmitting data to a specialty registry. These requirements can be used as an opportunity for wound care and hyperbaric medicine to obtain much-needed cost-effectiveness data. The incorporation of specialty-specific decision support rule offers another opportunity for wound care clinicians to harness the practice guidelines in this textbook to improve the care of wound and hyperbaric patients.

As we approach what will surely be a paradigm shift in the delivery of health care, we are reminded of an 1834 news article in the *London Times* describing the invention of the stethoscope: "That it will ever come into general use, notwithstanding its value, is extremely doubtful because its beneficial application requires much time and gives a good bit of trouble."[23] It seems that clinicians have always been slow to adopt new technology whenever the technology is "a good bit of trouble." While point-of-care charting using an EHR may be more challenging to adopt than the stethoscope, it can result in greater efficiency and improved patient care, as well as provide much-needed data for clinical research in the field of wound care and hyperbaric medicine. Since it is clearly here to stay, our focus should now be on how to best utilize electronic documentation on behalf of our patients and our specialty.

Review questions

1. **Which of the following statements about point-of-care charting are true?**
    a. Patients have been accepting because doctors tend to spend more time in the exam room with them.
    b. It makes point-of-care reminders possible that can drive better practice standards.
    c. If electronic prescribing is used, clinicians are warned of possible drug interactions while still in the examination room with the patient.
    d. It reduces charting errors.
    e. all of the above

2. **Which of the following statements correctly describe some potentially serious privacy and security issues relating to wound photographs?**
    a. There is unencrypted patient protected health information (PHI) in the camera.
    b. If the camera is lost or stolen, the hospital has committed a HIPAA violation, probably on multiple patients.
    c. If a doctor has patient photos containing PHI on his or her laptop, and the computer is lost or stolen, he or she has committed a serious HIPAA violation.
    d. Tattoos, date of service, and faces of family members are PHI.
    e. All are correct.

3. ***True/False:*** The hospital-based outpatient department (HOPD) is a provider-based setting with all care provided "incident to" the advanced practitioner.

4. ***True/False:*** As a result of the unique supervision rules surrounding the HOPD, the nurses should be able to chart completely independently of the doctor.

5. **Which of these EHR features increase the risk of litigation for the advanced practitioner?**
    a. a feature allowing him or her to sign all the unsigned charts without reading each one
    b. a feature allowing him or her to cut and paste from one chart to another
    c. a feature allowing the nurses and other staff members to chart completely independently from him or her so that he or she never has to review their documentation
    d. a feature allowing the nurses and other staff members to change their documentation after the advanced practitioner has signed the chart
    e. all of the above

ANSWERS: 1) e
2) e
3) True
4) False
5) e

References

1. McGlynn EA, Asch SM, Adams J, Keesey J, Hicks J, DeCristofaro A, Kerr EA. The quality of health care delivered to adults in the United States. N Engl J Med. 2003 Jun 2;348 (26):2635-45.
2. Asch SM, Kerr EA, Keesey J, Adams JL, Setodji CM, Malik S, McGlynn EA. Who is at greatest risk for receiving poor-quality health care? N Engl J Med. 2006 Mar 16;345(11):1147-56.
3. O'Kane M. Opening remarks at Health Care Summit, National Committee for Quality Assurance [Internet]. National Committee for Quality Assurance; 2010 Jul. Available from: http://www.ncqa.org/Portals/0/Public%20 Policy/Triple_Aim_Speech_Transcript.pdf.
4. HHS.gov [Internet]. U.S. Department of Health and Human Services, Office for Civil Rights. HITECH Act Enforcement Interim Final Rule. Available from: http://www.hhs.gov/ocr/privacy/hipaa/administrative/enforcementrule/hitechenforcementifr.html.
5. Hillestad R, Bigelow J, Bower A, Girosi F, Meili R, Scoville R, Taylor R. Can electronic medical record systems transform health care? Potential health benefits, savings, and costs. Health Aff. 2005;24(5):1103-17.
6. CMS.gov, Centers for Medicare & Medicaid Services [Internet]. U.S. Department of Health and Human Services, Centers for Medicare and Medicaid Services. MACRA: Delivery System Reform, Medicare Payment Reform. Available from: https://www.cms.gov/Medicare/Quality-Initiatives-Patient-Assessment-Instruments/Value-Based-Programs/MACRA-MIPS-and-APMs/MACRA-MIPS-and-APMs.html.
7. HHS.gov [Internet]. U.S. Department of Health and Human Services. About the Affordable Care Act. Available from: http://www.hhs.gov/healthcare/about-the-law/read-the-law/#.
8. Health Level Seven International [Internet]. Health Level Seven International. HL7/ASTM Implementation Guide for CDA® R2 – Continuity of Care Document (CCD®) Release 1. Available from: http://www.hl7.org/implement/standards/product_brief.cfm?product_id=6.
9. HealthIT.gov [Internet]. U.S. Department of Health and Human Services, Office of the National Coordinator for Health Information Technology. What are the advantages of electronic health records? Available from: https://www.healthit.gov/providers-professionals/faqs/what-are-advantages-electronic-health-records.
10. Fife CE, Eckert KA, Carter M. An update on the appropriate role for hyperbaric oxygen: indications and evidence. Plast Reconstr Surg [Internet]. 2016 Sep;138(3S):107S-16S. Available from: http://journals.lww.com/plasreconsurg/Fulltext/2016/09001/An_Update_on_the_Appropriate_Role_for_Hyperbaric.15.aspx.
11. Health Resources & Services Administration [Internet]. U.S. Department of Health and Human Services, Health Resources & Services Administration. Electronic prescribing. Available from: http://www.hrsa.gov/healthit/toolbox/HealthITAdoptiontoolbox/ElectronicPrescribing/elecprescribing.html.
12. HIMSS.org [Internet]. Healthcare Information and Management Systems Society. HIMSS Standards. Available from: http://www.himss.org/ASP/topics_FocusDynamic.asp?faid=39.
13. Fife CE, Walker D, Farrow W, Otto G. Wound center facility billing: a retrospective analysis of time, wound size, and acuity scoring for determining facility level of service. Ostomy Wound Manage. 2007;53(1):34-44.

14. Fife CE, Wall V, Carter MJ, Walker D, Thomson B. Examining the relationship between physician and facility level-of-service coding in outpatient wound centers: results of a multicenter study. Ostomy Wound Manage. 2012;58(3):20-8.
15. HHS.gov [Internet]. U.S. Department of Health and Human Services. Health Insurance Portability and Accountability Act of 1996 (HIPAA). Public Law 104-191, 110 Stat. 1936 (Aug. 21, 1996). Available from: http://www.hhs.gov/ocr/hipaa/.
16. Privacy rule: standards for privacy of individually identifiable health information. 45 Code of Federal Regulations, parts 160 and 164 [Internet]. U.S. Department of Health and Human Services; 2003 Apr 14. Available from: http://www.hhs.gov/ocr/privacy/hipaa/administrative/privacyrule/prdecember2000all8parts.pdf.
17. Medicare program integrity manual chapter 3 – verifying potential errors and taking corrective actions [Internet]. U.S. Department of Health and Human Services, Centers for Medicare and Medicaid Services. Available at: http://www.cms.gov/manuals/downloads/pim83c03.pdf.
18. AHIMA HIM Body of Knowledge [Internet]. The American Health Information Management Association. AHIMA guidelines for EHR documentation to prevent fraud. Available from: http://library.ahima.org/xpedio/groups/public/documents/ahima/bok1_033097.hcsp?dDocName=bok1_033097.
19. AHIMA HIM Body of Knowledge [Internet]. The American Health Information Management Association. Copying and pasting in the EHR-S: an HIM perspective. Available from: http://library.ahima.org/doc?oid=60164#.V1SnM2bmoyA.
20. U.S. Wound Registry [Internet]. U.S. Wound Registry. Available from: https://www.uswoundregistry.com/.
21. Fife CE, Gelly H, Walker D, Eckert KA. Rapid analysis of hyperbaric oxygen therapy registry data for reimbursement purposes: technical communication. UHM. 2016;43(6). Available from: https://www.uhms.org/publications/uhm-journal/uhm-journal-ahead-of-print-public.html?task=document.viewdoc&id=1072.
22. Quality Payment Program [Internet]. U.S. Department of Health and Human Services [cited 2017 Mar 18]. Available from: https://qpp.cms.gov/.
23. Grais IM. Proper use of the stethoscope: three heads and one tale. Tex Heart Inst J. 2013;40(2):120-2.

Chapter 30

MOVING FROM VOLUME TO VALUE IN WOUND CARE

Caroline E. Fife, MD, FAAFP, CWS, FUHM

KEY CONCEPTS

1. MACRA, the Medicare Access and Chip Reauthorization Act, was passed by Congress on April 1, 2015, and ushered in Medicare's Quality Payment Program (QPP) which seeks to transition practitioners away from a payment system based on volume to one based on value.

2. MACRA consists of two payment tracks: the Merit-based Incentive Payment System (MIPS) and Advanced Alternative Payment Models (APM).

3. MIPS defines four weighted categories of clinical performance that contribute to a composite performance score (CPS) of 100 points: Quality, Advancing care information, Clinical Practice Information Activities (CPIA) and Resource Use.

4. All providers' quality performance data is now available on the Physician Compare website.

5. Clinicians who succeed in the new QPP will be those who: 1) utilize their electronic health record effectively, 2) successfully report practice relevant quality measures, and 3) participate in a qualified clinical data registry

CONTENTS

Introduction to MIPS and MACRA

In 2014, Medicare covered 53.8 million people. Its total expenditures were $613.3 billion, but its total income was $599.3 billion.(1) This unsustainable math will result in the depletion of the Hospital Insurance Trust Fund by the year 2030. Of note, in 2014, $8.1 billion in trust fund assets were redeemed to help cover the shortfall of income that year. Medicare was able to return this money to the trust fund through a variety of recoupment activities targeting fraud and improper use programs. These recoupment activities directly affect wound care and hyperbaric medicine providers who are experiencing unprecedented scrutiny, driven in part by the urgent need to balance Medicare's budget. It is estimated that by the year 2089, Medicare costs will represent 6% of gross domestic product (GDP), assuming the cost savings of health-care reform are realized. However, if the payment reductions for physicians and other health services do not take full effect, Medicare spending will represent roughly 9.1% percent of GDP in 2089, putting an untenable strain on the U.S. economy and the American worker. We must reduce health-care spending, but how?

The commitment of such massive resources to health care for the elderly and disabled might be justified if there were universal agreement that the quality of care they receive is high. Frustratingly, some researchers have found a perverse relationship between quality of care and Medicare spending,(2) with states like Louisiana and Texas, which spend the most per patient (nearly $8,000 per beneficiary), providing lower quality care by some metrics than Utah, which spends about 60% as much (about $5,000 per beneficiary). Others have refuted these findings, suggesting that the issue is far more nuanced and profoundly affected by physician availability, population demographics, and other variables.(3) Nevertheless, overall there seems to be a lack of correlation between utilization of services (spending) and either health-care outcomes or quality of care. It also seems likely that the providers in the highest-spending regions are overusing services. Evidence suggests that these regions could provide equal or even better care at lower cost if they eliminated unneeded services. We already know that patients in general, and wound care patients in particular, often do not receive basic evidence-based care such as offloading or compression, even though they do receive expensive advanced therapeutics like cellular products and hyperbaric oxygen therapy (HBO_2 therapy).(4-5) It was this disconnect which provided impetus for Medicare's prior authorization program of hyperbaric oxygen therapy to ensure that appropriate conservative care was performed prior to HBO_2 therapy. Despite legitimate frustrations with the prior authorization program for hyperbaric oxygen (as only one example), there seem to be substantial opportunities for improving both the efficiency and the quality of medical care in the United States in general, and wound care services in particular. Both of these goals could be accomplished by providing better and consistent evidence-based care, while decreasing unnecessary and improper use of resources. If we do not succeed, simple math tells us that Medicare will not be available to our children.

To control spending on physician services, the Sustainable Growth Rate (SGR) formula was enacted by the Balanced Budget Act of 1997. The goal was to ensure that the annual increase in expenses per Medicare beneficiary did not exceed the growth in GDP. Every year following its passage, the Centers for Medicare & Medicaid Services (CMS) sent a report to the Medicare Payment Advisory Commission which advises Congress on the previous year's expenditures. If expenditures exceeded the target, the report provided a conversion factor to decrease physician payments for the following year in order to match the target SGR. However, this decrease in the physician fee schedule could be suspended or adjusted by Congress, often referred to as the annual doc fix. These temporary fixes had been enacted by Congress for 17 consecutive years, resulting in an ever-widening gap between the Medicare budget and the physician payment rate to the point that by 2015, a reduction of 21% in Medicare Part B physician compensation was needed to bring expenditures into alignment with the SGR. This crisis was averted by a surprising bipartisan move on April 1, 2015, when Congress passed MACRA, the Medicare Access and CHIP Reauthorization Act,[6] which established an entirely new framework for practitioner payment. It is the hope of CMS that MACRA will reward better care rather than just more care. Now being called the Quality Payment Program (QPP), MACRA consists of two payment tracks: the Merit-based Incentive Payment System (MIPS) and Advanced Alternative Payment Models (APMs). Most Part B clinicians will be subject to MIPS unless they are participating in an advanced APM (e.g., an Accountable Care Organization).

Under MACRA, professionals will receive an annual update of 0.5% in each of the years 2015 through 2019. Then, in 2019, it establishes an improved incentive payment program that will focus on providing value and quality. This incentive payment program, referred to as the Merit-based Incentive Payment System (MIPS), streamlines and consolidates previous incentive programs including the Physician Quality Performance System (PQRS) and the Meaningful Use (MU) of an Electronic Health Record (renamed Advancing Care Information or ACI). MIPS defines four categories of clinician performance that contribute to a composite performance score (CPS) of up to 100 points according to their performance in four weighted categories: Quality, Advancing Care Information, Clinical Practice Improvement Activities (IAs) and Resource Use (meaning, cost). Each year CMS changes the weighting of these categories so that relative importance of the categories changes annually. At least in the first few years, Quality contributes the largest percentage.

Clinicians with the worst MIPS scores in the first year (2017) will see as much as a 4% downward adjustment in their Medicare Part B payments in 2019. Adjustments lag two years behind the reporting of data. The highest performers could see a maximum base payment increase of as much as 12%. The program is budget neutral, which means that the money available for incentives comes from the money assessed as penalties. However, Congress set aside an additional $500 million as separate bonus money for exceptional performers to realize an additional 10% bonus, making a 22% increase in Medicare Part B payments possible for the top tier. Thus, it is possible for a few clinicians to earn very high bonuses because a larger pool of clinicians will experience penalties. A provider's MIPS score can cause a rapid and profound change to a clinician's revenue in either a positive or a negative direction. Penalties for poor performers continue to increase over time so that in 2021, practitioners could experience as much as a 7% loss of Medicare Part B payments.

I. The cost of chronic wounds to Medicare

Little has been written on the category of Resource Use (cost) with regard to the wound care practitioner. As it now stands, MACRA is not well targeted to identify resource use in patients with chronic nonhealing wounds even though this category (the importance of which increases over time) will be used to adjust physician payment. Resource use calculations are triggered either by the presence of a medical condition that CMS has identified as a major cost contributor or by the performance a specific surgical procedure also identified as common and costly. Sadly, the morbidity and associated costs of chronic wounds, which include amputation and death, have been largely ignored by CMS. Furthermore, thanks to Medicare policies directed at cost containment, chronic wounds are very likely to be treated in the outpatient or subacute setting and do not necessarily begin with a sentinel inpatient event or surgery. The Alliance of Wound Care Stakeholders, an association of clinical associations that advocates for patients with wounds, commissioned a study of the cost of wound care as part of its comments to CMS on MACRA. That analysis revealed that hospital outpatient services represented the largest share of wound care costs (36%), a finding not previously reported in the literature.[7] Costs within Medicare Advantage constituted 28% of resource use for wound care, whereas hospital *inpatient* costs accounted for only 18% of Medicare spending on wound care. The remaining service types (home health, skilled nursing, durable medical equipment, physician billing) represented only 1%–9%.[7] Chronic wounds impact nearly 20% of Medicare beneficiaries (over 11 million persons) and in 2014 alone, as a conservative estimate were responsible as much as $35 billion dollars in Medicare expenditures, including both fee-for-service and Medicare Advantage. If we include wounds as a secondary diagnosis, this cost of chronic wounds in 2014 may have reached $151.7 billion, with dehisced surgical wounds being the most expensive and most prevalent category. Currently, under MACRA, CMS is proposing 41 episode-based resource use measures for care areas including cardiovascular, gastrointestinal, and neurology, none of which include wound care. The Alliance analysis reveals that the care of patients with chronic wounds represents a far greater portion of the Medicare trust fund than previously understood and that these costs largely occur in the outpatient or subacute setting. Wound care stakeholders must work with CMS to ensure that this financial reality is reflected in the resource use measures developed as part of MIPS.

Because some provisions of the QPP continue to be a work in progress, this chapter will focus on quality reporting in general and its implications for wound care providers. It appears that at least 75% of the provider's MIPS score will be determined by performance in categories similar to PQRS and MU. This chapter will focus on how these initiatives can be harnessed to benefit wound care clinicians to improve the outcome of wound care patients and to preserve the revenue of wound care practitioners as MIPS is implemented.

II. Quality reporting

The Physician Quality Reporting System actually began in 2008 as a bonus program called PQRI (Physician Quality Reporting Initiative). Eligible providers (EPs) include almost any practitioner who bills under the Medicare Physician Fee Schedule, which includes podiatrists and nurse practitioners, as well as many other advanced practitioners. Although there are several hundred quality measures available for reporting under MIPS,[8] none are directly relevant to wound care or hyperbaric medicine. Some quality measures (QMs) are relevant to the care of the comorbid conditions that impact wound healing including the control of hemoglobin A1C, screening for tobacco use and counseling tobacco cessation, and assessing diabetics for appropriate footwear. It is certainly possible for a wound care practitioner to pass the quality portion of MIPS using measures that are not directly relevant to the care of patients with wounds. However, it must be remembered that all the providers' quality performance data will be publicly available on Physician Compare website[9] (and later, on social media sites like Yelp), so consumers will be able to see the scores of all eligible providers rated on a scale of 0 to 100 and how they compare to their peers nationally. This creates an interesting issue for wound care practitioners. Would a wound care practitioner wish to have his or her expertise in wound care judged publicly, based on the measures listed in Table 1? Knowing that private payers will use quality measures to set reimbursement rates and decide where to refer their beneficiaries in need of wound care, and that employers may use these QM performance rates to develop incentive packages for physician employees, will it be acceptable to "just report any measures" in order to pass, or do wound care providers need to demonstrate more than that?

III. The role of qualified clinical data registries (QCDR)

A QCDR is a CMS-approved entity that collects medical and/or clinical data for the purpose of patient and disease tracking to foster improvement in the quality of care provided to patients. In 2008, CMS began the program now called PQRS and created a reporting mechanism by which specialized registries could transmit quality data on behalf of providers in order to get credit for PQRS participation. In 2014, CMS introduced a new reporting mechanism called a Qualified Clinical Data Registry (QCDR). Just like the qualified data registries that existed previously, QCDRs complete the collection and submission of PQRS quality measures data on behalf of EPs. However, an important

TABLE 1. USWR quality measures

Risk-stratified Wound Outcome Measures (High Value)
• DFU outcome: healing or closure (risk-stratified)
• Venous leg ulcer outcome measure: healing or closure (risk-stratified)
• Major amputation in Wagner Grade 3, 4, or 5 DFUs treated with HBO_2 therapy (risk-stratified)
Appropriate Use Measures (High Value)
• Appropriate use of HBO_2 therapy for DFUs
• Appropriate use of cellular- or tissue-based products (CTP) DFUs or VLUs
Patient Reported Measures (High Value)
• Patient reported wound outcome
• Patient reported nutritional screen
Process Measures
• Adequate offloading of DFUs
• Adequate compression of VLUs
• Arterial screening of leg ulcer patients
• Nutritional screening of patients with wounds
• Checking vital signs and blood glucose (in diabetics) prior to HBO_2 therapy

distinction about a QCDR in comparison to other quality measure reporting registries is that QCDRs can actually *develop* quality measures which EPs can report for MIPS credit, even though the QCDR measures are not, strictly speaking, inside MIPS. The U.S. Wound Registry (USWR)[10] has been recognized by CMS as a QCDR for MIPS reporting. Quality measures that capture outcome, appropriate use, patient experience, and safety are considered by CMS to be high priority measures and there are relatively few of these measures in any area of medicine or surgery. Reporting these measures earns the EP bonus points under MIPS. The USWR, in conjunction with the Alliance of Wound Care Stakeholders and its member organizations, has developed high-priority measures for wound care and hyperbaric medicine, as well as several safety measures for wound patients including the Nutritional Screening measure for patients with wounds, many of which were approved by CMS for reporting under MIPS (see Table 1). USWR quality measure specifications are available as electronic clinical quality measures (eCQMs) that can be downloaded free of charge from the USWR website and installed into any certified EHR, enabling EPs to report wound-care-relevant quality measures via any certified EHR so participation is vendor neutral.[11] More importantly, by 2018, as EHRs comply with the Open API initiative, QCDR measures will be available as apps for installation into any EHR certified to the 2015 Meaningful Use standard, which obviates the need to have programmers install eCQMs.

CMS also provides bonus points for appropriate use measures. Medicare has increased its scrutiny of hyperbaric oxygen therapy (HBO_2 therapy) utilization through a variety of programs including requiring prior authorization of services or prepayment review. The USWR has encapsulated most of the elements of the prior authorization requirements for providing HBO_2 therapy to a patient with a diabetic foot ulcer within an Appropriate Use quality measure. Clinicians who perform well on this measure will likely do well with HBO_2 therapy prior authorization for that indication.

Currently, a major problem with our health-care system is that payment is not linked to patient outcome. Incentivizing clinicians based on the volume of services provided, unrelated to whether these interventions benefit patients is contributing to rapidly escalating health-care costs without an appreciable improvement in health-care quality. The first step to linking payment to patient outcome is being able to accurately report patient outcome, and doing so requires a method to risk stratify patients. Risk stratification is a corrective tool to level the playing field, adjusting for the differences in risk among patients so that clinicians who care for the sickest patients are not penalized by having outcomes that appear to be different than their peers. Risk stratification makes it possible to compare performance fairly. Data from the USWR were used to create a series of mathematical models called the Wound Healing Index (WHI) which can be used to predict the likelihood that a wound of a given type would heal.[12-14] The USWR has several risk stratified diabetic foot ulcer and venous ulcer outcome measures. It is no longer acceptable for clinicians to artificially inflate healing rates by simply not reporting the outcome of patients who fail to heal. Healing rates better than 90% are almost never observed even in randomized, controlled trials that invariably target uncomplicated wounds among unrealistically healthy patients. Clinicians who tout real world healing rates greater than 90% can only do so by ignoring a large percentage of patients who have failed to heal. In the real world, only about 66% of patients heal.[15] It is possible to use the WHI to report provider specific wound healing outcomes in relation to the predicted *likelihood* of healing. Risk stratified outcome reporting allows a clinician to show they are successful with the most difficult cases, and provides a mechanism to demonstrate the effectiveness of interventions like HBO_2 therapy.

For some unknown period of time it will still be possible for EPs to participate in MIPS via claims. However, this reporting avenue will eventually close and clinicians will be driven to report quality data through a QCDR. At some point, hyperbaric medicine and wound care practitioners should identify a few standard quality measures as well as some *practice relevant QCDR quality measures* that they feel represent quality care in their own practice, and get ready to report those measures via a QCDR using data entered into their EHR.

IV. Registry reporting and advancing care information

Meaningful Use and its reincarnation as ACI emphasize the use of the electronic health record for a variety of activities including: electronic prescribing, patient electronic access (e.g. patient portal), coordination of care through patient engagement, health information exchange of data, and the transmission of clinical data to a specialty registry. The laborious process of secondary data entry (e.g. entering data by hand into a Web form) to participate in a registry is a thing of the past. As discussed before, all certified EHRs are able to create and display a patient Continuity of Care Document (CCD) which summarizes key elements including: demographics, medications, allergies, past history, procedures, treatments, labs and studies. This vast amount of data would once have taken hours of time to enter into a registry, but now, once it exists inside the EHR as part of the patient record, the CCD can be transmitted to a registry like the USWR without the need for any special computer interfaces or secondary data entry.

With near universal hospital EHR adoption, the time is right for the opportunities and efficiencies inherent in EHRs to be realized, particularly for the field of hyperbaric medicine. The USWR sponsors a number of meaningful use registries including the Hyperbaric Oxygen Therapy Registry (HBOTR), the Negative Pressure Wound Therapy Registry, the Cellular and Tissue based Product Registry, the US Podiatry Registry, the Diabetic Foot Ulcer Registry, and the Venous Leg Ulcer Registry, all of which are listed on the National Institute of Health (NIH) Clinical Trials website. In 2016, US Hyperbaric Oxygen Therapy Registry data was vital during the analysis of the physician work component of the CPT code for supervision of hyperbaric oxygen therapy. The American Medical Association Relative Value Committee (RUC) needed data to understand the average number of comorbid medical conditions present among hyperbaric patients as well as the average number of medications taken. Using HBOTR data, within three hours, it was determined that the average number of comorbid conditions was 10 and the average number of medications was 12, among 11,240 unique hyperbaric patients.[16] Had HBOTR data not been readily available, reimbursement for hyperbaric chamber supervision would likely have been dramatically reduced. The number of clinicians submitting data to HBOTR is growing as a result of MU mandates, but it is not clear whether the impetus provided by MIPS will be sufficient motivation to expand participation in HBOTR in the absence of any additional CMS reporting requirements.

Unfortunately, CCDs do not provide any information on wound or hyperbaric patient *outcome* which is necessary if data are to be used for effectiveness research. However, risk stratified outcome data can be obtained from clinicians who report the USWR outcome measures. The eCQM structure of those measures facilitates the collection of outcome data in a structured way for clinical research.

V. Registry reporting and clinical practice improvement activities

QCDRs are also needed for the majority of the projects CMS has defined in the category of Clinical Practice Improvement Activities. As part of a clinicians' IA, the QCDR will provide benchmarking reports that will compare patient and practice data with aggregate national data so providers can use this information for quality improvement (QI) activities. The USWR has crafted IAs which can be achieved through the USWR to ensure that wound care and hyperbaric medicine practitioners make a smooth transition to MIPS.[17]

VI. Resource use and bundled payments

While many clinicians worry that health-care reform will mean cutbacks to necessary services, CMS estimates that fully half of all Medicare spending is wasted from overuse or misuse. CMS's move to package price cellular- and tissue-based products (CTPs) and the preauthorization of nonemergent hyperbaric oxygen therapy (HBO_2 therapy) are both aimed at what CMS perceives as over delivery of those services. Ultimately, wound care practitioners must demonstrate that an intervention reduces total cost of care and the only way to do that is by tracking the cost of an episode of care. Eventually CMS will transition outpatient payment to a system much like the current inpatient diagnosis related groups (DRGs) which bundle charges together for the treatment of a condition. If we are to make a successful transition to the QPP, we must ensure that we are providing consistent evidence based care that improves outcome, and we must demonstrate that this improved outcome saves resources over time. Other clinicians are already collaborating in the reporting of quality measures to demonstrate improved patient outcomes by focusing on quality. For example, a composite measure has been created for diabetes management which nearly all physicians in the city of Cincinnati agreed to report. After the data are validated, a community average is generated for each measured condition, a score is given for each physician practice, and then the scores are reported on a patient-focused website (www.yourhealthmatters.org). That is why it is vital that all wound care practitioners report the same quality measures so that their performance can be compared against the aggregate. For example, if one group of wound care practitioners reports a diabetic foot ulcer (DFU) offloading quality measure defined as the percentage of DFUs prescribed *any offloading one time* in 12 months, but another group reports the USWR measure which is defined as, the percentage of DFUs prescribed *evidence-based offloading* at *every visit*, the providers are not reporting the same standard of care. The second quality measure is the better measure of quality and also, harder to pass. More physicians may score 100% passing if they use the easy but not meaningful measure. However, which group of physicians is most likely to have the best healing rates in the shortest period of time at the lowest total cost of care?

Which measures we report does matter and we must develop corresponding episode of care measures that determine resource use.

This brings us to a discussion of episode of care or cost of care measures. CMS wants to understand the return on investment for various interventions. How is that possible using quality measures? One example is that of HealthPartners, the largest nonprofit health-care organization in the U.S. which provides insurance coverage for patients in Minnesota. At the time of this writing, it had also developed the most complex quality measure ever endorsed by the National Quality Forum. This measure allows a payer to understand the costs contributed by various sites of service for a given episode of care (e.g., a total knee replacement), as well as how various patient comorbid conditions contribute to cost. A comparison in wound care would be a quality measure that captures all the data from all sites of care pertaining to a DFU. That measure would include hospitalization charges, medications, physician charges, home nursing charges, and outpatient wound center charges (including HBO_2 therapy and cellular products). Remember that the results of such a quality measure would be posted publicly on the internet. It would then be possible for CMS and individual patients to determine where they could go to get the most cost-efficient care for a DFU (and the best outcome). Patients and payers could determine which providers and which wound centers (in conjunction with the associated hospital and health-care systems) provide the most efficient care.

CMS has already begun to develop payment bundles for orthopedic procedures and cardiac procedures which include all the related costs including the physician charges, the acute care stay and rehabilitation costs. This means that the silos in which we have previously provided wound care must come down. It will be necessary to provide wound care services across the continuum of care including the acute care hospital, the outpatient wound center, the long-term care hospital (LTCH), home nursing, and the nursing home. This will be challenging since the same wound care clinicians usually do not follow patients at all of these sites of care, some sites of care do not yet have access to EHRs, if they use EHRs the data are not shared between these sites, and no quality measures exist that are relevant to wound care across all these sites. Driving this process forward will be difficult because even the measure development process occurs in siloes linked to those sites of care and their data collection methods. For the time being, the best plan is a two-pronged approach: 1) develop more QCDR wound care measures and attempt to get them recognized in other sites of care and 2) work with CMS to develop episode of care measures for wound care.

Consider that in 2017 there were 33 quality measures for hospital outpatient departments, but none of them were directly relevant to hospital based outpatient wound centers.[18] Wound care clinicians forget that the majority of services delivered in the outpatient payment system are delivered in the emergency department (ED), outpatient surgery, or imaging suites. Of the available hospital outpatient quality measures, there are really only three measures that a hospital based outpatient wound center might report: 1) the ability for providers to receive lab data electronically into the EHR system as discreet searchable data, 2) tracking clinical results between visits, and 3) influenza vaccination coverage among health-care personnel. Obviously, none of these are directly relevant to wound care. New measures have been proposed for hospital outpatient departments such as using the Consumer Assessment of Healthcare Providers and Systems (CAHPS) surveys which ask consumers and patients to evaluate their experiences with health care. Of the CHAPS measures proposed for outpatient hospital departments, there are probably two that a wound center could use including the patient surveys of the facilities and staff and whether the patient would recommend the facility. Although there are no wound care quality measures that a hospital based outpatient wound clinic can report to CMS, many hospital-based outpatient wound centers are now using the USWR quality measures designed for eligible providers and reporting them internally to hospital-wide quality programs. The USWR QCDR measures can be used successfully to develop quality programs for outpatient wound centers.

The quality measures that skilled nursing facilities (SNFs) report to CMS offer an excellent opportunity to observe the sausage making that is quality measure reporting.[19] It is one thing to talk about quality in an abstract way and another thing to attempt to measure it precisely. SNFs report whether patients underwent an admission and discharge functional care plan assessment and whether residents experienced a fall with a major injury. Each of these parameters must be exhaustively defined. SNFs also report the one wound care relevant quality measure that exists other than those within a QCDR: The Percent of Residents or Patients with Pressure Ulcers That Are New or Worsened (NQF #0678). This quality measure reports the percent of patients or short-stay residents with Stage 2, 3 or 4 pressure ulcers that are new or worsened since admission. The measure is calculated using data from the Minimum Data Set (MDS) 3.0 assessment instrument for SNF residents, and the LTCH CARE Data Set. Data reporting for this measure affects payment for SNFs and LTCHs. This measure has previously been successfully implemented in Nursing Homes (NHs) and is currently publicly reported on CMS's Nursing Home Compare website.[20] The measure is intended to encourage SNF/Nursing Homes, and LTCHs to prevent pressure ulcer development or worsening and to closely monitor and appropriately treat existing pressure ulcers so the motivation behind it is laudable. However, the measure itself is not focused on any intervention that would actually prevent or treat pressure ulcers (e.g. improved nutrition or offloading), and it uses the deeply flawed NPUAP pressure ulcer staging system as its basis. This results in many problematic and unintended consequences such as holding a facility responsible for the worsening of an unstageable pressure ulcer when it is finally able to undergo staging. While pressure ulcers are a worthy target for a measure across all sites of care, this flawed pressure ulcer measure is a poor candidate. We are much in need of wound care relevant quality measures that can transition across all sites of care and which ideally will facilitate improved care processes. At this time, these providers have no wound care measures at all within MIPS excepting those in a QCDR, outpatient hospital departments (wound centers) have no wound care measures to report at all, and all other sites of care have only one deeply flawed pressure ulcer measure that focuses only on counting, staging, and measuring pressure ulcers (without a mechanism to define medically unpreventable ulcers). If wound care reimbursement is going to be tied to outcome and quality, with payment ultimately bundled for an entire episode of care, we have a long way to go to build a workable system that incentivizes caregivers properly and actually improves the quality of care among patients with wounds.

Although MIPS is a program specific to Medicare Part B payments, private payers have been clear that they intend to implement the same payment system, even using the same quality measures. In fact, the private payers may be ahead of CMS in shifting physician payment away from volume based payment. Even CMS is ahead of schedule in its speed of transition. CMS plans to have more than 50% of payment linked to quality or outcome by 2018. Providers participating in alternative payment models like ACOs will use quality measures. The challenge will be for the ACO to adopt quality measures that capture metrics relevant to wound care. An ongoing challenge for ACOs and bundled payment programs will be how to apportion physician and facility payments as providers increasingly strive to pay a global fee.[21] This will likely drive more wound care practitioners to become employees of various entities such as provider networks or hospital systems. Data suggest that MIPS will result in a decrease in payment to about 80% of solo practitioners and small group practices, so pressure will increase for clinicians to form real or virtual networks in which they can demonstrate improved patient outcomes at lower cost in order to maintain high reimbursement rates.

VII. A new way of allocating resources

At the beginning of this chapter we discussed the data suggesting that providers who spend the most Medicare dollars per capita are likely overusing services and that substantial savings could be realized by eliminating wasted care without resorting to the rationing of needed services. Advanced therapeutics like HBO_2 therapy or cellular products are wasted when they are provided to patients whose wounds would get well with conservative management, when patients are provided with more of these treatments than needed, or when patients who cannot benefit receive advanced therapeutics. There are three opportunities to limit waste: 1) identifying patients who will heal with conservative care, 2) identifying the point at which patients have had the optimal amount of an advanced treatment, and 3) identifying patients who cannot be helped by advanced therapeutics because their prognosis is so poor.

Currently, Medicare's method of allocating resources is via extremely blunt tools. In order to identify patients who will heal with conservative care, Medicare or its various Medicare Administrative Carriers (MACs) have crafted policies requiring that patients undergo 30 days of conservative care and show no evidence of healing before HBO_2 therapy (for example) is indicated. The problem with this requirement is that it delays hyperbaric treatment for all patients for at least a month, possibly reducing the effectiveness of HBO_2 therapy when it is finally initiated, after which HBO_2 therapy is then covered even for patients who may not be able to benefit because their condition is too severe. No data have been analyzed to assess the reliability of this approach. However, the WHI can predict which patients are not likely to heal spontaneously based on variables collected at the initial consultation, without the need to wait 30 days. A predictive model which can be used to estimate the likelihood that HBO_2 therapy will be of benefit for a given patient with a DFU has been available for nearly a decade.[22] Private payers appear willing to use predictive models to allocate resources, and these models have already been installed in one EHR and are available as apps. A paradigm for a new method of allocating HBO_2 therapy has been proposed.[23] It seems likely that predictive models could be used to allocate resources more fairly and with better outcomes than current Medicare policies which have not been subjected to any analysis. This approach would seem the logical way forward for our field as Medicare and private payers begin to develop the equivalent of outpatient diagnosis related groups or capitated payment for various types of wounds. Patients want to know their odds of benefitting from costly and/or time-consuming treatments. Furthermore, as hospitals and providers begin to share the financial risk of these decisions, all parties will seek data driven decisions.

VIII. The future of comparative effectiveness research in wound care and hyperbaric medicine

Randomized controlled trials (RCTs) are simply not possible for all interventions in medicine and surgery, particularly for underfunded areas like wound care and hyperbaric medicine. Furthermore, the design of most RCTs requires that patients with complex problems be excluded.[24] There is value in using real world data for comparative effectiveness research, but to do that successfully, it is necessary to create matched cohorts of patients. The WHI risk stratification tool can be used to create matched cohorts for comparative effectiveness research. This is a powerful argument for hyperbaric medicine practitioners to report risk stratified quality measures to the USWR. It would be nice to think that the effort and challenges providers experienced in adopting a certified EHR could be used for the benefit of patients and the field of hyperbaric medicine and wound care. The future of wound care and hyperbaric medicine will be linked to registry data and the best way to obtain provider support for that is to harness existing regulatory requirements.[25]

Summary

The Medicare Access and Chip Reauthorization Act went into effect January 1, 2017, and affects all advanced practitioners who accept Medicare Part B payments (with a few exceptions for very low volume practices, etc.). Nearly all wound care practitioners will be subject to MIPS which grades practitioners on a 0 to 100-point scale based on four weighted activities including quality reporting, clinical practice improvement activities, advancing care information, and resource use. In this zero-sum game, the bonus money experienced by a few practitioners are contributed by the majority who are penalized. Initially the penalty is only 4% but the maximum potential bonus is 22%. The details are extremely complicated and it is easy to feel overwhelmed. The bigger plan is to move all practitioners into advanced alternative payment models as quickly as possible.

It is important for wound care and hyperbaric medicine practitioners to remember four points: 1) all cost and quality data will eventually be public, 2) thanks to the existence of QCDRs, clinicians themselves can develop the quality measures they feel best represent quality practices, 3) CMS is going to analyze provider cost and quality data, and 4) with broad-based participation in a specialty specific QCDR, practitioners can provide and analyze their own cost and quality data in order to refute any CMS conclusions that might have negative implications for the wound care industry. We must continue to develop quality measures that demonstrate cost effective wound care technology and the skill level of the practitioners who use them. To survive the transition to a new method of health-care payment, EPs will need to practice evidence-based medicine, be efficient with resources, ensure that patients are satisfied with their care, and reduce the total cost of patient care. However, that will not be sufficient. They will need to do all those things, AND have the data to prove it.

Review questions

1. **MACRA actually is relatively good news for physician payment, compared to the alternative, for the following reasons (pick all that are correct):**

    a. Under the SGR rule it replaced, physicians would have had a 21% cut in Medicare Part B payments in 2015.

    b. Under the previous quality programs (PQRS and MU), by 2016 the best a practitioner could do was avoid a penalty; there were no bonuses.

    c. In 2016, practitioners who failed PQRS and MU lost up to 8% of their Medicare Part B payments.

    d. Under MACRA in 2017, the worst penalty is -4%.

    e. all of the above

2. **Which of the following are correct statements about why Congress passed MACRA (with bipartisan support)?**

    a. The Medicare trust fund is going bankrupt and cost savings are needed.

    b. There is no clear relationship between cost and quality of medical care in the U.S.

    c. It was hoped that linking payment to quality reporting would decrease cost and improve quality of care.

    d. It facilitated the focus on patient-reported outcomes and the focus on patient-centered care.

    e. all of the above

3. **Which statements about quality measures are true in relation to wound care practitioners?**

    a. They are now publicly reported on Physician Compare.

    b. Quality performance data will be available on sites like Yelp in the near future.

    c. Payers use them to set reimbursement rates for health-care plans.

    d. Employers use them in contract negotiations with physicians.

    e. all of the above

4. **Which statements about Qualified Clinical Data Registries (QCDRs) are true?**
    a. They can facilitate quality reporting on behalf of practitioners for MIPS.
    b. They can develop their own quality measures for MIPS.
    c. They can develop Clinical Practice Improvement Activities for MIPS.
    d. Providers get credit for transmitting data to them under Advancing Care information.
    e. all of the above

5. ***True or False.*** Although hospital-based outpatient wound centers have several quality measures to choose from when they report to CMS (as hospital outpatient departments), there are NO quality measures for HOPDs that have anything to do with wound care.

ANSWERS: 1) e
2) e
3) e
4) e
5) True

References

1. 2015 Annual Report of the Boards of Trustees of the Federal Hospital Insurance and Federal Supplementary Medical Insurance Trust Funds. [cited 2016 September 16]. Available from: https://www.cms.gov/research-statistics-data-and-systems/statistics-trends-and-reports/reportstrustfunds/downloads/tr2015.pdf.
2. Baicker K, Chandra A. Medicare spending, the physician workforce, and beneficiaries quality of care. Health Aff (Millwood). 2004; w184–w197. doi: 10.1377/hlthaff.w4.184. Published online 2004 April 7.
3. Cooper RA. States with more physicians have better-quality health care. Health Affairs. 2009;28(1):w91–w102. doi: 10.1377/hlthaff.28.1.w91.
4. Fife CE, Carter MJ, Walker D. Why is it so hard to do the right thing in wound care? Wound Repair Regen. 2010; 18:154–158.
5. Fife CE, Carter MJ, Walker D, Thomson B, Eckert K. Diabetic foot ulcer off-loading: the gap between evidence and practice. Data from the US Wound Registry. Adv Skin Wound Care. 2014; Jul;27(7):310-6. doi: 10.1097/01.ASW.0000450831.65667.89.
6. MACRA and MIPS. [cited 2017 Aug 21]. Available from: https://www.cms.gov/Medicare/Quality-Initiatives-Patient-Assessment-Instruments/Value-Based-Programs/MACRA-MIPS-and-APMs/MACRA-MIPS-and-APMs.html).
7. Value in Health. JVAL. Article 1928.
8. Quality Measure instructions for 2017 MIPS. [cited 2017 Aug. 21]. Available from: https://qpp.cms.gov/mips/quality-measures.
9. Physician Compare. [cited 2016 July 31]. Available from: https://www.medicare.gov/physiciancompare/search.html.
10. US Wound Registry. [cited 2016 July 31]. Available from: https://www.uswoundregistry.com/.
11. USWR Measure Specifications. [cited 2016 July 13]. Available from: https://www.uswoundregistry.com/Specifications.aspx.
12. Horn SD, Fife CE, Smout RJ, Barrett RS, Thomson B. Development of a wound healing index for patients with chronic wounds. WWR. 2013; 21(6): 823–832.
13. Horn SD, Barrett RS, Fife CE, Thomson B. A predictive model for pressure ulcer outcome: the wound healing index. Adv Skin Wound Care. 2015;28(12):560-72.
14. Fife CE, Horn SD, Smout RJ, Barrett RS, and Thomson B. A predictive model for diabetic foot ulcer outcome: the wound healing index. Adv in Wound Care. 2015; open access.
15. Fife, CE, Carter MJ, Walker D, Thomson B. Wound care outcomes and associated cost among patients treated in U.S. outpatient wound centers: data from the U.S. Wound Registry. Wounds. 2012;24(1) 10-17.
16. Fife CE, Gelly H, Walker D, Eckert KA. Rapid analysis of hyperbaric oxygen therapy registry data for reimbursement purposes, Undersea and Hyperbaric Medicine [in press].
17. Examples of CPIA in the U.S. Podiatry Registry. [cited 2016 July 31]. Available from: http://uspodiatryregistry.com/practiceimprovement.
18. Hospital Outpatient Measures.[cited 2016 July 31]. Available from: http://www.qualitynet.org/dcs/ContentServer?c=Page&pagename=QnetPublic%2FPage%2FQnetTier2&cid=1191255879384.
19. Skilled Nursing Facilities Technical Expert Panel Report. [cited 2016 July 31]. Available from: https://www.cms.gov/Medicare/Quality-Initiatives-Patient-Assessment-Instruments/NursingHomeQualityInits/Downloads/Development-of-the-Skilled-Nursing-Facility-Readmission-Measure-SNFRM-August-2012-Technical-Expert-Panel-Report.pdf.

20. Nursing Home Compare. [cited 2016 July 31]. Available from: http://www.medicare.gov/nursinghomecompare/search.html.
21. Fife CE, Wall V, Carter MJ, Walker D, Thomson D, Turner T, Revenue in U.S. hospital based outpatient wound centers: implications for creating accountable care organizations. J of Hospital Administration. 2013;2(3).
22. Fife CE, Buyukcakir C, Warriner R, Sheffield P, Love T, Otto G. Factors influencing the outcome of lower extremity of diabetic ulcers treated with hyperbaric oxygen therapy. Wound Repair Regen. 2007;15:322-331.
23. Fife CE, Eckert KA, Carter M. An update on the appropriate role for hyperbaric oxygen: indications and evidence. Plast Reconstr Surg. 2016;138.
24. Carter MJ, Fife CE, Walker D, Thomson B. Estimating the applicability of wound-care randomized controlled trials to general wound care populations by estimating the percentage of individuals excluded from a typical wound care population in such trials. Adv Skin Wound Care. 2009;22:316-24.
25. Fife C, Walker D, Thomson B. Electronic health records, registries, and quality measures: what? why? how? Adv Wound Care. 2013;2(10): 598–604. doi:10.1089/wound.2013.0476.

Chapter 31

PATIENT-CENTERED DECISION MAKING IN WOUND CARE AND HYPERBARIC MEDICINE

Caroline E. Fife, MD, FAAFP, CWS, FUHM

KEY CONCEPTS

1. Patient-centered care changes the focus of health care away from the disease and onto the patient. It is responsive to individual patient preferences, needs and values, ensuring that patient values guide all clinical decision making.

2. Practitioners are expected to always act in the patient's best interest, both from a medical and a fiduciary standpoint. This includes avoiding unnecessary treatments and charges.

3. Ethical use of off-label HBO_2 therapy does not require that all patients be enrolled in an IRB approved trial but it does require adequate informed consent, including specific elements defined by Chan and Brody in 2001 to better enable patient-centered decision making.

4. A major focus of the move to value based payment is an emphasis on patient reported outcomes although, sadly, few have been created for wound care or hyperbaric medicine.

5. The relationship between the patient and provider should be a collaborative partnership that includes respect for patient values, coordinated care, involvement of family and friends if desired by the patient, and access to care.

CONTENTS

Introduction

Patient-centered care has been identified by the Institute of Medicine (IOM) as one of the fundamental approaches needed to improve the quality of U.S. health care.[1] It is defined as care that is respectful of and responsive to individual patient preferences, needs, and values and which ensures that patient values guide all clinical decisions. The goal is to shift the focus of our health-care system away from *the disease*, and focus instead on *the patient*. The hope is that the patient will be actively engaged in deciding which path to take whenever the crossroads of an important health-care decision is reached. That philosophy presupposes that the patient is *able* to engage in this process and is capable of understanding the choices before him or her if presented with clear information. The practice of wound care often involves life-changing decisions, such as whether a limb should be amputated, and wound care practitioners often encounter patients near the end of life when the skin begins to break down due to the failure of multiple organ systems. Decisions regarding the use of advanced technology should be undertaken only after obtaining a clear understanding of the goals and expectations of the patient and family. Framing these choices can be difficult under the best of circumstances. All aspects of medicine are complex, but hyperbaric oxygen therapy (HBO_2 therapy) poses a special challenge since it may require an explanation of the physics of gas laws which, as will be discussed below, seem to have confused even some investigators in the field. As the U.S. health-care system undergoes a highly publicized restructuring around principles like patient centeredness, access to HBO_2 therapy for accepted indications (e.g., radiation proctitis and failing flaps) is diminishing just as the availability of HBO_2 therapy for off-label use is increasing. New therapies enter the wound care market almost weekly, but their effectiveness among compromised patients is unclear. How can we keep the best interests of the patient at the center of the decision-making process in these changing times?

I. Patient-centered wound care practice

The nature of the doctor-patient relationship is an unequal one. Patients are vulnerable in part because they may be ill but also because the difference in education creates a knowledge gap between the physician and the patient. As a result, for many generations, the model of medical practice was a paternalistic one. However, dramatic societal changes have altered patient expectations, technological advances make it impossible for the physician to be knowledgeable about everything, and changes in payment models often require patients to make difficult financial decisions pertaining to health-care choices. As a result of these and many other factors, collaboration between the physician and the patient regarding health-care decisions is the expected norm.

The technological advances of the past century have come with definite trade-offs. The Internet allows information (including inaccurate information) to spread rapidly. Unproven therapies are available if the patient wishes to pay for them. Patient expectations of technology are high, overuse of (or overreliance on) technology is a common temptation, and profit motives can drive therapeutic decisions. We need a framework to guide us. Nothing should change the practitioner's commitment to the principle of nonmaleficence which is often referred to as "First do no harm." Preventing harm is more important philosophically, morally, and legally than doing good. Practitioners should also maintain their commitment to beneficence, or always acting in the patient's best interest. This is required because patients often cannot act on their own for a variety of reasons, including ignorance, illness, or fear. Although these commitments are a valuable ethical infrastructure, they don't provide an approach to patient-centered practice.

The Picker Institute, in partnership with patients and families, identified eight indicators which define patient-centered, quality medical care from the perspective of patients:

1. respect for the patient's values, preferences, and expressed needs;
2. coordinated and integrated care;
3. clear, high-quality information and education for the patient and family;
4. physical comfort, including pain management;
5. emotional support and alleviation of fear and anxiety;
6. involvement of family members and friends, as appropriate;
7. continuity, including through care-site transitions;
8. and access to care.[(2)]

As an illustration, two patient vignettes are provided and then Table 1 describes the manner in which these eight principles were addressed.

Mrs. A is a 78-year-old woman with adult-onset diabetes who is on hospice care due to end-stage cardiac disease, with a life expectancy of less than six months. She has severe peripheral arterial and cerebrovascular disease, is status post-stroke with residual left-sided paralysis, and is not ambulatory. She has a recurrent first metatarsal head lesion on her right foot. Sometimes the toe joint is visible, and this is distressing to her family. Osteomyelitis is likely, based on X-ray findings. The wound is not painful, but she has ischemic leg pain. Transcutaneous oximetry values suggest that she would require an above-the-knee amputation to reach a level where healing would be likely, but she is not a candidate for general anesthesia.

Mr. B is a 70-year-old man who lives alone and has no family. He has poorly controlled insulin-dependent diabetes and severe peripheral arterial disease. He also is a paraplegic due to a motor vehicle accident 15 year earlier which left him wheelchair bound. He presents to the wound center with multiple bilateral lower-extremity leg ulcers that expose tendons and bone. Today he has cellulitis and a fever. Transcutaneous oximetry values below the knee are less than 20 mmHg on both legs. He has no pain in his legs due to his spinal cord injury. His cardiac status is good, and he is mentally alert and highly independent.

These cases illustrate the way in which two patients may be best managed with completely different treatment plans, based on their preferences and needs. Mrs. A is best served with comfort care; Mr. B is best served with bilateral amputations. While an amputation might have been medically reasonable for Mrs. A due to her osteomyelitis, it was not a patient-centered decision. Although limb salvage is usually the goal and is usually desired by most patients, for Mr. B, who was paralyzed and whose ischemic limbs represented only a source of infection and difficulty with transfers, amputation offered the ideal management plan.

II. Fiduciary ethics

Practitioners also have a fiduciary responsibility to patients. This means they are expected to be parsimonious with the patient's resources and trustworthy with matters involving billing. Both wound care and hyperbaric medicine continue to

TABLE 1. Patient-centered approach to wound care

Patient-Centered Principle [2]	Mrs. A	Mr. B
Respect for the patient's values, preferences, and expressed needs: "What can I do that would help you the most?"	"Stop my pain."	"Make it so that I don't have sores on my legs and can go home."
Emotional support and alleviation of fear and anxiety: "What is the thing you are most concerned about?"	"I don't want an amputation."	"I want to keep living independently in my apartment – not have to go to a nursing home."
Coordinated and integrated care	Discussed management with orthopedics and hospice as well as family. Conservative care seems the most reasonable plan with suppressive antibiotics.	Discussed management plan with orthopedics and patient. Admitted to the hospital for bilateral through-the-knee "guillotine" amputations so that he can perform transfers easily.
Physical comfort, including pain management	Pain management plan put in place.	Arranged social services, rehab therapy.
Involvement of family members and friends, as appropriate	Family decided to fund an arterial assist device as a trial to see if it improved pain and agreed to help her use it at home.	Called pastoral care. Arranged for Meals on Wheels.
Continuity of care	Arranged follow-up every two weeks or more often if needed.	Arranged follow-up every two weeks or more often if needed.
Access to care	Hospice nurses can access wound care on-call physician with questions.	Arranged van service for wound care appointments.
Clear, high-quality information and education for the patient and family	Explained aggressive versus conservative options to patient and family: amputation versus conservative care, risks versus benefits.	Explained options to the patient – not a good revascularization candidate, and, if limb salvage was attempted, he would need plastic surgery and long recovery with questionable outcome.

be scrutinized by various U.S. government agencies responsible for overseeing the Medicare trust fund. In 2004, when the Office of the Inspector General (OIG) performed a review of 368 medical records,[3] it found that 64% of surgical debridement services did not meet Medicare program requirements, resulting in approximately $64 million in improper payments. The main issues found by the OIG were as follows: 1) billing the debridement at a higher level than actually provided, 2) billing a nondebridement service as surgical debridement (e.g., callous paring), 3) insufficient documentation to justify the billed service, and 4) wound documentation that was inconsistent with the level of debridement billed (e.g., a wound documented as having healthy granulation tissue but debrided of muscle).

The improper use of HBO_2 therapy was the target of the OIG in 2000.[4] The OIG report concluded that 32% of the hyperbaric-related charges from hospitals and physicians could not be supported adequately with the documentation provided, 28% were paid in error, and 10% were paid for services that did not meet Medicare's medical necessity criteria. The OIG suspected that 74% of inappropriate payments did not have an attending physician present during the HBO_2 therapy session as required. It is likely that this report was partly responsible for the implementation by Medicare of a prior authorization program for HBO_2 therapy,[5] active in three states as of this writing but likely to expand nationally. The program requires hospitals to obtain approval before initiating HBO_2 therapy by submitting the patient's chart to their Medicare Administrative Carrier (MAC) for an exhaustive chart review. Private payers have begun requiring a similarly stringent authorization processes.

In a much-publicized retrospective analysis of HBO_2 therapy from a large dataset,[6] Margolis found that HBO_2 therapy was not effective in the treatment of diabetic foot ulcers (DFUs). However, a large portion of the DFUs treated with HBO_2 therapy were Wagner Grade 2, substantiating the OIG finding that Medicare is being improperly billed for patients who do not meet coverage criteria. The dataset did not include the necessary information to determine whether the other Medicare criteria for HBO_2 therapy had been met among the Wagner Grade 3 patients (e.g., had undergone vascular testing, had infection controlled, or had received offloading). In any case, the paper seems to underscore that HBO_2 therapy is not effective if used improperly and that it continues to be used improperly. If HBO_2 therapy is provided according to appropriate guidelines to save a diabetic limb from amputation, there is abundant data to support the assertion that patients are more likely to have limb salvage and thus to survive for five years and have a dramatically improved quality of life. Nevertheless, HBO_2 therapy is not cost-effective when provided 1) to patients who were going to get well anyway (unnecessary), 2) to patients who can't be helped (futile), or 3) in excess of the number needed to achieve the desired benefit (wasteful). These questions are relevant to a discussion on patient-centered care because of the following: Medicare is funded by everyone's tax dollars; Medicare beneficiaries are responsible for 20% of their Medicare-covered expenses which can be substantial; privately insured patients may be responsible for very high deductible payments; there are risks to HBO_2 therapy treatment even if they are rare; and patients and their family members devote considerable time and energy to attending treatment. Thus, clinicians are ethically obliged to be parsimonious with costly advanced therapeutics like HBO_2 therapy.

Unnecessary HBO_2 therapy can be reduced by screening patients with sea level air breathing transcutaneous oximetry ($TcPO_2$). Although $TcPO_2$ is unreliable at predicting which wounds *will* heal, it can be used to predict which wounds *will not* heal spontaneously due to tissue hypoxia and thus selecting which patients may need revascularization if it has not been performed.[7] If patients have undergone revascularization and their $TcPO_2$ remains low, in-chamber $TcPO_2$ is 75% accurate at predicting which DFUs will benefit from HBO_2 therapy.[8] A retrospective study demonstrated that when the $TcPO_2$ in-chamber was greater than 200 mmHg, 78.3% of DFUs benefited; when the $TcPO_2$ in-chamber was less than 100 mmHg, only 18% benefited.[8] Among renal failure patients with two or more DFUs, only 30% improved with HBO_2 therapy, raising questions as to the value of HBO_2 therapy for these unfortunate patients.[9] The incremental benefit of providing more than 40 HBO_2 therapy sessions for DFUs is questionable, based on retrospective data and mathematical modeling. Late effects of radiation likely have a quite different response curve.

It is possible that the advent of point-of-care electronic health records will also usher in a new era of patient-centered decision making. Predictive models like the Wound Healing Index already exist[10] which can estimate with greater accuracy than simple air breathing $TcPO_2$ whether a wound will heal with conservative care. Another mathematical model can predict the likelihood of success of HBO_2 therapy for a DFU, without the need for a hyperbaric exposure to obtain in-chamber $TcPO_2$, using only a few basic metrics (patient age, years of diabetes, transcutaneous value breathing air at sea level, pack/year smoking history, Wagner Grade of the ulcer).[9] These two models could be combined to create a patient-centered decision-making paradigm for the use of HBO_2 therapy in the diabetic foot which would be more accurate than the method currently used by Medicare.[11] Currently, the process by which the Centers for Medicare & Medicaid Services (CMS) selects DFUs to undergo HBO_2 therapy is to have all DFU patients wait 30 days and then allow all Wagner 3 DFUs that have failed to show any improvement to be treated with HBO_2 therapy. This method delays HBO_2 therapy for all patients (likely reducing its effectiveness), excludes some patients who need HBO_2 therapy and who could also benefit from it, and then allows HBO_2 therapy for some patients who cannot benefit. Although the use of mathematical models for such decisions is relatively new, they are part of the movement toward precision medicine and are certainly a more patient-centered decision process because they enable calculations based on the likelihood of benefit *for each specific patient*. This enables the clinician to have a more informed conversation with the patient as he or she weighs the predicted benefit *in his or her specific case* against the known risks. Certainly, even better predictive models could be developed using the data currently available in the Hyperbaric Oxygen Therapy Registry (HBOR). Sadly, analyses like these (which could significantly reduce wasted resources and improve the effectiveness of HBO_2 therapy) have not been supported by the hyperbaric industry, CMS, PCORI (the Patient-Centered Outcomes Research Institute), or any other organization. Despite a lack of ongoing support, the rich data available in the HBOR was able to provide critical information regarding the acuity level of patients treated with HBO_2 therapy, demonstrating they have an average of 10 comorbid conditions and take an average of 12 medications per patient.[12]

In its document reviewing the improper use of HBO_2 therapy,[4] the OIG's top five compliance issues could be summarized as follows: 1) billing Medicare for a noncovered condition, 2) inadequate documentation to support the medical necessity of HBO_2 therapy, 3) giving patients more hyperbaric treatments than medically necessary, 4) failing to perform the appropriate tests or treatment before instituting HBO_2 therapy, and 5) not having a physician in attendance during the hyperbaric treatment. Some of the compliance issues on the OIG's above list could be attributed to sloppy medical practice, but some of these behaviors are more nefarious. Improper billing of HBO_2 therapy has now become the focus of criminal investigations by a joint task force between the Department of Justice (DOJ) and CMS. Since its launch in 2007, the Medicare Fraud Strike Force, comprised of federal, state, and local investigators in nine U.S. cities, has specifically targeted fraud in many areas, including hyperbaric medicine, under the enforcement arm of the DOJ.[13] One hyperbaric operator found guilty of serious Medicare fraud has received a prison sentence. While much concern has been raised regarding the off-label use of HBO_2 therapy, unethical standards in the delivery of hyperbaric medicine for *approved* indications may have done more to jeopardize the availability HBO_2 therapy than unsubstantiated claims over off-label indications. The increasingly draconian measures the U.S. health-care system is employing to limit overuse and improper use of HBO_2 therapy could create a scenario in which the proven indications are no longer covered by payers, and HBO_2 therapy is primarily provided on a cash basis for off-label indications. At the very least, there is increasing pressure for facilities to use HBO_2 therapy for off-label indications, so reasonable guidance is needed.

III. A patient-centered approach to off-label use of HBO_2 therapy

For many years, the United States Food and Drug Administration (FDA) has deferred to the Undersea and Hyperbaric Medical Society (UHMS) to establish the list of indications for which HBO_2 therapy has sufficient evidence to support its use.[14-15] In the United States, the FDA, which regulates the marketing of both medical devices and drugs, classifies hyperbaric chambers as Class II medical devices because they do not support or sustain human life (Class III) but are not as innocuous as, for example, a tongue depressor (Class I).[16] The Food, Drug, and Cosmetic Act requires medical device manufacturers to notify the FDA of their intent to market a new medical device at least 90 days in advance using a process known as Premarket Notification, often referred to by the name of the subsection of the act in which it is found, "510(k)."[16] This process allows the FDA to determine whether a new device (not in commercial distribution prior to May 28, 1976) is substantially equivalent to a device which has already been classified. The 510(k) clearance process is relatively uncomplicated for hyperbaric chambers that have not undergone substantial changes in design or composition when compared to predecessor chambers. In the 510(k) process, manufacturers must also stipulate that there are no substantial changes to the *intended use* of the chamber. This means that, since 1978, all hyperbaric chambers cleared by the FDA can be promoted only for those conditions that are listed as approved in the *UHMS Hyperbaric Oxygen Therapy Committee Report.*[14] In order for a chamber to be approved to treat an indication that is not listed by the UHMS, the manufacturer must provide the FDA with compelling evidence to support the use of HBO_2 therapy for that condition. A health-care entity which advertises or promotes the off-label use of HBO_2 therapy is in breach of FDA regulations,[16] even if promoting an IRB-approved research protocol, and the FDA is within its purview to seize its assets, including the hyperbaric chamber. An entity wishing to use a hyperbaric chamber for an unapproved indication must request an investigational device exemption (IDE) from the FDA. In other words, if the facility is performing research on an indication that is not currently on the FDA approved list of uses, even if the research protocol is approved by an Institutional Review Board, it is still not possible to advertise or otherwise promote the use of HBO_2 therapy for this off-label indication. Updated guidelines regarding the promotion of off-label uses are pending from the FDA in the wake of several lawsuits successfully arguing that off-label promotion is protected as free speech and thus allowable as long as the information provided is truthful and not misleading.[17-18]

The above explanation notwithstanding, it is obvious from perusing the Internet that purveyors of hyperbaric therapy completely ignore restrictions on the promotion of its off-label use. HBO_2 therapy is widely promoted for autism, cerebral palsy, chronic neurological deficits due to stroke, Lyme disease, Meniere's disease, migraine, multiple sclerosis, Parkinson's disease, and chronic fatigue syndrome, among many others.[19] The FDA has released a statement strongly cautioning health-care consumers that HBO_2 therapy is not clinically proven to be an effective treatment for these conditions,[15] has filed complaints against centers using HBO_2 therapy for off-label conditions,[20] and has issued warning letters to the manufacturers of inflatable, low-pressure hyperbaric chambers for misbranding their devices.[21]

The UHMS reviewed the ethics of off-label use in 2001 in response to growing interest in the use of HBO_2 therapy for cerebral palsy. Fifteen years later, the framework of this ethics review remains current.[22] The lack of enforcement resources by the FDA, the desperation of patients suffering from otherwise untreatable conditions, and the decreasing revenue experienced by many hyperbaric centers are creating the ideal environment for a new model of HBO_2 therapy delivery. This new model of HBO_2 therapy delivery might be patient-centered in that it meets a demand for low-cost, available HBO_2 therapy, but it could also set the stage for a safety disaster and allow vulnerable patients to be exploited. In this new and unregulated marketplace, mandated safety standards for equipment and properly trained personnel are far less likely to be in place. Individuals are enticed to undergo off-label HBO_2 therapy treatment by convincing testimonials readily available online touting the benefits of HBO_2 therapy for conditions without successful alternative options (e.g., autism), and most consumers do not have the necessary scientific background to critically evaluate the evidence provided.[23-24]

The complete text of the Chan and Brody paper[22] is available from the UHMS Rubicon Foundation and is a valuable resource. The authors concluded that it is not unethical to treat a patient for an unproven or off-label indication. Nearly every day, clinicians utilize a drug or device for an indication different than the one for which the FDA originally cleared or approved it. This practice is not considered unethical simply because a device or drug proven to work for one indication is used for a different one, although patients should be informed of the off-label use. Case-by-case medical decisions to use HBO_2 therapy for off-label indications do not require IRB approval, but, if data are being collected with the intention of using that information to direct the care of future patients, then the activity should be considered research, and IRB approval should be sought. It is also not unethical to charge a patient for off-label use. Charges must be reasonable and transparent, and patients must understand in advance what the charges are. The focus of the patient-centered approach to off-label use is in the process of informed consent.

IV. Guidelines for off-label informed consent

Physicians routinely obtain informed consent from patients about to undergo HBO_2 therapy for approved indications. No less is expected for those receiving HBO_2 therapy for off-label use. Informed consent may be oral or written but must be documented, so it is generally easier to craft a written informed consent. Anecdotal reports raise concern that some patients treated for off-label indications do not undergo an appropriate consent process. For example, a news article reported the success of HBO_2

therapy for a stroke patient at a local hyperbaric center.[25] The radiologist who provided the hyperbaric treatment was quoted as saying that HBO_2 therapy had been proven effective in treating (among other off-label conditions) chronic obstructive pulmonary disease and emphysema. It seems highly unlikely that, as part of a consent process, the patient was informed of the risk of pulmonary overpressurization if the hyperbaric physician believed that HBO_2 therapy is a *treatment* for this malady rather than a potential contraindication to it.

When it pertains to off-label indications, ethicists[22] suggest that informed consent address five specific areas:

1. **Are there alternative medical treatments to HBO_2 therapy for this off-label use?**

   It is advisable that the informed consent clearly state that the indication for which the patient is being provided HBO_2 therapy is unproven or off-label and the patient understands this. If the patient is requesting HBO_2 therapy treatment for a condition for which some alternative treatment is available, then the cost, risk, and relative benefit of HBO_2 therapy should be compared to that treatment.

2. **What is the level and type of scientific data to support the use of HBO_2 therapy for this condition?**

   In 2001, Chan and Brody urged the UHMS to develop a better mechanism for rating the evidence that underpins the treatments the UHMS considers proven, and the UHMS responded by dramatically improving the *Hyperbaric Oxygen Therapy Committee Report*,[14] clearly identifying the evidence basis for each condition. That process is now continuing with the UHMS Guidelines project that includes evidence ratings on guidelines.gov.[26] For off-label indications, even animal data can be informative. There are some conditions for which no data exist that would suggest benefit from HBO_2 therapy (e.g., wrinkles or longevity).

3. **Are the risks of HBO_2 therapy acceptable?**

   HBO_2 therapy, while a relatively safe treatment overall, is not without risks. Although the risks are low and usually acceptable for life- and limb-threatening conditions, any risk is hard to justify if the possible benefit is unknown or nonexistent. For most of the approved indications, the likelihood of benefit can be easily estimated from published data and weighed against the known incidence of side effects such as hyperoxic seizures, allowing the clinician to have an informed conversation with the patient about risk versus benefit. What is not known when HBO_2 therapy is used for off-label treatment is how to balance these risks with possible benefit since the possible benefit is not known. This makes it even more imperative for patients to be clearly informed of the possible risks they may be incurring without any assurance of commensurate benefit. Poor fire safety practices may pose the greatest risk of patient endangerment with regard to HBO_2 therapy if the facility is not operated by trained personnel. Since 1967, there have been only 101 fatalities reported worldwide (only two in the United States) caused by fires in clinical hyperbaric chambers, an extraordinary safety record given the hundreds of thousands of hyperbaric exposures.[27] However, the most recent of these fires in the United States occurred in conjunction with the off-label use of HBO_2 therapy at a poorly maintained facility. Multiple violations of safety standards led to criminal convictions of the individuals involved.

Most chamber fires were caused by prohibited ignition sources such as electronics, cigarettes, and mobile phones that were brought inside the chamber by the occupants.[27-28] It is, therefore, particularly distressing to see Internet advertisements for off-label use of HBO_2 therapy featuring children inside of hyperbaric chambers using laptop computers or other prohibited electronic devices. Advertisements like this send a clear message that those chamber operators do not understand hyperbaric safety regulations or the risks associated with oxygen use. Portable hyperbaric chambers, developed originally for altitude sickness and capable of achieving only approximately half an atmosphere of pressure, are in common use in independent clinics, medical spas, and private homes. Promoters offer a quick step-by-step user video which substitutes for any formal technical safety training.[21,23] Does the patient understand that he or she is responsible for the cost?

Even if HBO_2 therapy treatments are offered at a much-reduced rate, vulnerable people may pay relatively large amounts of money for an unproven treatment administered in a potentially unsafe environment. Patients need to be clearly informed of all costs relating to the treatment and that their insurance will not cover these costs. The clinician cannot defraud the insurance company by attesting that the patient has a different (covered) indication in order to get HBO_2 therapy paid for by insurance for an uncovered indication. Decisions surrounding the off-label use of HBO_2 therapy can be particularly difficult when indications with insufficient data intersect patients with desperate medical situations. For example, online advocacy groups target the parents of children with autism and cerebral palsy, encouraging them to seek treatment with HBO_2 therapy.[19] Parents may pay out of pocket for hundreds of treatments and have a sense of guilt if they discontinue treatments.

4. **Physician disclosure of any financial issues which might affect the physician-patient relationship**

   If the physician recommending the HBO_2 therapy stands to receive direct financial gain from the treatment, this should be disclosed to the patient. There is normally a charge for the physician supervision of HBO_2 therapy treatments. However, if the physician also owns the hyperbaric chamber equipment (or benefits from the sale or distribution of the hyperbaric chambers), he or she may be receiving additional monies beyond the usual charge for treatment supervision. The patient has the right to know of any monetary considerations that could affect the physician's recommendation that he or she undergo treatment. It may be helpful for the hyperbaric physician to involve an independent expert (e.g., a traumatic brain injury specialist) to perform an independent medical evaluation and follow the patient's progress with HBO_2 therapy. The independent physician can provide an assessment of whether the patient is benefitting from treatment and whether continued treatments might be valuable.

V. The controversy of low-pressure oxygen

HBO_2 therapy is defined by the UHMS as the administration of oxygen at pressures ≥ 1.4 ATA, so breathing 100% oxygen at the equivalent of 1 atmosphere of pressure (sea level) is not hyperbaric oxygen. The use of low-pressure oxygen is a conundrum. In the randomized trial of cerebral palsy by Collet et al.,[29] the experimental subjects were breathing 100% oxygen at 1.75 ATA, which is a total of 1,330 mmHg. The control subjects breathed air at 1.3 ATA, a total of 988 mmHg pressure. When multiplied by 0.21 (the percentage of oxygen in air), the control subjects were respiring a partial pressure of oxygen of approximately 207 mmHg, which is equivalent to 27% O_2 at sea level (normobaric pressure). There was no difference in the outcome of the two groups, randomized to either hyperbaric oxygen or a sham treatment that was only slightly more oxygen than room air. Rather than concluding that HBO_2 therapy was ineffective (which was the obvious reason to design a randomized trial this way), the study concluded that since both groups of children improved somewhat, oxygen was beneficial to both groups. The Rossingol study is widely cited by advocates of HBO_2 therapy for autism. In this prospective trial, 62 young children with autism spectrum disorder (ASD) were treated with HBO_2 therapy at 1.3 ATA in a traditional hyperbaric chamber either with 24% oxygen or with a sham involving pressurized air (21% oxygen) at 1.03 ATA.[30] Because the hyperbaric oxygen group was receiving only 24% oxygen, their inspired pO_2 was only 237 mm Hg, which is equivalent to 31% O_2 at sea level. The authors found that the hyperbaric group significantly improved in their overall functioning, language and social skills, eye contact, and cognitive behavior compared to the control group. The control subjects in the Collette study who received the equivalent of 27% oxygen, and the "hyperbaric oxygen" subjects in Rossingol who received the equivalent of 31% oxygen, could both easily have been provided with this concentration of oxygen via a nasal cannula or oxygen mask and a bottle of oxygen in the comfort of their own home. Emotional debate continues to rage regarding whether some additional beneficial effect occurs simply because the patient has gone into the hyperbaric chamber. There does appear to be a placebo effect from simply going inside a hyperbaric chamber.[31] Inflatable chambers, originally designed for the treatment of acute mountain sickness, can achieve atmospheric pressures of only 1.3 ATA. They are now heavily marketed for home use and are often found in health spas. When compressed with air, they provide about the same percentage of oxygen as the Collet or Rossingol studies but at much greater expense, in addition to incurring the risk of otic barotrauma and fire. However, if our focus is on patient-centered care (including the ethical principles of nonmaleficence and beneficence), the benefits of simply providing oxygen by mask at sea level need to be pursued with the same vigor as mild hyperbaric oxygen using inflatable chambers since it provides exactly the same oxygen partial pressure and is both cheaper and safer.[32]

VI. Patient-reported outcomes and registry participation

It is not possible to have a patient-centered health-care system without obtaining patient-reported data. While there is much discussion about the value of patient-reported data, manufacturers and professional associations support patient-reported outcomes in the same way that beauty pageant contestants support world peace: Everyone is in favor of it, but no one actually contributes to it. The U.S. Wound Registry (USWR) is a 501(c)[3] nonprofit organization[33] which exists to improve the quality of care of patients with chronic nonhealing wounds and to increase the use of evidence-based treatment by their providers. To accomplish these goals, as a Qualified Clinical Data Registry (QCDR), the USWR collaborates with wound care stakeholders (e.g., the Alliance of Wound Care Stakeholders, the Undersea and Hyperbaric Medical Society) in the development of wound-care and hyperbaric-oxygen-specific quality measures.

In 2014, the USWR was among the first group of QCDRs recognized by CMS. Among the 21 measures developed by the USWR and recognized by CMS[34] are a patient-reported wound-related quality of life measure, a patient-reported wound outcome measure, and a patient-reported nutritional screening measure. Eligible providers (EPs) can download the specifications from the USWR website free of charge and install them into any certified EHR, enabling them to report these measures for credit in the Merit-Based Incentive Payment System (MIPS).

Patients with chronic wounds are likely to be members of vulnerable populations (e.g., minority races, the disabled, patients with dementia or at the extremes of age). These patients are almost never enrolled in wound care or HBO_2 therapy clinical trials. To obtain data on the effectiveness or the safety of wound care products or HBO_2 therapy among these disproportionately affected individuals, the best (and perhaps the only) mechanism will be through registry reporting of real world data. Clinicians who report wound care and hyperbaric specific quality measures are committed to providing the best possible care for their patients, as well as contributing to the learning health-care system that will provide better data in the future. That is the epitome of patient-centered health care.

Summary

In a system that values patient-centered care, the patient's values should guide clinical decisions and the relationship between the patient and the provider should be a collaborative partnership. Key indicators of patient-centered care include: respect for patient values, coordinated care, the availability of high-quality patient information, physical comfort (including pain management, emotional support, the involvement of family and friends, continuity throughout care transitions), and access to care. The ethical obligations of clinicians include the fiduciary responsibility not to bill for unnecessary care. The off-label use of FDA approved or cleared drugs and/or devices is not inherently unethical, and this applies to the off-label use of HBO_2 therapy. Guidelines exist for the off-label use of HBO_2 therapy. An IRB-approved research protocol is not required if no data are being collected for research purposes. However, patients must undergo informed consent, the elements of which must include the risks of HBO_2 therapy, the fact that HBO_2 therapy is unproven for the indication, information regarding any accepted alternative medical treatments, and disclosure of any financial incentives that the practitioner might have in recommending HBO_2 therapy. The use of low pressure oxygen (e.g. less than 1.4 ATA of oxygen), which may involve inflatable chambers, is increasingly promoted on social media. In many cases, the inspired oxygen partial pressure is less than can be achieved when administering 100% oxygen at sea level, but patients and at times, even clinicians, fail to understand this. Promotional materials often show lack of adherence to accepted fire safety regulations, raising concern that purveyors of such treatments are not properly trained to provide it. Patient-reported data may provide valuable insight into the use of HBO_2 therapy and is an area of considerable interest on the part of CMS. HBO_2 therapy practitioners can report some patient- reported quality measures for credit under MIPS through the HBOR, but more measure development is much needed in the field of hyperbaric medicine.

Review questions

1. **Using a patient-centered approach to care, a wound care practitioner would have the following approach to a major amputation in a limb salvage situation (below or above the knee). Choose the correct answer.**

    a. It is never acceptable because it is so disabling.

    b. The ideal way to determine if amputation is necessary is to have a surgeon evaluate a wound photo, as in the Fedorko study in Canada.

    c. It should be performed if the wound care practitioner thinks that it is necessary.

    d. A decision like major amputation should be a collaborative one based on the values and goals of the patient.

2. **Improper use of HBO_2 therapy, per the OIG report, includes all of the following except:**

    a. providing HBO_2 therapy without sufficient documentation to support medical necessity

    b. failing to obtain prior authorization of HBO_2 therapy from Medicare

    c. not having a physician in attendance

    d. providing HBO_2 therapy for a condition not covered by Medicare

    e. failing to perform the appropriate tests before starting HBO_2 therapy

3. **Correct statements about the FDA and HBO_2 therapy include the following:**

    a. During the 510(k) process, manufacturers stipulate that there are no substantial changes to the intended use of their chamber, so all hyperbaric chambers cleared by the FDA can be promoted only for those conditions that are listed as approved in the *UHMS Hyperbaric Oxygen Therapy Committee Report.*

    b. A health-care entity, which advertises or promotes the off-label use of HBO_2 therapy is in breach of FDA regulations and the FDA is within its purview to seize the assets of the organization, including the HBO_2 therapy chamber(s).

    c. An entity wishing to use a hyperbaric chamber for an unapproved indication must request an investigational device exemption (IDE) from the FDA.

    d. The promotion of off-label use is being reconsidered by the FDA as a result of litigation relating to free speech.

    e. All of the above are true.

4. **Per the Chan and Brody paper on the ethical use of HBO_2 therapy, which of the following statements regarding the off-label use of HBO_2 therapy is FALSE?**

    a. It is not unethical to treat a patient for an unproven or off-label indication.

    b. Case-by-case medical decisions to use HBO_2 therapy for off-label indications do not require IRB approval.

    c. Informed consent that includes the risks of HBO_2 therapy is NOT required for off-label use.

    d. If data are being collected with the intention of using that information to direct the care of future patients, then the activity is considered research, and IRB approval should be sought.

    e. It is also not unethical to charge a patient for off-label use.

5. ***True/False.*** One of the most confusing issues surrounding low pressure oxygen is that the inspired oxygen levels achieved are often less than can be provided by breathing 100% oxygen at sea level, making the use of a chamber unnecessary.

ANSWERS: 1) d
2) b
3) e
4) c
5) True

References

1. National Research Council. Crossing the quality chasm: a new health system for the 21st century. Washington (DC): National Academies Press; 2001.
2. Gerteis M, Edgman-Levitan S, Daley J, Delbanco T. Through the patient's eyes. San Francisco: Jossey-Bass; 1993.
3. Medicare payments for surgical debridement services in 2004 [Internet]. U.S. Department of Health and Human Services, Office of the Inspector General; 2007 May. 27 p. OEI-02-05-00390. Available from: http://oig.hhs.gov/oei/reports/oei-02-05-00390.pdf.
4. Hyperbaric oxygen therapy: its use and appropriateness [Internet]. U.S. Department of Health and Human Services, Office of Inspector General; 2000 Oct [cited 2015 Sep 30]. OEI 06-99-00090. Available from: http://oig.hhs.gov/oei/reports/oei-06-99-00090.pdf.
5. CMS.gov: Centers for Medicare & Medicaid Services [Internet]. Baltimore (MD): U.S. Centers for Medicare & Medicaid Services. Prior authorization of non-emergent hyperbaric oxygen [cited 2016 Oct 6]; [about 2 screens]. Available from: https://www.cms.gov/Research-Statistics-Data-and-Systems/Monitoring-Programs/Medicare-FFS-Compliance-Programs/Prior-Authorization-Initiatives/Prior-Authorization-of-Non-emergent-Hyperbaric-Oxygen.html.
6. Margolis DJ, Gupta J, Hoffstad O, Papdopoulos M, Glick HA, Thom SR, Mitra N. Lack of effectiveness of hyperbaric oxygen therapy for the treatment of diabetic foot ulcer and the prevention of amputation. Diabetes Care [Internet]. 2013 Feb; DC_122160. Available from: http://dx.doi.org/10.2337/dc12-2160.
7. Fife CE, Smart DR, Sheffield PJ, Hopf HW, Hawkins G, Clarke D. Transcutaneous oximetry in clinical practice: consensus statements from an expert panel based on evidence. Undersea Hyperb Med. 2009;36(1):43-53.
8. Fife CE, Buyukcakir C, Otto GH, Sheffield PJ, Warriner RA, Love TL, Mader J. The predictive value of transcutaneous oxygen tension measurement in diabetic lower extremity ulcers treated with hyperbaric oxygen therapy: a retrospective analysis of 1,144 Patients. Wound Repair Regen. 2002;10:198-207.
9. Fife CE, Buyukcakir C, Warriner R, Sheffield P, Love T, Otto G. Factors influencing the outcome of lower-extremity diabetic ulcers treated with hyperbaric oxygen therapy. Wound Repair Regen. 2007;15:322-31.
10. Horn SD, Fife CE, Smout RJ, Barrett RS, Thomson B. Development of a wound healing index for patients with chronic wounds. Wound Repair Regen. 2013;21:823-32.
11. Fife CE, Eckert KA, Carter MJ. An update on the appropriate role for hyperbaric oxygen: indications and evidence. Plast Reconstr Surg [Internet]. 2016;138(3 Suppl):107S-116S. Available from: http://journals.lww.com/plasreconsurg/Fulltext/2016/09001/An_Update_on_the_Appropriate_Role_for_Hyperbaric.15.aspx.
12. Fife CE, Gelly H, Walker D, Eckert KA. Rapid analysis of Hyperbaric Oxygen Therapy Registry data for reimbursement purposes: technical communication. Undersea Hyperb Med [Internet]. 2016;43(6):627-34. Available from: https://www.uhms.org/publications/uhm-journal/uhm-journal-ahead-of-print.html.
13. Le PJ. Lessons to learn from federal convictions of HBOT fraud. Today's Wound Clinic [Internet]. 2015 Mar [cited 2015 Jul 20];9(2). Available from: http://www.todayswoundclinic.com/articles/lessons-learn-federal-convictions-hbot-fraud.

14. Undersea & Hyperbaric Medical Society [Internet]. North Palm Beach (FL): Undersea and Hyperbaric Medical Society. Indications for hyperbaric oxygen therapy; 2015 [cited 2015 Jul 23]; [about 2 screens]. Available from: https://www.uhms.org/resources/hbo-indications.html.

15. FDA: U.S. Food & Drug Administration [Internet]. Silver Spring (MD): U.S. Food and Drug Administration. Hyperbaric oxygen therapy: don't be misled; 2013 [updated 2015 May 15; cited 2015 Jul 20]. Available from: http://www.fda.gov/ForConsumers/ConsumerUpdates/ucm364687.htm.

16. FDA: U.S. Food & Drug Administration [Internet]. Silver Spring (MD): U.S. Food and Drug Administration. Regulatory information. FD&C Act Chapter V: drugs and devices; [updated 2015 Sep 25; cited 2015 Sep 30]; [about 4 screens]. Available from: http://www.fda.gov/RegulatoryInformation/Legislation/FederalFoodDrugandCosmeticActFDCAct/FDCActChapterVDrugsandDevices/default.htm.

17. Boumil MM. Off-label marketing and the First Amendment. N Engl J Med. 2013;368:103-5.

18. Federal judge lets Amarin promote Vascepa off-label, says FDA policies violate 1st Amendment. Inside Health Policy [Internet]. 2015 Aug 7 [cited 2015 Aug 10]. Available from: http://insidehealthpolicy.com/login-redirect-no-cookie?n=84883&destination=node/84883.

19. Healing-arts.org [Internet]. Hyperbaric oxygen therapy providers and treatment centers in the United States treating autism, cerebral palsy and other neurological disorders; 2008 [cited 2015 Aug 15]. Available from: http://www.healing-arts.org/children/hyperbaric oxygen therapy_hbot.htm.

20. Gaffney A. FDA says medical device popular with elite athletes regularly misbranded [Internet]. Regulatory Focus: Healthcare Product Regulation. In Focus.; 2013 Aug 22 [cited 2015 Nov 30]. Available from: http://www.raps.org/focus-online/news/news-article-view/article/3980/.

21. Portable Hyperbaric Chambers Australia [Internet]. Portable Hyperbaric Holdings Pty Ltd; 2014. The Salus 36 [cited 2015 Jul 20]. Available from: http://02hyperbaricchambers.com/salus36-chamber/.

22. Chan EC, Brody B. Ethical dilemmas in hyperbaric medicine. Undersea Hyperb Med. 2001;28:123-30.

23. OmLife: Fitness Wellness Sports Science [Internet]. Souk Al Bahar, Dubai: OmLife. Mild hyperbaric oxygen chambers; 2012 May 12 [cited 2015 Jul 20]; [about 3.5 screens]. Available from: http://www.omlifeme.com/hyperbaric/.

24. Walker J. Hyperbaric oxygen therapy gets more popular as unapproved treatment. The Wall Street Journal [Internet]. 2015 Jan 5 [cited 2015 Jul 20]. Available from: http://www.wsj.com/articles/hyperbaric-oxygen-therapy-gets-more-popular-as-unapproved-autism-treatment-1420496506.

25. Libov C. Oxygen therapy heals stroke damage [Internet]. Newsmax.com; 2014 Mar 25 [cited 2015 Oct 30]. Available from: http://www.newsmax.com/Health/Headline/stroke-treatment-hyperbaric-oxygen-therapy-HBOT-COPD-Valerie-Green/2014/03/25/id/561674/.

26. A clinical practice guideline for the use of hyperbaric oxygen therapy in the treatment of diabetic foot ulcers [Internet]. Undersea and Hyperbaric Medical Society [cited 2016 Oct 6]. Available from: https://www.guideline.gov/summaries/summary/49353/undersea-and-hyperbaric-medical-society?q=hyperbaric+oxygen+therapy.

27. Sheffield PJ. Clinical chamber fires: to what extent is the problem? In: Workman WT, editor. Hyperbaric facility safety: a practical guide. 2nd ed. Best Publishing Co. Forthcoming 2018.

28. Newton J. Patient killed after blowing up hospital ward when he decided to smoke a cigarette while undergoing treatment in high pressure oxygen chamber. Daily Mail [Internet]. 2014 Jul 31 [updated 2014 Jul 31; cited 2015 Nov 30]. Available from: http://www.dailymail.co.uk/news/article-2711646/Patient-killed-blowing-hospital-ward-decided-smoke-cigarette-undergoing-treatment-high-pressure-oxygen-chamber.html#ixzz3szv6pHqM.

29. Collet JP, Vanasse M, Marois P, Amar M, Goldberg J, Lambert J, et al. Hyperbaric oxygen for children with cerebral palsy: a randomised multicentre trial. HBO-CP Res Group. Lancet. 2001;357:582-6.

30. Rossignol DA, Rossignol LW, Smith S, Schneider C, Logerquist S, Usman A, et al. Hyperbaric treatment for children with autism: a multicenter, randomized, double-blind, controlled trial. BMC Pediatr. 2009;9:21.

31. Bennett MH. Hyperbaric medicine and the placebo effect. Diving Hyperb Med. 2014;44:235-40.

32. Heuser G, Heuser SA, Rodelander D, Aguilera O, Uszler M. Treatment of neurologically impaired adults and children with "mild" hyperbaric oxygen (1.3 ATA and 24% oxygen) [Internet]. In: The Proceedings of the 2nd International Symposium on Hyperbaric Oxygenation in Cerebral Palsy and the Brain-Injured Child. [cited 2015 Sep 11]. 7 p. Available from: http://hyperbaricstudies.com/wp-content/uploads/Treatment-of-Neurologically-Impaired-Adults-and-Children-with-Mild-Hyperbaric-Oxygen.pdf.

33. U.S. Wound Registry [Internet]. The Woodlands (TX): U.S. Wound Registry [cited 2016 Oct 6]. Available from: https://www.uswoundregistry.com/.

34. U.S. Wound Registry [Internet]. The Woodlands (TX): U.S. Wound Registry. [cited 2016 Oct 6]. Available from: https://www.uswoundregistry.com/Specifications.aspx .

SECTION 8

WOUND CARE IN OTHER COUNTRIES

Editor - Julio E. Garcia, RN, MD, AAPWCA

Chapter 32

WOUND CARE PRACTICE IN INDIA

Tarun Sahni, MD
Arun Prasad, MD
Abhishek Tiwari, MD

CONTENTS

Introduction

- The knowledge of wounds and healing is possibly as old as humanity itself, since ancient humans must have sustained injuries which in the normal course of events would heal themselves. Over time, some of these wounds possibly did not heal due to foreign bodies, infection, poor circulation, and/or profuse bleeding, and the quest for wound healing mechanisms and methods gained importance.
- The use of turmeric moistened with oil still remains the primary form of treatment of small wounds as a "grandmother's remedy" in India. All methods of traditional Indian medicine such as Unani, homeopathy, and Siddha have various remedies to help wounds heal. The Chinese, Egyptians, and Greeks have used animal grease, lint, and honey for wound healing. Many antibacterial ointments have used honey for its efficacy in preventing infection in wounds.[1]
- Various online resources indicated the global market for advanced wound management totaled USD$8.6 billion in 2013, and by 2018, this market is likely to reach $11.3 billion compound annual growth rate (CAGR of 5.6%.) The Indian wound care market (traditional and advanced) was valued at USD$9.11 billion in 2008 and showing a CAGR of 15%. More than 90% of wound treatment in India currently involves traditional wound care. Another assessment predicts the Indian market for wound care products is expected to reach Indian rupee (INR) $22 billion by 2019.

I. Case studies

A review of literature shows many traditional methods used for wound healing in India. Placed below are some publications and two case studies, one showing a traditional Indian method of wound care and the second using advanced wound care modalities.

The *Indian Journal of Research in Homoeopathy* (2015) lists five case studies of gangrene, whose amputation were prevented through the use of Arsenicum album 12C, five times a day for one month, leading to complete healing.[2]

The *International Quarterly Journal of Research in Ayurveda* (AYU 2012) carries a report on the use of honey for wound healing. The study concludes that honey is a useful dressing material, and it renders economical when compared with conventional dressing materials. Honey is an ideal first-aid dressing material, especially for patients in remote areas.[3]

A. Case study 1 (use of Ayurveda formulation in wound healing)[4]

A 40-year-old female presented with a nonhealing, infected wound on her right gluteal region with a history of two months. On examination, there was a rounded wound having a black color, necrosed tissue, and foul-smelling slough, measuring about 3 inch × 3 inch × 1 inch in diameter caused by a pyogenic local infection (Figure 1). The characteristics of Dushta vrana like Ativivrita (broad base), Bhaira*va* (ugly look), Putipuyaman*sa* (pus discharge), Durgandh*a* (foul smell), Vedana (pain), *and* Dirghakalanubandhi (chronic) were noted in the wound. There was deep-seated, blackish slough at the base of the wound which was hard to remove initially.

The wound was cleaned daily with Panchawalkala kwatha, and then the paste made up of dried leaves powder of Katupila with sesame oil (Securinega leucopyrus) was applied in

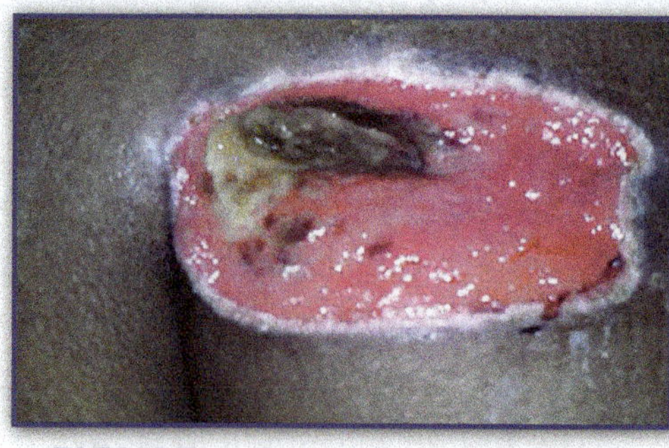

FIGURE 1. Dushta vrana (infected, nonhealing wound) at right gluteal region on day 1 of treatment

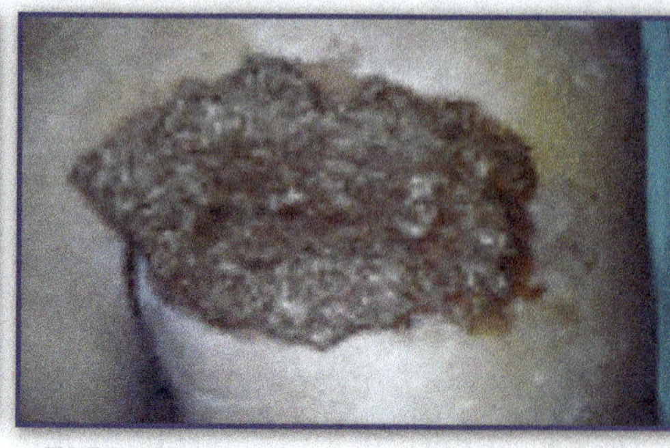

FIGURE 2. After application of Securinega leucopyrus paste

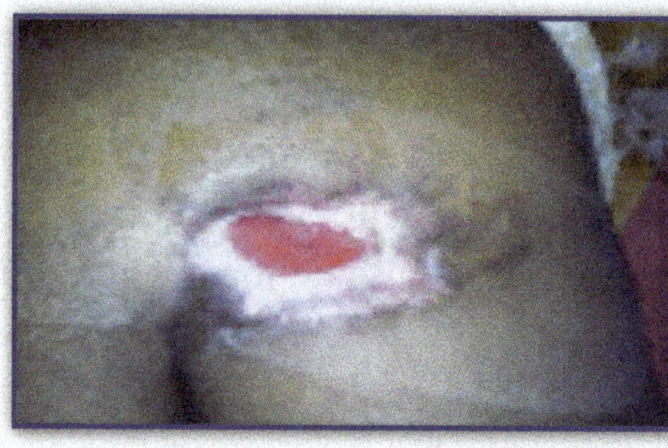

FIGURE 3. Wound status on the 21st day after treatment

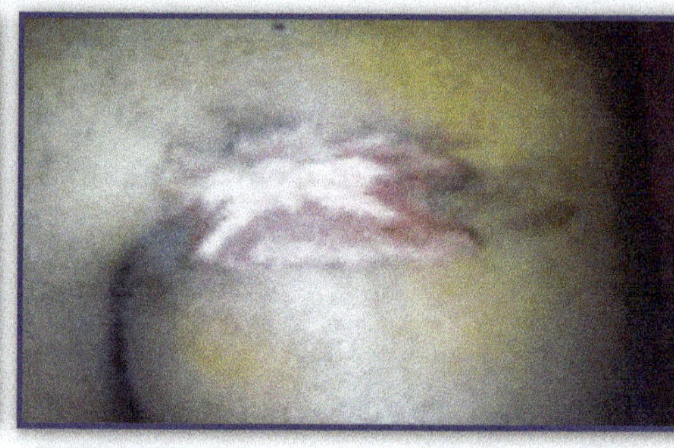

FIGURE 4. Completely healed wound with minimum scar on the 35th day

adequate quantity (Figure 2). Note: Panchavalkala is a combination of five astringent drugs which has a wide range of usage in Ayurveda:

1. Vata (Ficus Bengaenesis)
2. Udumbara (Ficus Glomerata)
3. Ashwatha (Ficus Religiosa)
4. Pakur (Ficus Infectoria)
5. Azadarachta Indica.

Numbers 1-4 are the root barks of the four species of Ficus. The wound was bandaged after covering with sterilized gauze and cotton pads for a month leading to complete healing (Figures 3-4). This case study showed effective wound healing by topical application of Katupila paste and sesame oil.

B. Case study 2 (use of advanced wound healing methods)[5]

A 23-year-old diver sustained accidental water jet injury to the left shoulder (Figure 5). The injury was severe with deep tissue penetration in the deltoid with pneumothorax and pneumomediastinum and extensive surgical emphysema (Figure 6).

High-pressure water jet injuries are surgical emergencies. A high index of suspicion of associated internal injuries and aggressive surgical intervention are required. These injuries pose a serious risk of bacterial infections and include gram-positive and gram-negative bacteria, fungi, and uncommon pathogens including Aeromonos hydrophia. The water used in high-pressure jet devices may be contaminated with sewage or oil lubricants. For these reasons, these injuries can have high mortality and morbidity.

He was managed with a combination of two

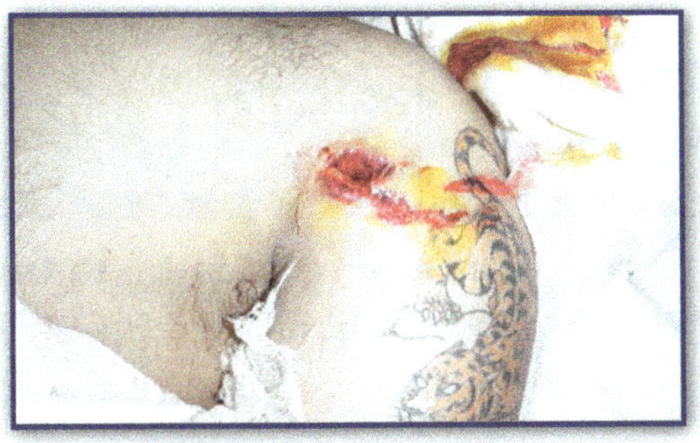

FIGURE 5. External wound

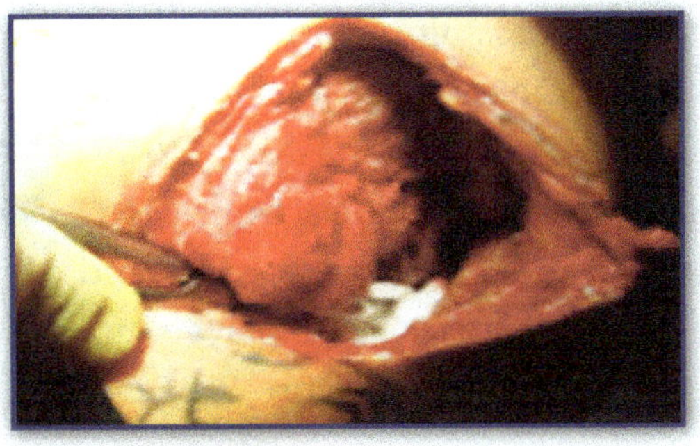

FIGURE 6. Internal wound

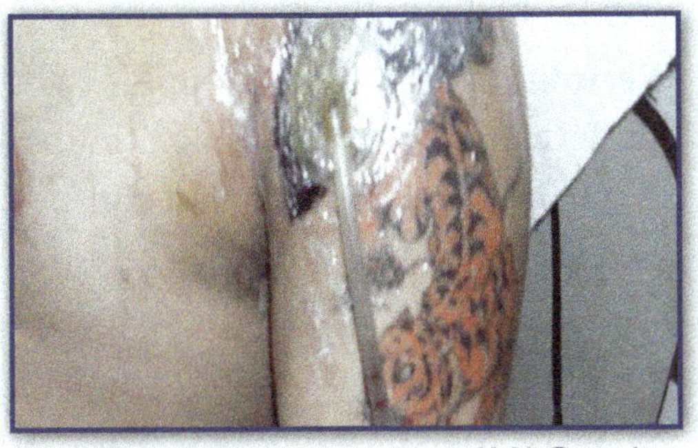

FIGURE 7. Application of VAC and hyperbaric oxygen

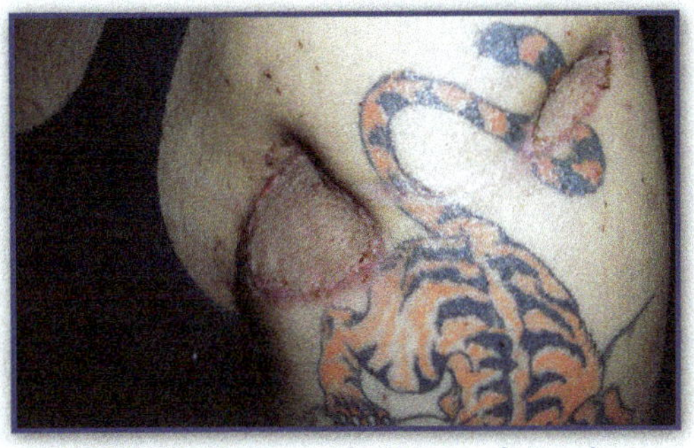

FIGURE 8. Day 10 skin graft in place

advanced wound management techniques: VAC and hyperbaric oxygen therapy in addition to the standard surgical practices of debridements and antibiotics (Figure 7). The patient responded well, leading to skin graft and was discharged within three weeks of injury (Figure 8).

Subsequent investigations showed absence of air in tissue cavities and normal pulmonary function. He had residual weakness of the left shoulder, which was actively rehabilitated two weeks after surgery. He recovered well enough to join his duty within 8-10 weeks after date of injury. He was found fit for diving after 24 weeks of the injury.

II. Wound care modalities used in India

- The maximum prevalence of wound care products in India fall under the "conventional" or "traditional" wound care products. Products like cotton and gauze are a major part of this, and swabs, dressings, and tapes make up the rest of it. The medical bandages and plaster segments have mostly orthopedic products like crepe and elastic adhesive bandages and immobility products.[6]
- In a stark contrast to developed markets, the smallest segment in the Indian wound care market is advanced wound care. The majority of advanced wound care is in four areas: diabetic wounds (40%–60%), pressure wounds (15%–20%), skin burn (40%–60%), posttraumatic ulcers (30%–50%), and general surgery (10%–15%).
- The AWC (advanced wound care) market in India comprises of hydrogel, collagens, and foam dressing and major brands include the following: hydrogel (Smith & Nephew, 3M, Dr. Reddy), collagen (Johnson & Johnson,

Dr. Reddy), foam dressing (Johnson & Johnson, S & N), film dressing Johnson & Johnson; active dressing (skin replacement - Beiserdorf and Johnson & Johnson); and calcium alginate dressing (3M). Hospitals are mostly using products from MNC brands like Johnson & Johnson, 3M, and Smith & Nephew. Many more players are entering the country with more range of products.[7]

- Another report shows the advanced wound care market to have expanded to 36% in hospitals; however, the actual figure may be lower (Figure 9).
- In an independent sample study of 30 multispecialty hospitals in India, collagen, hydrogels, and foam dressings form a major chunk of market share of the Indian AWC market (Figure 10).

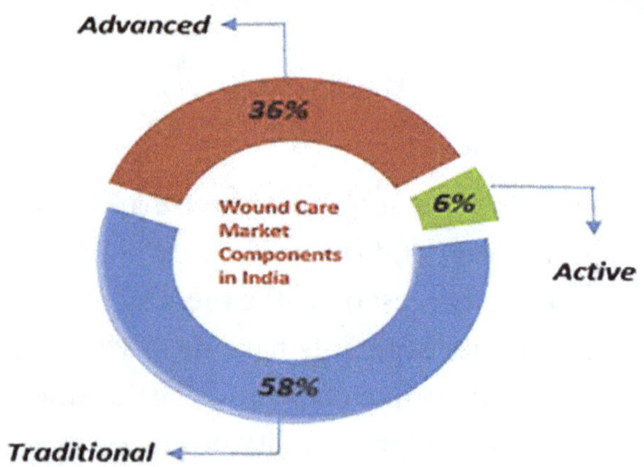

FIGURE 9. Wound care components in India

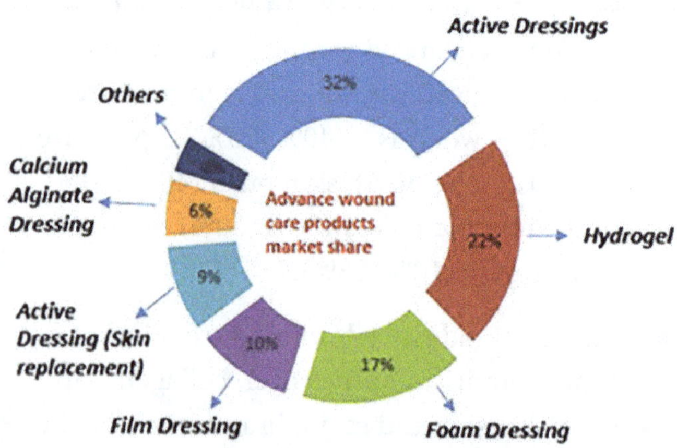

FIGURE 10. Advanced wound care products market share

III. Diagnostic services used for wound care in India

- **Transcutaneous oxygen measurement:** $TcpO_2$ measures the nutritive flow in the capillaries as well as oxygen and carbon dioxide levels at the wound site for wound-healing assessment and hyperbaric medicine.
- **Peripheral vascular Doppler with photoplethysmograph:** Photoplethysmography is an optical technique that can be used to detect blood volume changes in the microvascular bed of tissue. It is often used noninvasively to make measurements at the skin surface. When combined with Doppler, peripheral vascular disease can be diagnosed immediately.
- **Biothesiometer and SW monofilament:** They are inexpensive devices recommended for neurosensory testing.
- **Emed pressure scan:** Emed pressure scans collect and display the plantar pressure measurement.
- **Noncontact infrared foot thermometer**: It is used for measuring the dermal temperature to detect increases in thermometer due to some inflammation, which is one of earliest signs of tissue injury and ulceration.
- **Wound measurement camera:** They measure wounds more accurately than traditional wound measurement techniques. It is more reliable and makes it easier to properly document and measure wounds in hard-to-reach places, improving patient comfort.
- **Skin perfusion pressure mapper/device:** Skin perfusion pressure (SPP) is the pressure required for restoring microcirculatory

blood flow following release of carefully controlled occlusion. The measurement of SPP with laser Doppler is a noninvasive test. It has proven useful in the assessment of peripheral arterial disease (PAD) both for critical ischemia and also for the determination of optimal levels for amputation.

- **Podiatry Chair**: A podiatry chair offers the practitioner better assessment and management of wounds. It is strong, stable, and comfortable for patients suffering from wounds.

IV. Therapeutic devices used in wound care in India

- **Ultrasound wound debrider:** It applies low frequency, cavitational ultrasound to gently remove dead and diseased tissue cells, kills harmful bacteria and biofilm, and leaves healthy and prehealing granulation tissue intact.
- **Hyperbaric oxygen therapy:** Hyperbaric oxygen therapy is a form of treatment in which a patient breathes 100% oxygen while inside a special treatment chamber where the ambient pressure is higher than normal atmospheric pressure. This is useful for the treatment of medical illnesses such as gas gangrene, traumatic ischemia, and diabetic wound and many others.
- **Vacuum-assisted closure (VAC):** VAC therapy promotes wound healing through negative-pressure wound therapy. By delivering negative pressure (a vacuum) at the wound site through a patented dressing, this helps draw wound edges together, remove infectious materials, and actively promote granulation at the cellular level.
- **Intermittent compression therapy devices:** It is a therapeutic technique used in medical devices that include an air pump and inflatable auxiliary sleeves, gloves, or boots in a system designed to improve venous circulation in the limbs of patients who suffer edema or the risk of deep vein thrombosis (DVT).
- **Advanced wound dressings:** Advanced wound care products and treatments accelerate healing while maximizing patient comfort throughout treatment.
- **Electrical pedicure file system:** These tools are used for pedicure, that is, trimming and shaping toenails, as well as grinding and smoothing rough skin like corns and calluses. It helps in managing cracks as well. It helps to debride the foot in an outpatient setup.

V. Reimbursement issues in India[7-8]

- The reimbursement for wound care has to be seen in the overall health-care reimbursement and insurance sector in India.
- The health insurance sector hovers around 10% in density calculations. One of the main reasons for the low penetration and coverage of health insurance is the lack of competition in the sector. Health insurance in India typically pays only for inpatient hospitalization and for treatment at hospitals in India. Outpatient services were not payable under health policies in India.
- The Insurance Regulatory Authority of India (IRDA) is responsible for insurance policies in India. Until recently, to improve the awareness and reduce the procrastination for buying health insurance, the General Insurance Corporation of India and the Insurance Regulatory and Development Authority had launched an awareness campaign for all segments of the population. According to the World Bank, by 2010, 25% of India's population had access to some form

of health insurance. There are standalone health insurers along with government-sponsored health insurance providers.

- Traditional wound care in outpatient departments is usually paid for out of pocket and wounds treated as part of a surgical intervention are usually paid for by insurance during inpatient care.

VI. Wound care associations in India

There are three prominent wound care associations in India.

- **The Indian Society of Wound Management** (http://indiansocietyofwoundmanagement.org), which was established in September 1996. ISWM aims to bring together clinicians and practitioners of varied fields with a common interest in wound healing. Its ultimate goal is to establish wound care centers with state-of-the-art clinical and research facilities. Due to its efforts, dedicated wound clinics have been created in the teaching hospitals at Varanasi, Chennai, Mumbai, Nagpur, New Delhi, and Chandigarh. Presently, ISWM has over 150 life members.
- **The Diabetic Foot Society of India (DFSI)** (http://diabeticfootsocietyofindia.org), founded on March 30, 2002, is one of the few societies all over the world dedicated only to the diabetic foot. DFSI has been at the vanguard of training and sensitizing numerous medical and paramedical personnel through highly structured, innovative, and state-of-the-art educational programs to guide therapy, measure outcomes, and precisely identify risks associated with the ulceration of the diabetic foot.
- **The Indian Podiatry Association** (http://www.ipafootcare.org) was founded on April 1, 2009, with the objectives to disseminate and impart knowledge and promote awareness of diabetic and nondiabetic foot care, cures, and prevention. It uses a multidisciplinary approach to spread awareness among the general population by imparting education, interactive talks, holding seminars and refresher courses, publishing articles in magazines and newspapers, and distributing literature.

Summary

- India is a country with a complex mix of population, training of doctors, and health systems, with each segment being at a different stage of maturation. While the large population will provide a large pool of patients in all segments, the affordability and knowledge to use the latest technologies will vary in different parts of the country and even have contrasting standards within the same city.
- A wound can have a significant impact on a person's life. Wounds can lead to prolonged periods of disability in addition to pain and discomfort and may even prevent a person from performing everyday activities such as walking and bathing. This inactivity may in itself lead to further health problems. Some wounds are associated with odor and excessive drainage and require frequent attention that may impede social interactions. A nonhealing wound may prevent a return to work, which can have psychological as well as economic ramifications.
- The demand for high-quality health-care products such as advanced wound care products exists, but there is also a large

population that can only afford traditional wound products.

- The advanced wound care market in India definitely has many mountains to climb before it can overtake the huge traditional wound care market, as in developed countries. Vendors will need to educate the medical fraternity to make inroads. But only a reimbursement system can bring about the penetration levels seen in developed economies, and, while that is happening, the pace with which it is progressing is slow, and it will be a while before it has an impact in the foreseeable future.

References

1. Subramanian R. The growth of the Indian wound care market [Internet]. Morulaa Health Tech. Available from: (http://www.morulaa.com/download/indian_market_information/Indian%20Wound%20Care%20Market%20Overview%20Morulaa%20HealthTech.pdf?22d67d).
2. Mahesh S, Mallappa M, Vithoulkas G. Five case studies of gangrene, preventing amputation through homoeopathic therapy. Indian J Res Homoeopath. 2015.
3. Vijaya KK, Nistheshwar K. Wound healing activity of honey. A pilot study. Int Q J Res Ayurveda. 2012 Jul-Sep;33(3):374-7.
4. Ajmeer AS, Dudhamal TS, Gupta SK, Mahanta V. Topical application of Katupila (Securinega leucopyrus) in Dushta Vrana (chronic wound) showing excellent healing effect: a case study. Int Q J Res Ayurveda. 2014 Apr-Jun;35(2):175-8.
5. Sahni T. Advanced Wound Healing Methods, High-pressure water jet injury (L) shoulder with extensive surgical emphysema and pneumomediastinum. Forthcoming.
6. Khetan V. The Indian wound care market: a review. Frost & Sullivan; 2004 Dec.
7. Advanced wound care: portfolio extension (discussion document). Redseer Consulting; 2011 Jan.

Additional Resources

1. IBEF: India Brand Equity Foundation: www.ibef.org [Internet]. India Brand Equity Foundation. Available from: http://www.ibef.org.
2. Wikipedia [Internet]. Health insurance in India. Available from: https://en.wikipedia.org/wiki/Health_insurance_in_India.

Chapter 33

THE CURRENT STATE OF WOUND CARE IN AUSTRALIA

Iestyn Marc Lewis, BS, MB, FACEM, DHM

CONTENTS

Introduction

Australia spent 9.1% GDP on health care in 2011–2. This ranks favorably with similar OECD (Organisation for Economic Co-operation and Development) countries, such as the UK, Norway, and Sweden.(1) About 3% of this amount is spent on wound care each year. At any given time, it is estimated 450,000 people will require wound care, ¾ of which have chronic wounds (2% of Australia's 23 million population).(2-3) A complex public/private health-care model, general acceptance of suboptimal wound management, and physical geography means the provision of care within Australia is highly variable.(4-5)

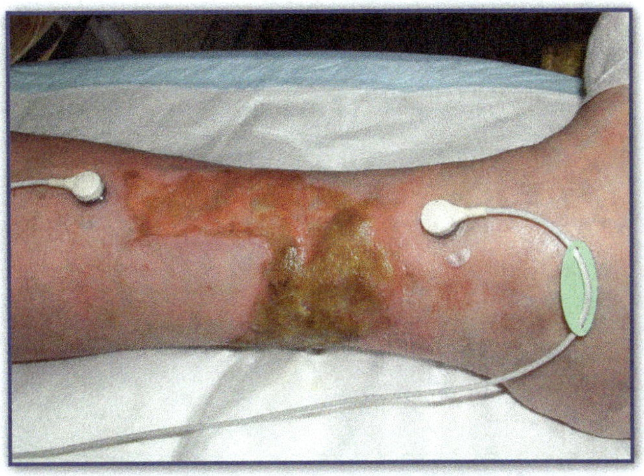

FIGURE 1. Mr. T on initial assessment

I. Case study

Mr. T is an example, albeit extreme, of how even in a universal health-care system there are barriers to receiving optimum care. Mr. T was 58 years old and steroid dependent with a long history of rheumatoid arthritis (RA), complicated by bilateral knee replacements, which became infected resulting in bilateral lower leg osteomyelitis with discharging sinuses. Combined with severe RA in his shoulders, Mr. T had limited mobility and was dependent on his family as carers. Despite these disabling complications, Mr. T's biggest complaint was a large ulcer on his left leg. For five years this almost circumferential lesion covered most of his lower leg, made walking incredibly painful, and affected his ability to sleep (Figure 1).

A number of barriers prevented Mr. T receiving specialist care. The regional town (population 20,000) where he lived is five hours from the nearest tertiary hospital with a multidisciplinary wound care team. Consultations with a visiting infectious disease specialist had been sporadic; his rheumatologist was based in a city two hours away, and his disabilities made attending appointments difficult. A local specialist wound care nurse had been treating Mr. T for about six months with little effect when he was referred to the regional complex wound care team. Not unwell enough to require inpatient hospital care, but too physically dependent to live in a hostel, it took a further three months to arrange for a nursing home to care for Mr. T for the six weeks of intensive treatment the team planned for him. The primary aim was to heal his ulcer, but we took this opportunity to bring his pain and osteomyelitis under control.

The treatment plan was multidisciplinary, including specialists in wound management, hyperbaric medicine, infectious diseases, plastic surgery, and complex pain. Mr. T received 30 hyperbaric oxygen treatments and frequent sharp debridement, additional to larval therapy. Compression garments were fitted while further investigations allowed the infectious disease team to optimize the antibiotic regimen. A persisting pain physician implemented a complex multimodal analgesia regimen facilitating Mr. T to sleep and mobilize more easily. Finally, with an optimized wound bed, a plastic surgeon placed a skin graft over the ulcer. At three weeks, 90% of the graft had taken. The remaining ulcerated area healed over the next six weeks

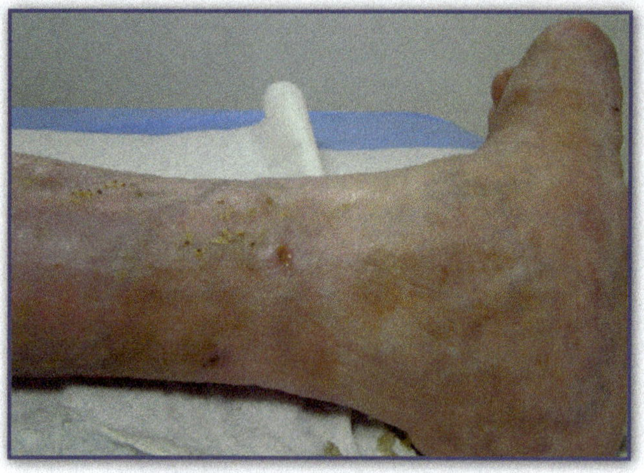

FIGURE 2. Mr. T after treatment

(Figure 2). While many of Mr. T's chronic health problems are ongoing, they are controlled and the healing of a large painful ulcer has improved his quality of life immeasurably.

II. Health-care delivery of wound care in Australia

Health care is universal in Australia; its provision is a complex web of public and private providers supported by Medicare, the national public health insurance scheme.[6] While everyone is entitled to the same care, those with private health insurance are usually able to access nonemergent treatment more quickly. Specialist services are often only available in cities, which may be hundreds of kilometers away from the 30% of the population living in rural areas.[7]

Wound management is provided in both community and hospital settings, with the bulk of the work being carried out in the community. While there is no strict division of labor, acute wounds are usually managed by family health physicians, particularly in younger patients. Older patients and those with chronic wounds tend to be managed by community nurses, with wound management making up around 50% of their workload.[8] Nurses will treat patients in their homes, a community clinic, or, in some areas, a Leg Club. Ellie Lindsay developed the Leg Club model in the UK to encourage peer support between patients. As well as providing expert wound management, this support group model reduces social isolation and improves psychological well-being and treatment compliance.[9] Frequency of visits and dressing changes will be dictated by those managing the wound; this may be community nurses, a family health physician, a specialist wound clinic, or wound care nurse practitioner.

Wound management in the hospital is predominantly postoperative wounds, particularly those beset by complications, burns, and recalcitrant or high-risk wounds, such as pressure injuries and diabetic foot ulcers. Many of these areas will have specialist multidisciplinary teams to manage patients in a holistic manner. Complex wound management clinics are expensive to run and tend to be held in public hospitals; an appointment will cost 10–20 times more than a community nurse visit. The aim in treating complex wounds aggressively is to reduce inpatient admissions by preventing complications, such as amputation and severe infections. Additional clinics such as the diabetic high-risk foot clinic include an endocrinologist, podiatrist, a specialist wound nurse, an infectious diseases physician, a vascular or orthopedic surgeon, an orthotist, and a dietician.[10-11] Unfortunately these services are only available in larger cities. In regional areas, community providers attempt to replicate the treatment but lack the resources to do so consistently.

Wound management is not yet a recognized medical specialty in Australia, and currently its practitioners cover a range of health disciplines, including medicine and podiatry. The greatest number is found within nursing. Specialist nurses have evolved out of the recognition that wound management has become more sophisticated and wound patients increasingly complex.

Wound Care Nurse Practitioners (WCNP) work independently, prescribe selective medications, request diagnostics tests, and perform invasive procedures, such as biopsies or sharp wound debridement.[12] The contrast to this specialization in a small group of dedicated professionals is that there is no, or at best minimal, teaching on complex wound management in the undergraduate curriculums of medical or nursing students. Without further dedicated study, this leaves many doctors and nurses underqualified and overwhelmed when faced with providing wound care.[13]

III. Wound care modalities

Modalities for wound management in Australia cover the spectrum from simple dressings to complex surgical interventions. The popularity of particular products will depend on local practice and who is paying for the product. Specialist wound care teams will often have access to treatments like negative pressure wound therapy, larval therapy, ultrasonic debridement, and hyperbaric oxygen, in addition to surgical interventions, such as skin grafting or revascularization.[14]

IV. Reimbursement issues

Visits to health professionals are usually provided at either no or minimal cost via the Medicare scheme which offers a system of reimbursements. Medications are mostly subsidized by the pharmaceutical benefits scheme (PBS). This limits the cost of medications to $1,120 per year, or $280 for concession cardholders. (US dollars)[15] Unfortunately wound products are only subsidized for Australian Defence Force Veterans. The remainder of the general population must pay for products, unless they are subsidized by a hospital or its clinics. This potentially creates an unfavorable environment for best-practice wound management, as many patients, particularly elderly pensioners, cannot afford wound products. While some providers are able to subsidize appropriate products, the cost of the product may be more than the reimbursement for the health professional's visit.[16] This creates a false economy where nonhealing wounds result in increased visits to health practitioners, increased number of prescriptions, and repeat inpatient admissions.[5]

V. Wound care associations

Wounds Australia, formerly the Australian Wound Management Association (AWMA), is Australia's peak body for wound management consultation and representation.

Wound Management Innovation CRC (Cooperative Research Centre) is a public/private venture to bring academics, industry, wound management professionals, and patient organizations together to provide research, development, and education.

Summary

Wound management continues to evolve in Australia and has yet to reach maturity. There are pockets of excellent practice, yet many patients are shortchanged, at least initially, by a system that is currently failing to train and reimburse its providers to provide what is known to be best practice. The future challenges in Australia will be to address the lack of subsidy for wound care products and raise awareness that the chronic wounds are an epidemic with proven and effective treatments. There are sound health economic reasons to do this, and, given the aging population, we will not be lacking for patients.[5,16]

References

1. OECD Health Statistics 2014. How does Australia compare [Internet]? Organisation for Economic Co-operation and Development [cited 2016 Aug 1]. Available from: http://www.oecd.org/els/health-systems/Briefing-Note-AUSTRALIA-2014.pdf.
2. Graves N, Zheng H. Modelling the direct health care costs of chronic wounds in Australia. Wound Pract Res. 2014;1:20-33.
3. Graves N, Zheng H. The prevalence and incidence of chronic wounds: a literature review. Wound Pract Res. 2014;1:4-19.
4. Prentice JL, Strachan V, Carville K, et al. Wounds West: delivering comprehensive strategies in improve wound management in Western Australian Health Services. Wound Pract Res. 2009;17(3):122-32.
5. Graves N, Finlayson K, Gibb M, et al. Modelling the economic benefit of gold standard care for chronic wound in a community setting. Wound Pract Res. 2014;22(3):163-8.
6. Australian Institute of Health and Welfare [Internet]. Australian Institute of Health and Welfare. Australia's Health 2014 [cited 2016 Aug 2]. Available from: http://www.aihw.gov.au/australias-health/2014/health-system/.
7. Australian atlas of healthcare variation [Internet]. Australian Commission on Safety and Quality in Health Care; 2015 Nov [cited 2016 Aug 2]. Available from: http://www.safetyandquality.gov.au/atlas/.
8. Rayner R. The role of nurse-led clinic in the management of chronic leg wounds. Prim Intent. 2006;14(4):150-67.
9. Shuter P, Finlayson K, Edwards H, et al. Leg Clubs – beyond the ulcers. Wound Pract Res. 2011;1:16-20.
10. Standards for high risk foot services (HRFS) in NSW. NSW Agency for Clinical Innovation [cited 2016 Aug 1]. Available from: http://www.aci.health.nsw.gov.au/__data/assets/pdf_file/0004/248323/ACI_Standards_for_High_Risk_Foot_Services.pdf.
11. Department of Health, Western Australia. High risk foot model of care. Perth (Australia): Health Networks Branch, Department of Health, Western Australia; 2010.
12. MacLellan L, Gardner G, Gardner A. Designing the future in wound care – the role of the nurse practitioner. Prim Intent. 2002;10(3):97-112.
13. Swanson T, Asimus M, McGuiness B. Wound management for the advanced practitioner. IP Communications; 2014. p. 505-22.
14. Swanson T, Asimus M, McGuiness B. Wound management for the advanced practitioner. IP Communications; 2014. p. 238-69.
15. Australian Government Department of Health [Internet]. Australian Government Department of Health. The Pharmaceutical Benefits Scheme [cited 2016 Aug 1]. Available from: http://www.pbs.gov.au/info/about-the-pbs#What_is_the_PBS.
16. Whitlock E, Morcom J, Spurling G, et al. Wound care costs in general practice – a cross-sectional study. Aust Fam Physician. 2014;43(3):143-6.

Chapter 34

PRESSURE ULCERS AND OTHER CHRONIC WOUNDS IN SPAIN

A Living Epidemic in the Twenty-First Century

J. Javier Soldevilla Agreda, RN, MsG, BAsc, PhD
Translated by Julio Garcia, RN, MD, AAPWCA

CONTENTS

Introduction

Chronic wounds in general, with special emphasis on pressure ulcers (PUs) have for too long been considered as banal, secondary, unavoidable, and especially silent processes and are in few circumstances considered sufficiently relevant so as to be treated as true health-care problems worthy of an appropriate response. However, with primary differences between the different types of skin ulcers, pressure and moisture ulcers, and lower-extremity ulcers, (which principally include venous, arterial, and neuropathic ulcers), they represent a severe problem to individuals, society, and our health-care system itself in Spain.

Problems for individuals:

- Impact on quality of life
- Reduction in autonomy and self-esteem
- Heightened risk of direct and indirect complications in state of health of the patients
- Potentially incapacitating states of health, which generate conditions of disability resulting in states of dependency or institutionalization
- Increase in risk of death and thus possibility of premature death

Problems for society:

- Workplace disabilities
- Threats against the rights of citizens by in some cases allowing the development of these conditions (while knowing how to prevent the vast majority of them) or their unnecessary prolongation due to inadequate medical care

Problems for the health-care system:

- Increased cost of care (human and material resources, physical space, hospitalizations, interventions, rehabilitation, etc.)
- Possible public health problems derived from the dissemination of multidrug-resistant pathogens
- Legal, personal, and institutional repercussions due to inadequate or nonexistent prevention and treatment.

I. Dimension of the problem of chronic wounds in Spain

In Spain, up to the beginning of the twenty-first century, we have not been able to avail ourselves of epidemiological information about pressure and lower-extremity ulcers that transcends concrete local realities and often generates the desired information with methodologies that make comparisons difficult.

The National Group for the Study and Advisement of Pressure Ulcers and Chronic Wounds (GNEAUPP) channeled this perceived need, developing since 2001, and every four years thereafter conducted national studies on the prevalence of pressure ulcers. The last findings in 2013 were as follows:

- adult inpatient: 7.87% (CI 95% 7.31%–8.47%)
- pediatric inpatient: 3.36% (CI 95% 1.44%–7.61%)
- community health centers: 13.41% (CI 95% 2.60%–14.2%) and in primary care settings from 0.44% (CI 95% 0.41-0.47%) in patients >65 years old and 8.51% (CI 95% 7.96- 9.10%) in patients in home-health programs

The prevalence was higher in ICUs, reaching 18%. Nosocomial PUs were 65.6% of the total, and just 29.4% were developed in domiciliary settings.[(1)]

The majority of the lesions were Stage 2 with a median onset time of 30 days and a median size of 6 cm^2.

Taking into account the estimated prevalences in this study and their projections, we must assume that close to 100,000 patients with pressure ulcers are cared for daily in Spain, of which over 80% are more than 65 years old.

Based on the British study by Bennet, Dealey, and Posnett,[2] undoubtedly the largest and most methodologically accurate in the calculation of treatment costs of pressure ulcers in a European country, Drs. Posnett and Torra extrapolated the data to the economic reality of Spain using available epidemiological data and determined treatment costs per episode of 211 Euros (233 USD) for a Stage I and 16,600 Euros (18,304 USD) for a Stage 4 pressure ulcer. The global annual cost to our health-care system was estimated at 1.687 million Euros, (1,860 million USD), which translates to 5.2% of the total health expenditures of our country.[3]

The first national study on the prevalence of leg ulcers in Spain was done by the GNEAUPP (National Group for the Study and Advisement of Pressure Ulcers and Chronic Wounds) in 2002[4] and revealed that the total prevalence of lower-extremity ulcers in patients over 14 was 0.165%.

It is believed that approximately 25% of diabetics present with foot pathology at some point during the history of their disease process, as this is the most common cause of hospital admissions (25%) and amputations and one of the causes of longer hospital stays.

The prevalence and incidence of these lower-extremity lesions is triplicated when one considers groups aged over 75; their chronicity (40–50% exceed a year of evolution); and recidivism (between 25% and 30% recidivism in the 12-month period following wound closure).

II. Wound care in Spain: health policy, management, and involved professionals

Health-care in Spain is universal and free. Citizens afflicted with any type of wound are taken care of by the health system in either a primary care or hospital setting during the whole disease process. This is a generous and high-quality health system, although perhaps with some doubts about its sustainability.

A persistent and as yet unanswered question pertains to preventive supplies in the home health setting, as these supplies are not entirely subsidized by the health system as happens with in-hospital supplies. This question must be answered in order to improve the system's efficacy.

It must be pointed out that it has only been a decade since Spain's Ministry of Health incorporated projects that set forth and evaluated safe practices in specific areas, among which, preventing pressure ulcers in at-risk patients was addressed for the first time and in writing. The development of joint strategies between all the country's health administrations resulted in better global results in the prevention of pressure ulcers, but above all in better parity, equality, and universality of health-care delivery in Spain. The Declaration of Rio de Janeiro regarding the prevention of pressure ulcers as a universal right, promoted by the Ibero-Latin-American Society for the Prevention of Ulcers and Chronic Wounds in 2011, espouses the same concept.[5]

Although with manifested differences among the regions comprising our country and especially among the different types of lesions (the diabetic foot seems to have more participative and multidisciplinary interest than PUs), the brunt of the load in caring for pressure ulcers and other chronic wounds in Spain rests primarily on nurses. This is a practice that has been tacitly in effect for years, although not sanctioned by the present legal environment (pending a reform of the country's Nurse Practice Act).

A majority of the nursing professionals in Spain from different clinical backgrounds have been selecting, and applying with scientific criteria, techniques for preparation of the wound bed of different chronic wounds (removal of non-viable tissue, control of exudate, management of localized inflammation and infection, etc.). They have been compiling an ample catalog of materials developed for their local and regional treatment (cleansing solutions, debridement procedures, bandages, dressings, etc.).

In Spain, there does not exist a specific specialty in wound management although GNEAUPP (National Group for the Study and Advisement of Pressure Ulcers and Chronic Wounds [www.gneaupp.org]) has for years granted a certificate of Expert in the Care of Pressure Ulcers, which, with the implicit limitations of its issuance by a scientific society, helps to guarantee the responsibility of health-care providers, validate their professional competency, and certify health-care practices.

Multidisciplinary chronic wound or wound care units in Spain are still a minority, but present experiences reveal the value of what has been achieved, making possible an efficient pathway to optimizing the resources for the attention, prevention, diagnosis, and treatment of persons with chronic wounds. These units, mainly led by advanced practice nurses, but with the participation of a great number of health-care specialists (specialists in vascular surgery, infectious diseases, microbiologists, podologists, etc.), comprise the academic and research activities related to chronic wounds within their spheres of influence.(6) Along the same lines, the development of Nursing Consultants in Chronic Wounds(7) is a professional field to be expanded. It has proven its effectiveness not only on a clinical level for patients having chronic wounds, but also with patient satisfaction.

III. Scientific associations in Spain related to chronic wounds

Although some related movements with lesser impact exist in the country, GNEAUPP, born in 1994 as a not-for-profit multidisciplinary scientific society, is distinguished by its specificity. It is composed at present by close to 6,000 health-care professionals, the majority of which are nurses.

Its objectives have been and always will be to provide evidence-based tools to health-care clinicians, to foster the implementation of clinical practice guidelines and preventive and therapeutic protocols throughout the various health-care delivery levels, and to homogenize the high diversity of therapeutic modalities by stimulating specialized clinical and investigational actions from within its ranks. A special mission since its inception was to establish a permanent epidemiologic data bank on these lesions and, as noted, five national studies on the prevalence of PUs and one national study on DFUs have been developed. These figures are presently considered "official" in the description of chronic wounds in Spain.

From that lonely and tortuous road initiated by few in a lowly considered discipline, a slow recognition was achieved. In conjunction with other societies in other European countries, we founded the European Pressure Ulcers Advisory Panel (EPUAP), have for many years been on the Executive Board of the European Wound Management Association (EWMA), and since 2008 have been actively participating in the development and direction of the Ibero-Latin-American Society on Ulcers and Wounds (SILAUHE).

Summary

The unavoidable inclusion of cost-effectiveness in the delivery of wound management health-care delivery in Spain, the greater awareness in the prevention of pressure ulcers and other chronic wounds, the more specific and rigorous undergraduate and postgraduate academic formation of health-care professionals, the generalized implementation of wound care clinics and nurse consultants, and the strength, investment, and growth in clinical research in the field of wound management will hold the key when the next chapter of the history of wound care in Spain is written.

References

1. Pancorbo-Hidalgo PL, García-Fernandez FP, Torra-Bou JE, Verdú-Soriano J, Soldevilla-Agreda JJ. Epidemiology of pressure ulcers in Spain in 2013: 4th national prevalence study. Gerokomos. 2014;25(4):162-70.
2. Bennett G, Dealey C, Posnett J. The cost of pressure ulcers in the UK. Aging. 2004;33:230-5.
3. Soldevilla-Agreda JJ, Torra-Bou JE, Posnnett J, Verdú-Soriano J, San Miguel L, Mayán-Santos JM. An approximation of the impact of the economic cost of the treatment of pressure ulcers. Gerokomos. 2007;18(4):201-10.
4. Torra-Bou JE, Soldevilla-Agreda JJ, Rueda-López J, Verdú-Soriano J, Roche E, Arboix-Perejamo M. MCF. First national study on the prevalence of legs in Spain. GNEAUPP-UIFC-Smith & Nephew, 2002-2003. Epidemiology of venous, arterial and mixed etiology ulcers and the diabetic foot Gerokomos. 2004;15(4):230-47.
5. SILAUHE. Declaration of Rio de Janeiro. Rio de Janeiro: Iberolatinamerican Society on Ulcers and Wounds; 2011.
6. Garcia-Fernández FP, López-Casanova P, Segovia-Gómez T, Soldevilla-Agreda JJ, Verdú-Soriano J. Multidisciplinary chronic wound units: wound clinics series: position papers GNEAUPP nº 10. Chronicles: national studies and advisory group on pressure ulcers and chronic wounds; 2012.
7. Soldevilla-Ágreda JJ, García-Fernández FP, López-Casanova P. Nurse consultants on chronic wounds. Series: position papers GNEAUPP nº 13. Logroño: national studies and advisory group on pressure ulcers and chronic wounds 2016.

Chapter 35

WOUND CARE IN THAILAND

Supaporn Opasanon, MD, FRCST, FICS, FACS
Apirag Chuangsuwanich, MD

CONTENTS

Introduction

At any given time, there are a large number of patients suffering from chronic nonhealing wounds in Thailand. For most people, wound healing is a natural process. But for some, it becomes a complex medical problem and needs to be treated on an individual basis. There are many different types of wounds including diabetic and pressure ulcers, radiation wounds, traumatic wounds, and ulcers caused by vascular problems. Estimates in 2015 indicate that 7% of the adult Thai population has diabetes. This is equivalent to 4 million people living with diabetes.[1] The incidence of diabetic foot ulcer is about 1.7% and lower extremity amputation about 0.1%. It can be time- and money-consuming to heal these wounds. Siriraj Hospital, the largest public hospital in Thailand, has spent on average of $2,300 (USD)/one admission (maximum cost of $25,000 [USD]) on the direct cost of amputation associated with DM foot ulcer.[2] Today, our country focuses on the cost-effectiveness to basic wound management and the advanced wound modalities which we believe to have the potential to remarkably decrease the overall costs of wound treatment.

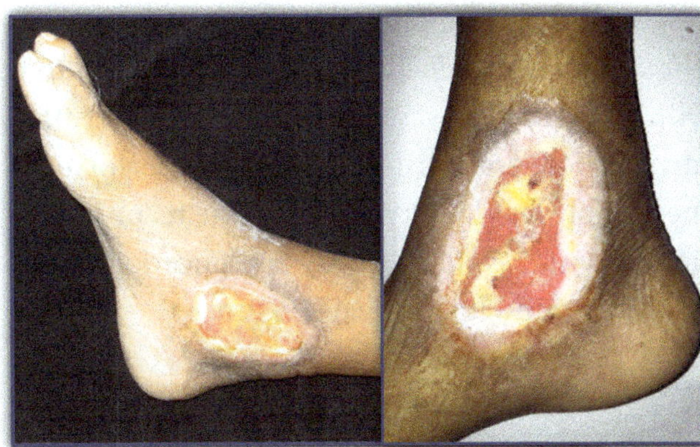

FIGURE 1. Chronic ulcer with bone exposure, right ankle

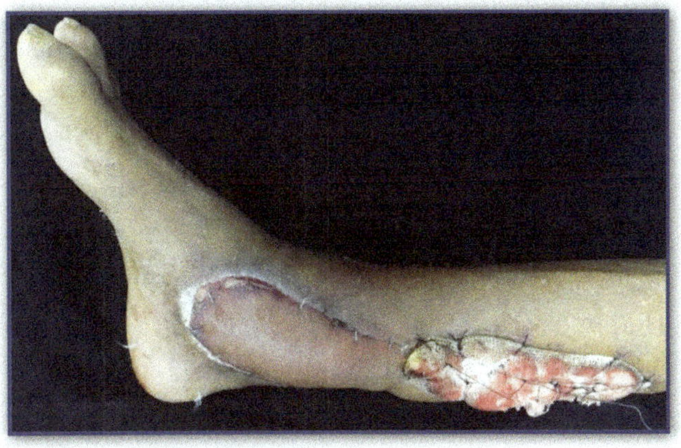

FIGURE 2. Posterior tibial artery perforator-based propeller flap

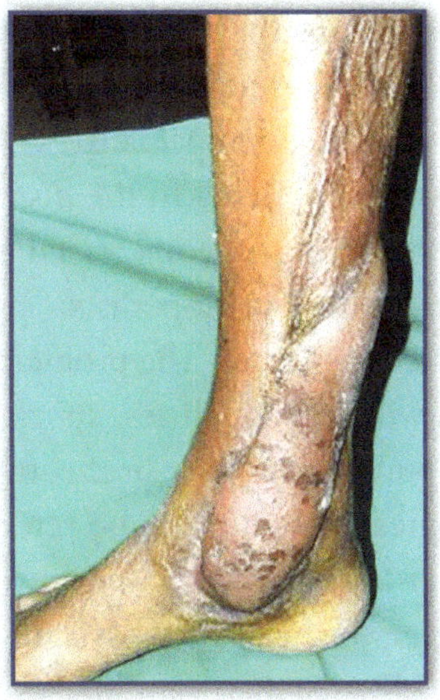

FIGURE 3. Wound heals with successful propeller flap

I. Case study

An 84-year-old male came to the hospital with chronic ulcer at his right ankle due to motorcycle exhaust burns. He was treated for this wound in a province hospital for two months. His underlying diseases were diabetes and hypertension. Wound at right malleolar area, size 5 x 3.5 cm, with exposed medial malleolus, talus and joint was found. The presence of granulation tissue, hyperkeratotic wound edge, with excess exudate was identified (Figure 1). Ankle brachial index (ABI) was 0.95. Peripheral pulse was full, but there was loss of sensation. Plain film right ankle showed no osteolytic lesion. Wound was debrided and negative pressure wound therapy was performed. Leg defect was reconstructed with the posterior tibial artery perforator-based *propeller flap*. Flap was rotated to 180 degrees to cover the defect as propeller fashion (Figure 2). The secondary defect at right calf was grafted with STSG that harvested from left thigh in 1.010 inches thickness. Bolster dressing was performed then. Short leg slab was applied. The reconstruction was *successful* with no complications and chronic wound finally heals (Figure 3).

II. Health-care delivery for wound care in Thailand

In Thailand, there is a concern with regard to the cost, access, quality and the system of health-care delivery. Access to health-care services is selectively based on insurance coverage. There are two main health-care delivery systems: public health sector and private health sector. Public health sector is complex. Regarding wound care, Thai people rely on community hospital work as their primary care. Basically, only general practitioners (GPs) work in the *community hospitals.* Primary physicians arrange patient access to hospital admissions and diagnostic testing and prescription drug therapy. However, there are the problems of limitation of wound product cost and wound care specialist. GPs can refer difficult wound patients to the *district hospital,* which has general surgeons, vascular surgeons, plastic surgeons, orthopedists, psychiatrists, and wound care nurses. The problem *is* a lack of advanced wound modalities, special investigations and equipment. In case of complex wound patients, these patients can be referred to specialists in a *tertiary hospital or university hospital.* However, the health-care system comes with serious problems that vary in severity across the region involving funding, service, and staff. Some tertiary hospitals cannot afford advanced wound products, so the patients need to pay them without reimbursement.

The private health sector is less complex. Some Thai people can afford to buy insurance out of their own private funds or they can pay for services privately. In case of emergency, Thai patients can visit any hospital. The Ministry of Public Health pays for emergency patients for the first 72 hours.

Although there is no official wound center in Thailand, there is an effective multidisciplinary wound care team. Multidisciplinary primary care teams have a fundamental role in the prevention and identification of wound types as well as in routine care at a level that fits with their competencies. Specialist teams comprise general surgeons, physicians with advanced training in wound management, vascular surgeons, plastic surgeons, orthopedists, and psychiatrists, who will also collaborate with many other specialists incorporated into the team. In addition, there are wound care nurses, nutritionists, clinical psychologists, technicians who perform noninvasive studies, and various therapies and experienced staff to assist with appointments, medical records, and health insurance processing.

III. Wound care modalities used in Thailand

In Thailand, the wound care team follows treatment protocols specifically established for each type of wound. Wound treatment modalities are selected based on patient factors, past treatment, and provider choice. Regarding wound care in Thailand, traditional treatment with normal saline solution, antiseptic solution, gauze and bandage is used. However, up-to-date approaches to wound healing are used and remain current in new scientific advances in wound care. Today, wound bed preparation concept is well accepted. The TIME principles, consisting of tissue debridement, infection or inflammation, moisture balance, and edge effect provide a systematic approach to the assessment and management of wounds. If standard wound care has failed, advanced wound care modalities may be required.

IV. Advanced wound care product categories in Thailand

1. Biophysical Agents - Hyperbaric Oxygen Therapy (HBOT), Ultrasound Therapy
2. Cellular and/or Tissue-Based Products for Wounds
   - Non-Viable Cells, Tissue-Based: Animal-Integra, Kerecis™ Omega3 Wound[3]
3. Compression
   - Dynamic Compression: Pumps
   - Static Compression: Stockings, Tubular Elastic Compression, Wraps
4. Debridement
   - Debridement Devices – Hydrosurgery (Versajet), Ultrasonic Wound Care System, Medical Maggots
5. Dressings
   - Alginates - Aquacel Ag, Algisite, Durafiber, Kaltostat
   - Antimicrobial Dressings - Iodiflex, Acticoat, Silver Products
   - Contact Layers - Mepitel, Urgotul
   - Foam Dressings -Allevyn, Easyfoam, Mepilex, Betaplast, Askina Calgitrol Ag, Aquacel foam
   - Hydrocolloids – Duoderm
   - Hydrogels: Amorphous -Intrasite Gel, Askina Gel, Duoderm Gel
   - Impregnated Dressings – Bactigras
   - Silicone Gel Sheets - Cica Care, Mepiform
   - Silver Products - Acticoat, Askina Calgitrol Ag, Aquacel Ag
   - Transparent Films - Tegaderm, Opsite
6. Growth Factors
   - Recombinant Human Epidermal Growth Factor (Easyef®)
   - Epidermal Growth Factor (Regend D)
7. Negative Pressure Wound Therapy (NPWT)
8. Offloading Devices
   - Offloading Footwear and Total Contact Cast
9. Wound Care Diagnostics
   - Angiography
   - Vascular Testing Devices – Transcutaneous Oxygen Tension ($TcPO_2$) Monitoring Device (TCOM), Segmental Blood Pressures, Ankle Brachial Index (ABI)

V. Reimbursement issues in Thailand

Most hospitals in Thailand are operated by the Ministry of Public Health. Other government units and public organizations also operate hospitals, including the military, universities, local governments and the Red Cross.[4] Private hospitals are regulated by the Medical Registration Division.

Public health insurance is provided through three systems:

1. Civil service welfare system for civil servants and their families. The Comptroller General's Department, Ministry of Finance directly controls this funding.

2. Social Security scheme for private employees. The Office of Social Security is attached to the Ministry of Labor and Social Welfare.

3. Universal Coverage System is available to all other Thai nationals. The National Health Security Office (NHSO) allocates funding through the Universal Coverage System. People were allowed to access services in their health district, and, if necessary, be referred for specialist treatment elsewhere.[5]

Some people buy private health insurance on their own. Some private hospitals are participants in these public health-care systems. According to the World Bank, under Thailand's health schemes, 99.5% of the population have health protection coverage.[5]

VI. Wound care association in Thailand

Established in 2005, the *Thai Society* of *Wound Healing (TSWH)* is a nonprofit medical society welcoming medical providers from all disciplines involved in theprevention and treatment of complex wounds. This society provides the Annual Wound Care Conference for wound care providers. Since then, TSWH has joined hands with the Burn Injury Society of Thailand to form a new association, Burn and Wound Healing Association (Thailand) (BWAT), a nonprofit medical association dedicated to advancing burn and wound management in Thailand. The Association's focus is on education, public policy, and the application of evidence-based wound care practice. The Asian Wound Healing Association and Asia Pacific Burns Association are the umbrella organizations under which all are united. In September 2011, BWAT held the 8th Asia Pacific Burn Congress and the 3rd Congress of The Asian Wound Healing Association (8th APBC and 3rd AWHA) in Thailand.

References

1. Bureau of Non-Communicable Disease [Internet]. Ministry of Public Health, Bureau of Non-Communicable Disease Control Department. Non-communicable disease data [cited 2016 Jul 16]. Available from: http://www.thaincd.com/information-statistic/non-communicable-disease-data.php.
2. Thirapatarapong W, Srisawasdi G. Epidemiology and direct cost of diabetes-related lower extremity amputations at Siriraj hospital. J Thai Rehabil Med. 2008;18(2):65-9.
3. WoundSource [Internet]. Kestrel Health Information. Kerecis™ Omega3 Wound. Available from: http://www.woundsource.com/product/kerecis-omega3-wound.
4. Wikipedia: the free encyclopedia [Internet]. Wikimedia Foundation, Inc. Health in Thailand. Available from: https://en.wikipedia.org/wiki/Health_in_Thailand.
5. The World Bank [Internet]. The World Bank Group. Thailand: sustaining health protection for all [cited 2012 Aug 29]. Available from: http://www.worldbank.org/en/news/feature/2012/08/20/thailand-sustaining-health-protection-for-all.

Chapter 36

WOUND CARE IN MALAYSIA

Harikrishna K. R. Nair, MD, FMSWCP

CONTENTS

Introduction

In Malaysia there was a renaissance in the field of wound care whereby the National Technical Committee on Wound Care was formed in 2009 under the Ministry of Health, and subsequently the 10th Circular of the Director General of Malaysia was released on the October 16, 2011. This circular is the first of its kind in the world whereby 146 hospitals under the ministry have to form the wound care teams and committees in their respective hospitals. This was a great top-down approach for wound management involving a multidisciplinary team with the usage of advanced wound care dressings and other modalities. Trainings are conducted at the zonal level which is North, East, South, Central, and the Malaysian states of Sabah, and Sarawak. Teams are functional. Surveillance to note the burden of the wound care terms and units are collected continuously from the hospitals and sent to the Medical Quality Branch of the Ministry of Health which is the secretariat for the National Committee.

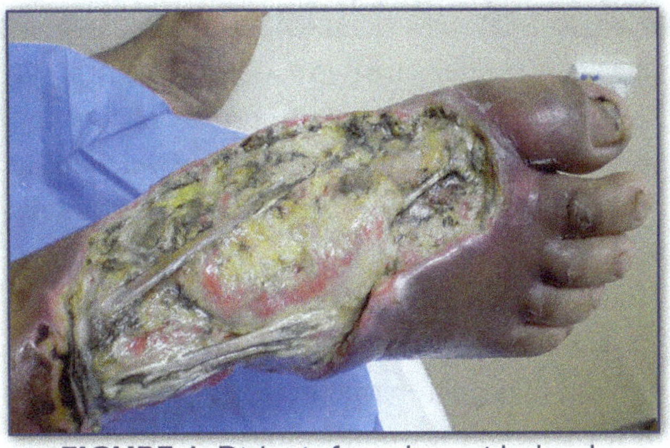

FIGURE 1. Diabetic foot ulcer with slough and tendon exposed

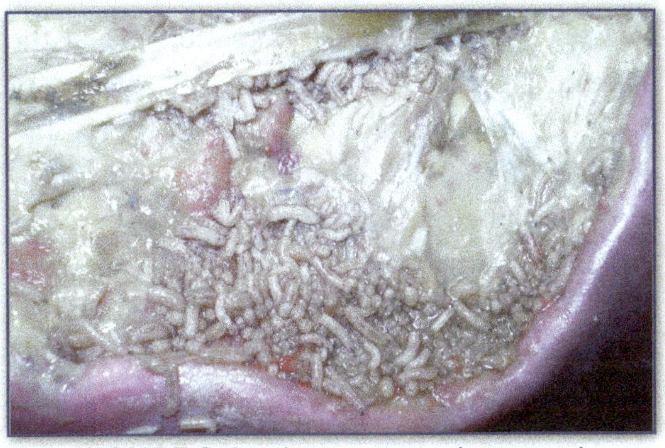

FIGURE 2. Lucilia cuprina in the wound

I. Case study

A 65-year-old Malay gentleman who is a known case of type 2 diabetes mellitus presented to us with a right dorsal aspect infected diabetic foot ulcer with tendons exposed. He discharged himself from the Orthopaedic Ward because they were planning for a below-knee amputation. He came to the Wound Care Clinic, and we used maggot debridement therapy to manage the slough. Opposite are the pictures of the wounds (Figures 1-3).

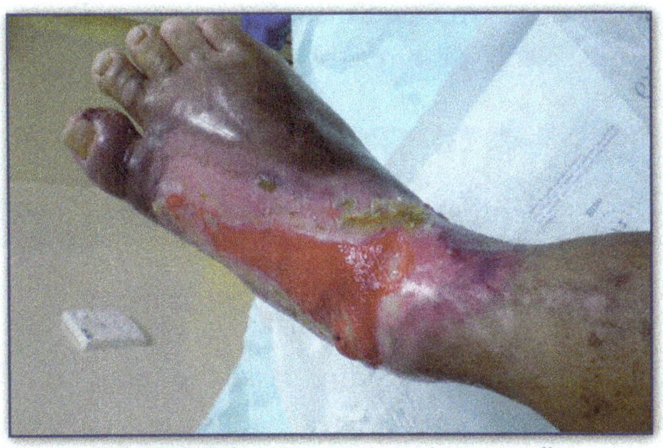

FIGURE 3. Wound granulating well

II. Health-care delivery for wound care in Malaysia

In Malaysia, there are two systems in health. We have the private setting with private clinics and private hospitals and the government setting with 1,000 government clinics and hospitals, which are divided into specialist and state hospitals and the district hospital.

Cases are seen at the government health clinics, and they are referred to the specialist clinics or the wound clinic in the hospital. In Malaysia, there is a top-down approach whereby the 10th Circular of the Director General's office, which was released on October 16, 2011, stated that all government hospitals have to form a wound care team and a wound care committee at the hospital level. The wound committee is comprised of doctors from the different specialities and is chaired by the deputy director (medical) of the hospital. The committee is in charge of procuring human resources and budgets as well as discussing the different aspects of multidisciplinary wound management. The wound team manages the wound cases.

The wound teams cover outpatients and inpatients. The stakeholders who champion the wound management are different in various hospitals whereby some are wound doctors and some are orthopaedic surgeons, general surgeons, or plastic surgeons.

III. Wound care modalities used in Malaysia

Many advanced wound dressings are available from all over the world, which includes silver dressings, collagen, iodine based products, polymer, keratin, and others. We also use maggot debridement therapy utilizing Lucilia cuprina, which are sterilized maggots for debridement. Negative pressure wound therapy is also used. Topical oxygen therapy, microcurrent therapy, monochromatic infrared therapy, and various other modalities are available including hyperbaric oxygen therapy in different centers but mainly in the Wound Care Unit, Department of Internal Medicine, Hospital Kuala Lumpur, which is the premier center and the center for training in Malaysia. Dermal skin substitutes are also available.

IV. Reimbursement issues in Malaysia

In the private setting, the patients have to pay, or they have insurance which covers the dressings and wound management. In the government setting, the services are subsidized whereby patients only pay USD.25 for each consultation and dressing. Meanwhile, the government specialist charges are USD1.25 for each consultation which includes blood tests, swabs, procedures, dressings, and etc. This is hugely subsidized by the Ministry of Health. However, patients buy their own advanced dressings, etc., by local purchase order or departmental budget. General products are supplied by the surgical stores and the pharmacy.

V. Wound care association

The Malaysian Society of Wound Care Professionals (MSWCP) was formed in the year 2011. MSWCP has organized five different Asia Pacific and International level conferences. The MSWCP also supplies wound care kits equipped with advanced wound care dressings for free to all the health clinics with family medicine specialists and also all the wound teams in the hospitals.

The society also sends kits and dressings during disasters such as during the typhoon Yolanda, which hit Tacloban, Philippines; the bomb blast in the Erawan shrine, Bangkok, Thailand; and during the floods in North Malaysia. MSWCP is also responsible for setting up a free wound clinic in the Indira Gandhi Memorial Hospital in Male, Maldives. MSWCP also publishes pamphlets, brochures, and posters as well as books such as the *Compendium of Wound Care Dressings, Maggot Debridement Therapy, Diabetic Foot – the Asian Perspective*, etc.

Summary

Wound care in Malaysia is still at the level of infancy but expanding dramatically. In the future, there is hope that all health facilities will have trained personnel with advanced wound care products and modalities available so that patients with wounds can be managed in a multidisciplinary approach with no or minimal complications.

References

1. Ministry of Health Malaysia. Malaysia. Available from: www.moh.gov.my.
2. Harikrishna, Nazni WA, Lee HL. Maggot debridement therapy – the Malaysian experience. 2014. Heal Digest. MSWCP.

Chapter 37

TREATMENT OF WOUNDS IN AFRICA

Terry Treadwell, MD, FACS

CONTENTS

Introduction

Wound management differs all over the world depending on the available resources and the training of the people providing the care. Unfortunately, in Africa, both the availability of resources to treat wounds and the people trained to treat them vary tremendously from country to country. There is a lack of understanding that the effective treatment of wounds will benefit people by improving their lives and helping them to become productive and self-sufficient. It is critical that the mission in Africa be to teach the importance of caring for wounds and how to do it appropriately and effectively. The concept of the team approach to care for patients with wounds is unknown in Africa but also must be stressed if there is to be improvement in wound management.(1) Unfortunately, the attitude among many government officials and health-care providers is one of disinterest and unconcern. Even the health-care providers who are willing to attempt to treat wounds are left with ancient or rarely effective therapies.(2) As a result, many people try to treat their wounds themselves or turn to traditional healers for help.(3) Teaching the concepts of modern wound care in Africa is a challenge that must be met before progress can be made in wound management.

I. Case studies

A. Case 1

A 54-year-old lady was seen in the Emergency Department of St. Martin's Hospital in Agroysum, Ghana, with the story that she had suffered a poisonous snake bite on her foot about eight hours prior. When asked why it took her so long to come for help, she replied that she had sought immediate help from the local traditional healer who had given her a "healing rock" to put on the bite on the foot (Figure 1). He assured her she would suffer no effect from the bite. With the passage of a few hours, she began to notice the leg was swelling, and she was not feeling well. It was then that she thought she should seek help at the hospital. After being evaluated, treatment was begun with the appropriate antivenom, antibiotics, and IV fluids. She began to feel better. Despite her improvement at the hospital, she refused to let us remove the rock from the bite site and debride the wound. Fortunately, she did well and had a full recovery. As she was leaving the hospital, her only comment to me was, "I told you the rock would make me well!"

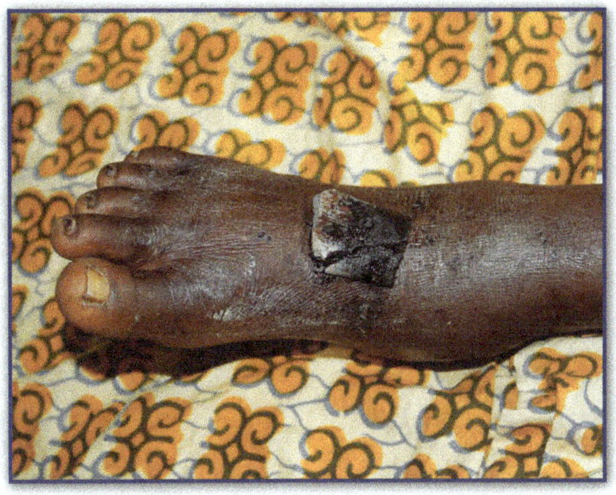

FIGURE 1. Snakebite treated with "healing" rock

B. Case 2

A two-year-old child was brought to the main teaching hospital in Kumasi, Ghana, after falling into a fire on which her mother was cooking. The child suffered second- and third-degree burns over the left chest and abdomen. When she arrived at the hospital, the wound was debrided and fine-mesh gauze soaked in Betadine solution was placed on the wound. This was covered with gauze pads. The next morning I was asked to see the child and make recommendations regarding her care. When I arrived at the bedside, the nurses were in the process of removing the dressing. The child was screaming as the nurses were peeling the tightly adherent gauze off the wound (Figure 2). It took nearly 20 minutes for them to remove the dressing. To watch that child suffer needlessly was almost more than I could manage. After the dressing was removed, the burns were inspected and found to be doing as well as possible after being abused as they had been. We had a long discussion about nonadherent dressings. Since they apparently had none, I showed them how to put petrolatum on gauze to make a nonadherent dressing. The next day the child had essentially no reaction to removal of the dressings.

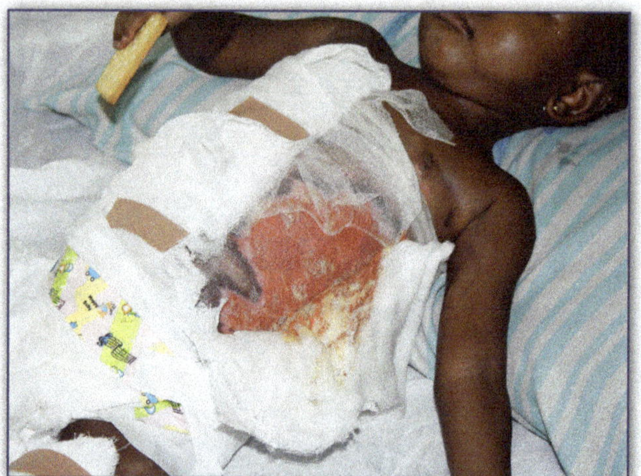

FIGURE 2. Third-degree burn of baby with gauze stuck to wound

II. Wound care in Africa

As one can imagine, care of wounds in Africa can vary widely depending on the person providing the care and the resources available to treat the wounds. As noted in the first case, a traditional healer practicing what he was taught by previous traditional healers may provide wound care by using techniques that he learned by trial and error. There are situations where the only health-care provider in an area is someone with no medical training but an interest in helping others. In areas where there are hospitals, there may be nurses and physicians providing care, but their training and dedication may be suspect. As noted above, many feel that wounds are the patient's problem to manage for themselves. As one can imagine, even in the best of hospitals and clinics, there are no treatment protocols for anything, much less wounds!

How are wounds treated in areas with few resources? It can be very interesting because treatments and dressings usually utilize what is available and not what is best for healing. The most common solutions used on wounds are the old standbys – povidone iodine, hydrogen peroxide, and acetic acid. These are used in various combinations with gauze dressings. There is no thought given to what these products might be doing to the wound and its ability to heal. Compression bandages are basically unknown in Africa. There are no attempts made to manage edema or lymphedema. Many local remedies are routinely used without any basic knowledge of how the treatment works or if it works.

One of our more interesting tasks has been to develop wound treatments and bandages that maintain the moist wound healing environment we recommend and do not do more harm than good.[4] Just one example is the need for a nonadherent dressing. We addressed this in two ways. Petrolatum is readily available in most African countries as is gauze. We taught the providers how to make petrolatum gauze and use it to prevent dressings from sticking to the wound.[5-6] The second approach was to find something available locally that could be used. The solution was almost all around us – banana leaves! It is known that banana leaves have a waxy coating on them, which will not stick to a wound bed. The banana leaves just need to be cut to size, cleaned, and applied to the wound. They not only provide a nonadherent wound dressing but also stimulate healing![7-9] We have been able to teach practitioners the importance of treating edema and lymphedema with compression bandages and how to provide that treatment with a modified short-stretch compression bandage they can make with local products. Other useful treatments and techniques have been outlined by Dr. Linda Benskin after spending many years in Ghana, Africa, working with local providers teaching wound care.[10] Many challenges still exist in trying to convince practitioners to use evidence-based wound treatment techniques and helping them find the treatments, dressings, and bandages to accomplish that goal.

As would be expected in any country with minimal resources, reimbursement is entirely dependent on the patient and what he or she can pay. Dressings and bandages have to be purchased by the patient or family and brought to the provider to apply them. As you can imagine, many dressings are used multiple times, which is not the ideal situation. Some of the African countries are beginning to consider some type of government-sponsored health-care funding program, but at this time resources are few and far between. Mission hospitals provide the only sponsored health care, and there are limits on those resources.

The introduction of modern wound care to Africa is in its infancy. There are training programs being developed by organizations such as the Pan African Academy of Christian Surgeons and the World Alliance of Wound and Lymphedema Care. Hopefully, with persistence and time, patients in Africa with wounds will have improved care of their wounds with better healing rates and fewer major amputations.[11] Our work is just beginning.

References

1. Treadwell TA. Integrating the concept of wound care, the importance of wound treatment, wound treatment education, and the wound care "team" in underdeveloped areas around the world. In: Macdonald JM, Geyer MJ, editors. WHO white paper: best practice recommendations for wound & lymphedema management. 2007.
2. Treadwell TA. The why and how of creating a wound treatment centre. World Counc Enteros Ther J. 2006;26(3):32-43.
3. Werner D, Thuman C, Maxwell J. Where there is no doctor: a village health care handbook. Berkeley (CA): The Hesperian Foundation; 1992. p. W1.
4. Treadwell TA. You are using what to treat what? Wounds. 2016;28(2):A6-7.
5. Treadwell TA, Walker DJ. The basics of wound care and how to make a non-adherent dressing wound training video. World Health Organization [video]. 2011.
6. Treadwell TA, Walker DJ. How to make a non-adherent wound dressing [poster]. World Health Organization; 2014.
7. Guenova E, Hoetzenecker W, et al. Banana leaves as an alternative wound dressing. Dermatol Surg. 2013;39:290-7.
8. Gore MA, Akolekar D. Evaluation of banana leaf dressing for partial thickness burn wounds. Burns. 2003;29(5):487-92.
9. Gore MA, Akolekar D. Banana leaf dressings for skin graft donor areas. Burns. 2003;29(5):483-6.
10. Benskin L. Handbook for health care in developing countries: a guide for promoting health in your community. Searcy (AK): International Health Care Foundation; 2002.
11. Treadwell TA, Macdonald J. Buruli ulcer: its impact and treatment worldwide, an interval report. Wounds. 2012;24(9 Suppl):19-20.

Chapter 38

WOUND CARE IN KOREA

Hyunsuk (Peter) Suh, MD, PhD
JoonPio (JP) Hong, MD, PhD, MMM

CONTENTS

Introduction

As Korea is moving toward an aged society, there is a large number of patients suffering from chronic diseases such as hypertension and diabetes. A report from the Korea Institute for Health and Social Affairs (KIHASA) in 2010 shows that more than 53% of people aged over 65 suffer from hypertension, and more than 19% of people have diabetes.[(1)] By the report from the Health Insurance Review and Assessment Service (HIRA), more than 2.5 million people visit hospitals because of diabetes, and the medical costs for treating diabetes were larger than 735 billion KRW (Korean won) in 2014.[(2)] As people become more aged, and more patients are bedridden, medical cost increases, quality of life is getting worse, and also mortality rate increases. Nowadays, our country is building bases for health maintenance in aged people. We are building a preventive health-care system throughout the lifetime, substantiating a health-care security system in old age, and activating a physical exercise system for health promotion of older persons.

In caring for chronic wounds, we cannot consider the wound apart from the patient. The condition of the patient and the status of the chronic disease have important roles in wound healing and recurrence of the wound. By an integrated patient care system and multidisciplinary approach, we work as a team with internal medicine, orthopedic surgery, vascular surgeons, rehabilitation medicine, and also with wound care nurses, nutritionists, and other medical personnel to not only heal the wound but also change the lifestyle to prevent recurrence of the ulcer and chronic wound.

I. Case study

A 65-year-old female with diabetes visited the emergency department for a foot ulcer with infection. The patient had a high fever, and there was severe inflammation in the wound (Figure 1). After stabilizing the vital signs, emergency debridement was performed by a plastic surgeon. After debridement, negative-pressure wound therapy with instillation was applied. After the patient was admitted to internal medicine for general care and blood sugar control, CT angiogram was checked based on the suspicion of limb ischemia. We found severe atherosclerosis of the peripheral vessels (Figure 2). Balloon angioplasty was done by a

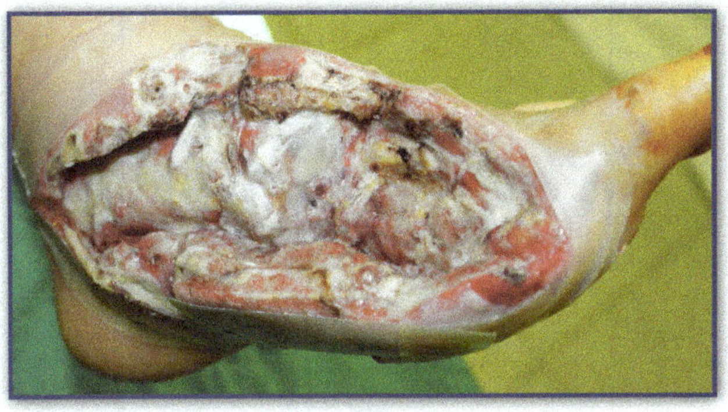

FIGURE 1.
Courtesy of Hyunsuk (Peter) Suh, MD

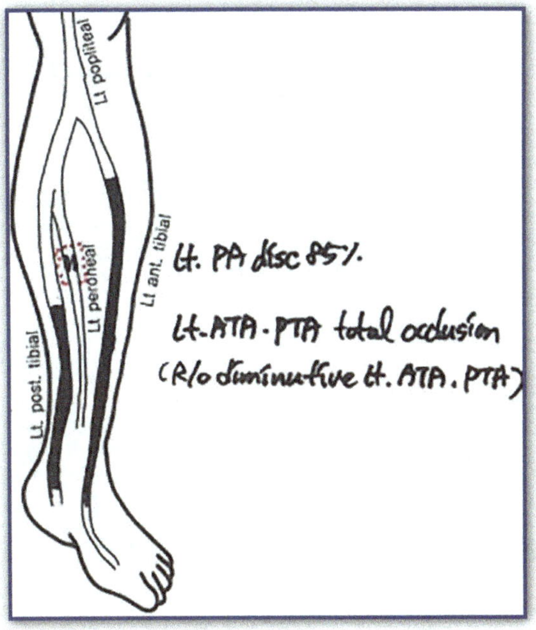

FIGURE 2.
Courtesy of Hyunsuk (Peter) Suh, MD

cardiologist with serial debridement for the infected wound. There was increased blood flow from the peroneal artery to the posterior tibial artery after ballooning the peroneal artery (Figure 3). Between the debridements, negative-pressure wound therapy was used. After two weeks of wound preparation (Figure 4), an anterolateral free flap was done to cover the defect. One month after surgery (Figure 5), the patient started ambulation with her usual shoe. The patient had no recurrence after one year of wound care.

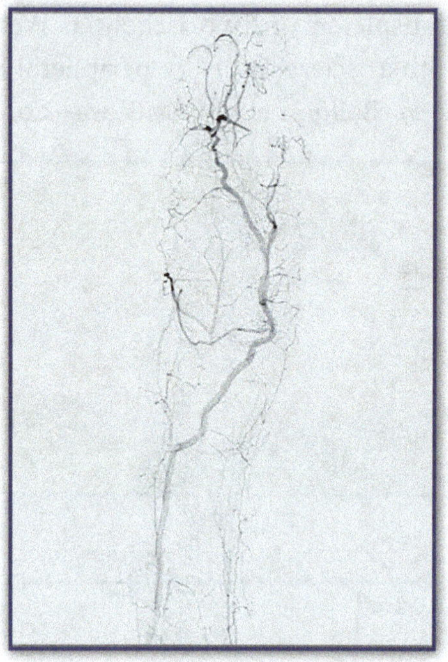

FIGURE 3.
Courtesy of Hyunsuk (Peter) Suh, MD

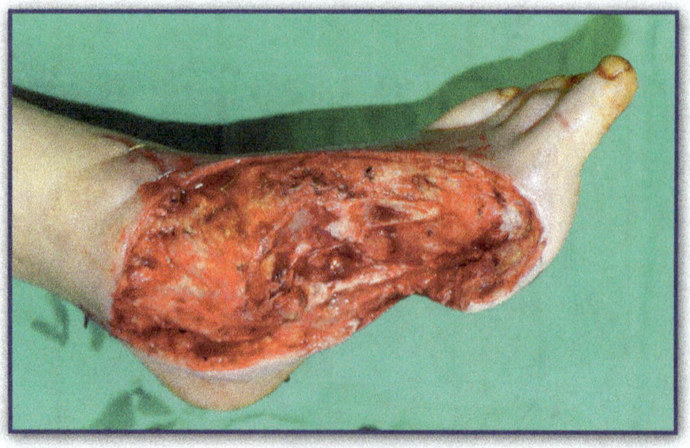

FIGURE 4.
Courtesy of Hyunsuk (Peter) Suh, MD

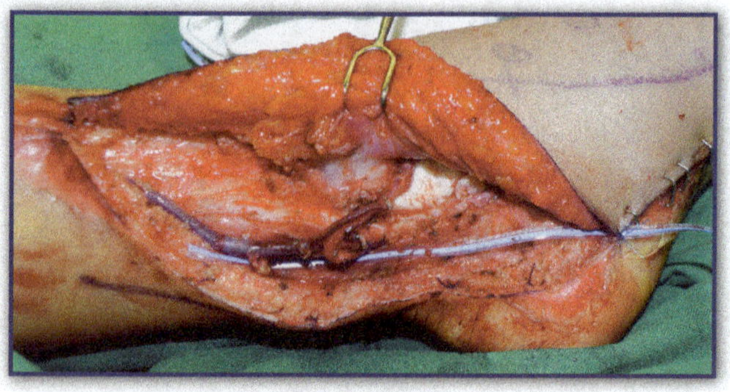

FIGURE 5.
Courtesy of Hyunsuk (Peter) Suh, MD

II. Health-care delivery for wound care in Korea

All hospitals in Korea are working under the regulation of the National Health Insurance Program. Every patient can go to any doctor or any medical institute whether it is public or private. The referral arrangement system is divided into two steps. The patient can go to a primary health-care service for the wound care or primary physicians may want to refer the patient to a secondary or tertiary service by simply writing a slip. Even in the private hospitals, medical cost is the same as with the public hospitals.

III. Wound care modalities used in Korea

New therapeutic *modalities* such as bioactive extracellular matrices, cellular and tissue products, negative-pressure wound therapy, and microvascular perfusion assessment devices are available in Korea.

By the report from the Korea Health Industry Development Institute,[(3)] our market of wound management materials is growing annually up to 19.7% every year during 2008–2013. By the same report, the annual increase of domestic materials is more than 38% every year during the same period, and 57% of the wound care materials were domestic products in 2013.[(3)]

Advanced wound materials

1. Hyperbaric oxygen therapy (HBO_2 therapy)
2. Negative-pressure wound therapy

Debridement devices

1. Hydrosurgery
2. Ultrasonic wound debridements

Cellular products/artificial dermis

1. Allogenic dermis
2. Autologous cultured epithelium
3. HolodermR

Cell therapy
Cell therapy is widely used in Korea to heal acute and chronic ulcers or for cosmetic purposes.

1. Autologous adipose-derived stromal vascular fraction (SVF) cells
2. Autologous bone marrow stromal stem cells
3. Autologous platelet-rich plasma
4. Many allogenic stem cells materials are under development (doing clinical studies)

Biological dressing material

1. Allogenic keratinocyte
2. KalodermR

Growth factors

1. bFGF (basic fibroblast growth factor)
2. rhEGF (recombinant human growth factor)
3. PDGF (platelet-derived growth factor)

Various dressing materials

Offloading devices/preventive surgery

1. Total contact cast, removable walker cast, removable walker boot
2. Ostectomy, resection arthroplasty, tendon lengthening
3. Nerve decompression surgery

Soft tissue covering surgery

1. Graft, local flap including propeller flap, free flaps

IV. Reimbursement issues in Korea

The health-care system in Korea has two components: health insurance and medical aid. The national health insurance system provides coverage for most of the citizens, and it is managed as a form of social insurance. On the other hand, the medical aid component provides support to lower-income groups and is funded by general revenue. One hundred percent of people in Korea are eligible for coverage under the National Health Insurance Program (NHIP) in two components. One hundred percent of hospitals are covered by the National Health Insurance Service (NHIS). But most of the cost for medical service is not all reimbursed by the program. Patients are required to pay a certain portion of the health-care cost. The co-payments differ according to the level of medical institute, type of disease, and whether they are in health insurance or medical aid, but not by the publicity of the hospitals.

V. Wound care associations in Korea

There are several wound care associations in Korea. The Korean Wound Management Society (KWMS) was established in 2002 as a nonprofit medical society, with a vision of integrating all realms of wound care to become a leader in wound management. The society has grown to become the large organization that it is now, with about 1,500 diverse members ranging from doctors and nurses to engineers, researchers, and industrial members. Medical personnel come from diverse backgrounds and include nurses working in acute care hospitals, home care, intensive care units, and wound care, as well as orthopedic surgeons, burn specialists, physicians working in rehabilitation medicine, dermatologists, and emergency department doctors. The Society sponsors a diverse array of academic symposia and forums. Korean Burn Society (KBS) is also a nonprofit medical society and was established in 1997. There are diverse members from emergency medicine doctors, general surgeons, plastic surgeons, internists, nutritionists, emergency medical technicians, and many other medical personnel. Also there is the Korean Society for Diabetic Foot, which was founded in 2013 as a nonprofit organization. The Korean Society for Diabetic Foot was organized by professionals in various fields such as endocrinology, orthopedics, plastic surgery, rehabilitation medicine, vascular surgery, and nursing. The aims of the society are to promote or carry out the knowledge of professionals and to apply such knowledge to the prevention and treatment of diabetic foot. These three organizations are coworkers in many ways towards wound care and prevention in Korea.

References

1. Sik CY. Korea's Health and Welfare Trends: 2010 [Internet]. Korea Institute for Health and Social Affairs; 2010 Dec. Available from: https://www.kihasa.re.kr/web/publication/research/view.do?menuId=44&tid=71&bid=12&division=001&keyField=title&searchStat=2017&key=2010&ano=987.

2. General statistics in health insurance 2014 [Internet]. Health Insurance Review and Assessment Service. Available from: http://opendata.hira.or.kr/op/opc/selectStcPblc.do?sno=10700&odPblcTpCd=002&searchCnd=&searchWrd=&pageIndex=1.

3. KHIDI brief [Internet]. Korea Health Industry Development Institute (KHIDI); 2014. Available from: https://www.khidi.or.kr/fileDownload?titleId=121295&fileId=1.

APPENDIX

CLINICAL DECISION-MAKING PATHWAYS IN CHRONIC WOUND CARE

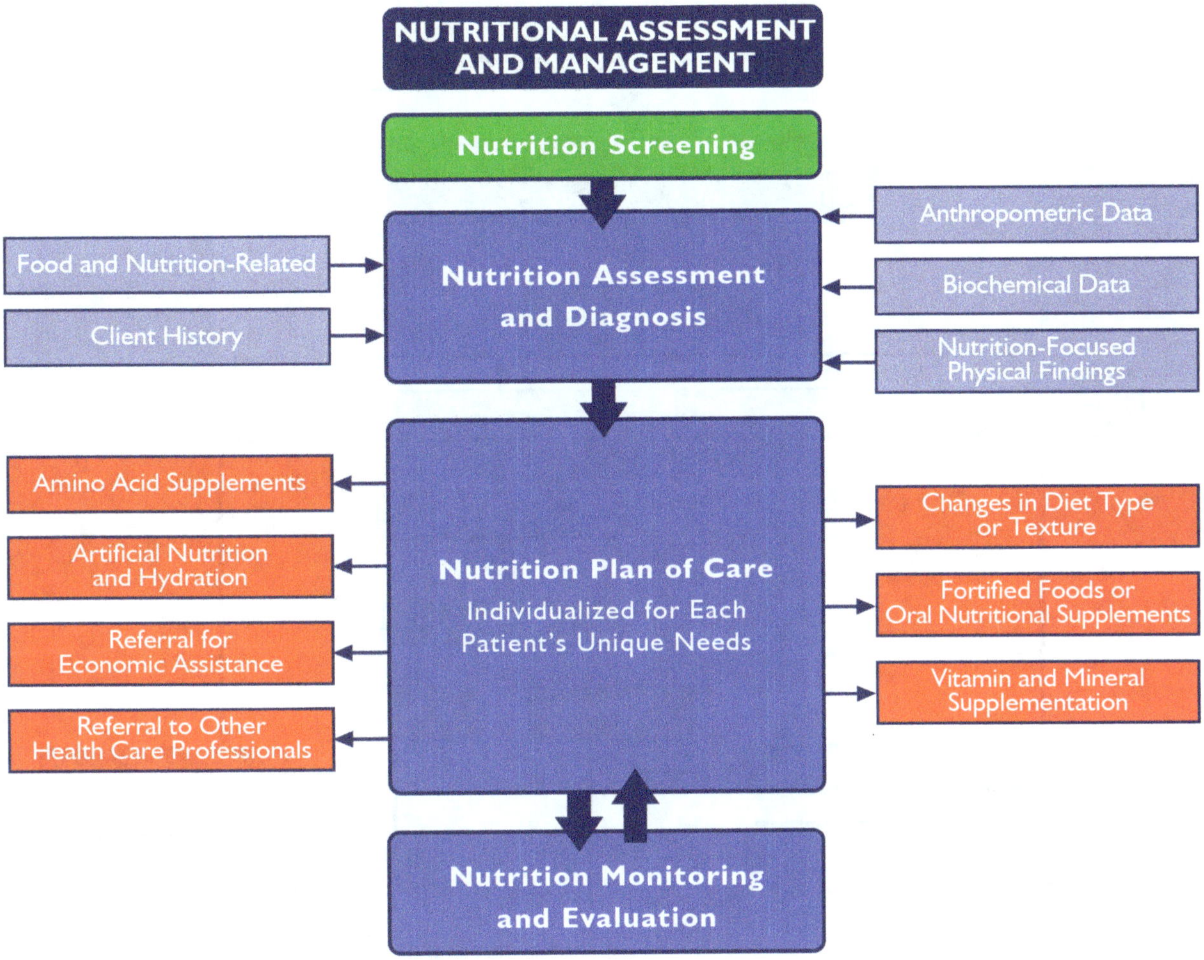

Printed with permission by Elizabeth Friedrich, MD
(Chapter 4: Nutritional Assessment and Management)

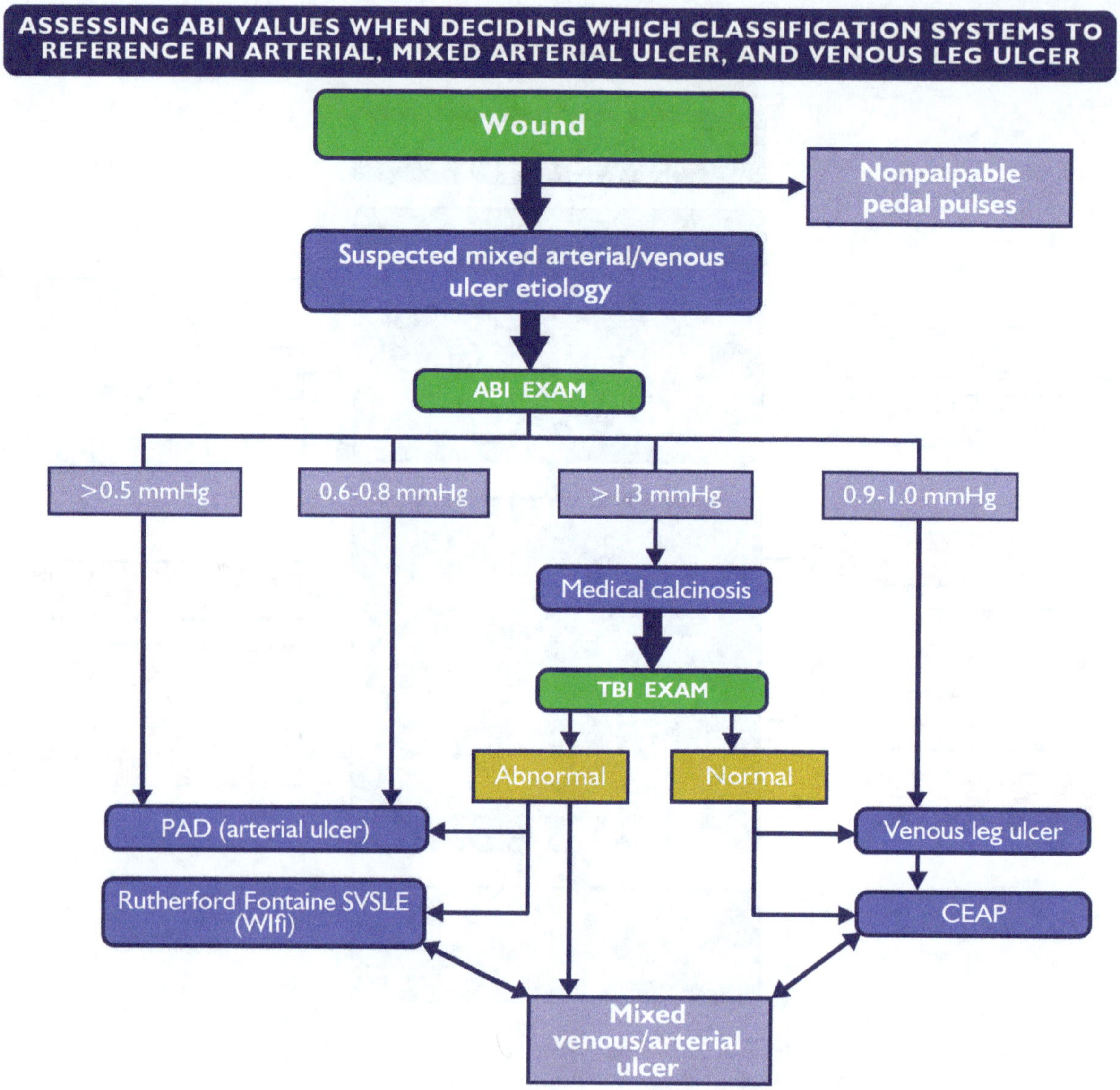

Printed with permission by Robert J. Snyder, MD
(Chapter 5: Wound Assessment)

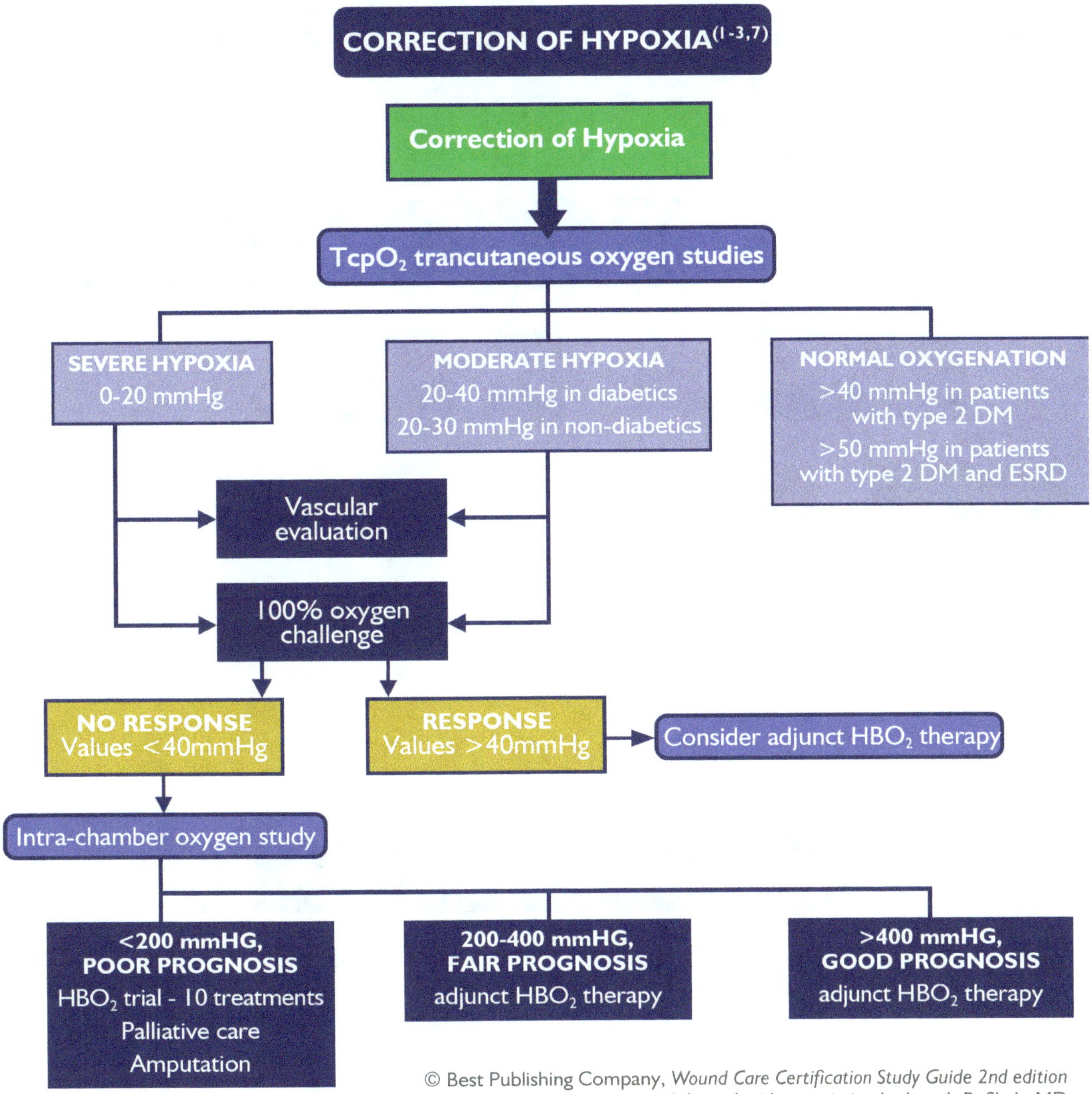
CORRECTION OF HYPOXIA(1-3,7)
Correction of Hypoxia
TcpO2 trancutaneous oxygen studies
SEVERE HYPOXIA
0-20 mmHg
MODERATE HYPOXIA
20-40 mmHg in diabetics
20-30 mmHg in non-diabetics
NORMAL OXYGENATION
>40 mmHg in patients with type 2 DM
>50 mmHg in patients with type 2 DM and ESRD
Vascular evaluation
100% oxygen challenge
NO RESPONSE
Values <40mmHg
RESPONSE
Values >40mmHg
Consider adjunct HBO2 therapy
Intra-chamber oxygen study
<200 mmHG,
POOR PROGNOSIS
HBO2 trial - 10 treatments
Palliative care
Amputation
200-400 mmHG,
FAIR PROGNOSIS
adjunct HBO2 therapy
>400 mmHG,
GOOD PROGNOSIS
adjunct HBO2 therapy

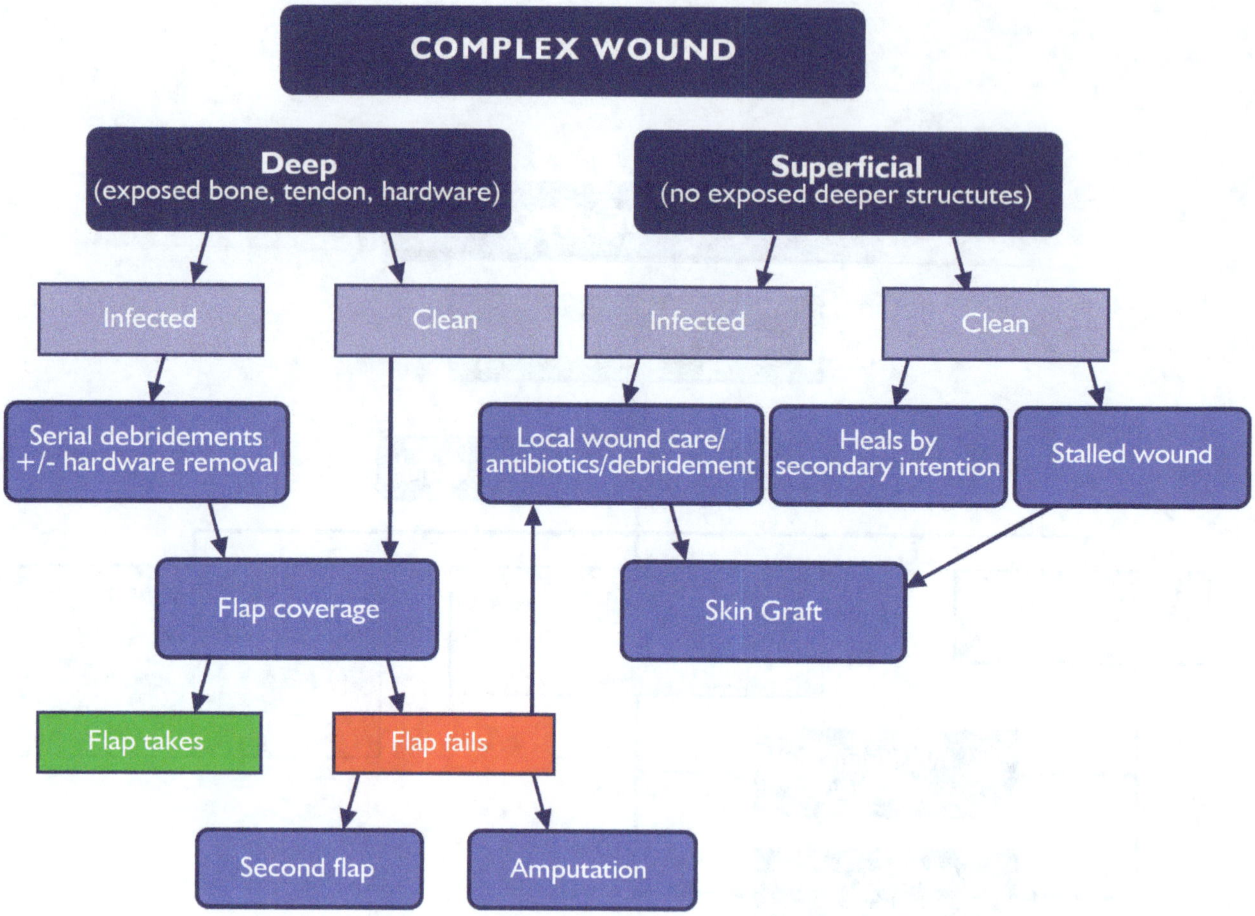

Printed with permission by Regina M. Fearmonti, MD
(Chapter 9: Plastic Surgery Approach to Wound Management and Closure)

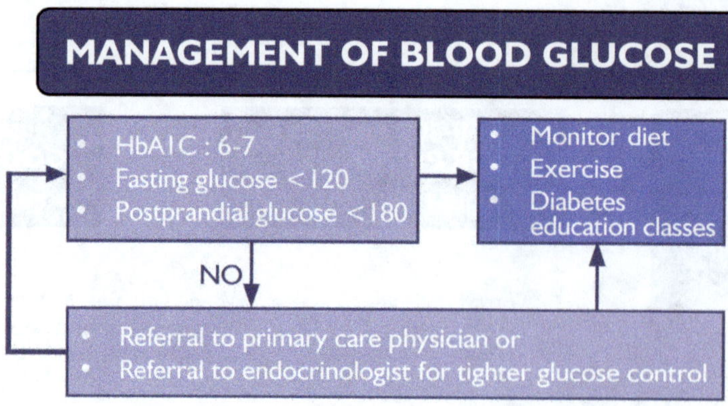

Adapted with permission by Jayesh B. Shah, MD
(Chapter 10: Diabetic Foot Ulcers)

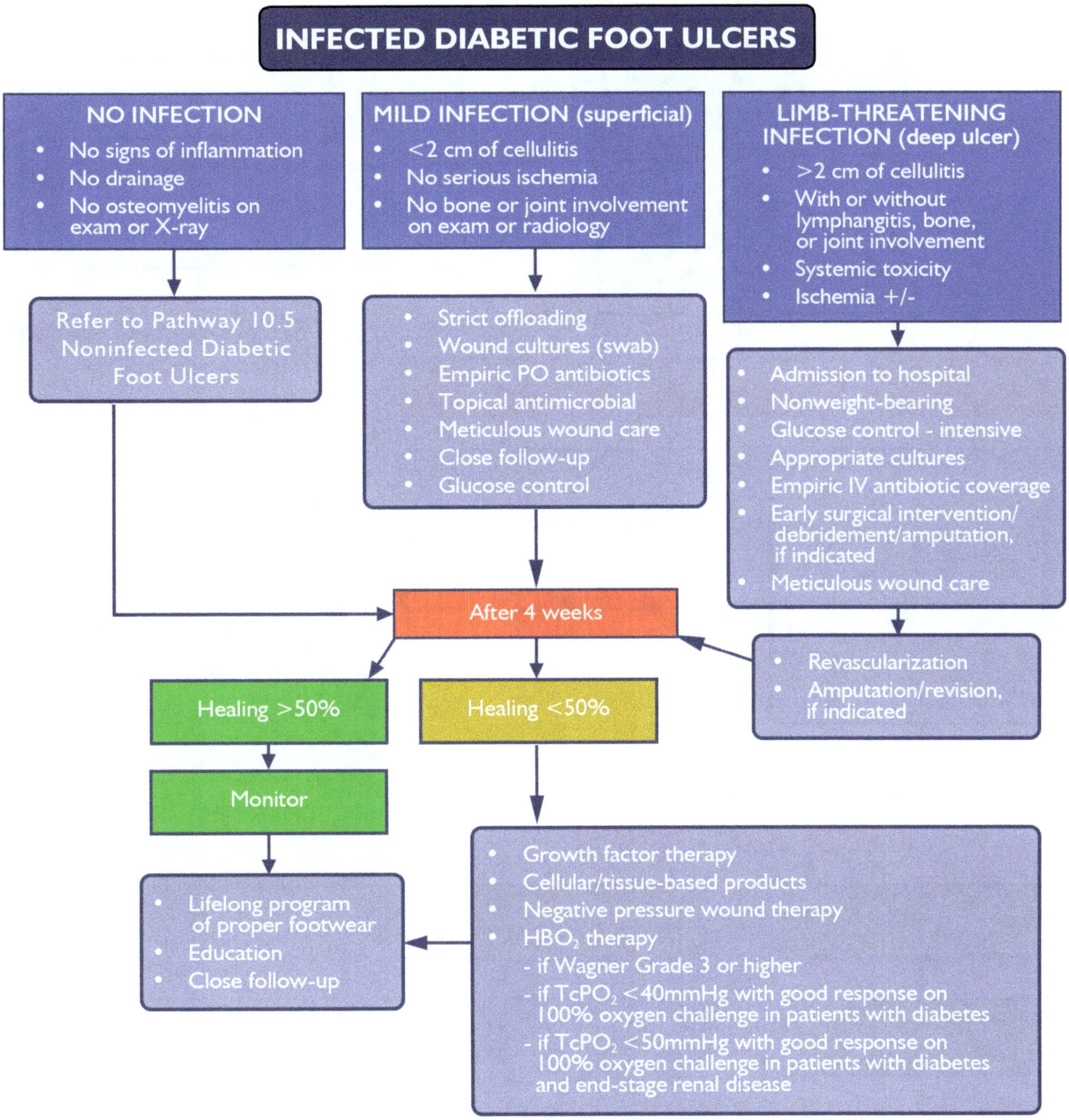
INFECTED DIABETIC FOOT ULCERS
NO INFECTION
• No signs of inflammation
• No drainage
• No osteomyelitis on exam or X-ray
MILD INFECTION (superficial)
• <2 cm of cellulitis
• No serious ischemia
• No bone or joint involvement on exam or radiology
LIMB-THREATENING INFECTION (deep ulcer)
• >2 cm of cellulitis
• With or without lymphangitis, bone, or joint involvement
• Systemic toxicity
• Ischemia +/-
Refer to Pathway 10.5 Noninfected Diabetic Foot Ulcers
• Strict offloading
• Wound cultures (swab)
• Empiric PO antibiotics
• Topical antimicrobial
• Meticulous wound care
• Close follow-up
• Glucose control
• Admission to hospital
• Nonweight-bearing
• Glucose control - intensive
• Appropriate cultures
• Empiric IV antibiotic coverage
• Early surgical intervention/ debridement/amputation, if indicated
• Meticulous wound care
After 4 weeks
• Revascularization
• Amputation/revision, if indicated
Healing >50%
Healing <50%
Monitor
• Lifelong program of proper footwear
• Education
• Close follow-up
• Growth factor therapy
• Cellular/tissue-based products
• Negative pressure wound therapy
• HBO₂ therapy
- if Wagner Grade 3 or higher
- if TcPO₂ <40mmHg with good response on 100% oxygen challenge in patients with diabetes
- if TcPO₂ <50mmHg with good response on 100% oxygen challenge in patients with diabetes and end-stage renal disease

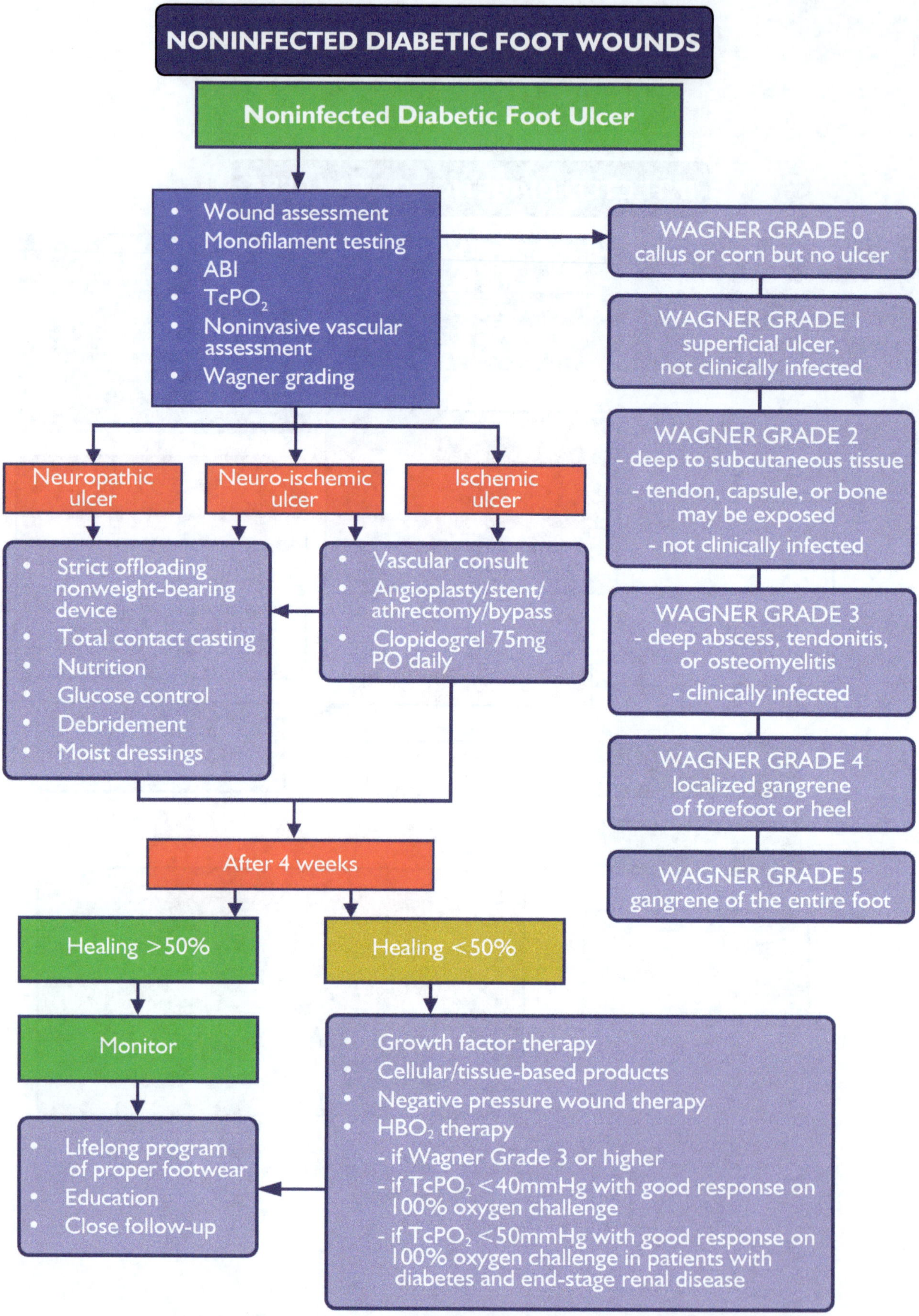

Adapted with permission by Jayesh B. Shah, MD
(Chapter 10: Diabetic Foot Ulcers)

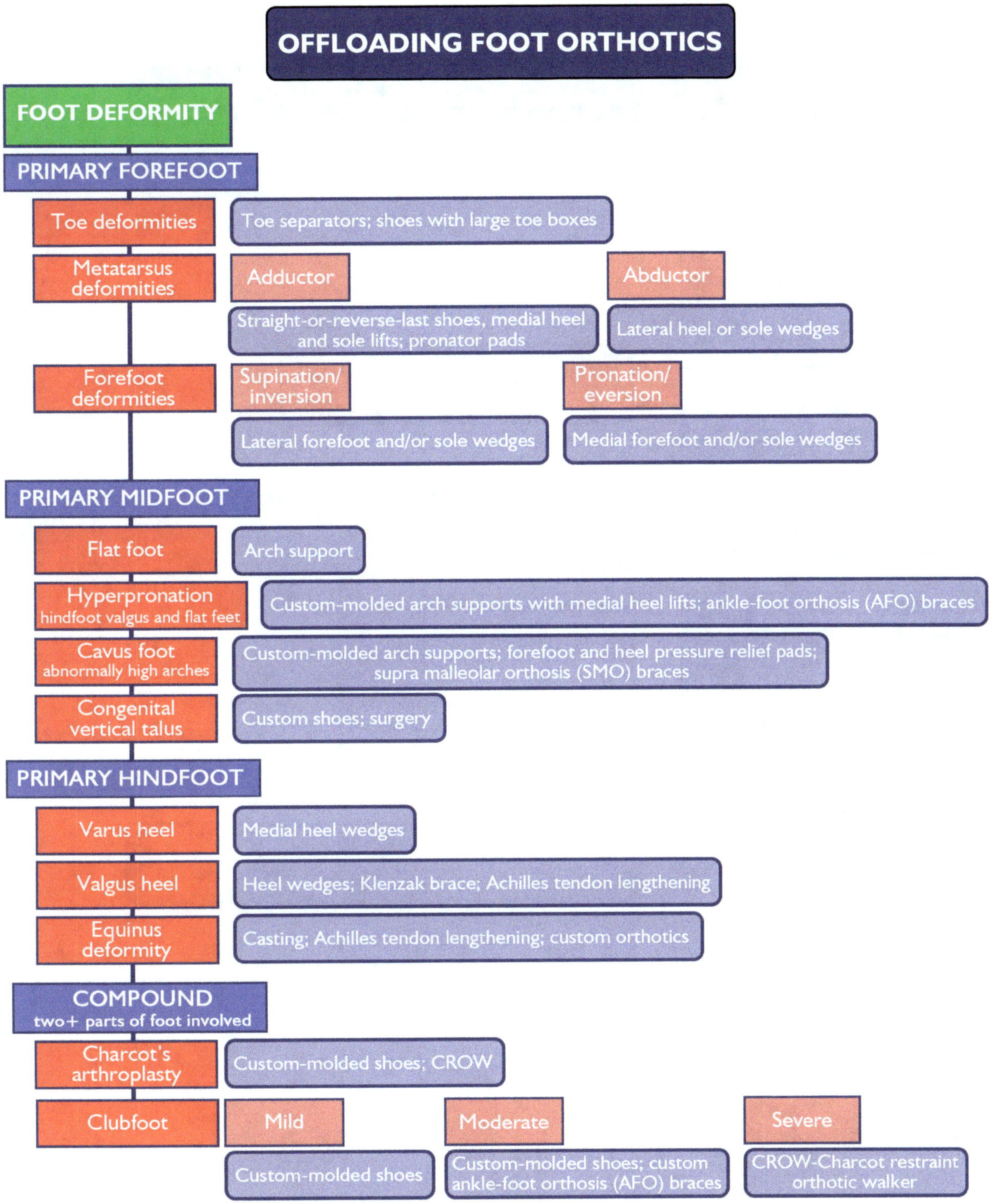

Adapted with permission by Jayesh B. Shah, MD
(Chapter 10: Diabetic Foot Ulcers)

PRESCRIPTION OFFLOADING SHOE ADJUSTMENTS[4]

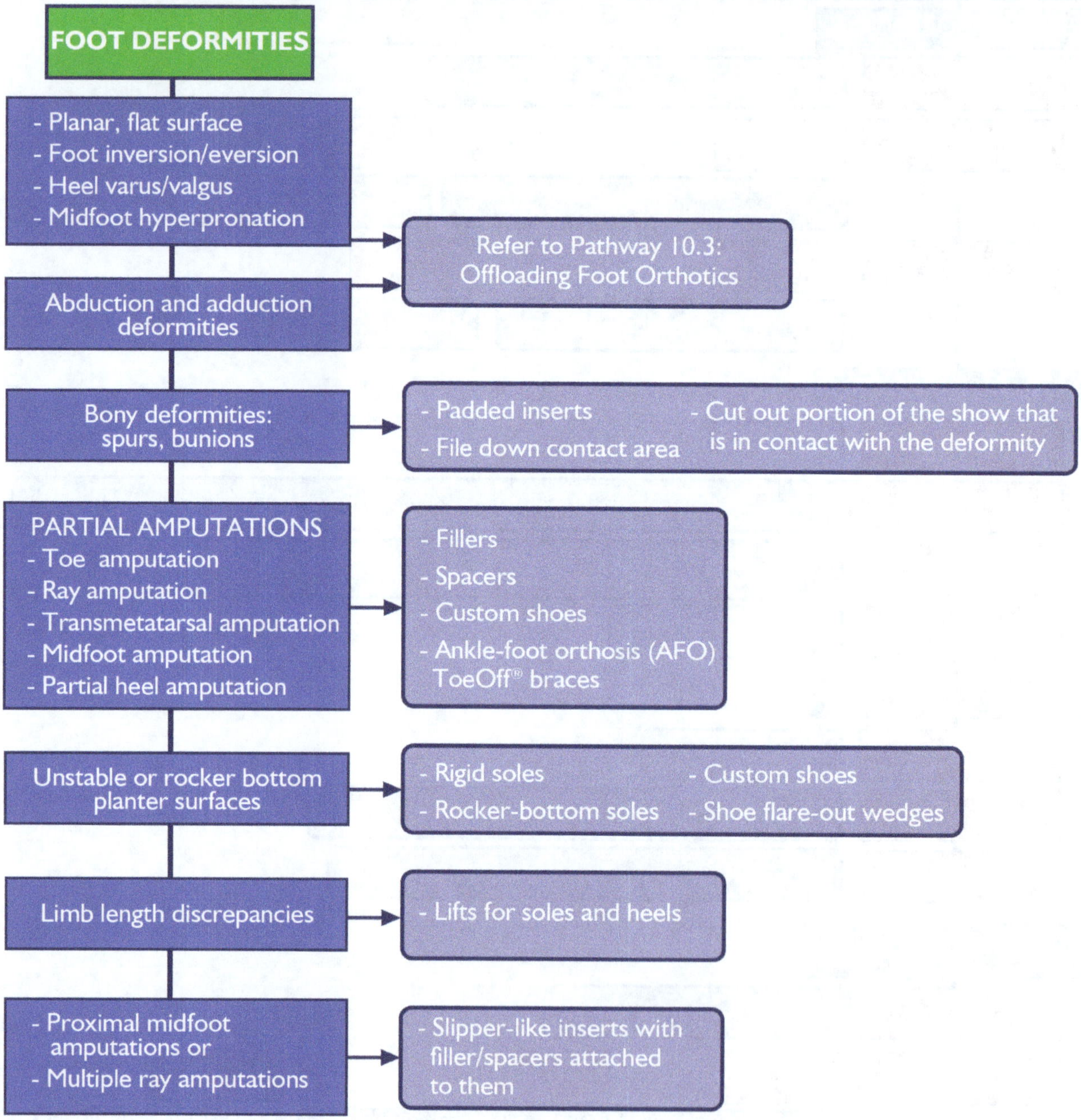

Adapted with permission by Jayesh B. Shah, MD
(Chapter 10: Diabetic Foot Ulcers)

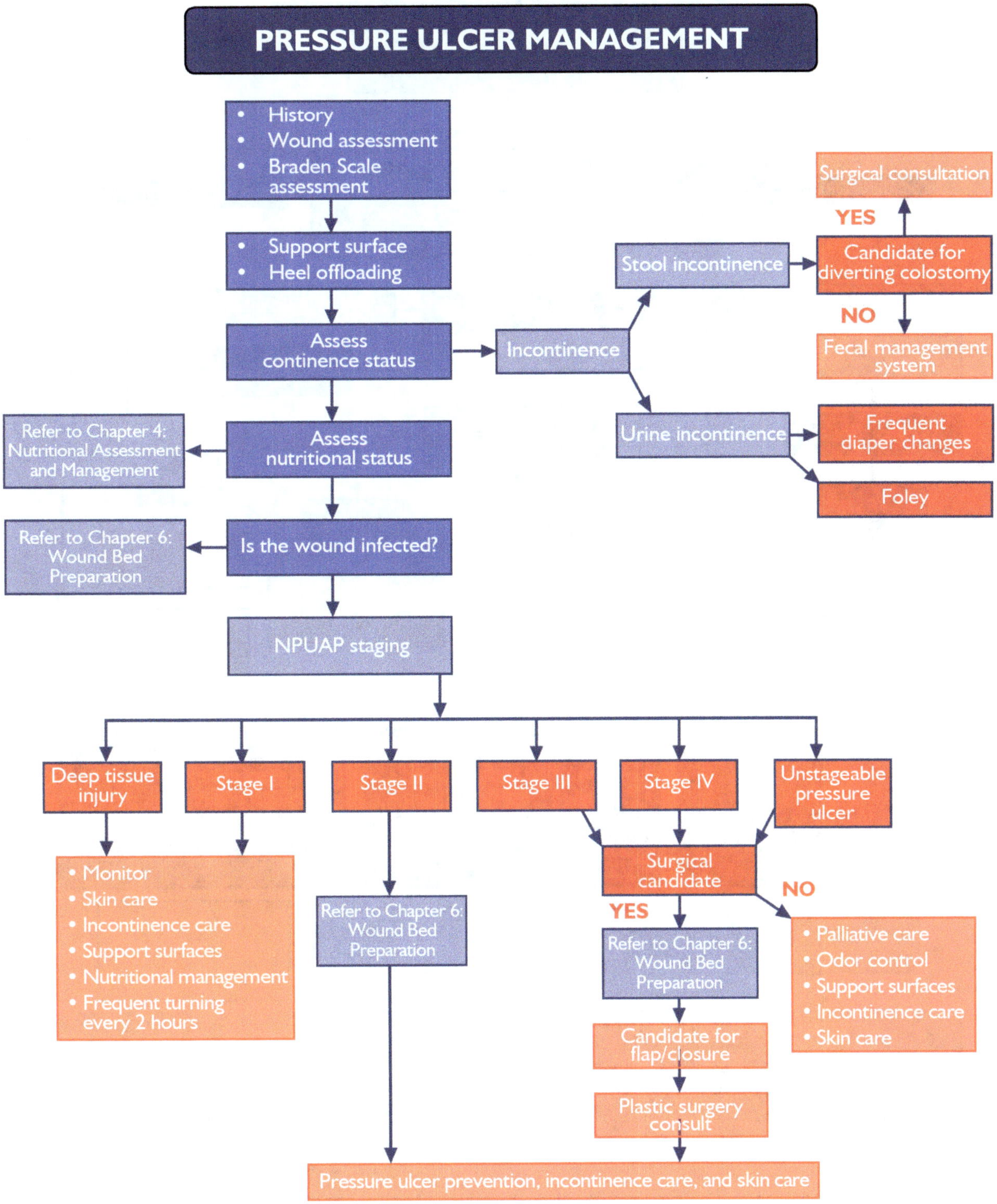

Adapted with permission by Jayesh B. Shah, MD
(Chapter 11: Pressure Ulcers)

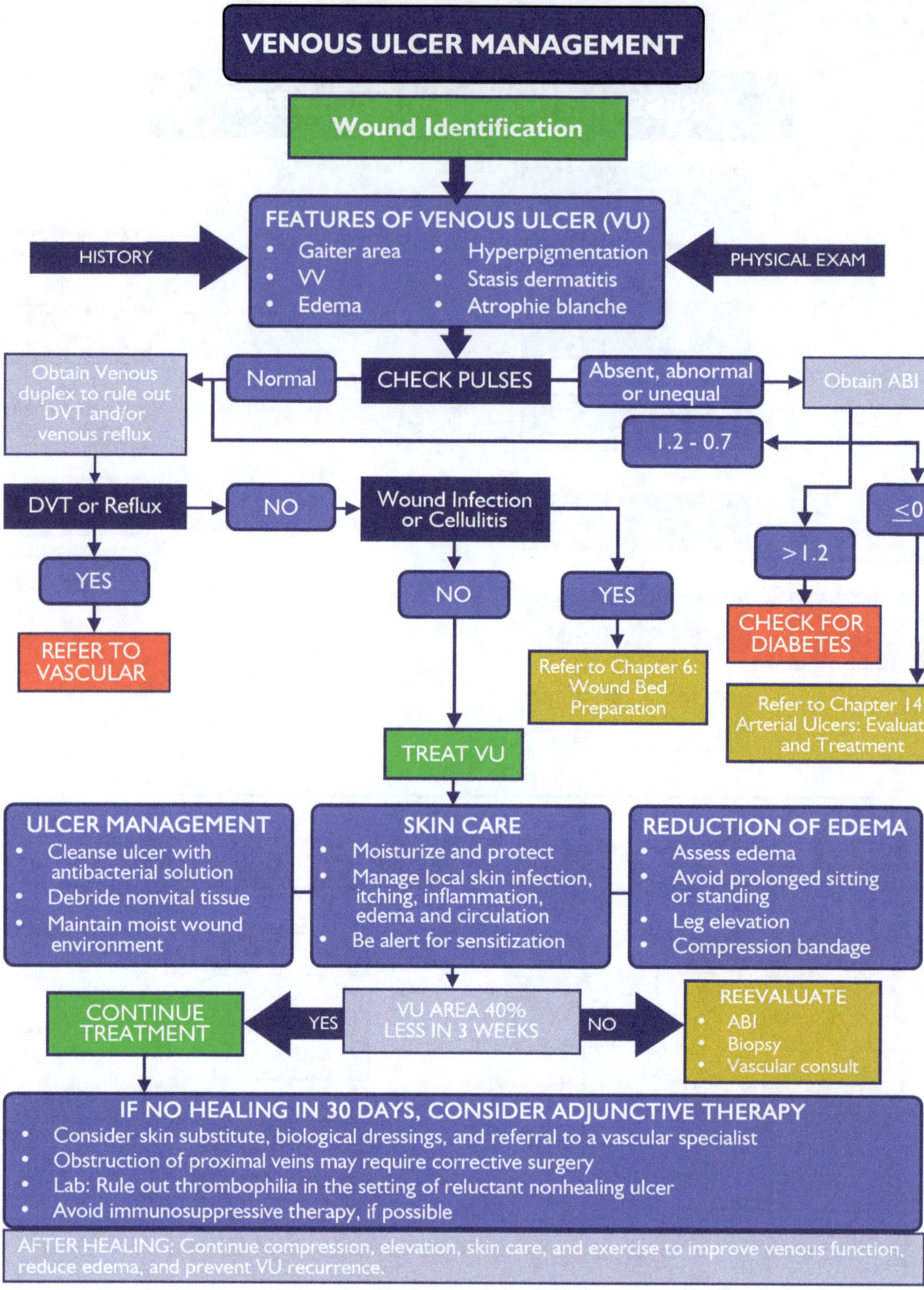

(Chapter 12: Venous Insufficiency Ulcer)

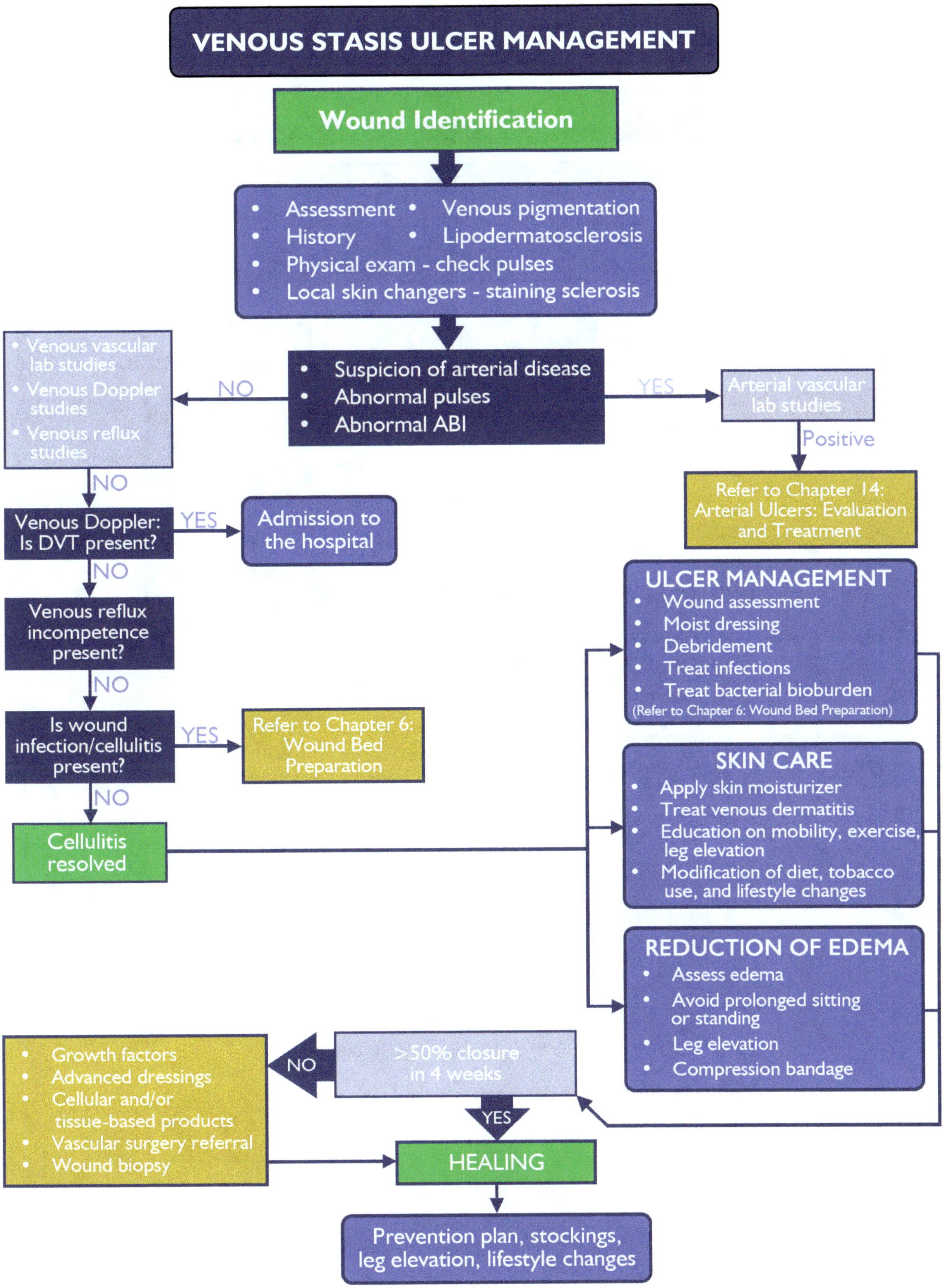
VENOUS STASIS ULCER MANAGEMENT
Wound Identification
• Assessment • Venous pigmentation
• History • Lipodermatosclerosis
• Physical exam - check pulses
• Local skin changers - staining sclerosis
• Suspicion of arterial disease
• Abnormal pulses
• Abnormal ABI
NO
YES
• Venous vascular lab studies
• Venous Doppler studies
• Venous reflux studies
Arterial vascular lab studies
Positive
Refer to Chapter 14: Arterial Ulcers: Evaluation and Treatment
NO
Venous Doppler: Is DVT present?
YES
Admission to the hospital
NO
Venous reflux incompetence present?
NO
Is wound infection/cellulitis present?
YES
Refer to Chapter 6: Wound Bed Preparation
NO
Cellulitis resolved
ULCER MANAGEMENT
• Wound assessment
• Moist dressing
• Debridement
• Treat infections
• Treat bacterial bioburden
(Refer to Chapter 6: Wound Bed Preparation)
SKIN CARE
• Apply skin moisturizer
• Treat venous dermatitis
• Education on mobility, exercise, leg elevation
• Modification of diet, tobacco use, and lifestyle changes
REDUCTION OF EDEMA
• Assess edema
• Avoid prolonged sitting or standing
• Leg elevation
• Compression bandage
• Growth factors
• Advanced dressings
• Cellular and/or tissue-based products
• Vascular surgery referral
• Wound biopsy
NO
>50% closure in 4 weeks
YES
HEALING
Prevention plan, stockings, leg elevation, lifestyle changes

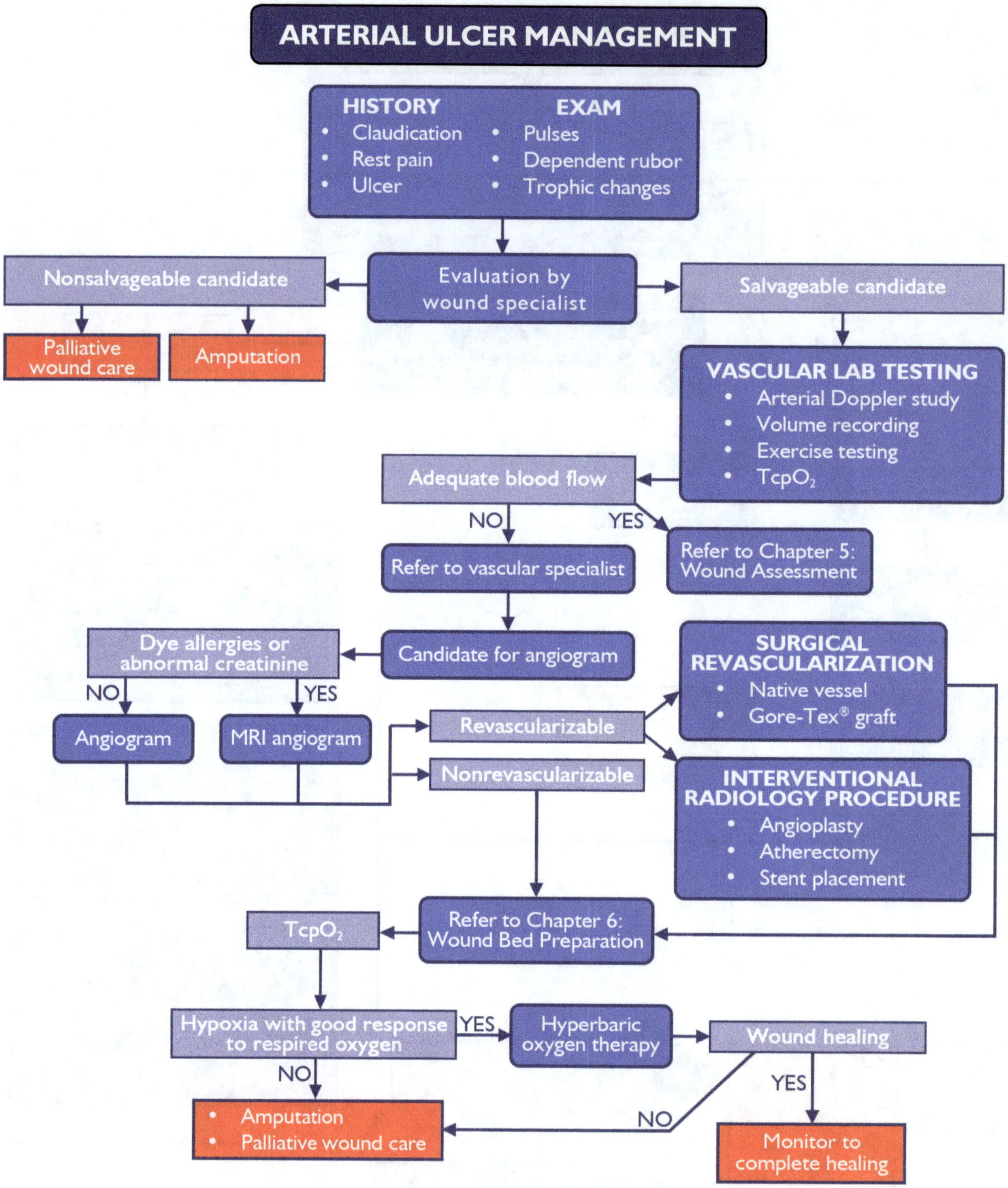

Adapted with permission by Jayesh B. Shah, MD
(Chapter 14: Arterial Ulcers: Evaluation and Treatment)

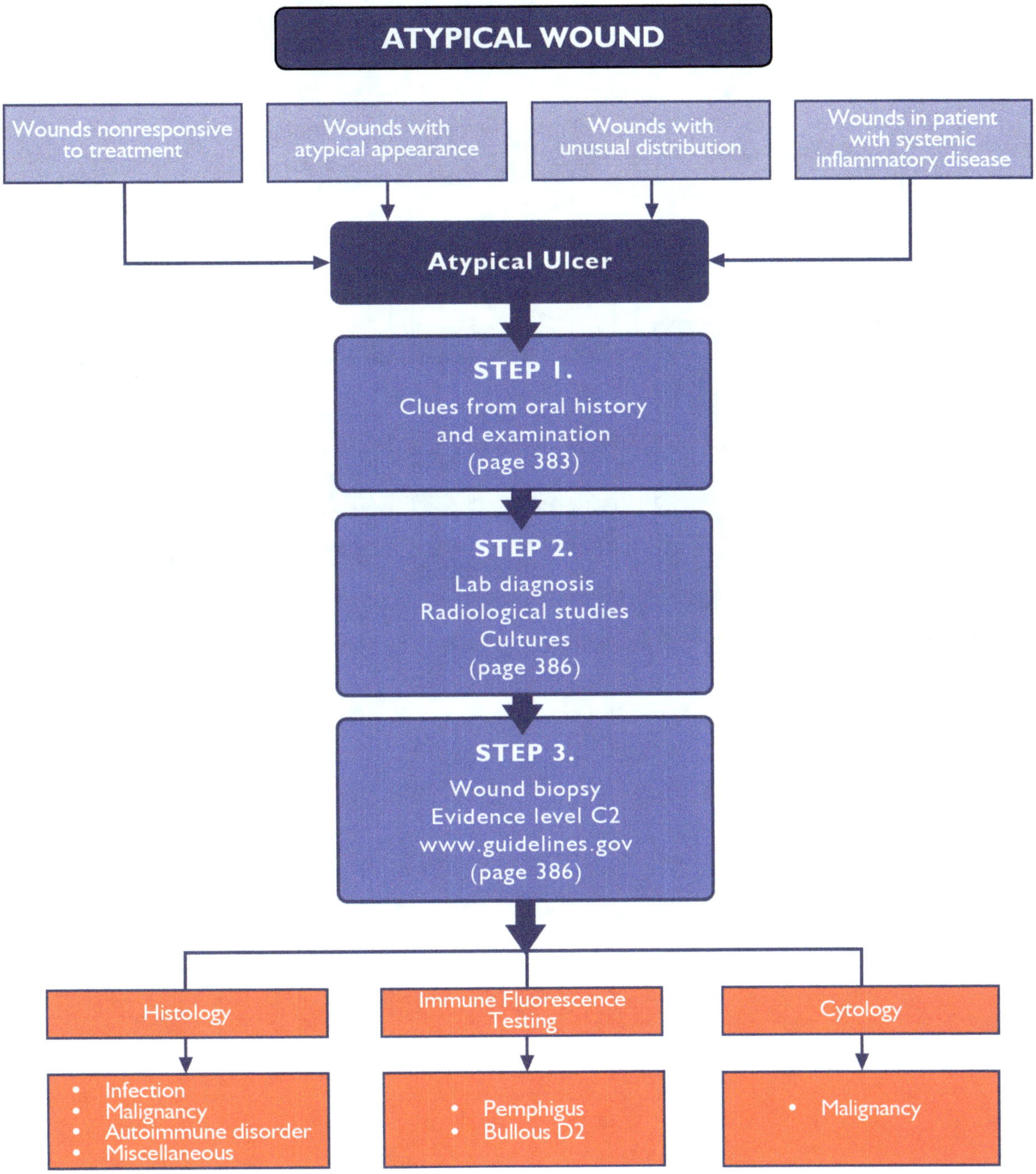

© Best Publishing Company, *Wound Care Certification Study Guide 2nd edition*
Adapted with permission by Jayesh B. Shah, MD
(Chapter 15: Commonly Misdiagnosed Ulcers and Atypical Ulcers)

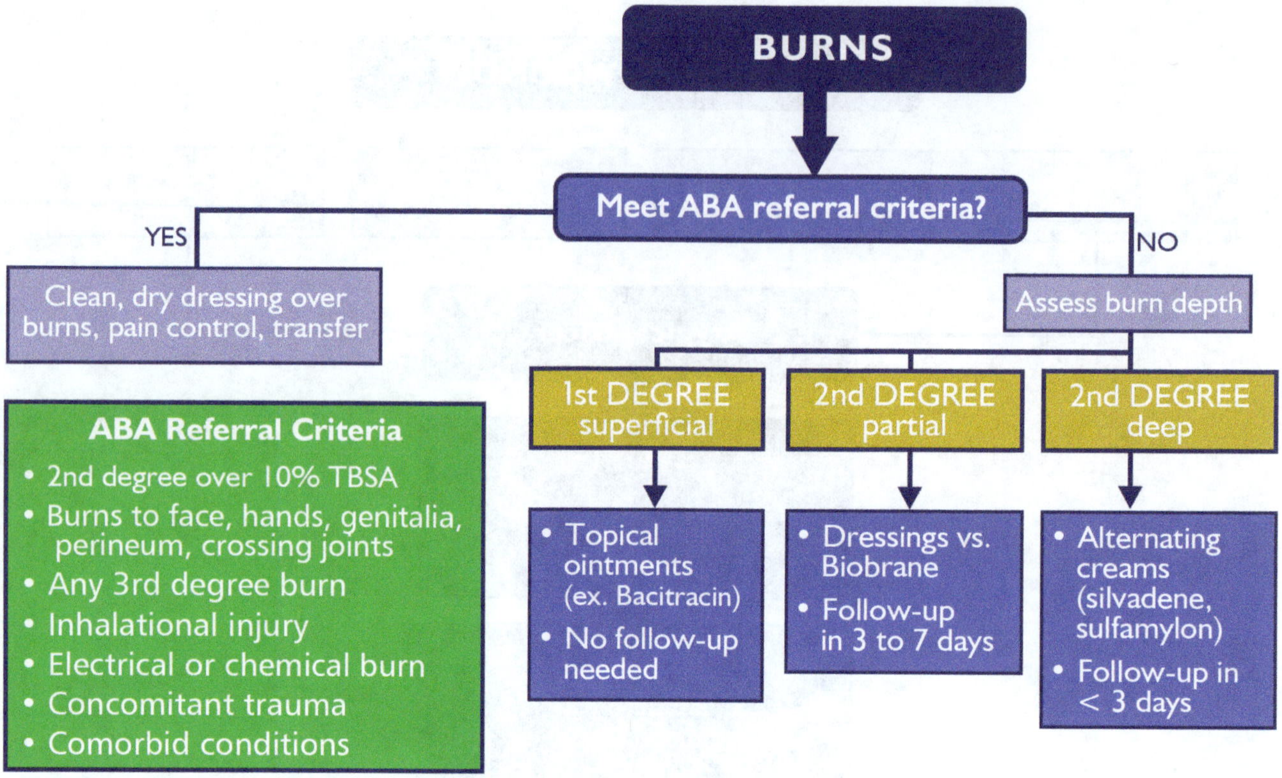

Printed with permission by Kevin Chung, MD, Julie A. Rizzo, MD, and Matthew P. Rowan, PhD (Chapter 18: Practical Approach to Burns).

INDEX

B

C

D

L

M

Q

R

S

T

X

www.ingramcontent.com/pod-product-compliance
Lightning Source LLC
LaVergne TN
LVHW081343011026
849161LV00013BB/2996